Nursing
Procedures

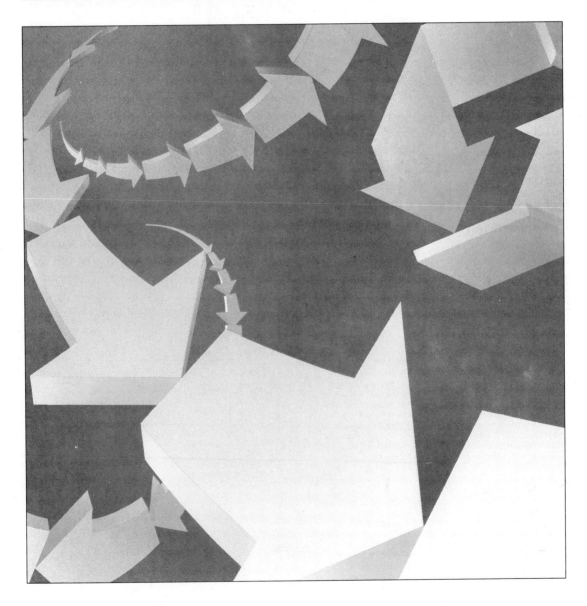

Springhouse Corporation
Springhouse, Pennsylvania

STAFF

Executive Director, Editorial
Stanley Loeb

Editorial Director
Matthew Cahill

Clinical Director
Barbara F. McVan, RN

Art Director
John Hubbard

Clinical Project Director
Patricia Dwyer Schull, RN, MSN

Senior Editor
Catherine E. Harold

Clinical Editors
Linda Roy, RN, MSN, CCRN; Julie N. Tackenberg, RN, MA, CNRN; Beverly Ann Tscheschlog, RN; Nina Poorman Welsh, RN

Drug Information Editor
George J. Blake, RPh, MS

Editors
Stephen Daly, Rafaela Ellis, Doris Falk, Karla Harby, Peter H. Johnson, Edith McMahon, June Norris, Gale Sloan, Mary Lou Webster

Copy Editors
Jane V. Cray (supervisor), Christina A. Price, Priscilla DeWitt, Terri Goshko, Nancy Papsin

Designers
Stephanie Peters (associate art director), Anita Curry (book designer), Kevin Curry, Darcy Feralio, Kristina Gabage, Susan Hopkins Rodzewich

Illustrators
John Carlance, Kevin Curry, Jacalyn Facciolo, Jean Gardner, Bob Jackson, Nancy Lou Makris, Bob Neuman, Judy Newhouse, Greg Purdon (cover), Mary Stangl, Larry Ward

Art Production
Robert Perry (manager), Heather Bernhardt, Donald Knauss, Robert Wieder

Typography
David Kosten (director), Diane E. Paluba (manager), Elizabeth Bergman, Joyce Rossi Biletz, Phyllis Marron, Robin Rantz, Valerie Rosenberger

Manufacturing
Deborah Meiris (manager), T.A. Landis, Jennifer Suter, Anna Brindisi

Production Coordination
Colleen M. Hayman

Editorial Assistants
Maree DeRosa, Beverly Lane, Mary Madden

Library of Congress Cataloging-in-Publication Data

Nursing procedures
    p.   cm.
    Includes bibliographical references and index.
    1. Nursing   I. Springhouse Corporation.
    [DNLM: 1. Nursing Care. WY 100 N9755]
RT41.N886   1992
610.73—dc20
DNLM/DLC   91-5081
ISBN 0-87434-392-5   CIP

Printed in the United States of America.
PROC-010192

CONTENTS

CONTRIBUTORS

Debra Arnow, RN, BSN, CNA
Nurse coordinator
Vanderbilt University Medical Center
Nashville, Tenn.

Ruth E. Blauer, RN, MS, CNA
Director, Education Department
Rutland (Vt.) Regional Medical Center

Barbara K. Blue, RN, MSN
Pediatric pulmonary nurse specialist
Phoenix (Ariz.) Children's Hospital

Valeria Brannon, RN, BSN
Nurse manager
Texas Children's Hospital
Houston

Cynthia Browder, RN, BSN
Assistant director of nursing
Texas Children's Hospital
Houston

Vicki L. Buchda, RN, MS
Director, Special Care
Maryvale Samaritan Medical Center
Phoenix, Ariz.

Sherry Buffington, RN, CCRN, CLA (ASCP)
Staff nurse, ICCU
Doylestown (Pa.) Hospital

Dorothy A. Calabrese, RN, MSN, CURN
Clinical nurse specialist, urology/oncology
Cleveland Clinic Foundation

Liz Chullino, RN, BSN
Nurse manager
Texas Children's Hospital
Houston

Carla M. Clark, RN, MS
Nurse research clinician
Good Samaritan Regional Medical Center
Phoenix, Ariz.

Bonita Gail Largent Cloyd, RN, BSN, CETN
Enterostomal therapist
Western Baptist Hospital
Paducah, Ky.

Peggy Coleman, RN, MSN, CNA
Nurse manager
Warren Grant Magnuson Clinical Center
National Institutes of Health
Bethesda, Md.

Catherine M. Collin, RN, MSN, CANP
Assistant professor of clinical nursing
University of Medicine and Dentistry of New Jersey
Newark, N.J.

Huberta Cozart, RN, BSN
Quality assurance coordinator
St. Luke's Episcopal Hospital
Houston

Jane Dolin, RN, BSN, ET
Patient education specialist
Allentown Hospital-Lehigh Valley Hospital Center
Allentown, Pa.

Shirley J. Edwards, RN, MSN, OCN
Clinical nurse specialist, oncology
Saint John's Hospital and Health Center
Santa Monica, Calif.

Marsha L. England, RN, CRNI, AA
Charge nurse, I.V. therapy
Saint John's Hospital and Health Center
Santa Monica, Calif.

Nina M. Fielden, RN, MSN, CNN
Clinical instructor, Critical Care Nursing Department
Cleveland Clinic Foundation

Marina Villano Flecksteiner, RN, BSN, CNN
Clinical instructor
Allentown Hospital-Lehigh Valley Hospital Center
Allentown, Pa.

Marilyn A. Folcik, RN, BA, MPH, ONC
Instructor, staff development
Hartford (Conn.) Hospital

Paul N. Franquist, RN, MSN
Clinical nurse specialist, medical/surgical
Desert Samaritan Medical Center
Mesa, Ariz.

Diane Broadbent Friedman, RN, MSN, CS
Research nurse coordinator
Milton S. Hershey Medical Center
Hershey, Pa.

Jan Fuchs, RN, MS, CNN
Head nurse
Peritoneal Dialysis Unit
Cleveland Clinic Foundation

Ellen D. Goodner, RN, BSN
Education instructor
Western Baptist Hospital
Paducah, Ky.

Jean B. Gordon, RN, OCN
Oncology clinical instructor
Saint Barnabas Medical Center
Livingston, N.J.

JoAnn Gruber, RN, BSN, CCRN
Coordinator, continuing education
Allentown Hospital-Lehigh Valley Hospital Center
Allentown, Pa.

Susan J. Hart, RN,C, MSN, CCRN
Clinical nurse specialist, critical care
Saint Barnabas Medical Center
Livingston, N.J.

Dianna C. Hayden, RN, BSN
Infection control practitioner
Western Baptist Hospital
Paducah, Ky.

Connie S. Heflin, RN, MSN
Associate professor of nursing
Paducah (Ky.) Community College

Christie Hoffman, RN
Staff nurse
Texas Children's Hospital
Houston

Marian J. Hoffman, RN, MSN, CNSN
Clinical nurse specialist, nutrition
Allentown Hospital-Lehigh Valley Hospital Center
Allentown, Pa.

Florence Jones, RN, MSN
Director of education
Western Baptist Hospital
Paducah, Ky.

John A. Kays, RN, MSN
Nurse manager, special surgery
Milton S. Hershey Medical Center
Hershey, Pa.

Marilyn Knoth, RN, MSN
Associate professor
Paducah (Ky.) Community College

Laura Kotagal, RN, BSN
Former clinical instructor, neuroscience nursing
Cleveland Clinic Foundation

Charles Krozek, RN, BA, MN
Nursing education coordinator
Saint John's Hospital and Health Center
Santa Monica, Calif.

Kathleen M. Malloch, RN, BS, MBA, CNA
Clinical nursing administrator
Maryvale Samaritan Medical Center
Phoenix, Ariz.

Clara Martin, RN
Infection control assistant
Texas Children's Hospital
Houston

Rebecca M. McCaskey, RN, BA, MEd
Clinical nurse educator
Warren Grant Magnuson Clinical Center
National Institutes of Health
Bethesda, Md.

Karen M.J. McCleave, RN, MS, CFNP, CIC
Supervisor, employee health/infection control
Maryvale Samaritan Medical Center
Phoenix, Ariz.

Debra McGeehin, RN, BSN
Clinical instructor
Allentown Hospital-Lehigh Valley Hospital Center
Allentown, Pa.

Kimberley W. McKinney, RN, BSN
Education instructor
Western Baptist Hospital
Paducah, Ky.

Cheryl Milford, RN, MS, CCRN
Nursing staff development specialist
Ohio State University, Columbus

Mary Beth Modic, RN, MSN
Quality monitor, nursing quality management
Cleveland Clinic Foundation

Carolyn J. Montgomery, MDiv, ThM
Chaplain
Doylestown (Pa.) Hospital

Deirdre P. Mountjoy, RN, MS
Staff development instructor
Maryvale Samaritan Medical Center
Phoenix, Ariz.

M. Louise Nix, RN,C, MSN, PNP
Staff development specialist
Texas Children's Hospital
Houston

Tena B. Payne, RN, MSN
Associate professor
Paducah (Ky.) Community College

Jody Pelusi, RN, MSN, OCN, RT
Clinical nurse specialist, oncology
Maryvale Samaritan Medical Center
Phoenix, Ariz.

Anna Pignanelli, BSN
Clinical instructor, surgical/oncology nursing
Cleveland Clinic Foundation

Marla J. Prizant-Weston, RN, MS, CCRN
Clinical nurse specialist, critical care
Desert Samaritan Medical Center
Phoenix, Ariz.

Frances W. Quinless, RN, PhD
Chair, Department of Nursing Education and Services
University of Medicine and Dentistry of New Jersey
Newark, N.J.

Lisa Rioux, RN, BSN, OCN
Clinical nurse II
Saint John's Hospital and Health Center
Santa Monica, Calif.

Carol F. Robinson, RN, MS, RRT, CNA
Pediatric pulmonary nurse specialist
Phoenix (Ariz.) Children's Hospital

Teresa Rodriguez-Wargo, RN, MSN, PNP
Staff development specialist
Texas Children's Hospital
Houston

Susan F. Rudy, RN, BSN
Clinical coordinator, oral surgery/otolaryngology
Warren Grant Magnuson Clinical Center
National Institutes of Health
Bethesda, Md.

Pat Sanderson, RN, BSN
Clinical educator
Saint John's Hospital and Health Center
Santa Monica, Calif.

Rhea C. Sanford, RN, MSN, CS
Clinical nurse specialist
John Dempsey Hospital
Farmington, Conn.

Ann Schneidman, RN, MS, NS
Pulmonary nurse consultant
Phoenix, Ariz.

Sonya Scott, RN, BSN
Clinical educator
Texas Children's Hospital
Houston

Daniele Shollenberger, RN, MSN
Clinical nurse specialist
Allentown Hospital-Lehigh Valley Hospital Center
Allentown, Pa.

Susan Simon, RN, MA
Home care coordinator
Medical Personnel Pool
Shaker Heights, Ohio

Marylou Nesbitt Snow, RN, MS, OCN
Clinical nurse specialist, oncology
Desert Samaritan Medical Center
Mesa, Ariz.

Nancy J. Stefan, RN, BSN
Nurse manager
Warren Grant Magnuson Clinical Center
National Institutes of Health
Bethesda, Md.

Dori Taylor, RN, PhD, CNA
Director, nursing education and research
Assistant clinical professor
John Dempsey Hospital
University of Connecticut, Farmington

Susan D. Taylor, RN, MSN
Associate professor of nursing
Paducah (Ky.) Community College

Freda Thompson, RN, MSN
Education instructor
Western Baptist Hospital
Paducah, Ky.

Kathryn I. Weber, RN
Staff nurse, I.V. Therapy Department
Saint John's Hospital and Health Center
Santa Monica, Calif.

Sarah E. Whitaker, RN, MSN
Lecturer
University of Texas at El Paso

Myrtle Taylor Williams, RN, MSN
Director, The Center for Nursing Development
Texas Children's Hospital
Houston

M. Catherine Wollman, RN, MSN, CRNP
Gerontologic clinical nurse specialist
University of Pennsylvania School of Nursing
Philadelphia

Pamela Peters Youngs, RN, BA, CCRN
Clinical nurse II
Saint John's Hospital and Health Center
Santa Monica, Calif.

CONSULTANTS

Madeline P. Albanese, RN, MSN, ONC
Manager, patient education
Thomas Jefferson University Hospital
Philadelphia

Kathleen C. Byington, RN, MSN
Pediatric clinical nurse specialist
Vanderbilt University
Nashville, Tenn.

Jeanette K. Chambers, RN, PhD, CS
Renal/medicine clinical nurse specialist
Riverside Methodist Hospitals
Adjunct instructor, College of Nursing
Ohio State University, Columbus

Karen K. Charland, RN, MSN
Clinical coordinator
The Graduate Hospital Wound Care Center
Philadelphia

Susan Dalton, RN, CCRN
High tech staff nurse
Home visiting nurse
Howell, N.J.

Betsy Eimer, RN, BSN
Independent nurse consultant
Staff nurse
Buffalo (N.Y.) General Hospital

Nancy Evans, RN, BSN, CGRN
Nurse manager
Gastroenterology Department
Daniel Freeman Memorial and Marina Hospitals
Inglewood, Calif.

Elizabeth A. Henneman, RN, MS, CCRN
Clinical nurse specialist
Medical Intensive Care Unit
UCLA Medical Center
Los Angeles

Patricia Holmes, RN, BSN
Independent nurse consultant
Ambler, Pa.

Flerida A. Imperial, RN, MN
Clinical nurse specialist
Cardiothoracic ICU
UCLA Medical Center
Los Angeles

Jeanne D. Kenna, RN, CRNI
I.V. staff nurse
Doylestown (Pa.) Hospital

Nancy A. McConaughy, RN, MSN, CNRN
Neuroscience clinical nurse specialist
University Medical Center
Tucson, Ariz.

Mary Jane McDevitt, RN, BS
Staff nurse, Oncology Unit 35
Fitzgerald-Mercy Hospital
Darby, Pa.

Doris Millam, BSN, MS, CRNI
I.V. therapy clinical nurse specialist
Holy Family Hospital
Des Plaines, Ill.

Rita Short Monahan, RN, MSN, EdD
Associate professor
Oregon Health Sciences University School of Nursing, La Grande

Lois A. Piano, RN,C, MSN
Assistant professor of nursing
Gwynedd Mercy College
Gwynedd Valley, Pa.

Kathleen B. Powell, RN, MSN
Hospital education coordinator
UAB Hospital
Birmingham, Ala.

Patricia L. Radzewicz, RN, BSN
Claims analyst
University of Illinois Office of University Counsel, Chicago

Sally Russell, RN, MN, CS
Instructor
St. Elizabeth Hospital School of Nursing
Lafayette, Ind.

Rosemary Theroux, RN,C, MS
Director, Women's Health Network
Leonard Morse Hospital
Natick, Mass.

FOREWORD

Whether you're a new nurse performing your first urinary catheter insertion or an experienced nurse monitoring a patient's hemodynamic status, you need clear, current, and complete information to help you carry out the procedure correctly and safely. Unfortunately, you often have to hunt for this information in hospital procedure manuals, in manufacturers' manuals, in professional journals, or in specialized publications. Unfortunately, too, these sources usually don't provide all the information you need.

Fortunately, *Nursing Procedures* does. This definitive one-volume resource explains and shows how to perform virtually every nursing procedure — more than 325 in all. What's more, the volume uses the nursing process to provide you with the basic and advanced concepts essential for today's nursing practice.

Nursing Procedures opens with six chapters devoted to broad nursing topics: fundamental procedures (including comprehensive guidelines for a systematic head-to-toe patient assessment), infection control, specimen collection, diagnostic testing, physical treatments, drug administration, and intravascular therapy. The next eight chapters cover procedures related to specific body systems. The final three chapters cover the special needs of pediatric, maternal-neonatal, and geriatric patients. Throughout all of the chapters, more than 500 drawings, photographs, and charts enhance the text. In fact, several common procedures, such as nasogastric tube insertion and cardiopulmonary resuscitation, contain step-by-step photographic or illustrated directions.

To help you use this book, each procedure appears in the same easy-to-follow format. Each starts with an introduction that defines and briefly describes the procedure, explains its purpose, and points out any contraindications. This section also summarizes other useful information, such as any special skills required to perform the procedure and the procedure's anticipated effectiveness.

Next, *Equipment* lists all the items you'll need to perform the procedure and, where appropriate, identifies the items available as kits. *Preparation of equipment*, which follows, explains all the steps that must be taken to ensure the procedure's effectiveness.

Implementation takes you step-by-step through the procedure in clear, concise style. Rationales, highlighted by *italicized type*, explain why each major step is performed.

Where necessary, you'll also find suggestions for patient teaching and discharge planning. Next, *Special considerations* lists additional important concerns related to the procedure, such as ways to avoid common problems, variations in performing the procedure, warnings and, where appropriate, insights from the latest medical and nursing research.

When appropriate, the *Complications* section alerts you to possible patient problems resulting from the procedure. Finally, *Documentation* tells you about procedure-specific items that should be included in your notes or on the patient's medical record. Besides fostering professional responsibility and accountability, accurate and complete documentation is essential for meeting regulatory standards and determining accurate reimbursement. And it helps you avoid potential legal problems.

Throughout the book, special graphic devices called logos draw your attention to important recurring topics. For example, all emergency procedures in the book, such as cardiopulmonary resuscitation, are identified by a special symbol at their start. Another logo identifies subject matter related to home care and how a procedure may be performed in the patient's home. Still another logo, *equipment,* explains and sometimes shows devices, such as the gastrostomy feeding button. *Troubleshooting* alerts you to equipment problems that may arise and explains how to prevent or correct them.

Nursing Procedures is an essential addition to your professional library, whether you're a nursing student, an experienced clinical nurse, a nurse educator, or an administrator. It's also indispensable for any nurse returning to active practice. Designed to save you time and improve your skills and confidence, this book will help you give quality patient care in any setting.

Marguerite K. Schlag, RN, MSN, EdD
  Director, Nursing Education and Development
  Robert Wood Johnson University Hospital
  New Brunswick, N.J.

NURSING PROCEDURES

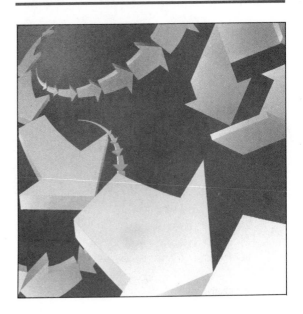

CHAPTER 1

FUNDAMENTAL PROCEDURES

FRANCES W. QUINLESS, RN, PhD
RUTH E. BLAUER, RN, MS, CNA

Introduction

Patients come to hospitals because they need skilled clinical observation and treatment. According to the American Hospital Association, about 37 million people undergo hospitalization each year, and for most, it's a trying experience. After all, hospitalization challenges the patient's sense of privacy and control of his life. He must relinquish at least part of his normal routine. He must rely on you and your co-workers to meet his fundamental needs. Depending on the complexity of his health problem, he and his family may also require teaching, counseling, coordination of services, development of community support systems, and help in coping with health-related changes in his life.

In many hospitals, staff nurses, primary nurses, and clinical nurse specialists deliver all these vital services. This chapter serves as a starting point to help you understand and perform many of these tasks confidently and effectively. It thoroughly covers all the fundamentals: admission, transfer and discharge procedures; assessment (including a section on writing a nursing care plan); ensuring patient safety and mobility (including proper use of restraints and assistive devices); practicing correct body mechanics and patient transfer techniques; and using special orthopedic beds. The chapter also includes a comprehensive review of personal hygiene and comfort measures, nutrition, elimination, surgical care, spiritual care, and postmortem care.

Before turning to these nursing care specifics, however, review the broader aims of your care, such as helping the patient cope with restricted mobility; giving him a comfortable, stimulating environment; making sure his hospital stay is free of hazards; promoting an uneventful recovery; and helping him return to his normal life.

Dealing with restricted mobility

Whenever a patient's condition impairs or prevents mobility, your nursing goals are to promote his independence by motivating him and helping him set goals, to prevent injury and the complications of immobility, to teach him needed skills, and to foster a positive body image, especially if he faces long-term or permanent immobility.

Promoting a comfortable environment

By manipulating physical factors in the patient's environment — temperature, humidity, lighting — you can af-
fect his comfort, condition, and at times, his response to treatment. For example, a room temperature of 68° to 72° F (20° to 22° C) and a relative humidity of 30% to 60%, although comfortable for most patients, may be too cold for elderly patients. Also, proper artificial or natural lighting helps duplicate the day-night cycle.

Providing sensory stimulation

Sensory stimulation (such as therapeutic touch) contributes to patient well-being. Although the amount and type of required stimulation varies with each patient, you can prevent sensory overload or deprivation by accurately assessing his needs. When evaluating stimuli in the patient's environment, remember that illness is a stressor that may intensify the patient's responses, especially to noise and odors.

Promoting safety

Besides weakening the patient, illness and any accompanying treatment may impair his judgment and contribute to accidents. Be alert to hazards in the patient's environment and teach him and his family to recognize them. When caring for a patient with restricted mobility, you must help him as he is moved, lifted, and transported. By using proper body mechanics and appropriate assistive devices, you can prevent injury, fatigue, and discomfort for your patient and yourself.

Preventing complications

For the bedridden patient, immobility poses special hazards, such as pressure on bony prominences; venous, pulmonary, and urinary stasis; and disuse of muscles and joints. These can lead to such complications as pressure ulcers, thrombi, phlebitis, pneumonia, urinary calculi, and contractures. To prevent complications, be sure to use correct positioning, meticulous skin care, assistive devices, and regular turning and range-of-motion exercises.

Promoting rehabilitation

The first step toward rehabilitation typically is progressive ambulation, which should begin as soon as possible — if necessary, using such assistive devices as a cane, crutches, or a walker. Effective rehabilitation also may require you to teach positioning, transfer, and mobilization techniques to the patient and his family. Demonstrating a technique — such as transfer from bed to wheelchair — during hospitalization helps the patient and his family to understand it. Allowing them to practice it under your supervision gives them the confidence to perform it at home. Encourage them to provide positive reinforcement to motivate the patient to work toward his goals.

ADMISSION, TRANSFER, AND DISCHARGE PROCEDURES

Admission

Admission to the nursing unit prepares the patient for his hospital stay. Whether the admission is scheduled or follows emergency treatment, effective admission procedures should accomplish the following goals: verify the patient's identity and assess his clinical status, make him as comfortable as possible in his new and potentially threatening environment, introduce him to roommates and staff, orient him to the physical environment and routine activities, and provide supplies and special equipment needed for daily care.

Because admission procedures can color the patient's perception of the hospital environment, they have a significant impact on subsequent treatment. Admission routines that are efficient and show appropriate concern for the patient ease his anxiety and promote cooperation and receptivity to treatment. Conversely, admission routines that the patient perceives as careless or excessively impersonal can heighten anxiety, reduce cooperation, impair his response to treatment, and perhaps aggravate symptoms.

Equipment

Hospital gown ▪ personal property form ▪ valuables envelope ▪ admission form ▪ nursing assessment form, if appropriate ▪ thermometer ▪ emesis basin ▪ bedpan or urinal ▪ bath basin ▪ water pitcher, cup, and tray ▪ urine specimen container, if needed.

An admission pack usually contains soap, comb, toothbrush, toothpaste, mouthwash, water pitcher, cup, tray, lotion, facial tissues, and thermometer (if you won't be using an electronic thermometer). Because the patient's pack is included in his hospital bill, he can take it home at the end of his stay. An admission pack helps prevent cross-contamination and increases nursing efficiency by providing basic items at each patient's bedside.

Implementation

• Obtain a gown and an admission pack for the patient.
• Position the bed as the patient's condition requires. If the patient is ambulatory, place the bed in the low position; if he is arriving on a stretcher, place the bed in the high position. Fold down the top linens.
• Adjust the lights, temperature, and ventilation in the room. If the patient requires emergency or special equipment, such as oxygen or suction, prepare it for use.

Admitting the adult patient

• When the patient arrives on the unit, greet him by his proper name and introduce yourself and any staff present. Be sure to speak slowly and clearly.
• Compare the name and hospital number on the patient's identification bracelet with that listed on the admission form. Verify the name and its spelling with the patient. Notify the admission office of any corrections.
• Quickly review the admission form and the doctor's orders. Note the reason for admission, any restrictions on activity or diet, and any orders for diagnostic tests requiring specimen collection.
• Escort the patient to his room and, if he's not in great distress, introduce him to his roommate. Then wash your hands and help him change into a hospital gown or pajamas; if the patient is sharing a room, provide privacy. Itemize all valuables, clothing, and prostheses on the nursing assessment form; if your hospital doesn't use such a form, itemize the patient's belongings in your notes. Encourage the patient to store valuables or money in the hospital safe or, preferably, to send them home along with any medications he may have brought. Show the ambulatory patient where the bathroom and closets are located.
• Take and record the patient's vital signs, and collect specimens if ordered. Measure the patient's height and weight if his condition allows it. If the patient can't stand, use a chair or bed scale and ask him his height. *Knowing the patient's height and weight is important for planning treatment and diet and for calculating medication and anesthetic dosages.*
• Show the patient how to use the equipment in his room. Be sure to include the call system, bed controls, TV controls, telephone, and lights.
• Explain the hospital routine. Tell the patient when to expect meals, vital sign checks, and medications. Inform him of the visiting hours and of any restrictions on visiting.
• Take a complete patient history. Include all previous hospitalizations, illnesses, and surgeries; current drug therapy; and food or drug allergies. Ask the patient to tell you why he came to the hospital. Record the answers (in the patient's own words) as the chief complaint. Follow up with a physical assessment, emphasizing complaints. If you discover any marks, bruises, or discolorations, record them on the nursing assessment form.
• After assessing the patient, inform him of any tests that have been ordered and when they're scheduled. Describe what he should expect.
• Before leaving the patient's room, make sure he's comfortable and safe. Adjust his bed, and place the call button and other equipment (such as water pitcher and cup,

emesis basin, and facial tissues) within easy reach. Raise the side rails.
• Post patient care reminders (concerning such topics as allergies or special needs) at the patient's bedside *to notify co-workers.* (See *Using patient care reminders* for examples.)

Admitting the pediatric patient
• Your initial goal will be to establish a friendly, trusting relationship with the child and his parents *to help relieve fears and anxiety, which can hinder treatment.* Remember that a child under age 3 may fear separation from his parents; an older child may worry about what will happen to him in the hospital.
• Speak directly to the child, and allow him to answer questions before obtaining more information from his parents.
• While orienting the parents and child to the unit, describe the layout of the room and bathroom, and tell them the location of the playroom, television room, and snack room, if available.
• Teach the child how to call the nurse. Stress that she will be available at all times to take care of all his needs, such as getting him a drink or helping him to the bathroom.
• Explain the institution's rooming-in and visiting policies *so the parents can take every opportunity to be with their child.*
• Inquire about the child's usual routine *so that favorite foods, bedtime rituals, toileting, and adequate rest can be incorporated into the hospital routine.*
• Encourage the parents to bring some of their child's favorite toys, blankets, or other items to the hospital *to make the child feel more at home amid unfamiliar surroundings.*

Special considerations
If the patient doesn't speak English and isn't accompanied by a bilingual family member, contact the appropriate resource (usually the social services department) to secure an interpreter.

Keep in mind that the patient admitted to the emergency department (ED) requires different procedures than the patient admitted to other departments. (See *Managing emergency admissions,* page 6.)

If the patient brings medication from home, take an inventory and record this information on the nursing assessment form. Instruct the patient not to take any medication unless authorized by the doctor. Send authorized medication to the hospital pharmacy for identification and relabeling. Send other medication home with a responsible family member, or store it in the designated area outside the patient's room until he's discharged. *Use*

Using patient care reminders

When placed at the head of the patient's bed, care reminders call attention to the patient's special needs and help ensure consistent care by communicating these needs to the hospital staff, the patient's family, and other visitors.

You can use a specially designed card or a plain piece of paper to post *important information* about the patient, such as the following:
• Allergies
• Dietary restrictions
• Fluid restrictions
• Specimen collection
• Patient deaf or hearing-impaired in right or left ear
• Foreign-language speaker

You can also use care reminders to post *special instructions,* such as the following:
• Complete bed rest
• No BP on right arm
• Turn q 1 hour
• NPO
• I & O

Never violate the patient's privacy by posting his diagnosis, details about surgery, or any information he might find embarrassing.

---

of unauthorized medication may interfere with treatment or cause an overdose.*

Find out the patient's normal routine, and ask him if he would like to make any adjustments to the hospital regimen; for instance, he may prefer to shower at night instead of in the morning. *By accommodating the patient with such adjustments whenever possible, you can ease his anxiety and help him feel more in control of his potentially threatening situation.*

Documentation
After leaving the patient's room, complete the nursing assessment form or your notes, as specified by your institution. The completed form should include the patient's vital signs, height, weight, allergies, and drug and health history; a list of his belongings and those that he sent home with family members; the results of your physical assessment (see "Physical assessment" elsewhere in this chapter); and a record of specimens collected for diagnostic tests.

Managing emergency admissions

For the patient admitted through the emergency department (ED), treating his immediate needs overshadows routine admission procedures. After ED treatment, the patient arrives on the nursing unit with a temporary identification bracelet, a doctor's order sheet, and a record of treatment. Read this record and talk to the nurse who cared for the patient in the ED to ensure continuity of care and to gain insight into the patient's condition and behavior.

Next, record any ongoing treatment, such as an I.V. infusion, in your notes. Take and record the patient's vital signs, and follow the doctor's orders for treatment. If the patient is conscious and not in great distress, explain any treatment orders. Otherwise, delay your explanation. If family members accompany the patient, ask them to wait in the lounge while you assess the patient and begin treatment. Permit them to visit the patient after he's settled in his room. When the patient's condition allows, proceed with routine admission procedures.

Transfer

Patient transfer—either within the hospital or to another care facility—requires thorough preparation and careful documentation. Preparation includes an explanation of the transfer to the patient and his family, discussion of the patient's condition and care plan with the staff at the receiving unit or facility, and arrangements for transportation if necessary. Documentation of the patient's condition before and during transfer and adequate communication between nursing staffs ensure continuity of nursing care and provide legal protection for the transferring hospital and its staff.

Equipment
Admission inventory of belongings ■ patient's chart, medication record, and nursing Kardex ■ medications ■ bag or suitcase.

Implementation
• Explain the transfer to the patient and his family. Assess his physical condition *to determine the means of transfer,* such as a wheelchair or a stretcher.

• Using the admissions inventory of belongings as a checklist, collect the patient's property. Be sure to check the entire room, including the closet, bedside stand, over-bed table, and bathroom. If the patient is being transferred to another facility, don't forget valuables or personal medications that have been stored.
• Gather the patient's medications from the cart and the refrigerator. If the patient is being transferred to another unit, send them to the receiving unit; if he's being transferred to another facility, return them to the hospital pharmacy.
• Notify the hospital's business office and other appropriate departments of the transfer.
• Have a staff person notify the dietary department, the pharmacy, and the hospital telephone operator of the transfer (if within the hospital).
• Contact the nursing staff on the receiving unit, and review the patient's condition, drug regimen, and nursing care plan with them *to ensure continuity of care.*

Transfer within the hospital
• If the patient is being transferred from or to an intensive care unit, your hospital may require new care orders from the patient's doctor. If so, review the new orders with the nursing staff at the receiving unit.
• Send the patient's chart, laboratory request slips, Kardex, special equipment, and other required materials to the receiving unit.
• Use a wheelchair to transport the ambulatory patient to the newly assigned room unless it's on the same unit as his present one, in which case he may be allowed to walk. Use a stretcher to transport the bedridden patient.
• Introduce the patient to the nursing staff at the receiving unit. Then take the patient to his room and, depending on his condition, place him in the bed or seat him in a chair. Introduce him to his new roommate, if appropriate, and tell him about any unfamiliar equipment in the room.

Transfer to an extended care facility
• Make sure the patient's doctor has written the transfer order on his chart and has completed the special transfer form. This form should include the patient's diagnosis, care summary, drug regimen, and special care instructions, such as diet and physical therapy.
• Complete the nursing summary, including the patient's assessment, progress, required nursing treatments, and special needs, *to ensure continuity of care.*
• Keep one copy of the transfer form and the nursing summary with the patient's chart, and forward the other copies to the receiving facility. However, don't send the patient's medications, Kardex, or chart.

Transfer to an acute care facility
• Make sure the doctor has written the transfer order on the patient's chart and has completed the transfer form as discussed above. Then complete the nursing summary.
• Depending on the doctor's instructions, send one copy of the transfer form and the nursing summary and photocopies of the pertinent excerpts from the patient's chart — such as laboratory test and X-ray results, patient history and physical progress notes, and vital sign records — to the receiving facility with the patient. Or, following your facility's policy, substitute a written summary of the patient's condition and hospital history for the excerpts from the patient's chart. *This information legally protects the transferring hospital and its staff and completes the patient's chart.*

Special considerations
If the patient requires an ambulance to take him to another facility, arrange transportation with the hospital's social services department. Ensure that the necessary equipment is assembled to provide care during transport.

Documentation
Record the time and date of transfer, the patient's condition during transfer, the name of the receiving unit or facility, and the means of transportation.

 # Discharge

Although discharge from the hospital is usually considered routine, effective discharge requires careful planning and continuing assessment of the patient's needs during his hospitalization. Ideally, discharge planning begins shortly after admission. Discharge planning aims to teach the patient and his family about his illness and its effect on his life-style; to provide instructions for home care; to communicate dietary or activity instructions; and to explain the purpose, adverse effects, and scheduling of drug treatment. It can also include arranging for transportation, follow-up care if necessary, and coordination of outpatient or home health care services.

Equipment
Wheelchair, unless the patient leaves by ambulance ■ patient's chart ■ patient instruction sheet ■ discharge summary sheet ■ plastic bag or patient's suitcase for personal belongings.

Implementation
• Before the day of discharge, inform the patient's family of the time and date of discharge. If his family can't arrange transportation, notify the social services department. (Always confirm arranged transportation on the day of discharge.)
• Obtain a written discharge order from the doctor. If the patient discharges himself against medical advice, obtain the appropriate hospital form. (See *Dealing with a discharge against medical advice.)*
• If the patient requires home medical care, confirm arrangements with the appropriate community agency or hospital department.
• On the day of discharge, review the patient's discharge care plan, initiated on admission and modified during his hospitalization, with the patient and his family. List prescribed drugs on the patient instruction sheet along with the dosage, prescribed time schedule, and adverse reactions that he should report to the doctor. Ensure that the drug schedule is consistent with the patient's life-style *to prevent improper administration and to promote patient compliance.* (See *Discharge teaching goals,* page 8.)
• Review procedures the patient or his family will perform at home. If necessary, demonstrate these procedures, provide written instructions, and check performance with a return demonstration.
• List dietary and activity instructions, if applicable, on the patient instruction sheet, and review the reasons for them. If the doctor orders bed rest, make sure the patient's family can provide daily care and will obtain necessary equipment.

Discharge teaching goals

Your discharge teaching should aim to ensure that
the patient:
☐ understands his illness
☐ complies with his drug therapy
☐ carefully follows his diet
☐ manages his activity level
☐ understands his treatments
☐ recognizes his need for rest
☐ knows about possible complications
☐ knows when to seek follow-up care.
   Remember that your discharge teaching must include the patient's family or other caregivers to ensure that the patient receives proper home care.

• Check with the doctor about the patient's next office
appointment; if the doctor hasn't yet done so, inform the
patient of the date, time, and location. If scheduling is
your responsibility, make an appointment with the doctor,
outpatient clinic, physical therapy, X-ray department, or
other health services, as needed. If the patient can't
arrange transportation, notify the social services department.
• Retrieve the patient's valuables from the hospital safe
and review each item with him. Then obtain the patient's
signature *to verify receipt of his valuables.*
• Obtain from the pharmacy any drugs the patient brought
to the hospital. Return these to the patient if drug therapy is unchanged. If giving a new prescription, provide
an explanation of the dosage, schedule, and adverse effects.
• If appropriate, take and record the patient's vital signs
on the discharge summary form. Notify the doctor if any
signs are abnormal, such as an elevated temperature. *If
necessary, the doctor may alter the patient's discharge plan.*
• Help the patient get dressed if necessary.
• Collect the patient's personal belongings from his room,
compare them with the admission inventory of belongings, and help place them in his suitcase or a plastic bag.
• After checking the room for misplaced belongings, help
the patient into the wheelchair, and escort him to the
hospital's exit; if the patient is leaving by ambulance,
help him onto the litter. If the patient's family hasn't
already made arrangements for payment, contact the
business office.
• After the patient has left the area, strip the bed linens
and notify the housekeeping staff that the room is ready
for terminal cleaning.

Special considerations
Whenever possible, involve the patient's family in discharge planning *so they can better understand and perform
patient care procedures.* Before the patient is discharged,
perform a physical assessment. If you detect abnormal
signs or the patient develops new symptoms, notify the
doctor and delay discharge until he has seen the patient.

Documentation
Although hospital policy determines the extent and form
of discharge documentation, you'll usually record the
time and date of discharge, the patient's physical condition, special dietary or activity instructions, the type
and frequency of home care procedures, the patient's drug
regimen, the dates of follow-up appointments, the mode
of departure and name of the patient's escort, and a
summary of the patient's hospitalization if necessary.

ASSESSMENT
Temperature

Body temperature represents the balance between heat
produced by metabolism, muscular activity, and other
factors and heat lost through the skin, lungs, and body
wastes. A stable temperature pattern promotes proper
function of cells, tissues, and organs; a change in this
pattern usually signals the onset of illness.
   Temperature can be measured with a mercury, a digital electronic, or a chemical-dot thermometer. Oral temperature in adults normally ranges from 97° to 99.5° F
(36.1° to 37.5° C); rectal temperature, the most accurate
reading, is usually 1° F higher; axillary temperature, the
least accurate, reads 1° to 2° F (0.6° to 1.1° C) lower.
   Temperature normally fluctuates with rest and activity. Lowest readings typically occur between 4 and 5
a.m.; the highest readings occur between 4 and 8 p.m.
Other factors also influence temperature, including sex,
age, emotional condition, and environment. Keep the following principles in mind. Women normally have higher
temperatures than men, especially during ovulation. Normal temperature is highest in neonates and lowest in
elderly persons. Heightened emotions raise temperature;
depressed emotions lower it. A hot external environment
can raise temperature; a cold environment lowers it.

Equipment
Mercury or electronic thermometer for oral or rectal use,
or chemical-dot thermometer ▪ water-soluble lubricant or
petroleum jelly (for rectal temperature) ▪ facial tissue ▪

EQUIPMENT

 Types of thermometers

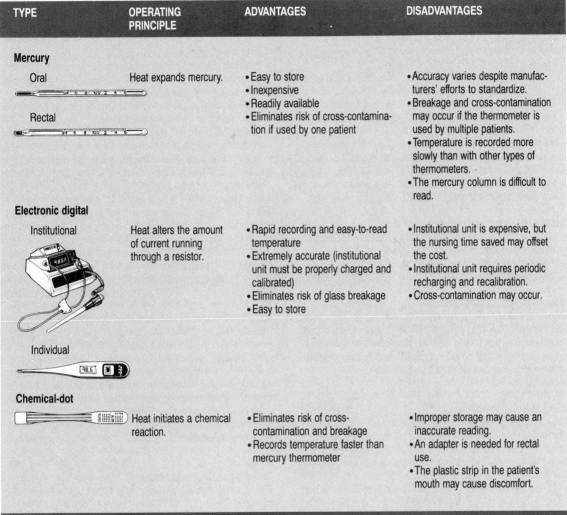

TYPE	OPERATING PRINCIPLE	ADVANTAGES	DISADVANTAGES
Mercury			
Oral	Heat expands mercury.	• Easy to store • Inexpensive • Readily available • Eliminates risk of cross-contamination if used by one patient	• Accuracy varies despite manufacturers' efforts to standardize. • Breakage and cross-contamination may occur if the thermometer is used by multiple patients. • Temperature is recorded more slowly than with other types of thermometers. • The mercury column is difficult to read.
Rectal			
Electronic digital			
Institutional	Heat alters the amount of current running through a resistor.	• Rapid recording and easy-to-read temperature • Extremely accurate (institutional unit must be properly charged and calibrated) • Eliminates risk of glass breakage • Easy to store	• Institutional unit is expensive, but the nursing time saved may offset the cost. • Institutional unit requires periodic recharging and recalibration. • Cross-contamination may occur.
Individual			
Chemical-dot	Heat initiates a chemical reaction.	• Eliminates risk of cross-contamination and breakage • Records temperature faster than mercury thermometer	• Improper storage may cause an inaccurate reading. • An adapter is needed for rectal use. • The plastic strip in the patient's mouth may cause discomfort.

disposable thermometer sheath or probe cover (except for chemical-dot thermometer) ▪ alcohol sponge.

Preparation of equipment
A thermometer may be included as part of the admission pack. If it is, keep it at the patient's bedside and, on discharge, allow him to take it home. Otherwise, obtain a thermometer from the nurse's station or central supply department, and bring it to the patient's bedside. If you use an electronic thermometer, make sure it has been recharged. (See *Types of thermometers.*)

Implementation
• Explain the procedure to the patient, and wash your hands.

Using a mercury thermometer

• Hold the thermometer between your thumb and index finger at the end opposite the bulb.

• If the thermometer has been soaking in a disinfectant, rinse it in cold water. *Rinsing removes chemicals that may irritate oral or rectal mucous membranes or axillary skin.* Avoid using hot water *because it expands the mercury, which could break the thermometer.* Using a twisting motion, wipe the thermometer from the bulb upward.

• Then quickly snap your wrist several times while holding the thermometer to shake it down. *Shaking causes the mercury to descend into the bulb.* The mercury will then expand in response to the patient's body temperature and be forced upward.

• To use a disposable sheath over the mercury thermometer, disinfect the thermometer with an alcohol sponge. Insert it into the disposable sheath opening, then twist to tear the seal at the dotted line. Pull it apart. *Using a sheath decreases contamination and reduces cleaning time.*

Using an electronic thermometer

• Insert the probe into a disposable probe cover. If taking a rectal temperature, lubricate the probe cover *to reduce friction and ease insertion.* Leave the probe in place until the maximum temperature appears on the digital display.

Using a chemical-dot thermometer

• Remove the thermometer from its protective dispenser case by grasping the handle end with your thumb and forefinger, moving the handle up and down to break the seal, and pulling the handle straight out. Be sure to keep the thermometer sealed until use *because opening it activates the dye dots.*

Taking an oral temperature

• Position the tip of the thermometer under the patient's tongue, as far back as possible, on either side of the frenulum linguae. *Placing the tip in this area promotes contact with abundant superficial blood vessels and contributes to an accurate reading.*

• Instruct the patient to close his lips but to avoid biting down with his teeth. *Biting can break a mercury thermometer, cutting the mouth or lips or causing ingestion of broken glass or mercury.*

• Leave a mercury thermometer in place for at least 2 minutes or a chemical-dot thermometer for 45 seconds *to register temperature,* or wait until the maximum temperature is displayed on the electronic thermometer. (With some electronic units, a buzzer sounds when the maximum temperature is reached; with others, a light appears.)

• For a mercury thermometer, remove and discard the disposable sheath, then read the temperature at eye level,

noting it before shaking down the thermometer. For an electronic thermometer, note the temperature, then remove and discard the probe cover. For the chemical-dot thermometer, read the temperature as the last dye dot that has changed color, or fired, then discard the thermometer and its dispenser case.

Taking a rectal temperature

• Position the patient on his side with his top leg flexed, and drape him to provide privacy. Then fold back the bed linens to expose the anus.

• Squeeze the lubricant onto a facial tissue *to prevent contamination of the lubricant supply.*

• Lubricate about ½" (1.3 cm) of the thermometer tip for an infant or about 1½" (3.8 cm) for an adult. *Lubrication reduces friction and thus eases insertion.* This step may be unnecessary when using disposable rectal sheaths *because they're prelubricated.*

• Lift the patient's upper buttock, and insert the thermometer about ½" for an infant or 1½" for an adult. Gently direct the thermometer along the rectal wall toward the umbilicus. *This will avoid perforating the anus or rectum or breaking the thermometer. It also will help ensure an accurate reading because the thermometer will register hemorrhoidal artery temperature instead of fecal temperature.* Feces may increase the patient's apparent temperature *because of the heat given off during decomposition.*

• Hold the mercury thermometer in place for 2 to 3 minutes or the electronic thermometer until the maximum temperature is displayed. *Holding it prevents damage to rectal tissues caused by displacement or loss of the thermometer into the rectum.* Note: Electronic thermometers usually provide a separate rectal probe that may be color coded to distinguish it more easily from the oral probe.

• Carefully remove the thermometer, wiping it as necessary.

• Wipe the patient's anal area *to remove any lubricant or feces.*

Taking an axillary temperature

• Position the patient comfortably with the axilla exposed.

• Gently pat the axilla dry with a facial tissue *because moisture conducts heat.* Avoid harsh rubbing, *which generates heat.*

• Ask the patient to place his hand over his chest and to grasp his opposite shoulder, lifting his elbow.

• Position the thermometer in the axilla, with the tip pointing toward the patient's head.

• Tell the patient to continue grasping his shoulder and to lower his elbow and hold it against his chest. *This promotes skin contact with the thermometer.*

• Leave a mercury thermometer in place for 10 minutes; leave an electronic thermometer in place until it displays the maximum temperature. Axillary temperature takes longer to register than oral or rectal temperature *because the thermometer isn't enclosed in a body cavity.*
• Grasp the end of the thermometer and remove it from the axilla.

Special considerations
Oral measurement is contraindicated in patients who are unconscious, disoriented, or seizure-prone; in young children and infants; and in patients with oral or nasal impairment that necessitates mouth breathing. Rectal measurement is contraindicated in patients with diarrhea, recent rectal or prostatic surgery or injury *because it may injure inflamed tissue,* or recent myocardial infarction *because anal manipulation may stimulate the vagus nerve, causing bradycardia or another rhythm disturbance.*

Drinking hot or cold liquids, chewing gum, or smoking may alter oral temperature readings. Wait 15 minutes after these activities before taking a temperature. Bathing may alter axillary temperature.

Use the same thermometer for repeated temperature taking *to avoid spurious variations caused by equipment differences.* Store chemical-dot thermometers in a cool area *because exposure to heat activates the dye dots.*

Don't avoid taking an oral temperature when the patient is receiving nasal oxygen *because oxygen administration raises oral temperature by only about 0.3° F (0.17° C).*

Documentation
Record the time, route, and temperature on the patient's chart.

Pulse

Blood pumped by the heart into an already-full aorta during ventricular contraction creates a fluid wave that travels from the heart to the peripheral arteries. This recurring wave — called a pulse — can be palpated at locations on the body where an artery crosses over bone or firm tissue. (See *Pulse points.*) In adults and children over age 3, the radial artery in the wrist is the most common palpation site because it's easily accessible and the artery can be compressed readily against the radius. In infants and children under age 3, a stethoscope is used to listen to the heart itself rather than palpating a pulse. Because auscultation is done at the heart's apex, this is called the apical pulse.

Pulse points

Shown below are anatomic locations where an artery crosses bone or firm tissue and can be palpated for a pulse.

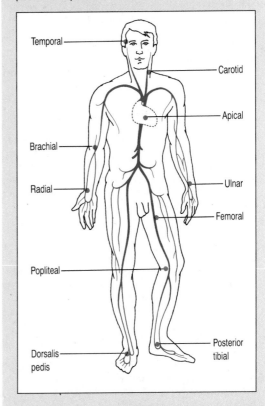

An apical-radial pulse is taken by simultaneously counting apical and radial beats — the first by auscultation at the apex of the heart, the second by palpation at the radial artery. Some heartbeats detected at the apex aren't strong enough to be detected at peripheral sites. When this occurs, the apical pulse rate is higher than the radial; the difference between the two rates is the pulse deficit.

Pulse taking involves determining the rate (number of beats per minute), rhythm (pattern or regularity of the beats), and volume (amount of blood pumped with each beat). If the pulse is faint or weak, use a Doppler ultrasound blood flow detector if available. (See *Detecting blood flow with Doppler ultrasound,* page 12.)

Detecting blood flow with Doppler ultrasound

More sensitive than palpation for determining pulse rate, the Doppler ultrasound blood flow detector is especially useful when a pulse is faint or weak. Unlike palpation, which detects arterial wall expansion and retraction, this instrument detects the motion of red blood cells.

Doppler probe with amplifier

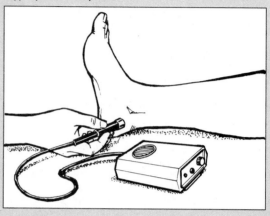

To use the Doppler device
• Apply a small amount of coupling gel or transmission gel (not water-soluble lubricant) to the ultrasound probe.
• Position the probe on the skin directly over the selected artery. In the top illustration, the probe is over the posterior tibial artery.
• When using a Doppler model like the one in the top illustration, turn the instrument on and, moving counterclockwise, set the volume control to the lowest setting. If your model doesn't have a speaker, plug in the earphones and slowly raise the volume. The Doppler ultrasound stethoscope shown at lower right is basically a stethoscope fitted with an audio unit, volume control, and transducer, which amplifies the movement of red blood cells.
• To obtain the best signals with either device, tilt the probe 45 degrees from the artery, making sure to put gel between the skin and the probe. Slowly move the probe in a circular motion to locate the center of the artery and the Doppler signal—a hissing noise at the heartbeat. Avoid moving the probe rapidly because this distorts the signal.
• Count the signals for 60 seconds to determine the pulse rate.
• After you've measured the pulse rate, clean the probe with a soft cloth soaked in antiseptic solution or soapy water. Don't immerse the probe or bump it against a hard surface.

Doppler ultrasound stethoscope

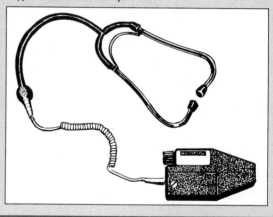

Equipment
Watch with second hand ■ stethoscope (for auscultating apical pulse) ■ Doppler ultrasound blood flow detector if necessary.

Preparation of equipment
If you're not using your own stethoscope, disinfect the earpieces with an alcohol sponge before and after use *to prevent cross-contamination.*

Implementation
• Wash your hands, and tell the patient that you intend to take his pulse.

• Make sure the patient is comfortable and relaxed *because an awkward, uncomfortable position may affect the heart rate.*

Taking a radial pulse
• Place the patient in a sitting or supine position, with his arm at his side or across his chest.
• Gently press your index, middle, and ring fingers on the radial artery, inside the patient's wrist. You should feel a pulse with only moderate pressure; *excessive pressure may obstruct blood flow distal to the pulse site.* Don't use your thumb to take the patient's pulse *because its own strong pulse may be confused with the patient's.*

Identifying pulse patterns

TYPE	RATE	RHYTHM (PER 3 SECONDS)	CAUSES AND INCIDENCE
Normal	60 to 80 beats/minute; in neonates, 120 to 140 beats/minute	● ● ● ●	• Varies with such factors as age, physical activity, and sex (men usually have lower pulse rates than women)
Tachycardia	Above 100 beats/minute	●●●●●●● ●	• Accompanies stimulation of the sympathetic nervous system by emotional stress – anger, fear, anxiety – or certain drugs, such as caffeine • May result from exercise and from certain health conditions, such as congestive heart failure, anemia, and fever (which increases oxygen requirements and therefore pulse rate)
Bradycardia	Below 60 beats/minute	● ● ●	• Accompanies stimulation of the parasympathetic nervous system by drugs – especially digitalis – and such conditions as cerebral hemorrhage and heart block • May also be present in fit athletes
Irregular	Uneven time intervals between beats (for example, periods of regular rhythm interrupted by pauses or premature beats)	●●●● ●●●	• May indicate cardiac irritability, hypoxia, digitalis overdose, potassium imbalance, or sometimes more serious arrhythmias if frequent premature beats • Occasional premature beats normal

• After you've located the pulse, count the beats for 60 seconds, or, if it's more convenient, count for 30 seconds and multiply by 2. *Counting for a full minute provides a more accurate picture of irregularities.* While counting the rate, assess pulse rhythm and volume by noting the pattern and strength of the beats. If you detect an irregularity, repeat the count, *because pulse irregularities are important signs.* Note if the irregularity occurs in a pattern or randomly. If doubt remains, take an apical pulse. (See *Identifying pulse patterns.*)

Taking an apical pulse
• Help the patient to a supine position and drape him if necessary.
• Warm the diaphragm or bell of the stethoscope in your hand before applying it to the patient's chest. *Placing a cold stethoscope against the skin may startle the patient and momentarily increase the heart rate.* Keep in mind that the bell transmits low-pitched sounds more effectively than the diaphragm.
• Place the diaphragm or bell of the stethoscope over the apex of the heart, which normally is located at the fifth intercostal space left of the midclavicular line. Then insert the earpieces into your ears. Count the beats for 60 seconds (or count for 30 seconds and multiply by 2) and note their rhythm and volume. Also evaluate the intensity (loudness) of heart sounds.
• Remove the stethoscope and make the patient comfortable.

Taking an apical-radial pulse
• Two nurses work together to obtain the apical-radial pulse; one palpates the radial pulse while the other auscultates the apical pulse with a stethoscope. Both must use the same watch when counting beats.

• Help the patient to a supine position and drape him if necessary.
• Locate the apical and radial pulses.
• Determine a time to begin counting. Then each nurse should count beats for 60 seconds.

Special considerations
When the peripheral pulse is irregular, take an apical pulse to measure the heartbeat more directly. If the pulse is faint or weak, use a Doppler ultrasound blood flow detector if available.

If a second nurse is not available to help take an apical-radial pulse, you can hold the stethoscope in place with the hand that holds the watch while palpating the radial pulse with the other hand. You can then feel any discrepancies between the apical and radial pulses.

Documentation
Record pulse rate, rhythm, and volume and the time of measurement. "Full" or "bounding" describes a pulse of increased volume; "weak" or "thready," decreased volume. When recording apical pulse, include intensity of heart sounds. When recording apical-radial pulse, chart the rate according to the pulse site—for example, A/R pulse of 80/76.

Respiration

Controlled by the respiratory center in the lateral medulla oblongata, respiration is the exchange of oxygen and carbon dioxide between the atmosphere and body cells. External respiration, or breathing, is accomplished by the diaphragm and chest muscles and delivers oxygen to the lower respiratory tract and alveoli.

Four measures of respiration—rate, rhythm, depth, and sound—reflect the body's metabolic state, diaphragm and chest-muscle condition, and airway patency. Respiratory rate is recorded as the number of cycles (with inspiration and expiration comprising one cycle) per minute; rhythm, as the regularity of these cycles; depth, as the volume of air inhaled and exhaled with each respiration; and sound, as the audible digression from normal, effortless breathing.

Equipment
Watch with second hand.

Implementation
• The best time to assess your patient's respirations is immediately after taking the pulse rate. Keep your fin-gertips over the radial artery, and don't tell the patient you're counting respirations. If you tell him, *he'll become conscious of his respirations and the rate may change.*
• Count respirations by observing the rise and fall of the patient's chest as he breathes. Or position the patient's opposite arm across his chest and count respirations by feeling its rise and fall. Consider one rise and one fall as one respiration.
• Count respirations for 30 seconds and multiply by 2 or count for 60 seconds if respirations are irregular *to account for variations in respiratory rate and pattern.* As you count respirations, be alert for and record such breath sounds as stertor, stridor, wheezing, and an expiratory grunt. *Stertor* is a snoring sound resulting from secretions in the trachea and large bronchi. Listen for it in patients with neurologic disorders and in those who are comatose. *Stridor* is an inspiratory crowing sound that occurs with upper airway obstruction in laryngitis, croup, or the presence of a foreign body. When listening for stridor in infants and children with croup, also observe for sternal, substernal, or intercostal retractions. *Wheezing* is caused by partial obstruction in the smaller bronchi and bronchioles. This high-pitched, musical sound is common in patients with emphysema or asthma. In infants, an *expiratory grunt* indicates imminent respiratory distress. In older patients, it may result from partial airway obstruction or neuromuscular reflex.
• To detect other breath sounds—such as crackles and rhonchi—or the lack of sound in the lungs, you will need a stethoscope.
• Observe chest movements for depth of respiration. If the patient inhales a small volume of air, record this as shallow; if he inhales a large volume, record this as deep.
• Watch chest movements and listen to breathing *to determine the rhythm and sound of respiration.* (See *Identifying respiratory patterns.*)

Special considerations
Respiratory rates below 8 and above 40 breaths/minute usually are considered abnormal; report the sudden onset of such rates promptly. Observe for signs of dyspnea, such as an anxious facial expression, flaring nostrils, a heaving chest wall, and cyanosis. To detect cyanosis, look for characteristic bluish discoloration in the nail beds or the lips, under the tongue, in the buccal mucosa, or in the conjunctiva.

In assessing the patient's respiratory status, consider his personal and family history. Ask if he smokes and, if so, for how many years and how many packs a day.

A child's respiratory rate may double in response to exercise, illness, or emotion. Normally, the rate for newborns is 30 to 80 breaths/minute; for toddlers, 20 to 40;

Identifying respiratory patterns

TYPE	CHARACTERISTICS	PATTERN	POSSIBLE CAUSES
Apnea	Periodic absence of breathing		• Mechanical airway obstruction • Conditions affecting the brain's respiratory center in the lateral medulla oblongata
Apneustic	Prolonged, gasping inspiration, followed by extremely short, inefficient expiration		• Lesions of the respiratory center
Bradypnea	Slow, regular respirations of equal depth		• Normal pattern during sleep • Conditions affecting the respiratory center: tumors, metabolic disorders, respiratory decompensation; use of opiates and alcohol
Cheyne-Stokes	Fast, deep respirations of 30 to 170 seconds punctuated by periods of apnea lasting 20 to 60 seconds		• Increased intracranial pressure, severe congestive heart failure, renal failure, meningitis, drug overdose, cerebral anoxia
Eupnea	Normal rate and rhythm		• Normal respiration
Kussmaul's	Fast (over 20 breaths/minute), deep (resembling sighs), labored respirations without pause		• Renal failure or metabolic acidosis, particularly diabetic ketoacidosis
Tachypnea	Rapid respirations. Rate rises with body temperature—about four breaths/minute for every degree Fahrenheit above normal		• Pneumonia, compensatory respiratory alkalosis, respiratory insufficiency, lesions of the respiratory center, and salicylate poisoning

and for children of school age and older, 15 to 25. Children usually reach the adult rate (12 to 20) at about age 15.

Documentation
Record the rate, depth, rhythm, and sound of the patient's respirations.

Blood pressure

Defined as the lateral force exerted by blood on the arterial walls, blood pressure depends on the force of ventricular contractions, arterial wall elasticity, peripheral vascular resistance, and blood volume and viscosity. Systolic, or maximum, pressure occurs during left ventricular contraction and reflects the integrity of the heart, arteries, and arterioles. Diastolic, or minimum, pressure occurs during left ventricular relaxation and directly indicates blood vessel resistance.

Pulse pressure, the difference between systolic and diastolic pressures, varies inversely with arterial elasticity. Rigid vessels, incapable of distention and recoil, produce high systolic pressure and low diastolic pressure. Normally, systolic pressure exceeds diastolic pressure by about 40 mm Hg. Narrowed pulse pressure—a difference of less than 30 mm Hg—occurs when systolic pressure falls and diastolic pressure remains constant, when diastolic pressure rises and systolic pressure stays constant, or when systolic pressure falls and diastolic pressure rises. These changes reflect reduced stroke volume, increased peripheral resistance, or both. Widened pulse pressure—a difference of more than 50 mm Hg between systolic and diastolic blood pressures—occurs when systolic pressure rises and diastolic pressure remains constant, when diastolic pressure falls and systolic pressure remains constant, or when systolic pressure rises and diastolic pressure falls. These changes reflect increased stroke volume, decreased peripheral resistance, or both.

Blood pressure is measured in millimeters of mercury with a sphygmomanometer and a stethoscope, usually at the brachial artery (less often at the popliteal or radial artery). Lowest in the neonate, blood pressure rises with age, weight gain, prolonged stress, and anxiety. (See *Effects of age on blood pressure.*)

Frequent blood pressure measurement is critical after serious injury, surgery, or anesthesia and during any illness or condition that threatens cardiovascular stability. (This may be done with an automated vital signs monitor.) Regular measurement is indicated for patients with a history of hypertension or hypotension, and yearly screening is recommended for all adults.

Equipment

Mercury or aneroid sphygmomanometer ▪ stethoscope ▪ alcohol sponge ▪ automated vital signs monitor (if available).

The sphygmomanometer consists of an inflatable compression cuff linked to a manual air pump and a mercury manometer or an aneroid gauge. The mercury sphygmomanometer is more accurate and requires calibration less frequently than the aneroid model but is larger and heavier. To obtain an accurate reading, you must rest its gauge on a level surface and view the meniscus at eye level; you can rest an aneroid gauge in any position but must view it directly from the front. Some mercury manometers have specially designed cases that open to form a level surface; others must be attached to a wall or to a base unit that stands on the floor.

Hook, bandage, snap, or Velcro cuffs come in six standard sizes ranging from newborn to extra-large adult. Disposable cuffs are available.

The automated vital signs monitor is a noninvasive device that measures pulse rate, systolic and diastolic pressures, and mean arterial pressure at preset intervals. (See *Using an electronic vital signs monitor.*)

Preparation of equipment

Carefully choose a cuff of appropriate size for the patient. *An excessively narrow cuff may cause a falsely high pressure reading; an excessively wide one, a falsely low reading.* If you're not using your own stethoscope, disinfect the earpieces with an alcohol sponge before placing them in your ears *to avoid cross-contamination.*

To use an automated vital signs monitor, collect the monitor, dual air hose, and pressure cuff. Then make sure the monitor unit is firmly positioned near the patient's bed.

Implementation

• Tell the patient that you're going to take his blood pressure.
• The patient can lie supine or sit erect during blood pressure measurement. His arm should be extended at

Effects of age on blood pressure

AGE	BLOOD PRESSURE (mm Hg)
Neonate	systolic: 50 to 52 diastolic: 25 to 30 mean: 35 to 40
3 years	systolic: 78 to 114 diastolic: 46 to 78
10 years	systolic: 90 to 132 diastolic: 56 to 86
16 years	systolic: 104 to 108 diastolic: 60 to 92
Adult	systolic: 95 to 140 diastolic: 60 to 90
Older adult	systolic: 140 to 160 diastolic: 70 to 90

Using an electronic vital signs monitor

An electronic vital signs monitor allows you to track a patient's vital signs continually, without having to reapply a blood pressure cuff each time. What's more, the patient won't need an invasive arterial line to gather similar data. The machine shown here is a Dinamap VS Monitor 8100, but these steps can be followed with most other monitors.

Some automated vital signs monitors, such as the Dinamap, are lightweight and battery-operated, and can be attached to an I.V. pole for continual monitoring, even during patient transfers. Make sure you know the capacity of the monitor's battery, and plug the machine in whenever possible to keep it charged.

Before using any monitor, check its accuracy. Determine the patient's pulse rate and blood pressure manually, using the same arm you'll use for the monitor cuff. Compare your results when you get initial readings from the monitor. If the results differ, call your supply department or the manufacturer's representative.

Preparing the device
• Explain the procedure to the patient. Describe the alarm system *so he won't be frightened if it's triggered.*
• Make sure the power switch is off. Then plug the monitor into a properly grounded wall outlet. Next, secure the dual air hose to the front of the monitor.
• Connect the pressure cuff's tubing into the other ends of the dual air hose, and tighten connections *to prevent air leaks.* Keep the air hose away from the patient *to avoid accidental dislodgment.*
• Squeeze all air from the cuff, and wrap it loosely around the patient's arm or leg, allowing 2 finger-breadths between cuff and arm or leg. Never apply the cuff to a limb that has an I.V. line in place. Position the cuff's "artery" arrow over the palpated brachial artery. Then secure the cuff for a snug fit.

Selecting parameters
• When you turn on the monitor, it will default to a manual mode. (In this mode, you can obtain vital signs yourself before switching to the automatic mode.) Press the "auto/manual" button to select the automatic mode. The monitor will give you baseline data for the pulse rate, systolic and diastolic pressures, and mean arterial pressure.
• Compare your previous manual results with these baseline data. If they match, you're ready to set the

alarm parameters. Press the "select" button to blank all displays except systolic pressure.
• Use the "high" and "low" limit buttons to set the specific parameters for systolic pressure. (These limits range from a high of 240 to a low of 0.) You'll also do this three more times for mean arterial pressure, pulse rate, and diastolic pressure. After you've set the parameters for diastolic pressure, press the "select" button again to display all current data. Even if you forget to do this last step, the monitor will automatically display current data 10 seconds after you set the last parameters.

Collecting data
• You also need to tell the monitor how often to obtain data. Press the "set" button until you reach the desired time interval in minutes. If you've chosen the automatic mode, the monitor will display a default cycle time of 3 minutes. You can override the default cycle time to set the interval you prefer.
• You can obtain a set of vital signs at any time by pressing the "start" button. Also, pressing the "cancel" button will stop the interval and deflate the cuff. You can retrieve stored data by pressing the "prior data" button. The monitor will display the last data obtained along with the time elapsed since then. Scrolling backward, you can retrieve data from the previous 99 minutes.

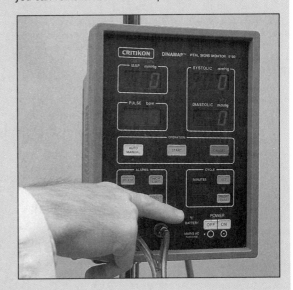

Positioning the blood pressure cuff

Wrap the cuff snugly around the upper arm above the antecubital area (the inner aspect of the elbow). When measuring an adult, place the lower border of the cuff about 1″ (2.5 cm) above the antecubital space. The center of the bladder should rest directly over the medial aspect of the arm. Most cuffs have an arrow for you to position over the brachial artery. Then, place the bell of the stethoscope on the brachial artery at the point where you hear the strongest beats.

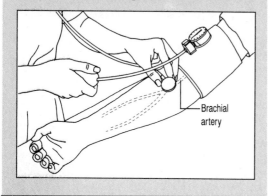

Brachial artery

heart level and be well supported. *If the artery is below heart level, the blood pressure may read falsely high.* Be sure the patient is relaxed and comfortable when you take his blood pressure *so it stays at its normal level.*
• Wrap the deflated cuff snugly around the upper arm. (See *Positioning the blood pressure cuff* for specific instructions.)
• If necessary, connect the appropriate tube to the rubber bulb of the air pump and the other tube to the manometer. Then insert the stethoscope earpieces into your ears.
• Locate the brachial artery by palpation. Center the bell of the stethoscope over the part of the artery where you detect the strongest beats, and hold it in place with one hand. *The bell of the stethoscope transmits low-pitched arterial blood sounds more effectively than the diaphragm.*
• Using the thumb and index finger of your other hand, turn the thumbscrew on the rubber bulb of the air pump clockwise to close the valve.
• Then pump air into the cuff while auscultating the sound over the brachial artery *to compress and, eventually, occlude arterial blood flow.* Pump air until the mercury column or aneroid gauge registers 160 mm Hg or at least 10 mm Hg above the level of the last audible sound.

• Carefully open the valve of the air pump and slowly deflate the cuff—no faster than 5 mm Hg/second. While releasing air, watch the mercury column or aneroid gauge and auscultate the sound over the artery.
• When you hear the first beat or clear tapping sound, note the pressure on the column or gauge. This is the systolic pressure. (The beat or tapping sound is the first of five Korotkoff sounds. The second sound resembles a murmur or swish; the third sound, crisp tapping; the fourth sound, a soft, muffled tone; and the fifth, the last sound heard.)
• Continue to release air gradually while auscultating the sound over the artery.
• Note the diastolic pressure—the fourth Korotkoff sound. If you continue to hear sounds as the column or gauge falls to zero (common in children), record the pressure at the beginning of the fourth sound. This is important *because, in some patients, a distinct fifth sound is absent.*
• Rapidly deflate the cuff. Record the pressure, wait 15 to 30 seconds, then repeat the procedure and record the pressures *to confirm your original findings.* After doing so, remove and fold the cuff, and return it to storage.

Special considerations

If you can't auscultate blood pressure, you may estimate systolic pressure. To do this, first palpate the brachial or radial pulse. Then inflate the cuff until you no longer detect the pulse. Slowly deflate the cuff and, when you detect the pulse again, record the pressure as the palpated systolic pressure. When measuring blood pressure in the popliteal artery, position the patient on his abdomen; wrap a cuff around the middle of the thigh, and proceed with blood pressure measurement.

Palpation of systolic blood pressure also may be important *to avoid underestimating blood pressure in patients with an auscultatory gap.* This gap is a loss of sound between the first and second Korotkoff sounds that may be as great as 40 mm Hg. You may find this in patients with venous congestion or hypotension.

If your patient is crying or anxious, delay blood pressure measurement, if possible, until the patient becomes calm *to avoid falsely elevated readings.*

If your hospital considers the fourth and fifth Korotkoff sounds as the first and second diastolic pressures, record both pressures.

Remember that malfunction in an aneroid sphygmomanometer can be identified only by checking it against a mercury manometer of known accuracy. Be sure to check your aneroid manometer this way periodically. Malfunction in a mercury manometer is evident in abnormal behavior of the mercury column. Don't attempt to repair either type of sphygmomanometer yourself; instead, send

Correcting problems of blood pressure measurement

PROBLEM AND POSSIBLE CAUSE	NURSING ACTION
False-high reading	
• Cuff too small	• Make sure the cuff bladder is 20% wider than the circumference of the arm or leg being used for measurement.
• Cuff wrapped too loosely, reducing its effective width	• Tighten the cuff.
• Slow cuff deflation, causing venous congestion in the arm or leg	• Never deflate the cuff more slowly than 2 mm Hg/heartbeat.
• Tilted mercury column	• Read pressures with the mercury column vertical.
• Poorly timed measurement—after patient has eaten, ambulated, appeared anxious, or flexed arm muscles	• Postpone blood pressure measurement or help the patient relax before taking pressures.
False-low reading	
• Incorrect position of arm or leg	• Make sure the arm or leg is level with the patient's heart.
• Mercury column below eye level	• Read the mercury column at eye level.
• Failure to notice auscultatory gap (sound fades out for 10 to 15 mm Hg, then returns)	• Estimate systolic pressure by palpation before actually measuring it. Then check this pressure against the measured pressure.
• Inaudible low-volume sounds	• Before reinflating the cuff, instruct the patient to raise the arm or leg to decrease venous pressure and amplify low-volume sounds. After inflating the cuff, tell the patient to lower the arm or leg. Then deflate the cuff and listen. If you still fail to detect low-volume sounds, chart the palpated systolic pressure.

it to the appropriate service department. (See *Correcting problems of blood pressure measurement.)*

Occasionally, blood pressure must be measured in both arms or with the patient in two different positions (such as lying and standing, or sitting and standing). In such cases, observe and record any significant difference between the two readings and record the blood pressure, the extremity, and the position used.

Complications
Don't take blood pressure in the arm on the affected side of a mastectomy *because it may decrease already compromised lymphatic circulation, worsen edema, and damage the arm.* Likewise, don't take blood pressure on the same arm of an arteriovenous fistula or hemodialysis shunt *because blood flow through the vascular device may be compromised.*

Documentation
On the patient's chart, record blood pressure as systolic over diastolic pressures, such as 120/78 mm Hg; if necessary, record systolic over the two diastolic pressures, such as 120/78/20 mm Hg. Chart an auscultatory gap if present. If required by your hospital, chart blood pressures on a graph, using dots or checkmarks. Also, document the extremity used and the patient's position.

Types of scales

For ambulatory patients | **For acutely ill or debilitated patients**

Standing scale

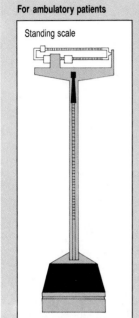

Chair scale   Bed scale

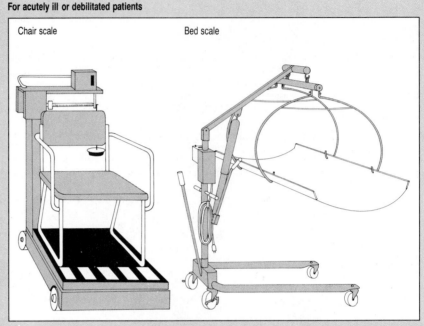

 # Height and weight

Height and weight are routinely measured for most patients during admission to the hospital. An accurate record of the patient's height and weight is essential for calculating dosages of drugs, anesthetics, and contrast agents; assessing the patient's nutritional status; and determining the height-weight ratio. And because body weight provides the best overall picture of fluid status, monitoring it daily proves important for patients receiving sodium-retaining or diuretic medications. Rapid weight gain may signal fluid retention; rapid weight loss may indicate diuresis.

Weight can be measured with a standing scale, chair scale, or bed scale; height can be measured with the measuring bar on a standing scale or with a tape measure for a supine patient.

Equipment
Scale—standing (with measuring bar), chair, or bed ■ wheelchair (if needed to transport patient) ■ tape measure if needed.

Preparation of equipment
Select the appropriate scale—usually, a standing scale for an ambulatory patient or a chair or bed scale for an acutely ill or debilitated patient. (See *Types of scales.*) Then check scale balance. Standing scales and, to a lesser extent, bed scales may become unbalanced when transported.

Implementation
• Explain the procedure to the patient. Refer to a chart of suggested healthy weight ranges *to determine norms for your patient's height and weight. (See Suggested weights for adults.)*

Suggested weights for adults

This chart provides a guideline for determining healthy weights. Higher weights in each category typically apply to men, who average more muscle and bone; lower weights usually apply to women, who have less muscle and bone. Suggested weights for people age 35 and over are higher than those for younger adults because recent research shows that older people can carry somewhat more weight without impairing their health. Height is measured without shoes; weight is measured without clothes.

HEIGHT	WEIGHT (LB)		HEIGHT	WEIGHT (LB)	
	Age 19 to 34	**Age 35 and over**		**Age 19 to 34**	**Age 35 and over**
5'0"	97 to 128	108 to 138	5'10"	132 to 174	146 to 188
5'1"	101 to 132	111 to 143	5'11"	136 to 179	151 to 194
5'2"	104 to 137	115 to 148	6'0"	140 to 184	155 to 199
5'3"	107 to 141	119 to 152	6'1"	144 to 189	159 to 205
5'4"	111 to 146	122 to 157	6'2"	148 to 195	164 to 210
5'5"	114 to 150	126 to 162	6'3"	152 to 200	168 to 216
5'6"	118 to 155	130 to 167	6'4"	156 to 205	173 to 222
5'7"	121 to 160	134 to 172	6'5"	160 to 211	177 to 228
5'8"	125 to 164	138 to 178	6'6"	164 to 216	182 to 234
5'9"	129 to 169	142 to 183			

Source: U.S. Department of Agriculture, U.S. Department of Health and Human Services. *Nutrition and Your Health: Dietary Guidelines for Americans*, 3rd ed. Washington, D.C., 1990.

Using a standing scale
• Place a paper towel on the scale's platform.
• Tell the patient to remove his robe and slippers or shoes *to ensure accurate measurement of height and weight.* If the scale has wheels, lock them before the patient steps on. Assist the patient onto the scale *to prevent falls.* Remain close to the patient *so you can steady him if necessary.*
• If you're using an upright balance (gravity) scale, slide the lower rider to the groove representing the largest increment below the patient's estimated weight. Grooves represent 50, 100, 150, and 200 lb (23, 45, 68, and 91 kg). Then slide the small upper rider until the beam balances. Add the upper and lower rider figures *to de-termine the weight.* (The upper rider is calibrated to eighths of a pound.)
• If you're using a multiple-weight scale, move the appropriate ratio weights onto the weight holder to balance the scale; ratio weights are labeled 50, 100, and 200 lb. Add ratio weights until the next weight causes the main beam to fall. Then adjust the main beam poise until the scale balances. Next, add the sum of the ratio weights to the figure on the main beam *to obtain the patient's weight.*
• Return ratio weights to their rack and the weight holder to its proper place.

• If you use a scale with a digital display, make sure the display reads 0 before use. Read the display with the patient on the scale and standing as still as possible.

• If you're measuring height, tell the patient to stand erect on the platform of the scale. Raise the measuring bar beyond the top of the patient's head, extend the horizontal arm, and lower the bar until it touches the top of the patient's head. Then read the patient's height.

• Help the patient off the scale, and give him his robe and slippers or shoes. Then return the measuring bar to its initial position.

Using a chair scale

• Transport the patient to the weighing area or the scale to the patient's bedside.

• Lock the scale in place *to prevent it from moving accidentally.*

• If you're using a scale with a swing-away chair arm, unlock the arm. When unlocked, the arm swings back 180 degrees to permit easy patient access.

• Position the scale beside the patient's bed or wheelchair with the chair arm open. Transfer the patient onto the scale, swing the chair arm to the front of the scale, and lock it in place.

• Weigh the patient by adding ratio weights and adjusting the main beam poise. Then unlock the swing-away chair arm as before, and transfer the patient back to his bed or wheelchair.

• Lock the main beam *to avoid damaging the scale during transport.* Unlock the wheels and remove the scale from the patient's room.

Using a multiple-weight bed scale

• Provide privacy, and tell the patient that you're going to weigh him on a special bed scale.

• Position the scale next to the patient's bed and lock the scale's wheels. Then turn the patient on his side, facing away from the scale.

• Release the stretcher frame to the horizontal position, and pump the hand lever until the stretcher is positioned over the mattress. Lower the stretcher onto the mattress, and roll the patient onto the stretcher.

• Raise the stretcher 2″ (5 cm) above the mattress. Then add ratio weights, and adjust the main beam poise as for the standing and chair scales.

• After weighing the patient, lower the stretcher onto the mattress, turn the patient on his side, and remove the stretcher. Be sure to leave the patient in a comfortable position.

Using a digital bed scale

• Provide privacy, and tell the patient that you're going to weigh him on a special bed scale. If the patient is being weighed for the first time, demonstrate the scale's operation.

• Release the stretcher to the horizontal position, then lock it in place. Turn the patient on his side, facing away from the scale.

• Roll the base of the scale under the patient's bed. Adjust the lever *to widen the base of the scale, providing stability.* After doing so, lock the scale's wheels.

• Center the stretcher above the bed, lower it onto the mattress, and roll the patient onto the stretcher. Then position the circular weighing arms of the scale over the patient, and attach them securely to the stretcher bars.

• Pump the handle with long, slow strokes *to raise the patient a few inches off the bed.* Ensure that the patient doesn't lean on or touch the headboard, side rails, or other bed equipment *because this will affect weight measurement.*

• Depress the operate button, and read the patient's weight on the digital display panel. Then press in the scale's handle *to lower the patient onto the bed.*

• Detach the circular weighing arms from the stretcher bars, roll the patient off the stretcher and remove it, and position him comfortably in bed.

• Release the wheel lock and withdraw the scale. Return the stretcher to its vertical position for storage.

Special considerations

Reassure and steady patients who are at risk for losing their balance on a scale.

Weigh the patient at the same time each day (usually before breakfast), in similar clothing, and using the same scale. If the patient uses crutches, weigh him with the crutches. Then weigh the crutches and any heavy clothing and subtract their weight from the total to determine the patient's weight. If the patient is markedly obese, check scale capacity. (Although some newer scales can measure up to 600 lb [272 kg], most scales can measure a maximum of 250 lb [113 kg].) You may have to weigh the patient on a large commercial scale (usually located on the loading dock or in the dietary department).

Before using a bed scale, cover its stretcher with a drawsheet *to avoid stains from perspiration, drainage, or excretions.* Balance the scale with the drawsheet in place *to ensure accurate weighing.*

When rolling the patient onto the stretcher, be careful not to dislodge I.V. lines, indwelling catheters, and other supportive equipment.

Documentation

Record the patient's height and weight on the nursing assessment form and other medical records, as required by your hospital.

Assessment techniques

To perform physical assessment, a nurse uses four basic techniques: inspection, palpation, percussion, and auscultation. Performing these techniques correctly helps elicit valuable information about the patient's condition.

Inspection requires the use of vision, hearing, touch, and smell. Special lighting and various equipment — such as an otosocope, a tongue blade, or an ophthalmoscope — may be used to enhance vision or examine an otherwise hidden area. Inspection begins during the first patient contact and continues throughout the assessment.

Palpation usually follows inspection, except when examining the abdomen or assessing infants and children. Palpation involves touching the body to determine the size, shape, and position of structures; to detect and evaluate temperature, pulsations, and other movement; and to elicit tenderness.

The four palpation techniques include light palpation, deep palpation, light ballottement, and deep ballottement. Ballottement is the palpation technique used to evaluate a floating or movable structure; the nurse gently bounces the structure being assessed by applying pressure against it; she then waits to feel it rebound. This technique may be used, for example, to check the position of an organ or a fetus.

Percussion uses quick, sharp tapping of the fingers or hands against body surfaces to produce sounds, detect tenderness, or assess reflexes. Percussing for sound helps locate organ borders, identify organ shape and position, and determine if an organ is solid or filled with fluid or gas.

Organs and tissues produce sounds of varying loudness, pitch, and duration, depending on their density. For example, air-filled cavities, such as the lungs, produce markedly different sounds from those produced by the liver and other dense tissues. Percussion techniques include indirect percussion, direct percussion, and blunt percussion.

Auscultation involves listening to various body sounds — particularly those produced by the heart, lungs, vessels, stomach, and intestines. Most auscultated sounds result from the movement of air or fluid through these structures.

Usually, the nurse auscultates after performing the other assessment techniques. When examining the abdomen, however, auscultation should occur after inspection but before percussion and palpation. This way, bowel sounds can be heard before palpation disrupts them. Auscultation is best performed first on infants and young children, who may start to cry when palpated or percussed. Auscultation is most successful when performed in a quiet environment with a properly fitted stethoscope.

Equipment
Flashlight or gooseneck lamp, as appropriate ▪ ophthalmoscope ▪ otoscope ▪ stethoscope.

Implementation
• Explain the procedure to the patient, have him undress, and drape him appropriately.
• Make sure the room is warm and adequately lit *to make the patient comfortable and aid visual inspection.*
• Warm your hands and the stethoscope.

Inspection
• Focus on areas related to the patient's chief complaint. Use your eyes, ears, and sense of smell to observe the patient.
• To inspect a specific body area, first make sure the area is sufficiently exposed and adequately lit. Then survey the entire area, noting key landmarks and checking its overall condition. Next, focus on specifics — color, shape, texture, size, and movement. Note any unusual findings as well as predictable ones.

Palpation
• Explain the procedure to the patient, and tell him what to expect, such as occasional discomfort as pressure is applied. Encourage him to relax *because muscle tension or guarding can interfere with performance and results of palpation.*
• Choose the area of your hands and fingers that will provide the best assessment *because all areas aren't equally sensitive to all sensations.* For example, use the fingertips to assess the texture of a rash, or the back of the hand to assess the temperature of a joint. (See *Using your hands in palpation,* page 24.)
• Provide just enough pressure to assess the tissue beneath one or both hands. Then release pressure and gently move to the next area, systematically covering the entire surface to be assessed.
• To perform light palpation, depress the skin, indenting it ½″ to ¾″ (1 to 2 cm). Use the lightest touch possible *because excessive pressure blunts your sensitivity.*
• If the patient tolerates light palpation and you need to assess deeper structures, increase your fingertip pressure, indenting the skin about 1½″ (4 cm). Place your other hand on top of the palpating hand *to control and guide your movements.*
• To perform light ballottement, apply light, rapid pressure from quadrant to quadrant on the patient's abdomen. Keep your hand on the skin to detect tissue rebound.

Using your hands in palpation

To enhance palpation technique, take advantage of the tactile sensitivity specific to each hand region. You can use your whole hand to test handgrip strength.

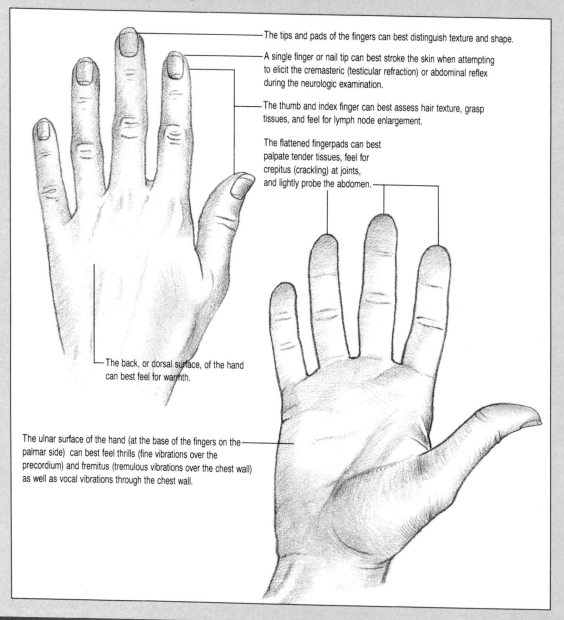

The tips and pads of the fingers can best distinguish texture and shape.

A single finger or nail tip can best stroke the skin when attempting to elicit the cremasteric (testicular refraction) or abdominal reflex during the neurologic examination.

The thumb and index finger can best assess hair texture, grasp tissues, and feel for lymph node enlargement.

The flattened fingerpads can best palpate tender tissues, feel for crepitus (crackling) at joints, and lightly probe the abdomen.

The back, or dorsal surface, of the hand can best feel for warmth.

The ulnar surface of the hand (at the base of the fingers on the palmar side) can best feel thrills (fine vibrations over the precordium) and fremitus (tremulous vibrations over the chest wall) as well as vocal vibrations through the chest wall.

• To perform deep ballottement, apply abrupt, deep pressure and then release it. Maintain fingertip contact.
• Use both hands (bimanual palpation) to trap a deep, underlying, hard-to-palpate organ (such as the kidney or spleen) or to fix or stabilize an organ (such as the uterus) with one hand while you palpate it with the other.

Percussion
• First, decide which of the percussion techniques best suits your assessment needs. Indirect percussion helps reveal the size and density of underlying thoracic and abdominal organs and tissues. Direct percussion helps assess an adult's sinuses for tenderness and elicits sounds in a child's thorax. Blunt percussion aims to elicit tenderness over organs such as the kidneys, gallbladder, or liver. When percussing, note the characteristic sounds produced. (See *Identifying percussion sounds.*)
• To perform indirect percussion, place one hand on the patient and tap the middle finger with the middle finger of the other hand. (See *Performing indirect percussion*, page 26.)
• To perform direct percussion, tap your hand or fingertip directly against the body surface.
• To perform blunt percussion, strike the ulnar surface of your fist against the body surface. Or place the palm of one hand against the body, make a fist with the other hand, and strike the back of the first hand.

Auscultation
• First, determine whether to use the bell or diaphragm of your stethoscope. Use the diaphragm to detect high-pitched sounds, such as breath and bowel sounds. Use the bell to detect lower-pitched sounds, such as heart and vascular sounds.
• Place the diaphragm or bell of the stethoscope over the appropriate area of the patient's body. Place the earpieces in your ears, listen intently to individual sounds, and try to identify their characteristics. Determine the intensity, pitch, and duration of each sound, and check the frequency of recurring sounds.

Special considerations
Avoid palpating or percussing an area of the body known to be tender at the start of your examination. Instead, work around the area; then gently palpate or percuss it at the end of the examination. *This progression minimizes your patient's discomfort and apprehension.*

To pinpont an inflamed area deep within the patient's body, perform a variation on deep palpation: Press firmly with one hand over the area you suspect is involved, and then lift your hand away quickly. If the patient reports that pain increases when you release the pressure, then you have identified rebound tenderness. (Suspect peritonitis if you elicit rebound tenderness when examining the abdomen.)

If you cannot palpate because the patient fears pain, try distracting him with conversation. Then perform aus-

Identifying percussion sounds

Percussion produces sounds that vary according to the tissue being percussed. This chart lists important percussion sounds along with their characteristics and typical sources.

SOUND	INTENSITY	PITCH	DURATION	QUALITY	SOURCE
Resonance	Moderate to loud	Low	Long	Hollow	Normal lung
Tympany	Loud	High	Moderate	Drumlike	Gastric air bubble, intestinal air
Dullness	Soft to moderate	High	Moderate	Thudlike	Liver, full bladder, pregnant uterus
Hyperresonance	Very loud	Very low	Long	Booming	Hyperinflated lung (as in emphysema)
Flatness	Soft	High	Short	Flat	Muscle

Performing indirect percussion

To perform indirect percussion, use the middle finger of your nondominant hand as the pleximeter (the mediating device used to receive the taps) and the middle finger of your dominant hand as the plexor (the device used to tap the pleximeter).
Place the pleximeter finger firmly against a body surface, such as the upper back. With your wrist flexed loosely, use the tip of your plexor finger to deliver a crisp blow just beneath the distal joint of the pleximeter. Be sure to hold the plexor perpendicular to the pleximeter. Tap lightly and quickly, removing the plexor as soon as you have delivered each blow. Move your nondominant hand to cover the entire area to be percussed.

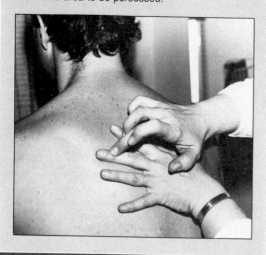

cultation and gently press your stethoscope into the affected area *to try to elicit tenderness.*

Complications
Palpation may cause an enlarged spleen or infected appendix to rupture.

Documentation
Document your assessment findings and the technique used to elicit those findings—for example, "right lower quadrant tenderness on deep palpation, no rebound tenderness."

 # Physical assessment

Nurses perform a complete physical assessment when the patient is admitted to the hospital and partial reassessments as the patient's condition warrants. A complete assessment includes a thorough health history and physical examination. The health history includes the chief complaint, a history of the present illness, general medical and surgical histories, a family history, a social history, and a review of systems.

Typically, physical examination follows a methodical, head-to-toe format. Patient preparation includes a clear explanation of the examination, and proper positioning and draping before and during the examination. During this procedure, the nurse must make every effort to recognize and respect the patient's feelings (particularly of embarrassment and anxiety) as well as to provide comfort measures and follow appropriate safety precautions.

Equipment
Although equipment varies with the examination's focus, the following may be included: scale with height measurement bar ■ urine specimen container and laboratory request form (if ordered) ■ sphygmomanometer ■ watch with second hand ■ stethoscope ■ thermometer ■ gown (for patient) ■ examining table (with stirrups if necessary) ■ gloves ■ drapes (sheet, bath blanket, or towel, as needed) ■ adhesive tape ■ spotlight or gooseneck lamp ■ flashlight ■ laryngeal mirror ■ tongue blades ■ percussion (reflex) hammer ■ otoscope ■ tuning fork ■ ear specula ■ tape measure ■ visual acuity chart ■ ophthalmoscope ■ test tubes of hot and cold water ■ containers of odorous materials (such as coffee, chocolate) ■ substances for taste assessment (sugar, salt, vinegar) ■ coin ■ pin and cotton ■ paper clip ■ fecal occult blood test kit ■ linen-saver pad ■ water-soluble lubricant ■ facial tissues ■ cotton-tipped applicators ■ nursing assessment form.

Preparation of equipment
Adjust the temperature in the examining room and close the doors *to prevent drafts.* Cover the examining table with a clean sheet or disposable paper. Then assemble the appropriate equipment for the examination.

Implementation
● Review the patient's health history *to obtain subjective data about the patient and insight into problem areas and subtle physical changes.* Investigate the patient's chief complaint. (See *Exploring a patient's symptoms.*)
● Obtain biographical data, including the patient's name; address; telephone number; contact person; sex; age and

Exploring a patient's symptoms

Essential to a complete physical assessment is a clear understanding of your patient's symptoms. One method for gaining that understanding involves using the mnemonic device PQRST as a guide.

Provocative or palliative
What causes the symptom? What makes it better or worse?
• What were you doing when you first noticed it?
• What seems to trigger it? Stress? Position? Certain activities? An argument? (For a sign, such as an eye discharge: What seems to cause it or make it worse? For a psychological symptom such as depression: Does the depression occur after specific events?)
• What relieves the symptom? Changing diet? Changing position? Taking medication? Being active?
• What makes the symptom worse?

Quality or quantity
How does the symptom feel, look, or sound? How much of it are you experiencing now?
• How would you describe the symptom—how it feels, looks, or sounds?
• How much are you experiencing now? Is it so much that it prevents you from performing any activities? Is it more or less than you experienced at any other time?

Region or radiation
Where is the symptom located? Does it spread?
• Where does the symptom occur?
• In the case of pain, does it travel down your back or arms, up your neck, or down your legs?

Severity
How does the symptom rate on a scale of 1 to 10, with 10 being the most severe?
• How bad is the symptom at its worst? Does it force you to lie down, sit down, or slow down?
• Does the symptom seem to be getting better, getting worse, or staying about the same?

Timing
When did the symptom begin? How often does it occur? Is it sudden or gradual?
• On what date and time did the symptom first occur?
• How did the symptom start? Suddenly? Gradually?
• How often do you experience the symptom? Hourly? Daily? Weekly? Monthly?
• When do you usually experience the symptom? During the day? At night? In the early morning? Does it awaken you? Does it occur before, during, or after meals? Does it occur seasonally?
• How long does an episode of the symptom last?

birth date; birthplace; Social Security number; race, nationality, and cultural background; marital status and names of persons living with the patient; education; religion; and occupation.
• Ask about health and illness patterns, the reason for seeking health care, current and past health status, family health status, and condition of body systems.
• Ask about health promotion and protection patterns, including health beliefs, personal habits, sleep and wake cycles, exercise, recreation, nutrition, stress level and coping skills, socioeconomic status, environmental health conditions, and occupational health hazards.
• Explore the patient's role and relationship patterns, including self-concept, cultural and religious influences, family roles and relationships, sexuality and reproductive patterns, social support systems, and any other psychosocial considerations.
• Explain the physical examination and answer questions.
• Instruct the patient to void if possible. Collect a urine specimen if ordered. *Emptying the bladder increases patient comfort during the examination.*

• Help the patient undress, and provide a gown. Then measure and record height, weight, and vital signs.
• Assist the patient onto the examination table. Requirements for positioning and draping vary with the body system and region being assessed. To examine the head, neck, and anterior and posterior thorax, have the patient sit on the edge of the examination table or the bed. For the abdomen and cardiovascular system, place the patient in a supine position and stand to his right. For a female patient, place a towel over her breasts and upper thorax during abdominal assessment. Pull the sheet down as far as her symphysis pubis, but no farther.
• Perform a physical examination as outlined in *Performing a head-to-toe assessment,* pages 28 to 38.

Documentation
Document significant normal and abnormal findings in an organized manner according to body systems.
(Text continues on page 39.)

Performing a head-to-toe assessment

The chart on the following pages provides guidelines for a systematic head-to-toe assessment. It groups assessment techniques by body region and nurse-patient positioning to make the assessment as efficient as possible and to avoid tiring the patient. The first column describes the assessment technique to use for each body system or region. The second column lists normal findings for adults. The third column reviews special considerations, including the purpose of the technique as well as nursing and developmental considerations.

TECHNIQUE	NORMAL FINDINGS	SPECIAL CONSIDERATIONS
Head and neck		
Inspect the patient's head. Note hair color, texture, and distribution. Palpate from the forehead to the posterior triangle of the neck for the posterior cervical lymph nodes.	Symmetrical, rounded normocephalic head positioned at midline and erect with no lumps or ridges	• This technique can detect asymmetry, size changes, enlarged lymph nodes, and tenderness. • Wear gloves for palpation if the patient has scalp lesions. • Inspect and gently palpate the fontanels and sutures in an infant.
Palpate in front of and behind the ears, under the chin, and in the anterior triangle for the anterior cervical lymph nodes.	Nonpalpable lymph nodes or small, round, soft, mobile, nontender lymph nodes	• This technique can detect enlarged lymph nodes. • Palpable lymph nodes may be normal in a patient under age 12.
Palpate the left and then the right carotid artery.	Bilateral equality in pulse amplitude and rhythm	• This technique evaluates circulation through the carotid pulse.
Auscultate the carotid arteries.	No bruit on auscultation	• Auscultation in this area can detect a bruit, a sign of turbulent blood flow.
Palpate the trachea.	Straight, midline trachea	• This technique evaluates trachea position.
Palpate the suprasternal notch.	Palpable pulsations with an even rhythm	• Palpation in this area allows evaluation of aortic arch pulsations.
Palpate the supraclavicular area.	Nonpalpable lymph nodes	• This technique can detect enlarged lymph nodes.
Palpate the thyroid gland and auscultate for bruits.	Thin, mobile thyroid isthmus; nonpalpable thyroid lobes	• Palpation detects thyroid enlargement, tenderness, or nodules.
Have the patient touch his chin to his chest and to each shoulder, each ear to the corresponding shoulder, then tip his head back as far as possible.	Symmetrical strength and movement of neck muscles	• These maneuvers evaluate range of motion (ROM) in the neck.

Performing a head-to-toe assessment *(continued)*

TECHNIQUE	NORMAL FINDINGS	SPECIAL CONSIDERATIONS
Head and neck *(continued)*		
Place your hands on the patient's shoulders while the patient shrugs them against resistance. Then place your hand on the patient's left cheek, then the right, and have the patient push against it.	Symmetrical strength and movement of neck muscles	• This procedure checks cranial nerve XI (accessory nerve) functioning and trapezius and sternocleidomastoid muscle strength.
Have the patient smile, frown, wrinkle the forehead, and puff out the cheeks.	Symmetrical smile, frown, and forehead wrinkles; equal puffing out of the cheeks	• This maneuver evaluates the motor portion of cranial nerve VII (facial nerve).
Occlude one nostril externally with your finger while the patient breathes through the other. Repeat on the other nostril.	Patent nostrils	• This technique checks the patency of the nasal passages.
Inspect the internal nostrils using a nasal speculum or an ophthalmoscope handle with a nasal attachment.	Moist, pink to red nasal mucosa without deviated septum, lesions, or polyps	• This technique can detect edema, inflammation, and excessive drainage. • Use only a flashlight to inspect an infant's or toddler's nostrils; a nasal speculum is too sharp.
Palpate the nose.	No bumps, lesions, edema, or tenderness	• This technique assesses for structural abnormalities in the nose. • An infant's nose usually is slightly flattened.
Palpate and percuss the frontal and maxillary sinuses. If palpation and percussion elicit tenderness, assess further by transilluminating the sinuses.	No tenderness on palpation or percussion	• These techniques are used to elicit tenderness, which may indicate sinus congestion or infection. • In a child under age 8, frontal sinuses commonly are too small to assess.
Palpate the temporomandibular joints as the patient opens and closes the jaws.	Smooth joint movement without pain; correct approximation	• This action assesses the temporomandibular joints and the motor portion of cranial nerve V (trigeminal nerve).
Inspect the oral mucosa, gingivae, teeth, and salivary gland openings, using a tongue blade and a penlight.	Pink, moist, smooth oral mucosa without lesions or inflammation; pink, moist slightly irregular gingivae without sponginess or edema; 32 teeth with correct occlusion	• This technique evaluates the condition of several oral structures. • A child may have up to 20 temporary (baby) teeth. • Slight gingival swelling may be normal during pregnancy.

Performing a head-to-toe assessment *(continued)*

TECHNIQUE	NORMAL FINDINGS	SPECIAL CONSIDERATIONS
Head and neck *(continued)*		
Observe the tongue and the hard and soft palates.	Pink, slightly rough tongue with a midline depression; pink to light red palates with symmetrical lines	• Observation provides information about the patient's hydration status and the condition of these oral structures.
Ask the patient to stick out his tongue.	Midline tongue without tremors	• This procedure tests cranial nerve XII (hypoglossal nerve).
Ask the patient to say "Ahh" while sticking out his tongue. Inspect the visible oral structures.	Symmetrical rise in soft palate and uvula during phonation; pink, midline, cone-shaped uvula; +1 tonsils (both tonsils behind the pillars)	• Phonation ("Ahh") checks portions of cranial nerves IX and X (glossopharyngeal and vagus nerves). Lowering the tongue aids viewing.
Test the gag reflex using a tongue blade.	Gagging	• Gagging during this procedure indicates that cranial nerves IX and X are intact.
Place the tongue blade at the side of the tongue while the patient pushes it to the left and right with the tongue.	Symmetrical ability to push tongue blade to left and right	• This action tests cranial nerve XII.
Test the sense of smell using a test tube of coffee, chocolate, or another familiar substance.	Correct identification of smells in both nostrils	• This action tests cranial nerve I (olfactory nerve). • Make sure the patient keeps both eyes closed during the test.
Eyes and ears		
Perform a visual acuity test using the standard Snellen eye chart or another visual acuity chart, with the patient wearing corrective lenses if needed.	20/20 vision	• This test assesses the patient's distance vision (central vision) and evaluates cranial nerve II (optic nerve).
Ask the patient to identify the pattern in a specially prepared page of color dots or plates.	Correct identification of pattern	• This test assesses the patient's color perception.
Test the six cardinal positions of gaze.	Bilaterally equal eye movement without nystagmus	• This test evaluates the function of each of the six extraocular muscles and tests cranial nerves III, IV, and VI (oculomotor, trochlear, and abducens nerves).
Inspect the external structures of the eyeball (eyelids, eyelashes, and lacrimal apparatus).	Bright, clear, symmetrical eyes free of nystagmus; eyelids close completely; no lesions, scaling, or inflammation	• This inspection allows detection of such problems as ptosis, ectropion (outward-turning eyelids), entropion (inward-turning eyelids), and styes.

Performing a head-to-toe assessment *(continued)*

TECHNIQUE	NORMAL FINDINGS	SPECIAL CONSIDERATIONS
Eyes and ears *(continued)*		
Inspect the conjunctiva and sclera.	Pink palpebral conjunctiva and clear bulbar conjunctiva without swelling, drainage, or hyperemic blood vessels; white, clear sclera	• Inspection detects conjunctivitis and the scleral color changes that may occur with systemic disorders.
Inspect the cornea, iris, and anterior chamber by shining a penlight tangentially across the eye.	Clear, transparent cornea and anterior chamber; illumination of total iris	• This technique assesses anterior chamber depth and the condition of the cornea and iris. • An elderly patient may exhibit a thin, grayish ring in the cornea (called arcus senilis).
Examine the pupils for equality of size, shape, reaction to light, and accommodation.	Pupils equal, round, reactive to light and accommodation (PERRLA), directly and consensually	• Testing the pupillary response to light and accommodation assesses cranial nerves III, IV, and VI.
Observe the red reflex using an ophthalmoscope.	Sharp, distinct orange-red glow	• Presence of the red reflex indicates that the cornea, anterior chamber, and lens are free from opacity and clouding.
Inspect the ear. Perform an otoscopic examination if indicated.	Nearly vertically positioned ears that line up with the eye, match the facial color, are similarly shaped, and are in proportion to the face; no drainage, nodules, or lesions	• A dark-skinned patient may have darker orange or brown cerumen (earwax); a fair-skinned patient typically will have yellow cerumen.
Palpate the ear and mastoid process.	No pain, swelling, nodules, or lesions	• This assessment technique can detect inflammation or infection. It may also uncover other abnormalities, such as nodules or lesions.
Perform the whispered voice test or the watch-tick test on one ear at a time.	Whispered voice heard at a distance of 1′ to 2′ (30 to 61 cm); watch-tick heard at a distance of 5″ (13 cm)	• This test grossly assesses cranial nerve VIII (acoustic nerve).
Perform Weber's test using a 512 or 1024 Hertz (Hz) tuning fork.	Tuning fork vibrations heard equally in both ears or in the middle of the head	• This test differentiates conductive from sensorineural hearing loss. • The sound is heard best in the ear with a conductive loss.
Perform the Rinne test using a 512 or 1024 Hz tuning fork.	Tuning fork vibrations heard in front of the ear for as long as they are heard on the mastoid process	• This test helps differentiate conductive from sensorineural hearing loss.

(continued)

Performing a head-to-toe assessment *(continued)*

TECHNIQUE	NORMAL FINDINGS	SPECIAL CONSIDERATIONS
Posterior thorax		
Observe the skin, bones, and muscles of the spine, shoulder blades, and back as well as symmetry of expansion and accessory muscle use.	Even skin tone; symmetrical placement of all structures; bilaterally equal shoulder height; symmetrical expansion with inhalation; no accessory muscle use	• Observation provides information about lung expansion and accessory muscle use during respiration. It may also detect a deformity that can alter ventilation, such as scoliosis.
Assess the anteroposterior and lateral diameters of the thorax.	Lateral diameter up to twice the anteroposterior diameter (2:1)	• This assessment may detect abnormalities, such as an increased anteroposterior diameter (barrel chest may be as low as 1:1). • Normal anteroposterior diameters vary with age. • Measure an infant's chest circumference at the nipple line.
Palpate down the spine.	Properly aligned spinous processes without lesions or tenderness; firm, symmetrical, evenly spaced muscles	• This technique detects pain in the spine and paraspinous muscles. It also evaluates the muscles' consistency.
Palpate over the posterior thorax.	Smooth surface; no lesions, lumps, or pain	• This technique helps detect musculoskeletal inflammation.
Assess respiratory excursion.	Symmetrical expansion and contraction of the thorax	• This technique checks for equal expansion of the lungs.
Palpate for tactile fremitus as the patient repeats the word "ninety-nine."	Equally intense vibrations of both sides of the chest	• Palpation provides information about the content of the lungs; vibrations increase over consolidated or fluid-filled areas and decrease over gas-filled areas.
Percuss over the posterior and lateral lung fields.	Resonant percussion note over the lungs that changes to a dull note at the diaphragm	• This technique helps identify the density and location of the lungs, diaphragm, and other anatomic structures. • Percussion may produce hyperresonant sounds in a patient with chronic obstructive pulmonary disease or an elderly patient because of hyperinflation of lung tissue.
Percuss for diaphragmatic excursion on each side of the posterior thorax.	Excursion from 1¼″ to 2¼″ (3 to 6 cm)	• This technique evaluates diaphragm movement during respiration.

Performing a head-to-toe assessment *(continued)*

TECHNIQUE	NORMAL FINDINGS	SPECIAL CONSIDERATIONS
Posterior thorax *(continued)*		
Auscultate the lungs through the posterior thorax as the patient breathes slowly and deeply through the mouth. Also auscultate lateral areas.	Bronchovesicular sounds (soft, breezy sounds) between the scapulae; vesicular sounds (soft, swishy sounds about two notes lower than bronchovesicular sounds) in the lung periphery	• Lung auscultation helps detect abnormal fluid or mucus accumulation as well as obstructed passages. • Auscultate a child's lungs before performing other assessment techniques that may cause crying, which increases the respiratory rate and interferes with clear auscultation. • A child's breath sounds are normally harsher or more bronchial than an adult's.
Anterior thorax		
Observe the skin, bones, and muscles of the anterior thoracic structures as well as symmetry of expansion and accessory muscle use during respiration.	Even skin tone; symmetrical placement of all structures; symmetrical costal angle of less than 90 degrees; symmetrical expansion with inhalation; no accessory muscle use	• Observation provides information about lung expansion and accessory muscle use. It may also detect a deformity that can prevent full lung expansion, such as pigeon chest.
Inspect the anterior thorax for lifts, heaves, or thrusts. Also check for the apical impulse.	No lifts, heaves, or thrusts; apical impulse not usually visible	• Apical impulse may be visible in a thin or young patient.
Palpate over the anterior thorax.	Smooth surface; no lesions, lumps, or pain	• This technique helps detect musculoskeletal inflammation.
Assess respiratory excursion.	Symmetrical expansion and contraction of the thorax	• This technique checks for equal expansion of the lungs.
Palpate for tactile fremitus as the patient repeats the word "ninety-nine."	Equally intense vibrations of both sides of the chest, with more vibrations in the upper chest than in the lower chest	• Palpation provides information about the content of the lungs.
Percuss over the anterior thorax.	Resonant percussion note over lung fields that changes to a dull note over ribs and other bones	• This technique helps identify the density and location of the lungs, diaphragm, and other anatomic structures. • Percussion is unreliable in an infant because of the infant's small chest size. • Percussion may produce hyperresonant sounds in an elderly patient because of hyperinflation of lung tissue.

(continued)

Performing a head-to-toe assessment *(continued)*

TECHNIQUE	NORMAL FINDINGS	SPECIAL CONSIDERATIONS
Anterior thorax *(continued)*		
Auscultate the lungs through the posterior thorax as the patient breathes slowly and deeply through the mouth. Also auscultate lateral areas.	Bronchovesicular sounds (soft, breezy sounds) between the scapulae; vesicular sounds (soft, swishy sounds about two notes lower than bronchovesicular sounds) in the lung periphery	• Lung auscultation helps detect abnormal fluid or mucus accumulation. • Auscultate a child's lungs before performing other assessment techniques that may cause crying. • Breath sounds are normally harsher or more bronchial in a child.
Inspect the breasts and axillae with the patient's hands resting at the sides of the body, placed on the hips, and raised above the head.	Symmetrical, convex, similar-looking breasts with soft, smooth skin and bilaterally similar venous patterns; symmetrical axillae with varying amounts of hair, but no lesions; nipples at same level on chest and of same color	• This technique evaluates the general condition of the breasts and axillae and detects such abnormalities as retraction, dimpling, and flattening. • Expect to see enlarged breasts with darkened nipples and areolae and purplish linear streaks if the patient is pregnant.
Palpate the axillae with the patient's arms resting against the side of the body.	Nonpalpable nodes	• This technique detects nodular enlargements and other abnormalities.
Palpate the breasts and nipples with patient lying supine.	Smooth, relatively elastic tissue without masses, cracks, fissures, areas of induration (hardness), or discharge	• This technique evaluates the consistency and elasticity of the breasts and nipples and may detect nipple discharge. • The premenstrual patient may exhibit breast tenderness, nodularity, and fullness. • A pregnant patient may discharge colostrum from the nipple and may exhibit nodular breasts with prominent venous patterns.
Inspect the neck for jugular vein distention with patient lying supine at a 45-degree angle.	No visible pulsations	• This technique assesses right-sided heart pressure.
Palpate the precordium for the apical impulse.	Apical impulse present in the apical area (fifth intercostal space at the midclavicular line)	• This action evaluates the size and location of the left ventricle.

Performing a head-to-toe assessment *(continued)*

TECHNIQUE	NORMAL FINDINGS	SPECIAL CONSIDERATIONS
Anterior thorax *(continued)*		
Auscultate the aortic, pulmonic, tricuspid, and mitral areas for heart sounds.	S_1 and S_2 heart sounds with a regular rhythm and an age-appropriate rate	• Auscultation over the precordium evaluates the heart rate and rhythm and can detect extra sounds, murmurs, and other abnormal heart sounds. • A child may have functional (innocent) heart murmurs.
Abdomen		
Observe the abdominal contour.	Symmetrical flat or rounded contour	• This technique determines whether the abdomen is distended or scaphoid. • An infant or a toddler will have a rounded abdomen.
Inspect the abdomen for skin characteristics, symmetry, contour, peristalsis, and pulsations.	Symmetrical contour with no lesions, striae, rash, or visible peristaltic waves	• Inspection can detect an incisional or umbilical hernia, or an abnormality caused by bowel obstruction.
Auscultate all four quadrants of the abdomen.	Normal bowel sounds in all four quadrants; no bruits	• Abdominal auscultation can detect abnormal bowel sounds.
Percuss from below the right breast to the inguinal area down the right midclavicular line.	Dull percussion note over the liver; tympanic note over the rest of the abdomen	• Percussion in this area helps evaluate the size of the liver.
Percuss from below the left breast to the inguinal area down the left midclavicular line.	Tympanic percussion note	• Percussion in this area that elicits a dull note can detect an enlarged spleen.
Palpate all four abdominal quadrants.	Nontender organs without masses	• Palpation provides information about the location, size, and condition of the underlying structures.
Palpate for the kidneys on each side of the abdomen.	Nonpalpable kidneys or solid, firm, smooth kidneys (if palpable)	• This technique evaluates the general condition of the kidneys.
Palpate the liver at the right costal border.	Nonpalpable liver or smooth, firm, nontender liver with a rounded, regular edge (if palpable)	• This technique evaluates the general condition of the liver.
Palpate for the spleen at the left costal border.	Nonpalpable spleen	• This procedure detects any splenomegaly (spleen enlargement).
Palpate the femoral pulses in the groin.	Strong, regular pulse	• Palpation assesses vascular patency.

(continued)

Performing a head-to-toe assessment *(continued)*

TECHNIQUE	NORMAL FINDINGS	SPECIAL CONSIDERATIONS
Upper extremities		
Observe the skin and muscle mass of the arms and hands.	Uniform color and texture with no lesions; elastic turgor; bilaterally equal muscle mass	• The skin provides information about hydration and circulation. Muscle mass provides information about injuries and neuromuscular disease.
Ask the patient to extend the arms forward and then rapidly turn the palms up and down.	Steady hands with no tremor or pronator drift	• This maneuver tests proprioception and cerebellar function.
Place your hands on the patient's upturned forearms while the patient pushes up against resistance. Then place your hands under the forearms while the patient pushes down.	Symmetrical strength and ability to push up and down against resistance	• This procedure checks the muscle strength of the arms.
Inspect and palpate the fingers, wrists, and elbow joints.	Smooth, freely movable joints with no swelling	• An elderly patient may exhibit osteoarthritic changes.
Palpate the patient's hands to assess skin temperature.	Warm, moist skin with bilaterally even temperature	• Skin temperature assessment provides data about circulation to the area.
Palpate the radial and brachial pulses.	Bilaterally equal rate and rhythm	• Palpation of pulses helps evaluate peripheral vascular status.
Inspect the color, shape, and condition of the patient's fingernails, and test for capillary refill.	Pink nail beds with smooth, rounded nails; brisk capillary refill; no clubbing	• Nail assessment provides data about the integumentary, cardiovascular, and respiratory systems.
Place two fingers in each of the patient's palms while the patient squeezes your fingers.	Bilaterally equal hand strength	• This maneuver tests muscle strength in the hands.
Lower extremities		
Inspect the legs and feet for color, lesions, varicosities, hair growth, nail growth, edema, and muscle mass.	Even skin color; symmetrical hair and nail growth; no lesions, varicosities, or edema; bilaterally equal muscle mass	• Inspection assesses adequate circulatory function.
Test for pitting edema in the pretibial area.	No pitting edema	• This test assesses for excess interstitial fluid.
Palpate for pulses and skin temperature in the posterior tibial, dorsalis pedis, and popliteal areas.	Bilaterally even pulse rate, rhythm, and skin temperature	• Palpation of pulses and temperature in these areas evaluates the patient's peripheral vascular status.

Performing a head-to-toe assessment *(continued)*

TECHNIQUE	NORMAL FINDINGS	SPECIAL CONSIDERATIONS
Lower extremities *(continued)*		
Perform the straight leg test on one leg at a time.	Painless leg lifting	• This test checks for vertebral disk problems.
Palpate for crepitus as the patient abducts and adducts the hip. Repeat on the opposite leg.	No crepitus; full ROM without pain	• Perform Ortolani's maneuver on an infant to assess hip abduction and adduction.
Ask the patient to raise his thigh against the resistance of your hands. Repeat this procedure on the opposite thigh.	Each thigh lifts easily against resistance	• This maneuver tests the motor strength of the upper legs.
Ask the patient to push outward against the resistance of your hands.	Each leg pushes easily against resistance	• This maneuver tests the motor strength of the lower legs.
Ask the patient to pull backward against the resistance of your hands.	Each leg pulls easily against resistance	• This maneuver tests the motor strength of the lower legs.
Nervous system		
Lightly touch the ophthalmic, maxillary, and mandibular areas on each side of the patient's face with a cotton-tipped applicator and a pin.	Correct identification of sensation and location	• This test evaluates the function of cranial nerve V (trigeminal nerve).
Touch the dorsal and palmar surfaces of the arms, hands, and fingers with a cotton-tipped applicator and pin.	Correct identification of sensation and location	• This test evaluates the function of the ulnar, radial, and medial nerves.
Touch several nerve distribution areas on the legs, feet, and toes with a cotton-tipped applicator and pin.	Correct identification of sensation and location	• This test evaluates the function of the dermatome areas randomly.
Place your fingers above the patient's wrist and tap them with a reflex hammer. Repeat on the other arm.	Normal reflex reaction	• This procedure elicits the brachioradialis deep tendon reflex (DTR).
Place your fingers over the antecubital fossa and tap them with a reflex hammer. Repeat on the other arm.	Normal reflex reaction	• This procedure elicits the biceps DTR.
Place your fingers over the triceps tendon area and tap them with a reflex hammer. Repeat on the other arm.	Normal reflex reaction	• This procedure elicits the triceps DTR.

(continued)

Performing a head-to-toe assessment (continued)

TECHNIQUE	NORMAL FINDINGS	SPECIAL CONSIDERATIONS
Nervous system (continued)		
Tap just below the patella with a reflex hammer. Repeat this procedure on the opposite patella.	Normal reflex reaction	• This procedure elicits the patellar DTR.
Tap over the Achilles tendon area with a reflex hammer. Repeat this procedure on the opposite ankle.	Normal reflex reaction	• This procedure elicits the Achilles DTR.
Stroke the sole of the patient's foot with the end of the reflex hammer handle.	Plantar reflex	• This procedure elicits plantar flexion of all toes. • Expect Babinski's sign in children age 2 and under.
Ask the patient to demonstrate dorsiflexion by bending both feet upward against resistance.	Both feet lift easily against resistance	• This procedure tests foot strength and ROM.
Ask the patient to demonstrate plantar flexion by bending both feet downward against resistance.	Both feet push down easily against resistance	• This procedure tests foot strength and ROM.
Inspect the feet and toes for lesions and lumps.	No lesions or lumps	• Condition of the feet and toes helps evaluate peripheral vascular status.
Using your finger, trace a one-digit number in the palm of the patient's hand.	Correct identification of number	• This procedure evaluates the patient's tactile discrimination through graphesthesia.
Place a familiar object, such as a key or a coin, in the patient's hand.	Correct identification of object	• This procedure evaluates the patient's tactile discrimination.
Observe the patient while he walks with a regular gait, on the toes, on the heels, and heel-to-toe.	Steady gait, good balance, and no signs of muscle weakness or pain in any style of walking	• This technique evaluates the cerebellum and motor system and checks for vertebral disk problems.
Inspect the scapulae, spine, back, and hips as the patient bends forward, backward, and from side to side.	Full ROM, easy flexibility, and no signs of scoliosis or varicosities	• Inspection evaluates the patient's ROM and detects musculoskeletal abnormalities, such as scoliosis.
Perform the Romberg test. Ask the patient to stand straight with both eyes closed and both arms extended, with hands palms up.	Steady stance with minimal weaving	• This test checks cerebellar functioning and evaluates balance and coordination.

Preparation of a nursing care plan

A care plan directs the patient's nursing care from admission to discharge. This written action plan is based on nursing diagnoses that have been formulated after reviewing assessment findings. (See *Elements of a nursing diagnosis.*) The care plan consists of three parts: *goals* or *expected outcomes*, which describe behaviors or results to be achieved within a specified time; appropriate *nursing actions* or *interventions* needed to achieve these goals; and *evaluations* of the established goals.

A nursing care plan should be written for each patient, preferably within 24 hours of admission. It's usually begun by the patient's primary nurse or the nurse who admits the patient. If the care plan contains more than one nursing diagnosis, the nurse must assign priorities to each one and implement those with the highest priority first. Nurses update and revise the plan throughout the patient's stay, and the document becomes part of the permanent patient record.

Some health care facilities use standardized care plans that can be modified to serve many patients. Others use computer programs to facilitate nursing care plan development. Most have preprinted care plan forms, often on the nursing Kardex, that can be filled in as needed.

Besides guiding patient care, a nursing care plan serves as a database when planning assignments, giving change-of-shift reports, conferring with the doctor or other members of the health care team, planning patient discharge, and documenting patient care. In addition, the care plan can be used as a management tool to determine staffing needs and assignments.

Equipment
Preprinted nursing care plan form ▪ computer program for nursing care plan development if appropriate ▪ patient record, including nursing assessment.

Implementation
● Review the patient record, especially the nursing assessment completed on admission. Obtain from the patient any additional subjective or objective information needed to complete your assessment. Review diagnostic test results, the medical plan, and other information that may affect patient care. If the patient has just been admitted, complete a nursing history and physical assessment and add it to the patient's record.
● Based on an analysis of the data, determine which nursing diagnoses will guide your patient care. Be sure to address all of the patient's significant needs when determining nursing diagnoses.

Elements of a nursing diagnosis

The following summary presents the key elements of a nursing diagnosis.

Human response or problem
After analyzing the patient's condition, choose a diagnostic label from a hospital-sanctioned list or create a label specific to the patient. For consistency, most hospitals use NANDA's list of nursing diagnoses. An example of a diagnostic label is *Fluid volume excess.*

Related factors
The second part of the nursing diagnosis lists factors that seem to influence the patient in a way that pertains to the diagnostic label. Connect these factors to the diagnostic label with the phrase *related to* or the abbreviation *R/T.* The previous example could read, *Fluid volume excess R/T increased sodium intake.*

Signs and symptoms
To complete the nursing diagnosis, list signs and symptoms uncovered during assessment that help define the diagnostic label. You may list them beneath the diagnosis and related factors. Or you may add them to the diagnostic statement and connect them with the phrase *as evidenced by* or the abbreviation *AEB.* The example could read, *Fluid volume excess R/T increased sodium intake AEB edema, weight gain, shortness of breath, and S_3 heart sounds.*

● Work with the patient to identify individualized short-term and long-term goals (expected outcomes) for each nursing diagnosis. Short-term goals include those of immediate concern that can be achieved quickly. Long-term goals take more time to achieve and usually involve prevention, patient teaching, and rehabilitation.

A correctly written goal expresses the desired patient behavior, criteria for measurement, appropriate time, and conditions under which the behavior will occur. For example, a goal containing all these elements might read: "Using crutches, Mary Ballin will walk to the end of the hall and back by Monday." *Goals (or expected outcomes) serve as the basis for evaluating the effectiveness of your nursing interventions.*
● Select interventions that will help the patient achieve the stated goals for each nursing diagnosis. Include spe-

Tips for writing an effective patient care plan

How do you write a care plan that's realistic, accurate, and helpful? Here are some guidelines.

Be systematic
Avoid setting an initial goal that's impossible to achieve. For example, suppose the goal for a newly admitted patient with a cerebrovascular accident was "Patient will ambulate without assistance." Although this goal is certainly appropriate in the long term, several short-term goals, such as "Patient maintains joint range-of-motion," need to be achieved first.

Be realistic
The nursing intervention should match staff resources and capabilities. For example, "Passive range-of-motion exercises to all extremities every 2 hours" may not be reasonable given the unit's staffing pattern and care requirements. The goals you set to correct a patient's problem should reflect what's reasonably possible in your setting—for example, "Passive range-of-motion exercises with a.m. care, p.m. care, and once at night."

Be clear
Remember, you'll use goals to evaluate the effectiveness of the care plan, so it's important to express them clearly.

Be specific
"Give plenty of fluids" doesn't indicate much; the directive is nonspecific. In contrast, an intervention that says "Force fluids—1,000 ml/day shift, 1,000 ml/evening shift, 500 ml/night shift" allows another nurse to carry out the intervention with some assurance of having done what you ordered.

Be brief
An intervention that says "Follow turning schedule posted at bedside" is more readable and useful than having the entire schedule written on the nursing care plan.

---

cific information, such as the frequency or particular intervention technique. *Goals specify what you and your patient would like to have happen and establish criteria against which you'll judge further nursing actions.* (See *Tips for writing an effective patient care plan.)*

Special considerations
Always fill out the nursing care plan in ink *because the document is part of the permanent medical record.* If you must revise your plan as the patient's condition changes, fill out a new care plan and add it to the medical record.

Sign and date the care plan whenever you make new entries *to keep the plan current and to maintain accountability for planning the patient's care.*

Be aware that using a standardized care plan risks "standardizing" your patient's care, too. Customize the standardized plan as needed *to address your patient's individual concerns.*

Because long-term goals may not be met during hospitalization, your planning should address postdischarge and home care needs as well. Interventions may include coordinating home care services.

Documentation
Documentation of the patient's progress (or lack of it) is required by the Joint Commission on Accreditation of

Health Care Organizations and other regulatory agencies that monitor health care quality. Document all pertinent nursing diagnoses, expected outcomes, nursing interventions, and evaluations of expected outcomes. Write the care plan clearly and concisely, so other members of the health care team can understand it.

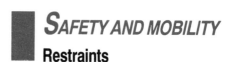

SAFETY AND MOBILITY
Restraints

Various soft restraints limit movement to prevent the confused, disoriented, or combative patient from injuring himself or others. Vest and belt restraints, used to prevent falls from a bed or a chair, permit full movement of arms and legs. Limb restraints, used to prevent removal of supportive equipment—such as I.V. lines, indwelling catheters, and nasogastric tubes—allow only slight limb motion. Like limb restraints, mitts prevent removal of supportive equipment, keep the patient from scratching rashes or sores, and prevent the combative patient from injuring himself or others. Body restraints, used to control the combative or hysterical patient, immobilize all or most of the body.

When soft restraints aren't sufficient and sedation is dangerous or ineffective, leather restraints can be used. Depending on the patient's behavior, leather restraints may be applied to all limbs (four-point restraints) or to one arm and one leg (two-point restraints). The duration of such restraint is governed by state law and by hospital policy.

Because a patient rarely submits readily to leather restraints, safe and speedy application requires teamwork by several staff members, the availability of all equipment, proper patient positioning, and a brief, clear explanation of the procedure to the patient.

Restraints must be used cautiously in seizure-prone patients because they increase the risk of fracture and trauma. And because restraints can cause skin irritation and restrict blood flow, they shouldn't be applied directly over wounds or I.V. catheters. Vest restraints should be used with caution in patients who have congestive heart failure or respiratory disorders. Such restraints can tighten with movement, further limiting circulation and respiratory function.

Equipment
For soft restraints: restraint (vest, limb, mitt, belt, or body, as needed) ▪ gauze pads if needed.

For leather restraints: two wrist and two ankle leather restraints ▪ four straps ▪ key ▪ large gauze pads to cushion each extremity.

Preparation of equipment
Before entering the patient's room, make sure the restraints are the correct size, using the patient's build and weight as a guide. (For children, who typically are too small for standard restraints, see *Types of child restraints*, page 42.) If the restraints are too loose and you can't obtain smaller ones, build them up with gauze pads or washcloths and tape them down securely. If you use leather restraints, be sure the straps are unlocked and the key fits the locks.

Implementation
• Obtain a doctor's order for the restraint if required. However, never leave a confused or combative patient unattended or unrestrained while attempting to secure the order.
• If necessary, obtain adequate assistance to restrain the patient before entering his room. Enlist the aid of several co-workers and organize their effort, giving each person a specific task; for example, one person explains the procedure to the patient and applies the restraints while the others immobilize the patient's arms and legs.

• Tell the patient what you're about to do and describe the restraints to him. Assure him that they are being used to protect him from injury rather than to punish him.

Applying a vest restraint
• Assist the patient to a sitting position if his condition permits. Then slip the vest over his gown. Crisscross the cloth flaps at the front, placing the V-shaped opening at the patient's throat. Never crisscross the flaps in the back *because this may cause the patient to choke if he tries to squirm out of the vest.*
• Pass the tab on one flap through the slot on the opposite flap. Then adjust the vest for the patient's comfort. You should be able to slip your fist between the vest and the patient. Avoid wrapping the vest too tightly *because it may restrict respiration.*
• Tie all restraints securely to the frame of the bed, chair, or wheelchair and out of the patient's reach. Use a bow or a knot that can be released quickly and easily in an emergency. (See *Knots for securing soft restraints,* page 43.) Never tie a regular knot to secure the straps. Leave 1″ to 2″ (2.5 to 5 cm) of slack in the straps *to allow room for movement.*
• After applying the vest, check the patient's respiratory rate and breath sounds regularly. Be alert for signs of respiratory distress. Also, make sure the vest hasn't tightened with the patient's movement. Loosen the vest frequently, if possible, *so the patient can stretch, turn, and breathe deeply.*

Applying a limb restraint
• Wrap the patient's wrist or ankle with gauze pads *to reduce friction between the patient's skin and the restraint, helping to prevent irritation and skin breakdown.* Then wrap the restraint around the gauze pads.
• Pass the strap on the narrow end of the restraint through the slot in the broad end, and adjust for a snug fit. Or fasten the buckle or Velcro cuffs to fit the restraint. You should be able to slip one or two fingers between the restraint and the patient's skin. Avoid applying the restraint too tightly *because it may impair circulation distal to the restraint.*
• Tie the restraint as above.
• After applying limb restraints, be alert for signs of impaired circulation in the extremity distal to the restraint. If the skin appears blue or feels cold, or if the patient complains of a tingling sensation or numbness, loosen the restraint. Perform range-of-motion (ROM) exercises regularly *to stimulate circulation and prevent contractures and resultant loss of mobility.*

Types of child restraints

You may need to restrain an infant or a child to prevent injury or to facilitate examination, diagnostic tests, or treatment. If so, follow these steps:
• Provide a simple explanation, reassurance, and constant observation to minimize the child's fear.
• Explain the restraint to the parents and enlist their help. Reassure them that it will not hurt the child.
• Make sure restraint ties or safety pins are secured outside the child's reach to prevent injury.
• When using a mummy restraint, secure the infant's arms in proper alignment with the body to avoid dislocation and other injuries.

Vest

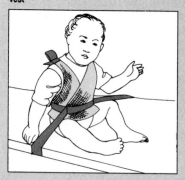

Elbow

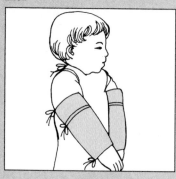

Mummy

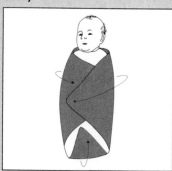

Belt

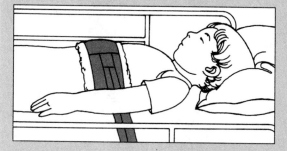

Limb

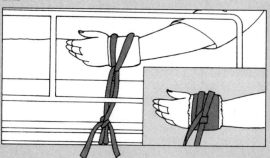

Crib with net

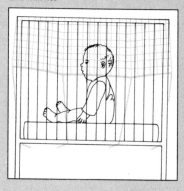

Mitt

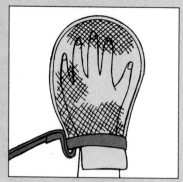

Restraining board

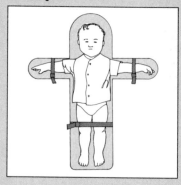

Applying a mitt restraint
• Wash and dry the patient's hands.
• Roll up a washcloth or gauze pad, and place it in the patient's palm. Have him form a loose fist, if possible, then pull the mitt over it and secure the closure.
• *To restrict the patient's arm movement,* attach the strap to the mitt and tie it securely, using a bow or a knot that can be released quickly and easily in an emergency.
• When using mitts made of transparent mesh, check hand movement and skin color frequently *to assess circulation.* Remove the mitts regularly *to stimulate circulation,* and perform passive ROM exercises *to prevent contractures.*

Applying a belt restraint
• Center the flannel pad of the belt on the bed. Then wrap the short strap of the belt around the bed frame and fasten it under the bed.
• Position the patient on the pad. Then have him roll slightly to one side while you guide the long strap around his waist and through the slot in the pad.
• Wrap the long strap around the bed frame and fasten it under the bed.
• After applying the belt, slip your hand between the patient and the belt *to ensure a secure but comfortable fit. A loose belt can be raised to chest level; a tight one can cause abdominal discomfort.*

Applying a body (Posey net) restraint
• Place the restraint flat on the bed, with arm and wrist cuffs facing down and the V at the head of the bed.
• Place the patient in the prone position on top of the restraint.
• Lift the V over the patient's head. Thread the chest belt through one of the loops in the V *to ensure a snug fit.*
• Secure the straps around the patient's chest, thighs, and legs. Then turn the patient on his back.
• Secure the straps to the bed frame *to anchor the restraint.* Then secure the straps around the patient's arms and wrists.

Applying leather restraints
• Position the patient supine on the bed, with each arm and leg securely held down *to minimize combative behavior and to prevent injury to the patient and others.* Immobilize the patient's arms and legs at the joints—knee, ankle, shoulder, and wrist—*to minimize his movement without exerting excessive force.*
• Apply pads to the patient's wrists and ankles *to reduce friction between his skin and the leather, preventing skin irritation and breakdown.*
• Wrap the restraint around the gauze pads. Then insert the metal loop through the hole that gives the best fit.

Knots for securing soft restraints

When securing soft restraints, use knots that can be released quickly and easily, like those shown below. Remember, never secure restraints to the bed's side rails.

Magnus hitch

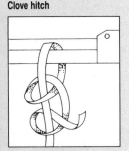

Clove hitch

Loop

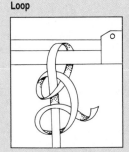

Reverse clove hitch

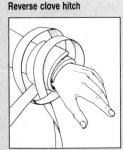

Apply the restraints securely but not too tightly. You should be able to slip one or two fingers between the restraint and the patient's skin. *A tight restraint can compromise circulation; a loose one can slip off or move up the patient's arm or leg, causing skin irritation and breakdown.*
• Thread the strap through the metal loop on the restraint, close the metal loop, and secure the strap to the bed frame, out of the patient's reach.
• Lock the restraint by pushing in the button on the side of the metal loop, and tug it gently to be sure it's secure. Once the restraint is secure, a co-worker can release the arm or leg. Flex the patient's arm or leg slightly before locking the strap *to allow room for movement and to prevent frozen joints and dislocations.*
• Place the key in an accessible location at the nurse's station.
• After applying leather restraints, observe the patient regularly *to give emotional support and to reassess the need*

for continued use of the restraint. Check his pulse rate and vital signs at least every 2 hours. Remove or loosen the restraints one at a time, every 2 hours, and perform passive ROM exercises if possible. Watch for signs of impaired peripheral circulation, such as cool, cyanotic skin. To unlock the restraint, insert the key into the metal loop, opposite the locking button. This releases the lock, and the metal loop can be opened.

Special considerations
Because the authority to use restraints varies among hospitals, you should know your hospital's policy. You may be able to apply restraints without a doctor's order in an emergency. Also, be sure to know your state's regulations governing such restraints. For example, some states prohibit the use of four-point restraints.

When the patient is at high risk for aspiration, restrain him on his side. Never secure all four restraints to one side of the bed *because the patient may fall out of bed.*

When loosening restraints, have a co-worker on hand to assist in restraining the patient if necessary.

After assessing the patient's behavior and condition, you may decide to use a two-point restraint, which should restrain one arm and the opposite leg—for example, the right arm and the left leg. Never restrain the arm and leg on the same side *because the patient may fall out of bed.*

Don't apply a limb restraint above an I.V. site *because the constriction may occlude the infusion or cause infiltration into surrounding tissue.*

Never secure restraints to the side rails *because someone might inadvertently lower the rail before noticing the attached restraint. This may jerk the patient's limb or body, causing him discomfort and trauma.*

Don't restrain a patient in the prone position. *This position limits his field of vision, intensifies feelings of helplessness and vulnerability, and impairs respiration, especially if the patient has been sedated.*

Because the restrained patient has limited mobility, his nutrition, elimination, and positioning become your responsibility. *To prevent pressure ulcers,* reposition the patient regularly, and massage and pad bony prominences and other vulnerable areas.

When using washable restraints, place them in the laundry as your hospital directs. Many hospitals separate restraints from other linens to avoid losing them.

Complications
Excessively tight limb restraints can reduce peripheral circulation; tight vest restraints can impair respiration. Apply restraints carefully and check them regularly.

Skin breakdown can also occur under limb restraints. To prevent this, pad the patient's wrists and ankles, loosen or remove the restraints frequently, and provide regular skin care.

Long periods of immobility can predispose the patient to pneumonia, urine retention, constipation, and sensory deprivation. Reposition the patient and attend to his elimination requirements as needed.

Some patients resist restraints by biting, kicking, scratching, or head butting, possibly injuring themselves or others.

Documentation
Record the behavior that necessitated restraints, when the restraints were applied and removed, and the type of restraints used. If you expect a continued need for restraints, document their use in the Kardex.

Record vital signs, skin condition, respiratory status, peripheral circulation, and mental status.

Devices to maintain alignment and reduce pressure

Various assistive devices can be used to maintain correct body positioning and to help prevent complications that commonly arise when a patient must be on prolonged bed rest. These devices include cradle boots to protect the heels and help prevent skin breakdown, footdrop, and external hip rotation; abduction pillows to help prevent internal hip rotation after femoral fracture, hip fracture, or surgery; trochanter rolls to help prevent external hip rotation; and hand rolls to help prevent hand contractures.

Several of these devices—cradle boots, trochanter rolls, and hand rolls—are especially useful when caring for patients who have a loss of sensation, mobility, or consciousness.

Equipment
Cradle boots or substitute ■ abduction pillow ■ trochanter rolls ■ hand rolls. (See *Common preventive devices.*)

Cradle boots are made of sponge rubber and have space cut out to enclose the ankle and foot. Other commercial boots are available, but not all help to prevent external hip rotation. Footboards with antirotation blocks help prevent footdrop and external hip rotation but don't prevent heel pressure. High-topped sneakers may be used to help prevent footdrop, but they don't prevent external hip rotation or heel pressure.

The abduction pillow is a wedge-shaped piece of sponge rubber with lateral indentations for the patient's thighs.

EQUIPMENT

Common preventive devices

Hand roll: prevents hand contractures

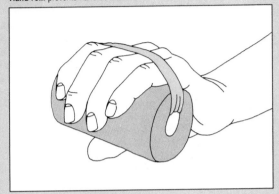

Cradle boot: prevents footdrop, skin breakdown, and external hip rotation

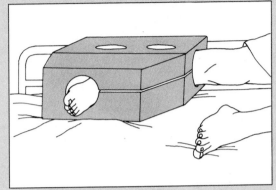

Abduction pillow: prevents internal hip rotation

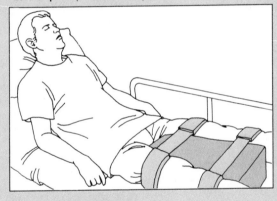

Trochanter roll: prevents external hip rotation

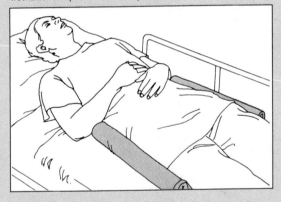

Its straps wrap around the thighs to maintain correct positioning. Although a properly shaped bed pillow may temporarily substitute for the commercial abduction pillow, it's difficult to apply and fails to maintain the correct lateral alignment.

The commercial trochanter roll is made of sponge rubber but can also be improvised from a rolled blanket or towel. The hand roll, available in hard and soft materials, is held in place by fixed or adjustable straps. It can be improvised from a rolled washcloth secured with roller gauze and adhesive tape.

Preparation of equipment

If you're using a device that's available in different sizes, select the appropriate size for the patient.

Implementation

• Explain the purpose and steps of the procedure to the patient.

Applying cradle boots

• Open the slit on the superior surface of the boot. Then place the patient's heel in the circular cutout area. If the patient is positioned laterally, you may apply the boot only to the bottom foot and support the flexed top foot with a pillow.

• If appropriate, insert the other heel in the second boot.

• Position the patient's legs properly *to prevent strain on hip ligaments and pressure on bony prominences.*

Applying an abduction pillow

• Place the pillow between the supine patient's legs. Slide it toward the groin so that it touches the legs all along its length.
• Place the upper part of both legs in the pillow's lateral indentations, and secure the straps *to prevent the pillow from slipping.*

Applying trochanter rolls

• Position one roll along the outside of the thigh, from the iliac crest to midthigh. Then place another roll along the other thigh. Make sure neither roll extends as far as the knee *to avoid peroneal nerve compression and palsy, which can lead to footdrop.*
• If you've fashioned trochanter rolls from a towel, leave several inches unrolled and tuck this under the patient's thigh *to hold the device in place and maintain the patient's position.*

Applying hand rolls

• Place one roll in the patient's hand to maintain the neutral position. Then secure the strap, if present, or apply roller gauze and secure with nonallergenic or adhesive tape.
• Place another roll in the other hand.

Special considerations

Remember that the use of assistive devices doesn't preclude regularly scheduled patient positioning, range-of-motion exercises, and skin care.

Home care

Explain the use of appropriate devices to the patient and caregiver. Demonstrate how to use each device, emphasizing proper alignment of extremities, and have the patient or caregiver give a return demonstration so you can check for proper technique. Emphasize measures needed to prevent pressure ulcers.

Complications

Contractures and pressure ulcers may occur with use of a hand roll and possibly with other assistive devices. To avoid these problems, remove a soft hand roll every 4 hours (every 2 hours if the patient has hand spasticity); remove a hard hand roll every 2 hours.

Documentation

Record the use of these devices in the patient's chart and the nursing care plan, and indicate assessment for complications. Reevaluate your patient care goals as needed.

 # Passive range-of-motion exercises

Used to move the patient's joints through as full a range of motion as possible, passive range-of-motion (ROM) exercises improve or maintain joint mobility and help prevent contractures. Performed by a nurse, a physical therapist, or a caregiver of the patient's choosing, these exercises are indicated for the patient with temporary or permanent loss of mobility, sensation, or consciousness. Performed properly, passive ROM exercises require recognition of the patient's limits of motion and support of all joints during movement.

Passive ROM exercises are contraindicated in patients with septic joints, acute thrombophlebitis, severe arthritic joint inflammation, or recent trauma with possible hidden fractures or internal injuries.

Implementation

• Determine the joints that need ROM exercises, and consult the doctor or physical therapist about limitations or precautions for specific exercises. The exercises below treat all joints, but they don't have to be performed in the order given or all at once. You can schedule them over the course of a day, whenever the patient is in the most convenient position. Remember to perform all exercises slowly, gently, and to the end of the normal range of motion or to the point of pain, but no further. (See *Glossary of joint movements* to review ROM terminology.)
• Before you begin, raise the bed to a comfortable working height.

Exercising the neck

• Support the patient's head with your hands and extend the neck, flex the chin to the chest, and tilt the head laterally toward each shoulder.
• Rotate the head from right to left.

Exercising the shoulders

• Support the patient's arm in an extended, neutral position, then extend the forearm and flex it back. Abduct the arm outward from the side of the body, and adduct it back to the side.
• Rotate the shoulder so that the arm crosses the midline, and bend the elbow so that the hand touches the opposite shoulder, then touches the mattress of the bed for complete internal rotation.
• Return the shoulder to a neutral position and, with elbow bent, push the arm backward so that the back of the hand touches the mattress for complete external rotation.

Glossary of joint movements

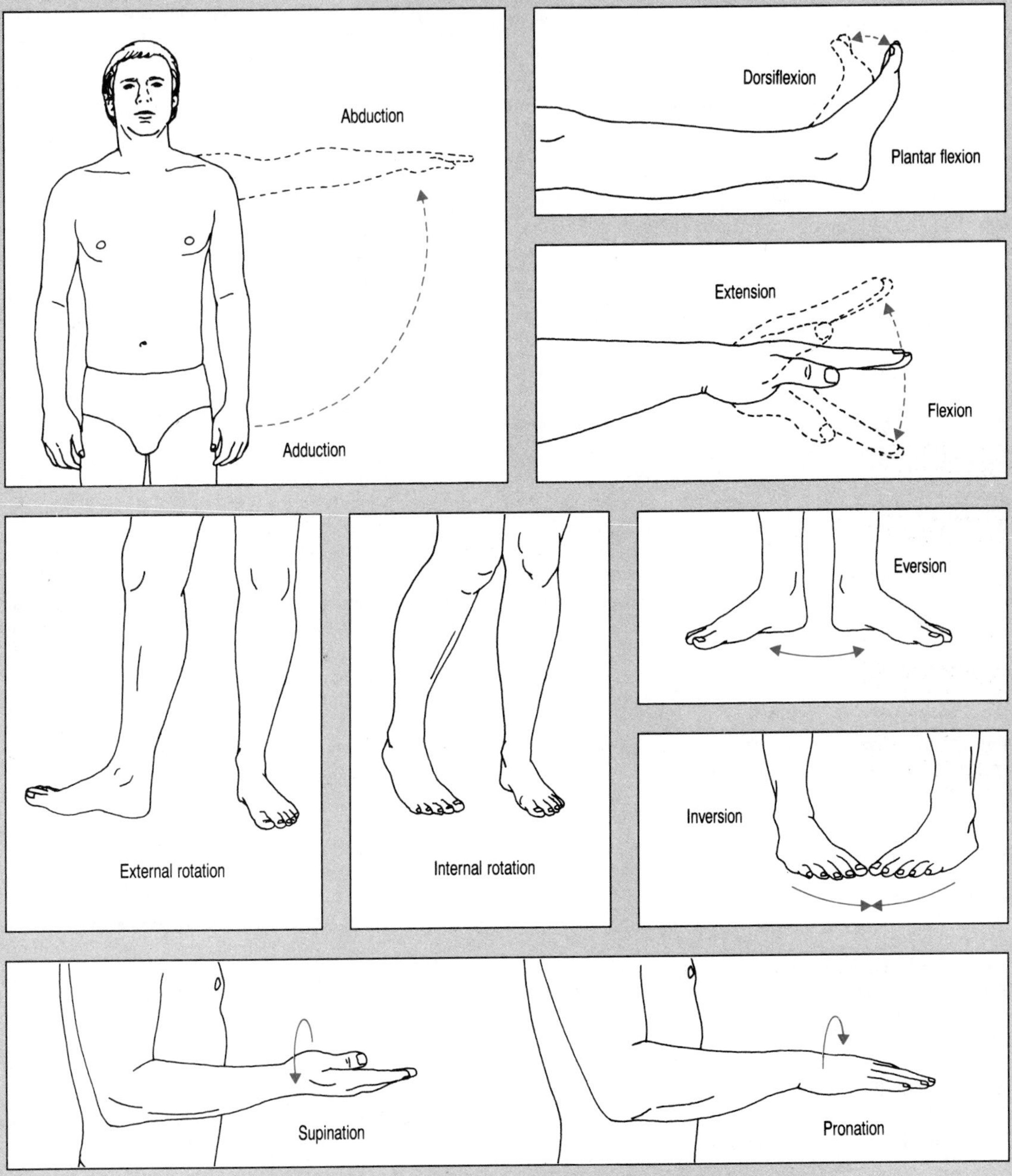

Abduction

Adduction

Dorsiflexion

Plantar flexion

Extension

Flexion

External rotation

Internal rotation

Eversion

Inversion

Supination

Pronation

Exercising the elbow
● Place the patient's arm at his side with his palm facing up.
● Flex and extend the arm at the elbow.

Exercising the forearm
● Stabilize the patient's elbow, and then twist the hand to bring the palm up (supination).
● Twist it back again to bring the palm down (pronation).

Exercising the wrist
● Stabilize the forearm and flex and extend the wrist.
● Then rock the hand sideways for lateral flexion and rotate the hand in a circular motion.

Exercising the fingers and thumb
● Extend the patient's fingers, and then flex the hand into a fist; repeat extension and flexion of each joint of each finger and thumb separately.
● Spread two adjoining fingers apart (abduction) and then bring them together (adduction).
● Oppose each fingertip to the thumb, and rotate the thumb and each finger in a circle.

Exercising the hip and knee
● Fully extend the patient's leg, and then bend the hip and knee toward the chest, allowing full joint flexion.
● Next, move the straight leg sideways, out and away from the other leg (abduction), and then back, over, and across it (adduction).
● Rotate the straight leg internally toward the midline, and then externally away from the midline.

Exercising the ankle
● Bend the patient's foot so that the toes push upward (dorsiflexion), and then bend the foot so that the toes push downward (plantar flexion).
● Rotate the ankle in a circular motion.
● Invert the ankle so that the sole of the foot faces the midline, and evert the ankle so that the sole faces away from the midline.

Exercising the toes
● Flex the patient's toes toward the sole of the foot, and then extend them back toward the top of the foot.
● Spread two adjoining toes apart (abduction) and bring them together (adduction).

Special considerations
Because joints begin to stiffen within 24 hours of disuse, start passive ROM exercises as soon as possible, and perform them at least once a shift, particularly while bathing or turning the patient. Use proper body mechanics, and repeat each exercise at least three times.

Patients who experience prolonged bed rest or limited activity without profound weakness can also be taught to perform ROM exercises on their own (called active ROM) or may benefit from isometric exercises. (See *Learning about isometric exercises.*)

If the disabled patient requires long-term rehabilitation after discharge, consult with a physical therapist and teach a family member or caregiver to perform passive ROM exercises.

Documentation
Record the joints exercised, the presence of edema or pressure areas, any pain resulting from the exercises, any limitation of ROM, and the patient's tolerance of the exercises.

 Progressive ambulation

After surgery or a period of bed rest, patients must begin the gradual return to full ambulation. When begun promptly and properly, this process—called progressive ambulation—thwarts many of the complications of prolonged inactivity.

Complications prevented by early progressive ambulation include respiratory stasis and hypostatic pneumonia; circulatory stasis, thrombophlebitis, and emboli; urine retention, urinary tract infection, and urinary stasis and calculus formation; abdominal distention, constipation, and decreased appetite; and sensory deprivation. Progressive ambulation also helps restore the patient's sense of equilibrium and enhances his self-confidence and self-image.

Progressive ambulation begins with dangling the patient's feet over the edge of the bed and progresses to seating him in an armchair or wheelchair, walking around the room with him, and then walking with him in the halls until he can walk by himself. The patient's progress depends on his physical condition and his tolerance. Successful return to full ambulation requires correct body mechanics, careful patient observation, and open communication between patient, doctor, and nurse.

Equipment
Robe ■ chair or wheelchair ■ slippers for sitting, hard-soled shoes for walking ■ assistive device (cane, crutches, walker) if necessary ■ optional: walking belt.

Learning about isometric exercises

Patients can strengthen and increase muscle tone by contracting muscles against resistance (from other muscles or from a stationary object, such as a bed or a wall) without joint movement. These exercises require only a comfortable position—standing, sitting, or lying down—and proper body alignment. For each exercise, instruct the patient to hold each contraction for 2 to 5 seconds and to repeat it three to four times daily, below peak contraction level for the first week and at peak level thereafter.

Neck rotators
The patient places the heel of his hand above one ear. Then he pushes his head toward the hand as forcefully as possible, without moving the head, neck, or arm. He repeats the exercise on the other side.

Neck flexors
The patient places both palms on his forehead. Without moving his neck, he pushes the head forward while resisting with the palms.

Neck extensors
The patient clasps his fingers behind his head, then pushes the head against the clasped hands without moving his neck.

Shoulder elevators
Holding the right arm straight down at the side, the patient grasps his right wrist with his left hand. He then tries to shrug his right shoulder, but prevents it from moving by holding his arm in place. He repeats this exercise, alternating arms.

Shoulder, chest, and scapular musculature
The patient places his right fist in his left palm and raises both arms to shoulder height. He pushes the fist into the palm as forcefully as possible without moving either arm. Then, with his arms in the same position, he clasps the fingers and tries to pull the hands apart. He repeats the pattern, beginning with the left fist in the right palm.

Elbow flexors and extensors
With his right elbow bent 90 degrees and his right palm facing upward, the patient places his left fist against his right palm. He tries to bend the right elbow further while resisting with the left fist. He repeats the pattern, bending the left elbow.

Abdomen
The patient assumes a sitting position and bends slightly forward, with his hands in front of the middle of his thighs. He tries to bend forward further, resisting by pressing the palms against the thighs.

Alternatively, in the supine position, he clasps his hands behind his head. Then he raises his shoulders about 1″ (2.5 cm), holding this position for a few seconds.

Back extensors
In a sitting position, the patient bends forward and places his hands under his buttocks. He tries to stand up, resisting with both hands.

Hip abductors
While standing, the patient squeezes his inner thighs together as tightly as possible. Placing a pillow between the knees supplies resistance and increases the effectiveness of this exercise.

Hip extensors
The patient squeezes his buttocks together as tightly as possible.

Knee extensors
The patient straightens his knee fully. Then he vigorously tightens the muscle above the knee so that it moves the kneecap upward. He repeats this exercise, alternating legs.

Ankle flexors and extensors
The patient pulls his toes upward, holding briefly. Then he pushes them down as far as possible, again holding briefly.

Preparation of equipment
If the patient requires an assistive device, the physical therapist usually selects the appropriate one and teaches its use.

Implementation
• Check the patient's history, diagnosis, and therapeutic regimen. Ask him if he feels pain or weakness; if necessary, give medication for pain and wait 30 to 60 minutes for it to take effect before attempting ambulation. Re-

Helping the patient regain mobility

Dangling legs
To help the patient support himself in a dangling position, move an overbed table in front of him and place a pillow on it.

Sitting
Seat the patient in a chair with armrests and a straight back, with his lower back against the rear of the chair, feet flat on the floor, hips and knees at right angles, and upper body straight. Rest his forearms on the armrests.

Walking
Provide a path unimpeded by equipment and other objects, and avoid overexertion. If necessary, hold the patient so you can control his upper and lower body and any lateral movements.

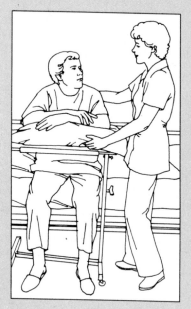
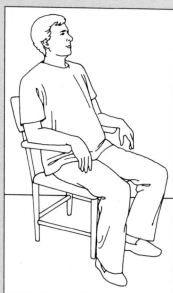
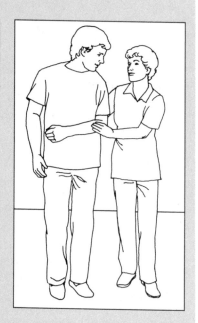

member that the medicated patient may overestimate his capabilities or develop hypotension, dizziness, or drowsiness.
• Explain the immediate goal of ambulation and the way you'll help him achieve it. (See *Helping the patient regain mobility.*) Provide encouragement *because he may be hesitant or fearful;* reassure him that he need not attempt more than he can reasonably do. If he fears pain in an incision, show him how to support it by placing a hand alongside or gently over the dressing site, or splint the incision for him.
• Remove equipment or other objects *to provide a clear path and prevent falls.*

Dangle the patient's legs
• Position the bed horizontally and the patient laterally, facing you. Move his legs over the side of the bed and grasp his shoulders, standing with your feet apart so you have a wide base of support. Ask the patient to help by pushing up from the bed with his arms. Then shift your weight from the foot closest to the patient's head to the other foot as you steadily and deliberately raise the patient to the sitting position. Pull with your whole body, not just your arms, *to avoid straining your back and jostling the patient.*

Alternatively, you can raise the head of the bed to a 45-degree angle *to allow easier elevation of the patient.* Don't use this method if the patient has trouble balancing himself while sitting *because he could fall.* Ask a co-worker for assistance whenever necessary.

• While the patient adjusts to an upright position, continue to stand facing him *to keep him from falling,* and observe him closely. Be alert for signs and symptoms of orthostatic hypotension, such as fainting, dizziness, and complaints of blurred vision. If desired, check the patient's pulse rate and blood pressure. If the pulse rate increases more than 20 beats/minute, allow the patient to rest before progressing slowly.

Assist the patient to stand

• After the patient can dangle his legs successfully and can support his weight on them, attempt the standing position.

• Help the patient put on a robe and slippers or shoes. If you plan to use a walking belt, apply it now. Do not allow a robe, a urinary catheter's drainage tube, or anything else to dangle around the patient's feet.

• If the patient is alert and has fair to good strength, place his feet flat on the floor and allow him to stand by himself. As he stands, place one hand under his axilla and the other hand around his waist *to prevent falls.* Help him stand fully erect *to promote good balance and correct breathing.* Encourage him to look forward and not at the floor *to help maintain his balance.*

• If the patient needs help standing up, position your knees at either side of his. Bend your knees, put your arms around his waist, and instruct him to push up from the bed with his arms. Then straighten your knees and pull the patient with you while rising to an erect position. *This technique helps you avoid back muscle strain.*

Help the patient sit or walk

• Once the patient stands, you can pivot and lower him into an armchair or wheelchair, or you can begin to walk with him.

• If you've decided to seat him, make sure the chair is secure and won't slip as you lower the patient into it. Place his lower back against the rear of the chair and his feet flat on the floor. Position his hips and knees at right angles, and keep his upper body straight. Then flex his elbows and place his forearms on the arms of the chair.

• If the patient can walk safely only with your assistance, stand behind him, placing one hand under his axilla and the other hand around his waist. *This allows you to control the upper and lower body as well as lateral deviation.*

• If you can't support the patient, ask a co-worker to help you. Stand to one side of the patient and place your hand under his arm or on his elbow, or grasp the walking belt. Standing on the other side of the patient, the assisting co-worker should support the patient in the same way.

• Give the patient verbal and tactile cues *to encourage him during walking.* Stay close to a railed wall or another supportive structure and, if necessary, allow the patient to rest in a chair before attempting to walk back to his room. If he can't walk back, tell him to remain seated while you summon assistance or obtain a wheelchair. Don't leave the patient unattended if you have any reason to think he may fall. If you can't find a chair nearby, have the patient lean against the wall and call for assistance as you help support him. If necessary, steady him as he slides down the wall to sit on the floor.

Special considerations

If early ambulation is impossible, encourage bed exercises. Don't let the use of catheters and infusion bottles discourage ambulation; secure these devices so they are easily portable, and check dressings and tubes carefully afterward for proper position and changes in drainage. If appropriate, measure pulse, respiratory rate, and blood pressure. When leaving the patient sitting up in a chair, make certain he has a call button or signal device. Restrain the confused patient to prevent falls.

If the patient begins to fall, don't try to catch him. Instead, do your best to break his fall by easing him to the bed, chair, or floor, making sure he doesn't strike his head. Then summon help. Don't leave the patient alone—he needs your comfort and reassurance.

If the patient experiences dyspnea, diaphoresis, or orthostatic hypotension, stabilize his position and take vital signs. Place him in semi-Fowler's position to facilitate breathing. If his condition doesn't improve rapidly, notify the doctor.

Documentation

Record the type of transfer and assistance required; the duration of sitting, standing, or walking; the distance walked, if appropriate; the patient's response to ambulation; and any significant changes in blood pressure, pulse, and respiration.

 Tilt table

The tilt table, a padded table or bed-length board that can be raised gradually from a horizontal to a vertical position, can help prevent the complications of prolonged bed rest. Used for the patient with a spinal cord injury, brain damage, orthostatic hypotension, or any other condition that prevents free standing, the tilt table increases tolerance of the upright position, conditions the cardiovascular system, stretches muscles, and helps prevent contractures, bone demineralization, and urinary calculus formation.

Equipment

Tilt table with footboard and restraining straps ▪ sphygmomanometer ▪ stethoscope ▪ antiembolism stockings or elastic bandages ▪ optional: abdominal binder.

Preparation of equipment

Common types of tilt tables include the electric table, which moves at a slow, steady rate; the manual table, which is raised by a handle; and the spring-assisted table, which is raised by a pedal. Familiarize yourself with operating instructions for the model you'll be using.

Implementation

• Explain the use and benefits of the tilt table to the patient.
• Apply antiembolism stockings *to restrict vessel walls and help prevent blood pooling and edema.* If necessary, apply an abdominal binder *to avoid pooling of blood in the splanchnic region, which contributes to insufficient cerebral circulation and orthostatic hypotension.*
• Make sure the tilt table is locked in the horizontal position. Then summon assistance and transfer the patient to the table, placing him in the supine position with feet flat against the footboard.
• If the patient can't bear weight on one leg, place a wooden block between the footboard and the weight-bearing foot, permitting the non-weight-bearing leg to dangle freely.
• Fasten the safety straps, then take the patient's blood pressure and pulse rate.
• Tilt the table slowly in 15- to 30-degree increments, evaluating the patient constantly. Take his blood pressure every 3 to 5 minutes *because movement from the supine to the upright position decreases systolic pressure.* Be alert for signs and symptoms of insufficient cerebral circulation: dizziness, nausea, pallor, diaphoresis, tachycardia, or a change in mental status. If the patient experiences any of these signs or symptoms, or hypotension or seizures, return the table immediately to the horizontal position.
• If the patient tolerates the position shift, continue to tilt the table until reaching the desired angle, usually between 45 degrees and 80 degrees. A 60-degree tilt gives the patient the physiologic effects and sensations of standing upright.
• Gradually return the patient to the horizontal position, and check his vital signs. Then obtain assistance and transfer the patient onto the stretcher for transport back to his room.

Special considerations

Let the patient's response determine the angle of tilt and duration of elevation, but avoid prolonged upright positioning *because it may lead to venous stasis.*
◆ *Nursing alert.* Never leave the patient unattended on the tilt table *because marked physiologic changes, such as hypotension or severe headache, can occur suddenly.* ◆

Complications

Use of a tilt table can lead to sudden hypotension, severe headache, and other dramatic physiologic changes.

Documentation

Record the angle and duration of elevation; changes in the patient's pulse rate, blood pressure, and physical and mental status; and his response to treatment.

 Canes

Indicated for the patient with one-sided weakness or injury, occasional loss of balance, or increased joint pressure, a cane provides balance and support for walking and reduces fatigue and strain on weight-bearing joints. Available in various sizes, the cane should extend from the greater trochanter to the floor and have a rubber tip to prevent slipping. Canes are contraindicated for the patient with bilateral weakness; such a patient should use crutches or a walker.

Equipment

Rubber-tipped cane ▪ optional: walking belt.

Although wooden canes are available, three types of aluminum canes are used most frequently. The standard aluminum cane—used by the patient who needs only slight assistance to walk—provides the least support; its half-circle handle allows it to be hooked over chairs. The T-handle cane—used by the patient with hand weakness—has a straight, shaped handle with grips and a bent shaft. It provides greater stability than the standard cane. The quad (broad-based) cane is used by the patient with poor balance or one-sided weakness and an inability to hold onto a walker with both hands stemming from a cerebrovascular accident. The base of this type of cane splits into four short, splayed legs in a rectangular array. The quad cane provides greater stability than a standard cane but considerably less than a walker.

Preparation of equipment

Ask the patient to hold the cane on the uninvolved side 4″ to 6″ (10 to 15 cm) from the base of the little toe. If the cane is made of aluminum, adjust its height by pushing in the metal button on the shaft and raising or lowering the shaft; it it's wood, the rubber tip can be removed and excess length sawed off. At the correct height, the handle of the cane is level with the greater trochanter and allows approximately 15-degree flexion at the elbow. If the cane is too short, the patient will have to drop his shoulder to lean on it; if it's too long, he'll have to raise his shoulder and will have difficulty supporting his weight.

Implementation
• Explain the mechanics of cane walking to the patient. Demonstrate the technique, then have the patient return the demonstration. Coordinate practice sessions in the physical therapy department if necessary.
• Tell the patient to hold the cane on the uninvolved side *to promote a reciprocal gait pattern and to distribute weight away from the involved side.*
• Instruct the patient to hold the cane close to his body *to prevent leaning,* and to move the cane and the involved leg simultaneously, followed by the uninvolved leg.
• Encourage the patient to keep the stride length of each leg and the timing of each step (cadence) equal.

Negotiating stairs
• Instruct the patient to always use a railing, if present, when going up or down stairs. Tell him to hold the cane with the other hand or to keep it in the hand grasping the railing. To ascend stairs, the patient should lead with the uninvolved leg and follow with the involved leg; to descend, he should lead with the involved leg and follow with the uninvolved one. Help the patient remember by telling him to use this mnemonic device: "The good goes up, and the bad goes down."
• To negotiate stairs without a railing, the patient should use the walking technique to ascend and descend the stairs but should move the cane just before the involved leg. Thus, to ascend stairs, the patient should hold the cane on the uninvolved side, step with the uninvolved leg, advance the cane, then move the involved leg. To descend, he should hold the cane on the uninvolved side, lead with the cane, then advance the involved leg and, finally, the uninvolved leg.

Using a chair
• To teach the patient to sit down, stand by his affected side and tell him to place the backs of his legs against the edge of the chair seat. Then tell him to move the cane out from his side and to reach back with both hands to grasp the chair's armrests. Supporting his weight on the armrests, he can then lower himself onto the seat. While he's seated, he should keep the cane hooked on the armrest or the chair back.

• To teach the patient to get up, stand by his affected side and tell him to unhook the cane from the chair and hold it in his stronger hand as he grasps the armrests. Then tell him to move his uninvolved foot slightly forward, to lean slightly forward, and to push against the armrests to raise himself upright.
• Warn the patient not to lean on the cane when sitting or rising from the chair *to prevent falls.*
• Supervise your patient each time he gets in or out of a chair until you're both certain he can do it alone.

Special considerations
To prevent falls during the learning period, guard the patient carefully by standing behind him slightly to his stronger side and putting one foot between his feet and your other foot to the outside of the uninvolved leg. If necessary, use a walking belt.

Complications
A poorly fitted cane can cause the patient to lose his balance and fall.

Documentation
Record the type of cane used, the amount of guarding required, the distance walked, and the patient's understanding and tolerance of cane walking.

 # Crutches

Crutches remove weight from one or both legs, enabling the patient to support himself with his hands and arms. Typically prescribed for the patient with lower-extremity injury or weakness, crutches require balance, stamina, and upper-body strength for successful use. Crutch selection and walking gait depend on the patient's condition. The patient who can't use crutches may be able to use a walker.

Equipment
Crutches with axillary pads, handgrips, and rubber suction tips ■ optional: walking belt.

Three types of crutches are commonly used. Standard aluminum or wooden crutches are used by the patient with a sprain, strain, or cast. They require stamina and upper-body strength. Aluminum forearm crutches are used by the paraplegic or other patient using the swing-through gait. They have a collar that fits around the forearm and a horizontal handgrip that provides support. Platform crutches are used by the arthritic patient who has an upper-extremity deficit that prevents weight bear-

Fitting a patient for a crutch

Position the crutch so that it extends from a point 4" to 6" (10 to 15 cm) to the side and 4" to 6" in front of the patient's feet to 1½" to 2" (4 to 5 cm) below the axillae (about the width of two fingers). Then adjust the handgrips so that the patient's elbows are flexed at a 15-degree angle when he's standing with the crutches in the resting position.

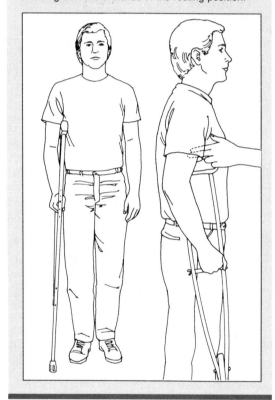

ing through the wrist. They provide padded surfaces for the upper extremities.

Preparation of equipment

After choosing the appropriate crutches, adjust their height with the patient standing or, if necessary, recumbent. (See *Fitting a patient for a crutch* for specific instructions.)

Implementation

• Consult with the patient's doctor and physical therapist *to coordinate rehabilitation orders and teaching.*
• Describe the gait you will teach and the reason for your choice. Then demonstrate the gait, as necessary. Have the patient give a return demonstration.
• Place a walking belt around the patient's waist, if necessary, *to help prevent falls.* Tell the patient to position the crutches and to shift his weight from side to side. Then place the patient in front of a full-length mirror *to facilitate learning and coordination.*
• Teach the four-point gait to the patient who can bear weight on both legs. Although this is the safest gait, *because three points are always in contact with the floor,* it requires greater coordination than others *because of its constant shifting of weight.* Use this sequence: right crutch, left foot, left crutch, right foot. Suggest counting *to help develop rhythm,* and make sure each short step is of equal length. If the patient gains proficiency at this gait, teach the faster two-point gait.
• Teach the two-point gait to the patient with weak legs but good coordination and arm strength. This is the most natural crutch-walking gait *because it mimics walking, with alternating swings of the arms and legs.* Instruct the patient to advance the right crutch and left foot simultaneously, followed by the left crutch and right foot.
• Teach the three-point gait to the patient who can bear only partial or no weight on one leg. Instruct him to advance both crutches 6" to 8" (15 to 20 cm) along with the involved leg. Then tell him to bring the uninvolved leg forward and to bear the bulk of his weight on the crutches but some of it on the involved leg, if possible. Stress the importance of taking steps of equal length and duration with no pauses.
• Teach the swing-to or swing-through gaits—the fastest ones—to the patient with complete paralysis of the hips and legs. Instruct the patient to advance both crutches simultaneously and to swing the legs parallel to (swing-to) or beyond the crutches (swing-through).
• To teach the patient who uses crutches to get up from a chair, tell him to hold both crutches in one hand, with the tips resting firmly on the floor. Then instruct him to push up from the chair with his free hand, supporting himself with the crutches.
• To sit down, the patient reverses the process: Tell him to support himself with the crutches in one hand and to lower himself with the other.
• To teach the patient to ascend stairs using the three-point gait, tell him to lead with the uninvolved leg and to follow with both the crutches and the involved leg. To descend stairs, he should lead with the crutches and the involved leg and follow with the good leg. He may find

it helpful to remember "The good goes up, the bad goes down."

Special considerations
Encourage arm- and shoulder-strengthening exercises to prepare the patient for crutch walking. If possible, teach two techniques—one fast and one slow—*so the patient can alternate between them to prevent excessive muscle fatigue and can adjust more easily to various walking conditions.*

Complications
When used with chronic conditions, the swing-to and swing-through gaits can lead to atrophy of the hips and legs if appropriate therapeutic exercises are not performed routinely. Warn the patient against habitually leaning on his crutches *because prolonged pressure on the axillae can damage the brachial nerves, causing brachial nerve palsy.*

Documentation
Record the type of gait the patient used, the amount of assistance required, the distance walked, and the patient's tolerance of the crutches and gait.

Walkers

A walker consists of a metal frame with handgrips and four legs that buttresses the patient on three sides. One side remains open. Because this device provides greater stability and security than other ambulatory aids, it's recommended for the patient with insufficient strength and balance to use crutches or a cane, or with weakness requiring frequent rest periods. Attachments for standard walkers and modified walkers help meet special needs.

Equipment
Walker ∎ platform or wheel attachments, as necessary.

Various types of walkers are available. The standard walker is used by the patient with unilateral or bilateral weakness or an inability to bear weight on one leg. It requires arm strength and balance. Platform attachments may be added to this walker for the patient with arthritic arms or a casted arm, who can't bear weight directly on his hand, wrist, or forearm. With the doctor's approval, wheels may be placed on the front legs of the standard walker to allow the extremely weak or poorly coordinated patient to roll the device forward, instead of

lifting it. However, wheels are applied infrequently *because they may be a safety hazard.*

The stair walker—used by the patient who must negotiate stairs without bilateral handrails—requires good arm strength and balance. Its extra set of handles extends toward the patient on the open side. The rolling walker—used by the patient with very weak legs—has four wheels and a seat. The reciprocal walker—used by the patient with very weak arms—allows one side to be advanced ahead of the other.

Preparation of equipment
Obtain the appropriate walker with the advice of a physical therapist, and adjust it to the patient's height: His elbows should be flexed at a 15-degree angle when standing comfortably within the walker with his hands on the grips. To adjust the walker, turn it upside down, and change the leg length by pushing in the button on each shaft and releasing it when the leg is in the correct position. Make sure the walker is level before the patient attempts to use it.

Implementation
• Help the patient stand within the walker, and instruct him to hold the handgrips firmly and equally. Stand behind him, closer to the involved leg.
• If the patient has one-sided leg weakness, tell him to advance the walker 6″ to 8″ (15 to 20 cm) and to step forward with the involved leg and follow with the uninvolved leg, supporting himself on his arms. Encourage him to take equal strides. If he has equal strength in both legs, instruct him to advance the walker 6″ to 8″ and to step forward with either leg. If he can't use one leg, tell him to advance the walker 6″ to 8″ and to swing onto it, supporting his weight on his arms.
• If the patient is using a reciprocal walker, teach him the two-point or four-point gait (see "Crutches" in this chapter). If the patient is using a wheeled or stair walker, reinforce the physical therapist's instructions. Stress the need for caution when using a stair walker.
• Teach the patient how to use a chair safely. (See *Teaching safe use of a walker,* page 56.)

Special considerations
If the patient starts to fall, support his hips and shoulders *to help maintain an upright position if possible.*

Documentation
Record the type of walker and attachments used, the degree of guarding required, the distance walked, and the patient's tolerance of ambulation.

Teaching safe use of a walker

Sitting down
• First, tell the patient to stand with the back of his stronger leg against the front of the chair, his weaker leg slightly off the floor, and the walker directly in front.
• Tell him to grasp the armrests on the chair one arm at a time while supporting most of his weight on the stronger leg. (In the illustrations below, the patient has left leg weakness.)
• Tell the patient to lower himself into the chair and slide backward. After he is seated, he should place the walker beside the chair.

Getting up
• After bringing the walker back to the front of his chair, tell the patient to slide forward in the chair. Placing the back of his stronger leg against the seat, he should then advance the weaker leg.
• Next, with both hands on the armrests, the patient can push himself to a standing position. Supporting himself with the stronger leg and the opposite hand, the patient should grasp the walker's handgrip with his free hand.
• Then have the patient grasp the free handgrip with his other hand.

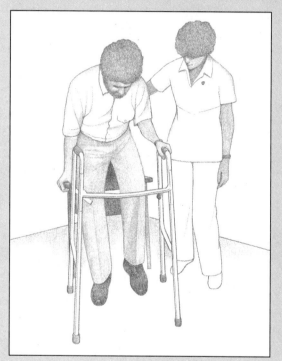

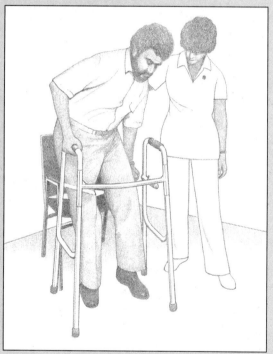

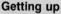

Supplemental bed equipment

Certain equipment can promote the bedridden patient's comfort and help prevent pressure ulcers and other complications of immobility. A wood or hard plastic footboard prevents footdrop by maintaining proper alignment. It also raises bed linens off of the patient's feet. The foot cradle — a horizontal or arched bar over the end of the bed — keeps bed linens off of the patient's feet, preventing skin irritation and breakdown, especially in patients with peripheral vascular disease or neuropathy. The bed board, made of wood or wood covered with canvas, firms the mattress and is especially useful for the patient with spinal injuries. The metal basic frame and the metal trapeze (a triangular piece attached to this frame) allow the patient with arm mobility and strength to lift himself off the bed, facilitating bed making and bedpan positioning. The metal overbed cradle, a cagelike frame positioned on top of the mattress, keeps bed linens off of the patient with burns, open wounds, or a wet cast.

The vinyl water mattress and the foam mattress, used to prevent or treat pressure ulcers, exert less pressure on the skin than the standard hospital mattress. Although the alternating pressure pad (a vinyl pad divided into chambers filled with air or water and attached to an electric pump) serves the same purpose, it also stimulates circulation by alternately inflating and deflating its chambers.

All supplemental bed equipment is optional, depending on the patient's needs. Reusable and disposable water mattresses are available. The reusable water mattress replaces the standard hospital mattress and rests on a sheet of heavy cardboard placed over the bedsprings; the smaller, less bulky disposable mattress rests on top of the standard hospital mattress. (See *Types of supplemental bed equipment,* page 58.)

Equipment

Footboard and cover ■ drawsheet ■ bath blanket ■ foot cradle ■ bed board ■ basic frame with trapeze ■ overbed cradle ■ roller gauze ■ water mattress ■ stretcher ■ alternating pressure pad ■ pump and tubing ■ footstool ■ linen-saver pad ■ foam mattress (such as a convoluted foam mattress) ■ safety pins ■ plastic protective sleeve for foam mattress (partial or full length).

Preparation of equipment

If you're preparing a footboard for use, place a cover over it to provide padding. Or pad it with a folded drawsheet or bath blanket: Bring the top and side edges of the sheet or blanket to the back of the footboard, miter the corners, and secure them at the center with safety pins. *Padding cushions the patient's feet against pressure from the hard footboard, helping to prevent skin irritation and breakdown.* Avoid wrinkles *to prevent skin irritation.*

Implementation

• Tell the patient what you're going to do and describe the equipment.
• Wash your hands.

Using a footboard

• Move the patient up in bed *to allow room for the footboard.* Loosen the top linens at the foot of the bed, and then fold them back over the patient *to expose his feet.*
• Lift the mattress at the foot of the bed, and place the lip of the footboard between the mattress and the bedsprings. Or secure the footboard under both sides of the mattress.

• Adjust the footboard so that the patient's feet rest comfortably against it. If the footboard isn't adjustable, tuck a folded bath blanket between the board and the patient's feet.
• Unless the footboard has side supports, place a sandbag, a folded bath blanket, or a pillow alongside each foot *to maintain 90-degree foot alignment.*
• Fold the top linens over the footboard, tuck them under the mattress, and miter the corners.

Using a foot cradle

• Loosen the top linens at the foot of the bed, and fold them over the patient or to one side.
• When using a one-piece cradle, place one side arm under the mattress, carefully extend the arch over the bed, and place the other side arm under the mattress on the opposite side. Then adjust the tension rods *so that they rest securely over the edge of the mattress.*
• When using a sectional cradle with two side arms, first place the side arms under the mattress. Secure the tension rods over the edge of the mattress. Then carefully place the arch over the bed and connect it to the side arms.

When using a sectional cradle with one side arm, connect the side arm and horizontal cradle bar before placement. Then place the side arm under the mattress on one side of the bed.

• Cover the cradle with the top linens, tuck them under the mattress at the foot of the bed, and miter the corners.

Using a bed board

• Transfer the patient from his bed to a stretcher or a chair. Obtain assistance if necessary.
• Strip the linens from the bed. If you plan to reuse them, fold each piece neatly and hang it over the back of a chair. Otherwise, place soiled linens in a laundry bag.
• If the bed board consists of wooden slats encased in canvas, lift the mattress at the head of the bed and center the board over the bedsprings *to prevent it from jutting out and causing accidental injury.* Unroll the slats to cover the bedsprings at the head of the bed. Then lift the mattress at the foot of the bed and unroll the remaining slats.

If the bed board consists of one solid or two hinged pieces of wood, lift the mattress on one side of the bed and center the board over the bedsprings.

• After positioning the bed board, replace the linens. Then return the patient to bed.

Using a basic frame with trapeze

• If an orthopedic technician isn't available to secure the frame and trapeze to the patient's bed, get assistance to

Types of supplemental bed equipment

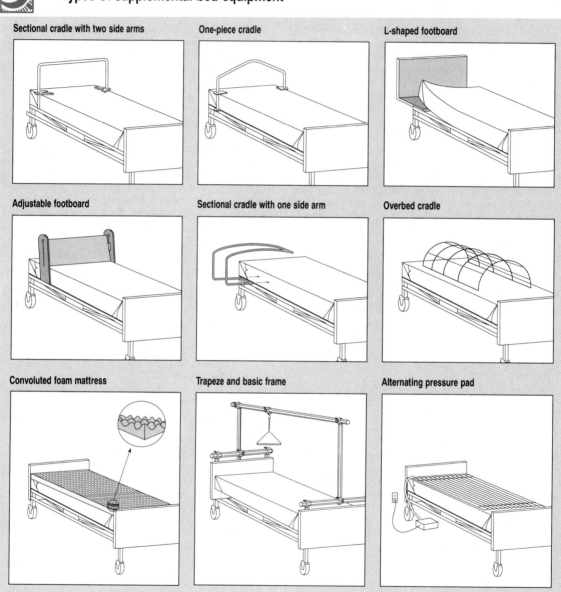

Sectional cradle with two side arms

One-piece cradle

L-shaped footboard

Adjustable footboard

Sectional cradle with one side arm

Overbed cradle

Convoluted foam mattress

Trapeze and basic frame

Alternating pressure pad

attach these devices to the bed, as necessary. Be sure to hang the trapeze within the patient's easy reach so he won't need to strain to reach it.

Using an overbed cradle
• Loosen and remove the top linens.
• Carefully lower the cradle onto the patient's bed and secure it in place. Wrap roller gauze around both sides

of the cradle. Then pull the gauze taut and attach it to the bedsprings.

• Cover the cradle with the top linens, tuck them under the mattress at the foot of the bed, and miter the corners.

Using a portable water mattress

• This mattress is heavy and bulky, so you'll need several co-workers *to help you transfer it from the stretcher to the patient's bed.* Check with the maintenance department before transferring the mattress *because its weight may rule out use on some electric beds.* Also, ensure that the patient isn't prone to motion sickness *because the movement of the water in the mattress may cause nausea.*

• Position the mattress on the bed, and place the protective cover over it. Then place a bottom sheet over the cover and tuck it in loosely.

• Place a sheepskin, linen-saver pad, or drawsheet over the bottom sheet, as needed. Adding these items doesn't decrease the effectiveness of this mattress.

• Position the patient comfortably on the mattress. Then cover him with the top linens, and tuck them in loosely.

• Check the water mattress daily *to ensure adequate flotation.* To do so, place your hand under the patient's thighs. If you can feel the bottom of the mattress, arrange to have water added.

Using an alternating pressure pad

• If possible, transfer the patient from his bed to a chair or stretcher. Get help if necessary.

• Strip the linens from the bed. Then inspect the plug and electrical cord of the alternating pressure pad for defects. Don't use the unit if it appears damaged.

• Unfold the pad on top of the mattress with the appropriate side facing up.

• Place the motor on a linen-saver pad on the floor or on a footstool near the mattress outlets. Connect the tubing securely to the motor and to the mattress outlets, and plug the cord into an electrical outlet. Turn the motor on.

• After several minutes, observe the emptying and filling of the pad's chambers, and check the tubing for kinks *because they could interfere with the pad's function.*

• Place a bottom sheet over the pad, and tuck it in loosely. *To avoid tube constriction,* don't miter the corner where the tubing is attached.

• Position the patient comfortably on the pad, cover him with the top linens, and tuck them in loosely.

• If the pad becomes soiled, clean it with a damp cloth and mild soap, then dry it well. *To avoid damaging the pad's surface,* don't use alcohol.

• When the patient no longer needs the pad or is discharged, turn the motor off, disconnect the tubing, and unplug the cord from the wall outlet. Remove the pad

from the patient's bed, and fold and discard it. Or, if applicable, give the pad to the patient to take home. Inform him that the motor needed to power the pad can usually be rented from a surgical supply store. Explain to the patient or a caregiver how to operate the pad at home.

• Coil the tubing and electrical cord, and then strap them to the motor. Return the motor unit to the central supply department.

Using a convoluted foam mattress

• If possible, transfer the patient from his bed to a chair or stretcher. Get help if necessary.

• Strip the linens from the bed. Then place the foam mattress on top of the standard mattress, wavy side up.

• Slip the protective sleeve over the foam mattress at the patient's buttock level *to prevent leakage of excretions into the mattress.* If necessary, use a full-length sleeve.

• Place a bottom sheet over the foam mattress, and tuck it in loosely. *Tucking it too tightly can decrease the cushioning effect.*

• Position the patient comfortably on the mattress. Then cover him with the top linens and tuck them in loosely.

• When the patient no longer needs the mattress or is discharged, discard the mattress or let him take it home. (See *Helping patients improvise assistive devices at home,* page 60.)

Special considerations

Place the patient in bed before positioning and securing an overbed or foot cradle *to ensure its proper placement and to prevent patient injury.* Similarly, remove the cradle before the patient gets out of bed. When turning or positioning the patient on his side, be sure the foot cradle's tension rod doesn't rest against his skin *because this may cause pressure and predispose him to skin breakdown.*

Exercise caution when turning the obese patient on a water mattress *because turning displaces a large volume of water.* Be sure to keep the side rails raised during turning *to prevent falls.*

Avoid placing excessive layers of drawsheets or linen-saver pads between the alternating pressure pad and the patient, *because these decrease the pad's effectiveness.* Avoid using pins or sharp instruments near an alternating pressure pad or water mattress *to prevent accidental puncture.*

Use up to three foam mattresses on the bed, as the patient's condition requires. Place one mattress on the bed to prevent pressure ulcers, two or three mattresses to treat them. You can decrease the pressure exerted on the bony prominences by increasing the number of mattresses.

♦ *Nursing alert.* Because a plastic-covered mattress slides off a bed board easily, be sure a co-worker is standing

Helping patients improvise assistive devices at home

Assistive devices can increase patient comfort and improve care given in the home. This equipment need not be expensive. If the patient's illness is brief or financial constraints exist, teach patients and caregivers to improvise assistive devices with common household items. For example:
• Side rails can be made by placing kitchen chairs along the sides of a bed and securing their legs to the bed frame.
• Linen-saver pads can be fashioned from shower curtains, plastic tablecloths, a plastic raincoat, or trash bags.
• Absorbent pads can be made by placing sheets of newspaper and a bottom layer of plastic inside a pillowcase. When damp, discard the newspaper and wash the pillowcase.
• An ironing board, a wooden crate with two sides removed, a child's table, or a sturdy cardboard box can serve as an over-the-bed table or a bed cradle.
• Backrests can be fashioned from a large item such as a cutting board padded on top and supported underneath by pillows.
• A pull rope to assist the patient in turning or sitting up can be made by braiding nylon stockings together and fastening the rope to the side or end of the bed.

on the opposite side of the bed when you're transferring the patient from stretcher to bed. ♦

If the bottom sheet isn't wide enough to cover both the standard and foam mattresses, use two bottom sheets. Cover the standard mattress with one sheet, then cover the foam mattress with a second sheet and tuck it between the standard and foam mattresses. Two top sheets may be needed to cover the patient when using a footboard, foot cradle, or bed cradle.

Because a foam mattress is tightly rolled for storage, it may need to be unrolled on a clean empty bed and allowed to recover its original springiness before use.

Don't use a foam mattress to lift the patient *because the mattress may tear, causing the patient to fall.*

Documentation

In your notes and care plan, record the type of supplemental bed equipment used, the time and date of use, and the patient's response to treatment.

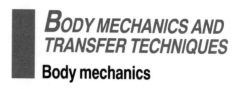

BODY MECHANICS AND TRANSFER TECHNIQUES

Body mechanics

Many patient care activities require the nurse to push, pull, lift, and carry. By using proper body mechanics, the nurse can avoid musculoskeletal injury and fatigue, and reduce the risk of injuring patients. Correct body mechanics can be summed up in three principles, as presented below.

Keep a low center of gravity by flexing the hips and knees instead of bending at the waist. This position distributes weight evenly between the upper and lower body and helps maintain balance.

Create a wide base of support by spreading the feet apart. This tactic provides lateral stability and lowers the body's center of gravity.

Maintain proper body alignment and keep the body's center of gravity directly over the base of support by moving the feet rather than twisting and bending at the waist.

Implementation

Follow the directions below to push, pull, stoop, lift, and carry correctly.

Pushing and pulling correctly

• Stand close to the object and place one foot slightly ahead of the other, as in a walking position. Tighten the leg muscles and set the pelvis by simultaneously contracting the abdominal and gluteal muscles.
• To push, place your hands on the object and flex your elbows. Lean into the object by shifting weight from the back leg to the front leg, and apply smooth, continuous pressure.
• To pull, grasp the object and flex your elbows. Lean away from the object by shifting weight from the front leg to the back leg. Pull smoothly, avoiding sudden, jerky movements.
• After you've started to move the object, keep it in motion; *stopping and starting uses more energy.*

Stooping correctly

• Stand with your feet 10″ to 12″ (25 to 30 cm) apart and one foot slightly ahead of the other *to widen the base of support.*
• Lower yourself by flexing your knees, and place more weight on the front foot than on the back foot. Keep the upper body straight by not bending at the waist.

• To stand up again, straighten the knees and keep the back straight.

Lifting and carrying correctly
• Assume the stooping position directly in front of the object *to minimize back flexion and avoid spinal rotation when lifting.*
• Grasp the object, and tighten your abdominal muscles.
• Stand up by straightening the knees, using the leg and hip muscles. Always keep your back straight *to maintain a fixed center of gravity.*
• Carry the object close to your body at waist height — near the body's center of gravity — *to avoid straining the back muscles.*

Special considerations
Wear shoes with low heels, flexible nonslip soles, and closed backs *to promote correct body alignment, facilitate proper body mechanics, and prevent accidents.* When possible, pull rather than push an object *because the elbow flexors are stronger than the extensors.* When doing heavy lifting or moving, remember to use assistive or mechanical devices, if available, or obtain assistance from co-workers; know your limitations and use sound judgment.

 Patient transfer from bed to stretcher

Transfer from bed to stretcher, one of the most common transfers, can require the help of one or more co-workers, depending on the patient's size and condition and the primary nurse's physical abilities. Techniques for achieving this transfer include the straight lift, carry lift, lift sheet, and roller board.

In the straight (or patient-assisted) lift — used to move the pediatric or very light patient, or the patient who can assist transfer — the members of the transfer team place their hands and arms beneath the patient's buttocks and, if necessary, his shoulders. Other patients may require a four-person straight lift, detailed below. In the carry lift, team members roll the patient onto their upper arms and hold him against their chests. In the lift sheet transfer, they place a sheet under the patient and lift or slide him onto the stretcher. In the roller board transfer, two team members slide the patient onto the stretcher.

Equipment
Stretcher ▪ roller board or lift sheet if necessary.

Preparation of equipment
Adjust the bed to the same height as the stretcher.

Implementation
• Tell the patient that you're going to move him from the bed to the stretcher and place him in the supine position.
• Ask team members to remove their rings and watches *to avoid scratching the patient during transfer.*

Four-person straight lift
• Place the stretcher parallel to the bed, and lock the wheels of both *to ensure the patient's safety.*
• Stand at the center of the stretcher, and have another team member stand at the patient's head. The two other team members should stand next to the bed, on the other side — one at the center and the other at the patient's feet.
• Slide your arms, palms up, beneath the patient, while the other team members do the same. In this position, you and the team member directly opposite support the patient's buttocks and hips; the team member at the head of the bed supports the patient's head and shoulders; the one at the foot supports the patient's legs and feet.
• On a count of three, the team members lift the patient several inches, move him onto the stretcher, and slide their arms out from under him. Keep movements smooth *to minimize patient discomfort and avoid muscle strain by team members.*

Four-person carry lift
• Place the stretcher perpendicular to the bed, with the head of the stretcher at the foot of the bed. Lock the bed and stretcher wheels *to ensure the patient's safety.*
• Raise the bed to a comfortable working height.
• Line up all four team members on the same side of the bed as the stretcher, with the tallest member at the patient's head and the shortest at his feet. The member at the patient's head is the leader of the team and gives the lift signals.
• Tell the team members to flex their knees and slide their hands, palms up, under the patient until he rests securely on their upper arms. Make sure the patient is adequately supported at the head and shoulders, buttocks and hips, and legs and feet.
• On a count of three, the team members straighten their knees and roll the patient onto his side, against their chests. *This reduces strain on the lifters* and allows them to hold the patient for several minutes if necessary.
• Together the team members step back, with the member supporting the feet moving the farthest, to bring the patient's legs around to the foot of the stretcher. On a count of three, the team members lower the patient onto

the stretcher by bending at the knees and sliding their arms out from under the patient.

Four-person lift sheet transfer

• Position the bed, stretcher, and team members for the straight lift. Then instruct the team to hold the edges of the sheet under the patient, grasping them close to the patient *to obtain a firm grip, provide stability, and spare the patient undue feelings of instability.*
• On a count of three, the team members lift or slide the patient onto the stretcher in a smooth, continuous motion *to avoid muscle strain and minimize patient discomfort.*

Roller board transfer

• Place the stretcher parallel to the bed, and lock the wheels of both *to ensure the patient's safety.*
• Stand next to the bed, and instruct a co-worker to stand next to the stretcher.
• Reach over the patient and pull the far side of the bedsheet toward you to turn the patient slightly on his side. Your co-worker then places the roller board beneath the patient, making sure the board bridges the gap between stretcher and bed.
• Ease the patient onto the roller board and release the sheet. Your co-worker then grasps the near side of the sheet at the patient's hips and shoulders and pulls him onto the stretcher in a smooth, continuous motion. She then reaches over the patient, grasps the far side of the sheet, and logrolls him toward her.
• Remove the roller board as your co-worker returns the patient to the supine position.

After all transfers

• Position the patient comfortably on the stretcher, apply safety straps, and raise and secure the side rails.

Special considerations

When transferring a helpless or markedly obese patient from bed to stretcher, first lift and move the patient, in increments, to the edge of the bed. Then rest for a few seconds, repositioning the patient if necessary, and lift him onto the stretcher. If the patient can bear weight on his arms or legs, two or three co-workers can perform this transfer: One co-worker can support the buttocks and guide the patient, another can stabilize the stretcher by leaning over it and guiding the patient into position, and a third can transfer any attached equipment. If a team member isn't available to guide equipment, move I.V. lines and other tubing first *to make sure they're out of the way and not in danger of pulling loose,* or disconnect tubes if possible. If the patient is light, three co-workers can perform the carry lift; however, no matter how many team members are present, one must stabilize the head

if the patient can't support it himself, has cervical instability or injury, or has undergone surgery.

Depending on the patient's size and condition, lift sheet transfer can require two to seven co-workers.

Documentation

Record the time and, if necessary, the type of transfer in your notes. Complete other required forms, as necessary.

Patient transfer from bed to wheelchair

For the patient with diminished or absent lower-body sensation or one-sided weakness, immobility, or injury, transfer from bed to wheelchair may require partial support to full assistance — initially by at least two persons. Subsequent transfer of the patient with generalized weakness may be performed by one nurse. After transfer, proper positioning helps prevent excessive pressure on bony prominences, which predisposes the patient to skin breakdown.

Equipment

Wheelchair with locks (or sturdy chair) ■ pajama bottoms (or robe) ■ shoes or slippers with nonslip soles ■ optional: transfer board if appropriate. (See *Teaching the patient to use a transfer board.)*

Implementation

• Explain the procedure to the patient and demonstrate his role.
• Place the wheelchair parallel to the bed, facing the foot of the bed, and lock its wheels. Make sure the bed wheels are also locked. Raise the footrests *to avoid interfering with the transfer.*
• Check pulse rate and blood pressure with the patient supine *to obtain a baseline.* Then help him put on the pajama bottoms and slippers or shoes with nonslip soles *to prevent falls.*
• Raise the head of the bed and allow the patient to rest briefly *to adjust to posture changes.* Then, bring him to the dangling position (see "Progressive ambulation" in this chapter). Recheck pulse rate and blood pressure if you suspect cardiovascular instability. Don't proceed until the patient's pulse rate and blood pressure are stabilized *to prevent falls.*
• Tell the patient to move toward the edge of the bed and, if possible, to place his feet flat on the floor. Stand

Teaching the patient to use a transfer board

For the patient who can't stand, a transfer board allows safe transfer from bed to wheelchair. To perform this transfer, take the following steps.

• First explain and demonstrate the procedure. Eventually, the patient may become proficient enough to transfer himself independently or with some supervision.

• Help the patient put on pajama bottoms or a robe, and shoes or slippers.

• Place the wheelchair parallel to and facing the foot of the bed. Lock the wheels, and remove the armrest closest to the patient. Make sure the bed is flat, and adjust its height so that it's level with the wheelchair seat.

• Assist the patient to a sitting position on the edge of the bed, with his feet resting on the floor. Make sure the front edge of the wheelchair seat is aligned with the back of the patient's knees as shown in the illustration below. *Although it's important that the patient have an even surface on which to transfer, he may find it easier to transfer to a slightly lower surface.*

• Ask the patient to lean away from the wheelchair while you slide one end of the transfer board under him.

• Now place the other end of the transfer board on the wheelchair seat, and help the patient return to the upright position.

• Stand in front of the patient *to prevent him from sliding forward.* Tell him to push down with both arms, lifting the buttocks up and onto the transfer board. The patient then repeats this maneuver, edging along the board, until he's seated in the wheelchair. If the patient can't use his arms to assist with the transfer, stand in front of him, put your arms around him, and—if he's able—have him put his arms around you. Gradually slide him across the board until he's safely in the chair as shown below.

• Once the patient is in the chair, fasten a seat belt, if necessary, *to prevent falls.*

• Then remove the transfer board, replace the wheelchair armrest, and reposition the patient in the chair.

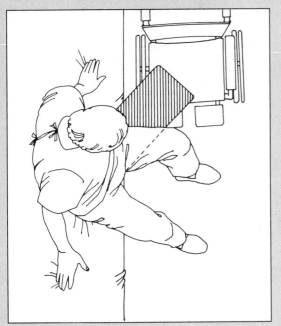

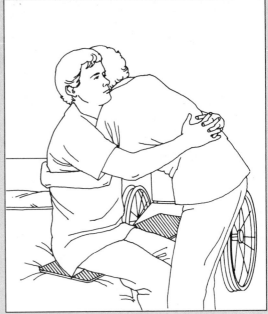

in front of the patient, blocking his toes with your feet and his knees with yours *to prevent his knees from buckling.*

• Flex your knees slightly, place your arms around the patient's waist, and tell him to place his hands on the edge of the bed. Avoid bending at your waist *to prevent back strain.*

• Ask the patient to push himself off the bed and to support as much of his own weight as possible. At the same time, straighten your knees and hips, raising the patient as you straighten your body.

• Supporting the patient as needed, pivot toward the wheelchair, keeping your knees next to his. Tell the patient to grasp the farthest armrest of the wheelchair with his closest hand.

• Help the patient lower himself into the wheelchair by flexing your hips and knees, but not your back. Instruct him to reach back and grasp the other wheelchair armrest as he sits *to avoid abrupt contact with the seat.* Fasten the seat belt *to prevent falls* and, if necessary, check pulse rate and blood pressure *to assess cardiovascular stability.* If the pulse rate is 20 beats or more above baseline, stay with the patient and monitor him closely until it returns to normal *because he is experiencing orthostatic hypotension.*

• If the patient can't position himself correctly, help him move his buttocks against the back of the chair *so the ischial tuberosities, not the sacrum, provide the base of support.*

• Place the patient's feet flat on the footrests, pointed straight ahead. Then position the knees and hips with the correct amount of flexion and in appropriate alignment. If appropriate, use elevating leg rests to flex the patient's hips at more than 90 degrees; *this position relieves pressure on the popliteal space and places more weight on the ischial tuberosities.*

• Position the patient's arms on the wheelchair's armrests with shoulders abducted, elbows slightly flexed, forearms pronated, and wrists and hands in the neutral position. If necessary, support or elevate the patient's hands and forearms with a pillow *to prevent dependent edema.*

Special considerations

If the patient starts to fall during transfer, ease him to the closest surface — bed, floor, or chair. Never stretch to finish the transfer. Doing so can cause loss of balance, falls, muscle strain, and other injuries — to you and the patient.

If the patient has one-sided weakness, follow the preceding steps, but place the wheelchair on the patient's unaffected side. Instruct the patient to pivot and bear as much weight as possible on the unaffected side. Support the affected side *because the patient will tend to lean*

to this side. Use pillows to support the hemiplegic patient's affected side *to prevent slumping in the wheelchair.*

Documentation

If necessary, record the time of transfer and the extent of assistance in your notes, and note how the patient tolerated the activity.

Patient transfer with a hydraulic lift

Using a hydraulic lift to raise the immobile patient from the supine to the sitting position allows safe, comfortable transfer between bed and chair. It's indicated for the obese or immobile patient for whom manual transfer poses the potential for nurse or patient injury. Although most hydraulic lift models can be operated by one person, it's better to have two staff members present during transfer to stabilize and support the patient.

Equipment

Hydraulic lift, with sling, chains or straps, and hooks ■ chair or wheelchair.

Preparation of equipment

Because hydraulic lift models may vary in weight capacity, check the manufacturer's specifications before attempting patient transfer. Make sure the bed and wheelchair wheels are locked before beginning the transfer.

Implementation

• Explain the procedure to the patient, and reassure him that the hydraulic lift can safely support his weight and won't tip over.

• Make sure the side rail opposite you is raised and secure. Then roll the patient toward you, onto his side, and raise the side rail. Walk to the opposite side of the bed and lower the side rail.

• Place the sling under the patient's buttocks with its lower edge below the greater trochanter. Then fanfold the far side of the sling against the back and buttocks.

• Roll the patient toward you onto the sling, and raise the side rail. Then lower the opposite side rail.

• Slide your hands under the patient and pull the sling from beneath him, smoothing out all wrinkles. Then roll the patient onto his back and center him on the sling.

• Place the appropriate chair next to the head of the bed, facing the foot.

• Lower the side rail next to the chair, and raise the bed only until the base of the lift can extend under the bed.

Using a hydraulic lift

After placing the patient supine in the center of the sling, position the hydraulic lift above him, as shown here. Then attach the chains to the hooks on the sling.

Turn the lift handle clockwise to raise the patient to the sitting position. If he's positioned properly, continue to raise him until he's suspended just above the bed.

After positioning the patient above the wheelchair, turn the lift handle counterclockwise to lower him onto the seat. When the chains become slack, stop turning and unhook the sling from the lift.

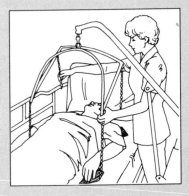
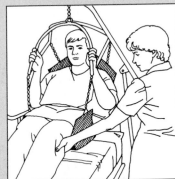
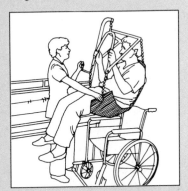

To avoid alarming and endangering the patient, don't raise the bed completely.

• Set the lift's adjustable base to its widest position *to ensure the highest level of stability.* Then move the lift so that its arm lies perpendicular to the bed, directly over the patient.

• Connect one end of the chains (or straps) to the side arms on the lift; connect the other, hooked end to the sling. Face the hooks away from the patient *to prevent them from slipping and to avoid the risk of their pointed edges injuring the patient.* The patient may place his arms inside or outside the chains (or straps) or he may grasp them once the slack is gone (to avoid injury). (See *Using a hydraulic lift.*)

• Tighten the turnscrew on the lift. Then, depending on the type of lift you're using, pump the handle or turn it clockwise until the patient has assumed a sitting position and his buttocks clear the bed surface by 1″ or 2″ (2.5 or 5 cm). Momentarily suspend the patient above the bed *until he feels secure in the lift and sees that it can bear his weight.*

• Steady the patient as you move the lift or, preferably, have another co-worker guide the patient's body while you move the lift. Depending on the type of lift you're using, the arm should now rest in front or to one side of the chair.

• Release the turnscrew. Then depress the handle or turn it counterclockwise *to lower the patient into the chair.* While lowering the patient, push gently on his knees *to maintain the correct sitting posture.* After lowering the patient into the chair, fasten the seat belt *to ensure his safety.*

• Remove the hooks or straps from the sling, but leave the sling in place under the patient so you'll be able to transfer him back to the bed from the chair. Then move the lift away from the patient.

• To return the patient to bed, reverse the procedure.

Special considerations

If the patient has an altered center of gravity (caused by a halo vest or a lower-extremity cast, for example), obtain help from a co-worker before transferring him with a hydraulic lift.

If the patient will require use of a hydraulic lift for transfers after discharge, teach his family how to use this device correctly and allow them to practice with supervision.

Documentation

If necessary, record the time of transfer in your notes.

Operating a Stryker wedge frame

First, obtain the help of a co-worker. Then remove the armboards from the frame. Arrange the anterior frame over the patient and lock it at the head end. Replace the anterior half of the ring, if removed, and close it over the patient until it locks automatically.

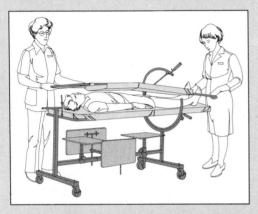

Then place the patient's arms around the anterior frame if he is able to grasp it. Otherwise, use safety straps to keep his arms in place. Pull out the locking pin, release the lock and, with a co-worker's help, turn the patient. Always turn the patient in the direction of the narrow wedge to minimize his risk of falling.

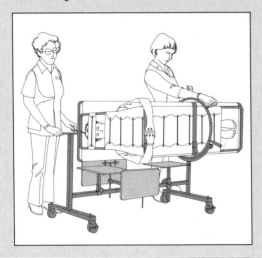

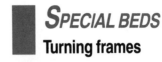

SPECIAL BEDS
Turning frames

When a patient must remain immobile, such as after spinal injury or surgery, use of a turning frame allows repeated changes between the supine and prone positions without disturbing spinal alignment. The turning frame includes an anterior section and a posterior section, with the patient secured between them. The anterior and posterior sections pivot as one unit; the patient lies on the anterior frame in the prone position and on the posterior frame in the supine position.

One type of turning frame, the Stryker frame, accommodates cervical traction. (See *Operating a Stryker wedge frame.)* Another type, made by the Orthopedic Equipment Company, accommodates cervical and pelvic traction.

Operating either frame requires training and experience for at least one member of the turning team. Use of these frames may be contraindicated in obese patients.

Equipment
Turning frames with safety straps ■ armboards ■ special sheets (with ties) for each frame ■ fresh linens ■ pillow or sheepskin ■ hand rolls or cradle boots ■ footboard.

Preparation of equipment
Place sheets on the anterior and posterior frames. Tie the sheet corners to the frame, and secure the remainder of each sheet to the nearest fastener. Make sure the posterior frame's perineal opening is in the correct position. Secure the posterior frame to the bed and lock it in place. Then, turn the bed *to check that it's working properly.* Next, lock its wheels.

Implementation
• Obtain assistance from several co-workers for the initial transfer of the patient to the frame.
• Explain the use of the turning frame to the patient. Tell him that he may feel confined when the frames are in place, and that he may experience a floating sensation during turning. Reassure him that the frames will hold him securely and that the top frame will be removed after he is turned.
• Check to see that the posterior frame is locked into position.
• Transfer the patient in the supine position to the posterior frame, taking care to maintain spinal alignment. Attach and adjust the armboards *for comfort and support.* Make sure the patient's hands are in a functional position *to prevent deformity.*

• Support the patient's feet in the correct position with a footboard *to prevent footdrop.*
• Make sure all tubes are positioned properly *to maintain their function.*
• Retain the help of one or more co-workers before you turn the patient.
• To turn the patient from supine to prone, remove the top sheet, if present. Then, place a pillow or sheepskin lengthwise over the patient's legs, chest, or other areas *to promote comfort and act as a pad during turning.*
• Detach the armboards and store them on the shelf under the bed.
• Carefully remove the nuts at both ends of the posterior frame, and position the anterior frame so its face support fits over the patient's face and its upper portion extends from the shoulders to the symphysis pubis, with the 4″ (10 cm) opening over the perineum. Make sure the lower portion of the frame extends to the ankles, allowing the feet to extend over the end of the frame in the prone position. Check that the patient is in proper alignment.
• After adjusting the anterior frame, securely lock it in place at both ends.
• Place the patient's arms at his sides or, if possible, have him put them around and grasp the anterior frame *for a sense of security during turning.*
• Place two or three safety straps around the turning frames *to promote the patient's safety and prevent his arms and legs from slipping during turning.* If necessary, reposition the I.V., indwelling urinary catheter, or chest tubing appropriately *to prevent dislodgement or entanglement during turning.*
• In wedge-shaped frames, always turn the patient in the direction of the narrow wedge *to minimize the risk of falling.* Tell the patient which direction he'll be turning.
• With one co-worker positioned at each end of the bed, simultaneously remove the locking pins and release the bed turning locks. Then, on the count of three, turn the patient quickly and smoothly, maintaining cervical traction. If extra co-workers are present, ask them to stand beside the frame during the turn *to reassure the patient, who may be anxious and afraid of falling.*
• Close both locks and replace the pins before releasing your grip on the frame. Then remove the safety straps and the posterior frame.
• Position the patient properly. Make sure all tubing and equipment are properly positioned and adjusted.
• Replace and adjust the armboards and change the linens if necessary.
• Assess the patient's level of consciousness, mobility, and sensation. Assess the skin for redness or pressure areas, and provide skin care or other prescribed treatments.

• Evaluate the patient's tolerance for the prone and supine positions.
• Follow the same procedure to return the patient to the supine position.

Special considerations
Turn the patient at least every 2 hours. Between turnings, perform appropriate range-of-motion exercises, as ordered. If the patient finds the prone position uncomfortable, administer prescribed pain medication before turning. If he has skull tongs in place, turn him cautiously *to avoid dislodging them.* If he's connected to a mechanical ventilator, disconnect the device immediately before turning and reconnect it immediately afterward. Hand rolls and cradle boots can be used during turning *to help keep the patient's hands and feet comfortable.*

Remove the perineal section of the frame for bedpan use, but always replace it immediately afterward *to prevent spinal misalignment from inadequate support of the patient's buttocks in the supine position.* Provide appropriate diversion and encourage the patient's family and friends to do so *to counteract boredom.* Adjust the reading board for meals and reading, and provide adequate light *to prevent eyestrain.*

Documentation
Record the time of turning, the patient's reaction during turning, any treatments administered, and your observations concerning the patient's skin condition and overall status.

 ## CircOlectric bed

This bed permits frequent turning of the severely injured or immobilized patient with minimal trauma or extraneous movement. Its multiple intermediate positions help prevent and treat pressure ulcers and respiratory and circulatory complications. The bed's narrow mattress permits close proximity between patient and nurse, allowing better body mechanics and preventing back strain. Because this bed is portable, it eliminates potentially traumatic patient transfer. Safe operation requires at least two persons. (See *Using the CircOlectric bed,* page 68.)

Equipment
CircOlectric bed ▪ fitted sheets ▪ sheepskin ▪ bedpan.

Preparation of equipment
In some hospitals with low doorways, you may need to remove the upper half of the frame to get the bed into

Using the CircOlectric bed

This type of bed allows you to rotate the patient 180 degrees to a prone or supine position. It is fitted with safety stops that prevent it from being rotated more than 210 degrees. During operation, one nurse reassures the patient and ensures his safety while the other turns the bed.

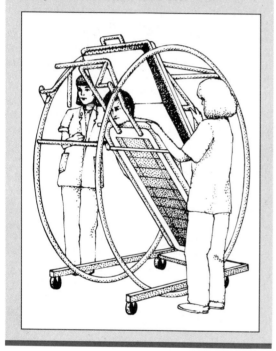

an elevator or the patient's room. To do so, simply remove the connecting bolts; after the bed is in the patient's room, reassemble the frame.

Place a specially fitted sheet over the turning frame and the bottom mattress *to ensure the patient's comfort and help prevent pressure ulcers.* If necessary, secure a bedpan below the perineal opening of the bottom mattress.

Before placing the patient in the bed, examine its electrical cord and plug for defects, and place the cord where it won't be caught or severed during turning. Then plug the cord into an electrical outlet and check the bed's mechanical function. Lock the bed's wheels before transferring the patient.

Implementation

• *Because the size and appearance of the CircOlectric bed may initially alarm the patient,* describe the bed's advantages and the turning procedure to the patient beforehand. Reassure him that the bed will hold him securely.
• After obtaining assistance from co-workers, transfer the patient to the bed, taking care to position him correctly over the perineal opening.
• Position the bed's footboard against his feet *to help prevent footdrop and promote body alignment.* To secure the footboard, press the buttons and slide the unit toward his feet until it reaches the desired position. When turning the frame, press the buttons and slide the footboard toward the end of the bed.
• Place sheepskin under the patient's heels *to help prevent pressure ulcers.* If necessary, place supports under the patient's lower legs *to raise his heels off the bed.*
• Install the canvas-covered side rails *to ensure the patient's safety and promote a sense of security.* Loosen the stabilizing bolts in the square holders on either side of the bed. Then select the correct counterpiece on the side rail: The straight counterpiece keeps the side rail upright for protection at night and during supine positioning, while the 90-degree angle counterpiece keeps it level for prone positioning and for use as an armrest. After each side rail is in position, tighten its stabilizing bolt.

Turning to the prone position

• Before turning the patient, straighten the bed and its wheels as needed *to prevent unwanted movement.* Then release the footboard and move it away from the patient's feet. Leave enough room for placement of a footboard on the turning frame.
• If the patient is in traction, secure the traction guide equipment to the mobile portion of the frame. Because the weights will hang freely on the side of the circular frame, they won't be affected by turning.
• With the assistance of a co-worker, lift the turning frame over the patient. Remove the nuts on the bolts at both ends of the mattress. Slip the holes in the turning frame over the bolts and replace the nuts, turning them as tightly as possible. If you can't secure the nuts tightly by hand, place a turning key in the small holes of the nuts and then tighten them.
• Pad and position the footboard on the turning frame. Depress the buttons to adjust it properly. Be sure the footboard rests securely against the patient's feet *because it will bear his weight when he's upright.*
• Apply the head restraint *to support and immobilize the head during the turning and prone positioning.* Make sure the restraint is sufficiently padded *to help prevent facial pressure ulcers. Check for pressure areas to determine the best position for the head support because some beds have*

slings instead of metal bars. Secure the headrest by adjusting the clamps.
• Tuck in the sheets at the head of the mattress *so they don't rub against the patient's neck, causing ulcerations or occluding a tracheostomy.* Tell the patient to cross his hands over his chest or to grasp the sides of the turning frame *to protect his hands.* If the patient is paralyzed, place his arms at the sides and fasten the safety straps around the turning and posterior frames. *This promotes the patient's safety and keeps his arms at his sides and between the frames during turning.*
• Remove the bedpan if it's in place. Free I.V. lines, traction weights, any indwelling catheter drainage bag, or other attachments, and reposition them *to prevent dislodgement, entanglement, or complications during turning.*
• Unclamp the control switch from the bed frame. Hold it so you can operate the switch with your thumb. While a co-worker watches and reassures the patient, turn the bed using steady, continuous pressure on the control switch *to minimize the patient's nausea and vertigo.* Safety latches prevent the bed from turning too far in either direction.
• After the patient is positioned correctly, release the nut from the front of the main mattress. Free the mattress frame from the bolt and replace the nut. Pull forward on the release bar at the top of the frame. A series of springs raises the mattress up and off the patient's back, and a catch in the frame locks the mattress in the raised position. While the patient is prone, provide back care and change the sheets on the main mattress. If the patient's feet are lower than his head, check his feet and ankles for dependent edema.

Returning to the supine position
• Release the catch by pulling the release bar forward. Pull the mattress into place and bolt it.
• Remove the armrests and bedpan. Correctly position I.V. lines, traction weights, any indwelling catheter drainage bag, and other tubing or attachments before turning. Hold the control switch in the reverse position until the bed is level.
• When the bed is in position, release the nuts, remove the turning frame, and replace the nuts. Position the patient comfortably and adjust the footboard appropriately.
• If the patient is at a stage of rehabilitation requiring periodic standing, flip the safety latch forward *to stop the bed in the upright position.* Be sure to release the latch before returning the patient to horizontal.
• If the patient needs to sit up periodically, push forward on the lever at the side of the mattress. Apply safety belts, if necessary. To return the patient to the supine position, pull back on the lever.

Special considerations
Provide extra skin care and padding for the feet, occiput, chin, and forehead *because these areas endure added pressure.* If the patient has a tracheostomy and is connected to a mechanical ventilator, use a hand-held resuscitation bag, such as an Ambu bag, during turning. If the patient is receiving oxygen, temporarily disconnect it during turning.

The patient may experience nausea, vertigo, fear of falling, or spatial disorientation during turning. *To minimize nausea and vertigo,* be sure to complete the turn slowly and without interruption. *To minimize spatial disorientation,* place an overbed table within the patient's field of vision.

Watch carefully for signs of cardiac arrest, particularly during the patient's first few turnings. If the patient has neurologic damage, a doctor should be present the first few times.

After turning and positioning are completed, provide prism glasses or attach a mirror to the upper part of the bed *to increase the patient's field of vision.*

If the electricity fails, you can turn the bed with the hand crank stored in the tray at the head of the bed. Keep the end stud nuts on the appropriate frame bar when not in use *to avoid misplacing them.*

Complications
Pressure ulcers may form on the feet, occiput, chin, and forehead after a prolonged period, and on the heels of a patient with diminished sensation in his legs.

Documentation
Record the date and time the patient was transferred to the bed, the frequency of turning, and the patient's response to the maneuver.

Rotation beds

Because of their constant motion, rotation beds—such as the Roto Rest—promote postural drainage and peristalsis and help prevent the complications of immobility, including pressure ulcers, deep vein thrombi, orthostatic hypotension, bone demineralization, and formation of renal calculi. The bed rotates from side to side in a cradlelike motion, achieving a maximum elevation of 62 degrees and full side-to-side turning approximately every 4½ minutes.

Because the bed holds the patient motionless, it's especially helpful for patients with spinal cord injury, multiple trauma, cerebrovascular accident, multiple scle-

Understanding the Roto Rest bed

Driven by a silent motor, this bed turns the immobilized patient slowly and continuously, more than 300 times daily. The motion provides constant passive exercise and peristaltic stimulation without depriving the patient of sleep or risking further injury. The bed is radiolucent, permitting X-rays to be taken through it without moving the patient. It also has a built-in cooling fan, and allows access for surgery on multiple-trauma patients without disrupting spinal alignment or traction.

The bed's hatches give access to various parts of the patient's body. Arm hatches permit full range of motion and have holes for chest tubes. Leg hatches allow full hip extension. The perineal hatch provides access for bowel and bladder care, the thoracic hatch for chest auscultation and lumbar puncture, and the cervical hatch for wound care, bathing, and shampooing.

Top view

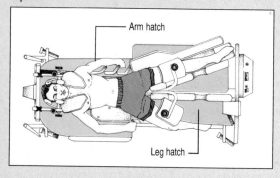

Back view

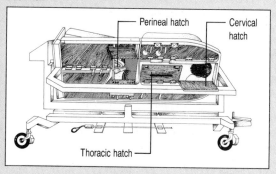

rosis, coma, severe burns, hypostatic pneumonia, atelectasis, or other unilateral lung involvement causing poor ventilation and perfusion.

Rotation beds can accommodate cervical traction devices and tongs. One type of Roto Rest bed has an access hatch underneath for the perineal area; another type has access hatches for the perineal, cervical, and thoracic areas. Both have arm and leg hatches that fold down to allow range-of-motion exercises. Other features include variable angles of rotation, a fan, access for X-rays, and supports and clips for chest tubes, catheters, and drains. Racks beneath the bed hold X-ray plates in place for chest and spinal films. (See *Understanding the Roto Rest bed.*)

Rotation beds are contraindicated for the patient who has severe claustrophobia or who has an unstable cervical fracture without neurologic deficit and the complications of immobility. Patient transfer and positioning on the bed should be performed by at least two persons to ensure his safety.

The instructions given below apply to the Roto Rest bed.

Equipment
Rotation bed with appropriate accessories ▪ pillowcases or linen-saver pads ▪ flat sheet or padding.

Preparation of equipment
When using the Roto Rest bed, carefully inspect the bed and run it through a complete cycle in both automatic and manual modes *to ensure that it's working properly.* If you're using the Mark I model, check the tightness of the set screws at the head of the bed.

To prepare the bed for the patient, remove the counterbalance weights from the keel and place them in the base frame's storage area. Release the connecting arm by pulling down on the cam handle and depressing the lower side of the footboard. Next, lock the table in the horizontal position, and place all side supports in the extreme lateral position by loosening the cam handles on the underside of the table. Slide the supports off the bed. Note that all supports and packs are labeled *right* or *left* on the bottom *to facilitate reassembly.*

Remove the knee packs by depressing the snap button and rotating and pulling the packs from the tube. Then remove the abductor packs (the Mark III model has only one) by depressing and sliding them toward the head of the bed. Next, loosen the foot and knee assemblies by lifting the cam handle at its base, and slide them to the foot of the bed. Finally, loosen the shoulder clamp assembly and knobs, swing the shoulder clamps to the vertical position, and retighten them.

If you're using the Mark I model, remove the cervical, thoracic, and perineal packs. Cover them with pillowcases or linen-saver pads, smooth all wrinkles, and replace the packs. If you're using the Mark III model, remove the perineal pack, cover, and replace. Cover the upper half of the bed, which is a solid unit, with padding or a sheet. Install new disposable foam cushions for the patient's head, shoulders, and feet.

Implementation

• If possible, show the patient the bed before use. Explain and demonstrate its operation and reassure the patient that the bed will hold him securely.
• Before positioning the patient on the bed, make sure it's turned off. Then, place and lock the bed in horizontal position, out of gear. Latch all hatches and lock the wheels.
• Obtain assistance and transfer the patient. Move him gently to the center of the bed *to prevent contact with the pillar posts and to ensure proper balance during bed operation.* Smooth the pillowcase or linen-saver pad beneath his hips. Then, place any tubes through the appropriate notches in the hatches and ensure that any traction weights hang freely.
• Insert the thoracic side supports in their posts. Adjust the patient's longitudinal position to allow a 1" (2.5 cm) space between the axillae and the supports, *thereby avoiding pressure on the axillary blood vessels and the brachial plexus.* Push the supports against his chest and lock the cam arms securely *to provide support and ensure patient safety.*
• Place the disposable supports under his legs *to remove pressure from his heels and prevent pressure ulcers.*
• Install and adjust the foot supports so his feet lie in the normal anatomic position, *thereby helping to prevent footdrop.* The foot supports should be in position for only 2 hours of every shift *to prevent excessive pressure on the soles and toes.*
• Place the abductor packs in the appropriate supports, allowing a 6" (15 cm) space between the packs and the

patient's groin. Tighten the knobs on the bed's underside at the base of the support tubes.
• Install the leg side supports snugly against the patient's hips, and tighten the cam arms. Position the knee assemblies slightly above his knees and tighten the cam arms. Then place your hand on the patient's knee and move the knee pack until it rests lightly on the top of your hand. Repeat for the other knee.
• Loosen the retaining rings on the crossbar, and slide the head and shoulder assembly laterally. *The retaining rings maintain correct lateral position of the shoulder clamp assembly and head support pack.*
• Carefully lower the head and shoulder assembly into place and slide it to touch the patient's head.
• Place your hand on the patient's shoulder, and move the shoulder pack until it touches your hand. Tighten it in place. Repeat for the other shoulder. *The 1" clearance between the shoulders and the packs prevents excess pressure, which can lead to pressure ulcers.*
• Place the head pack close to, but not touching, the patient's ears (or tongs).
• Tighten the head and shoulder assembly securely *so it won't lift off the bed.* Position the restraining rings next to the shoulder assembly bracket and tighten them.
• Place the patient's arms on the disposable supports. Install the side arm supports and secure the safety straps, placing one across the shoulder assembly and the other over the thoracic supports. If necessary, cover the patient with a flat sheet.

Balancing the bed

• Place one hand on the footboard *to prevent the bed from turning rapidly if it's unbalanced.* Then remove the locking pin. If the bed rotates to one side, reposition the patient in its center; if it tilts to the right, gently turn it slightly to the left and slide the packs on the right side toward the patient; if it tilts to the left, reverse the process. If a large imbalance exists, you may have to adjust the packs on both sides.
• After the patient is centered, gently turn the bed to the 62-degree position.
• Measure the space between the patient's chest, hip, and thighs and the inside of the packs. If this space exceeds ½" (1.3 cm) for the Mark III model or 1" for the Mark I, return the bed to horizontal position, lock it in place, and slide the packs inward on both sides. If the space appears too tight, proceed as above but slide both packs outward. *Excessively loose packs cause the patient to slide from side to side during turning, possibly resulting in unnecessary movement at fracture sites, skin irritation from shearing force, and bed imbalance. Overly tight packs can place pressure on the patient during turning.*

• After adjusting the packs, check the bed; balance it and make any necessary adjustments.
• If you're using the Mark III model bed and the patient weighs more than 160 lb (72 kg), the bed may become top-heavy. To correct this, place counterbalance weights in the appropriate slots in the keel of the bed. Add one weight for every 20 lb (9 kg) over 160, but remember that placement of weights doesn't replace correct patient positioning.
• If you're using the Mark I model, it may be necessary to add weights for the patient weighing less than 160 lb. Place one weight for each 20 lb less than 160 in the proper bracket at the foot of the bed.

Initiating automatic bed rotation

• Ensure that all packs are securely in place. Then hold the footboard firmly and remove the locking pin *to start the bed's motor.* The bed will continue to rotate until the pin is reinserted.
• Raise the connecting arm cam handle until the connecting assembly snaps into place, locking the bed into automatic rotation.
• Remain with the patient for at least three complete turns from side to side *to evaluate his comfort and safety.* Observe his response and offer him emotional support.

Special considerations

If the patient develops cardiac arrest while on the bed, perform cardiopulmonary resuscitation after taking the bed out of gear, locking it in horizontal position, removing the side arm support and the thoracic pack, lifting the shoulder assembly, and dropping the arm pack. Doing all these steps takes only 5 to 10 seconds. *You won't need a cardiac board because of the bed's firm surface.*

If the electricity fails, lock the bed in horizontal or lateral position and rotate it manually every 30 minutes *to prevent pressure ulcers.* If cervical traction causes the patient to slide upward, place the bed in reverse Trendelenburg's position; if extremity traction causes the patient to migrate toward the foot of the bed, use Trendelenburg's position.

Lock the bed in the extreme lateral position for access to the back of the head, thorax, and buttocks through the appropriate hatches. Clean the mattress and nondisposable packs during patient care, and rinse them thoroughly *to remove all soap residue.* When replacing the packs and hatches, take care not to pinch the patient's skin between the packs. *This can cause pain and tissue necrosis.*

Expect increased drainage from any pressure ulcers for the first few days the patient is on the bed *because the motion helps debride necrotic tissue and improves local circulation.*

Perform or schedule daily range-of-motion exercises, as ordered, *because the bed allows full access to all extremities without disturbing spinal alignment.* Drop the arm hatch for shoulder rotation, remove the thoracic packs for shoulder abduction, and drop the leg hatch and remove leg and knee packs for hip rotation and full leg motion.

For female patients, tape an indwelling urinary catheter to the thigh before bringing it through the perineal hatch. For the male patient with spinal cord lesions, tape the catheter to the abdomen and then to the thigh *to facilitate gravity drainage.* Hang the drainage bag on the clips provided, and make sure it doesn't become caught between the bed frames during rotation.

If the patient has a tracheal or endotracheal tube and is on mechanical ventilation, attach the tube support bracket between the cervical pack and the arm packs. Tape the connecting T tubing to the support and run it beside the patient's head and off the center of the table *to help prevent reflux of condensation.* For a patient with pulmonary congestion or pneumonia, suction secretions more often during the first 12 to 24 hours on the bed *because the motion will increase drainage.* A vibrator is available for use under the thoracic hatch of the Mark I to help mobilize pulmonary secretions more quickly.

Documentation

Record changes in the patient's condition and his response to therapy in your progress notes. Note turning times and ongoing care on the flowchart.

 ## Clinitron therapy bed

Originally called the air-fluidized bed and designed for managing burns, the Clinitron therapy bed is now used for patients with various debilities. The bed is actually a large tub that supports the patient on a thick layer of silicone-coated microspheres of lime glass. A monofilament polyester filter sheet covers the microsphere-filled tub. Warmed air, propelled by a blower beneath the bed, passes through it. The resulting fluidlike surface reduces pressure on the skin sufficiently to avoid obstructing capillary blood flow, thereby helping to prevent pressure ulcers and to promote wound healing. The bed's air temperature can be adjusted to help control hypothermia and hyperthermia. (See *A look at the Clinitron therapy bed.*)

Small amounts of wound drainage can flow into the microspheres, eliminating the need for most dressings. In addition, use of this therapy permits harmless contact between the bed's surface and grafted sites, promoting comfort and healing. In addition, when the air pressure

A look at the Clinitron therapy bed

The Clinitron therapy bed is a large tub filled with microspheres that are suspended by air pressure and give the patient fluidlike support. The bed provides the advantages of flotation without the disadvantages of instability, patient positioning difficulties, and immobility.

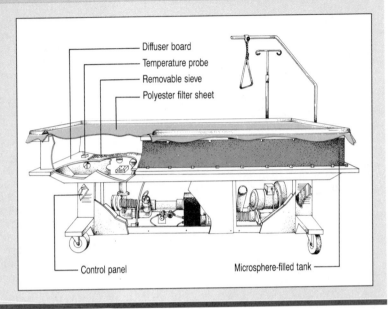

- Diffuser board
- Temperature probe
- Removable sieve
- Polyester filter sheet

Control panel

Microsphere-filled tank

---

is turned off, the bed forms a firm surface that molds to the shape of the patient's body, allowing the nurse to move the patient or change his position.

The Clinitron therapy bed may be contraindicated for the patient unable to mobilize and expel pulmonary secretions because the lack of back support impairs productive coughing. Patients who have skin problems may benefit from an air therapy bed instead of a Clinitron bed. (See *Air therapy beds*, page 74.) Because operation of the Clinitron therapy bed is complex, it requires special training.

Equipment

Clinitron therapy bed with microspheres (about 1,650 lb [750 kg]) ▪ filter sheet ▪ six aluminum rails (for restraining and sealing filter sheet) ▪ flat sheet ▪ elastic cord.

Preparation of equipment

Normally, a manufacturer's representative or a trained hospital staff member prepares the bed for use. If you must help with the preparation, be sure the microspheres reach to within ½″ (1.3 cm) of the top of the tank. Then position the filter sheet on the bed with its printed side facing up. Match the holes in the sheet to the holes in the edge of the bed's frame. Place the aluminum rails on

the frame, with the studs in the proper holes. Depress the rails firmly, and secure them by tightening the knurled knobs to seal the filter sheet. Place a flat hospital sheet over the filter sheet, and secure it with the elastic cord *to prevent billowing.* Turn on the air current *to activate the microspheres.* Then turn it off *to ensure that the bed's working properly.*

Implementation

- Explain and, if possible, demonstrate the operation of the Clinitron therapy bed for the patient. Tell him the reason for its use and that he'll feel as though he's floating on air. Then turn off the air pressure.
- With the help of three or more co-workers, transfer the patient to the bed using a lift sheet.
- Turn on the air pressure to activate the bed, and remove the lift sheet.
- Adjust the air temperature as necessary. Because the bed usually operates within 10° to 12° F (5.5° to 6.7° C) of ambient air temperature, set the room temperature to 75° F (24° C). If microsphere temperature reaches 105° F (41° C), the bed automatically shuts off. It restarts automatically after 30 minutes.

Air therapy beds

Patients who have or risk skin breakdown may benefit from an alternative to the Clinitron therapy bed: an air therapy bed without the microspheres. This type of bed has air-filled compartments that can be inflated to varying degrees, thus providing different levels of support to different body parts.

Optional in some air therapy beds is a pulsating or rotating motion that stimulates capillary blood flow, prevents venous stasis, increases peristalsis, and improves pulmonary hygiene. Because ordinary linen-saver pads block air flow, you'll need to use air-permeable pads that are available from the manufacturer.

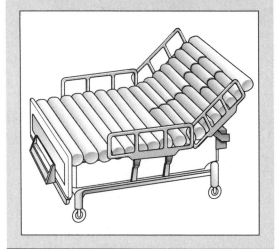

Special considerations

Monitor the patient's fluid and electrolyte status *because the warm, dry air circulated by the Clinitron therapy bed increases evaporative water loss, possibly requiring modifications in oral or I.V. fluid intake.* Because of this drying effect, always cover a mesh graft for the first 2 to 8 days, as ordered. If the patient experiences excessive dryness of the upper respiratory tract, use a humidifier and mask, as ordered. Encourage coughing and deep breathing *to help prevent pulmonary complications.* After prolonged use of a Clinitron therapy bed, watch for hypocalcemia and hypophosphoremia.

Any copiously draining wound should be covered with a porous dressing *to absorb some of the drainage.* Cover petroleum-jelly or silver-based topical applications with an impervious dressing *to minimize or prevent their ab-*

sorption by the microspheres. Avoid using wet dressings or soaks *because the excess fluid causes the microspheres to clump, impairing the fluid support effect.* The bed restarts automatically if shut off for 30 minutes, so unplug it to perform longer procedures.

To position a bedpan, roll the patient away from you, place the bedpan on the flat sheet, and push it into the microspheres. Then reposition the patient. To remove the bedpan, hold it steady and roll the patient away from you. Turn off the air pressure and remove the bedpan. Then turn the air on and reposition the patient.

Don't wear a watch when handling the microspheres *because they are small enough to penetrate the watch and damage the mechanism.* Don't secure the filter sheet with pins or clamps, *which may puncture the sheet and release microspheres.* Take care to avoid puncturing the bed when giving injections. Repair any holes or tears with iron-on patching tape. Sieve the microspheres monthly or between patients *to remove any clumped microspheres.* Handle them carefully to avoid spills, because they will make floors slippery and may cause falls. Treat a soiled filter sheet and clumped microspheres as contaminated items and handle according to hospital policy. Change the filter sheet and operate the unit unoccupied for 24 hours between patients.

Documentation

Record the duration of therapy and the patient's response to it. Document the condition of the patient's skin, pressure ulcers, and any other wounds.

PERSONAL HYGIENE AND COMFORT

Making an unoccupied bed

Although considered routine, daily changing and periodic straightening of bed linens promotes patient comfort and prevents skin breakdown. When preceded by thorough hand washing, performed using clean technique, and followed by proper handling and disposal of soiled linens, this procedure helps control nosocomial infections. In *open-bed technique,* performed during the ambulatory patient's hospitalization, bedmaking entails folding top linens to the foot of the bed to permit easy patient access. In *closed-bed technique,* performed after the patient's discharge, bedmaking entails keeping top linens unfolded and even with the top of the mattress until the next patient's admission.

Equipment

Two sheets (one fitted, if available) ▪ pillowcase ▪ bedspread ▪ gloves, if the patient has open lesions or has been incontinent ▪ optional: bath blanket, laundry bag, linen-saver pads, drawsheet.

Preparation of equipment

Obtain clean linen, which should be folded in half lengthwise and then folded again, creating a center crease that makes it easier to position the sheet on the bed. If the linen is folded incorrectly, refold it before attempting to make the bed. The bottom sheet should be folded so the rough side of the hem is facedown when placed on the bed; *this helps prevent skin irritation caused by the rough hem edge rubbing against the patient's heels.* The top sheet should be folded similarly, so the smooth side of the hem is faceup when folded over the spread, *giving the bed a finished appearance.*

Implementation

• Wash your hands thoroughly, don gloves if the patient has lesions or has been incontinent, and bring clean linen to the patient's bedside. If the patient is present, tell him that you're going to change his bed. Help him to a chair if necessary.

• Move any furniture away from the bed *to provide ample working space.*

• Lower the head of the bed *to make the mattress level and ensure tight-fitting, wrinkle-free linens.* Then, raise the bed to a comfortable working height *to prevent back strain.*

• When stripping the bed, watch for the patient's eyeglasses, dentures, or other belongings that may have fallen among the linens.

• Remove the pillowcase and place it in the laundry bag, or use the pillowcase, hooked over the back of a chair, as a laundry bag. Set the pillow aside.

• Lift the mattress edge slightly and work around the bed, untucking the linens. If you plan to reuse the top linens, fold the top hem of the spread down to the bottom hem. Then pick up the hemmed corners, fold the spread into quarters, and hang it over the back of the chair. Do the same for the top sheet. Otherwise, carefully remove and place the top linens in the laundry bag or pillowcase. *To avoid spreading microorganisms,* don't fan the linen, hold it against your clothing, or place it on the floor.

• Remove the soiled bottom linens, and place them in the laundry bag.

• If the mattress has slid downward, push it to the head of the bed; *adjusting it after bedmaking loosens the linens.*

• Place the bottom sheet with its center fold in the middle of the mattress. For a fitted sheet, secure the top and bottom corners over the mattress corners on the side of the bed nearest you. For a flat sheet, align the end of the sheet with the foot of the mattress, and miter the top corner *to keep the sheet firmly tucked under the mattress.* To miter the corner, first tuck the top end of the sheet evenly under the mattress at the head of the bed. Then lift the side edge of the sheet about 12″ (30 cm) from the mattress corner and hold it at a right angle to the mattress. Tuck in the bottom edge of the sheet hanging below the mattress. Finally, drop the top edge and tuck it under the mattress.

• After tucking under one side of the bottom sheet, place the drawsheet (if needed) about 15″ (38 cm) from the top of the bed, with its center fold in the middle of the bed. Then tuck in the entire edge of the drawsheet on the side of the bed nearest you.

• Place the top sheet with its center fold in the middle of the bed and its wide hem even with the top of the bed. Position the rough side of the hem faceup, *so the smooth side shows after folding.* Allow enough sheet at the top of the bed to form a cuff over the spread.

• Place the spread over the top sheet, with its center fold in the middle of the bed. (If the patient will be returning from surgery, follow an alternate technique as described in *Making a surgical bed,* page 76.)

• Make a 3″ (7.6 cm) toe pleat, or vertical tuck, in the top linens *to allow room for the patient's feet and to prevent pressure that can cause discomfort, skin breakdown, and footdrop.*

• Tuck the top sheet and spread under the foot of the mattress. Then, miter the bottom corners.

• Move to the opposite side of the bed and repeat the procedure.

• After fitting all corners of the bottom sheet or tucking them under the mattress, pull the sheet at an angle from the head toward the foot of the bed. *This tightens the linens, making the bottom sheet taut and wrinkle-free and promoting patient comfort.*

• Fold the top sheet over the spread at the head of the bed *to form a cuff and to give the bed a finished appearance.* When making an open bed, fanfold the top linens to the foot of the bed *to allow easy patient access.* If a linen-saver pad is needed, place it on top of the bottom sheets.

• Slip the pillow into a clean case, tucking its corners well into the case *to ensure a smooth fit.* Then place the pillow with its seam toward the top of the bed *to prevent it from rubbing against the patient's neck, causing irritation,* and its open edge facing away from the door *to give the bed a finished appearance.*

• Lower the bed and lock its wheels *to ensure patient safety.*

• Return furniture to its proper place, and place the call button within the patient's easy reach. Carry soiled linens from the room in outstretched arms *to avoid contaminating your uniform.*

Making a surgical bed

Preparation of a surgical bed permits easy patient transfer from surgery and promotes cleanliness and comfort. To make such a bed, take the following steps:
• Assemble linens as you would for making an unoccupied bed, including two clean sheets (one fitted, if available), a drawsheet, a bath blanket, a spread or sheet, a pillowcase, facial tissues, a trash bag, and linen-saver pads. Raise the bed to a comfortable working height *to prevent back strain.*
• Slip the pillow into a clean pillowcase and place it on a nearby table or chair.
• Make the foundation of the bed using the bottom sheet and drawsheet.
• Place an open bath blanket about 15″ (38 cm) from the head of the bed with its center fold positioned in the middle of the bed. *The blanket warms the patient and counteracts the decreased body temperature caused by anesthesia.*
• Place a top sheet or spread on the bath blanket, and position it as you did the blanket. Then fold the blanket and sheet back from the top, so that the blanket shows over the sheet. Similarly, fold the sheet and blanket up from the bottom, as shown below.

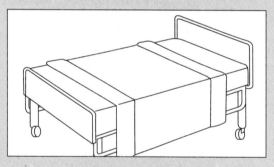

• On the side of the bed where you'll receive the patient (usually nearest the door), fold up the two outer corners of the sheet and blanket so they meet in the middle of the bed, as shown at the top of the next column.

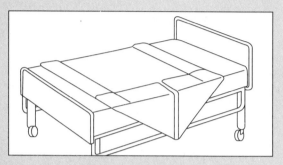

• Pick up the point hanging over this side of the bed, and fanfold the linens back to the opposite side of the bed *so the linens won't interfere with patient transfer from the stretcher to the bed.*

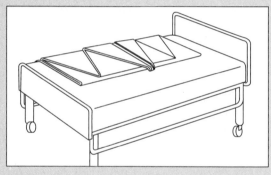

• Raise the bed to the high position if you haven't already. Then lock the wheels and lower the side rails. Be sure the side rails work properly. Move the bedside stand and other objects out of the stretcher's path *to facilitate easy transfer when the patient arrives.*
• After the patient is transferred to the bed, position the pillow for his comfort and safety. Cover him by pulling the top point of the sheet and blanket over him and opening the folds. After covering the patient, tuck in the linens at the foot of the bed and miter the corners.

• After disposing of the linens, remove gloves if used and wash your hands thoroughly *to prevent the spread of microorganisms.*

Special considerations

Because a hospital mattress is usually covered with plastic to protect it and to facilitate cleaning between patients, a flat bottom sheet tends to loosen and become untucked. Use a fitted sheet, if available, to prevent this.

If a fitted sheet is not available, the top corners of a flat sheet may be tied together under the top of the mattress to prevent the sheet from becoming dislodged. A bath blanket placed on top of the mattress, under the bottom sheet, helps to absorb moisture and prevent dislodgement of the bottom sheet.

Documentation
Although linen changes aren't usually documented, record their dates and times in your notes for patients with incontinence, excessive wound drainage, or diaphoresis.

 # Making an occupied bed

For the bedridden patient, daily linen changes promote comfort and help prevent skin breakdown and nosocomial infection. Such changes necessitate the use of side rails to prevent the patient from rolling out of bed and, depending on his condition, the use of a turning sheet to move him from side to side.

Making an occupied bed may require more than one person. It also entails loosening the bottom sheet on one side and fanfolding it to the center of the mattress instead of loosening the bottom sheet on both sides and removing it, as in an unoccupied bed. Also, the foundation of the bed must be made before applying the top sheet instead of making both the foundation and top on one side before completing them on the other side. (See *Making a traction bed*, page 78, for a specialized technique.)

Equipment
Two sheets (one fitted, if available) ▪ pillowcase ▪ one or two drawsheets ▪ spread ▪ one or two bath blankets ▪ gloves, if the patient has open lesions or has been incontinent ▪ sheepskin or other comfort-enhancing device, as needed ▪ optional: laundry bag, linen-saver pad.

Preparation of equipment
Obtain clean linen and be sure it's folded properly, as for an unoccupied bed.

Implementation
• Wash your hands, don gloves if necessary, and bring clean linen to the patient's room.
• Identify the patient and tell him you will be changing his bed linens. Explain how he can help if he is able, adjusting the plan according to his abilities and needs. Provide privacy.
• Move any furniture away from the bed *to ensure ample working space.*
• Raise the side rail on the far side of the bed *to prevent falls.* Adjust the bed to a comfortable working height *to prevent back strain.*

• If the patient's condition permits, lower the head of the bed *to ensure tight-fitting, wrinkle-free linens.*
• When stripping the bed, watch for the patient's eyeglasses, dentures, and other belongings that may have fallen among the linens.
• Cover the patient with a bath blanket *to avoid exposure and provide warmth and privacy.* Then fanfold the top sheet and spread from beneath the bath blanket, and bring them back over the blanket. Loosen the top linens at the foot of the bed and remove them separately. If you plan to reuse the top linens, fold each piece neatly and hang it over the back of the chair. Otherwise, place it in the laundry bag. *To avoid dispersing microorganisms,* don't fan the linens, hold them against your clothing, or place them on the floor.
• If the mattress slides down when the head of the bed is raised, pull it up toward the head of the bed. *Adjusting the mattress after the bed is made loosens the linens.* If the patient is able, ask him to grasp the head of the bed and pull with you; otherwise, ask a co-worker to help you.
• Roll the patient to the far side of the bed, and position the pillow lengthwise under his head *to support his neck.* Ask the patient to help (if he's able) by grasping the far side rail as he turns *so that he's positioned at the far side of the bed.*
• Loosen the soiled bottom linens on the side of the bed nearest you. Then roll the linens toward the patient's back in the middle of the bed.
• Place a clean bottom sheet on the bed, with its center fold in the middle of the mattress. If you're using a fitted sheet, secure the top and bottom corners over the side of the mattress nearest you. If you're using a flat sheet, place its end even with the foot of the mattress. Miter the top corner as you would for an unoccupied bed *to keep linens firmly tucked under the mattress, preventing wrinkling.*
• Fanfold the remaining clean bottom sheet toward the patient, and place the drawsheet, if needed, about 15″ (38 cm) from the top of the bed, with its center fold in the middle of the mattress. Tuck in the entire edge of the drawsheet on the side nearest you. Fanfold the remaining drawsheet toward the patient.
• If necessary, position a linen-saver pad on the drawsheet *to absorb excretions or surgical drainage,* and fanfold it toward the patient.
• Raise the other side rail, and roll the patient over the soiled and fanfolded linen to the clean side of the bed. Ask the patient to help (if he's able) by grasping the rail.
• Move to the unfinished side of the bed and lower the side rail nearest you. Then loosen and remove the soiled bottom linens separately and place them in the laundry bag.

Making a traction bed

For a patient in traction, obtain help from a co-worker to make the bed. Work from head to toe *to minimize the risk of traction misalignment.*

Preparation
• Wash your hands. Put on gloves if the patient has open lesions or has been incontinent. Bring clean linen to the patient's room, and arrange the linen in the order of use on the bedside stand or a chair.
• Explain the procedure to the patient, provide privacy, and remove unnecessary furniture and equipment from around the bed.

Change the linens
• Lower the side rails on both sides of the bed. Stand near the headboard on one side, and have a co-worker stand near the headboard on the opposite side, facing you.
• Gently pull the mattress to the head of the bed. Avoid sudden movements *because they can misalign traction and cause patient discomfort.*
• Remove the pillow from the bed. Loosen the bottom linens, and roll them from the headboard toward the patient's head. Then, remove the soiled pillowcase and replace it with a clean one.
• Fold a clean bottom sheet crosswise with the rough side of the hem facedown. Then place the sheet across the head of the bed. Tell the patient to raise her head and upper shoulders by grasping the trapeze above the bed. With your co-worker, quickly fanfold the bottom

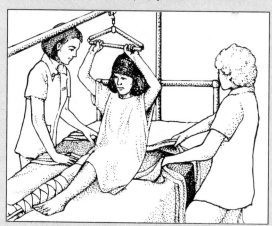

sheet from the head of the bed under the patient's shoulders, so that it meets the soiled linen. Tuck at least 12″ (30 cm) of the bottom sheet tightly under the head of the mattress. Miter the corners and tuck in the sides as far down as possible.
• Tell the patient to raise her buttocks by grasping the trapeze. As a team, move toward the foot of the bed and, in one movement, quickly and carefully roll soiled linens and clean linens under the patient's buttocks, as shown in the illustration.
• Instruct the patient to release the trapeze and to rest. Place a pillow under her head for comfort.
• If allowed, remove any pillows from under the patient's extremity. If pillow removal is contraindicated, continue to move linens toward the foot of the bed and under the patient's legs and traction while your co-worker lifts the pillows and supports the patient's extremity.
• Put soiled linens in a laundry bag or pillowcase.
• Tuck the remaining loose linens securely under the mattress. To ensure a tight-fitting bottom sheet, have the patient raise her weight off the bed by simultaneously grasping the trapeze and raising her buttocks while you pull the sheet tight. As needed, place a drawsheet, linen-saver pad, or sheepskin under the patient's buttocks. After the foundation is made, you can complete the bedmaking alone.
• If the bottom sheet doesn't cover the foot of the mattress, use a drawsheet to cover it. Miter its corners and tuck in the sides.
• Replace the pillows under the patient's extremity, then cover her with a clean top sheet. Fold over the top hem of the sheet approximately 8″ (20 cm). If one or both legs are in traction, fit the lower end of the sheet loosely over the traction apparatus; avoid applying unnecessary pressure to the traction ropes. To secure the sheet, tuck in the corner opposite the traction under the foot of the bed and miter the corner. Neatly tuck in the lower corner of the sheet on the traction side *to expose the leg and foot.*
• If the traction equipment exposes the patient's sides, place a drawsheet across the bed. Avoid using a full sheet or spread *because either one will be too cumbersome.*
• Lower the bed but don't allow the traction weights to touch the floor. Raise the side rails *to prevent falls.* If allowed, leave one side rail down so the patient can reach the bedside stand.

• Pull the clean bottom sheet taut. Secure a fitted sheet over the mattress corners or place the end of a flat sheet even with the foot of the bed, and miter the top corner. Pull the drawsheet taut and tuck it tightly under the mattress. Unfold and smooth the linen-saver pad, if used.
• Assist the patient to the supine position if his condition permits.
• Remove the soiled pillowcase, and place it in the laundry bag. Then slip the pillow into a clean pillowcase, tucking its corners well into the case *to ensure a smooth fit.* Place the pillow beneath the patient's head, with its seam toward the top of the bed *to prevent it from rubbing against the patient's neck, causing irritation.* Place the pillow's open edge away from the door *to give the bed a finished appearance.*
• Unfold the clean top sheet over the patient with the rough side of the hem facing away from the bed *to avoid irritating the patient's skin.* Allow enough sheet at the top of the bed to form a cuff over the spread.
• Remove the bath blanket from beneath the sheet, and center the spread over the top sheet.
• Make a 3" (7.6 cm) toe pleat, or vertical tuck, in the top linens *to allow room for the patient's feet and prevent pressure that can cause discomfort, skin breakdown, and footdrop.*
• Tuck the top sheet and spread under the foot of the bed, and miter the bottom corners. Fold the top sheet over the spread *to give the bed a finished appearance.*
• Raise the head of the bed to a comfortable position for the patient, make sure both side rails are raised, and then lower the bed and lock its wheels *to ensure the patient's safety.* Assess the patient's body alignment and his mental and emotional status.
• Return furniture to its proper place, and place the call button within the patient's easy reach. Remove the laundry bag from the room.
• Remove and discard gloves, if used, and wash your hands thoroughly *to prevent the spread of nosocomial infections.*

Special considerations
Use a fitted bottom sheet, when available, because a flat sheet slips out from under the mattress easily, especially if the mattress is plastic-coated.

Prevent the patient from sliding down in bed by tucking a tightly rolled pillow under the top linens at the foot of the bed. Provide additional comfort for the diaphoretic or bedridden patient by folding a bath blanket in half lengthwise and placing it between the bottom sheet and the plastic mattress cover; the blanket acts as a cushion and helps absorb moisture. *To help prevent sheet burns on the heels, elbows, and bony prominences,* center a bath blanket or sheepskin over the bottom sheet, and tuck the blanket securely under the mattress.

If the patient can't help you to move or turn him, devise a turning sheet *to facilitate bedmaking and repositioning.* To do this, first fold a drawsheet or bath blanket and place it under the patient's buttocks. Make sure the sheet extends from shoulders to knees *so that it supports most of the patient's weight.* Roll the sides of the sheet to form handles. Next, ask a co-worker to help you lift and move the patient. With one person holding each side of the sheet, you can move the patient without wrinkling the bottom linens. If you can't get help and must turn the patient yourself, stand at the side of the bed. Turn the patient toward the rail and, if he's able, ask him to grasp the rail to assist in turning. Then reach over the patient and firmly grasp the opposite rolled edge of the turning sheet. Pull the rolled edge carefully toward you and turn the patient.

Documentation
Although linen changes aren't usually documented, record their dates and times in your notes for patients with incontinence, excessive wound drainage, pressure ulcers, or diaphoresis.

 Bed bath

A complete bed bath cleans the skin, stimulates circulation, provides mild exercise, and promotes comfort. Bathing also allows assessment of skin condition, joint mobility, and muscle strength. Depending on the patient's overall condition and duration of hospitalization, he may have a complete or partial bath daily. A partial bath — including hands, face, axillae, back, genitalia, and anal region — can replace the complete bath for the patient with dry, fragile skin or extreme weakness, and can supplement the complete bath for the diaphoretic or incontinent patient.

Equipment
Bath basin ■ bath blanket ■ soap ■ towel ■ washcloth ■ skin lotion ■ orangewood stick ■ gloves, if the patient has open lesions or has been incontinent ■ deodorant ■ optional: bath oil, perineal pad, ABD pad, linen-saver pad.

Preparation of equipment
Adjust the temperature of the patient's room, and close any doors or windows to prevent drafts. Determine the patient's preference for soap or other hygiene aids *because*

some patients are allergic to soap or prefer bath oil or lotions. Assemble the equipment on an overbed table or bedside stand.

Implementation

• Tell the patient you'll be giving him a bath, and provide privacy. If the patient's condition permits, encourage him to assist with bathing *to provide exercise and promote independence.*

• Raise the patient's bed to a comfortable working height *to avoid back strain.* Offer him a bedpan or urinal.

• Fill the bath basin two-thirds full of warm water (about 115° F [46° C]) and bring it to the patient's bedside. If a bath thermometer isn't available, test the water temperature carefully with your elbow *to avoid scalding or chilling the patient;* the water should feel comfortably warm.

• If the bed will be changed after the bath, remove the top linen. If not, fanfold it to the foot of the bed.

• Don gloves if necessary. Position the patient supine, if possible.

• Remove the patient's gown and other articles, such as elastic stockings, elastic bandages, and restraints (as ordered). Cover him with a bath blanket *to provide warmth and privacy.*

• Place a towel under the patient's chin. To wash his face, begin with the eyes, working from the inner to the outer canthus without soap. Use a separate section of the washcloth for each eye *to avoid spreading ocular infection.*

• If the patient tolerates soap, apply it to the cloth, and wash the rest of his face, ears, and neck, using firm, gentle strokes. Rinse thoroughly *because residual soap can cause itching and dryness.* Then dry the area thoroughly. Observe the skin for irritation, scaling, or other abnormalities.

• Turn down the bath blanket, and drape the patient's chest with a bath towel. While washing, rinsing, and drying the chest and axillae, observe the patient's respirations. Use firm strokes *to avoid tickling the patient.* If the patient tolerates deodorant, apply it.

• Place a bath towel beneath the patient's arm farthest from you. Then bathe his arm, using long, smooth strokes and moving from wrist to shoulder, *to stimulate venous circulation.* If possible, soak the patient's hand in the basin *to remove dirt and soften nails.* Clean the patient's fingernails with the orangewood stick, if necessary. Observe the color of his hand and nail beds to *assess peripheral circulation.* Follow the same procedure for the other arm and hand.

• Turn down the bath blanket to expose the patient's abdomen and groin, keeping a bath towel across his chest *to prevent chills.* Bathe, rinse, and dry the abdomen and groin while checking for abdominal distention or tenderness. Then turn back the bath blanket to cover the patient's chest and abdomen.

• Uncover the leg farthest from you, and place a bath towel under it. Flex this leg and bathe it, moving from ankle to hip *to stimulate venous circulation.* Do not massage the leg, however, *to avoid dislodging any existing thrombus, possibly causing a pulmonary embolus.* Rinse and dry the leg.

• If possible, place a basin on the patient's bed, flex the leg at the knee, and place the foot in the basin. Soak the foot, and then wash and rinse it thoroughly. Remove the foot from the basin, dry it, and clean the toenails. Observe skin condition and color during cleaning *to assess peripheral circulation.* Repeat the procedure for the other leg and foot.

• Cover the patient with the bath blanket *to prevent chilling.* Then lower the bed and raise the side rails *to ensure patient safety* while you change the bath water.

• When you return, roll the patient on his side or stomach, place a towel beneath him, and cover him *to prevent chilling.* Bathe, rinse, and dry his back and buttocks.

• Massage the patient's back with lotion, giving attention to bony prominences. Check for redness, abrasions, and pressure ulcers.

• Bathe the anal area from front to back *to avoid contaminating the perineum.* Rinse and dry the area well.

• After lowering the bed and raising the side rails *to ensure the patient's safety,* change the bath water again. Then turn the patient on his back and bathe the genital area thoroughly but gently, using a different section of the washcloth for each downward stroke. Bathe from front to back, avoiding the anal area. Rinse thoroughly and pat dry.

• If applicable, perform indwelling catheter care. Apply perineal pads or scrotal supports, as needed.

• Dress the patient in a clean gown, and reapply any elastic bandages, elastic stockings, or restraints removed before the bath.

• Remake the bed or change the linens, and remove the bath blanket.

• Place a bath towel beneath the patient's head *to catch loose hair,* and then brush and comb his hair.

• Return the bed to its original position and make the patient comfortable.

• Carry soiled linens to the hamper with outstretched arms. *To avoid spreading microorganisms,* don't let soiled linens touch your clothing. Remove gloves, if applicable.

Special considerations

Fold the washcloth around your hand to form a mitt while bathing the patient. *This keeps the cloth warm longer and avoids dribbling water on the patient from the cloth's loose ends.* Change the water as often as necessary to keep it warm and clean.

Carefully dry creased skin-fold areas — for example, under breasts, in the groin area, and between fingers, toes, and buttocks. Dust these areas lightly with powder after drying *to reduce friction.* Use powder sparingly *to avoid caking and irritation, and to avoid provoking coughing in patients with respiratory disorders.*

If the patient has very dry skin, use bath oil instead of soap. No rinsing is necessary. Warm the lotion before using it for back massage *because cold lotion can startle the patient and induce muscle tension and vasoconstriction.* (See "Back care" in this chapter.) *To improve circulation, maintain joint mobility, and preserve muscle tone,* move the body joints through their full range of motion during the bath.

If the patient is incontinent, loosely tuck an ABD pad between his buttocks and place a linen-saver pad under him *to absorb fecal drainage.* Together these pads will help prevent skin irritation and reduce the number of linen changes.

Documentation
Record the date and time of the bed bath on the flowchart. Note the patient's tolerance for the bath, his range of motion, and his self-care abilities, and report any unusual findings.

 Tub baths and showers

Tub baths and showers provide personal hygiene, stimulate circulation, and reduce tension for the patient. They also allow you to observe skin conditions and assess joint mobility and muscle strength. If not precluded by the patient's condition or safety considerations, privacy during bathing promotes the patient's sense of well-being by allowing him to assume responsibility for his own care.

Patients who are recovering from recent surgery, who are emotionally unstable, or who have casted extremities or dressings in place usually require the doctor's permission for a tub bath or shower. (For an alternate bathing method, see *Using the hydraulic bath lift.)*

Equipment
One or two washcloths ■ bath towel ■ bath blanket ■ soap (or nonallergenic equivalent) ■ nonskid bath mat, if tub lacks nonskid strips ■ towel mat ■ bath thermometer ■ clean clothing or hospital gown ■ optional: chair, shower cap, bath oil, shampoo, or mild castile soap.

Using the hydraulic bath lift

For the debilitated patient who is unable to ambulate to the shower or tub, a hydraulic bath lift can facilitate transfer and eliminate strain on the nurse's back. The bath lift typically is used in a rehabilitation or geriatric setting.

To accomplish patient transfer, lower the lift (a chair or stretcher) to the patient's bed level. Suspend the patient, position him above a height-adjustable tub set to your most comfortable working height, and then lower him into the tub. Because the patient remains on the lift throughout his bath, simply reverse the procedure when taking the patient out of the tub.

When using a hydraulic lift for the first time, most patients feel somewhat insecure and fearful. With experience, however, most find the bathing system comfortable and relaxing.

Preparation of equipment
Prepare the bathing area before the patient arrives. Close any doors or windows and adjust the room temperature *to avoid chilling the patient.* Check that the bathtub or shower is clean. Then assemble bathing articles and observe appropriate safety measures.

For a bath: Position a chair next to the tub *to help the patient get in and out and to provide a seat if he becomes weak.* Place a bath blanket over the chair *to cover the patient if he becomes chilled.* Fill the tub halfway with water, and test the temperature with a bath thermometer. The temperature should range from 100° to 110° F (38° to 43° C). If you don't have a bath thermometer, test the temperature by immersing your elbow in the water; it should feel comfortable to the touch. Besides the obvious risk of scalding the patient, excessively hot water can cause cutaneous vasodilation, *which alters blood flow to the brain and may lead to dizziness or fainting.*

For a shower: Place a nonskid chair in the shower *to provide support.* The chair also allows the patient to sit down while washing his legs and feet, *reducing the risk of falling.*

Cover the floor of the shower with a nonskid mat unless it already has nonskid strips. Next, place a towel mat next to the bathing area. Remove electrical appliances, such as hair driers and heaters, from the patient's reach *to prevent electrical accidents.* Adjust water flow and temperature just before the patient gets into the shower.

Implementation

• Escort the patient to the bathing area, explain the procedure, and help him undress as necessary. Offer him a shower cap if he wants to keep his hair dry. Otherwise, provide shampoo or mild castile soap.

• Help the patient into the tub or shower. Provide washcloths and soap. If he has dry skin, add bath oil to the water. Wait until after he gets into the tub before adding bath oil *because oil makes the tub slick and increases the risk of falling.*

• Taking care to respect his privacy, help the patient bathe, as needed; he may appreciate help washing his back. If you can safely leave the patient alone, place the call button within easy reach and show him how to use it.

• Tell the patient to leave the door unlocked for his own safety, but assure him that you'll post an OCCUPIED sign on the door. Stay nearby in case of emergency, and check on the patient every 5 to 10 minutes.

• When the patient finishes bathing, drain the tub or turn off the shower.

• Assist the patient onto the bath mat *to prevent him from falling.* Then help him to dry off and don a clean gown or other clothing, as appropriate.

• Escort the patient to his room or to his bed.

• Dry the floor of the bathing area well *to prevent slipping.* Ensure that the tub or shower is cleaned and disinfected.

• Dispose of soiled towels and return the patient's personal belongings to his bedside.

Special considerations

If you're giving a tub bath to a patient with a cast or dressing on an arm or leg, wrap the extremity in a clear plastic bag. Secure the bag with tape, being careful not to constrict circulation. Instruct the patient to dangle the arm or leg over the edge of the tub, and keep it out of the water.

Encourage the patient to use safety devices, bars, and rails when bathing. *Because bathing in warm water causes vasodilation,* the patient may feel faint. If so, open the drain or turn off the shower. Cover the patient's shoulders and back with a bath towel, and instruct him to lean forward in the tub and to lower his head. Alternatively, assist him out of the shower onto a chair, lower his head, and summon help. If you have an ampule of aromatic spirits of ammonia readily available, break it open and wave it under the patient's nostrils. Never leave the patient unattended to obtain an ampule. When the patient recovers, escort him to bed and monitor vital signs.

Documentation

Describe the patient's skin condition and record any discoloration or redness in your notes.

Hair care

Hair care includes combing, brushing, and shampooing. Combing and brushing stimulates scalp circulation, removes dead cells and debris, and distributes hair oils to produce a healthy sheen. Shampooing removes dirt and old oils and helps prevent skin irritation.

Frequency of hair care depends on the length and texture of the patient's hair, the duration of hospitalization, and the patient's condition. Usually, hair should be combed and brushed daily, and shampooed according to the patient's normal routine. Typically, no more than 1 week, or perhaps 2, should elapse between washings. Shampooing is contraindicated in patients with recent craniotomy, depressed skull fracture, conditions necessitating intracranial pressure monitoring, or other cranial involvement.

Equipment

Comb and brush ▪ hand towel ▪ liquid shampoo (or mild soap, such as castile) ▪ shampoo tray with tubing ▪ washcloth ▪ three bath towels ▪ two bath blankets ▪ cotton ▪ pail or plastic wastebasket ▪ two large pitchers or other large containers ▪ one small pitcher or beaker ▪ basin ▪ linen-saver pads ▪ gloves, if the patient has open scalp lesions ▪ optional: hair conditioner or rinse, alcohol, oil, hair ties, footstool, drawsheet.

Preparation of equipment

The comb and brush should be clean. If necessary, wash them in hot, soapy water. The comb should have dull, even teeth *to prevent scratching the scalp.* The brush should have stiff bristles *to enhance vigorous brushing and stimulation of circulation.*

Before shampooing the patient's hair, adjust room temperature and eliminate drafts *to prevent chilling the patient.* Next, obtain a shampoo tray or devise a trough, if necessary. (For instructions, see *How to make a shampoo trough.)*

Implementation

• Assemble the equipment on the patient's bedside stand.

Combing and brushing

• Tell the patient you're going to comb and brush his hair. If possible, encourage him to do this himself, assisting him as necessary.

• Adjust the bed to a comfortable working height *to prevent back strain.* If the patient's condition allows, help him to a sitting position by raising the head of the bed.

• Provide privacy, and drape a bath towel over the patient's pillow and shoulders *to catch loose hair and dirt.* Don gloves if the patient has open scalp lesions.

• For short hair, comb and brush one side at a time. For long or curly hair, turn the patient's head away from you, and then part his hair down the middle from front to back. If the hair is tangled, rub alcohol or oil on the hair strands to loosen them. Comb and vigorously brush the hair on the side facing you. Then turn the patient's head and comb and brush the opposite side. Part hair into small sections for easier handling. Comb one section at a time, working from the ends toward the scalp to remove tangles. Anchor each section of hair above the area being combed *to avoid hurting the patient.* After combing, brush vigorously.

• Style the hair as the patient prefers. Braiding long or curly hair helps prevent snarling. To braid, part hair down the middle of the scalp and begin braiding near the face. Don't braid too tightly *to avoid patient discomfort.* Fasten the ends of the braids with hair ties. Pin the braids across the top of the patient's head or let them hang, as the patient desires, *so the finished braids don't press against the patient's scalp.*

• After styling the hair, carefully remove the towel by folding it inward. *This prevents loose hairs and debris from falling onto the pillow or into the patient's bed.*

Shampooing a bedridden patient's hair

• Cover the patient with a bath blanket. Then fanfold the linens to the foot of the bed, or remove them if they're scheduled to be changed.

• Place a wastebasket on a linen-saver pad on the floor or on a footstool near the head of the bed. The pail or container catches wastewater from the shampoo tray.

• Fill large pitchers or containers with comfortably warm water and place them on the overbed table.

• Lower the head of the bed until it's horizontal, and remove the patient's pillow, if allowed.

• Fold the second bath blanket and tuck it under the patient's shoulders *to improve water drainage.*

• Cover the bath blanket and the head of the bed with a linen-saver pad *to protect them from moisture.*

• Place a bath towel and linen-saver pad together, and position them around the patient's neck and over his shoulders. *This protects the patient from moisture and pads his neck against the pressure of the shampoo tray.*

• Place the shampoo tray under the patient's head with his neck in the U-shaped opening. Arrange the bath blanket and towel so the patient is comfortable.

• Adjust the shampoo tray to carry wastewater away from the patient's head, and place the drainage tubing in the pail. Tuck a folded towel or drawsheet under the opposite

How to make a shampoo trough

To make a trough, roll a bath blanket, towel, or drawsheet into a log. Shape the log into a "U" and place it in a large plastic bag. Arrange the bag under the patient's head, with the end of the bag extending over the edge of the bed and into a bucket on the floor, as shown below. Proceed with the shampooing as you would with a shampoo tray.

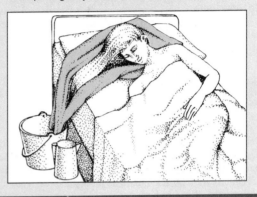

side of the shampoo tray *to promote drainage, if necessary.* Don gloves if the patient has open scalp lesions.

• When shampooing, place cotton in the patient's ears *to prevent moisture from collecting in the ear canals.*

• Fill the small pitcher or beaker by dipping it into the large pitcher. Carefully pour water over the patient's hair. *To avoid spills,* don't overfill the shampoo tray.

• Then, with your fingertips, rub shampoo into the patient's hair. Massage his scalp well *to emulsify hair oils. Vigorous rubbing stimulates the scalp and also helps the patient relax.*

• Using the small pitcher or beaker, pour water over the patient's hair until it's free of shampoo. Then reapply shampoo and rinse again. Apply conditioner or a rinse, if desired.

• Remove the shampoo tray, and wrap the patient's hair in a towel. Remove the linen-saver pad from the bed, and return the bed to its original position.

• Dry the patient's hair by gently rubbing it with a towel. Then comb, brush, and style it.

• Remake the bed or change the linens, if needed, and remove the bath blanket.

• Reposition the patient comfortably.

• Remove and empty the pail. Clean the shampoo tray, and return it to storage. Remove pitchers from the bedside, and return the shampoo to the bedside stand.

Special considerations

When giving hair care, check the patient's scalp carefully for signs of scalp disorders or skin breakdown, particularly if the patient is bedridden. Make sure each patient has his own comb and brush *to avoid cross-contamination.*

If you don't have a shampoo tray and can't devise a trough, place pillows under the patient's shoulders to elevate his head, and use a basin. Because a standard basin doesn't have a drainage spout, empty it frequently *to prevent overflow.*

Documentation

Record the date, time, and patient's response to the shampoo on the flowchart. Describe any scalp abnormalities in your notes.

 # Shaving

Performed with a straight, safety, or electric razor, shaving is part of the male patient's usual daily care. Besides reducing bacterial growth on the face, shaving promotes patient comfort by removing whiskers that can itch and irritate the skin and produce an unkempt appearance. Because nicks and cuts occur most frequently with a straight or a safety razor, shaving with an electric razor is indicated for the patient with a clotting disorder or the patient undergoing anticoagulant therapy. Shaving may be contraindicated in the patient with a facial skin disorder or wound.

Equipment

For a straight or a safety razor: Shaving kit containing a straight razor and soap container, or a safety razor ∎ gloves ∎ soap or shaving cream ∎ towel ∎ washcloth ∎ basin ∎ optional: after-shave lotion, talcum powder.

For an electric razor: Bath towel ∎ optional: pre-shave and after-shave lotions, mirror, grounded three-pronged plug.

Preparation of equipment

With a straight or a safety razor, make sure the blade is sharp, clean, even, and rust-free. If necessary, insert a new blade securely into the razor. A razor may be used more than once, but only by the same patient. If the patient is bedridden, assemble the equipment on the bedside stand or overbed table; if he's ambulatory, assemble it at the sink. When the patient is ready to shave, fill the basin or sink with warm water.

If you're using an electric razor, check its cord for fraying or other damage that could create an electrical

hazard. If the razor isn't double-insulated or battery-operated, use a grounded three-pronged plug. Examine the razor head for sharp edges and dirt. Read the manufacturer's instructions, if available, and assemble the equipment at the bedside.

Implementation

• Tell the patient that you're going to shave him, and provide privacy. Ask him to assist you as much as possible *to promote his independence.*

• Unless contraindicated, place the conscious patient in the high Fowler's or semi-Fowler's position. If the patient is unconscious, elevate his head *to prevent soap and water from running behind it.*

• Direct bright light onto the patient's face, but not into his eyes.

Using a straight or a safety razor

• Drape a bath towel around the patient's shoulders, and tuck it under his chin *to protect the bed from moisture and to catch falling whiskers.*

• Put on gloves, and fill the basin with warm water. Using the washcloth, wet the patient's entire beard with warm water. Let the warm cloth soak the beard for at least 1 minute *to soften whiskers.*

• Apply shaving cream to the beard. Or, if you're using soap, rub to form a lather.

• Gently stretch the patient's skin taut with one hand and shave with the other, holding the razor firmly. Ask the patient to puff his cheeks or turn his head, as necessary, to shave hard-to-reach areas.

• Begin at the sideburns and work toward the chin using short, firm, downward strokes in the direction of hair growth. *This reduces skin irritation and helps prevent nicks and cuts.*

• Rinse the razor often *to remove whiskers.* Apply more warm water or shaving cream to the face, as needed, *to maintain adequate lather.*

• Shave across the chin and up the neck and throat. Use short, gentle strokes for the neck and the area around the nose and mouth *to avoid skin irritation.*

• Change the water, and rinse any remaining lather and whiskers from the patient's face. Then dry his face with a bath towel and, if the patient desires, apply after-shave lotion or talcum powder.

• Rinse the razor and basin, and then return the razor to its storage area.

Using an electric razor

• Plug in the razor, and apply pre-shave lotion, if available, *to remove skin oils.* If the razor head is adjustable, select the appropriate setting.

• Using a circular motion and pressing the razor firmly against the skin, shave each area of the patient's face until smooth.
• If the patient desires, apply talcum powder or after-shave lotion.
• Clean the razor head, and return the razor to its storage area.

Special considerations
If the patient is conscious, find out his usual shaving routine. Although shaving in the direction of hair growth is most common, the patient may prefer the opposite direction.

Don't interchange patients' shaving equipment *to prevent cross-contamination.*

Complications
Cuts and abrasions are the most common complications of shaving and can require application of antiseptic lotion.

Documentation
If applicable, record nicks or cuts resulting from shaving.

 # Eye care

When paralysis or coma impairs or eliminates the corneal reflex, frequent eye care aims to keep the exposed cornea moist, preventing ulceration and inflammation. Application of saline-saturated gauze pads over the eyelids moistens the eyes. Commercially available eye ointments and artificial tears also lubricate the corneas, but a doctor's order is required for their use.

Although eye care isn't a sterile procedure, asepsis should be maintained as much as possible.

Equipment
Sterile basin ■ gloves ■ sterile towel ■ sterile normal saline solution ■ sterile cotton balls ■ mineral oil ■ artificial tears or eye ointment (if ordered) ■ gauze or eye-pads ■ nonallergenic tape.

Preparation of equipment
Assemble the equipment at the patient's bedside. Pour a small amount of saline solution into the basin.

Implementation
• Wash your hands thoroughly, put on gloves, and tell the patient what you're about to do, even if he is comatose or appears unresponsive.

• To remove secretions or crusts adhering to the eyelids and eyelashes, first soak a cotton ball in sterile normal saline solution. Then gently wipe the patient's eye with the moistened cotton ball, working from the inner canthus to the outer canthus *to prevent debris and fluid from entering the nasolacrimal duct.*
• *To prevent cross-contamination,* use a fresh cotton ball for each wipe until the eye is clean. *To prevent irritation,* avoid using soap for cleaning the eyes. Repeat the procedure for the other eye.
• After cleaning the eyes, instill artificial tears or apply eye ointment, as ordered, *to keep them moist.*
• Close the patient's eyelids. Dab a small amount of mineral oil on each lid *to lubricate and protect fragile skin.*
• Soak gauze or eyepads in sterile normal saline solution, place them over the eyelids, and secure with nonallergenic tape. Change gauze pads, as necessary, *to keep them well saturated.*
• After giving eye care, cover the basin with a sterile towel and dispose of gloves. Change the eye care setup (basin, towel, and normal saline solution) at least daily.

Documentation
Record the time and type of eye care in your notes. If applicable, chart administration of eyedrops or ointment in the patient's medication record. Document unusual crusting or excessive or colored drainage.

 # Contact lens care

Illness or emergency treatment may require that you insert or remove and store a patient's contact lenses. Proper handling and lens care techniques help prevent eye injury and infection as well as lens loss or damage. Appropriate lens-handling techniques depend in large part on what type of lenses the patient wears.

All contact lenses float on the corneal tear layer. Rigid lenses typically have a smaller diameter than the cornea; soft lens diameter typically exceeds that of the cornea. Because they're larger and more pliable, soft lenses tend to mold themselves more closely to the eye for a more stable fit than rigid lenses.

Modes of lens wear vary widely. Although most patients remove and clean their lenses daily, some wear lenses overnight or for several days (sometimes up to a month) without removing them for cleaning. Still other patients wear disposable lenses, which means that they replace old lenses with new ones at regular intervals (a few days to a few months), possibly without removing them for cleaning between replacements.

Keep in mind that lenses handled improperly can provide a direct source of contamination to the eye.

Equipment
Lens storage case or two small medicine cups and adhesive tape ■ gloves ■ patient's equipment for contact lens care, if available ■ sterile normal saline solution or soaking solution ■ flashlight, if needed ■ optional: suction cup.

Preparation of equipment
If a commercial lens storage case isn't available, place enough sterile normal saline solution into two small medicine cups to submerge a lens in each one. To avoid confusing the left and right lenses, which may have different prescriptions, mark one cup "L" and the other cup "R" and place the corresponding lens in each cup.

Implementation
• Tell the patient what you're about to do, wash your hands, and put on gloves *to help prevent ocular infection.*

Inserting rigid lenses
• Wet one lens with solution, and gently rub it between your thumb and index finger, or place it on your palm and rub it with your opposite index finger. Rinse well with the solution, leaving a small amount in the lens.
• Place the lens, convex side down, on the tip of the index finger of your dominant hand.
• Instruct the patient to gaze upward slightly. Separate the eyelids with your other thumb and index finger, and place the lens directly and gently on the cornea. You need not press it to the eye; the tear film will attract it naturally at the first touch. Using the same procedure, insert the opposite lens.

Inserting soft lenses
• To see if the lens is inside out, bend it between your thumb and index finger or fill it with saline or soaking solution. If the lens tends to roll inward or the edge points slightly inward, it's oriented correctly. If the edge points outward or the lens tends to collapse over your fingertip, it's probably inside out and should be reversed.
• Wet the lens with fresh normal saline solution, and rub it gently between your thumb and index finger, or place it on your palm and rub it with your opposite index finger. Rinse well.
• Place the lens, convex side down, on the tip of the index finger of your dominant hand.
• Instruct the patient to gaze upward slightly. Separate the eyelids with your other thumb and index finger, and place the lens on the sclera, just below the cornea. Then, slide the lens gently upward with your finger until it centers on the cornea. Using the same procedure, insert the opposite lens.

Removing rigid lenses
• Before removing a lens, position the patient supine *to prevent the lens from popping out onto the floor, risking loss or damage.*
• Place one thumb against the patient's upper eyelid and the other thumb against the lower eyelid. Move the lids toward each other while gently pressing inward against the eye *to trap the lens edge and break the suction.* Extract the lens from the patient's eyelashes. (See *Removing a patient's contact lenses.*)
• Depending on the lens type and thickness, it may pop out when the suction breaks. You may want to try to break the suction with one hand while cupping the other hand below the patient's eye *to catch the lens as it falls.*
• Sometimes the lens will pop out on its own if you ask the patient to blink after stretching the corner of the eyelids toward the temporal bone, thus tightening the lid edges against the globe of the eye.
• After removal, place the lens in the proper well of the storage case (L or R) with enough of the appropriate storage solution to cover it. Alternatively, place the lens in a labeled medicine cup with solution, and secure adhesive tape over the top of the cup *to prevent loss of the lens.*
• Remove and care for the opposite lens using the same technique.

Removing soft lenses
• Position the patient supine. Using your nondominant hand, raise the patient's upper eyelid and hold it against the orbital rim.
• Lightly place the forefinger of your other hand on the lens and move it down onto the sclera below the cornea. Then pinch the lens between your forefinger and thumb; it should pop off.
• Place the lens in the proper well of the storage case with enough of the appropriate storage solution to cover it. Alternatively, place the lens in a labeled medicine cup with solution, and secure adhesive tape over the top of the cup *to prevent loss of the lens.*
• Remove and care for the other lens using the same technique.

Cleaning lenses
• Because lens-cleaning steps vary with lens type and with each manufacturer's and doctor's instructions, ask the patient to guide you step-by-step through his normal cleaning routine.

Removing a patient's contact lenses

Contact lens removal techniques depend largely on the type of lenses the patient wears and how readily they come off the eye. For successful removal of soft and rigid lenses, follow the steps outlined below. If you have trouble removing lenses manually, try using a specially-made suction cup.

Soft lenses
With the patient looking up and her upper lid raised, use your dominant index finger to slide the lens onto the lower cornea. Pinch the lens between your index finger and thumb to remove it.

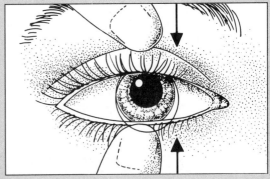

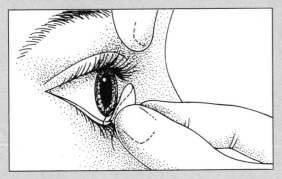

Using a suction cup
Separate the lids with your nondominant hand. Squeeze the suction cup with your dominant hand, and place it gently against the lens. Open your fingers slightly to create suction between the lens and the cup. Rock the lens gently to remove it.

Rigid lenses
Place one thumb on each eyelid and move the lids toward each other, pressing gently against the eyeball. When the lids meet the lens edges, the suction breaks and the lens is released, as shown at the top of the next column. Catch the lens in your lower hand or remove it from the patient's lashes.

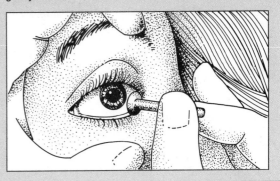

• If the patient is unable to tell you how to clean his lenses properly, remember that all lens types require two steps: cleaning and disinfection.
• Cleaning involves rubbing the lens with a surfactant solution designed to remove most surface deposits. For most patients, especially those who wear soft lenses, the cleaning step also may include use of an enzyme agent to remove protein deposits against which surfactant cleaners typically are ineffective. Enzyme cleaning involves soaking the lenses overnight in a solution in which you've dissolved special enzyme tablets.
• Disinfection, which doesn't require rubbing, may be accomplished through chemical means or by heat. This step aims to rid the lens of infectious organisms.

• If you must clean a patient's lenses, use only his own solutions. *This minimizes the risk of allergic reactions to substances included in other solution brands.* Never touch the nozzle opening of a solution bottle to the lens, your fingers, or anything else *to avoid contaminating solution remaining in the bottle.*

Special considerations
If the patient's eyes appear dry or you have trouble moving the lens on the eye, instill several drops of sterile normal saline solution, and wait a few minutes before trying again to remove the lens *to prevent corneal damage.* If you still can't remove the lens easily, notify the doctor. Avoid instillation of eye medication while the patient is

wearing lenses. The lenses can trap the medication, possibly causing eye irritation or lens damage.

Don't allow soft lenses, which are 40% to 60% water, to dry out. If they do, soak them in sterile normal saline solution and they may return to their natural shape.

If an unconscious patient is admitted to the emergency department, check for contact lenses by opening each eyelid and searching with a small flashlight. If you detect lenses, remove them immediately *because tears cannot circulate freely beneath the lenses with eyelids closed, possibly leading to corneal oxygen depletion or infection.*

Advise contact lens wearers to carry appropriate identification to speed lens removal and ensure proper care in an emergency.

If a patient cannot provide adequate care for his lenses during hospitalization, encourage him to send them home with a family member. If you aren't sure how to care for the lenses in the interim, store them in sterile normal saline solution until the family member can take them home.

Documentation
Record eye condition before and after removal of lenses; the time of lens insertion, removal, and cleaning; the location of stored lenses; and, if applicable, the removal of lenses from the hospital by a family member.

Mouth care

Given in the morning, at bedtime, or after meals, mouth care entails brushing and flossing the teeth and inspecting the mouth. It removes soft plaque deposits and calculus from the teeth, cleans and massages the gums, reduces mouth odor, and helps prevent infection. By freshening the patient's mouth, mouth care also enhances appreciation of food, thereby aiding appetite and nutrition.

Although the ambulatory patient can usually perform mouth care alone, the bedridden patient may require partial or full assistance. The comatose patient requires use of suction equipment to prevent aspiration during oral care.

Equipment
Towel or facial tissues ▪ emesis basin ▪ trash bag ▪ mouthwash ▪ toothbrush and toothpaste ▪ pitcher and glass ▪ drinking straw ▪ dental floss ▪ gloves ▪ dental floss holder, if available ▪ small mirror, if necessary ▪ optional: oral irrigating device.

For the comatose or debilitated patient, as needed:
Linen-saver pad ▪ bite-block ▪ petroleum jelly ▪ hydrogen peroxide ▪ mineral oil ▪ cotton-tipped mouth swab ▪ oral suction equipment or gauze pads ▪ optional: lemon-glycerin swabs or mouth-care kit, tongue blade, 4" × 4" gauze pads, adhesive tape.

Preparation of equipment
Fill a pitcher with water and bring it and other equipment to the patient's bedside. If you'll be using oral suction equipment, connect the tubing to the suction bottle and suction catheter, insert the plug into an outlet, and check for correct operation. If necessary, devise a bite-block to protect yourself from being bitten during the procedure. Wrap a gauze pad over the end of a tongue blade, fold the edge in, and secure it with adhesive tape.

Implementation
• Wash your hands thoroughly, put on gloves, explain the procedure to the patient, and provide privacy.

Supervising mouth care
• For the bedridden patient capable of self-care, encourage him to perform his own mouth care.
• If allowed, place the patient in Fowler's position. Place the overbed table in front of the patient, and arrange the equipment on it. Open the table and set up the built-in mirror, if available, or position a small mirror on the table.
• Drape a towel over the patient's chest to protect his gown. Instruct him to floss his teeth while looking into the mirror.
• Observe the patient *to be sure he's flossing correctly,* and correct him if necessary. Tell him to wrap the floss around the second or third fingers of both hands. Starting with his back teeth and without injuring the gums, he should insert the floss as far as possible into the space between each pair of teeth. Then he should clean the surfaces of adjacent teeth by pulling the floss up and down against the side of each tooth. After the patient flosses a pair of teeth, remind him to use a clean 1" (2.5-cm) section of floss for the next pair.
• After the patient flosses, mix mouthwash and water in a glass, place a straw in the glass, and position the emesis basin nearby. Then instruct the patient to brush his teeth and gums while looking into the mirror. Encourage him to rinse frequently during brushing, and provide facial tissues for him to wipe his mouth.

Performing mouth care
• For the comatose patient or the conscious patient incapable of self-care, you'll perform mouth care. If the patient wears dentures, clean them thoroughly. (See

Dealing with dentures

Prostheses made of plastic or vulcanite, dentures replace some or all of the patient's natural teeth. Dentures require proper care to remove soft plaque deposits and calculus and to reduce mouth odor. Such care involves removing and rinsing dentures after meals, daily brushing and removal of tenacious deposits, and soaking in a commercial denture cleaner. Dentures must be removed from the comatose or presurgical patient to prevent possible airway obstruction.

Preparation
Start by assembling the following equipment at the patient's bedside: emesis basin ■ labeled denture cup ■ toothbrush or denture brush ■ gloves ■ toothpaste ■ commercial denture cleaner ■ paper towel ■ cotton-tipped mouth swab ■ mouthwash ■ gauze ■ optional: adhesive denture liner.
    Wash your hands and put on gloves.

Removing dentures
• To remove a full upper denture, grasp the front and palatal surfaces of the denture with your thumb and forefinger. Position the index finger of your opposite hand over the upper border of the denture, and press *to break the seal between denture and palate.* Grasp the denture with gauze *because saliva can make it slippery.*
• To remove a full lower denture, grasp the front and lingual surfaces of the denture with your thumb and index finger, and gently lift up.
• To remove partial dentures, exert equal pressure on the border of each side of the denture. Avoid lifting the clasps, *which easily bend or break.*

Oral and denture care
• After removing dentures, place them in a properly labeled denture cup. Add warm water and a commercial denture cleaner *to remove stains and hardened deposits.* Follow package directions. Avoid soaking dentures overnight if they have metal parts *because corrosion may result.* Also, avoid soaking dentures in mouthwash *because it may pit the denture material.*
• Instruct the patient to rinse with mouthwash *to remove food particles and reduce mouth odor.* Then stroke the palate, buccal surfaces, gums, and tongue with a soft toothbrush or cotton-tipped mouth swab *to clean the mucosa and stimulate circulation.* Inspect for irritated areas or sores *because they may indicate a poorly fitting denture.*
• Carry the denture cup, emesis basin, toothbrush, and toothpaste to the sink. After lining the basin with a paper towel, fill it with water *to cushion the dentures in case you drop them.* Hold the dentures over the basin, wet them with warm water, and apply toothpaste to a denture brush or long-bristled toothbrush. Clean the dentures using only moderate pressure *to prevent scratches* and warm water *to prevent distortion.*
• Clean the denture cup, and place the dentures in it. Rinse the brush, and clean and dry the emesis basin. Return all equipment to the patient's bedside stand.

Inserting dentures
• If the patient desires, apply adhesive liner to the dentures. Moisten them with water, if necessary, *to reduce friction and ease insertion.*
• Encourage the patient to wear his dentures *to enhance his appearance, facilitate eating and speaking, and prevent changes in the gum line that may affect denture fit.*

Dealing with dentures.) Some patients may benefit from using an oral irrigating device, such as a Water Pik. (See *Using an oral irrigating device,* page 90.)
• Raise the bed to a comfortable working height *to prevent back strain.* Then lower the head of the bed, and position the patient on his side, with his face extended over the edge of the pillow *to facilitate drainage and prevent fluid aspiration.*
• Arrange the equipment on the overbed table or bedside stand, including the oral suction equipment, if necessary. Turn on the machine. If a suction machine isn't available, wipe the inside of the patient's mouth frequently with a gauze pad.

• Place a linen-saver pad under the patient's chin and an emesis basin near his cheek *to absorb or catch drainage.*
• Lubricate the patient's lips with petroleum jelly *to prevent dryness and cracking.* Reapply lubricant, as needed, during oral care.
• If necessary, insert the bite-block *to hold the patient's mouth open during oral care.*
• Using a dental floss holder, hold the floss against each tooth and direct it as close to the gum as possible without injuring the sensitive tissues around the tooth.
• After flossing the patient's teeth, mix mouthwash and water in a glass and place the straw in it.

Using an oral irrigating device

An oral irrigating device, such as the Water Pik, directs a pulsating jet of water around the teeth to massage gums and remove debris and food particles. It's especially useful for cleaning areas missed by brushing, such as around bridgework, crowns, and dental wires. Because this device enhances oral hygiene, it benefits patients undergoing head and neck irradiation, which can damage teeth and cause severe caries. The device also maintains oral hygiene in a patient with a fractured jaw or with mouth injuries that limit standard mouth care.

Equipment
To use the device, first assemble the following equipment: oral irrigating device ▪ towel ▪ emesis basin ▪ pharyngeal suction apparatus ▪ salt solution or mouthwash, if ordered ▪ soap.

Implementation
• Turn the patient to his side *to prevent aspiration of water*. Then, place a towel under his chin and an emesis basin next to his cheek *to absorb or catch drainage*.
• Insert the oral irrigating device's plug into a nearby electrical outlet. Remove the device's cover, turn it upside down, and fill it with lukewarm water or with a mouthwash or salt solution, as ordered. When using a salt solution, dissolve the salt beforehand in a separate container. Then pour the solution into the cover.
• Secure the cover to the base of the device. Remove the water hose handle from the base, and snap the jet tip into place. If necessary, wet the grooved end of the tip *to ease insertion*. Adjust the pressure dial to the setting most comfortable for the patient. If his gums are tender and prone to bleed, choose a low setting.
• Adjust the knurled knob on the handle *to direct the water jet*, place the jet tip in the patient's mouth, and

turn on the device. Instruct the alert patient to keep his lips partially closed *to avoid spraying water.*
• Direct the water at a right angle to the gum line of each tooth and between teeth. Avoid directing water under the patient's tongue *because this may injure sensitive tissue.*

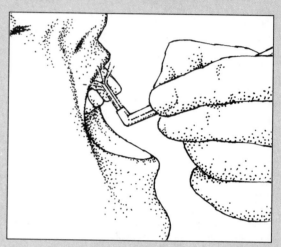

After irrigating each tooth, pause briefly and instruct the patient to expectorate the water or solution into the emesis basin. If he's unable to do so, suction it from the sides of the mouth with the pharyngeal suction apparatus. After irrigating all teeth, turn off the device, and remove the jet tip from the patient's mouth.
• Empty the remaining water or solution from the cover, remove the jet tip from the handle, and return the handle to the base. Clean the jet tip with soap and water, rinse the cover, and dry them both and return them to storage.

• Wet the toothbrush with water. If necessary, use hot water *to soften the bristles.* Apply toothpaste.
• Brush the patient's lower teeth from the gum line up; the upper teeth, from the gum line down. Place the brush at a 45-degree angle to the gum line, and press the bristles gently into the gingival sulcus. Using short, gentle strokes *to prevent gum damage,* brush the facial surfaces (toward the cheek) and the lingual surfaces (toward the tongue) of the bottom teeth. Use just the tip of the brush for the lingual surfaces of the front teeth. Then, using the same technique, brush the facial and lingual

surfaces of the top teeth. Next, brush the biting surfaces of the bottom and top teeth, using a back and forth motion. If possible, ask the patient to rinse frequently during brushing by taking the mouthwash solution through the straw. Hold the emesis basin steady under the patient's cheek, and wipe his mouth and cheeks with facial tissues, as needed.
• After brushing the patient's teeth, dip a cotton-tipped mouth swab into the mouthwash solution. Press the swab against the side of the glass to remove excess moisture. Gently stroke the gums, buccal surfaces, palate, and

tongue *to clean the mucosa and stimulate circulation.* Replace the swab as necessary for thorough cleaning. Avoid inserting the swab too deeply *to prevent gagging and vomiting.*

After mouth care
• Assess the patient's mouth for cleanliness and tooth and tissue condition. Then remove your gloves, rinse the toothbrush, and clean the emesis basin and glass. Empty and clean the suction bottle, if used, and place a clean suction catheter on the tubing. Return reusable equipment to the appropriate storage location and properly discard disposable equipment in the trash bag.

Special considerations
Use cotton-tipped mouth swabs to clean the teeth of a patient with sensitive gums. *These swabs produce less friction than a toothbrush but don't clean as well.*

Clean the mouth of a toothless comatose patient by wrapping a gauze pad around your index finger, moistening it with mouthwash, and gently swabbing the oral tissues. If necessary, moisten gauze pads in an equal mixture of hydrogen peroxide and water *to remove tenacious mucus.*

Remember that mucous membranes dry quickly in the patient breathing through his mouth or receiving oxygen therapy. Moisten his mouth and lips regularly with mineral oil, lemon-glycerin swabs, or water. If you use water as the lubricant, place a short straw in a glass of water and stop the open end with your finger. Remove the straw from the water and, with your finger in place, position it in the patient's mouth. Release your finger slightly to let the water flow out gradually. If the patient is comatose, suction excess water *to prevent aspiration.*

Documentation
Record the date and time of mouth care in your notes. Also document any unusual conditions, such as bleeding, edema, mouth odor, excessive secretions, or plaque on the tongue.

Back care

Regular bathing and massage of the neck, back, buttocks, and upper arms promotes patient relaxation and allows assessment of skin condition. Particularly important for the bedridden patient, massage causes cutaneous vasodilation, helping to prevent pressure ulcers caused by prolonged pressure on bony prominences or by perspiration. Gentle back massage can be performed after myo-

cardial infarction but may be contraindicated in patients with rib fractures, surgical incisions, or other recent traumatic injury to the back.

Equipment
Basin ■ soap ■ bath blanket ■ bath towel ■ washcloth ■ back lotion with lanolin base ■ gloves, if the patient has open lesions or has been incontinent ■ optional: talcum powder.

Preparation of equipment
Fill the basin two-thirds full with warm water. Place the lotion bottle in the basin to warm it. *Application of warmed lotion prevents chilling or startling the patient, thereby reducing muscle tension and vasoconstriction.*

Implementation
• Assemble the equipment at the patient's bedside.
• Explain the procedure to the patient, and provide privacy. Ask him to tell you if you're applying too much or too little pressure.
• Adjust the bed to a comfortable working height and lower the head of the bed, if allowed. Wash your hands and put on gloves, if applicable.
• Place the patient in the prone position, if possible, or on his side. Position him along the edge of the bed nearest you *to prevent back strain.*
• Untie the patient's gown, and expose his back, shoulders, and buttocks. Then drape the patient with a bath blanket *to prevent chills and minimize exposure.* Place a bath towel next to or under the patient's side *to protect bed linens from moisture.*
• Fold the washcloth around your hand to form a mitt. *This prevents the loose ends of the cloth from dripping water onto the patient, and also keeps the cloth warm longer.* Then, work up a lather with soap.
• Using long, firm strokes, bathe the patient's back, beginning at the neck and shoulders and moving downward to the buttocks. Rinse and dry well *because moisture trapped between the buttocks can cause chafing and predispose the patient to formation of pressure ulcers.* While giving back care, closely examine the patient's skin, especially the bony prominences of the shoulders, the scapulae, and the coccyx, for redness or abrasions.
• Remove the warmed lotion bottle from the basin, and pour a small amount of lotion into your palm. Rub your hands together *to distribute the lotion.* Then, apply the lotion to the patient's back, using long, firm strokes. *The lotion reduces friction, making back massage easier.*
• Massage the patient's back, beginning at the base of the spine and moving upward to the shoulders. For a relaxing effect, massage slowly; for a stimulating effect, massage quickly. Alternate the three basic strokes: ef-

How to give a back massage

Three strokes used commonly when giving a back massage are effleurage, friction, and petrissage. Start with effleurage and go on to friction and then to petrissage. Perform each stroke at least six times before moving on to the next, and then repeat the whole series if desired. When performing effleurage and friction, keep your hands parallel to the vertebrae to avoid tickling the patient. For all three strokes, maintain a regular rhythm and steady contact with the patient's back to help him relax.

Effleurage
Using your palm, stroke from the buttocks up to the shoulders, over the upper arms, and back to the buttocks. Use slightly less pressure on the downward strokes.

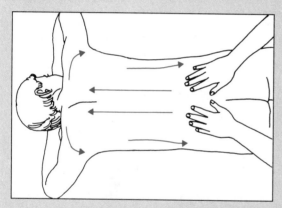

Friction
Use circular thumb strokes to move from buttocks to shoulders; then, using a smooth stroke, return to the buttocks, as shown at the top of the next column.

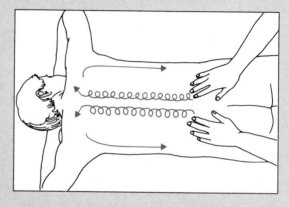

Petrissage
Using your thumb to oppose your fingers, knead and stroke half the back and upper arms, starting at the buttocks and moving toward the shoulder. Then knead and stroke the other half of the back, rhythmically alternating your hands.

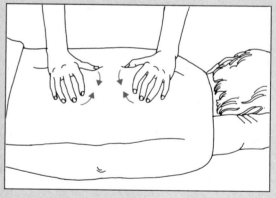

fleurage, friction, and petrissage, as shown in *How to give a back massage*. Add lotion, as needed, keeping one hand on the patient's back *to avoid interrupting the massage*.
• Compress, squeeze, and lift the trapezius muscle *to help relax the patient*.
• Finish the massage by using long, firm strokes, and blot any excess lotion from the patient's back with a towel. Then, retie the patient's gown and straighten or change the bed linens, as necessary.

• Return the bed to its original position, and make the patient comfortable. Empty and clean the basin. Dispose of gloves, if used, and return equipment to the appropriate storage area.

Special considerations
Before giving back care, assess the patient's body structure and skin condition, and tailor the duration and intensity of the massage accordingly. If you're giving back

care at bedtime, have the patient ready for bed beforehand, so the massage can help him fall asleep.

Use separate lotion for each patient *to prevent cross-contamination.* If the patient has oily skin, substitute a talcum powder or lotion of the patient's choice. However, don't use powder if the patient has an endotracheal or tracheal tube in place *to avoid aspiration.* Also, avoid using powder and lotion together *because this may lead to skin maceration.*

When massaging the patient's back, stand with one foot slightly forward and your knees slightly bent *to allow effective use of your arm and shoulder muscles.* Give special attention to bony prominences *because these areas are disposed to formation of pressure ulcers.* Don't massage the patient's legs unless ordered *because reddened legs can signal clot formation, and massage can dislodge the clot, causing an embolus.* Develop a turning schedule and give back care at each position change.

Documentation
Chart back care on the flowchart. Record redness, abrasion, or change in skin condition in your notes.

 # Foot care

Daily bathing of feet and regular trimming of toenails promotes cleanliness, prevents infection, stimulates peripheral circulation, and controls odor by removing debris from between toes and under toenails. It's particularly important for bedridden patients and those especially susceptible to foot infection. Increased susceptibility may be caused by peripheral vascular disease, diabetes mellitus, poor nutritional status, arthritis, or any condition that impairs peripheral circulation. In such patients, proper foot care should include meticulous cleanliness and regular observation for signs of skin breakdown. (See *Foot care for diabetic patients* for additional instructions.)

Toenail trimming is contraindicated in patients with toe infections, diabetes mellitus, neurologic disorders, renal failure, or peripheral vascular disease, unless performed by a doctor or podiatrist.

Equipment
Bath blanket ▪ large basin ▪ soap ▪ towel ▪ linen-saver pad ▪ pillow ▪ washcloth ▪ toenail clippers ▪ orangewood stick ▪ emery board ▪ cotton-tipped applicator ▪ cotton ▪ lotion ▪ water-absorbent powder ▪ bath thermometer ▪ gloves, if the patient has open lesions.

Foot care for diabetic patients

Because diabetes mellitus can reduce blood supply to the feet, normally minor foot injuries can lead to dangerous infection. When caring for a diabetic patient, keep these foot care guidelines in mind:
• Exercising the feet daily can help improve circulation. While the patient is sitting on the edge of the bed, ask him to point his toes upward, then downward, 10 times. Then have him make a circle with each foot 10 times.
• A diabetic's shoes must fit properly. Instruct the patient to break in new shoes gradually by increasing wearing time by 30 minutes each day. Also tell him to check his old shoes frequently in case they develop rough spots in the lining.
• Tell the patient to wear clean socks daily and to avoid socks with holes, darned spots, or rough, irritating seams.
• Advise the patient to see a doctor if he has corns or calluses.
• Tell the patient to wear warm socks or slippers and use extra blankets to avoid cold feet. He should not use heating pads and hot water bottles because these may cause burns.
• Teach the patient to regularly inspect the skin on his feet for cuts, cracks, blisters, or red, swollen areas. Even slight cuts on the feet should receive a doctor's attention. As a first-aid measure, tell him to wash the cut thoroughly and apply a mild antiseptic. Urge him to avoid harsh antiseptics, such as iodine, because they can damage tissue.
• Advise the diabetic patient to avoid tight-fitting garments or activities that can decrease circulation. The patient should especially avoid wearing elastic garters, sitting with knees crossed, picking at sores or rough spots on the feet, walking barefoot, or applying adhesive tape to the skin on his feet.

Preparation of equipment
Fill the basin halfway with warm water. Test water temperature with a bath thermometer *because patients with diminished peripheral sensation could burn their feet in excessively hot water (over 105° F [40.6° C]) without feeling any warning pain.* If a bath thermometer is unavailable, test the water by inserting your elbow. The water temperature should feel comfortably warm.

Implementation
• Assemble equipment at the patient's bedside. Wash your hands and put on gloves, if necessary.
• Tell the patient that you'll wash his feet and provide foot and toenail care.
• Cover the patient with a bath blanket. Fanfold the top linen to the foot of the bed.
• Place a linen-saver pad and a towel under the patient's feet *to keep the bottom linen dry.* Then position the basin on the pad.
• Insert a pillow beneath the patient's knee *to provide support,* and cushion the rim of the basin with the edge of the towel *to prevent pressure.*
• Immerse one foot in the basin. Wash it with soap, then allow it to soak for about 10 minutes. *Soaking softens the skin and toenails, loosens debris under toenails, and comforts and refreshes the patient.*
• After soaking the foot, rinse it with a washcloth, remove it from the basin, and place it on the towel.
• Dry the foot thoroughly, especially between the toes, *to avoid skin breakdown.* Blot gently to dry *because harsh rubbing may damage the skin.*
• Empty the basin, refill it with warm water, and clean and soak the other foot.
• While the second foot is soaking, give the first one a pedicure. Using the cotton-tipped applicator, carefully clean the toenails. Using an orangewood stick, gently remove any dirt beneath the toenails; avoid injuring subungual skin.
• Trim nails with toenail clippers, if needed, by cutting straight across *to prevent ingrown toenails.* Clip small sections of the nail at a time, starting at one edge and working across. File trimmed toenails with an emery board to smooth rough edges. *Keeping toenails trimmed and filed prevents scratching and injury to the skin on the opposite leg.*
• Rinse the foot that has been soaking, dry it thoroughly, and give it a pedicure.
• Apply lotion *to moisten dry skin,* or lightly dust water-absorbent powder between the toes *to absorb moisture.*
• Remove and clean all equipment and dispose of gloves.

Special considerations
While providing foot care, observe the color, shape, and texture of the toenails. If you see redness, drying, cracking, blisters, discoloration, or other signs of traumatic injury, especially in patients with impaired peripheral circulation, notify the doctor. *Because such patients are vulnerable to infection and gangrene, they need prompt treatment.*

If a patient's toenail grows inward at the corners, tuck a wisp of cotton under it *to relieve pressure on the toe.*

When giving the bedridden patient foot care, unless contraindicated, perform range-of-motion exercises *to stimulate circulation and prevent foot contractures or muscle atrophy.* Tuck folded 2″ × 2″ gauze pads between overlapping toes *to protect the skin from the toenails.* Apply heel protectors *to prevent skin breakdown.*

Documentation
Record the date and time of bathing and toenail trimming in your notes. Record and report any abnormal findings and any nursing actions you take.

Perineal care

Perineal care, including the external genitalia and the anal area, should be performed during the daily bath and, if necessary, at bedtime and after urination and bowel movements. The procedure promotes cleanliness and prevents infection. It also removes irritating and odorous secretions, such as smegma, a cheeselike substance that collects under the foreskin of the penis and on the inner surface of the labia. For the patient with perineal skin breakdown, frequent bathing followed by application of an ointment or cream aids healing.

Universal precautions must be followed when providing perineal care, with due consideration given to the patient's privacy.

Equipment
Gloves ▪ washcloths ▪ clean basin ▪ mild soap ▪ bath towel ▪ bath blanket ▪ toilet tissue ▪ linen-saver pad ▪ trash bag ▪ optional: bedpan, peri bottle, antiseptic soap, petroleum jelly, zinc oxide cream, vitamin A and D ointment, and an ABD pad.

Following genital or rectal surgery, you may need to use sterile supplies, including sterile gloves, gauze, and cotton balls.

Preparation of equipment
Obtain ointment or cream, as needed. Fill the basin two-thirds full with warm water. Also, fill the peri bottle with warm water, if needed.

Implementation
• Assemble equipment at the patient's bedside. Provide privacy.
• Wash your hands thoroughly, put on gloves, and tell the patient what you're about to do.
• Adjust the bed to a comfortable working height *to prevent back strain,* and lower the head of the bed, if allowed.

• Provide privacy and help the patient to a supine position. Place a linen-saver pad under the patient's buttocks *to protect the bed from stains and moisture.*

Perineal care for the female patient
• To minimize the patient's exposure and embarrassment, place the bath blanket over her with corners head to foot and side to side. Wrap each leg with a side corner, tucking it under the hip. Then fold back the corner between the legs to expose the perineum.
• Ask the patient to bend her knees slightly and to spread her legs. Separate her labia with one hand and wash with the other, using gentle downward strokes from the front to the back of the perineum *to prevent intestinal organisms from contaminating the urethra or vagina.* Avoid the area around the anus, and use a clean section of washcloth for each stroke by folding each used section inward. *This prevents the spread of contaminated secretions or discharge.*
• Using a clean washcloth, rinse thoroughly from front to back *because soap residue can cause skin irritation.* Pat the area dry with a bath towel *because moisture can also cause skin irritation and discomfort.*
• Apply ordered ointments or creams.
• Turn the patient on her side to Sims' position, if possible, *to expose the anal area.*
• Clean, rinse, and dry the anal area, starting at the posterior vaginal opening and wiping from front to back.

Perineal care for the male patient
• Drape the patient's legs *to minimize exposure and embarrassment* and expose the genital area.
• Hold the shaft of the penis with one hand and wash with the other, beginning at the tip and working in a circular motion from the center to the periphery *to avoid introducing microorganisms into the urethra.* Use a clean section of washcloth for each stroke *to prevent the spread of contaminated secretions or discharge.*
• Rinse thoroughly, using the same circular motion.
• For the uncircumcised patient, gently retract the foreskin and clean beneath it. Rinse well but don't dry *because moisture provides lubrication and prevents friction when replacing the foreskin.* Replace the foreskin *to avoid constriction of the penis, which causes edema and tissue damage.*
• Wash the rest of the penis, using downward strokes toward the scrotum. Rinse well and pat dry with a bath towel.
• Clean the top and sides of the scrotum; rinse thoroughly and pat dry. Handle the scrotum gently *to avoid causing discomfort.*
• Turn the patient on his side. Clean the bottom of the scrotum and the anal area. Rinse well and pat dry.

After providing perineal care
• Reposition the patient and make him comfortable. Remove the bath blanket and linen-saver pad, and then replace the bed linens.
• Clean and return the basin and dispose of soiled articles including gloves.

Special considerations
Give perineal care to a patient of the opposite sex in a matter-of-fact way *to minimize embarrassment.*

If the patient is incontinent, first remove excess feces with toilet tissue. Then position him on a bedpan, and add a small amount of antiseptic soap to a peri bottle *to eliminate odor.* Irrigate the perineal area *to remove any remaining fecal matter.*

After cleaning the perineum, apply ointment or cream (petroleum jelly, zinc oxide cream, or vitamin A and D ointment) *to prevent skin breakdown by providing a barrier between the skin and excretions.*

To reduce the number of linen changes, tuck an ABD pad between the patient's buttocks *to absorb oozing feces.*

Documentation
Record perineal care and any special treatment in your notes. Document the need for continued treatment, if necessary, in your care plan. Describe perineal skin condition and any odor or discharge.

 Hour of sleep care

Hour of sleep (h.s.) care meets the patient's physical and psychological needs in preparation for sleep. It includes providing for the patient's hygiene, making the bed clean and comfortable, and ensuring safety. For example, raising the bed's side rails can prevent the drowsy or sedated patient from falling out. Bedtime care also provides an opportunity to answer the patient's questions about the next day's tests and procedures and to discuss his worries and concerns.

Effective h.s. care prepares the patient for a good night's sleep. Ineffective care may contribute to sleeplessness, which can intensify patient anxiety and interfere with treatment and recuperation.

Equipment
Bedpan, urinal, or commode ■ basin ■ soap ■ towel ■ washcloth ■ toothbrush and toothpaste ■ denture cup and commercial denture cleaner, if necessary ■ lotion ■ clean linens, if necessary ■ blankets ■ facial tissues ■ soft restraints, if necessary.

Recording fluid intake and output

Accurate intake and output records help evaluate a patient's fluid and electrolyte balance, suggest various diagnoses, and influence the choice of fluid therapy. These records are mandatory for patients with burns, renal failure, electrolyte imbalance, recent surgical procedures, congestive heart failure, or severe vomiting and diarrhea, and for those patients receiving diuretics or corticosteroids. Intake and output records are also significant in monitoring patients with nasogastric tubes, drainage collection devices, or those receiving I.V. therapy.

Fluid intake comprises all fluid entering the patient's body, including beverages, fluids contained in solid foods taken by mouth, and foods that are liquid at room temperature, such as flavored gelatin, custard, ice cream, and some beverages. Additional intake includes G.I. instillations, bladder irrigations, and I.V. fluids.

Fluid output includes all fluid that leaves the patient's body, including urine, loose stools, vomitus, aspirated fluid loss, and drainage from surgical drains, nasogastric tubes, and chest tubes.

When recording fluid intake and output, enlist the patient's help if possible. Record amounts in cubic centimeters (cc) or milliliters (ml). Measure, don't estimate. For a small child, weigh diapers if appropriate. Monitor intake and output during each shift, and notify the doctor if amounts differ significantly over a 24-hour period. Document your findings in the appropriate location; describe any fluid restrictions and the patient's compliance.

Preparation of equipment

Assemble the equipment at the patient's bedside. For the ambulatory patient who is capable of self-care, assemble soap, a washcloth, a towel, and oral hygiene items at the sink.

Implementation

• Tell the patient you will help him prepare for sleep, and provide privacy.
• Offer the patient on bed rest a bedpan, urinal, or commode. Otherwise, assist the ambulatory patient to the bathroom.
• Fill the basin with warm water and bring it to the patient's bedside. Immerse the lotion in the basin *to warm it for back massage.* Then wash the patient's face and

hands and dry them well. Encourage the patient to do this himself, if possible, *to promote independence.*
• Provide toothpaste or a properly labeled denture cup and commercial denture cleaner. Assist the patient with oral hygiene, as necessary. (See "Mouth care" in this chapter.) If the patient prefers to wear dentures until bedtime, leave denture-care items within easy reach.
• After providing mouth care, turn the patient on his side or stomach. Wash, rinse, and dry the patient's back and buttocks. Massage well with lotion *to help relax the patient.* (See "Back care" in this chapter for complete information on massage.) While providing back care, observe the skin for redness, cracking, or other signs of breakdown. If the patient's gown is soiled or damp, provide a clean one and help him put it on, if necessary.
• Check dressings, binders, antiembolism stockings, or other aids, changing or readjusting them as needed.
• Refill the water container, and place it and a box of facial tissues within the patient's easy reach *to prevent falls if patient needs to reach for these items.*
• Straighten or change bed linens, as necessary, and fluff the patient's pillow. Cover him with a blanket or place one within his easy reach *to prevent chills during the night.* Then position him comfortably. If he appears distressed, restless, or in pain, give ordered drugs, as needed.
• After making the patient comfortable, evaluate his mental and physical condition. Then, if ordered and in accord with hospital policy, apply soft restraints *to prevent falls.* Place the bed in a low position and raise the side rails. Place the call button within the patient's easy reach, and instruct him to call you whenever necessary. Next, tidy the patient's environment: Move all breakables from the overbed table out of his reach, and remove any equipment and supplies that could cause falls should the patient get up during the night. Finally, turn off the overhead light and put on the night-light.

Special considerations

Ask the patient about his sleep routine at home and, whenever possible, let him follow it. Also try to observe certain rituals, such as a bedtime snack, *which can aid sleep.* A back massage, a tub bath, or a shower also help relax the patient and promote a restful night. If the patient normally bathes or showers before bedtime, let him do so in the hospital if his condition and doctor's orders permit it.

Documentation

Record the time and type of h.s. care in your notes. Include application of soft restraints or any other special procedures.

NUTRITION AND ELIMINATION
Feeding

Confusion, arm or hand immobility, injury, weakness, or restrictions on activities or positions may prevent a patient from feeding himself. Feeding the patient then becomes a key nursing responsibility. Injured or debilitated patients may experience depression and subsequent anorexia. Meeting such patients' nutritional needs requires determining food preferences, conducting the feeding in a friendly, unhurried manner, encouraging self-feeding to promote independence and dignity, and documenting intake and output. (See *Recording fluid intake and output.)*

Equipment
Meal tray ■ overbed table ■ linen-saver pad or towels ■ clean linens ■ flexible straws ■ basin of water ■ feeding syringe ■ assistive feeding devices, if necessary.

Implementation
● *Because many adults consider being fed demeaning,* be sure to allow the patient some control over mealtime. For example, let the patient set the pace of the meal or determine the order in which he eats the various foods.
● Raise the head of the bed if allowed. *Fowler's or semi-Fowler's position makes swallowing easier and reduces the risk of aspiration and choking.*
● Before the meal tray arrives, give the patient soap, a basin of water or a wet washcloth, and a hand towel *to clean his hands.* If necessary, you may wash his hands for him.
● Wipe the overbed table with soap and water or alcohol, especially if a urinal or bedpan had been placed on it.
● When the meal tray arrives, compare the name on the tray with the name on the patient's wristband. Check the tray to be sure it contains foods appropriate for the patient's condition.
● Encourage the patient to feed himself if he's able. If the patient is restricted to the prone or the supine position but can use his arms and hands, encourage him to try foods he can pick up, such as sandwiches. If he can assume the Fowler's or semi-Fowler's position but has limited use of his arms or hands, instruct him in the use of assistive feeding devices. (See *Using assistive feeding devices,* page 98.)
● If necessary, tuck a napkin or towel under his chin *to protect his gown from spills.* Use a linen-saver pad or towel *to protect bed linens.*
● Position a chair next to the patient's bed *so you can sit comfortably if you need to feed him yourself.*

Arranging food for the visually impaired patient

To help the blind or visually impaired patient feed himself, tell him that placement of various foods on his plate corresponds to the hours on a clock face. Maintain consistent placement for subsequent meals. The illustration shows meat at 12 o'clock, a vegetable at 6 o'clock, and rice at 9 o'clock.

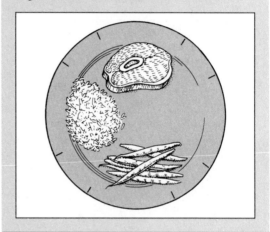

● Set up the patient's tray, remove the plate from the tray warmer, and discard all plastic wrappings. Then cut the food into bite-sized pieces and prepare it, as necessary. Arrange food on the plate, if necessary. (See *Arranging food for the visually impaired patient.)*
● Ask the patient which food he prefers to eat first *to promote his sense of control over the meal.* Some patients prefer to eat one food at a time, while others prefer to alternate foods.
● If the patient has difficulty swallowing, offer liquids carefully with a spoon or feeding syringe *to help prevent aspiration.* Pureed or soft foods, such as custard or flavored gelatin, may be easier to swallow than liquids. If the patient doesn't have difficulty swallowing, use a flexible straw *to reduce the risk of spills.*
● Ask the patient to indicate when he's ready for another mouthful. Pause between courses and whenever the patient wants to rest. During the meal, wipe the patient's mouth and chin, as necessary.
● When the patient finishes eating, remove the tray. If necessary, clean up spills and change the bed linens. Provide mouth care.

EQUIPMENT

Using assistive feeding devices

Various feeding devices can help the patient who has limited arm mobility, grasp, range of motion, or coordination. Before introducing your patient to an assistive feeding device, assess his ability to master it. Don't introduce a device he can't manage. If his condition is progressively disabling, encourage him to use the device only until his mastery of it falters.

Introduce the assistive device before mealtime, with the patient seated in a natural position. Explain its purpose, show the patient how to use it, and encourage him to practice. After meals, wash the device thoroughly and store it in the patient's bedside stand. Document the patient's progress and share it with staff and family members to help reinforce the patient's independence. Specific devices include the following:

Plate guard
This device blocks food from spilling off the plate. Attach the guard to the side of the plate opposite the hand the patient uses to feed himself. Guiding the patient's hand, show him how to push food against the guard to secure it on the utensil. Then have him try again with food of a different consistency. When the patient tires, feed him the rest of the meal. At subsequent meals, encourage the patient to feed himself for progressively longer periods until he can feed himself an entire meal.

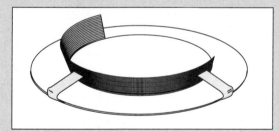

Swivel spoon
This utensil helps the patient with limited range of motion in his forearm and will fit in universal cuffs.

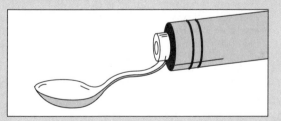

Universal cuffs
These flexible bands help the patient with flail hands or diminished grasp. Each cuff contains a slot that holds a fork or spoon. Attach the cuff to the hand the patient uses to feed himself. Then place the fork or spoon in the cuff slot. Bend the utensil to facilitate feeding.

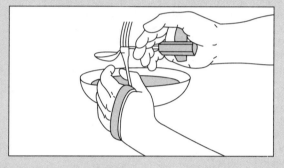

Long-handled utensils
These utensils have jointed stems to help the patient with limited range of motion in his elbow and shoulder.

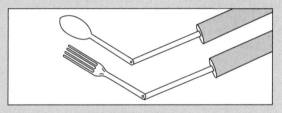

Utensils with built-up handles
These utensils can help the patient with diminished grasp. They can be purchased or can be improvised by wrapping tape around the handles.

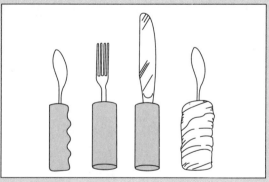

Special considerations

Don't feed the patient too quickly *because this can upset him and impair digestion.*

If the patient is restricted to the prone position, give foods that he can chew easily. If he's restricted to the supine position, feed him liquids carefully and only after he has swallowed any food in his mouth *to reduce the risk of aspiration.*

If the patient's food intake is inadequate because of chronic poor eating habits or anorexia, offer small, frequent meals *to provide a well-balanced diet.* If the patient won't eat, try to find out why. For example, confirm his food preferences. Also, make sure the patient isn't in pain at mealtimes or that he hasn't received any treatments immediately before a meal that could upset or nauseate him. Find out if any of his medications cause anorexia, nausea, or sedation. Of course, clear the bedside of emesis basins, urinals, bedpans, and similar distractions at mealtimes.

Establish a pattern for feeding the patient, and share this information with the rest of the nursing staff *so the patient doesn't need to repeatedly instruct staff members about the best way to feed him.*

If the patient and his family are willing, suggest that family members assist with feeding. This will make the patient feel more comfortable at mealtimes and may facilitate discharge planning.

Complications

Choking and aspiration of food can occur if the patient is fed too quickly or is given excessively large mouthfuls.

Documentation

Describe the feeding technique used in the nursing care plan to ensure continuity of care. In your notes, record the amount of food and fluid consumed; also note the fluids consumed on the intake and output record, if required. Note which foods the patient consistently fails to eat, then try to find the reason. Record the patient's level of independence. For the blind patient, record the pattern of feeding on the nursing care plan.

Bedpan and urinal

These devices permit elimination by the bedridden patient and accurate observation and measurement of urine and stool by the nurse. A bedpan is used by the female patient for defecation and urination and by the male patient for defecation; a urinal is used by the male patient for urination. Either device should be offered frequently — before meals, visiting hours, morning and evening care, and before any treatments or procedures. Whenever possible, allow the patient to use a bedpan or urinal in privacy.

Equipment

Bedpan or urinal with cover ▪ toilet tissue ▪ two washcloths ▪ soap ▪ gloves ▪ towel ▪ linen-saver pad ▪ bath blanket ▪ pillow ▪ optional: air freshener, talcum powder.

Available in adult and pediatric sizes, the bedpan may be disposable or reusable (the latter can be sterilized). The fracture pan, a type of bedpan, is used when spinal injuries, body or leg casts, or other conditions prohibit or restrict turning the patient. Like the bedpan, the urinal may be disposable or reusable.

Preparation of equipment

Obtain the appropriate bedpan or urinal. If you're using a metal bedpan, warm it under running water *to avoid startling the patient and stimulating muscle contraction, which hinders elimination.* Dry the bedpan thoroughly and test its temperature *because metal retains heat.* If necessary, lightly sprinkle talcum powder on the edge of the bedpan *to reduce friction during placement and removal.* For a thin patient, place a linen-saver pad at the edge of the bedpan *to minimize pressure on the coccyx.*

Implementation

• If the patient's condition permits, provide privacy. Put on gloves *to prevent contact with body fluids and comply with universal precautions.*

To place a bedpan

• If allowed, elevate the head of the bed slightly *to prevent hyperextension of the spine when the patient raises the buttocks.*

• Rest the bedpan on the edge of the bed. Then, turn down the corner of the top linens and draw up the patient's gown. Ask him to raise the buttocks by flexing his knees and pushing down on his heels. While supporting the patient's lower back with one hand, center the curved, smooth edge of the bedpan beneath the buttocks.

• If the patient cannot raise his buttocks, lower the head of the bed to horizontal and help the patient roll onto one side, with buttocks toward you. Position the bedpan properly against the buttocks, and then help the patient roll back onto the bedpan. Once the patient is positioned comfortably, raise the head of the bed as indicated.

• After positioning the bedpan, elevate the head of the bed further, if allowed, until the patient is sitting erect. *Because this position resembles the normal elimination posture, it aids in defecation and urination.* (See *Using a com-*

Using a commode

An alternative to a bedpan, a commode is a portable chair made of wood, plastic, or metal, with a large opening in the center of the seat. It may have a bedpan or bucket that slides underneath the opening, or it may slide directly over the toilet, adding height to the standard toilet seat. Unlike a bedpan, a commode allows the patient to assume his normal elimination posture, which aids in defecation.

Before the patient uses it, inspect the commode's condition and make sure it is clean. Roll or carry the commode to the patient's room. Place it parallel and as close as possible to the patient's bed, and secure its brakes or wheel locks. If necessary, block its wheels with sandbags. Assist the patient onto the commode, provide toilet tissue, and place the call button within his reach. Instruct the patient to push the call button when he has finished.

If necessary, assist the patient with cleaning. Help him into bed and make him comfortable. Offer the patient soap, water, and a towel to wash his hands. Then close the lid of the commode or cover the bucket. Roll the commode or carry the bucket to the bathroom or hopper room. If ordered, observe and measure the contents before disposal. Rinse and clean the bucket, and then spray or wipe the bucket and commode seat with disinfectant. Use an air freshener if appropriate.

mode for another implement that permits normal elimination posture.)
• If elevation of the head of the bed is contraindicated, tuck a small pillow or folded bath blanket under the patient's back *to cushion the sacrum against the edge of the bedpan and support the lumbar region.*
• If the patient can be left alone, place the bed in a low position and raise the side rails *to ensure his safety.* Place toilet tissue and the call button within the patient's reach, and instruct him to push the button after elimination. If the patient is weak or disoriented, remain with him.
• Before removing the bedpan, lower the head of the bed slightly. Then ask the patient to raise his buttocks off the bed. Support the lower back with one hand, and gently remove the bedpan with the other *to avoid skin injury caused by friction.* If the patient cannot raise his buttocks, ask him to roll off the pan while you assist with one

hand. Hold the pan firmly with the other hand to avoid spills. Cover the bedpan and place it on the chair.
• Assist with cleaning the anal and perineal area, as necessary, *to prevent irritation and infection.* Turn the patient on his side, wipe carefully with toilet tissue, clean the area with a damp washcloth and soap, and dry well with a towel. For the female patient, clean from front to back *to avoid introducing rectal contaminants into the vaginal or urethral openings.*

To place a urinal
• Lift the corner of the top linens, hand the urinal to the patient, and allow him to position it.
• If the patient can't position the urinal himself, spread his legs slightly and hold the urinal in place *to prevent spills.*
• After the patient voids, carefully withdraw the urinal.

After use of a bedpan or urinal
• Give the patient a clean, damp, warm washcloth for his hands. Check the bed linens for wetness or soiling, and straighten or change them, if needed. Make the patient comfortable. Place the bed in the low position and raise the side rails.
• Take the bedpan or urinal to the bathroom or hopper room. Observe the color, odor, amount, and consistency of its contents. If ordered, measure urine output or liquid stool, or obtain a specimen for laboratory analysis.
• Empty the bedpan or urinal into the toilet or hopper. Rinse with cold water and clean it thoroughly, using a disinfectant solution. Dry and return it to the patient's bedside stand.
• Use an air freshener, if necessary, *to eliminate offensive odors and reduce the patient's embarrassment.*
• Remove gloves and wash your hands.

Special considerations
Explain to the patient that drug treatment and changes in his environment, diet, and activities may disrupt his usual elimination schedule. Try to anticipate elimination needs, and offer the bedpan or urinal frequently *to help reduce embarrassment and minimize the risk of incontinence.* Avoid placing a bedpan or urinal on top of the bedside stand or overbed table *to avoid contamination of clean equipment and food trays.* Similarly, avoid placing it on the floor *to prevent the spread of microorganisms from the floor to the patient's bed linens when the device is used.*

If the patient feels pain during turning or feels uncomfortable on a standard bedpan, use a fracture pan. Unlike the standard bedpan, the fracture pan is slipped under the buttocks from the front rather than the side. Because it's shallower than the standard bedpan, you need only lift the patient slightly to position it. If the patient is obese or otherwise difficult to lift, ask a co-worker to help you.

If the patient has an indwelling urinary catheter in place, carefully position and remove the bedpan *to avoid tension on the catheter, which could dislodge it or irritate the urethra.* After the patient defecates, wipe, clean, and dry the anal region, taking care to avoid catheter contamination. If necessary, clean the urinary meatus with povidone-iodine solution.

Documentation

Record the time, date, and type of elimination on the flowchart and the amount of urine output or liquid stool on the intake and output record, as needed. In your notes, document the presence of blood, pus, or other abnormal characteristics in urine or stool.

 # Male incontinence device

Many patients don't require an indwelling urinary catheter to manage their incontinence. For male patients, a male incontinence device reduces the risk of urinary tract infection from catheterization, promotes bladder retraining when possible, helps prevent skin breakdown, and improves the patient's self-image. The device consists of a condom catheter secured to the shaft of the penis and connected to a leg bag or drainage bag. It has no contraindications, but can cause skin irritation and edema.

Equipment

Condom catheter ▪ drainage bag ▪ extension tubing ▪ nonallergenic tape or incontinence sheath holder ▪ commercial adhesive strip or skin-bond cement ▪ elastic adhesive or Velcro, if needed ▪ gloves ▪ razor, if needed ▪ basin ▪ soap ▪ washcloth ▪ towel.

Preparation of equipment

Fill the basin with lukewarm water. Then, bring the basin and the remaining equipment to the patient's bedside.

Implementation

● Explain the procedure to the patient, wash your hands thoroughly, put on gloves, and provide privacy.

Applying the device

● If the patient is circumcised, wash the penis with soap and water, rinse well, and pat dry with a towel. If the patient is uncircumcised, gently retract the foreskin and clean beneath it. Rinse well but don't dry *because moisture provides lubrication and prevents friction during foreskin*

replacement. Replace the foreskin *to avoid penile constriction.* Then, if necessary, shave the base and shaft of the penis *to prevent the adhesive strip or skin-bond cement from pulling pubic hair.*

● If you're using a precut commercial adhesive strip, insert the glans penis through its opening, and position the strip 1″ (2.5 cm) from the scrotal area. If you're using uncut adhesive, cut a strip to fit around the shaft of the penis. Remove the protective covering from one side of the adhesive strip and press this side firmly to the penis *to enhance adhesion.* Then remove the covering from the other side of the strip. If a commercial adhesive strip isn't available, apply skin-bond cement and let it dry for a few minutes.

● Position the rolled condom catheter at the tip of the penis, with its drainage opening at the urinary meatus.

● Unroll the catheter upward, past the adhesive strip on the shaft of the penis. Then gently press the sheath against the strip until it adheres. (See *How to apply a condom catheter,* page 102.)

● After the condom catheter is in place, secure it with hypoallergenic tape or an incontinence sheath holder.

● Using extension tubing, connect the condom catheter to the leg bag or drainage bag. Remove and discard your gloves.

Removing the device

● Don gloves and simultaneously roll the condom catheter and adhesive strip off the penis and discard them. If you've used skin-bond cement rather than an adhesive strip, remove it with solvent. Also remove and discard the nonallergenic tape or incontinence sheath holder.

● Clean the penis with lukewarm water, rinse thoroughly, and dry. Check for swelling or signs of skin breakdown.

● Remove the leg bag by closing the drain clamp, unlatching the leg straps, and disconnecting the extension tubing at the top of the bag. Discard your gloves.

Special considerations

If nonallergenic tape or an incontinence sheath holder isn't available, secure the condom with a strip of elastic adhesive or Velcro. Apply the strip snugly — but not too tightly — *to prevent circulatory constriction.*

Inspect the condom catheter for twists and the extension tubing for kinks *to prevent obstruction of urine flow, which could cause the condom to balloon, eventually dislodging it.*

Documentation

Record the date and time of application and removal of the incontinence device. Also note skin condition and the patient's response to the device, including voiding pattern, to assist with bladder retraining.

How to apply a condom catheter

Apply an adhesive strip to the shaft of the penis about 1″ (2.5 cm) from the scrotal area.

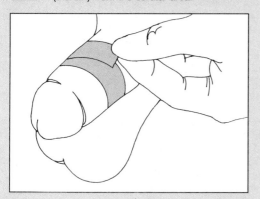

Then roll the condom catheter onto the penis past the adhesive strip, leaving about ½″ (1.3 cm) of clearance at the end. Press the sheath gently against the strip until it adheres.

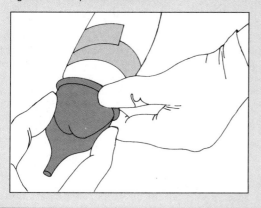

Credé's maneuver

When lower motor neuron damage impairs the voiding reflex, the urinary bladder may become flaccid or areflexic. Because the bladder fails to contract properly, urine collects inside it, causing distention. Credé's maneuver — application of manual pressure over the lower abdomen — promotes complete emptying of the bladder. After appropriate instruction, the patient can perform this maneuver himself, unless he cannot reach his lower abdomen or lacks sufficient strength and dexterity. Even when performed properly, however, Credé's maneuver isn't always successful and doesn't always eliminate the need for catheterization.

Credé's maneuver cannot be used after abdominal surgery if the incision is not completely healed. When using Credé's maneuver, close monitoring of urine output is necessary to help detect possible infection from accumulation of residual urine.

Equipment
Bedpan, urinal, or bedside commode.

Implementation
• Explain the procedure to the patient and wash your hands.
• If allowed, place the patient in Fowler's position and position the bedpan or urinal. Alternatively, if the patient's condition permits, assist him onto the bedside commode.
• Place your hands flat on the patient's abdomen just below the umbilicus. Ask the female patient to bend forward from the hips. Then, firmly stroke downward toward the bladder about six times *to stimulate the voiding reflex.*
• Place one hand on top of the other above the pubic arch. Press firmly inward and downward *to compress the bladder and expel residual urine.*

Special considerations
After the patient has learned the procedure and can use Credé's maneuver successfully, measuring the expelled urine may not be necessary. The patient may then use the maneuver to void directly into the toilet.

Documentation
Record the date and time of the procedure and the amount of urine expelled.

Digital removal of fecal impaction

Fecal impaction — a large, hard, dry mass of stool in the folds of the rectum and, at times, in the sigmoid colon — results from prolonged retention and accumulation of stool. Common causes include poor bowel habits, inactivity, dehydration, improper diet (especially inadequate fluid intake), constipation-inducing drugs, and incomplete bowel cleaning after a barium enema or barium swallow. Digital removal of fecal impaction, which is used when oil retention and cleansing enemas, suppositories, and laxatives fail to clear the impaction, may require a doctor's order.

This procedure is contraindicated during pregnancy; after rectal, genitourinary, abdominal, perineal, or gynecologic reconstructive surgery; in patients with myocardial infarction, coronary insufficiency, pulmonary embolus, congestive heart failure, heart block, and Stokes-Adams syndrome (without pacemaker treatment); and in patients with GI or vaginal bleeding, hemorrhoids, rectal polyps, or blood dyscrasias.

Equipment

Gloves (2 pairs) ■ linen-saver pad ■ bedpan ■ plastic disposal bag ■ soap ■ water-filled basin ■ towel ■ water-soluble lubricant ■ washcloth.

Implementation

• Explain the procedure to the patient and provide privacy.
• Position the patient on his left side and flex his knees *to allow easier access to the sigmoid colon and rectum.* Drape the patient, and place a linen-saver pad beneath the buttocks *to prevent soiling the bed linens.*
• Put on gloves, and moisten an index finger with water-soluble lubricant *to reduce friction during insertion, thereby avoiding injury to sensitive tissue.*
• Instruct the patient to breathe deeply *to promote relaxation.* Then gently insert the lubricated index finger beyond the anal sphincter until you touch the impaction. Rotate the finger gently around the stool *to dislodge and break it into small fragments.* Then work the fragments downward to the end of the rectum, and remove each one separately.
• Before removing the finger, gently stimulate the anal sphincter with a circular motion two or three times *to increase peristalsis and encourage evacuation.*
• Remove the finger and change your gloves. Then clean the anal area with soap and a basin of water and lightly pat dry with a towel.
• Offer the patient the bedpan or commode *because digital manipulation stimulates the urge to defecate.*
• Place disposable items in the plastic bag and discard properly. If necessary, clean the bedpan and return it to the bedside stand.
• Wash your hands.

Special considerations

If the patient experiences pain, nausea, rectal bleeding, changes in pulse rate or skin color, diaphoresis, or syncope, stop immediately and notify the doctor.

Complications

Digital removal of fecal impaction can stimulate the vagus nerve and may decrease heart rate and cause syncope.

Documentation

Record the time and date of the procedure, the patient's response, and stool color, consistency, and odor.

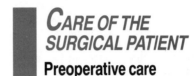

CARE OF THE SURGICAL PATIENT
Preoperative care

Preoperative care begins when the patient's surgery is planned and ends with the administration of anesthesia. This phase of care includes a preoperative interview and assessment to collect baseline subjective and objective data from the patient and his family; diagnostic tests such as urinalysis, electrocardiogram, and chest radiography; preoperative teaching; securing informed consent from the patient; and physical preparation.

Equipment

Gloves ■ thermometer ■ sphygmomanometer ■ stethoscope ■ watch with second hand ■ weight scale ■ tape measure.

Preparation of equipment

Assemble all equipment needed at the patient's bedside or in the admission area.

Implementation

• Obtain a health history and assess the patient's knowledge, perceptions, and expectations about his surgery. Ask about previous medical and surgical interventions. Also determine the patient's psychosocial needs; ask about occupational well-being, financial matters, support systems, mental status, and cultural beliefs. Use your institution's preoperative surgical assessment data base, if available, to gather this information. Obtain a drug history. Ask about current prescription and over-the-counter medications, and about known allergies to foods and drugs.
• Measure the patient's height, weight, and vital signs.
• Identify risk factors that may interfere with a positive expected outcome. Be sure to consider age, general health, medications, mobility, nutritional status, fluid and electrolyte disturbances, and life-style. Also consider the

Obtaining informed consent

Informed consent means that the patient is entitled to a full explanation of the procedure, its risks and complications, and the risk if the procedure isn't performed at this time. Although obtaining informed consent is the doctor's responsibility, the nurse is responsible for verifying that this step has been taken.

You may be asked to witness the patient's signature. However, if you didn't hear the doctor's explanation to the patient, you must sign that you are witnessing the patient's signature only.

Consent forms must be signed before the patient receives his preoperative medication because forms signed after sedatives are given are legally invalid. Adults and emancipated minors can sign their own consent forms. Children's consent forms, or those of adults with impaired mental status, must be signed by a parent or guardian.

primary disorder's duration, location, and nature, and the extent of the surgical procedure.

• Explain preoperative procedures to the patient. Include typical events that the patient can expect. Discuss equipment that may be used postoperatively, such as nasogastric tubes and I.V. equipment. Explain the typical incision, dressings, and staples or sutures that will be used. *Preoperative teaching can help reduce postoperative anxiety and pain, increase patient compliance, hasten recovery, and decrease length of hospital stay.*

• Talk the patient through the sequence of events from operating room to recovery room (postanesthesia care unit or PACU) back to patient's room. Some patients may be transferred from the PACU to an intensive care unit or surgical care unit. Your patient may also benefit from a tour of the areas he will see during the perioperative events.

• Tell the patient about exercises that he may be expected to perform after surgery, such as deep breathing, coughing (while splinting the incision if necessary), extremity exercises, and movement and ambulation *to minimize respiratory and circulatory complications.* If the patient will undergo ophthalmic or neurologic surgery, he won't be asked to cough *because coughing increases intracranial pressure.*

• If the patient is to receive patient-controlled anesthesia (PCA) postoperatively, teach him about the technique. Urge him to push the medication button on the unit only when he feels pain—not when he is tired, sleepy, or is

pain-free. (See "Use of I.V. controllers and pumps," Chapter 6, for more information on PCA.)

• On the day of surgery, important interventions include giving morning care, verifying that the patient has signed an informed consent form (see *Obtaining informed consent*), administering ordered preoperative medications, completing the preoperative checklist and chart, and providing support to the patient and his family.

• Other immediate preoperative interventions may include preparing the GI tract (restricting food and fluids for about 8 hours before surgery) *to reduce vomiting and the risk of aspiration,* cleaning the lower GI tract of fecal material by enemas before abdominal or GI surgery, and giving antibiotics for 2 or 3 days preoperatively *to prevent contamination of the peritoneal cavity by GI bacteria.*

• Just before the patient is moved to the surgical area, make sure he's wearing a hospital gown, has his identification band in place, and has his vital signs recorded. Check to see that hairpins, nail polish, and jewelry have been removed. Note whether dentures, contact lenses, or prosthetic devices have been removed or left in place.

Special considerations

Preoperative medications must be given on time *to enhance the effect of ordered anesthesia.* The patient should take nothing by mouth preoperatively. Do not give oral medications unless ordered. Be sure to raise the bed's side rails immediately after giving preoperative medications.

If family or others are present, direct them to the appropriate waiting area and offer support as needed.

Documentation

Complete the preoperative checklist used by your hospital. Record all nursing care measures and preoperative medications, results of diagnostic tests, and the time the patient is transferred to the surgical area. The chart and the surgical checklist must accompany the patient to surgery.

Skin preparation

Proper preparation of the patient's skin for surgery renders it as free as possible from microorganisms, thereby reducing the risk of infection at the incision site. It does not duplicate or replace the full sterile preparation that immediately precedes surgery. Rather, it may involve a bath, shower, or local scrub with an antiseptic detergent solution, and hair removal. (See *Where to remove hair for surgery,* pages 106 and 107.)

The Association of Operating Room Nurses (AORN) recommends that hair not be removed from the area surrounding the operative site unless it's thick enough to interfere with surgery because hair removal may increase the risk of infection. Each hospital has a hair removal policy.

The area of preparation always exceeds that of the expected incision to minimize the number of microorganisms in the areas adjacent to the proposed incision and to allow surgical draping of the patient without contamination.

Equipment

Antiseptic soap solution ▪ tap water ▪ bath blanket ▪ two clean basins ▪ linen-saver pad ▪ adjustable light ▪ sterile razor with sharp new blade, if needed ▪ scissors ▪ optional: 4″ × 4″ gauze pads, cotton-tipped applicators, acetone or nail polish remover, orangewood stick, trash bag, towel, gloves.

Preparation of equipment

Use warm tap water *because heat reduces the skin's surface tension and facilitates removal of soil and hair.* Dilute the antiseptic detergent solution with warm tap water in one basin *for washing,* and pour plain warm water into the second basin *for rinsing.*

Implementation

• Check the doctor's order and explain the procedure to the patient, including the reason for the extensive preparations *to avoid causing undue anxiety.* Provide privacy, wash your hands thoroughly, and don gloves.

• Place the patient in a comfortable position, drape him with the bath blanket, and expose the preparation area. For most surgeries, this area extends 12″ (30 cm) in each direction from the expected incision site. However, *to ensure privacy and avoid chilling the patient,* expose only one small area at a time while performing skin preparation.

• Position a linen-saver pad beneath the patient *to catch spills and avoid linen changes.* Adjust the light to illuminate the preparation area.

• Assess skin condition in the preparation area and report any rash, abrasion, or laceration to the doctor before beginning the procedure. *Any break in the skin increases the risk of infection and could cause cancellation of planned surgery.*

• Have the patient remove all jewelry in or near the operative site.

• As ordered, don gloves and begin removing hair from the preparation area by clipping any long hairs with scissors. If ordered, shave all remaining hair within the area *to remove microorganisms.* Perform the procedure as

near to the time of surgery as possible *so that microorganisms will have minimal time to proliferate.* Use only a sterilized or sterile disposable razor with a sharp new blade *to avoid the risk of infection from a contaminated razor.*

• Use a gauze pad to spread liquid soap over the shave site, or use the pad provided in the disposable kit.

• Pull the skin taut in the direction opposite the direction of hair growth *because this makes the hair rise and facilitates shaving.*

• Holding the razor at a 45-degree angle, shave with short strokes in the direction of hair growth *to avoid skin irritation and achieve a smooth clean shave.*

• If possible, avoid lifting the razor from the skin and placing it down again *to minimize the risk of lacerations.* Also avoid applying pressure *because this can cause abrasions, particularly over bony prominences.*

• Rinse the razor frequently and reapply liquid soap to the skin as needed *to keep the area moist.*

• Change the rinse water if necessary. Then rinse the soap solution and loose hair from the preparation area, and inspect the skin. Immediately notify the doctor of any new nicks, lacerations, or abrasions, and file a report if your institution requires it.

• Proceed with a 10-minute scrub *to ensure a clean preparation area.* Wash the area with a gauze pad dipped in the antiseptic soap solution. Using a circular motion, start at the expected incision site and work outward toward the periphery of the area *to avoid recontaminating the clean area.* Apply light friction while washing *to improve the antiseptic effect of the solution.* Replace the gauze pad as necessary.

• Carefully clean skin folds and crevices *because they harbor greater numbers of microorganisms.* Scrub the perineal area last, if it's part of the preparation area, for the same reason. Pull loose skin taut. If necessary, use cotton-tipped applicators to clean the umbilicus and an orangewood stick to clean under nails. Be sure to remove any nail polish *because the anesthetist uses nail bed color to determine adequate oxygenation and may place a probe on the nail to measure oxygen saturation.*

• Dry the area with a clean towel and remove the linen-saver pad.

• Give the patient any special instructions for care of the prepared area, and remind him to keep the area clean for surgery. Make sure the patient is comfortable.

• Properly dispose of solutions and trash bag, and clean or dispose of soiled equipment and supplies according to hospital policy.

Special considerations

Avoid shaving facial or neck hair on women and children unless ordered. Never shave eyebrows *because this dis-*

(Text continues on page 108.)

Where to remove hair for surgery

Shoulder and upper arm
On operative side, from fingertips to hairline and center chest to center spine, extending to iliac crest and including the axilla.

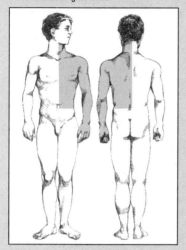

Forearm, elbow, and hand
On operative side, from fingertips to shoulder. Include the axilla unless surgery is for hand. Trim and clean fingernails.

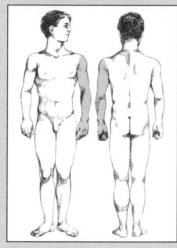

Thigh
On operative side, from toes to 3″ (7.6 cm) above umbilicus and from midline front to midline back, including pubis. Clean and trim toenails.

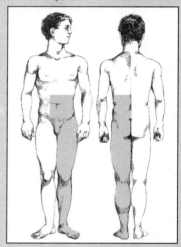

Chest
From chin to iliac crests and nipple on unaffected side to midline of back on operative side (2″ [5 cm] beyond midline of back for thoracotomy). Include axilla and entire arm to elbow on operative side.

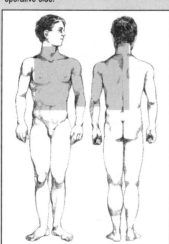

Abdomen
From 3″ above the nipples to upper thighs, including the pubis.

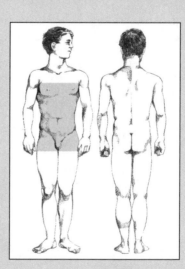

Lower abdomen
From 2″ above umbilicus to midthigh, including pubic area. For femoral ligation, to midline of thigh in back. For herniaplasty and embolectomy, to costal margin and down to knee.

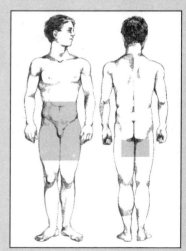

Where to remove hair for surgery *(continued)*

Hip

On operative side, from toes to nipples and at least 3″ (7.6 cm) beyond midline back and front, including the pubis. Clean and trim toenails.

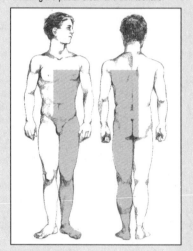

Knee and lower leg

On operative side, remove hair from toes to groin. Clean and trim toenails.

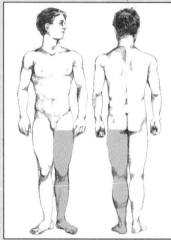

Ankle and foot

On operative side, remove hair from toes to 3″ above the knee. Clean and trim toenails.

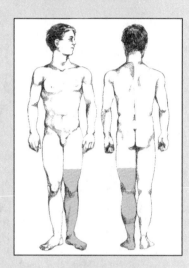

Flank

On operative side, remove hair from nipples to pubis, 3″ beyond midline in back, 2″ past abdominal midline. Include pubic area and, on affected side, upper thigh and axilla.

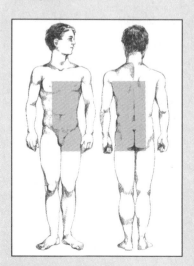

Perineum

From pubis, perineum, and perianal area, and from the waist to at least 3″ below the groin in front and at least 3″ below the buttocks in back.

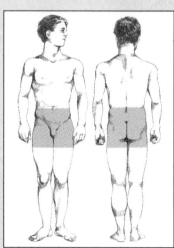

Spine

Remove hair from entire back, including shoulders and neck to hairline, and down to both knees. Include axillae.

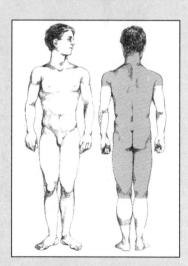

rupts normal hair growth and the new growth may prove unsightly. Scalp shaving is usually performed in the operating room, but if you're required to prepare the patient's scalp, put all hair in a plastic or paper bag and store with the patient's possessions.

If the patient won't hold still for shaving, remove hair with a depilatory cream. Although this method produces clean, intact skin without risking lacerations or abrasions, it can cause skin irritation or rash, especially in the groin area. If possible, cut long hairs with scissors before applying the cream *because removal of remaining hair then requires less cream.* Then use a glove to apply the cream in a layer ½" (1.3 cm) thick. After about 10 minutes, remove the cream with moist gauze pads. Next, wash the area with antiseptic soap solution, rinse, and pat dry.

Complications
Rashes, nicks, lacerations, and abrasions are the most common complications of skin preparation. They also increase the risk of postoperative infection.

Documentation
Record the date, time, and area of preparation; skin condition before and after preparation; any complications; and the patient's tolerance. If your hospital requires it, complete an incident report if the patient suffers nicks, lacerations, or abrasions during skin preparation.

 Postoperative care

This phase of care begins when the patient arrives in the post-anesthesia care unit (PACU) and continues as he moves on to the short procedure unit, medical-surgical unit, or critical care area. Postoperative care aims to minimize postoperative complications by early detection and prompt treatment. The patient recovering from anesthesia may be experiencing pain, inadequate oxygenation, or adverse physiologic effects of sudden movement.

Recovery from general anesthesia takes longer than induction because the anesthetic is retained in fat and muscle. Fat has a meager blood supply; thus, it releases the anesthetic slowly, providing enough anesthesia to maintain adequate blood and brain levels during surgery. The patient's recovery time varies with his amount of body fat, his overall condition, his premedication regimen, and the type, dosage, and duration of anesthesia.

Equipment
Thermometer ■ watch with second hand ■ stethoscope ■ sphygmomanometer ■ postoperative flowchart or other documentation tool.

Preparation of equipment
Assemble equipment at the patient's bedside.

Implementation
• Obtain the patient's record from the PACU nurse. This should include a summary of operative procedures and pertinent findings; type of anesthesia; vital signs (preoperative, intraoperative and postoperative); medical history; medication history, including preoperative, intraoperative, and postoperative medications; fluid therapy, including estimated blood loss, type and number of drains, catheters, and characteristics of drainage; and notes on the condition of the surgical wound. *If the patient had vascular surgery, for example , knowing the location and duration of blood vessel clamping is important for preventing postoperative complications.*

• Transfer the patient from the PACU stretcher to the bed and position him properly. Get a co-worker to help, if necessary. When moving the patient, keep transfer movements smooth *to minimize pain and postoperative complications and avoid back strain by team members.*

• If the patient has had orthopedic surgery, always get a co-worker to help transfer him. Ask the co-worker to move only the affected extremity.

• If the patient is in skeletal traction, you may have to follow special orders for moving him. If you must move him, have a co-worker move the weights as you and another co-worker move the patient.

• Make the patient comfortable and raise the bed's side rails *to ensure the patient's safety.*

• Assess the patient's level of consciousness, skin color, and mucous membranes.

• Monitor the patient's respiratory status by assessing his airway. Note breathing rate and depth, and auscultate breath sounds. Administer oxygen and initiate oximetry *to monitor oxygen saturation* if ordered.

• Monitor the patient's pulse rate. It should be strong and easily palpable. The postoperative heart rate should be within 20% of the preoperative heart rate.

• Compare postoperative blood pressure to preoperative blood pressure. It should be within 20% of the preoperative level unless the patient suffered a hypotensive episode during surgery.

• Assess the patient's temperature *because anesthesia lowers body temperature.* Body temperature should be at least 95° F (35° C). If it's lower, apply blankets *to warm the patient.*

• Assess the patient's infusion sites for redness, pain, swelling, or drainage.

• Assess surgical wound dressings. Dressings should be clean and dry. If they're soiled, assess the characteristics of the drainage and outline the soiled area. Note the date and time of assessment on the dressing. Assess the soiled area frequently; if it enlarges, reinforce the dressing and alert the doctor.

• Note the presence and condition of any drains and tubes. Note the color, type, odor, and amount of drainage. Make sure all drains are properly connected and free of kinks and obstructions.

• If the patient has had vascular or orthopedic surgery, assess the appropriate extremity — or all extremities, depending on the surgical procedure. Assess color, temperature, sensation, movement, and presence and quality of pulses, and notify the doctor of any abnormalities.

• As the patient recovers from anesthesia, monitor his respiratory and cardiovascular status closely. Be alert for signs of airway obstruction and hypoventilation caused by laryngospasm, or for sedation, which can lead to hypoxemia. Cardiovascular complications — such as arrhythmias and hypotension — may result from the anesthetic agent or the operative procedure.

• Encourage coughing and deep-breathing exercises. Don't encourage them if the patient has just had nasal, ophthalmic, or neurologic surgery *to avoid increasing intracranial pressure.*

• Administer postoperative medications, such as antibiotics, analgesics, antiemetics, or reversal agents, as ordered and appropriate.

• Remove all fluids from the patient's bedside until he is alert enough to eat and drink. Before giving him liquids, assess his gag reflex *to prevent aspiration.* To do this, lightly touch the back of the patient's throat with a cotton swab — the patient will gag if the reflex has returned. Do this test quickly *to prevent a vagal reaction.*

Special considerations

Fear, pain, anxiety, hypothermia, confusion, and immobility can upset the patient and jeopardize his safety and postoperative status. Offer emotional support to the patient and his family. Keep in mind that the patient who has lost a body part or who has been diagnosed with an incurable disease will need ongoing emotional support. Refer him and his family to appropriate clerical or psychological counseling.

As the patient recovers from general anesthesia, reflexes appear in reverse order to that in which they disappeared. Hearing recovers first, so avoid holding inappropriate conversations near the patient.

The patient under general anesthesia can't protect his own airway because of muscle relaxation. As he

recovers, his cough and gag reflexes reappear. If he can lift his head without assistance, he's usually able to breathe on his own and protect his airway.

If the patient received spinal anesthesia, he will need to remain supine with the bed adjusted to between 0 degrees and 20 degrees for at least 6 hours *to reduce the risk of spinal headache from leakage of cerebrospinal fluid.* The patient will also be unable to move his legs so be sure to explain this to him, and reassure him that sensation and mobility will return.

If patient has had epidural anesthesia for postoperative pain control, monitor his respiratory status closely. *Respiratory arrest may result from paralysis of the diaphragm by the anesthetic.* The patient may also experience nausea, vomiting, or itching.

If the patient will be using a patient-controlled anesthesia (PCA) unit, make sure he understands how to use it. Caution him to activate it only when he has pain, not when he feels sleepy or is pain-free. Review your hospital criteria for PCA.

Complications

Postoperative complications may include arrhythmias, hypotension, hypovolemia, septicemia, septic shock, atelectasis, pneumonia, thrombophlebitis, pulmonary embolism, urine retention, wound infection, wound dehiscence, evisceration, abdominal distention, paralytic ileus, constipation, altered body image, and postoperative psychosis.

Documentation

Document vital signs on the appropriate flowchart. Record the condition of dressings, and drains, and characteristics of drainage. Document all interventions taken to alleviate pain and anxiety and the patient's responses to them. Document any complications that may have occurred and interventions taken.

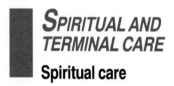

SPIRITUAL AND TERMINAL CARE

Spiritual care

Religious beliefs can profoundly influence a patient's recovery rate, attitude toward treatment, and overall response to hospitalization. In certain religious groups, beliefs can preclude diagnostic tests and therapeutic treatments, demand dietary restrictions, and prohibit organ donation and artificial prolongation of life. (See *Beliefs and practices of selected religions,* pages 110 to 112.)

Beliefs and practices of selected religions

A patient's religious beliefs can affect his attitudes toward illness and traditional medicine. By trying to accommodate the patient's religious beliefs and practices in your care plan, you can increase his willingness to learn and comply with treatment regimens. Because religious beliefs may vary within particular sects, individual practices may differ from those described here.

RELIGION	BIRTH AND DEATH RITUALS	DIETARY RESTRICTIONS	PRACTICES IN HEALTH CRISIS
Adventist	None (baptism of adults only)	Alcohol, coffee, tea, narcotics, stimulants; in many groups, meat prohibited also	Communion and baptism performed. Some members believe in divine healing, anointing with oil, and prayer. Some regard Saturday as the Sabbath.
Baptist	At birth, none (baptism of believers only); before death, counseling by clergy member and prayer	Alcohol; in some groups, coffee and tea prohibited also	Some believe in healing by laying on of hands. Resistance to medical therapy occasionally approved.
Christian Scientist	At birth, none; before death, counseling by a Christian Science practitioner	Alcohol, coffee, and tobacco prohibited	Many members refuse all treatment, including drugs, biopsies, physical examination, and blood transfusions and permit vaccination only when required by law. Alteration of thoughts is believed to cure illness. Hypnotism and psychotherapy are prohibited. (Christian Science nurses and nursing homes honor these beliefs.)
Church of Christ	None (baptism at age 8 or older)	Alcohol discouraged	Communion, anointing with oil, laying on of hands, and counseling by a minister.
Eastern Orthodox	At birth, baptism and confirmation; before death, last rites. For members of the Russian Orthodox Church, arms are crossed after death, fingers set in cross, and unembalmed body clothed in natural fiber.	For members of the Russian Orthodox Church and usually the Greek Orthodox Church, no meat or dairy products on Wednesday, Friday, and during Lent	Anointing of the sick. For members of the Russian Orthodox Church, cross necklace is replaced immediately after surgery and shaving of male patients is not allowed except in preparation for surgery. For members of the Greek Orthodox Church, communion and Sacrament of Holy Unction.
Episcopalian	At birth, baptism; before death, occasional last rites	For some members, abstention from meat on Friday, fasting before communion (which may be daily)	Communion, prayer, and counseling by a minister.

Beliefs and practices of selected religions *(continued)*

RELIGION	BIRTH AND DEATH RITUALS	DIETARY RESTRICTIONS	PRACTICES IN HEALTH CRISIS
Jehovah's Witnesses	None	Abstention from foods to which blood has been added	Typically, no blood transfusions are permitted; may require a court order for emergency transfusion.
Judaism	Ritual circumcision on eighth day after birth; burial of dead fetus; ritual washing of dead; burial (including organs and other body tissues) occurs as soon as possible; no autopsy or embalming	For Orthodox and Conservative Jews, kosher dietary laws (for example, pork and shellfish prohibited); for Reform Jews, usually no restrictions	Donation or transplantation of organs requires rabbinical consultation. For Orthodox and Conservative Jews, medical procedures may be prohibited on Sabbath – from sundown Friday to sundown Saturday – and special holidays.
Lutheran	Baptism usually performed 6 to 8 weeks after birth	None	Communion, prayer, and counseling by a minister.
Mormon	At birth, none (baptism at age 8 or older); before death, baptism and gospel preaching	Alcohol, tobacco, tea, and coffee prohibited; meat intake limited	Divine healing through the laying on of hands; communion on Sunday; some members may refuse medical treatment. Many wear a special undergarment.
Moslem	If abortion occurs before 130 days, fetus treated as discarded tissue; after 130 days, as a human being. Before death, confession of sins with family present; after death, only relatives or friends may touch the body.	Pork prohibited; daylight fasting during ninth month of Muhammadan calendar	Faith healing for the patient's morale only; conservative members reject medical therapy.
Orthodox Presbyterian	Infant baptism; scripture reading and prayer before death	None	Communion, prayer, and counseling by a minister.
Pentecostal Assembly of God, Foursquare Church	None (baptism only after age of accountability)	Abstention from alcohol, tobacco, meat slaughtered by strangling, any food to which blood has been added, and sometimes pork	Divine healing through prayer, anointing with oil, and laying on of hands.

(continued)

Beliefs and practices of selected religions *(continued)*

RELIGION	BIRTH AND DEATH RITUALS	DIETARY RESTRICTIONS	PRACTICES IN HEALTH CRISIS
Roman Catholic	Infant baptism, including baptism of aborted fetus without sign of clinical death (tissue necrosis); before death, anointing of the sick	Fasting or abstention from meat on Ash Wednesday and on Fridays during Lent; this practice usually waived for the hospitalized	Burial of major amputated limb (sometimes) in consecrated ground; donation or transplantation of organs allowed if the benefit to recipient outweighs the donor's potential harm.
United Methodist	None (baptism of children and adults only)	None	Communion before surgery or similar crisis; donation of body parts encouraged.

Consequently, effective patient care requires recognition and respect for the patient's religious beliefs. Recognizing his beliefs and need for spiritual care may require close attention to the patient's nonverbal cues or seemingly casual remarks that express his spiritual concerns. Respecting his beliefs may require setting aside one's own to help the patient follow his. Providing spiritual care may require contacting an appropriate member of the clergy in the hospital or community; assisting him in performing rites and administering sacraments by gathering the necessary equipment; and preparing the patient for the pastoral visit.

Equipment
Clean towels (one or two) ▪ teaspoon, or 1-oz (30 ml) medicine cup (for baptism) ▪ container of water (for emergency baptism).

Some hospitals, particularly those with a religious affiliation, provide baptismal trays. The clergy member may bring holy water, holy oil, or other religious articles to minister to the patient.

Preparation of equipment
For baptism, cover a small table with a clean towel. Fold a second towel and place it on the table, along with the teaspoon or medicine cup. For communion and anointing, cover the bedside stand with a clean towel. For religious circumcision, sterilize the ceremonial instruments, if requested to do so by the participating clergy member. (In Jewish practice, a *mohel* is a specialist certified by rabbinical authorities to perform circumcision.)

Implementation
● Check the patient's admission record *to determine religious affiliation.* Remember that the patient may claim no religious beliefs. If a patient states that he is agnostic, this may not rule out his desire for spiritual or pastoral care. Such patients may also wish to speak with a clergy member, so watch and listen carefully for subtle expressions of this desire.
● Evaluate the patient's behavior for signs of loneliness, anxiety, or fear—*emotions that may signal his need for spiritual counsel.* Also consider whether the patient is facing a health crisis, which may occur before childbirth, surgery, chronic illness, or impending death. Remember that a patient may feel acutely distressed because of his inability to participate in religious observances. Help such a patient verbalize his beliefs *to relieve stress.* Listen to the patient and let him express his concerns, but carefully refrain from imposing your beliefs on him *to avoid conflict and further stress.* If the patient requests, arrange a visit by an appropriate member of the clergy. Consult this clergy member if you need more information about the patient's beliefs.
● If your patient faces the possibility of abortion, amputation, transfusion, or other medical procedures with important religious significance or implications, try to discover his or her spiritual attitude. Also, try to determine your patient's attitude toward the importance of laying on of hands, confession, communion, observance of holy days (such as the Sabbath), and restrictions in diet or physical appearance. Helping the patient continue his normal religious practices during hospitalization *can help reduce stress.*

• If the patient is pregnant, find out her beliefs concerning infant baptism and circumcision, and comply with them after delivery.

• If a neonate is in critical condition, call an appropriate clergy member immediately. To administer emergency baptism, the official pours a small amount of holy water into a teaspoon or a medicine cup and sprinkles a few drops of water over the infant's head while saying, "(Name of child), I baptize you in the name of the Father, the Son, and the Holy Spirit. Amen." In an extreme emergency, you can perform a Roman Catholic baptism, using a container of any available water. If you do so, be sure to notify the priest *because this sacrament must be administered only once.*

• If a Jewish woman delivers a male infant prematurely or by cesarean birth, ask her if she plans to observe the rite of circumcision or *bris,* a significant ceremony performed on the eighth day after birth. (Because a patient who delivers a healthy, full-term baby vaginally is usually discharged quickly, this ceremony is normally performed outside the hospital.) For a *bris,* ensure privacy and, if requested, sterilize the instruments.

• If the patient requests communion, prepare him for it before the clergy member arrives. First, place him in Fowler's or semi-Fowler's position, if his condition permits. Otherwise, allow him to remain supine. Tuck a clean towel under his chin and straighten the bed linens.

• If a terminally ill patient requests the Sacrament of the Sick (Last Rites) or special treatment of his body after death, call an appropriate clergy member. For the Roman Catholic patient, call a Roman Catholic priest to administer the sacrament, even if the patient is unresponsive or comatose. To prepare the patient for this sacrament, uncover the arms and fold back the top linens to expose the feet. After the clergy member anoints the patient's forehead, eyes, nose, mouth, hands, and feet, straighten and retuck the bed linens.

Special considerations

Handle the patient's religious articles carefully to avoid damage or loss. Become familiar with religious resources in your hospital. Some hospitals employ one or more clergy members who counsel patients and staff and link patients to other pastoral resources.

If the patient tries to convert you to his personal beliefs, tell him that you respect his beliefs but are content with your own. Likewise, avoid attempts to convert the patient to your personal beliefs.

Documentation

Complete a baptismal form and attach it to the patient's record; send a copy of the form to the appropriate clergy member. Record the rites of circumcision and Last Rites in your notes. Also, record Last Rites in red on the Kardex so it won't be repeated unnecessarily.

Care of the dying patient

A patient needs intensive physical support and emotional comfort as he approaches death. Signs and symptoms of impending death include reduced respiratory rate and depth, decreased or absent blood pressure, weak or erratic pulse rate, lowered skin temperature, decreased level of consciousness (LOC), diminished sensorium and neuromuscular control, diaphoresis, pallor, cyanosis, and mottling.

Emotional support for the dying patient and his family most often means simple reassurance and the nurse's physical presence to help ease fear and loneliness. More intense emotional support is important at much earlier stages, especially for patients with long-term progressive illnesses, who can work through the stages of dying. (See *Five stages of dying,* page 114.)

Emotional care also requires respect for the patient's wishes about extraordinary means of supporting life. The patient may have signed a living will. This document, legally binding in most states, declares the patient's desire for a natural death unimpeded by the artificial support of defibrillators, respirators, auxiliary hearts, life-sustaining drugs, and so on. If the patient has signed such a document, the nurse must respect his wishes and communicate the doctor's "no code" order to all staff members.

Equipment

Clean bed linens ■ clean gowns ■ gloves ■ water-filled basin ■ soap ■ washcloth ■ towels ■ lotion ■ linen-saver pads ■ petroleum jelly ■ lemon-glycerin swabs ■ suction and resuscitation equipment, as necessary ■ optional: indwelling urinary catheter.

Implementation

• Assemble equipment at the patient's bedside, as needed.

Meeting physical needs

• Take vital signs often, and observe for pallor, diaphoresis, and decreased LOC.

• Reposition the patient in bed at least every 2 hours, *because sensation, reflexes, and mobility diminish first in the legs and gradually in the arms.* Make sure the bed sheets cover him loosely *to reduce discomfort caused by pressure on arms and legs.*

Five stages of dying

According to Elisabeth Kübler-Ross, author of *On Death and Dying,* the dying patient may progress through five psychological stages in preparation for death. Although each patient experiences these stages differently, and not necessarily in this order, understanding them will help you meet your patient's needs.

Denial
When the patient first learns of his terminal illness, he'll refuse to accept the diagnosis. He may experience physical symptoms similar to a stress reaction—shock, fainting, pallor, sweating, tachycardia, nausea, and GI disorders. During this stage, be honest with the patient but not blunt or callous. Maintain communication with him so he can discuss his feelings when he accepts the reality of death. Don't force the patient to confront this reality.

Anger
Once the patient stops denying his death, he may show deep resentment toward those who will live on after he dies—to you, to the hospital staff, and to his own family. Although you may instinctively draw back from the patient or even resent him for his behavior, remember that he is dying and has a right to be angry. After you accept his anger, you can help him find different ways to express it and can help his family to understand it.

Bargaining
Although the patient accepts impending death, he attempts to bargain for more time with God or fate. He will probably strike this bargain secretly. If he does confide in you, don't urge him to keep his promises.

Depression
First, the patient may experience regrets about his past; then he grieves about his current condition. He may withdraw from his friends, family, doctor, and from you. He may suffer from anorexia, increased fatigue, self-neglect. You may find him sitting alone, in tears. Accept the patient's sorrow, and if he talks to you, listen. Provide comfort by touch, as appropriate. Resist the temptation to make optimistic remarks or cheerful small talk.

Acceptance
In this last stage, the patient accepts the inevitability and imminence of his death—without emotion. He may simply desire the quiet company of a family member or friend. If, for some reason, a family member or friend can't be present, stay with the patient to satisfy his final need. Remember that many patients die before reaching this stage.

• When the patient's vision and hearing start to fail, turn his head toward the light and speak to him from near the head of the bed. *Because hearing may be acute despite loss of consciousness,* avoid whispering or speaking inappropriately about the patient in his presence.

• Change the bed linens and the patient's gown as needed. Provide skin care during gown changes, and adjust the room temperature for patient comfort, if necessary.

• Observe for incontinence or anuria, *the result of diminished neuromuscular control or decreased renal function.* If necessary, obtain an order to catheterize the patient, or place linen-saver pads beneath the patient's buttocks. Don gloves and provide perineal care with soap, a washcloth and towels *to prevent irritation and discomfort.*

• With suction equipment, suction the patient's mouth and upper airway *to remove secretions.* Elevate the head of the bed *to decrease respiratory resistance.* As the patient's condition deteriorates, he may breathe mostly through his mouth.

• Offer fluids frequently, and lubricate the patient's lips and mouth with petroleum jelly or lemon-glycerin swabs *to counteract dryness.*

• If the comatose patient's eyes are open, provide appropriate eye care *to prevent corneal ulceration.* Such ulceration can cause blindness and prevent the use of these tissues for transplantation should the patient die. (See *Understanding organ and tissue donation.)*

• Provide ordered pain medication as needed. Keep in mind that, as circulation diminishes, medications given intramuscularly will be poorly absorbed. Medications should be given intravenously, if possible, *for optimum results.*

Meeting emotional needs
• Fully explain all care and treatments to the patient even if he's unconscious *because he may still be able to hear.* Answer the conscious patient's questions as candidly as possible, without sounding calloused or blunt.

• Allow the patient to express his feelings, which may range from anger to loneliness. Take time to talk with the patient. When you do, sit near the head of the bed. Avoid looking rushed or unconcerned.

• Notify family members, if they're not present, when the patient wishes to see them. Let the patient and his family discuss death at their own pace. Give them opportunities to express their feelings, but avoid encouraging them if they seem unwilling.

• Offer to contact a member of the clergy or social services department, or other persons as the patient requests, if appropriate.

Special considerations

If the patient has signed a living will, the doctor will write a "no code" order on his progress notes and order sheets. Know your state's policy regarding the living will. If it's legal, transfer the "no code" order to the patient's chart or Kardex and, at the end of your shift, inform the incoming staff of this order.

If family members remain with the patient, show them the location of bathrooms, lounges, and cafeterias. Explain the patient's needs, treatments, and care plan to them. If appropriate, offer to teach them specific skills so they can take part in nursing care. Emphasize that their efforts are important and effective. As the patient's death approaches, give them emotional support.

At an appropriate time, ask the patient's family if they have considered organ and tissue donation. Check the patient's records *to determine if he completed an organ donor card.*

Documentation

Record changes in the patient's vital signs, intake and output, and LOC. Note the times of cardiac arrest and the end of respiration, and notify the doctor when these occur.

Postmortem care

After the patient dies, care includes preparing him for family viewing, arranging transportation to the morgue or funeral home, and determining the disposition of the patient's belongings. In addition, postmortem care entails comforting and supporting the patient's family and friends and providing for their privacy.

Postmortem care usually begins after a doctor certifies the patient's death. If the patient died violently or under suspicious circumstances, postmortem care may

---

Understanding organ and tissue donation

The federal Required Request Law, enacted in 1986, states that all acute care facilities that receive Medicare funds must ask about organ donation from every eligible donor. According to the American Medical Association, about 25 kinds of organs and tissues are being transplanted. Although donor organ requirements vary, the typical donor must be between ages 6 months and 50 years and free from transmissible disease, cancer, septicemia, diabetes, and hypertension.

Tissue donation requirements are less restrictive. Virtually any patient who dies free from contagious disease or systemic infection can donate tissue, such as skin, corneas, bone, and heart valves. Cancer patients are the exception, to avoid the risk of spreading metastatic cells.

Collection of most organs, such as the heart, liver, kidney, or pancreas, requires that the patient be pronounced brain dead and kept physically alive until the organs are harvested. Tissue such as eyes, skin, bone, and heart valves may be taken after death. Contact your regional organ procurement organization for specific organ donation criteria or to identify a potential donor. If you don't know the regional organ procurement organization in your area, call the United Network for Organ Sharing at (804) 330-8500.

---

be postponed until the medical examiner completes an autopsy.

Equipment

Gauze or soft string ties ■ gloves ■ chin straps ■ ABD pads ■ cotton balls ■ plastic shroud or body wrap ■ three identification tags ■ adhesive bandages to cover wounds or punctures ■ plastic bag for patient's belongings ■ water-filled basin ■ soap ■ towels ■ washcloths ■ stretcher.

A commercial morgue pack usually contains gauze or string ties, chin straps, a shroud, and identification tags.

Implementation

• Document any auxiliary equipment, such as a mechanical ventilator, still present. Put on gloves.

• Place the body in the supine position, arms at the sides and head on a pillow. Then elevate the head of the bed slightly *to prevent discoloration from blood settling in the face.*

• If the patient wore dentures and hospital policy permits, gently insert them; then close the mouth. Close the eyes by gently pressing on the lids with your fingertips. If they don't stay closed, place moist cotton balls on the eyelids for a few minutes, and then try again to close them. Place a folded towel under the chin *to keep the jaw closed.*

• Remove all indwelling catheters, tubes, and tape, and apply adhesive bandages to puncture sites. Replace soiled dressings.

• Collect all the patient's valuables *to prevent loss.* If you're unable to remove a ring, cover it with gauze, tape it in place, and tie the gauze to the wrist *to prevent slippage and subsequent loss.*

• Clean the body thoroughly, using soap, a basin and washcloths. Place one or more ABD pads between the buttocks *to absorb rectal discharge or drainage.*

• Cover the body up to the chin with a clean sheet.

• Offer comfort and emotional support to the family and intimate friends. Ask if they wish to see the body. If they do, allow them to do so in privacy. Ask if they would prefer to leave the patient's jewelry on the body.

• After the family leaves, remove the towel from under the chin of the deceased patient. Pad the chin, and wrap chin straps under the chin and tie them loosely on top of the head. Then, pad the wrists and ankles *to prevent bruises,* and tie them together with gauze or soft string ties.

• Fill out the three identification tags. Each tag should include the deceased patient's name, room and bed numbers, date and time of death, and doctor's name. Tie one tag to the deceased patient's hand or foot, but don't remove his hospital identification bracelet *to ensure correct identification.*

• Place the shroud or body wrap on the morgue stretcher and, after obtaining assistance, transfer the body to the stretcher. Wrap the body, and tie the shroud or wrap with the string provided. Then, attach another identification tag, and cover the shroud or wrap with a clean sheet. If a shroud or wrap isn't available, dress the deceased patient in a clean gown and cover the body with a sheet.

• Place the deceased patient's personal belongings, including valuables, in a bag and attach the third identification tag to it.

• If the patient died of an infectious disease, label the body according to your hospital's policy.

• Close the doors of adjoining rooms, if possible. Then take the body to the morgue. Use corridors that aren't crowded and, if possible, use a service elevator.

Special considerations

Give the deceased patient's personal belongings to his family or bring them to the morgue. If you give the family jewelry or money, make sure a co-worker is present as a witness. Obtain the signature of an adult family member *to verify receipt of valuables or to state their preference that jewelry remain on the patient.*

Offer emotional support to the deceased patient's family and friends, and to the patient's hospital roommate, if appropriate.

Documentation

Although the extent of documentation varies among hospitals, always record the disposition of the patient's possessions, especially jewelry and money. Also note the date and time the deceased patient was transported to the morgue.

Selected references

Association of Operating Room Nurses. *AORN Standards and Recommended Practices for Preoperative Nursing.* Denver: Association of Operating Room Nurses, Inc., 1989.

Barnum, B. *Nursing Theory: Analysis, Application, Evaluation.* Glenview, Ill.: Scott, Foresman & Co., 1990.

Barris, R., et al. *Occupational Therapy in Psychosocial Practice.* Thorofare, N.J.: Charles B. Slack, Inc., 1988.

Basmajian, J. *Therapeutic Exercise,* 5th ed. Baltimore: Williams & Wilkins Co., 1989.

Baum, C., et al. *Human Performance Deficits: Occupational Therapy Assessment and Intervention.* Thorofare, N.J.: Charles B. Slack, Inc., 1989.

Bomar, P. *Nurses and Family Health Promotions: Concepts, Assessment, and Interventions.* Baltimore: Williams & Wilkins Co., 1989.

Carpenito, L.J. *Nursing Diagnosis: Application to Clinical Practice,* 2nd ed. Philadelphia: J.B. Lippincott Co., 1988.

Doenges, M., et al. *Nursing Care Plans: Guidelines for Planning Patient Care,* 2nd ed. Philadelphia: F.A. Davis Co., 1989.

Doughty, D., et al. "Your Patient: Which Therapy?" *Journal of Enterostomal Therapy* 17(4):154-59, July-August 1990.

Fraulini, K. *After Anesthesia: A Guide for PACU, ICU and Medical-Surgical Nurses.* Norwalk, Conn.: Appleton & Lange, 1987.

Guzzetta, C. *Assessment Tools for Clinical Practice.* St. Louis: C.V. Mosby Co., March 1989.

Henderson, V. "Nursing Process — A Critique," *Holistic Nursing Practice* 1(3):7-18, 1987.

Illustrated Manual of Nursing Practice. Springhouse, Pa.: Springhouse Corp., 1991.

Kemp, B., et al. *Fundamentals of Nursing: A Framework for Practice,* 2nd ed. Glenview, Ill.: Scott, Foresman & Co., 1989.

Kneedler, J., and Dodge, G. *Perioperative Patient Care: The Nursing Perspective,* 2nd ed. St. Louis: C.V. Mosby Co., 1987.

Kozier, B., and Erb, G. *Techniques in Clinical Nursing,* 3rd ed. Reading, Mass.: Addison-Wesley Publishing Co., 1989.

Leuner, J., et al. *Mastering the Nursing Process: A Case Method Approach.* Philadelphia: F.A. Davis Co., 1989.

Lovell, H., and Anderson, C. "Put Your Patient on the Right Bed," *RN* 53(5):66-72, May 1990.

Morton, P. *Health Assessment in Nursing.* Springhouse, Pa.: Springhouse Corp., 1989.

Norton, D. "Helping Patients Give the Gift of Life," *RN* 53(12):30-34, December 1990.

Nurse's Handbook of Law and Ethics. Springhouse, Pa.: Springhouse Corp., 1992.

Pender, N. *Health Promotion in Nursing Practice,* 2nd ed. East Norwalk, Conn.: Appleton & Lange, 1987.

Potter, P., and Perry, A. *Fundamentals of Nursing: Concepts, Process and Practice,* 2nd ed. St. Louis: Mosby-Year Book, Inc., 1989.

Sparks, S., and Taylor, C. *Nursing Diagnosis Reference Manual.* Springhouse, Pa.: Springhouse Corp., 1991.

Stevens, S., and Becker, K. "A Simple, Step-by-Step Approach to Neurological Assessment," Part 1. *Nursing88* 18(9):53-61, September 1988.

Sutton, S. *Home Health Nursing: Clinical Procedures.* Baltimore: Williams & Wilkins Co., 1988.

Taylor, M., et al. *Fundamentals of Nursing: The Art and Science of Nursing Care.* Philadelphia: J.B. Lippincott Co., 1989.

Yura, H., and Walsh, M. *The Nursing Process: Assessing, Planning, Implementing, Evaluating,* 5th ed. Norwalk, Conn.: Appleton & Lange, 1987.

CHAPTER 2

INFECTION CONTROL

KAREN M.J. McCLEAVE, RN, MS, CFNP, CIC

Introduction

The mysteries of infection have been unfolding since Koch, Pasteur, and other microbiologists uncovered the link between bacteria and infection in the late 19th century. But despite our increased understanding of infectious diseases and the advent of programs to survey, prevent, identify, and control them, nosocomial infections occur more than 2 million times each year. They raise health care costs by about $2 billion, lengthen hospital stays, and lead directly or indirectly to about 25,000 patient deaths annually.

Not all nosocomial infections can be prevented. Immunodeficient patients, for example, or those receiving immunosuppressive therapy may succumb to nosocomial infection despite all precautions. However, studies have shown that about 400,000 infections could be prevented every year by faithful adherence to infection-control principles. This chapter contains detailed instructions for using these principles effectively.

Causes and incidence

Nosocomial infections result from aerobic and anaerobic bacteria, viruses, parasites, and fungi. The most common nosocomial infections involve the urinary tract, surgical wounds, the lower respiratory tract, and blood.

Urinary tract infections commonly result from catheter insertion or urogenital surgery. Surgical wound infections result from contamination during surgery, skin damage from preoperative hair removal, impaired blood supply, or coexisting medical problems. Lower respiratory tract infections can result from aspiration of oropharyngeal secretions, contaminated ventilation equipment (such as nebulizers), lung seeding by blood-borne pathogens, or airborne spread of pathogens from other patients. Bacteremia may arise as a complication of other nosocomial infections, such as pneumonia and surgical wound infections.

Nosocomial infections are three times more common among surgical patients than nonsurgical patients. The risk of such infections rises with the patient's age and duration of preoperative and total hospitalization.

Infection-control programs

According to recommendations issued in 1958 by the Joint Commission on Accreditation of Hospitals (now the Joint Commission on Accreditation of Healthcare Organiza-

tions) and the American Hospital Association, every accredited hospital must have an infection-control committee and a surveillance system as part of a formal infection-control program. Such a program aims to reduce the infection rate by emphasizing to the hospital staff the risk of contagion and by encouraging them to assume responsibility for preventing it. An effective infection-control program can reduce the incidence of nosocomial infections by about 20%.

To guide hospitals in their infection-control efforts, the Centers for Disease Control (CDC) in 1970 published a manual that detailed seven categories of isolation techniques. The recommendations were revised in 1983 to reduce unnecessary procedures and to adapt to the increased use of intensive care units, invasive procedures, and immunosuppressive treatments, and to counter the spread of drug-resistant pathogens. In 1984, a new approach to infection control, known as body substance isolation, called for health care workers to don gloves before contacting mucous membranes and broken skin, and before anticipated contact with any moist body substances. In 1988, the CDC refined this concept in its *universal precautions*, which recommend that health care workers wear gloves and other personal protective equipment (such as a mask, goggles, and a gown) to reduce exposure to blood and body fluids implicated in the transmission of blood-borne infections. Universal precautions may be implemented to replace diagnosis- and disease-specific isolation categories. Alternatively, these latter isolation categories may be used to supplement universal precautions.

In most hospitals, infection-control practitioners—usually registered nurses—assume daily responsibility for surveillance and other aspects of infection control. Although specific responsibilities may vary among hospitals, typical activities include:
- teaching the hospital staff the importance of correct hand washing between patient contacts (the most effective way to reduce infection risk)
- assessing patients for infection and taking proper precautions against contamination and contagion
- showing the staff how to collect and handle laboratory specimens
- developing infection-control guidelines, instructing the staff, and monitoring isolation procedures.

Isolation as prevention

Most isolation procedures aim to prevent transmission of disease from infected patients to other patients, hospital staff, and visitors. In contrast, isolation may also aim to protect immunocompromised patients from exogenous pathogens. Many mysteries must be solved before these and other procedures can reduce the incidence

Proper hand-washing technique

To minimize the spread of infection, follow these basic hand-washing instructions. With your hands angled downward under the faucet, adjust the water temperature until it's comfortably warm.

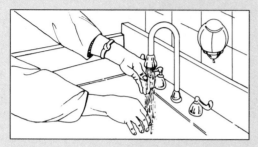

Work up a generous lather by scrubbing vigorously for 10 seconds. Be sure to clean beneath fingernails, around knuckles, and along the sides of fingers and hands.

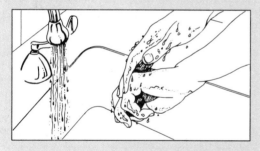

Rinse your hands completely to wash away suds and microorganisms. Pat dry with a paper towel. To prevent recontaminating your hands on the faucet handles, cover each one with a dry paper towel when turning off the water.

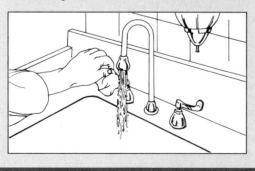

of nosocomial infections. But for now, strict adherence to your hospital's infection-control policies and the procedures outlined in this chapter can go far toward keeping infection at bay.

GENERAL PRINCIPLES
Hand washing

The hands serve as the conduit for almost every transfer of potential pathogens from one patient to another, from a contaminated object to the patient, or from hospital staff to the patient. Thus, hand washing is the single most important procedure in preventing contagion. To protect patients from nosocomial infections, hand washing must be performed routinely and thoroughly. In effect, clean and healthy hands with smooth skin, short fingernails, and no rings or false fingernails minimize the risk of contamination. Microorganisms are more difficult to remove from rough or chapped hands.

Equipment
Soap or detergent ▪ warm running water ▪ paper towels ▪ optional: antiseptic cleaning agent, fingernail brush, plastic sponge brush or plastic cuticle stick.

Implementation
• Remove rings or false fingernails as your hospital's policy dictates *because they harbor dirt and skin microorganisms.* Remove your watch or wear it well above the wrist.
• Wet your hands and wrists with warm water and apply soap from a dispenser. Don't use bar soap *because it allows cross-contamination.* Hold your hands below elbow level *to prevent water from running up your arms and back down, thus contaminating clean areas.* (See *Proper hand-washing technique.*)
• Work up a generous lather by rubbing your hands together vigorously for about 10 seconds. *Soap and warm water reduce surface tension and this, aided by friction, loosens surface microorganisms, which wash away in the lather.* The more vigorously you rub your hands when washing, the more microorganisms you remove.
• Pay special attention to the area under fingernails and around cuticles, and to the thumbs, knuckles, and sides of the fingers and hands *because microorganisms thrive in these protected or overlooked areas.* If you don't remove your wedding band, move it up and down your finger to clean beneath it.

• Avoid splashing water on yourself or the floor *because microorganisms spread more easily on wet surfaces and because slippery floors are dangerous.* Avoid touching the sink or faucets *because they're considered contaminated.*

• Rinse hands and wrists well *because running water flushes suds, soil, and microorganisms away.*

• Pat hands and wrists dry with a paper towel. Avoid rubbing, *which can cause abrasion and chapping.*

• If the sink is not equipped with knee or foot controls, turn off the faucets by gripping them with a dry paper towel *to avoid recontaminating your hands.*

Special considerations

Before participating in any sterile procedure or whenever your hands are grossly contaminated, wash your forearms also, and clean under the fingernails and in and around the cuticles with a fingernail brush, disposable sponge brush, or plastic cuticle stick. Use these softer implements *because brushes, metal files, or other hard objects may injure your skin and, if reused, may be a source of contamination.*

Follow your hospital's policy concerning when to wash with soap and when to use an antiseptic cleaning agent. Typically, you'll wash with *soap* before coming on duty; before and after direct or indirect patient contact; before and after performing any bodily functions, such as blowing your nose or using the bathroom; before preparing or serving food; before preparing or administering medications; after direct or indirect contact with a patient's excretions, secretions, or blood; and after completing your shift.

Use an *antiseptic* cleaning agent when *you must reliably eliminate microorganisms from your hands,* such as before and after handling invasive devices, performing wound care and dressing changes, and after your hands have been contaminated with virulent pathogens. Antiseptics are also recommended for hand washing in isolation rooms, newborn nurseries, and before caring for any highly susceptible patient. Even if you're putting on clean or sterile gloves, wash before and after with an antiseptic *so microorganisms will not grow under the gloves or in case the gloves are torn or punctured.*

Home care

If you're providing care in the patient's home, bring your own supply of soap and disposable paper towels. If there's no running water, disinfect your hands with alcohol sponges.

Complications

Because it strips natural skin oils, frequent hand washing may result in dryness, cracking, and irritation. These effects are probably more common after repeated use of antiseptic cleaning agents, especially in persons with sensitive skin. Be sure to remove antiseptic residues carefully to help minimize irritation.

If your hands are dry or cracked, or if you develop dermatitis, apply an emollient hand cream after each washing or switch to a different cleaning agent. Don't allow irritated skin to reduce your attention to hand washing; if that happens, your hands could become a conduit of infection.

Isolation equipment use

Isolation procedures may be implemented to prevent the spread of infection from patient to patient, from the patient to health care workers, or from health care workers to the patient. Isolation procedures may also lessen the risk of infection in immunocompromised patients. Central to the success of these procedures are the selection of proper equipment and adequate training of those who use it.

Equipment

Materials required for isolation typically include barrier clothing, an isolation cart or anteroom for storing equipment, and a door card notifying all who enter the room that isolation precautions are in effect.

Barrier clothing includes the following: gowns ■ gloves ■ caps ■ goggles ■ masks. Each staff member must be trained in the proper use of barrier clothing.

Isolation supplies may include the following: labels ■ tape ■ specially marked laundry bags (and water-soluble laundry bags, if used) ■ plastic trash bags.

An isolation cart may be used when the patient's room has no anteroom. The cart can be a covered, wheeled utility table, or it can be specially designed for use during isolation precautions. It should include a work area (such as a pull-out shelf), drawers or a cabinet area for holding isolation supplies and, possibly, a pole on which to hang coats or jackets.

Supplies for the cart or anteroom should be stocked according to the isolation category being used and the patient's individual needs.

Preparation of equipment

Remove the cover from the isolation cart, if necessary, and set up the work area. Check the cart or anteroom *to ensure that correct and sufficient supplies are in place for the designated isolation category.*

Donning a face mask

To avoid spreading airborne particles, wear a face mask—sterile or nonsterile, as indicated. Position the mask to cover your nose and mouth, and secure it high enough to ensure stability. Tie the bottom string first, then pull the mask up over your face and tie the top string.

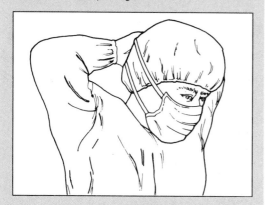

Adjust the metal nose strip if the mask has one.

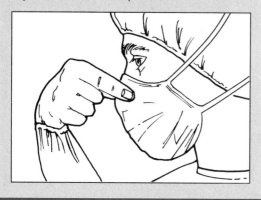

Implementation

• Remove your watch or push it well up your arm. Remove your rings according to hospital policy. *These actions help to prevent the spread of microorganisms hidden under your watch or rings.*

• Wash your hands with an antiseptic cleaning agent *to prevent growth of microorganisms under gloves.*

Putting on isolation garb

• Put the gown on and wrap it around the back of your uniform. Tie the strings or fasten the snaps or pressure-sensitive tabs at the neck. Make sure your uniform is completely covered, and secure the gown at the waist.

• Put on a cap and make sure it covers all your hair.

• Place the mask snugly over your nose and mouth. Secure ear loops around your ears or tie the strings behind your head high enough so the mask won't slip off. If the mask has a metal strip, squeeze it to fit your nose firmly but comfortably. (See *Donning a face mask.*) If you wear eyeglasses, tuck the mask under their lower edge.

• Put on the gloves. Cover the edges of the gown's sleeves by pulling the gloves over the cuffs.

Removing isolation garb

• Remember that the outside surfaces of your barrier clothes are contaminated.

• With the gloves on, untie the gown's waist strings, *which are considered contaminated.*

• With your gloved left hand, remove the right glove by pulling on the cuff, turning the glove inside out as you pull. Don't touch any skin with the outside of either glove. (See *Removing contaminated gloves.*) Then, remove the left glove by wedging one or two fingers of your right hand inside the glove and pulling it off, turning it inside out as you remove it. Discard the gloves in the trash container.

• Untie your mask, holding it only by the strings. Discard the mask and cap in the trash container. If the patient has a disease that is spread by airborne pathogens, you may prefer to remove the mask and cap last.

• Untie the neck straps of your gown. Grasp the outside of the gown at the back of the shoulders and pull the gown down over your arms, turning it inside out as you remove it *to ensure containment of the pathogens.*

• Holding the gown well away from your uniform, fold it inside out. Discard it in the laundry or trash container, depending on whether the gown is cloth or paper.

• If the sink is inside the patient's room, wash your hands and forearms with soap or antiseptic before leaving the room. Turn off the faucet using a paper towel and discard the towel in the room. Grasp the door handle with a clean paper towel to open it, and discard the towel in a trash container inside the room. Close the door from the outside with your bare hand.

• If the sink is in an anteroom, wash your hands and forearms with soap or antiseptic after leaving the room.

Special considerations

Use gowns, gloves, caps, goggles and masks only once, and discard them in the appropriate container before leaving a contaminated area. Isolation garb loses its ef-

Removing contaminated gloves

Proper removal techniques are essential for preventing the spread of pathogens from gloves to your skin surface. Follow these steps carefully.

1. Using your left hand, pinch the right glove near the top. Avoid allowing the glove's outer surface to buckle inward against your wrist.

2. Pull downward, allowing the glove to turn inside out as it comes off. Keep the right glove in your left hand after removing it.

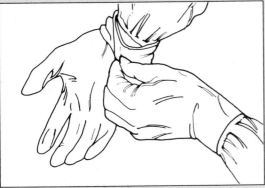

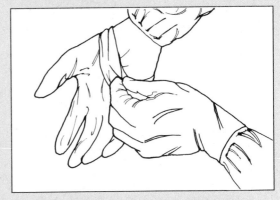

3. Now insert the first two fingers of your ungloved right hand under the edge of the left glove. Avoid touching the glove's outer surface or folding it against your left wrist.

4. Pull downward, so the glove turns inside out as it comes off. Continue pulling until the left glove completely encloses the right and has its uncontaminated inner surface facing out.

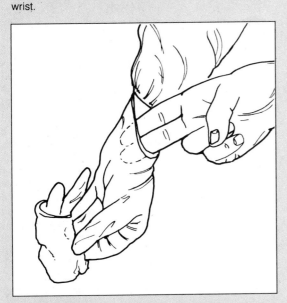

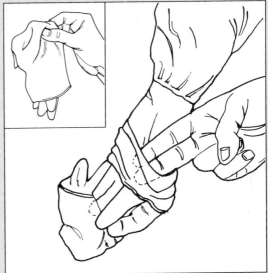

Defining infection-control terms

Although often used interchangeably, three terms have distinctive meanings of great importance in infection control.

Cleaning physically removes dirt and debris from a surface, usually with water and with or without detergents. Microorganisms removed by cleaning are not killed. Equipment must be cleaned before disinfection or sterilization.

Disinfecting serves as an intermediate state between clean and sterile because it kills certain kinds of microorganisms but not spores. Equipment can be disinfected by pasteurization, by exposure to ultraviolet rays, or by soaking in a disinfectant solution. Before disinfection, equipment must be clean of organic debris because disinfectants can't penetrate pus, blood, or other organic substances and may even be neutralized by them.

Sterilizing destroys all microorganisms — bacteria, viruses, fungi, parasites, and their spores — through the use of pressurized steam, gas (ethylene oxide), liquid (actuated glutaraldehyde), or dry heat. Because boiling water doesn't kill spores, it can't be used for sterilization.

fectiveness when wet *because moisture permits organisms to seep through the material.* Change masks and gowns as soon as moisture is noticeable or according to manufacturer's recommendations or hospital policy.

At the end of your shift, restock used items *to ensure an adequate supply for the next person.* When the patient is transferred to another unit or is discharged, return the isolation cart to the appropriate area for cleaning and restocking of supplies. An isolation room or other room prepared for isolation purposes must be thoroughly cleaned and disinfected before use by another patient. (See *Defining infection-control terms.*)

Reportable diseases

Certain contagious diseases must be reported to local and state public health officials and, ultimately, to the Centers for Disease Control (CDC). Typically, these diseases fit one of two categories: those reported individually on definitive or suspected diagnosis, and those reported by the number of cases per week. The most commonly reported diseases include hepatitis, measles, viral meningitis, salmonellosis, shigellosis, syphilis, and gonorrhea. (See *Checklist of reportable diseases* for an extensive listing.)

In most states, the patient's doctor must report communicable diseases to health officials. In hospitals, the infection-control practitioner or epidemiologist reports them. However, you should know the reporting requirements and procedure. Fast, accurate reporting helps identify and control infection sources, prevent epidemics, and guide public health planning and policy.

Equipment
Nursing procedure or infection-control manual ▪ disease-reporting form, if available.

Implementation
● Make sure reportable diseases are listed and that the list is available to all shifts.
● Know your hospital's protocol for reporting diseases. Typically, you'll contact the infection-control practitioner or epidemiologist. If this person isn't available, contact your supervisor or the infectious-disease doctor on call.

Documentation
Document any disease reported to the infection-control practitioner, the practitioner's name, and the date and time of the report.

*G*UIDELINES
Universal precautions

Universal precautions were developed by the Centers for Disease Control (CDC) in response to the increasing incidence of human immunodeficiency virus (HIV), hepatitis B virus (HBV), and other blood-borne diseases. CDC officials recommend that caregivers handle all blood and potentially bloody body substances and tissues as if they're infectious, regardless of the patient's diagnosis.

Universal precautions encompass most of the individual blood and body fluid isolation precautions previously recommended by the CDC for patients with known or suspected blood-borne pathogens. Universal precautions are meant to be combined with other category- or disease-specific isolation precautions, such as disease-specific isolation for highly contagious and resistant organisms (methicillin-resistant *Staphylococcus aureus,* for example).

Checklist of reportable diseases

Because disease reporting laws vary from state to state, this list isn't conclusive, and may be changed periodically. Local agencies report certain diseases to their state health departments, which in turn determine which diseases are reported to the CDC.

- ☐ Acquired immunodeficiency syndrome (AIDS)
- ☐ Amebiasis
- ☐ Animal bites
- ☐ Anthrax (cutaneous or pulmonary)
- ☐ Aseptic meningitis
- ☐ Botulism (food-borne, infant)
- ☐ Brucellosis
- ☐ Cholera
- ☐ Diphtheria (cutaneous or pharyngeal)
- ☐ Encephalitis (postinfectious or primary)
- ☐ Gastroenteritis (institutional outbreaks)
- ☐ Gonorrhea
- ☐ Group A beta-hemolytic streptococcal infections (including scarlet fever)
- ☐ Guillain-Barré syndrome
- ☐ Hepatitis A (include suspected source)
- ☐ Hepatitis B (include suspected source)
- ☐ Hepatitis C, also called non-A, non-B (include suspected source)
- ☐ Hepatitis, unspecified (include suspected source)
- ☐ Influenza
- ☐ Legionellosis (Legionnaires' disease)
- ☐ Leprosy
- ☐ Leptospirosis
- ☐ Malaria
- ☐ Measles (rubeola)
- ☐ Meningitis (specify etiology)
- ☐ Meningococcal disease
- ☐ Mumps
- ☐ Pertussis
- ☐ Plague (bubonic or pneumonic)
- ☐ Poliomyelitis (spinal paralytic)
- ☐ Psittacosis
- ☐ Rabies
- ☐ Reye's syndrome
- ☐ Rheumatic fever
- ☐ Rocky Mountain spotted fever
- ☐ Rubella (congenital syndrome)
- ☐ Rubella (German measles)
- ☐ Salmonellosis (excluding typhoid fever)
- ☐ Shigellosis
- ☐ Smallpox
- ☐ Staphylococcal infections (neonatal)
- ☐ Syphilis (congenital < 1 year)
- ☐ Syphilis (primary or secondary)
- ☐ Tetanus
- ☐ Toxic shock syndrome
- ☐ Trichinosis
- ☐ Tuberculosis
- ☐ Tularemia
- ☐ Typhoid fever
- ☐ Typhus (flea- and tick-borne)
- ☐ Varicella (chicken pox)
- ☐ Yellow fever

The specific body fluids covered by universal precautions include blood; semen; vaginal secretions; cerebrospinal, synovial, pleural, peritoneal, pericardial, and amniotic fluid; bloody saliva; breast milk; and any other body fluid that contains visible blood. Universal precautions don't apply to contact with feces, saliva, nasal secretions, sputum, sweat, tears, vomitus, or urine unless traces of blood are present.

To reduce the risk of spreading nosocomial infections through substances not included in universal precautions, many institutions have adopted an infection-control regimen that combines universal precautions with body substance isolation, a system developed before universal precautions to prevent the spread of nosocomial infections by cross-contamination. Universal precautions recommend donning gloves before any exposure to blood and body fluids; body substance isolation recommends donning gloves before contact with blood, all body secretions or excretions, mucous membranes and broken skin, and indwelling device insertion sites. With body substance isolation, respiratory and strict isolation procedures must still be used if an airborne disease is present. Each institution must establish an infection-control policy that lists specific barrier precautions. (See *Guidelines for minimizing infection*, pages 126 to 129, for an example.)

Equipment

Gloves ■ masks ■ goggles, glasses, or face shields ■ gowns or aprons ■ resuscitation masks ■ bags for specimens ■ 1:10 dilution of bleach to water (mixed daily) or hospital-

Guidelines for minimizing infection

The table below lists the minimum requirements for using gloves, gowns, masks, and eye protection to avoid contacting and spreading pathogens. It assumes that thorough hand washing is performed in all cases. Refer to your hospital's guidelines and use your own judgment when assessing the need for barrier protection in specific situations.

PROCEDURE	GLOVES	GOWN	MASK	EYE WEAR
Bathing, for patient with open lesions	✔	–	–	–
Bedding, changing visibly soiled	✔	If soiling likely	–	–
Bleeding or pressure application to control it	✔	If soiling likely	If splattering likely	If splattering likely
Blood glucose (capillary) testing	✔	–	–	–
Breathing treatment, routine	If soiling likely	–	–	–
Cardiopulmonary resuscitation	✔	–	–	–
Central venous line insertion and venesection	✔	–	–	–
Central venous pressure measurement	✔	–	–	–
Cervical cauterization	✔	–	–	–
Chest drainage system change	✔	If splattering likely	–	–
Chest tube insertion	✔	If soiling likely	If splattering likely	If splattering likely
Chest tube removal	✔	If soiling likely	If splattering likely	If splattering likely
Cleaning, anal	✔	–	–	–
Cleaning (feces, spilled blood or body substances, or surfaces contaminated by blood or body fluids)	✔	If soiling likely	–	–
Cleaning, urine	✔	–	–	–
Colonoscopy, flexible sigmoidoscope	✔	✔	–	–
Coughing, frequent and forceful by patient; direct contact with secretions	–	–	✔	✔

Note: ✔ indicates that barrier is necessary; – indicates that barrier typically is not necessary.

Guidelines for minimizing infection *(continued)*

PROCEDURE	GLOVES	GOWN	MASK	EYE WEAR
Dialysis, peritoneal				
Initiation of acute treatment	✓	✓	If splattering likely	If splattering likely
Performing an exchange	✓	✓	If splattering likely	If splattering likely
Termination of acute treatment	✓	✓	If splattering likely	If splattering likely
Dismantling tubing from cycler	✓	✓	If splattering likely	If splattering likely
Discarding peritoneal drainage	✓	✓	If splattering likely	If splattering likely
Irrigating peritoneal catheter	✓	✓	If splattering likely	If splattering likely
Specimen collection	✓	–	–	–
Tubing change	✓	✓	If splattering likely	If splattering likely
Skin care (catheter site)	✓	✓	✓	✓
Assisting with insertion of acute peritoneal catheter (outside sterile field)	✓	✓	If splattering likely	If splattering likely
Dressing change for burns	✓	✓	–	–
Dressing removal or change for wounds with little or no drainage	✓	–	–	–
Dressing removal or change for wounds with large amount of drainage	✓	If soiling likely	–	–
Emptying drainage receptacles, including suction containers, urine receptacles, bedpans, emesis basins	✓	If soiling likely	If splattering likely	If splattering likely
Emptying wastebaskets	✓	–	–	–
Enema	✓	If soiling likely	–	–
Fecal impaction, removal of	✓	–	–	–
Fecal incontinence, placement of indwelling urinary catheter for, and emptying bag	✓	If splattering likely	–	–
Gastric lavage	✓	If soiling likely	–	–
Incision and drainage of abscess	✓	If splattering likely	–	–
Intravenous or intra-arterial line				
Insertion	✓	–	–	–
Removal	✓	–	–	–
Tubing change at catheter hub	✓	–	–	–
Intubation or extubation	✓	If splattering likely	If splattering likely	If splattering likely

(continued)

Guidelines for minimizing infection *(continued)*

PROCEDURE	GLOVES	GOWN	MASK	EYE WEAR
Invasive procedures (lumbar puncture, bone marrow aspiration, paracentesis, liver biopsy) outside sterile field	✔	–	–	–
Irrigation				
Indwelling urinary catheter	✔	–	–	–
Vaginal	✔	If soiling likely	–	–
Wound	✔	If soiling likely	If splattering likely	If splattering likely
Joint or nerve injection	✔	–	–	–
Lesion biopsy or removal	✔	–	–	–
Medication administration				
Eye, ear, and nose drops	✔	–	–	–
I.M. or S.C.	✔	–	–	–
I.V. (direct or into hub of catheter or heparin lock)	✔	–	–	–
Oral	✔	–	–	–
Rectal or vaginal suppository	✔	–	–	–
Topical medication for lesion	✔	–	–	–
Nasogastric tube, insertion or irrigation	✔	If soiling likely	If splattering likely	If splattering likely
Oral and nasal care	✔	–	–	–
Ostomy care, irrigation, and teaching	✔	If soiling likely	–	–
Oxygen tubing, drainage of condensate	✔	–	–	–
Pelvic exam and Pap test	✔	–	–	–
Perineal cleaning	✔	–	–	–
Postmortem care	✔	If soiling likely	–	–
Pressure ulcer care	✔	–	–	–
Shaving	✔	–	–	–
Specimen collection (blood, stool, urine, sputum, wound)	✔	–	–	–

Note: ✔ indicates that barrier is necessary; – indicates that barrier typically is not necessary.

Guidelines for minimizing infection *(continued)*

PROCEDURE	GLOVES	GOWN	MASK	EYE WEAR
Suctioning				
Nasotracheal or endotracheal	✔	If soiling likely	If splattering likely	If splattering likely
Oral or nasal	✔	–	–	–
Temperature, rectal	✔	–	–	–
Tracheostomy suctioning and cannula cleaning	✔	If soiling likely	If splattering likely	If splattering likely
Tracheostomy tube change	✔	–	If splattering likely	If splattering likely
Urine and stool testing	✔	–	–	–
Wound packing	✔	If soiling likely	–	–

Adapted from Pugliese, G., ed. *Universal Precautions: Policies, Procedures, and Resources.* Chicago: American Hospital Publishing, Inc., 1991.

strength disinfectant certified effective against HBV and HIV.

Implementation
• Wash your hands immediately if they become contaminated with blood or body fluids; also wash your hands before and after patient care and after removing gloves. *Hand washing retards the growth of microorganisms on your skin.*
• Wear gloves if you will or could come in contact with blood, specimens, tissue, body fluids or excretions, or contaminated surfaces or objects.
• Change your gloves between patient contacts *to avoid cross-contamination.*
• Wear a gown, face shield, goggles, and a mask during procedures likely to generate droplets of blood or body fluids, such as surgery, endoscopic procedures, or dialysis.
• Handle used needles or other sharp implements carefully. Do not bend, break, reinsert them into their original sheaths, or unnecessarily handle them. Discard them intact immediately after use into an impervious disposal box. *These measures reduce the risk of accidental injury or infection.*
• Immediately notify your employee health provider of all needle-stick accidents, mucosal splashes, or contamination of open wounds with blood or body fluids *to allow investigation of the incident and appropriate care and documentation.*

• Properly label all specimens collected from patients and place them in plastic bags at the collection site.
• Promptly clean all blood and body fluid spills with a 1:10 dilution of bleach to water (mixed daily) or with an approved hospital-strength disinfectant effective against HBV and HIV.
• Disposable food trays and dishes aren't necessary.
• If you have an exudative lesion, avoid all direct patient contact until the condition has resolved and you've been cleared by the employee health provider.

Special considerations
Universal precautions are intended to supplement rather than replace recommendations for routine infection control, such as hand washing and use of gloves.

Keep mouthpieces, resuscitation bags, and other ventilation devices nearby *to minimize the need for emergency mouth-to-mouth resuscitation, thus reducing the risk of exposure to body fluids.*

◆ *Nursing alert.* Because precautions can't be specified for every clinical situation, you must use your judgment in individual cases. What's more, if your work requires you to be exposed to blood, you should receive an HBV vaccine. ◆

Complications
Failure to follow universal precautions may lead to exposure to blood-borne diseases and all the complications they may incur.

Documentation
Record any special needs for universal precautions on the nursing care plan.

 ## Respiratory isolation

This procedure prevents the spread of infectious diseases transmitted by airborne pathogens that are breathed, sneezed, or coughed into the environment. (See *Diseases requiring respiratory precautions.*) This isolation category includes the former categories of acid-fast bacillus (AFB) isolation and strict isolation.

Effective respiratory isolation requires a private room with the door kept closed, the use of masks by anyone entering the room, use of gloves, thorough hand-washing technique, and proper handling and disposal of articles contaminated by respiratory tract secretions. Patients with active tuberculosis or measles must be placed in a room with positive air pressure that is vented directly to the outside of the building.

When handling infants who require respiratory isolation, proper technique requires the use of masks, gloves, and gowns. These barriers prevent contamination of clothing by respiratory tract secretions.

Equipment
Masks ■ gowns, if necessary ■ gloves ■ plastic bags ■ isolation door card ■ isolation tape or labels.

Gather any additional supplies, such as a thermometer, stethoscope, and blood pressure cuff *so that you don't have to leave the isolation room unnecessarily.*

Preparation of equipment
Keep all respiratory isolation supplies outside the patient's room in a cart or anteroom.

Implementation
• Locate the patient in a private room with private toilet facilities and an anteroom, if possible. If necessary, two patients with the same infection may share a room. Explain isolation procedures to the patient *to ease his anxiety and promote cooperation.*
• Keep the patient's door closed at all times *to isolate the patient's airborne secretions.* Put a respiratory isolation card on the door *to notify anyone entering the room.*
• Wash your hands before entering and after leaving the room and during patient care if you handled respiratory tract secretions.
• Pick up your mask by the top strings, adjust it around your nose and mouth, and tie the strings for a comfortable

fit. If the mask has a flexible metal nose strip, adjust it to fit firmly but comfortably. Avoid touching the front of the mask during use *because its surface will have become contaminated.*
• Instruct the patient to cover his mouth with a facial tissue while coughing or sneezing *to control the spread of airborne droplets.*
• Tape an impervious bag to the patient's bedside *so he can dispose of facial tissues correctly.*
• Place all sputum specimens from respiratory isolation patients in impervious, labeled containers and send them to the laboratory.
• Ensure that all visitors wear masks and, if necessary, gowns.
• Place all items that have come in direct contact with the patient—such as linens, trash, and nondisposable utensils or instruments—in a single impervious bag before removal from the room *to prevent contagion.* Place this bag inside a second bag if there is visible outside contamination or if the bag may be punctured.

Special considerations
Before removing your mask, remove your gloves and wash your hands. Untie the strings and dispose of the mask, handling it by the strings only.

If the patient has a highly contagious respiratory disease, you may discard the mask and gloves in a lined, covered receptacle outside the patient's room. Thus, you'll be outside the room (with the door shut behind you) before removing your protective garb.

Remember to discard the mask and gloves right at the door. *Carrying them away from the patient's immediate area promotes contamination.*

Documentation
Record the need for respiratory isolation on the nursing care plan. Document initiation and maintenance of the procedure, the patient's tolerance of the procedure, and any patient teaching. Also document the date isolation was discontinued.

 ## Neutropenic isolation

Unlike other isolation procedures, neutropenic isolation (also known as protective or reverse isolation) guards the patient who is at increased risk of infection against contact with potential pathogens. This procedure is used primarily for patients with extensive noninfected burns and for those who have leukopenia, a depressed immune system, or who are receiving immunosuppressive treat-

Diseases requiring respiratory precautions

DISEASE	PRECAUTIONARY PERIOD
Chicken pox (varicella)	Until lesions become crusted
Diphtheria (pharyngeal)	When nose and throat cultures taken 24 hours after ending treatment are negative for causative organism
Epiglottitis, meningitis, and pneumonia caused by *Haemophilus influenzae*	4 hours after start of effective therapy
Erythema infectiosum	7 days after onset
Hemorrhagic fevers (such as Lassa fever, Marburg virus disease)	Duration of illness
Herpes zoster (shingles)	Duration of illness
Measles (rubeola)	4 days after start of rash (for duration of illness in immunocompromised patients)
Meningitis (*H. influenzae* or *Neisseria meningitidis* known or suspected)	4 hours after start of effective therapy
Meningococcemia	24 hours after start of effective therapy
Mumps	9 days after onset of swelling
Pertussis (whooping cough)	7 days after start of effective therapy or 3 weeks after onset of paroxysms, if untreated
Plague (pneumonic)	3 days after start of effective therapy
Pneumonia (*H. influenzae, N. meningitidis*)	4 hours after start of effective therapy
Rabies	Duration of illness
Rubella (congenital syndrome)	For first year after birth unless nasopharyngeal cultures are negative for causative organism after age 3 months
Rubella (German measles)	7 days after onset of rash
Smallpox (variola)	Duration of illness
Tuberculosis (pulmonary, confirmed or suspected)	Depends on clinical response; usually 10 to 21 days after start of effective therapy

Adapted from Pugliese, G., ed. *Universal Precautions: Policies, Procedures, and Resources.* Chicago: American Hospital Publishing, Inc., 1991.

ments. (See *Conditions or treatments requiring neutropenic isolation* for more information.)

Neutropenic isolation requires a private room equipped with positive air pressure, if possible, to force suspended particles down and out of the room. It also requires use of gowns, gloves, and masks by hospital staff and visitors, and thorough hand-washing technique using an antiseptic cleaning agent.

To care for patients who have temporarily increased susceptibility, such as those who have undergone bone marrow transplantation, neutropenic isolation may also require a patient-isolator unit and the use of sterile linens, gowns, gloves, and head and shoe coverings. In such cases, all other items taken into the room should be sterilized.

Equipment
Gowns ▪ gloves ▪ masks ▪ shoe covers, if required ▪ plastic bags ▪ neutropenic isolation door cards.

Gather any additional supplies, such as a thermometer, stethoscope, and blood pressure cuff *so you don't have to leave the isolation room unnecessarily.*

Preparation of equipment
Keep supplies in a clean enclosed cart or in an anteroom outside the room.

Implementation
• After placing the patient in a private room, explain isolation procedures to him *to ease his anxiety and promote cooperation.*

• Place neutropenic isolation cards on the door *to caution those entering the room.*

• Wash your hands with an antiseptic agent before putting on gloves *to prevent bacterial growth on gloved skin.* Wash your hands again after leaving the room.

• Put on a clean mask each time you enter the patient's room. Use gowns and gloves according to universal precaution recommendations.

• Don't allow visits by anyone known to be infected or ill. Show all visitors how to put on masks before entering the patient's room, and tell them to remove them only after leaving the room.

Special considerations
Don't perform invasive procedures, such as urethral catheterization, unless absolutely necessary *because these procedures risk serious infection in the patient with impaired resistance.* Avoid transporting the patient out of the room; if he must be moved, gown and mask him first.

Instruct the housekeeping staff to put on gowns, gloves, and masks before entering the patient's room; no ill or infected person should enter. The room should be

Conditions or treatments requiring neutropenic isolation

CONDITION OR TREATMENT	PERIOD OF ISOLATION
Acquired immunodeficiency syndrome	Until white blood cell count reaches 1000/mm³ or less, or according to hospital guidelines
Agranulocytosis	Until remission
Burns Noninfected, extensive	Until skin surface heals substantially

Dermatitis
    Noninfected vesicular, bullous, or eczematous disease
    (when severe and extensive)
	Until skin surface heals substantially

Immunosuppressive therapy	Until patient's immunity is adequate
Lymphomas and leukemia Especially in late stages of Hodgkin's disease or acute leukemia	Until clinical improvement is substantial

cleaned with new or scrupulously clean equipment. Because the patient does not have a contagious disease, materials leaving the room need no special precautions, and the room requires no special cleaning after the patient has been discharged.

Documentation
Record the need for neutropenic isolation on the nursing care plan.

Selected references

Centers for Disease Control. "Recommendations for Prevention of HIV Transmission in Health-Care Settings," in *Morbidity and Mortality Weekly Report* 36(Supp. 2S):3S-18S, August 21, 1987.

Centers for Disease Control. "Summary of Notifiable Diseases: United States," in *Morbidity and Mortality Weekly Report* 38(54):3, 10, October 5, 1990.

Centers for Disease Control. "Update: Universal Precautions for Prevention of Transmission of Human Immunodeficiency Virus, Hepatitis B Virus and Other Bloodborne Pathogens in Health-Care Settings," in *Morbidity and Mortality Weekly Report* 37(24):377-88, June 24, 1988.

Department of Labor, Occupational Safety and Health Administration. "Occupational Exposure to Hepatitis B Virus and Human Immunodeficiency Virus, Advance Notice of Proposed Rulemaking" *Federal Register* 52(228):45438-41, November 27, 1987.

Illustrated Manual of Nursing Practice. Springhouse, Pa.: Springhouse Corp., 1991.

Jackson, M.M., et al. "Why Not Treat All Body Substances as Infectious?" *AJN* 87(9):1137-39, September 1987.

Kozier, B., and Erb, G. *Techniques in Clinical Nursing,* 3rd ed. New York: Addison-Wesley Publishing Co., 1989.

Pugliese, Gina, ed. *Universal Precautions: Policies, Procedures, and Resources.* Chicago: American Hospital Publishing, 1991.

Wyngarden, J.B., and Smith, L.B. *Cecil Textbook of Medicine,* 18th ed. Philadelphia: W.B. Saunders Co., 1988.

CHAPTER 3

SPECIMEN COLLECTION AND TESTING

SHERRY BUFFINGTON, RN, CCRN, CLA (ASCP)

Introduction

Collecting specimens promptly and correctly can directly affect a patient's diagnosis, treatment, and recovery. In many cases, the nurse holds sole responsibility for collecting appropriate specimens.

However, even for tests that aren't the nurse's hands-on responsibility, you may be responsible for scheduling them, preparing the patient beforehand, assisting the doctor or other caregiver in performing the test, and caring for the patient afterward. For some tests, you'll teach the patient how to perform the procedure at home — for example, blood glucose tests or fecal occult blood tests. In every case, your nursing responsibilities depend on the clinical setting and your hospital's policies as well as the guidelines provided in your state's or province's nurse practice act.

No matter what part you play in a patient's diagnostic workup, your role always is pivotal in ensuring proper preparation, testing, and aftercare.

Patient preparation

A thorough working knowledge of diagnostic tests will help you prepare patients for them. If you can explain a test with clarity and compassion, you'll help put the patient at ease, gain his trust and cooperation, and thus ensure more accurate results. Helping him understand a procedure based on the doctor's explanations also paves the way for consent that's truly informed.

When preparing a patient, make your explanations clear, straightforward, and complete. For example, before a difficult or painful procedure, such as bone marrow biopsy, you should warn the patient about the type of discomfort he will probably feel. Letting him know exactly what to expect helps him tolerate such a procedure. Preparation should include telling the patient how long the procedure takes and how soon the results will be available.

If you're assisting the doctor with a test, talk to the patient throughout to comfort and encourage him. Prepare him for upcoming sensations, if necessary. Afterward, watch for adverse reactions or complications, and be prepared to implement appropriate care.

Some tests require more detailed instructions to promote cooperation and ensure accurate specimen collection, especially when the patient must modify his behavior before the test or when he will be collecting the specimen himself. For example, you may have to instruct him to observe a special diet, to suspend taking certain medications, or to learn a special collection technique.

Whenever possible, reinforce your verbal explanations with appropriate printed information. Make sure the patient has time to read the information before physical preparation for the test or procedure begins. Many institutions also have videocassettes, telelectures, and films available to augment the patient-teaching process.

Informed consent

Fundamental requirements have been established to protect a patient's rights while he's receiving care. One of the most important rights is informed consent, which states that the patient (or a responsible family member if the patient is legally incompetent) must fully understand what will be done during a test, surgery, or any medical procedure and must understand its risks and implications *before* he can legally consent to it.

Explaining a procedure, how it will be performed, and its potential benefits and risks is primarily the doctor's responsibility. The nurse typically reinforces the doctor's explanation, confirms that the patient comprehends it, and verifies that written consent has been given when necessary. Written consent isn't always necessary for individual tests; informed verbal consent may be adequate. The patient retains the legal right to withdraw consent — verbal or written — at any time and for any reason and to refuse care or treatment.

Safety measures

Keep in mind that proper specimen collection not only helps to ensure accurate results but also protects you and the patient. Use of gloves and other barriers has become routine in many heath care settings. Before you're exposed to a patient's body fluids, be sure you understand and comply with appropriate precautions.

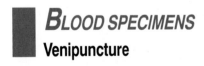

BLOOD SPECIMENS
Venipuncture

Performed to obtain a venous blood sample, venipuncture involves piercing a vein with a needle and collecting blood in a syringe or evacuated tube. Typically, venipuncture is performed using the antecubital fossa. If necessary, however, it can be performed on a vein in the wrist, the dorsum of the hand or foot, or another accessible location. Usually, laboratory personnel carry out the procedure in

Guide to color-top collection tubes

TUBE COLOR	DRAW VOLUME	ADDITIVE	PURPOSE
Red	2 to 20 ml	None	Serum studies
Lavender	2 to 10 ml	EDTA	Whole blood studies
Green	2 to 15 ml	Heparin (sodium, lithium, or ammonium)	Plasma studies
Blue	2.7 or 4.5 ml	Sodium citrate and citric acid	Coagulation studies on plasma
Black	2.7 or 4.5 ml	Sodium oxalate	Coagulation studies on plasma
Gray	3 to 10 ml	Glycolytic inhibitor, such as sodium fluoride, powdered oxalate, or glycolytic-microbial inhibitor	Glucose determinations on serum or plasma
Yellow	12 ml	Acid-citrate-dextrose (ACD)	Whole blood studies

the hospital setting; however, a nurse may perform it occasionally.

Equipment
Tourniquet ▪ gloves ▪ syringe or evacuated tubes and needle holder ▪ 70% ethyl alcohol or povidone-iodine sponges ▪ 20G or 21G needle for the forearm or 25G for the wrist, hand, ankle, or for children ▪ color-coded tubes containing appropriate additives (see *Guide to color-top collection tubes)* ▪ labels ▪ laboratory request form ▪ 2″ × 2″ gauze pads ▪ adhesive bandage.

Preparation of equipment
If you're using evacuated tubes, open the needle packet, attach the needle to its holder, and select the appropriate tubes. If you're using a syringe, attach the appropriate needle to it. Be sure to choose a syringe large enough to hold all the blood required for the test. Label all collection tubes clearly with the patient's name and room number, the doctor's name, and the date and time of collection.

Implementation
• Wash your hands thoroughly and don gloves *to prevent cross-contamination.*
• Tell the patient that you're about to take a blood sample, and explain the procedure *to ease his anxiety and en-*

courage his cooperation. Ask him if he's ever felt faint, sweaty, or nauseated when having blood drawn.
• If the patient is on bed rest, ask him to lie supine, with his head slightly elevated and his arms at his sides. Ask the ambulatory patient to sit in a chair and support his arm securely on an armrest or table.
• Assess the patient's veins *to determine the best puncture site.* (See *Possible venipuncture sites.)* Observe the skin for the vein's blue color, or palpate the vein for a firm rebound sensation.
• Tie a tourniquet 2″ (5 cm) proximal to the area chosen. *By impeding venous return to the heart while still allowing arterial flow, a tourniquet produces venous dilation.* If arterial perfusion remains adequate, you'll be able to feel the radial pulse. (If the tourniquet fails to dilate the vein, have the patient open and close his fist repeatedly. Then ask him to close his fist as you insert the needle and to open it again when the needle is in place.)
• Clean the venipuncture site with a povidone-iodine sponge or with an alcohol sponge. Don't wipe off the povidone-iodine with alcohol *because alcohol cancels the effect of povidone-iodine.* Wipe in a circular motion, spiraling outward from the site *to avoid introducing potentially infectious skin flora into the vessel during the procedure.* If you use alcohol, apply it with friction for 30 seconds, or until the final sponge comes away clean. Allow the skin to dry before performing venipuncture.

• Immobilize the vein by pressing just below the venipuncture site with your thumb and drawing the skin taut.

• Position the needle holder or syringe with the needle bevel up and the shaft parallel to the path of the vein and at a 30-degree angle to the arm. Insert the needle into the vein. If you're using a syringe, venous blood will appear in the hub; withdraw the blood slowly, pulling the plunger of the syringe gently *to create steady suction* until you obtain the required sample. *Pulling the plunger too forcibly may collapse the vein.* If you're using a needle holder and evacuated tube, a drop of blood will appear just inside the needle holder. Grasp the holder securely to stabilize it in the vein, and push down on the collection tube until the needle punctures the rubber stopper. Blood will flow into the tube automatically.

• Remove the tourniquet as soon as blood flows adequately *to prevent stasis and hemoconcentration, which can impair test results.* If the flow is sluggish, leave the tourniquet in place longer, but always remove it before withdrawing the needle.

• After you've drawn the sample, place a gauze pad over the puncture site, and slowly and gently remove the needle from the vein. When using an evacuated tube, remove it from the needle holder *to release the vacuum* before withdrawing the needle from the vein.

• Apply gentle pressure to the puncture site for 2 or 3 minutes or until bleeding stops. *This prevents extravasation into the surrounding tissue, which causes hematoma.*

• After bleeding stops, apply an adhesive bandage.

• If you've used a syringe, transfer the sample to a collection tube. Detach the needle from the syringe, open the collection tube, and gently empty the sample into the tube, being careful to avoid foaming, *which may cause hemolysis.*

• Finally, check the venipuncture site *to make sure a hematoma hasn't developed.* If it has, then apply warm soaks.

• Discard used gloves in the appropriate container.

Special considerations

Never draw a venous sample from an arm or leg already being used for I.V. therapy or blood administration *because this may affect test results.* Don't draw a venous sample from an infection site *because this risks introduction of pathogens into the vascular system.* Likewise, avoid drawing blood from edematous areas, arteriovenous shunts, or sites of previous hematoma or vascular injury.

If you use a blood pressure cuff as a tourniquet, inflate it to a level between the patient's systolic and diastolic pressures *to allow for venous distention without constricting arterial flow.* If the patient has large, distended, highly visible veins, perform venipuncture without a tourniquet *to minimize the risk of hematoma.*

Possible venipuncture sites

The illustrations below show the anatomic locations of veins that can be used for venipuncture. The most commonly used sites are on the forearm, followed by those on the hand. Keep in mind that using the leg veins raises the patient's risk of thrombophlebitis.

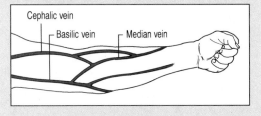

Cephalic vein

Basilic vein — Median vein

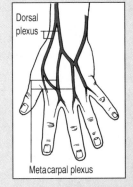

Dorsal plexus

Metacarpal plexus

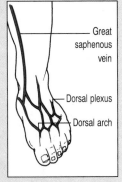

Great saphenous vein

Dorsal plexus

Dorsal arch

If the patient has a clotting disorder or is receiving anticoagulant therapy, maintain firm pressure on the venipuncture site for at least 5 minutes after withdrawing the needle *to prevent possible formation of a hematoma.* Perform venipuncture cautiously in patients who have clotting disorders or who are receiving anticoagulant therapy.

Avoid using veins in the patient's legs for venipuncture, if possible, *because this increases the risk of thrombophlebitis.*

Complications

Hematoma at the needle insertion site is the most common complication of venipuncture. Infection may result from poor technique.

Documentation

Record the date, time, and site of venipuncture; name of the test; the time the sample was sent to the laboratory; and any adverse effects the patient experiences, such as a hematoma or anxiety.

Blood culture

Normally bacteria-free, blood is susceptible to infection through infusion lines, as well as from thrombophlebitis, infected shunts, or bacterial endocarditis from prosthetic heart valve replacements. Bacteria may also invade the vascular system from local tissue infections through the lymphatic system and the thoracic duct.

Blood cultures are performed to detect bacterial invasion (bacteremia) and the systemic spread of such an infection (septicemia) through the bloodstream. In this procedure, a laboratory technician or a nurse collects a venous blood sample by venipuncture at the patient's bedside and then transfers it into two bottles, one containing an anaerobic medium and the other an aerobic medium. The bottles are incubated, encouraging any organisms present in the sample to grow in the media. Blood cultures allow identification of about 67% of pathogens within 24 hours and up to 90% within 72 hours. (See *Isolator blood-culturing system* for a description of another type of culturing procedure.)

Although some authorities consider the timing of culture collections debatable and possibly irrelevant, others advocate drawing three blood samples at least 1 hour apart. The first of these should be collected at the earliest sign of suspected bacteremia or septicemia. To check for suspected bacterial endocarditis, three or four samples may be collected at 5- to 30-minute intervals before starting antibiotic therapy.

Equipment

Tourniquet ■ gloves ■ alcohol sponges ■ povidone-iodine sponges ■ 10-ml syringe for an adult; 6-ml syringe for a child ■ three or four 20G 1½″ needles ■ two or three blood culture bottles (50-ml bottles for adults, 20-ml bottles for infants and children) with sodium polyethanol sulfonate added (one aerobic bottle containing a suitable medium, such as Trypticase soy broth with 10% carbon dioxide atmosphere; one anaerobic bottle with prereduced medium; and, possibly, one hyperosmotic bottle with 10% sucrose medium) ■ laboratory request form ■ small adhesive bandages ■ 2″ × 2″ gauze pads.

Preparation of equipment

Check culture bottle expiration dates and replace outdated bottles.

Implementation

• Tell the patient that you need to collect a series of blood samples to check for infection. Explain the procedure *to ease his anxiety and promote cooperation.* Explain that the procedure usually requires three separate blood samples drawn at different times.

• Wash your hands and put on gloves.

• Tie a tourniquet 2″ (5 cm) proximal to the area chosen. (See "Venipuncture" in this chapter.)

• Clean the venipuncture site with a povidone-iodine sponge or with an alcohol sponge. Don't wipe off the povidone-iodine with alcohol *because alcohol cancels the effect of povidone-iodine.* Start at the site and work outward in a circular motion. Wait 30 to 60 seconds for the solution to dry.

• Perform a venipuncture, drawing 10 ml of blood from an adult or 2 to 6 ml from a child.

Isolator blood-culturing system

A single-tube blood-culturing system, the Isolator uses lysis and centrifugation to help detect septicemia and monitor the effectiveness of antibacterial drug therapy.

The Isolator evacuated tube, used to collect the blood sample, contains a substance that lyses red blood cells. Then, centrifugation concentrates bacteria and other organisms in the sample onto an inert cushioning pad; the concentrate can then be applied directly onto four agar plates.

The Isolator has several advantages over conventional blood-culturing methods. This system:
• eliminates the bottle method's lengthy incubation period, providing faster results
• improves bacterial survival
• results in more valid positive results through direct application onto agar plates, which dilutes any antibiotic present in the sample to a greater degree
• detects more yeast and polymicrobial infections
• improves the laboratory's ability to detect organisms that are difficult to grow
• is easier to use at the patient's bedside and to transport because blood is drawn directly into the Isolator tube.

• Wipe the diaphragm tops of the culture bottles with a povidone-iodine sponge, and change the needle on the syringe used to draw the blood.
• Inject 5 ml of blood into each 50-ml bottle or 2 ml into a 20-ml pediatric culture bottle. (Bottle size may vary with the hospital's protocol, but the sample dilution should always be 1:10.)
• Label the culture bottles with the patient's name and room number, the doctor's name, and the date and time of collection. Indicate the suspected diagnosis and the patient's temperature, and note on the laboratory request form any recent antibiotic therapy. Send the samples to the laboratory immediately.
• Discard the gloves in the appropriate container.

Special considerations

Obtain each set of cultures from a different site. Avoid using existing blood lines for cultures unless the sample is drawn when the line is inserted or unless catheter sepsis is suspected.

Complications

The most common complication of venipuncture is formation of a hematoma. If a hematoma develops, apply warm soaks to the site.

Documentation

In your notes, record the date and time of blood sample collection, the name of the test, the amount of blood collected, the number of bottles used, the patient's temperature, and any adverse reactions to the procedure.

 # Blood glucose tests

Rapid, easy-to-perform reagent strip tests (such as Glucostix, Chemstrip bG, or Multistix) use a drop of capillary blood obtained by fingerstick, heelstick, or earlobe puncture as a sample. These tests can detect or monitor elevated blood glucose levels in patients with diabetes, screen for diabetes mellitus and neonatal hypoglycemia, and help distinguish diabetic coma from nondiabetic coma. In these tests, a reagent patch on the tip of a hand-held plastic strip changes color in response to the amount of glucose in the blood sample. Comparing the color change with a standardized color chart provides a semiquantitative measurement of blood glucose levels; inserting the strip in a portable blood glucose meter (such as a Glucometer II, Accu-Chek II, or One Touch) provides quantitative measurements that compare in accuracy with other laboratory tests. Some meters store successive

test results electronically to help determine glucose patterns.

These tests can be performed in the hospital, the doctor's office, or the patient's home.

Equipment

Reagent strips ■ gloves ■ portable blood glucose meter, if available ■ gauze pads ■ alcohol sponges ■ disposable lancets ■ small adhesive bandage ■ watch or clock with a second hand.

Implementation

• Explain the procedure to the patient or to the infant's parents.
• Select the puncture site — usually the fingertip or earlobe for an adult or the heel or great toe for an infant.
• Wash your hands and don gloves.
• If necessary, dilate the capillaries by applying warm, moist compresses to the area for about 10 minutes.
• Wipe the puncture site with an alcohol sponge and dry it thoroughly with a gauze pad.
• To draw a sample from the patient's fingertip with a disposable lancet (smaller than 2 mm), make the puncture on the side of the fingertip and position the lancet perpendicular to the lines of the patient's fingerprints. Pierce the skin sharply and quickly *to minimize the patient's anxiety and pain, and to increase blood flow.* Alternatively, you may want to use a mechanical bloodletting device, such as an Autolet, which uses a spring-loaded lancet.
• After puncturing the finger, wipe away the first drop of blood *to avoid diluting the sample with tissue fluid.* For the same reason, avoid squeezing the puncture site.
• Touch a drop of blood to the reagent patch on the strip; make sure you cover the entire patch.
• After collecting the blood sample, briefly apply pressure to the puncture site *to prevent painful extravasation of blood into subcutaneous tissues.* Ask the adult patient to hold a gauze pad firmly over the puncture site until bleeding stops.
• Leave the blood on the strip for exactly 60 seconds, and then quickly wash it off with a stream of water from a wash bottle. Don't hold the strip under a faucet *because a strong stream of water will wash off too much blood.* Some reagent strips require only that the blood be wiped off, without washing. Follow the manufacturer's instructions exactly *because results will influence insulin dosage.*
• Immediately after washing, compare the color change on the strip with the standardized color chart on the product container. If you're using a blood glucose meter, follow the manufacturer's instructions. Meter designs vary, but they all analyze a drop of blood placed on a

Oral and intravenous glucose tolerance tests

For monitoring trends in glucose metabolism, two tests may offer benefits over testing blood with reagent strips.

Oral glucose tolerance test

The most sensitive test for detecting borderline diabetes mellitus, the oral glucose tolerance test (OGTT) measures carbohydrate metabolism after ingestion of a challenge dose of glucose. The body absorbs this dose rapidly, causing plasma glucose levels to rise and peak within 30 minutes to 1 hour. The pancreas responds by secreting insulin, causing glucose levels to return to normal within 2 to 3 hours. During this period, plasma and urine glucose levels are monitored to assess insulin secretion and the body's ability to metabolize glucose.

Although you may not collect the blood and urine specimens (usually five of each) required for this test, you will be responsible for preparing the patient for the test and monitoring his physical condition during the test.

Begin by explaining the OGTT to the patient. Then, tell him to maintain a high-carbohydrate diet for 3 days and to fast for 10 to 16 hours before the test, as ordered. The patient must not smoke, drink coffee or alcohol, or exercise strenuously for 8 hours before or during the test. Inform him that he will then receive a challenge dose of 100 g of carbohydrate (usually a sweetened carbonated beverage or gelatin).

Tell the patient who will perform the venipunctures and when, and that he may feel slight discomfort from the needle punctures and the pressure of the tourniquet. Reassure him that collecting each blood sample usually takes less than 3 minutes. As ordered, withhold drugs that may affect test results. Remind him not to discard the first voided urine specimen on waking.

During the test period, watch for signs and symptoms of hypoglycemia—weakness, restlessness, nervousness, hunger, and sweating—and report these to the doctor immediately. Encourage the patient to drink plenty of water to promote adequate urine excretion. Provide a bedpan, urinal, or specimen container when necessary.

I.V. glucose tolerance test

This test may be chosen for patients unable to absorb an oral dose of glucose—for example, those with malabsorption disorders, short-bowel syndrome, or those who have had a gastrectomy. The I.V. glucose tolerance test measures blood glucose after an I.V. infusion of 50% glucose over 3 or 4 minutes. Blood samples are then drawn after 30 minutes, 1 hour, 2 hours, and 3 hours. After an immediate glucose peak of 300 to 400 mg/dl (accompanied by glycosuria), the normal glucose curve falls steadily, reaching fasting levels within 1 to 1¼ hours. Failure to achieve fasting glucose levels within 2 to 3 hours typically confirms diabetes.

reagent strip that comes with the unit, and they provide a digital display of the resulting glucose level.

• After bleeding has stopped, you may apply a small adhesive bandage to the puncture site.

Special considerations

Before using reagent strips, check the expiration date on the package and replace outdated strips. Also check for special instructions related to the specific reagent. The reagent area of a fresh strip should match the color on the "0" block on the color chart. Protect the strips from light, heat, and moisture.

Before using a blood glucose meter, calibrate it and run it with a control sample *to ensure accurate test results.* Follow the manufacturer's instructions for calibration.

Avoid selecting cold, cyanotic, or swollen puncture sites *to ensure an adequate blood sample.* If you can't obtain a capillary sample, perform venipuncture and place a large drop of venous blood on the reagent strip. If you

want to test blood from a refrigerated sample, allow the blood to return to room temperature before testing it.

To help detect abnormal glucose metabolism and diagnose diabetes mellitus, the doctor may order other blood glucose tests. (See *Oral and intravenous glucose tolerance tests.)*

Home care

If the patient will be using the reagent strip system at home, teach him the proper use of the lancet or Autolet, the reagent strips and color chart, and the portable blood glucose meter, as necessary. Also provide written guidelines.

Documentation

Record the reading from the reagent strip (using a portable blood glucose meter or a color chart) in your notes or on a special flowchart, if available. Also record the time and date of the test.

Arterial puncture for blood gas analysis

Obtaining an arterial blood sample requires percutaneous puncture of the brachial, radial, or femoral artery or withdrawal of a sample from an arterial line. Once drawn, the sample can be analyzed for arterial blood gases.

Arterial blood gas (ABG) analysis evaluates ventilation by measuring blood pH and the partial pressures of oxygen (PaO_2) and carbon dioxide ($PaCO_2$) in arterial blood. Blood pH measurement reveals the blood's acid-base balance. PaO_2 indicates the amount of oxygen that the lungs deliver to the blood, and $PaCO_2$ indicates the lungs' capacity to eliminate carbon dioxide. ABG samples can also be analyzed for oxygen content and saturation and for bicarbonate values.

ABG analysis is ordered commonly for patients who have chronic obstructive pulmonary disease, pulmonary edema, acute respiratory distress syndrome, myocardial infarction, or pneumonia. It's also performed during episodes of shock and after coronary artery bypass surgery, resuscitation from cardiac arrest, changes in respiratory therapy or status, and prolonged anesthesia.

Most ABG samples can be drawn by a respiratory technician or specially trained nurse. Collection from the femoral artery, however, is usually performed by a doctor. Before attempting a radial puncture, Allen's test should be performed to assess the adequacy of the blood supply to the patient's hand. (See *Performing Allen's test.*)

Equipment
10-ml glass syringe or plastic luer-lock syringe specially made for drawing blood gases ■ 1-ml ampule of aqueous heparin (1:1,000) ■ 20G 1¼″ needle ■ 22G 1″ needle ■ alcohol sponge ■ povidone-iodine sponge ■ two 2″×2″ gauze pads ■ gloves ■ rubber cap for syringe hub or rubber stopper for needle ■ ice-filled plastic bag ■ label ■ laboratory request form ■ adhesive bandage ■ optional: 1% lidocaine solution.

Many hospitals use a commercial ABG kit that contains all the equipment listed above (except the adhesive bandage and ice). If your hospital doesn't use such a kit, obtain a sterile syringe specially made for drawing blood gases and use a clean emesis basin filled with ice instead of the plastic bag to transport the sample to the laboratory.

Preparation of equipment
Prepare the collection equipment before entering the patient's room. Wash your hands thoroughly; then open the ABG kit and remove the specimen label and the plastic

---

Performing Allen's test

Rest the patient's arm on the mattress or bedside stand, and support his wrist with a rolled towel. Have him clench his fist. Then, using your index and middle fingers, press on the radial and ulnar arteries. Hold this position for a few seconds.

Without removing your fingers from the patient's arteries, ask him to unclench his fist and hold his hand in a relaxed position. The palm will be blanched because pressure from your fingers has impaired the normal blood flow.

Release pressure on the patient's ulnar artery. If the hand becomes flushed, which indicates blood filling the vessels, you can safely proceed with the radial artery puncture. If the hand doesn't flush, perform the test on the other arm.

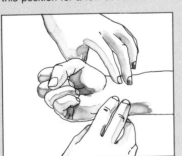
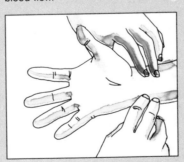
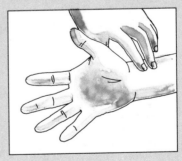

Arterial puncture technique

The angle of needle penetration in arterial blood gas sampling depends on the artery to be sampled. For the radial artery, which is used most commonly, the needle should enter bevel up at a 30- to 45-degree angle.

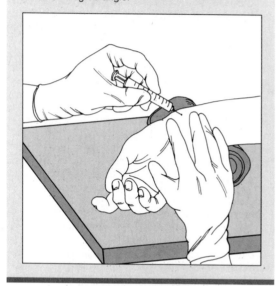

bag. Record on the label the patient's name and room number, the date and collection time, and the doctor's name. Fill the plastic bag with ice and set it aside.

To heparinize the syringe, first attach the 20G needle to the syringe. Then open the ampule of heparin. Draw all the heparin into the syringe *to prevent the sample from clotting.* Hold the syringe upright, and pull the plunger back slowly to about the 7-ml mark. Rotate the barrel while pulling the plunger back *to allow the heparin to coat the inside surface of the syringe.* Then, slowly force the heparin toward the hub of the syringe and expel all but about 0.1 ml of heparin.

To heparinize the needle, first replace the 20G needle with the 22G needle. Then, hold the syringe upright, tilt it slightly, and eject the remaining heparin. *Excess heparin in the syringe alters blood pH and PaO_2 values.*

Implementation

• Tell the patient you need to collect an arterial blood sample, and explain the procedure *to help ease anxiety and promote cooperation.* Tell him that the needle stick will cause some discomfort but that he must remain still during the procedure.

• After washing your hands and donning gloves, place a rolled towel under the patient's wrist *for support.* Locate the artery and palpate it for a strong pulse.

• Clean the puncture site with a povidone-iodine sponge or with an alcohol sponge. Don't wipe off the povidone-iodine with alcohol *because alcohol cancels the effect of povidone-iodine.*

• Using a circular motion, clean the area, starting in the center of the site and spiraling outward *to avoid introducing potentially infectious skin flora into the vessel during the procedure.* If you use alcohol, apply it with friction for 30 seconds or until the final sponge comes away clean. Allow the skin to dry.

• Palpate the artery with the index and middle fingers of one hand while holding the syringe over the puncture site with the other hand.

• Hold the needle bevel up at a 30- to 45-degree angle. When puncturing the brachial artery, hold the needle at a 60-degree angle. (See *Arterial puncture technique.*)

• Puncture the skin and the arterial wall in one motion, following the path of the artery.

• Watch for blood backflow in the syringe. Don't pull back on the plunger *because arterial blood should enter the syringe automatically.* Fill the syringe to the 5-ml mark.

• After collecting the sample, press a gauze pad firmly over the puncture site until bleeding stops—at least 5 minutes. If the patient is receiving anticoagulant therapy or has a blood dyscrasia, apply pressure for 10 to 15 minutes; if necessary, ask a co-worker to hold the gauze pad in place while you prepare the sample for transport to the laboratory. Don't ask the patient to hold the pad. *If he fails to apply sufficient pressure, a large, painful hematoma may form, hindering future arterial punctures at that site.*

• Check the syringe for air bubbles *because these can alter PaO_2 values.* If air bubbles appear, remove them by holding the syringe upright and slowly ejecting some of the blood onto a $2'' \times 2''$ gauze pad.

• Insert the needle into a rubber stopper, or remove the needle and place a rubber cap directly on the needle hub. *This prevents the sample from leaking and keeps air out of the syringe.*

• Put the labeled sample in the ice-filled plastic bag or emesis basin. Attach a properly completed laboratory request form, and send the sample to the laboratory immediately.

• When bleeding stops, apply a small adhesive bandage to the site.

• Monitor the patient's vital signs, and observe for signs of circulatory impairment, such as swelling, discoloration, pain, numbness, or tingling in the bandaged arm or leg. Watch for bleeding at the puncture site.

Special considerations
If the patient is receiving oxygen, make sure that his therapy has been underway for at least 15 minutes before drawing arterial blood.

Unless ordered, don't turn off existing oxygen therapy before drawing arterial blood samples. However, be sure to indicate the amount and type of oxygen therapy the patient is receiving on the laboratory request slip.

If the patient isn't receiving oxygen, indicate that he is breathing room air.

If the patient has just received a breathing treatment or nebulizer treatment, wait about 20 minutes before drawing the sample.

If necessary, you may anesthetize the puncture site with 1% lidocaine solution. Consider such use of lidocaine carefully *because it delays the procedure, the patient may be allergic to the drug, or the resulting vasoconstriction may prevent successful puncture.*

When filling out a laboratory request form for ABG analysis, be sure to include the following information *to help the laboratory staff calibrate the equipment and evaluate results correctly:* the patient's current temperature, most recent hemoglobin level, current respiratory rate, and fraction of inspired oxygen and tidal volume if the patient is on a ventilator.

Complications
If you use too much force when attempting to puncture the artery, the needle may touch the periosteum of the bone, causing the patient considerable pain; or you may advance the needle through the opposite wall of the artery. If this happens, slowly pull the needle back a short distance and check to see if get a blood return. If blood still fails to enter the syringe, withdraw the needle completely and start with a fresh heparinized needle. Do not make more than two attempts to withdraw blood from the same site. *Probing the artery may injure it and the radial nerve. Also, hemolysis will alter test results.*

If arterial spasm occurs, blood will not flow into the syringe and you won't be able to collect the sample. If this happens, replace the needle with a smaller one and attempt the puncture again. *A smaller-bore needle is less likely to cause arterial spasm.*

Documentation
Record the results of Allen's test, the time the sample was drawn, the patient's temperature, the site of the arterial puncture, the length of time pressure was applied to the site to control bleeding, and the type and amount of oxygen therapy the patient was receiving.

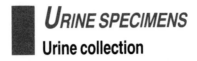

URINE SPECIMENS
Urine collection

A random urine specimen, usually collected as part of the physical examination or at various times during hospitalization, permits laboratory screening for urinary and systemic disorders, as well as for drug screening. A clean-catch midstream specimen, once used only to confirm urinary tract infection, is now replacing random collection for many other purposes because it provides a virtually uncontaminated specimen without the need for bladder catheterization.

An indwelling catheter specimen — obtained either by clamping the drainage tube and emptying the accumulated urine into a container or by aspirating a sample with a syringe — requires sterile technique to prevent catheter contamination and urinary tract infection. This method is contraindicated in patients who have recently undergone genitourinary surgery.

Equipment
For a random specimen: bedpan or urinal with cover, if necessary ▪ gloves ▪ graduated container ▪ specimen container with lid ▪ label ▪ laboratory request form.

For a clean-catch midstream specimen: basin ▪ soap and water ▪ towel ▪ gloves ▪ three sterile 2″ × 2″ gauze pads ▪ povidone-iodine solution ▪ sterile specimen container with lid ▪ label ▪ bedpan or urinal, if necessary ▪ laboratory request form. (Commercial clean-catch kits containing antiseptic towelettes, sterile specimen container with lid and label, and instructions for use in several languages are widely used.)

For an indwelling catheter specimen: 10-ml syringe ▪ 21G or 22G 1½″ needle ▪ tube clamp ▪ sterile specimen cup with lid ▪ gloves ▪ alcohol sponge ▪ label ▪ laboratory request form.

Implementation
• Tell the patient that you need a urine specimen for laboratory analysis. Explain the procedure to him and his family, if necessary, *to promote cooperation and prevent accidental disposal of specimens.*

Collecting a random specimen
• Provide privacy. Instruct the patient on bed rest to void into a clean bedpan or urinal, or ask the ambulatory patient to void into either one in the bathroom.
• Don gloves. Then pour at least 120 ml of urine into the specimen container, and cap the container securely. If the patient's urine output must be measured and re-

Aspirating a urine specimen

To aspirate a urine specimen from a rubber indwelling catheter that has no built-in sampling port, insert the syringe needle into the catheter just above where it connects to the drainage tube. This position prevents accidental puncture of the lumen that connects with the catheter balloon. Aspirating the water from this lumen can deflate the balloon and dislodge the catheter.

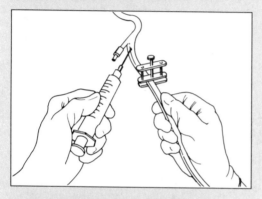

To aspirate a specimen from a built-in sampling port, wipe the port with an alcohol sponge and insert the needle perpendicular to the catheter.

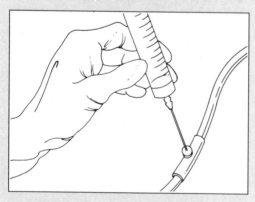

corded, pour the remaining urine into the graduated container. Otherwise, discard the remaining urine. If you inadvertently spill urine on the outside of the container, clean and dry it *to prevent possible cross-contamination.*
• Label the sample container with the patient's name and room number and the date and time of collection, attach the request form, and send it to the laboratory immediately. *Delaying the sample may alter test results.*
• Clean the graduated container and urinal or bedpan, and return these to their proper storage. Discard disposable items.
• Wash your hands thoroughly *to prevent cross-contamination.* Offer the patient a washcloth and soap and water to wash his hands.

Collecting a clean-catch midstream specimen
• Because the goal of this method is a virtually uncontaminated specimen, explain the procedure to the patient carefully. Provide illustrations to emphasize the correct collection technique, if possible.
• Tell the patient to remove all clothing from the waist down and to stand in front of the toilet as for urination or, if female, to sit far back on the toilet seat and spread her legs. Then have the patient clean the periurethral area (tip of the penis or labial folds, vulva, and urethral meatus) with soap and water and then wipe the area three times, each time with a fresh 2″ × 2″ gauze pad soaked in povidone-iodine solution, or with the wipes provided in a commercial kit. Instruct the female patient to separate her labial folds with the thumb and forefinger. Tell her to wipe down one side with the first pad and discard it, to wipe the other side with the second pad and discard it and, finally, to wipe down the center over the urinary meatus with the third pad and discard it. Stress the importance of cleaning from front to back *to avoid contaminating the genital area with fecal matter.* For the uncircumcised male patient, emphasize the need to retract his foreskin *to effectively clean the meatus* and to keep it retracted during voiding.
• Tell the female patient to straddle the bedpan or toilet *to allow labial spreading.* She should continue to keep her labia separated with her fingers while voiding.
• Instruct the patient to begin voiding into the bedpan, urinal, or toilet *because the urine stream washes bacteria from the urethra and urinary meatus.* Then, without stopping the urine stream, the patient should move the collection container into the stream, collecting about 30 to 50 ml at the midstream portion of the voiding. The patient can then finish voiding into the bedpan, urinal, or toilet.
• Don gloves before discarding the first and last portions of the voiding, and measure the remaining urine in a graduated cylinder for intake and output records, if necessary. Be sure to include the amount in the specimen container when recording the total amount voided.
• Take the sterile container from the patient, and cap it securely. Avoid touching the inside of the container or the lid. If the outside of the container is soiled, clean it and wipe it dry. Remove gloves and discard them properly.

• Wash your hands thoroughly *to prevent cross-contamination.* Tell the patient to wash his hands also.
• Label the container with the patient's name and room number, name of test, type of specimen, collection time, and suspected diagnosis, if known. If a urine culture has been ordered, note any current antibiotic therapy on the laboratory request form. Send the container to the laboratory immediately, or place it on ice *to prevent specimen deterioration and altered test results.*

Collecting an indwelling catheter specimen
• About 30 minutes before collecting the specimen, clamp the drainage tube *to allow urine to accumulate.*
• Put on gloves. If the drainage tube has a built-in sampling port, wipe the port with an alcohol sponge. Uncap the needle on the syringe, and insert the needle into the sampling port at a 90-degree angle to the tubing. Aspirate the specimen into the syringe. (See *Aspirating a urine specimen.)*
• If the drainage tube doesn't have a sampling port and the catheter is made of rubber, obtain the specimen from the catheter. *Other types of catheters will leak after you withdraw the needle.* To withdraw the specimen from a rubber catheter, wipe it with an alcohol sponge just above the point where it connects to the drainage tube. Insert the needle into the rubber catheter at a 45-degree angle and withdraw the specimen. Never insert the needle into the shaft of the catheter *because this may puncture the lumen leading to the catheter balloon.*
• Transfer the specimen to a sterile container, label it, and send it to the laboratory immediately or place it on ice. If a urine culture is to be performed, be sure to list any antibiotic therapy on the laboratory request form.
• If the catheter is not made of rubber or has no sampling port, wipe the area where the catheter joins the drainage tube with an alcohol sponge. Disconnect the catheter, and allow urine to drain into the sterile specimen container. Avoid touching the inside of the sterile container with the catheter, and don't touch anything with the catheter drainage tube *to avoid contamination.* When you have the specimen, wipe both connection sites with an alcohol sponge and join them. Cap the specimen container, label it, and send it to the laboratory immediately or place it on ice.
◆ *Nursing alert.* Make sure you unclamp the drainage tube after collecting the specimen *to prevent urine backflow that may cause bladder distention and infection.* ◆

Home care
Instruct the patient to collect the sample in a clean container with a tight-fitting lid, and to keep it on ice or in the refrigerator (separate from any food items) for up to 24 hours.

Documentation
Record the times of specimen collection and transport to the laboratory. Specify the test, and the appearance, odor, color, and any unusual characteristics of the specimen. If necessary, record the urine volume on the patient's intake and output record.

Timed urine collection

Because hormones, proteins, and electrolytes are excreted in small variable amounts in urine, specimens for measuring these substances must typically be collected over an extended time to yield quantities of diagnostic value.

A 24-hour specimen is used most commonly because it provides an average excretion rate for substances eliminated during this period. Timed specimens may also be collected for shorter periods, such as 2 or 12 hours, depending on the specific information needed.

A timed urine specimen may also be collected after administering a challenge dose of a chemical — inulin, for example — to detect various renal disorders.

Equipment
Large collection bottle with a cap or stopper, or a commercial plastic container ■ preservative, if necessary ■ gloves ■ bedpan or urinal, if patient does not have an indwelling catheter ■ graduated container, if patient is on intake and output measurement ■ gloves ■ ice-filled container, if a refrigerator isn't available ■ label ■ laboratory request form ■ four patient care reminders.

Check with the laboratory to see what preservatives may be needed in the urine specimen, or if a dark collection bottle is required.

Implementation
• Explain the procedure to the patient and his family members, as necessary, *to enlist their cooperation and prevent accidental disposal of urine during the collection period.* Emphasize that loss of even *one* urine specimen during the collection period invalidates the test and requires that it begin again.
• Place patient care reminders over the patient's bed, in his bathroom, on the bedpan hopper in the utility room, and on the urinal or indwelling catheter collection bag. Include the patient's name and room number, the date, and the collection interval.
• Instruct the patient to save all urine during the collection period, to notify you after each voiding, and to avoid contaminating the urine with stool or toilet tissue.

Explain any dietary or drug restrictions and be sure he understands and is willing to comply with them.

For 2-hour collection

• If possible, instruct the patient to drink two to four 8-oz glasses (480 to 960 ml) of water about 30 minutes before collection begins. After 30 minutes, tell him to void. Don gloves and discard this specimen *so the patient starts the collection period with an empty bladder.*

• If ordered, administer a challenge dose of medication (such as glucose solution or corticotropin), and record the time.

• If possible, offer the patient a glass of water at least every hour during the collection period *to stimulate urine production.* After each voiding, don gloves and add the specimen to the collection bottle.

• Instruct the patient to void about 15 minutes before the end of the collection period, if possible, and add this specimen to the collection bottle.

• At the end of the collection period, remove and discard gloves and send the appropriately labeled collection bottle to the laboratory immediately, along with a properly completed laboratory request form.

For 12- and 24-hour collection

• Put on gloves and ask the patient to void. Then discard this urine *so he starts the collection period with an empty bladder.* Record the time.

• After putting on gloves and pouring the first urine specimen into the collection bottle, add the required preservative. Then refrigerate the bottle or keep it on ice until the next voiding, as appropriate.

• Collect all urine voided during the prescribed period. Just before the collection period ends, ask the patient to void again, if possible. Add this last specimen to the collection bottle, pack it in ice *to inhibit deterioration of the specimen,* and remove and discard gloves. Send the specimen to the laboratory. Include a properly completed laboratory request form.

Special considerations

The patient should be hydrated before and during the test *to ensure adequate urine flow.*

Before collection of a timed specimen, make sure the laboratory will be open when the collection period ends *to help ensure prompt, accurate results.* Never store a specimen in a refrigerator containing food or medication *to avoid contamination.* If the patient has an indwelling catheter in place, put the collection bag in an ice-filled container at his bedside.

Instruct the patient to avoid exercise, ingestion of coffee or tea, or any drugs (unless otherwise directed by the doctor) before the test *to avoid altering test results.*

If you accidentally discard a specimen during the collection period, restart the collection. Accidentally discarding a specimen during the test period may result in an additional day of hospitalization, possibly causing the patient personal and financial hardship. Therefore, emphasize the need to save all the patient's urine during the collection period to all persons involved in his care, as well as to family or other visitors.

Home care

If the patient must continue collecting urine at home, provide written instructions for the appropriate method. Tell the patient he can keep the specimens in a brown bag in his refrigerator at home, separate from other refrigerator contents.

Documentation

In the Kardex and in your notes, record the date and interval of collection and that the specimen was sent to the laboratory.

Urine glucose and ketone tests

Reagent tablet and strip tests are used to monitor urine glucose and ketone levels and to screen for diabetes. *Urine ketone tests* monitor fat metabolism, help diagnose carbohydrate deprivation and diabetic ketoacidosis, and help distinguish between diabetic and nondiabetic coma. However, urine glucose tests are less accurate than blood glucose tests, and are now used less frequently because of the increasing convenience of blood self-testing.

The *copper reduction test* (Clinitest) measures the concentration of reducing substances in the urine through the reactions of these substances with a tablet composed of sodium hydroxide, cupric sulfate, and other reagents. When this tablet is added to a test tube containing drops of water and urine, the reaction generates heat. Simultaneously, reduction of cupric ions in the presence of glucose causes a color change. Comparison of this test color with a standardized color chart gives the approximate level of urine glucose. Similarly, the Acetest tablet test produces a color reaction that allows an estimate of urine ketone levels by comparison to a standardized chart.

Glucose oxidase tests (such as Diastix, Tes-Tape, and Chemstrip UG strips) produce color changes when patches of reagents implanted in hand-held plastic strips react with glucose in the patient's urine; *urine ketone strip tests* (such as Chemstrip K and Ketostix) are similar. All test results are read by comparing color changes against a standardized reference chart.

Equipment

For reagent tablet tests: specimen container ■ 10-ml test tube ■ medicine dropper ■ gloves ■ Clinitest or Acetest tablets ■ Clinitest or Acetest color chart.

   For reagent strip tests: specimen container ■ gloves ■ glucose or ketone test strips ■ reference color chart.

   Wear gloves as barrier protection when performing all urine tests.

Implementation

• Explain the test to the patient, and if he's a newly diagnosed diabetic, teach him to perform the test himself. Check his history for medications that may interfere with test results.
• Before each test, instruct the patient not to contaminate the urine specimen with stool or toilet tissue.
• Test the urine specimen immediately after the patient voids.

Clinitest tablet test

• Ask the patient to void, and then ask him to drink a glass of water, if possible. Don gloves and collect a second-voided urine specimen 30 to 45 minutes later.
• Perform the 5-drop test: With the medicine dropper, transfer 5 drops of urine from the specimen container to the test tube. Rinse the dropper and add 10 drops of water to the test tube. Then add one Clinitest tablet to the tube.
• Hold the test tube near the top during the reaction *because the test solution will come to a boil.* Observe the color change that occurs during the reaction.
• Fifteen seconds after effervescence subsides, shake the tube gently. Observe the solution's color and compare it with the Clinitest color chart.
• Remove and discard gloves, and record the test results. Ignore any changes that develop after 15 seconds.
• If the color changes rapidly in the 5-drop test, record the result as "over 2%" glucosuria.
• Alternately, perform the 2-drop test: Transfer 2 drops of urine from the specimen container to the test tube, and then add 10 drops of water and a Clinitest tablet. After the reaction, observe the color of the test solution, and compare it with the Clinitest color chart.
• Remove and discard your gloves, and record the test results.
• Rapid color change in the 2-drop test indicates glycosuria up to 5%.

Acetest tablet test

• Don gloves and collect a second-voided specimen, as for the Clinitest tablet test.
• Place the Acetest tablet on a piece of white paper, and add 1 drop of urine to the tablet.
• After 30 seconds, compare the tablet's color (white, lavender, or purple) with the Acetest color chart. Remove gloves and record the test results.

Glucose oxidase strip tests

• Explain the test to the patient and, if he's diagnosed as diabetic, teach him to perform it himself. Check his history for medications that may interfere with test results. Don gloves before collecting specimens for each of these tests, and remove them to record test results.
• Instruct the patient to void. Ask him to drink a glass of water, if possible, and collect a second-voided specimen after 30 to 45 minutes.
• If you're using Clinistix, dip the reagent end of the strip into the urine for 2 seconds. Remove excess urine by tapping the strip against the container's rim, wait for exactly 10 seconds, and then compare its color with the color chart on the container. Ignore color changes that occur after 10 seconds. Record the result.
• If you're using a Diastix strip, dip the reagent end of the strip into the urine for 2 seconds. Tap off excess urine, wait for exactly 30 seconds, and then compare its color with the standardized color chart on the container. Ignore color changes that occur after 30 seconds. Record the result.
• If you're using a Tes-Tape strip, pull about 1½″ (3.8 cm) of the reagent strip from the dispenser, and dip one end about ¼″ (0.6 cm) into the specimen for 2 seconds. Tap off excess urine, wait exactly 60 seconds, and then compare the darkest part of the tape with the standardized color chart. If the test result exceeds 0.5%, wait an additional 60 seconds and make a final comparison. Record the result.

Ketone strip tests

• Explain the procedure to the patient, and if he's diagnosed as diabetic, teach him to perform the test. Check his medication history. If he's receiving phenazopyridine or levodopa, use Acetest tablets instead *because reagent strips will give inaccurate results.*
• Don gloves and collect a second-voided midstream specimen.
• If you're using Ketostix, dip the reagent end of the strip into the specimen and remove it immediately. Wait exactly 15 seconds, and then compare the color of the strip with the standardized color chart on the container. Ignore color changes that occur after 15 seconds. Record the result.

• If you're using Keto-Diastix, dip the reagent end of the strip into the specimen and remove it immediately. Tap off excess urine, and hold the strip horizontally *to prevent mixing of chemicals between the two reagent squares.* Wait exactly 15 seconds, and then compare the color of the ketone part of the strip with the standardized color chart. After 30 seconds, compare the color of the glucose part of the strip with the chart. Record the results.

Special considerations
Keep reagent strips in a cool, dry place at a temperature below 86° F (30° C), but don't refrigerate them. Keep the containers tightly closed. Don't use discolored or outdated strips.

♦ *Nursing alert.* Because Clinitest tablets contain caustic soda, keep the container tightly closed and in a dry place. If you must handle these tablets, keep your fingers dry *to prevent the tablet from leaving a deposit, which could then be accidentally ingested or brought into contact with eyes, skin, mucous membranes, or clothing, causing caustic burns.* ♦

Documentation
In your notes, record color changes according to the information on the charts on the reagent containers, or use special flowcharts designed to record this information. If you're teaching a patient how to perform the test, keep a record of his progress.

 ## Urine specific gravity

The kidneys maintain homeostasis by varying urine output and its concentration of dissolved salts. Urine specific gravity measures the concentration of urine solutes, which reflects the kidneys' capacity to concentrate urine. The capacity to concentrate urine is among the first functions lost when renal tubular damage occurs.

Urine specific gravity is determined by comparing the weight of a urine specimen with that of an equivalent volume of distilled water, which is 1.000. Because urine contains dissolved salts and other substances, it's heavier than 1.000. Urine specific gravity ranges from 1.003 (very dilute) to 1.035 (highly concentrated); normal values range from 1.010 to 1.025. Specific gravity is commonly measured with a urinometer (a specially calibrated hydrometer designed to float in a cylinder of urine.) The more concentrated the urine, the higher the urinometer floats — and the higher the specific gravity. It may also be measured by a refractometer, which measures the re-

fraction of light as it passes through a urine sample, or by a reagent strip test.

Elevated specific gravity reflects an increased concentration of urine solutes, which occurs in conditions causing renal hypoperfusion, and may indicate congestive heart failure, dehydration, hepatic disorders, or nephrosis. Low specific gravity reflects failure to reabsorb water and concentrate urine; it may indicate hypercalcemia, hypokalemia, alkalosis, acute renal failure, pyelonephritis, glomerulonephritis, or diabetes insipidus.

Although urine specific gravity is commonly measured with a random urine specimen, more accurate measurement is possible with a controlled specimen collected after fluids are withheld for 12 to 24 hours.

Equipment
Calibrated urinometer and cylinder, refractometer, or reagent strips (Multistix) ▪ gloves ▪ graduated specimen container.

Implementation
• Explain the procedure to the patient, and tell him when you will need the specimen. Explain why you're withholding fluids and for how long *to ensure his cooperation.*

Measuring with a urinometer
• Don gloves and collect a random urine specimen. Allow it to come to room temperature (71.6° F [22° C]) before testing *because this is the temperature at which most urinometers are calibrated.*
• Fill the cylinder about three-fourths full of urine. Then, gently drop the urinometer into the cylinder.
• When the urinometer stops bobbing, read the specific gravity from the calibrated scale marked directly on the stem of the urinometer. Make sure the instrument floats freely and doesn't touch the sides of the cylinder. Read the scale at the lowest point of the meniscus *to ensure an accurate reading.* (For specific instructions, see *Using a urinometer.)*
• Discard the urine, and rinse the cylinder and urinometer in cool water. *Warm water coagulates proteins in urine, making them stick to the instrument.*
• Remove gloves and wash your hands thoroughly *to prevent cross-contamination.*

Measuring with a refractometer
• Don gloves and collect a random or controlled urine specimen.
• Place a single drop of urine on the refractometer slide.
• Turn on the light and look through the eyepiece, where you will see the specific gravity indicated on a scale. (Some instruments use a digital display.)

Measuring with a reagent strip

- Don gloves and obtain a random or controlled urine specimen.
- Dip the reagent end of the test strip into the specimen for 2 seconds.
- Tap the strip on the rim of the specimen container *to remove excess urine,* and compare the resultant color change with the color chart supplied with the kit.

Special considerations

Test the urinometer in distilled water at room temperature *to check that its calibration is 1.000.* If necessary, correct the urinometer reading for temperature effects; add 0.001 to your observed reading for every 5.4° F (3° C) above the calibration temperature of 71.6° F (22° C); subtract 0.001 for every 5.4° F below 71.6° F.

Documentation

Record the specific gravity, volume, color, odor, and appearance of the collected urine specimen.

Urine pH

The pH of urine—its alkalinity or acidity—reflects the ability of the kidneys to maintain a normal hydrogen ion concentration in plasma and extracellular fluids. The normal hydrogen ion concentration in urine varies, ranging from pH 4.6 to 8.0, but it usually averages around pH 6.0.

The simplest procedure for testing the pH of urine consists of dipping a reagent strip (such as a Combistix) into a fresh specimen of the patient's urine and comparing the resultant color change with a standardized color chart.

An alkaline pH (above 7.0), resulting from a diet low in meat but high in vegetables, dairy products, and citrus fruits, causes turbidity and formation of phosphate, carbonate, and amorphous crystals. Alkaline urine may also result from urinary tract infection and from metabolic or respiratory alkalosis.

An acid pH (below 7.0), resulting from a high-protein diet, also causes turbidity, with formation of oxalate, cystine, amorphous urate, and uric acid crystals. Acid urine may also result from renal tuberculosis, phenylketonuria, alkaptonuria, pyrexia, diarrhea, starvation, and all forms of acidosis.

Measuring urine pH can also help monitor some medications, such as methenamine, that are active only at certain pH levels.

Using a urinometer

With the urinometer floating in a cylinder of urine, position your eye at a level even with the bottom of the meniscus and read the specific gravity from the scale printed on the urinometer.

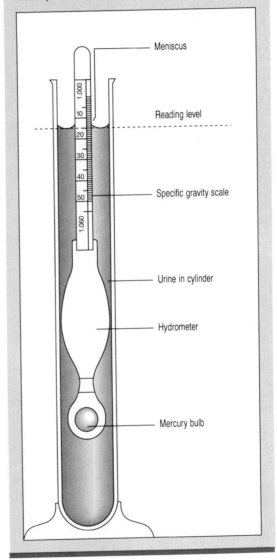

Meniscus

Reading level

Specific gravity scale

Urine in cylinder

Hydrometer

Mercury bulb

Equipment

Urine specimen container ▪ gloves ▪ reagent strips ▪ color chart. (The reagent strip has a pH indicator as part of a battery of indicators.)

Implementation

- Wash your hands thoroughly and don gloves.
- Provide the patient with a specimen container, and instruct him to collect a clean-catch midstream specimen (see "Urine collection" in this chapter). Dip the reagent strip into the urine, remove it, and tap off the excess urine from the strip.
- Hold the strip horizontally *to avoid mixing reagents from adjacent test areas on the strip*. Then, compare the color on the strip with the standardized color chart on the strip package. This comparison can be made up to 60 seconds after immersing the strip.
- Discard the urine specimen. If you're monitoring the patient's intake and output, measure the amount of urine discarded.
- Discard gloves and wash your hands thoroughly *to prevent cross-contamination*.

Special considerations

Use only a fresh urine specimen *because bacterial growth at room temperature changes urine pH*. Avoid letting a drop of urine run off the pH reagent onto adjacent reagent spots on the strip *because these other reagents will change the pH result*.

Urine collected at night is usually more acidic than urine collected during the day.

Documentation

Record the test results, the time of voiding, and the amount voided.

Straining urine for calculi

Renal calculi, or kidney stones, may develop anywhere in the urinary tract. They may be excreted with the urine or may become lodged in the urinary tract, causing hematuria, urine retention, renal colic and, possibly, hydronephrosis.

Ranging from microscopic to several centimeters in size, calculi are formed in the kidneys when mineral salts — principally calcium oxalate or calcium phosphate — collect around a nucleus of bacterial cells, blood clots, or other particles. Other substances involved in calculus formation may include uric acid, xanthine, and ammonia.

Renal calculi result from many causes, including hypercalcemia, which may occur with hyperparathyroidism, excessive dietary intake, prolonged immobility, abnormal urine pH levels, dehydration, hyperuricemia associated with gout, and some hereditary disorders. Most commonly, calculi form as a result of urine stasis stemming from dehydration (which concentrates urine), benign prostatic hyperplasia, neurologic disorders, or urethral stricture.

Testing for calculi requires careful straining of *all* the patient's urine through a gauze pad or fine-mesh sieve and, at times, quantitative laboratory analysis of questionable specimens. Such testing typically continues until the patient passes the calculi or until after surgery, as ordered.

Equipment

Fine-mesh sieve or 4" × 4" gauze pad ▪ graduated container ▪ urinal or bedpan ▪ gloves ▪ laboratory request form ▪ three patient care reminders ▪ specimen container (for use if calculi are found).

Implementation

- Explain the procedure to the patient and his family, if possible, *to ensure cooperation and to stress the importance of straining all his urine*.
- Post a patient care reminder stating STRAIN ALL URINE over his bed, in his bathroom, and on the collection container.
- Tell the patient to notify you after each voiding.
- If a commercial strainer isn't available, unfold a 4" × 4" gauze pad, place it over the top of a graduated measuring container, and secure it with a rubber band.
- Don gloves. With the strainer secured over the mouth of the collection container, pour the specimen through the strainer. If the patient has an indwelling catheter, strain all urine from the collection bag before discarding it.
- Examine the strainer for calculi. If you detect any calculi or if the filtrate looks questionable, notify the doctor, place the filtrate in a specimen container, and send it to the laboratory with a laboratory request form.
- If the strainer is intact, rinse it carefully and reuse it. If it has become damaged, discard it and replace it with a new strainer. Remove and discard gloves.

Special considerations

Save and send to the laboratory any small or suspicious-looking residue left in the specimen container *because even tiny calculi can cause hematuria and pain. Calculi may also appear in various colors, each of which has diagnostic value.*

Home care

If the patient will be straining his urine at home, teach him how to use a strainer and emphasize the importance of straining *all* his urine for the prescribed period.

Documentation

Chart the times of specimen collection and transport to the laboratory, if necessary. Describe any filtrate passed, and note any pain or hematuria that occurred during voiding.

STOOL SPECIMENS
Stool collection

Stool is collected to determine the presence of blood, ova and parasites, bile, fat, pathogens, or such substances as ingested drugs. Gross examination of stool characteristics, such as color, consistency, and odor, can reveal such conditions as GI bleeding and steatorrhea. Stool specimens are collected randomly or for specific periods, such as 72 hours. Because stool specimens can't be obtained on demand, their proper collection necessitates careful instructions to the patient to ensure an uncontaminated specimen.

Equipment

Specimen container with lid ▪ two tongue blades ▪ paper towel or paper bag ▪ bedpan or portable commode ▪ two patient care reminders (for timed specimens) ▪ laboratory request form ▪ gloves.

Implementation

• Explain the procedure to the patient and to family members, if possible, *to ensure their cooperation and prevent inadvertent disposal of timed stool specimens.*

Collecting a random specimen

• Tell the patient to notify you when he has the urge to defecate. Have him defecate into a clean, dry bedpan or commode. Instruct him not to contaminate the specimen with urine or toilet tissue *because urine inhibits fecal bacterial growth and toilet tissue contains bismuth, which interferes with test results.*
• Don gloves.
• Using a tongue blade, transfer the most representative stool specimen from the bedpan to the container, and cap the container. If the patient passes blood, mucus, or pus with the stool, be sure to include this with the specimen.

• Wrap the tongue blade in a paper towel and discard it. Remove your gloves, and wash your hands thoroughly *to prevent cross-contamination.*
• Label the specimen container with the patient's name and room number and the date and time of collection. Send it to the laboratory with a laboratory request form immediately *because a fresh specimen provides the most accurate results.* Refrigerate the specimen if it can't be transported to the laboratory immediately. *Note:* Some pathogens are killed by refrigeration. (Do not refrigerate stool collected to confirm the presence of ova and parasites; such a specimen must be examined immediately or discarded.)

Collecting a timed specimen

• Place a patient care reminder stating SAVE ALL STOOL over the patient's bed, in his bathroom, and in the utility room.
• After donning gloves, collect the first defecation, and include this in the total specimen.
• Obtain the timed specimen as you would a random specimen, but remember to transfer all stool to the specimen container.
• If stool must be obtained with an enema, use only tap water or normal saline solution.
• As ordered, send each specimen to the laboratory immediately with a laboratory request form or, if permitted, refrigerate the specimens collected during the test period and send them when collection is complete. Remove and discard gloves.
• Make sure the patient is comfortable after the procedure and that he has the opportunity to thoroughly clean his hands and perianal area. Perineal care may be necessary for some patients.

Special considerations

Never place a stool specimen in a refrigerator that contains food or medication *to prevent contamination.* Notify your nurse manager or the doctor if the stool appears unusual.

Home care

If the patient is to collect a specimen at home, instruct him to collect it in a clean container with a tight-fitting lid, wrap the container in a brown paper bag, and keep it in the refrigerator (separate from any food items) until it can be transported.

Documentation

Record the time of specimen collection and transport to the laboratory. Note stool color, odor, consistency, and any unusual characteristics; also note if the patient had difficulty passing the stool.

Fecal occult blood tests

Fecal occult blood tests are valuable for determining the presence of occult blood (hidden GI bleeding) and for distinguishing between true melena and melena-like stools. Certain medications, such as iron supplements and bismuth compounds, can darken stools so that they resemble melena.

Two common occult blood screening tests are Hematest (an orthotolidin reagent tablet) and the Hemoccult slide (filter paper impregnated with guaiac). Both tests produce a blue reaction in a fecal smear if occult

HOME CARE

Home tests for fecal occult blood

Most fecal occult blood tests require the patient to collect a sample of his stool and smear some of it on a slide. In contrast, some new tests don't require the patient to handle stool, making the procedure safer and simpler. One example is a test called Colocare.

If the patient will perform the Colocare test at home, tell him to avoid red meat and vitamin C supplements for 2 days before the test. He should check with his doctor about discontinuing any medications before the test. Some drugs that may interfere with test results include aspirin, indomethacin, corticosteroids, phenylbutazone, reserpine, dietary supplements, anticancer drugs, and anticoagulants.

Tell the patient to flush the toilet twice just before performing the test to remove any toilet-cleaning chemicals from the tank. Tell him to defecate into the toilet but to throw no toilet paper into the bowl. Within 5 minutes, he should remove the test pad from its pouch and float it printed side up on the surface of the water. Tell him to watch the pad for 15 to 30 seconds for any evidence of blue or green color changes, and have him record the result on the reply card.

Emphasize that he should perform this test with three consecutive bowel movements and then send the completed card to his doctor. However, he should call his doctor immediately if he notes a positive color change in the first test.

blood loss exceeds 5 ml in 24 hours. A newer test, Colocare, requires no fecal smear.

Occult blood tests are particularly important for early detection of colorectal cancer because 80% of patients with this disorder test positive. However, a single positive test result does not necessarily confirm GI bleeding or indicate colorectal cancer. For a confirmed positive result, the test must be repeated at least three times while the patient follows a meatless, high-residue diet. Still, a confirmed positive test doesn't necessarily indicate colorectal cancer. It does indicate the need for further diagnostic studies; GI bleeding can result from many causes other than cancer, such as ulcers and diverticula. These tests are easily performed on collected specimens or smears from digital rectal examination.

Equipment
Test kit ∎ glass or porcelain plate ∎ tongue blade or other wooden applicator ∎ gloves.

Implementation
• Put on gloves and collect a stool specimen.

Hematest reagent tablet test
• Use a wooden applicator to smear a bit of the stool specimen on the filter paper supplied with the kit. Or, after performing a digital rectal examination, wipe the finger you used for examination on a square of the filter paper.
• Place the filter paper with the stool smear on a glass plate.
• Remove a reagent tablet from the bottle, and immediately replace the cap tightly. Then, place the tablet in the center of the stool smear on the filter paper.
• Add one drop of water to the tablet, and allow it to soak in for 5 to 10 seconds. Add a second drop, letting it run from the tablet onto the specimen and filter paper. If necessary, tap the plate gently to dislodge any water from the top of the tablet.
• After 2 minutes, the filter paper will turn blue if the test is positive. Do not read the color that appears on the tablet itself or develops on the filter paper after the 2-minute period.
• Note the results, and discard the filter paper.
• Remove and discard your gloves, and wash your hands thoroughly.

Hemoccult slide test
• Open the flap on the slide packet, and use a wooden applicator to apply a thin smear of the stool specimen to the guaiac-impregnated filter paper exposed in box A. Or, after performing a digital rectal examination, wipe the finger you used for examination on a square of the filter paper.

• Apply a second smear from another part of the specimen to the filter paper exposed in box B *because some parts of the specimen may not contain blood.*

• Open the flap at the rear of the slide package, and place 2 drops of Hemoccult developing solution on the paper over each smear. A blue reaction will appear in 30 to 60 seconds if the test is positive.

• Record the results of the test and discard the slide package.

• Remove and discard your gloves, and wash your hands thoroughly.

Special considerations

Make sure stool specimens aren't contaminated with urine, soap solution, or toilet tissue, and test them as soon as possible after collection.

Test samples from several different portions of the same specimen *because occult blood from the upper GI tract isn't always evenly dispersed throughout the formed stool; likewise, blood from colorectal bleeding may occur mostly on the outer stool surface.*

Check the condition of the reagent tablets and note their expiration date. Use only fresh tablets and discard outdated ones. Protect Hematest tablets from moisture, heat, and light.

If repeated testing is necessary after a positive screening test, explain the test to the patient. Instruct him to maintain a high-fiber diet and to refrain from eating red meat, poultry, fish, turnips, and horseradish for 48 to 72 hours before the test as well as throughout the collection period *because these substances may alter test results.*

As ordered, have the patient discontinue use of iron preparations, bromides, iodides, rauwolfia derivatives, indomethacin, colchicine, salicylates, potassium, phenylbutazone, oxyphenbutazone, bismuth compounds, steroids, and ascorbic acid for 48 to 72 hours before the test and during it *to ensure accurate test results and to avoid possible bleeding that some of these compounds may cause.*

Home care

If the patient will be using the Hemoccult slide packet at home, advise him to complete the label on the slide packet before specimen collection. If he'll be using a Colocare test packet, advise him that this test is a preliminary screen for occult blood in his stool. Tell him he won't have to obtain a stool specimen to perform the test, but that he should follow your instructions carefully. (See *Home tests for fecal occult blood.)*

Documentation

Record the time and date of the test, the result, and any unusual characteristics of the stool tested. Report positive results to the doctor.

OTHER SPECIMENS
Sputum collection

Secreted by mucous membranes lining the bronchioles, bronchi, and trachea, sputum helps protect the respiratory tract from infection. When expelled from the respiratory tract, sputum carries with it saliva, nasal and sinus secretions, dead cells, and normal oral bacteria. Sputum specimens may be cultured for identification of respiratory pathogens.

The usual method of sputum specimen collection is expectoration, which may require ultrasonic nebulization, hydration, or chest percussion and postural drainage. Less common methods include tracheal suctioning and, rarely, bronchoscopy. Tracheal suctioning is contraindicated within 1 hour of eating and in patients with esophageal varices, nausea, facial or basilar skull fractures, laryngospasm, or bronchospasm. It should be performed cautiously in patients with cardiac disease, because it may precipitate cardiac arrhythmias.

Equipment

For expectoration: sterile specimen container with tight-fitting cap ■ label ■ laboratory request form ■ aerosol (10% sodium chloride, propylene glycol, acetylcysteine, or sterile or distilled water) to induce coughing, as ordered ■ facial tissues ■ emesis basin ■ gloves, if necessary.

For tracheal suctioning: #12 to #14 French sterile suction catheter ■ water-soluble lubricant ■ laboratory request form ■ sterile gloves ■ sterile in-line specimen trap (Lukens trap) ■ 3-ml syringe, if necessary ■ normal saline solution ■ portable suction machine, if wall unit is unavailable ■ oxygen therapy equipment. ■ optional: nasal airway, to obtain a nasotracheal specimen with suctioning, if needed. (Commercial suction kits are available containing all equipment except the suction machine and an in-line specimen container.)

Implementation

• Tell the patient you will collect a specimen of sputum (not saliva), and explain the procedure *to ease his anxiety and promote cooperation.* If possible, collect the specimen early in the morning, before breakfast, *to obtain an overnight accumulation of secretions.*

Attaching a specimen trap to a suction catheter

Wearing gloves, push the suction tubing onto the male adapter of the in-line trap.

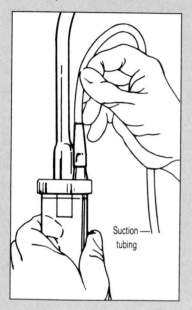

Suction tubing

Insert the suction catheter into the rubber tubing of the trap.

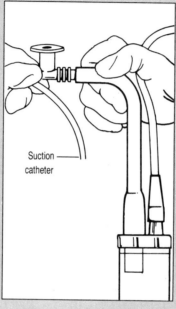

Suction catheter

After suctioning, disconnect the in-line trap from the suction tubing and catheter. To seal the container, connect the rubber tubing to the male adapter of the trap.

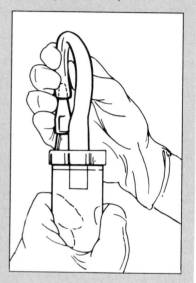

Collecting sputum by expectoration

• Instruct the patient to sit on a chair or at the edge of the bed. If he can't sit up, place him in high Fowler's position.
• Ask the patient to rinse his mouth with water *to reduce specimen contamination by oral bacteria and food particles.* (Avoid mouthwash or toothpaste *because they may affect the mobility of organisms in the sputum sample.)* Then tell him to cough deeply and expectorate directly into the specimen container. Ask him to produce at least 15 ml of sputum, if possible.
• Put on gloves.
• Cap the container and, if necessary, clean its exterior *to prevent cross-contamination.* Label the container with the patient's name and room number, the doctor's name, date and time of collection, and initial diagnosis. Also include on the laboratory request form whether the patient was febrile or was taking antibiotics, and whether sputum was induced *(because such specimens commonly appear watery and may resemble saliva).* Send the specimen to the laboratory immediately.

Collecting sputum by tracheal suctioning

• If the patient can't produce an adequate specimen by coughing, prepare to suction him to obtain the specimen. Explain the suctioning procedure to him and tell him that he may cough, gag, or feel short of breath during the procedure.
• Check the suction machine to be sure it's functioning properly. Then, place the patient in a high or semi-Fowler's position.
• Administer oxygen to the patient before beginning the procedure.
• Wash your hands thoroughly.
• Put on sterile gloves. Consider one hand sterile and the other hand clean *to prevent cross-contamination.*
• Connect the suction tubing to the male adapter of the in-line trap. Attach the sterile suction catheter to the rubber tubing of the trap. (See *Attaching a specimen trap to a suction catheter.)*
• Position a mask over your face *because the patient may cough violently during suctioning.* Tell the patient to tilt his head back slightly. Then lubricate the catheter with

normal saline solution, and gently pass it through the patient's nostril without suction.
• When the catheter reaches the larynx, the patient will cough. As he does, quickly advance the catheter into the trachea. Tell the patient to take several deep breaths through his mouth *to help ease insertion.*
• To obtain the specimen, apply suction for 5 to 10 seconds but never longer than 15 seconds *because prolonged suctioning can cause hypoxia.* If the procedure must be repeated, let the patient rest for four to six breaths. When collection is completed, discontinue the suction, gently remove the catheter, and administer oxygen.
• Detach the catheter from the in-line trap, gather it up in your dominant hand, and pull the glove cuff inside out and down around the used catheter to enclose it for disposal. Remove and discard the other glove and your mask.
• Detach the trap from the tubing connected to the suction machine. Seal the trap tightly by connecting the rubber tubing to the male adapter of the trap. Label the trap's container as an expectorated specimen, and send it to the laboratory immediately with a completed laboratory request form.
• Offer the patient a glass of water or mouthwash.

Special considerations
If you cannot obtain a sputum specimen through tracheal suctioning, perform chest percussion *to loosen and mobilize secretions,* and position the patient for optimal drainage. After 20 to 30 minutes, repeat the tracheal suctioning procedure.

Before sending the specimen to the laboratory, examine it to make sure it is actually sputum, not saliva, *because saliva will produce inaccurate test results.*

Because expectorated sputum is contaminated by normal mouth flora, tracheal suctioning provides a more reliable specimen for diagnosis.

If the patient becomes hypoxic or cyanotic during suctioning, remove the catheter immediately and administer oxygen.

If the patient has asthma or chronic bronchitis, watch for aggravated bronchospasms with use of more than a 10% concentration of sodium chloride or acetylcysteine in an aerosol. If he has suspected tuberculosis, don't use more than 20% propylene glycol with water when inducing a sputum specimen *because a higher concentration inhibits growth of the pathogen and causes erroneous test results.* If propylene glycol isn't available, use 10% to 20% acetylcysteine with water or sodium chloride.

Complications
Patients with cardiac disease may develop arrhythmias during the procedure as a result of coughing, especially when the specimen is obtained by suctioning.

Other complications may include tracheal trauma or bleeding, vomiting, aspiration, and hypoxemia.

Documentation
In your notes, record the method used to obtain the specimen, the time and date of collection, how the patient tolerated the procedure, the color and consistency of the specimen, and its proper disposition.

 # Lumbar puncture

This procedure involves insertion of a sterile needle into the subarachnoid space of the spinal canal, usually between the third and fourth lumbar vertebrae. The procedure may be performed for several reasons: to detect increased intracranial pressure (ICP) or the presence of blood in cerebrospinal fluid (CSF), which indicates cerebral hemorrhage; to obtain CSF specimens for laboratory analysis; or to inject dyes or gases for contrast in radiologic studies of the brain and spinal cord. Lumbar puncture is also used therapeutically to administer drugs or anesthetics and to relieve ICP by removing CSF.

Performed by a doctor with a nurse assisting, lumbar puncture requires sterile technique and careful patient positioning. This procedure is contraindicated in patients with lumbar deformity or infection at the puncture site. It should be performed cautiously in patients with increased ICP, because the rapid reduction in pressure that follows withdrawal of fluid can cause tonsillar herniation and medullary compression.

Equipment
Overbed table ■ one or two pairs of sterile gloves for the doctor ■ sterile gloves for the nurse ■ povidone-iodine solution ■ sterile gauze pads ■ alcohol sponges ■ sterile fenestrated drape ■ 3-ml syringe for local anesthetic ■ 25G ¾" sterile needle for injecting anesthetic ■ local anesthetic (usually 1% lidocaine) ■ 18G or 20G 3½" spinal needle with stylet (22G needle for children) ■ three-way stopcock ■ manometer ■ small adhesive bandage ■ three sterile collection tubes with stoppers ■ laboratory request forms ■ labels ■ light source, such as a gooseneck lamp.

Disposable lumbar puncture trays containing most of the needed sterile equipment are generally available.

Implementation
• Explain the procedure to the patient *to ease his anxiety and ensure cooperation.* Be sure a consent form has been signed.

Positioning for lumbar puncture

Have the patient lie on his side at the edge of the bed, with his chin tucked to his chest and his knees drawn up to his abdomen. Make sure the patient's spine is curved and his back is at the edge of the bed, as shown here. This position widens the spaces between the vertebrae, easing insertion of the needle.

To help the patient maintain this position, place one of your hands behind his neck and the other hand behind his knees, and pull gently. Hold the patient firmly in this position throughout the procedure to prevent accidental needle displacement.

Patient positioning

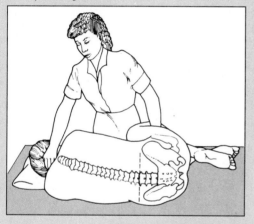

Typically, the doctor inserts the needle between the third and fourth lumbar vertebrae, as shown here.

Needle insertion

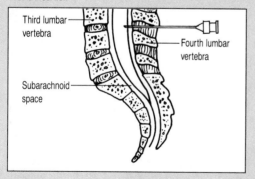

Third lumbar vertebra

Fourth lumbar vertebra

Subarachnoid space

• Inform the patient that he may experience headache after lumbar puncture, but reassure him that his cooperation during the procedure minimizes such an effect. (*Note:* Sedatives and analgesics are usually withheld before this test if there is evidence of a central nervous system disorder *because they may mask important symptoms.*)

• Immediately before the procedure, provide privacy and instruct the patient to void.

• Wash your hands thoroughly.

• Open the equipment tray on an overbed table, being careful not to contaminate the sterile field when you open the wrapper.

• Provide adequate lighting at the puncture site, and adjust the height of the patient's bed *to allow the doctor to perform the procedure comfortably.*

• Position the patient (see *Positioning for lumbar puncture*), and reemphasize the importance of remaining as still as possible *to minimize discomfort and trauma.*

• The doctor cleans the puncture site with sterile gauze pads soaked in povidone-iodine solution, wiping in a circular motion away from the puncture site; he uses three different pads *to prevent contamination of spinal tissues by the body's normal skin flora.* After allowing the skin to dry, he may wipe the area in a similar manner with alcohol sponges *to improve his view of the puncture site.* Next, he drapes the area with the fenestrated drape *to provide a sterile field.* (If the doctor uses povidone-iodine sponges instead of sterile gauze pads, he may remove his sterile gloves and put on another pair *to avoid introducing povidone-iodine into the subarachnoid space with the lumbar puncture needle.*)

• If there is no ampule of anesthetic on the equipment tray, clean the injection port of a multidose vial of anesthetic with an alcohol sponge. Then invert the vial 45 degrees so the doctor can insert a 25G needle and syringe and withdraw the anesthetic for injection.

• Before the doctor injects the anesthetic, tell the patient he'll experience a transient burning sensation and local pain. Ask him to report any other persistent pain or sensations *because these may indicate irritation or puncture of a nerve root, requiring repositioning of the needle.*

• When the doctor inserts the sterile spinal needle into the subarachnoid space between the third and fourth lumbar vertebrae, instruct the patient to remain still and breathe normally. If necessary, hold the patient firmly in position *to prevent sudden movement that may displace the needle.*

• If a lumbar puncture is being performed to administer contrast media for radiologic studies or spinal anesthetic, the doctor injects the dye or anesthetic at this time.

• When the needle is in place, the doctor attaches a manometer with a three-way stopcock to the needle hub

to read CSF pressure. If ordered, help the patient extend his legs *to provide a more accurate pressure reading.*
• The doctor then detaches the manometer and allows fluid to drain from the needle hub into the collection tubes. When he has collected approximately 2 or 3 ml in each tube, mark the tubes in sequence, stopper them securely, and label them properly.
• If the doctor suspects an obstruction in the spinal subarachnoid space, he may check for Queckenstedt's sign. He first takes an initial CSF pressure reading. Then, as ordered, compress the patient's jugular vein for 10 seconds. *This temporarily obstructs blood flow from the cranium, increasing ICP and — if no subarachnoid block exists — causes CSF pressure to rise as well.* The doctor then takes pressure readings every 10 seconds until the pressure stabilizes.
• After the doctor collects the specimens and removes the spinal needle, clean the puncture site with povidone-iodine and apply a small adhesive bandage.
• Send the CSF specimens to the laboratory immediately, with properly completed laboratory request forms.

Special considerations
During lumbar puncture, watch closely for signs of adverse reaction: elevated pulse rate, pallor, or clammy skin. Alert the doctor immediately to any significant changes.

The patient may be ordered to lie flat for 8 to 12 hours after the procedure. If necessary, place a patient care reminder on his bed to this effect.

Collected CSF specimens must be sent to the laboratory immediately; they cannot be refrigerated for later transport.

Complications
Headache is the most common adverse effect of lumbar puncture. Others may include a reaction to the anesthetic, meningitis, epidural or subdural abscess, bleeding into the spinal canal, CSF leakage through the dural defect remaining after needle withdrawal, local pain caused by nerve root irritation, edema or hematoma at the puncture site, transient difficulty in voiding, and fever. The most serious complications of lumbar puncture, although rare, are tonsillar herniation and medullary compression.

Documentation
Record the initiation and completion times of the procedure, the patient's response, the administration of drugs, the number of specimen tubes collected, the time of transport to the laboratory, and the color, consistency, and any other characteristics of the collected specimens.

Papanicolaou test

Also known as the Pap test or Pap smear, this cytologic test developed in the 1920s by George N. Papanicolaou allows early detection of cervical cancer. The test involves scraping secretions from the cervix, spreading them on a slide, and immediately coating the slide with fixative spray or solution to preserve specimen cells for nuclear staining. Cytologic evaluation then outlines cell maturity, morphology, and metabolic activity. Although cervical scrapings are the most common test specimen, the Pap test also permits cytologic evaluation of the vaginal pool, prostatic secretions, urine, gastric secretions, cavity fluids, bronchial aspirations, and sputum.

Equipment
Bivalve vaginal speculum ■ gloves ■ Pap stick (wooden spatula) ■ long cotton-tipped applicator ■ three glass microscope slides ■ fixative (a commercial spray or 95% ethyl alcohol solution) ■ adjustable lamp ■ drape ■ laboratory request forms.

Preparation of equipment
Select a speculum of the appropriate size and gather the equipment in the examining room. Label the glass slides with the patient's name and "E," "C," and "V" *to differentiate endocervical, cervical, and vaginal specimens.*

Implementation
• Explain the procedure to the patient and wash your hands.
• Instruct the patient to void *to relax the perineal muscles and facilitate bimanual examination of the uterus.*
• Provide privacy and instruct the patient to undress below the waist, but to wear her shoes, if desired, *to cushion her feet against the stirrups.* Then instruct her to sit on the examining table and to drape her genital region.
• Place the patient in the lithotomy position, with her feet in the stirrups and her buttocks extended slightly beyond the edge of the table. Adjust the drape.
• Adjust the lamp *to fully illuminate the genital area.* Then, fold back the corner of the drape *to expose the perineum.*
• If you're performing the procedure, first put on gloves. Then take the speculum in your dominant hand and moisten it with warm water *to ease insertion. Avoid using water-soluble lubricants, which can interfere with accurate laboratory testing.*
• Warn the patient that you're about to touch her *to avoid startling her.* Then, gently separate the labia with the thumb and forefinger of your nondominant hand.

• Instruct the patient to take several deep breaths, and insert the speculum into the vagina. Once it's in place, slowly open the blades *to expose the cervix.* Then lock the blades in place.

• Insert a cotton-tipped applicator through the speculum ⅕" into the cervical os. Rotate it 360 degrees *to obtain an endocervical specimen.* Then remove the cotton-tipped applicator and gently roll it in a circle across the slide marked "E." Refrain from rubbing the applicator on the slide *to prevent cell destruction.* Immediately place the slide in a fixative solution or spray it with a fixative *to prevent drying of the cells, which interferes with nuclear staining and cytologic interpretation.*

• Insert the small curved end of the Pap stick through the speculum and place it directly over the cervical os. Rotate the stick gently but firmly *to scrape cells loose.* Remove the stick, spread the specimen across the slide marked "C," and fix it immediately, as before.

• Insert the opposite end of the Pap stick or a cotton-tipped applicator through the speculum, and scrape the posterior fornix or vaginal pool — an area that collects cells from the endometrium, vagina, and cervix. Remove the stick or applicator, spread the specimen across the slide marked "V," and fix it immediately.

• Unlock the speculum *to ease removal and avoid accidentally pinching the vaginal wall.* Then withdraw the speculum.

• Remove the gloves from your nondominant hand to perform the bimanual exam, which usually follows the Pap test. Then remove and discard your other glove.

• Gently remove the patient's feet from the stirrups and assist her to a sitting position. Provide privacy for her to dress.

• Fill out the appropriate laboratory request forms, including the date of the patient's last menses.

Special considerations

Many preventable factors can interfere with the Pap test's accuracy, so provide appropriate patient teaching beforehand. For example, use of a vaginal douche in the 48-hour period before specimen collection washes away cellular deposits and prevents adequate sampling. Instillation of vaginal medications in the same period makes cytologic interpretation difficult. Collection of a specimen during menstruation prevents adequate sampling because menstrual flow washes away cells; ideally, such collection should take place 5 to 6 days before menses or 1 week after it. Application of topical antibiotics promotes rapid, heavy shedding of cells and requires postponement of the Pap test for at least 1 month.

If the patient has had a complete hysterectomy, collect test specimens from the vaginal pool and cuff.

Complications

Failure to unlock the speculum blades before removal can pinch vaginal tissue.

Although slight cramping normally accompanies this exam, rough handling of the speculum can cause severe cramping.

Scraping an inflamed cervix with the Pap stick can cause slight bleeding.

Documentation

On the patient's chart, record the date and time of specimen collection, any complications, and the nursing action taken.

 # Swab specimens

Correct collection and handling of swab specimens helps the laboratory staff identify pathogens accurately, with a minimum of contamination from normal bacterial flora. Collection normally involves sampling inflamed tissues and exudates from the throat, nasopharynx, wounds, eye, ear, or rectum with sterile swabs of cotton or other absorbent material. Such swabs are immediately placed in a sterile tube containing a transport medium and, in the case of sampling for anaerobes, an inert gas. These specimens are usually collected to identify pathogens and sometimes to identify asymptomatic carriers of certain easily transmitted disease organisms.

Equipment

For a throat specimen: sterile swab ■ tongue blade ■ sterile culture tube with transport medium (or commercial collection kit) ■ penlight ■ gloves ■ label ■ laboratory request form.

For a nasopharyngeal specimen: sterile, flexible cotton-tipped wire swab ■ gloves ■ tongue blade ■ sterile culture tube with transport medium ■ penlight ■ label ■ laboratory request form ■ optional: small open-ended Pyrex tube or nasal speculum.

For a wound specimen: sterile gloves ■ alcohol or povidone-iodine sponges ■ sterile swabs ■ sterile 10-ml syringe ■ sterile 21G needle ■ sterile forceps ■ sterile culture tube with transport medium (or commercial collection kit for aerobic culture) ■ labels ■ special anaerobic culture tube containing carbon dioxide or nitrogen ■ fresh dressings for the wound ■ laboratory request form ■ optional: rubber stopper for needle.

For an ear specimen: gloves ■ sterile swabs ■ sterile culture tube with transport medium ■ normal saline solution ■ two 2" × 2" gauze pads ■ label ■ 10-ml syringe and 22G 1″ needle (for tympanocentesis) ▪ label ▪ laboratory request form.

For an eye specimen: sterile gloves ▪ sterile swabs ▪ sterile wire culture loop (for corneal scraping) ▪ sterile culture tube with transport medium ▪ sterile normal saline solution ▪ two 2″ × 2″ gauze pads ▪ label ▪ laboratory request form.

For a rectal specimen: gloves ▪ sterile swab ▪ soap and water ▪ washcloth ▪ normal saline solution ▪ sterile culture tube with transport medium ▪ label ▪ laboratory request form.

Implementation
• Explain the procedure to the patient *to ease his anxiety and ensure cooperation.*

Collecting a throat specimen
• Tell the patient he may gag during the swabbing but that the procedure takes less than a minute.
• Instruct him to sit erect at the edge of the bed or on a chair, facing you. Wash your hands and don gloves.
• Ask the patient to tilt his head back. Depress his tongue with the tongue blade, and illuminate his throat with the penlight *to check for inflamed areas.*
• If the patient starts to gag, withdraw the tongue blade and tell him to breathe deeply. Once he's relaxed, reinsert the tongue blade but not as deeply as before.
• Using the cotton-tipped wire swab, wipe the tonsillar areas from side to side, including any inflamed or purulent sites. Don't touch the tongue, cheeks, or teeth with the swab *to avoid contaminating it with oral bacteria.*
• Withdraw the swab and immediately place it in the culture tube. If you're using a commercial kit, crush the ampule of culture medium at the bottom of the tube and push the swab into the medium *to keep the swab moist.*
• Discard gloves and wash your hands.
• Label the specimen with the patient's name and room number, the doctor's name, and the date, time, and site of collection. On the laboratory request form, indicate if any organism is strongly suspected, especially *Corynebacterium diphtheriae* (requires two swabs and special growth medium), *Bordetella pertussis* (requires a nasopharyngeal culture and special growth medium), and *Neisseria meningitidis* (requires enriched selective media).
• Send the specimen to the laboratory immediately *to prevent growth or deterioration of microbes.*

Collecting a nasopharyngeal specimen
• Tell the patient he may gag or feel the urge to sneeze during the swabbing but that the procedure takes less than 1 minute.
• Instruct him to sit erect at the edge of the bed or on a chair, facing you. Wash your hands and don gloves.

Obtaining a nasopharyngeal specimen

After you've passed the swab into the nasopharynx, *gently* but quickly rotate the swab to collect the specimen. Then remove the swab, taking care not to injure the nasal mucous membrane.

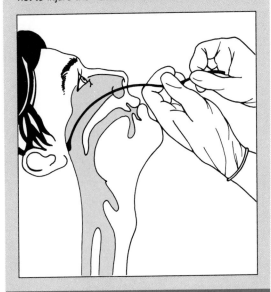

• Ask him to blow his nose *to clear his nasal passages.* Then check his nostrils for patency with a penlight.
• Tell the patient first to occlude one nostril and then the other as he exhales. Listen for the more patent nostril *because you'll insert the swab through it.*
• Ask the patient to cough *to bring organisms to the nasopharynx for a better specimen.*
• Bend the sterile wire swab in a curve and then open the package without contaminating the swab.
• Ask the patient to tilt his head back, and gently pass the swab through the more patent nostril about 3″ to 4″ (8 to 10 cm) into the nasopharynx, keeping the swab near the septum and the floor of the nose. (See *Obtaining a nasopharyngeal specimen.*) Rotate the swab quickly and remove it.
• Alternatively, depress the patient's tongue with a tongue blade, and pass the bent wire swab up behind the uvula. Rotate the swab and withdraw it.
• Remove the cap from the culture tube, insert the swab, and break off the contaminated end. Close the tube tightly, label it for throat culture, fill out laboratory request form, and send the specimen and form to the laboratory im-

Anaerobic specimen collection

Because most anaerobes die when exposed to oxygen, they must be transported in tubes filled with carbon dioxide or nitrogen. The anaerobic specimen collector shown here includes a rubber-stoppered tube filled with carbon dioxide, a small inner tube, and a swab attached to a plastic plunger.

Before specimen collection, the small inner tube containing the swab is held in place with the rubber stopper (as shown on the left). After collecting the specimen, quickly replace the swab in the inner tube and depress the plunger to separate the inner tube from the stopper (right), forcing it into the larger tube and exposing the specimen to a carbon dioxide-rich environment.

Before **After**

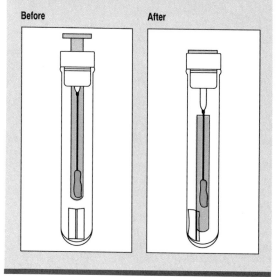

mediately. If you're collecting the specimen to isolate a possible virus, check with the laboratory for the recommended collection technique.
• Discard gloves and wash your hands.

Collecting a wound specimen
• Wash your hands, prepare a sterile field, and put on sterile gloves. With sterile forceps, remove the dressing to expose the wound. Dispose of the soiled dressings properly.

• Clean the area around the wound with an alcohol or povidone-iodine sponge *to reduce the risk of contaminating the specimen with skin bacteria.* Allow the area to dry.
• For an aerobic culture, use a sterile cotton-tipped swab to collect as much exudate as possible, or insert the swab deeply into the wound and gently rotate it. Remove the swab from the wound and immediately place it in the aerobic culture tube. Send the tube to the laboratory immediately with a completed laboratory request form. Never collect exudate from the skin and then insert the same swab into the wound; *this could contaminate the wound with skin bacteria.*
• For an anaerobic culture, insert the sterile cotton-tipped swab deeply into the wound, rotate it gently, remove it, and immediately place it in the anaerobic culture tube (see *Anaerobic specimen collection*). Or, insert a sterile 10-ml syringe, without a needle, into the wound, and aspirate 1 to 5 ml of exudate into the syringe. Then attach the 21G needle to the syringe, and immediately inject the aspirate into the anaerobic culture tube. If an anaerobic culture tube is unavailable, obtain a rubber stopper, attach the needle to the syringe, gently push all the air out of the syringe by pressing on the plunger. Stick the needle tip into the rubber stopper, and send the syringe of aspirate to the laboratory immediately with a completed laboratory request form.
• Apply a new dressing to the wound. (See Chapter 4, Physical treatments.)

Collecting an ear specimen
• Wash your hands and put on gloves.
• Gently clean excess debris from the patient's ear with normal saline solution and gauze pads.
• Insert the swab into the ear canal, and rotate it gently along the walls of the canal.
• Withdraw the swab, being careful not to touch other surfaces *to prevent contaminating the specimen.*
• Place the swab in the culture tube with transport medium.
• Remove the gloves and dispose of them properly. Wash your hands.
• Label the specimen for culture, complete a laboratory request form, and send the sample to the laboratory immediately.

Collecting a middle ear specimen
• Put on gloves and clean the outer ear with normal saline solution and gauze pads. After the doctor punctures the eardrum with a needle and aspirates fluid into the syringe, replace the cap on the needle, label the syringe, complete a laboratory request form, and send the sample to the laboratory immediately.

Collecting an eye specimen
• Wash your hands and put on sterile gloves.
• Gently clean excess debris from the outside of the eye with normal saline solution and gauze pads, wiping from the inner to the outer canthus.
• Retract the lower eyelid *to expose the conjunctival sac.* Gently rub the sterile swab over the conjunctiva, being careful not to touch other surfaces *to avoid contaminating the specimen.* Hold the swab parallel to the eye, rather than pointed directly at it, *to prevent accidental injury caused by sudden movement.* (If a corneal scraping is required, this procedure is performed by a doctor using a wire culture loop.)
• Immediately place the swab or wire loop in the culture tube with transport medium.
• Remove the gloves and dispose of them properly. Wash your hands.
• Label the specimen for culture, complete a laboratory request form, and send the specimen to the laboratory immediately.

Collecting a rectal specimen
• Wash your hands and put on gloves.
• Clean the area around the patient's anus using a washcloth and soap and water.
• Insert the swab, moistened with normal saline solution or sterile broth medium, through the anus and advance it about ⅜″ (1 cm) for infants or 1½″ (4 cm) for adults. While withdrawing the swab, gently rotate it against the walls of the lower rectum to sample a large area of the rectal mucosa.
• Place the swab in a culture tube with transport medium. Then, label the tube for rectal culture, complete a laboratory request form, and send the specimen to the laboratory immediately.
• Remove your gloves and dispose of them properly. Wash your hands.

Special considerations
Note recent antibiotic therapy on the laboratory request form.
For a nasopharyngeal specimen: Because certain organisms, such as *Corynebacterium diphtheriae* and *Bordetella pertussis,* require special growth media, inform the laboratory if you suspect these are present.
For a wound specimen: Although you would normally clean the area around a wound to prevent contamination by normal skin flora, don't clean a perineal wound with alcohol *to avoid irritating sensitive tissues.* Also make sure antiseptic doesn't enter the wound. *Because most anaerobes are destroyed by oxygen,* place the specimen in the culture tube quickly. Ensure that no air enters the tube

and that the double stoppers on the anaerobic collection tube are secure.
For an ear specimen: Insert the swab into the ear gently. Then rotate it carefully *to avoid damaging the eardrum.* Restrain a child or uncooperative patient *to prevent ear trauma from sudden movement.* When sending a specimen in a syringe to the laboratory, secure its cap.
For an eye specimen: Don't use an antiseptic before culturing *to avoid irritating the eye and inhibiting growth of organisms in culture.* Swab the eye carefully *to avoid corneal irritation or trauma.* If the patient is a child or an uncooperative adult, ask a co-worker to restrain the patient's head *to prevent eye trauma from sudden movement.*

Documentation
Record the time, date, and site of specimen collection and recent or current antibiotic therapy. Note any unusual appearance or odor of the specimen.

Bone marrow aspiration and biopsy

A specimen of bone marrow—the major site of blood cell formation—may be obtained by aspiration or needle biopsy. The procedure allows evaluation of overall blood composition by studying blood elements and precursor cells, as well as abnormal or malignant cells. Such aspiration removes cells through a needle inserted into the marrow cavity of the bone; a biopsy removes a small, solid core of marrow tissue through the needle. Both procedures are usually performed by a doctor, but some hospitals authorize specially trained chemotherapy nurses or nurse clinicians to perform them, with the aid of an assistant.

Aspirates are valuable in diagnosing various disorders and cancers, such as oat cell carcinoma, leukemia, and such lymphomas as Hodgkin's disease. Biopsies are often performed simultaneously to stage the disease and to monitor response to treatment.

Equipment
For aspiration: prepackaged bone marrow set, which includes: povidone-iodine sponges ■ two sterile drapes (one fenestrated, one plain) ■ ten 4″ × 4″ gauze pads ■ ten 2″ × 2″ gauze pads ■ two 12-ml syringes ■ 22G 1″ or 2″ needle ■ a scalpel ■ sedative ■ specimen containers ■ bone marrow needle ■ 70% isopropyl alcohol ■ 1% lidocaine (unopened bottle) ■ adhesive tape ■ sterile gloves ■ glass slides and cover slips ■ labels.

Common sites for bone marrow aspiration and biopsy

The *posterior superior iliac crest* is the preferred site for aspiration because it's free of nearby vital organs or vessels. For aspiration of bone marrow from this site, the patient is placed either in the lateral position with one leg flexed or in the prone position.

For aspiration or biopsy from the *anterior iliac crest,* the patient is placed in the supine or side-lying position. This site is used with patients who cannot lie prone because of severe abdominal distention. Aspiration from the *sternum* involves the greatest risk but may be used

because this site is near the surface, the cortical bone is thin, and the marrow cavity contains numerous cells and relatively little fat or supporting bone. The sternum is rarely used for biopsy, however, because of its small size and proximity to vital organs.

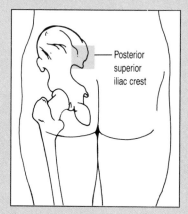

Posterior superior iliac crest

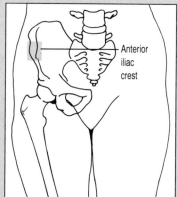

Anterior iliac crest

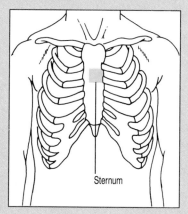

Sternum

For biopsy: all equipment listed above ▪ Vim-Silverman, Jamshidi, Illinois sternal, or Westerman-Jensen needle ▪ Zenker's fixative.

Implementation
• Tell the patient the doctor will collect a bone marrow specimen, and explain the procedure *to ease his anxiety and ensure cooperation.* Make sure the patient or a responsible family member understands the procedure and implications of this test and signs a consent form obtained by the doctor.
• Inform the patient that the procedure normally takes 5 to 10 minutes, that test results usually are available in 1 day, and that more than one marrow specimen may be required.
• Check the patient's history for hypersensitivity to the local anesthetic. Tell him which bone — sternum or posterior superior or anterior iliac crest — will be sampled. Inform him that he will receive a local anesthetic and will feel heavy pressure from insertion of the biopsy or aspiration needle, as well as a brief, pulling sensation on removal of the marrow specimen. Tell him the doctor may make a small incision to avoid tearing the skin.

• If the patient has osteoporosis, tell him needle pressure may be minimal; if he has osteopetrosis, inform him a drill may be needed.
• Provide a sedative, as ordered, before the test.
• Position the patient according to the selected puncture site. (See *Common sites for bone marrow aspiration and biopsy.*)
• Using sterile technique, the puncture site is cleaned with povidone-iodine solution and allowed to dry; then the area is draped.
• To anesthetize the site, the doctor infiltrates it with 1% lidocaine, first injecting a small amount intradermally, and then using a larger 22G 1" to 2" needle to anesthetize the tissue down to the bone.
• When the needle tip reaches the bone, the doctor anesthetizes the periosteum by injecting a small amount of lidocaine in a circular area about ¾" (2 cm) in diameter. The needle should be withdrawn from the periosteum after each injection.
• After allowing about 1 minute for the lidocaine to take effect, a scalpel may be used to make a small stab incision in the patient's skin to accommodate the bone marrow needle. *This technique avoids pushing skin into the bone*

marrow and also helps avoid unnecessary skin tearing to help reduce the risk of infection.

Bone marrow aspiration

• The doctor inserts the bone marrow needle at the selected site and lodges it firmly in the bone cortex. If the patient feels sharp pain instead of pressure when the needle first touches bone, the needle was probably inserted outside the anesthetized area. If this happens, the needle should be withdrawn slightly and moved to the anesthetized area.

• The needle is advanced by applying an even, downward force with the heel of the hand or the palm, while twisting it back and forth slightly. A crackling sensation means the needle has entered the marrow cavity.

• Next, the doctor removes the inner cannula, attaches the syringe to the needle, aspirates the required specimen (usually about 1 ml), and withdraws the needle.

• The nurse dons gloves and applies pressure to the aspiration site with a gauze pad for 5 minutes to control bleeding, while an assistant prepares the marrow slides. The area is then cleaned with alcohol to remove the povidone-iodine, the skin dried thoroughly with a 4″ × 4″ gauze pad, and a sterile pressure dressing applied.

Bone marrow biopsy

• The doctor inserts the biopsy needle into the periosteum and advances it steadily until the outer needle passes through the bone cortex into the marrow cavity.

• The biopsy needle is directed into the marrow cavity by alternately rotating the inner needle clockwise and counterclockwise. Then, a plug of tissue is removed, the needle assembly withdrawn, and the marrow specimen expelled into a properly labeled specimen bottle containing Zenker's fixative or formaldehyde.

• The nurse dons gloves and cleans the area around the biopsy site with alcohol to remove the povidone-iodine solution, firmly presses a sterile 2″ × 2″ gauze pad against the incision to control bleeding, and applies a sterile pressure dressing.

Special considerations

Faulty needle placement may yield too little aspirate. If the procedure fails to produce a specimen, the needle must be withdrawn from the bone (but not from the overlying soft tissue), the stylet replaced, and the needle reinserted into a second site within the anesthetized field.

Bone marrow specimens should not be collected from irradiated areas *because radiation may have altered or destroyed the marrow.*

Complications

Bleeding and infection are potentially life-threatening complications of aspiration or biopsy at any site. Complications of sternal needle puncture are uncommon but include puncture of the heart and major vessels, causing severe hemorrhage; puncture of the mediastinum, causing mediastinitis or pneumomediastinum; and puncture of the lung, causing pneumothorax.

If hematoma occurs around the puncture site, apply warm soaks. Give analgesics for site pain or tenderness.

Documentation

Chart the time, date, location, and patient's tolerance of the procedure and the specimen obtained.

Selected references

Clinical Laboratory Tests: Values and Implications. Springhouse, Pa.: Springhouse Corp., 1991.

DeGroot, K.D., and Damato, M.B. *Critical Care Skills.* Norwalk, Conn.: Appleton & Lange, 1987.

Diagnostic Test Implications. Clinical Skillbuilders. Springhouse, Pa.: Springhouse Corp., 1991.

Illustrated Manual of Nursing Practice. Springhouse, Pa.: Springhouse Corp., 1991.

Kee, J.L. *Laboratory and Diagnostic Tests with Nursing Implications,* 3rd ed. Norwalk, Conn.: Appleton & Lange, 1991.

Kinkade, S.L., and Lohrman, J. *Critical Care Nursing Procedures.* Philadelphia: B.C. Decker, Inc., 1990.

Kinney, M.R., et al. *AACN's Clinical Reference for Critical Care Nursing,* 2nd ed. New York: McGraw-Hill Book Co., 1988.

Luckmann, J., and Sorensen, K. *Medical-Surgical Nursing,* 3rd ed. Philadelphia: W.B. Saunders Co., 1987.

Oski, F.A. *Principles and Practices of Pediatrics.* Philadelphia: J.B. Lippincott Co., 1990.

Persons, C. *Critical Care Procedures and Protocols: A Nursing Process Approach.* Philadelphia: J.B. Lippincott Co., 1987.

Ryan, et al. *Kistner's Gynecology,* 5th ed. St. Louis: Mosby-Year Book, Inc., 1990.

Scott, J.R., et al. *Danforth's Obstetrics & Gynecology,* 6th ed. Philadelphia: J.B. Lippincott Co., 1990.

Tietz, N.W. *Clinical Guide to Laboratory Tests,* 2nd ed. Philadelphia: W.B. Saunders Co., 1990.

CHAPTER 4

PHYSICAL TREATMENTS

KATHLEEN MALLOCH, RN, BS, MBA, CNA

Introduction

Used effectively for centuries, many physical treatments have become fundamental nursing procedures. The principles behind such treatments as application of heat and cold—and often the techniques for performing them—remain essentially unchanged. But that doesn't make them any less important than more involved or specialized procedures created by new, high-tech medical treatments. In fact, physical treatments that many nurses might consider routine are those most responsible for maintaining patient comfort, decreasing anxiety, and reducing the risk of infection.

Proven effective

Most physical treatments have endured procedurally intact because of their effectiveness. Some treatments stimulate or support normal physiologic processes. For example, application of heat enhances healing because the warmth causes vasodilation, thereby increasing blood supply to the affected area and making more nutrients available for tissue growth. Antiembolism stockings support blood vessels, increasing venous return and thereby reducing the risk of deep vein thrombosis. Drains allow wound secretions to escape to the surface from underlying tissue, thus assisting the healing process.

Other physical treatments prevent a pathologic response or inhibit a full-blown response. For example, cold application produces vasoconstriction and increases blood viscosity, thereby reducing inflammation, bleeding, and localized tissue edema. Medicated baths relieve itching and reduce the irritation caused by various skin disorders. Wound irrigation performed with an antiseptic solution inhibits bacterial growth. And radiation treatments inhibit or destroy cancerous cells, offering patients palliation, control, or a cure. In all of these instances, nursing assessment and interventions are essential to the success of physical treatments.

Advances in equipment

Improvements in physical treatments have resulted in part from equipment advances. For example, single-use or single-patient disposable products have heightened efficiency and safety. Hot-water bottles and ice collars, sterile gauze dressings, presaturated sterile swabs, and aquamatic K pads are all available for single use. The number and types of disposable items and the variety of prepackaged procedure setup trays available continue to expand. One of the latest such products is the single-patient hyperthermia-hypothermia blanket. This disposable, lightweight vinyl blanket connects to a conventional control module for use both under and over the patient.

A portable fiberglass tub makes it possible to bathe rather than sponge patients on bed rest. The full-sized tub stands as high as the bed, rolls easily on casters, and fills and empties at the bedside through a hose that attaches to any faucet.

Vinyl pressure cuffs improve on the well-known and effective antiembolism stockings. This portable system simulates the normal pumping action of leg muscles by inflating progressively from the ankle to above the calf, assisting venous return and preventing blood backflow.

Nonallergenic adhesive gauze dressings cover an entire wound site with a single sheet of air- and exudate-permeable adhesive gauze. This type of occlusive dressing is particularly well suited for large or curved body areas and holds dressings securely without tape or straps. The gauze can be lifted off easily and painlessly for examination of the wound—even on sensitive or hairy skin—and then can be pressed back into place.

The silicone-foam dressing has improved the care of open, granulating wounds. Poured into the wound in liquid form, this new packing quickly congeals into an absorbent rubber pad with the exact contour of the wound, but it permits air circulation, doesn't cause irritation, and can be reused.

The new portable and disposable equipment saves nursing time because it's easier to use than the equipment it replaces. And nursing time saved means fewer delays in delivering patient care. What's more, disposables reduce the spread of nosocomial infection and—because they're new for each use—enhance patient comfort.

HEAT AND COLD
Direct heat application

Heat applied directly to the patient's body raises tissue temperature and enhances the inflammatory process by causing vasodilation and increasing local circulation. This promotes leukocytosis, suppuration, drainage, and healing. Heat also increases tissue metabolism, reduces pain caused by muscular spasm, and decreases congestion in deep visceral organs.

Direct heat may be dry or moist. Dry heat can be delivered at a higher temperature and for a longer time.

Devices for applying dry heat include the hot water bottle, electric heating pad, K pad, and chemical hot pack.

Moist heat softens crusts and exudates, penetrates deeper than dry heat, doesn't dry the skin, produces less perspiration, and usually is more comfortable for the patient. Devices for applying moist heat include warm compresses for small body areas and warm packs for large areas.

Direct heat treatment can't be used on a patient at risk for hemorrhage. It also is contraindicated if the patient has a sprained limb in the acute stage (because vasodilation would increase pain and swelling), or if he has a condition associated with acute inflammation, such as appendicitis. Direct heat should be applied cautiously to pediatric and elderly patients and to patients with impaired renal, cardiac, or respiratory function; arteriosclerosis or atherosclerosis; and impaired sensation. It should be applied with extreme caution to heat-sensitive areas, such as scar tissue or stomas. Because it raises the risk of burns and possible systemic effects, such as an increased respiratory rate and hypotension, direct heat should be used only when a doctor's order specifies it.

Equipment
Patient thermometer ▪ towel ▪ adhesive tape or roller gauze ▪ gloves, if the patient has an open lesion.

For a hot water bottle: hot tap water ▪ pitcher ▪ bath (utility) thermometer ▪ absorbent, protective cloth covering.

For an electric heating pad: absorbent, protective cloth covering.

For a K pad: distilled water ▪ temperature-adjustment key ▪ absorbent, protective cloth covering.

For a chemical hot pack (disposable): absorbent, protective cloth covering.

For a warm compress or pack: basin of hot tap water or container of sterile water, normal saline, or other solution, as ordered ▪ hot water bottle, K pad, or chemical hot pack ▪ linen-saver pad.

The following items may be sterile or nonsterile, depending on the type of procedure required: compress material (flannel, 4″ × 4″ gauze pads) or pack material (absorbent towels, ABD pads) ▪ petroleum jelly ▪ cotton-tipped applicators ▪ forceps ▪ bowl or basin ▪ bath (utility) thermometer ▪ waterproof covering ▪ towel ▪ dressing.

Preparation of equipment
Hot water bottle: Fill the bottle with hot tap water *to detect leaks and warm the bottle,* and then empty it. Run hot tap water into a pitcher and measure the water temperature with the bath thermometer. Adjust the temperature as ordered, usually to 115° to 125° F (46.1° to 51.7° C) for adults and 105° to 115° F (40.6° to 46.1° C)

for children under age 2 and elderly patients. Next, pour hot water into the bottle, filling it one-half to two-thirds full. *Partially filling the bottle keeps it lightweight and flexible to mold to the treatment area.* Squeeze the bottle until the water reaches the neck *to expel any air that would make the bottle inflexible and reduce heat conduction.* Fasten the top, and cover the bag with an absorbent, protective cloth *to provide insulation and absorb the patient's perspiration.* Secure the cover with tape or roller gauze.

Electric heating pad: Check the cord for frayed or damaged insulation. Then, plug in the pad and adjust the control switch to the desired setting. Wrap the pad in a protective cloth covering, and secure the cover with tape or roller gauze.

K pad: Check the cord for safety, as above, and fill the control unit two-thirds full with distilled water. Do not use tap water *because it leaves mineral deposits in the unit.* Check for leaks, and then tilt the unit in several directions *to clear the pad's tubing of air, which could interfere with even heat conduction.* Tighten the cap, and then loosen it a quarter turn *to allow heat expansion within the unit.* After making sure the hoses between the control unit and the pad are free of tangles, place the unit on the bedside table, slightly above the patient *so gravity can assist water flow.* If the central supply department has not preset the temperature on the control unit, use the key provided to make this adjustment. The usual temperature is 105° F. Then, place the pad in a protective cloth covering and secure the cover with tape or roller gauze. Plug in the unit, turn it on, and allow the pad to warm for 2 minutes.

Chemical hot pack: Select a pack of the correct size. Then, follow the manufacturer's directions (strike, squeeze, or knead) *to activate the heat-producing chemicals.* Place the pack in a protective cloth covering and secure the cover with tape or roller gauze.

Sterile warm compress or pack: Warm the container of sterile water or solution by setting it in a sink or basin of hot water. Measure the solution's temperature with a sterile bath thermometer. If a sterile thermometer is unavailable, pour some heated sterile solution into a clean container, check the temperature with a regular bath thermometer, and then discard the tested solution. Adjust the temperature of the sterile solution by adding hot or cold water to the sink or basin until the solution reaches 131° F (55° C) for adults or 105° F for children and elderly patients and for an eye compress. Pour the heated solution into a sterile bowl or basin. Then, using sterile technique, soak the compress or pack in the heated solution. If necessary, prepare a hot water bottle, K pad, or chemical hot pack *to keep the compress or pack warm.*

Nonsterile warm compress or pack: Fill a bowl or basin with hot tap water or other solution, and measure the temperature of the fluid with a bath thermometer. Adjust the temperature as ordered, usually to 131° F (55° C) for adults or 105° F (40.6° C) for children and elderly patients and for an eye compress. Then soak the compress or pack in the hot liquid. If necessary, prepare a hot water bottle, K pad, or chemical hot pack *to keep the compress or pack warm.*

Implementation
• Check the doctor's order and assess the patient's condition.
• Explain the procedure to the patient, and tell him not to lean or lie directly on the heating device *because this reduces air space and increases the risk of burns.* Warn the patient against adjusting the temperature of the heating device or adding hot water to a hot water bottle, even if he feels he can tolerate a higher temperature. Advise him to report pain or discomfort immediately and to remove the device himself if necessary.
• Provide privacy and make sure the room is warm and free of drafts. Wash your hands thoroughly.
• Take the patient's temperature, pulse, and respirations *to serve as a baseline.* If heat treatment is being applied to raise the patient's body temperature, monitor temperature, pulse, and respirations throughout the application.
• Expose only the treatment area *because vasodilation will make the patient feel chilly.*

To apply a hot water bottle, an electric heating pad, a K pad, or a chemical hot pack
• Before applying the heating device, press it against the inner aspect of your forearm *to test its temperature and heat distribution.* If it heats unevenly, obtain a new device.
• Apply the device to the treatment area, and if necessary, secure it with tape or roller gauze. Begin timing the application.
• Assess the patient's skin condition frequently, and remove the device if you observe increased swelling or excessive redness, blistering, maceration, or pronounced pallor, or if the patient reports pain or discomfort. Refill the hot water bottle as necessary *to maintain the correct temperature.*
• Remove the device after 20 to 30 minutes, or as ordered.
• Dry the patient's skin with a towel and re-dress the site, if necessary. Take the patient's temperature, pulse, and respirations *for comparison with the baseline.* Position him comfortably in bed.
• If the treatment is to be repeated, store the equipment in the patient's room, out of his reach; otherwise, return the equipment to its proper place.

To apply a warm compress or pack
• Place a linen-saver pad under the treatment area. Spread petroleum jelly (sterile, if necessary) over the affected area. Avoid applying it directly to any areas of skin breakdown or to eye tissues. (You may use sterile cotton-tipped applicators for a sterile procedure.) *The petroleum jelly reduces maceration and the risk of burns by decreasing the rate of heat penetration.*
• Remove the warm compress or pack from the bowl or basin. (Use sterile forceps for a sterile procedure.)
• Wring excess solution from the compress or pack (using sterile forceps for a sterile procedure). *Excess moisture increases the risk of burns.*
• Apply the compress gently to the affected site (using forceps, if warranted). After a few seconds, lift the compress (with forceps, if needed) and check the skin for excessive redness, maceration, or blistering. When you're sure the compress isn't causing a burn, mold it firmly to the skin *to keep out air, which reduces the temperature and effectiveness of the compress.* Work quickly *so the compress retains its heat.*
• Apply a waterproof covering (sterile, if warranted) to the compress. Secure the covering with tape or roller gauze *to prevent it from slipping.*
• Place a hot water bottle, K pad, or chemical hot pack over the compress and waterproof covering *to maintain the correct temperature.* Begin timing the application.
• Check the patient's skin every 5 minutes for signs of tissue intolerance. Remove the device if the skin shows excessive redness, maceration, or blistering or if the patient feels pain or discomfort. Change the compress as necessary to maintain the correct temperature.
• After 15 or 20 minutes or as ordered, remove the compress. (Use forceps, if warranted.) Discard the compress into a waterproof trash bag.
• Dry the patient's skin with a towel (sterile, if necessary). Note the condition of the skin and re-dress the area, if necessary. Take the patient's temperature, pulse, and respiration *for comparison with the baseline.* Then make sure the patient is comfortable.
• Discard liquids and disposable equipment. Return used sterile equipment to the central supply department for sterilization. Clean any remaining equipment and, if the treatment will be repeated, store it in the patient's room, out of his reach; otherwise, return it to storage.

Special considerations
Make sure the patient is positioned in proper alignment *to maintain his comfort during the procedure.* Keep the call button within easy reach, and make sure the patient can remove the heating device if he experiences discomfort.

Unless ordered otherwise, discontinue the heat treatment after 30 minutes *because, by this time, maximum*

Using moist heat to relieve muscle spasm

Tell patients to choose moist heat rather than dry heat when attempting to ease muscle tension or spasm. Moist heat is less drying to the skin, less apt to cause burns, less likely to cause excessive fluid and salt loss through sweating, and more likely to penetrate deeper tissues. Instruct the patient to apply heat for 20 to 30 minutes, as follows:
• Place a moist towel over the painful area.
• Cover the towel with a hot water bottle properly filled and at the correct temperature.
• Remove the hot water bottle and wet pack after 20 to 30 minutes. Don't continue application for longer than 30 minutes because therapeutic value decreases after that time.

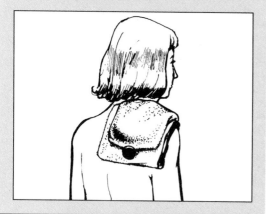

vasodilation has probably occurred; vasoconstriction then follows, reversing the effects of the heat treatment. Also, allow at least 1 hour between treatments *to avoid vasoconstriction*.

Because the temperature of a chemical hot pack varies from 101° to 114° F (38.3° to 45.6° C), use a different heating device for treatments requiring a specific or higher temperature.

Don't use an electric heating device near oxygen *because a spark from a frayed wire could cause explosion and fire. Also, to prevent electric shock*, avoid using an electric heating pad near liquid (including on a patient who is incontinent) and avoid handling any electric device with wet hands. When securing a heating device, don't use safety pins *because heated metal can cause burns or electric shock, and accidental puncture of a K pad or chemical hot*

pack can allow fluid to leak, resulting in burns. Avoid crushing or creasing the wires in an electric heating pad *because this may cause portions of the pad to overheat, leading to burns or fire.*

If the patient is unconscious, anesthetized, irrational, neurologically impaired, or insensitive to heat for any reason, stay with him throughout the treatment, and check the site frequently *to avoid such complications as edema, maceration, blotchy redness, and blisters.*

When direct heat is ordered to decrease congestion within internal organs, the application must cover a large enough area *to increase blood volume at the skin's surface*. For relief of pelvic organ congestion, for example, apply heat over the patient's lower abdomen, hips, and thighs. To achieve local relief, you may concentrate heat only over the specified area. (See *Using moist heat to relieve muscle spasm.*)

When applying moist heat to an open wound or to a lesion expected to open during treatment, use sterile technique. When applying moist heat to both eyes, use separate sterile equipment for each eye *to prevent cross-contamination.*

You may use sterile gloves instead of sterile forceps for application of sterile moist compresses or packs. As an alternative method of applying sterile moist compresses, use a bedside sterilizer to sterilize the compresses. Saturate the compress with tap water or other solution and wring it dry. Then place it in the bedside sterilizer at 275° F (135° C) for 15 minutes. Remove the compress with sterile forceps, and wring out the excess solution. Then place the compress in a sterile bowl and measure its temperature with a sterile thermometer. Apply the compress as instructed above when it reaches the correct temperature.

Commercial premoistened sterile compresses may be used as an alternative. Refer to the instructions on the package insert, and follow the same general observations and precautions mentioned above.

Complications
Because tissue damage may result from direct heat application, monitor the temperature of the compress carefully. Assess frequently the condition of the patient's skin under the heat application device.

Documentation
Record the time and date of heat application; the type, temperature or heat setting, duration, and site of application; the patient's temperature, pulse, respirations, and skin condition before, during, and after treatment; signs of complications; and the patient's tolerance of and reaction to treatment.

Radiant heat application

Radiant heat—dry heat shed onto a specific body area rather than applied directly to it—can improve circulation, decrease wound exudation, prevent maceration, and promote healing. Indicated for patients with stasis or slow-healing wounds, this treatment can be delivered during dressing changes and wound debridement.

No specific conditions contraindicate radiant heat treatment, but it must be used judiciously because it can dry the wound excessively; this, in turn, can impair healing. Scar tissue and stomas must be covered during radiant heat treatment, and heat-insensitive patients—such as the very young, elderly, and debilitated—require frequent monitoring to prevent burns.

Radiant heat is delivered by a heat lamp or heat cradle. The heat lamp, called a gooseneck lamp because of its long flexible neck, holds a single light bulb of 25 to 100 watts and conducts heat to a localized treatment site. Bulb wattage and the distance between the lamp and the patient regulate the amount of heat delivered. The heat cradle, a metal frame with one or more sockets for 25-watt bulbs, radiates heat to larger areas, such as the legs or abdomen. The cradle fits over the treatment site. Although its construction permits little control over the distance between the patient and the heat source, you can control the amount of heat delivered by manipulating the number of 25-watt bulbs used and the type and amount of covering tented over the cradle. Some cradles are equipped with thermostats that indicate the temperature and amount of heat projected.

Equipment
Patient thermometer ▪ gloves, if necessary ▪ heat lamp or heat cradle ▪ yardstick or measuring tape ▪ sheet ▪ one or more bath blankets.

Preparation of equipment
Check the doctor's order, and insert the prescribed wattage bulb in the heat lamp or heat cradle. If you're using the heat lamp, place it at the bedside, plug it into an outlet, and turn it on for a few minutes before exposing the patient *to warm the lamp and avoid chilling the patient.* If you're using the heat cradle, position it over the patient before turning it on *to avoid causing burns.*

Implementation
• Assess the patient's condition, explain the procedure to him, and help him into a comfortable position.
• Provide privacy and make sure the room is warm and free of drafts. Wash your hands thoroughly.

• Remove any metal objects from the patient, such as jewelry and orthopedic braces, before starting the treatment. *Metal objects heat rapidly and may cause discomfort or burns.*
• Record the patient's temperature, pulse, and respirations *to serve as a baseline.*
• Expose only the treatment site *to reduce body heat loss and to avoid chilling the patient.*
• Make sure the patient's skin is clean and dry *to reduce the risk of burns.*

Positioning the heat lamp
• Position the prewarmed lamp at the patient's side, not over him, *so if it falls, it won't strike or burn him.*
• Using a yardstick or measuring tape as a guide, adjust the neck of the lamp so the light bulb is the correct distance from the patient's skin. To determine the correct distance, consider the wattage of the bulb and the patient's physical condition, skin pigmentation, and ability to tolerate heat. In most cases, allow 14″ (35.6 cm) between the bulb and the patient's skin for a 25-watt bulb, 18″ (45.7 cm) for a 40-watt bulb, and 24″ to 30″ (61 to 76.2 cm) for a 60-watt or higher bulb.

Positioning the heat cradle
• Place the cradle on the bed, directly over or to the side of the treatment site. Plug in the cord and turn on the device.
• Cover the cradle with a sheet *to prevent drafts and to concentrate the heat on the treatment site. To prevent a fire,* make sure the sheet doesn't touch the bulbs.

Delivering the heat treatment
• With either heating device, time the application carefully.
• Check bulb position and the patient's skin every 5 minutes *to make sure the patient can tolerate the treatment.* If the patient can't tolerate the heat at the prescribed distance, discontinue the treatment and notify the doctor.
• For a cradle equipped with a thermostat, maintain the heat at 86° to 90° F (30° to 32.2° C) or as ordered.
• Turn off the heating device as ordered, usually after 10 to 15 minutes for the first treatment and 20 to 30 minutes for subsequent treatments.
• Dry the patient's skin, re-dress the treatment site if necessary, and obtain temperature, pulse, and respirations *for comparison with the baseline.* Make sure the patient is comfortable.
• If the treatment will be repeated, store the equipment in the patient's room, out of his reach; otherwise, return it to storage.

Special considerations

Avoid application of creams or ointments to the exposed area before the treatment *because they may increase the risk of burns.*

Never enclose a heat lamp and exposed body part under sheets or blankets. *Doing so increases heat intensity and the risk of burns or fire.* The heat cradle can safely support covers only if they don't touch any light bulbs.

To prevent fire or explosion, protect hot light bulbs from paper, cloth, liquids, sprays, and mists.

Caution the patient not to touch the heat lamp or heat cradle *to prevent burns.* If the patient is very young, elderly, unconscious, anesthetized, neurologically impaired, or otherwise insensitive to heat, stay with him during the treatment, and watch for signs of heat intolerance: redness, pain, extreme chills, and changes in vital signs.

Complications

Despite precautions, radiant heat treatment can burn a patient who has extremely sensitive skin.

Documentation

For heat lamp treatment, record the time, date, and duration of treatment; light bulb wattage; distance of the lamp from the patient's skin; the patient's temperature, pulse, and respirations before, during, and after treatment; appearance of the treatment site before and after; and the patient's tolerance for treatment. For heat cradle treatments, also record the number of light bulbs and the number and type of cradle covers used.

 Cold application

The application of cold constricts blood vessels; inhibits local circulation, suppuration, and tissue metabolism; relieves vascular congestion; slows bacterial activity in infections; reduces body temperature; and may act as a temporary anesthetic during brief, painful procedures. (See *Reducing pain with ice massage.)* Because treatment with cold also relieves inflammation, reduces edema, and slows bleeding, it may provide effective initial treatment after eye injuries, strains, sprains, bruises, muscle spasms, and burns. Cold does not reduce existing edema, however, because it inhibits reabsorption of excess fluid.

Cold may be applied in dry or moist forms, but ice should not be placed directly on a patient's skin because it may further damage tissue. Moist application is more penetrating than dry because moisture facilitates conduction. Devices for applying dry cold include an ice bag

or collar, K pad (which can produce cold or heat), and chemical cold packs and ice packs. Devices for applying moist cold include cold compresses for small body areas and cold packs for large areas.

Apply cold treatments cautiously on patients with impaired circulation, on children, and on elderly or arthritic patients because of the risk of ischemic tissue damage.

Equipment

Patient thermometer ▪ towel ▪ adhesive tape or roller gauze ▪ gloves, if necessary.

For an ice bag or collar: tap water ▪ ice chips ▪ absorbent, protective cloth covering.

For a K pad: distilled water ▪ temperature-adjustment key ▪ absorbent, protective cloth covering.

For a chemical cold pack: Single-use packs are available for applying dry cold. These lightweight plastic packs contain a chemical that turns cold when activated. Reusable, sealed cold packs, filled with an alcohol-based solution, are also available. These packs are stored frozen until use and, after exterior disinfection, may be refrozen and used again.

For a cold compress or pack: basin of ice chips ▪ container of tap water ▪ bath (utility) thermometer ▪ compress material (4″ × 4″ gauze pads or washcloths) or pack material (towels or flannel) ▪ linen-saver pad ▪ waterproof covering.

Preparation of equipment

Ice bag or collar: Select a device of the correct size, fill it with cold tap water, and check for leaks. Then, empty the device and fill it about halfway with crushed ice. *Using small pieces of ice keeps the device flexible for molding to the patient's body.* Squeeze the device *to expel air that might reduce conduction.* Fasten the cap and wipe any moisture from the outside of the device. Wrap the bag or collar in a cloth covering, and secure the cover with tape or roller gauze. *The protective cover prevents tissue trauma and absorbs condensation.*

K pad: Check the cord for frayed or damaged insulation. Then fill the control unit two-thirds full with distilled water. Do not use tap water *because it leaves mineral deposits in the unit.* Check for leaks, and then tilt the unit several times *to clear the pad's tubing of air, which could interfere with conduction.* Tighten the cap. After ensuring that the hoses between the control unit and pad are free of tangles, place the unit on the bedside table, slightly above the patient *so gravity can assist water flow.* If the central supply department has not preset the temperature on the control unit, use the key provided to adjust it to the lowest temperature. Cover the pad with an absorbent, protective cloth and secure the cover with tape or roller gauze. Plug in the unit and turn it on. Allow the pad to cool for 2 minutes before placing it on the patient.

Chemical cold pack: Select a pack of the appropriate size, and follow the manufacturer's directions (strike, squeeze, or knead) *to activate the cold-producing chemicals.* Make certain that the container has not been broken during activation; *such damage may allow the chemicals to leak out.* Wrap the pack in a cloth cover, and secure the cover with tape or roller gauze.

Cold compress or pack: Cool the tap water by placing the container of water in a basin of ice or by adding ice to the water. Using a bath thermometer for guidance, adjust the water temperature to 59° F (15° C) or as ordered. Immerse the compress material or pack material in the water.

Implementation
● Check the doctor's order and assess the patient's condition.
● Explain the procedure to the patient, provide privacy, and make sure the room is warm and free of drafts. Wash your hands thoroughly.
● Record the patient's temperature, pulse, and respirations *to serve as a baseline.*
● Expose only the treatment site *to avoid chilling the patient.*

To apply an ice bag or collar, K pad, or chemical cold pack
● Place the covered cold device on the treatment site and begin timing the application.
● Observe the site frequently for signs of tissue intolerance: blanching, mottling, graying, cyanosis, maceration, or blisters. Also, be alert for shivering and for the patient's complaints of burning or numbness. If any of these signs or symptoms develop, discontinue treatment and notify the doctor.
● Refill or replace the cold device as necessary *to maintain the correct temperature.* Change the protective cover if it becomes wet.
● Remove the device after the prescribed treatment period (usually 30 minutes).

To apply a cold compress or pack
● Place a linen-saver pad under the treatment area.
● Remove the compress or pack from the water, and wring it out *to prevent dripping.* Apply it to the treatment site and begin timing the application.
● Cover the compress or pack with a waterproof covering *to provide insulation and to keep the surrounding area dry.* Secure the covering with tape or roller gauze *to prevent it from slipping.*

Reducing pain with ice massage

Normally, ice should not be applied directly to a patient's skin because it risks damaging the skin surface and underlying tissues. However, when carefully performed, this technique – called ice massage – may help patients tolerate brief, painful procedures, such as biopsy under local anesthesia, bone marrow aspiration, catheterization, chest tube removal, injection into joints, lumbar puncture, and suture removal.

Prepare for ice massage by gathering the ice, a porous covering to hold it in (if desired), and a cloth for wiping water from the patient as the ice melts.

Just before the procedure begins, rub the ice over the appropriate area to numb it. Assess the site frequently; stop rubbing immediately if you detect signs of tissue intolerance.

As the procedure begins, rub the ice over a point near but not at the site. This distracts the patient from the procedure itself and gives him another stimulus on which to concentrate.

If the procedure lasts longer than about 10 minutes, or if you think tissue damage may occur, move the ice to a different site and continue the massage.

If you know in advance that the procedure probably will last longer than 10 minutes, massage the site intermittently – 2 minutes of massage alternating with a rest period until the skin regains its normal color. Alternatively, you can divide the area into several sites and apply ice to each one for several minutes at a time.

● Check the application site frequently for signs of tissue intolerance. Also note the patient's complaints of burning or numbness. If these signs or symptoms develop, discontinue treatment and notify the doctor.
● Change the compress or pack as necessary *to maintain the correct temperature.* Remove it after the prescribed treatment period (usually 20 minutes).

To conclude all cold applications
● Dry the patient's skin and re-dress the treatment site according to the doctor's orders. Then, position the patient comfortably, and take his temperature, pulse, and respirations *for comparison with the baseline.*
● Dispose of liquids and soiled materials properly. If treatment will be repeated, clean and store the equipment in

Using cold for a muscle sprain

Cold can help relieve pain and reduce edema during the first 24 to 72 hours after a sprain occurs. Tell the patient to apply cold to the area four times daily for 20 to 30 minutes each time.

For each application, instruct the patient to obtain enough crushed ice to cover the painful area, place it in a plastic bag, and place the bag inside a pillowcase or large piece of cloth, as shown below.

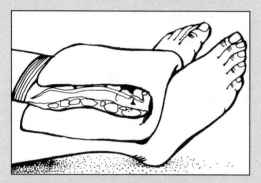

For later applications, the patient may wish to fill a paper cup with water, stand a tongue blade in the cup, and place it in the freezer. After the water freezes, he can peel the paper off the ice and hold it with the protruding handle. If he chooses this method, however, tell him to cover the area with a cloth before applying the ice. Applying ice directly to the skin could cause frostbite or cold shock.

Instruct the patient to rub the ice over the painful area for the specified treatment time. Warn him that, although ice eases pain in a joint that has begun to stiffen, he shouldn't let the analgesic effect encourage overuse of the joint.

After 24 to 72 hours, when heat, redness, and swelling have subsided or when cold no longer helps, the patient should switch to heat application.

the patient's room, out of his reach; otherwise, return it to storage.

Special considerations

Apply cold immediately after an injury *to minimize edema.* (See *Using cold for a muscle sprain.*) Although colder temperatures can be tolerated for a longer time when the treatment site is small, don't continue any application for longer than 1 hour *to prevent reflexive vasodilation.* Application of temperatures below 59° F (15° C) will also cause local reflex vasodilation.

When applying cold to an open wound or to a lesion that may open during treatment, use sterile technique. Also maintain sterile technique during eye treatment, with separate sterile equipment for each eye *to prevent cross-contamination.*

Avoid securing cooling devices with pins *because an accidental puncture may allow extremely cold fluids to leak out and burn the patient's skin.*

If the patient is unconscious, anesthetized, neurologically impaired, irrational, or otherwise insensitive to cold, stay with him throughout the treatment and check the application site frequently for complications. Warn the patient against placing ice directly on his skin *because the extreme cold can cause burns.*

Complications

Thrombi may result from hemoconcentration. Pain, burning, or numbness may result from intense cold.

Documentation

Record the time, date, and duration of cold application; type of device used (ice bag or collar, K pad, or chemical cold pack); site of application; temperature or temperature setting; patient's temperature, pulse, and respirations before and after application; skin appearance before, during, and after application; any signs of complications; and the patient's tolerance for treatment.

Hyperthermia-hypothermia blanket

A blanket-sized aquamatic K pad, the hyperthermia-hypothermia blanket raises, lowers, or maintains body temperature through conductive heat or cold transfer between the blanket and the patient. It can be operated manually or automatically.

In manual operation, the nurse or doctor sets the temperature on the unit. The blanket reaches and maintains this temperature regardless of the patient's temperature. The temperature setting must be manually adjusted to reach a different temperature setting. The nurse monitors the patient's body temperature using a conventional thermometer.

In automatic operation, the unit directly and continually monitors the patient's temperature by means of a thermistor probe (rectal, skin, or esophageal) and alternates heating and cooling cycles as necessary to achieve and maintain the desired body temperature. The thermistor probe also may be used in conjunction with manual operation but is not essential. The unit is equipped with an alarm to warn of abnormal temperature fluctuations, and a circuit breaker that protects against current overload.

The blanket is used most commonly to reduce high fever when more conservative measures — such as baths, ice packs, and antipyretics — are unsuccessful. Its other uses include maintaining normal temperature during surgery or shock; inducing hypothermia during surgery to decrease metabolic activity and thereby reduce oxygen requirements; reducing intracranial pressure; controlling bleeding and intractable pain in patients with amputations, burns, or cancer; and providing warmth in cases of severe hypothermia.

Equipment
Hyperthermia-hypothermia control unit ▪ operation manual ▪ fluid for the control unit (distilled water or distilled water and 20% ethyl alcohol) ▪ thermistor probe (rectal, skin, or esophageal) ▪ one or two hyperthermia-hypothermia blankets ▪ one or two disposable blanket covers (or one or two sheets or bath blankets) ▪ lanolin or a mixture of lanolin and cold cream ▪ patient thermometer (for manual mode) ▪ adhesive tape ▪ towel ▪ sphygmomanometer ▪ gloves, if necessary ▪ optional: protective wraps for the patient's hands and feet.

Disposable hyperthermia-hypothermia blankets are available for single-patient use.

Preparation of equipment
First, read the operation manual. Inspect the unit and each blanket for leaks and the plugs and the connecting wires for broken prongs, kinks, and fraying. If you detect or suspect malfunction, don't use the equipment.

Review the doctor's order, and prepare one or two blankets by covering them with disposable covers (or use a sheet or a bath blanket when positioning the blanket on the patient). *The cover absorbs perspiration and condensation, which could cause tissue breakdown if left on the skin.* Connect the blanket to the control unit, and set the controls for manual or automatic operation and for the desired blanket or body temperature. Make sure the machine is properly grounded before plugging it in. Turn on the machine and add liquid to the unit reservoir, if necessary, as fluid fills the blanket. Allow the blanket to preheat or precool *so the patient receives immediate thermal benefit.* Place the control unit at the foot of the bed.

Implementation
• Assess the patient's condition and explain the procedure to him. Provide privacy and make sure the room is warm and free of drafts. Check hospital policy and, if necessary, make sure the patient or a responsible family member has signed a consent form.

• Wash your hands thoroughly. If the patient is not already wearing a hospital gown, ask him to put one on. Use a gown with cloth ties, not metal snaps or pins *because these could cause heat or cold injury.*

• Take the patient's temperature, pulse, respirations, and blood pressure *to serve as a baseline,* and assess level of consciousness, pupil reaction, limb strength, and skin condition.

• Keeping the bottom sheet in place and the patient recumbent, roll him to one side and slide the blanket halfway under him, so its top edge aligns with his neck. Then roll the patient back, and pull and flatten the blanket across the bed. Place a pillow under the patient's head. Make sure the patient's head doesn't lie directly on the blanket *because the blanket's rigid surface may be uncomfortable and the heat or cold may lead to tissue breakdown.* If necessary, use a sheet or bath blanket as insulation between the patient and the blanket.

• Apply lanolin or a mixture of lanolin and cold cream to the patient's skin where it touches the blanket *to help protect the skin from heat or cold sensation.*

• In automatic operation, insert the thermistor probe in the patient's rectum and tape it in place *to prevent accidental dislodgment.* If rectal insertion is contraindicated, tuck a skin probe deep into the axilla, and secure it with tape. If the patient is comatose or anesthetized, insert an esophageal probe. Plug the other end of the probe into the correct jack on the unit's control panel.

• Place a sheet or, if ordered, the second hyperthermia-hypothermia blanket over the patient. *This increases thermal benefit by trapping cooled or heated air.*

• Wrap the patient's hands and feet, if he wishes, *to minimize chilling and promote comfort.* Monitor vital signs and perform a neurologic assessment every 5 minutes until the desired body temperature is reached; then every 15 minutes until temperature is stable or as ordered.

• Check fluid intake and output hourly or as ordered. Observe the patient regularly for color changes in skin, lips, and nail beds, and for edema, induration, inflammation, pain, or sensory impairment. If these occur, discontinue the procedure and notify the doctor.

• Reposition the patient every 30 minutes to 1 hour, unless contraindicated, *to prevent skin breakdown.* Keep the patient's skin, bedclothes, and blanket cover free of perspiration and condensation, and reapply cream to exposed body parts as needed.

• After turning off the machine, follow the manufacturer's directions. *Some units must remain plugged in for at least 30 minutes to allow the condenser fan to remove water vapor from the mechanism.* Continue to monitor the pa-

tient's temperature until it stabilizes *because body temperature can fall as much as 5° F (2.8° C) after this procedure.*
• Remove all equipment from the bed. Dry the patient and make him comfortable. Supply a fresh hospital gown, if necessary. Cover the patient lightly.
• Continue to perform neurologic checks and monitor vital signs, fluid intake and output, and general condition every 30 minutes for 2 hours and then hourly or as ordered.
• Return the equipment to the central supply department for cleaning, servicing, and storage.

Special considerations
If the patient shivers excessively during hypothermia treatment, discontinue the procedure and notify the doctor immediately. *By increasing metabolism, shivering elevates body temperature.*

Avoid lowering the temperature more than 1 degree every 15 minutes *to prevent premature ventricular contractions.*

Don't use pins to secure catheters, tubes, or blanket covers *because an accidental puncture can result in fluid leakage and burns.*

With hyperthermia or hypothermia therapy, the patient may experience a secondary defense reaction (vasoconstriction or vasodilation, respectively) that causes body temperature to rebound and thus defeat the treatment's purpose.

If the patient requires isolation, place the blanket, blanket cover, and probe in a plastic bag clearly marked with the type of isolation *so the central supply department can give it special handling.* If the blanket is disposable, discard it using appropriate precautions.

To avoid bacterial growth in the reservoir or blankets, always use sterile distilled water and change it monthly. Check to see if hospital policy calls for adding a bacteriostatic agent to the water. Avoid using de-ionized water, *because it may corrode the system.*

Complications
Use of a hyperthermia-hypothermia blanket can cause shivering, marked changes in vital signs, increased intracranial pressure, respiratory distress or arrest, cardiac arrest, oliguria, and anuria.

Documentation
Record the patient's pulse, respirations, blood pressure, neurologic signs, fluid intake and output, skin condition, and position change. Record the patient's temperature and that of the thermal pad every 30 minutes while the pad is in use. Also document the type of hyperthermia-hypothermia unit used; control settings (manual or automatic, and temperature settings); date, time, duration,

and patient's tolerance of treatment; and any signs of complications.

Sponge bath

The sponge bath—with tepid water, alcohol, or a mixture of the two—reduces fever by dilating superficial blood vessels, thus releasing heat and lowering body temperature. An alcohol sponge bath effects the fastest temperature reduction because alcohol evaporates faster than water and thus removes heat more rapidly from the skin surface. However, alcohol is also more drying to the skin, and the rapid temperature loss produced by an alcohol bath may cause chilling and a rebound rise in temperature. A tepid-water sponge bath, with or without alcohol, may lower systemic temperature when routine fever treatments fail, particularly for infants and children, whose temperatures tend to rise very high, very quickly.

Equipment
Basin of tepid water, approximately 80° to 93° F (26° to 34° C) ▪ 70% isopropyl (rubbing) alcohol, if prescribed ▪ bath (utility) thermometer ▪ bath blanket ▪ linen-saver pad ▪ washcloths ▪ patient thermometer ▪ hot water bottle and cover ▪ ice bag and cover ▪ towel ▪ emesis basin (if using alcohol) ▪ clean gown ▪ gloves, if the patient has open lesions or has been incontinent.

Preparation of equipment
Prepare a hot water bottle and an ice bag. Then place the bath thermometer in a basin, and run water over it until the temperature reaches the high end of the tepid range (93° F) *because the water will cool during the bath.* Add alcohol, if prescribed, at room temperature in a 1:1 proportion. Immerse the washcloths in the tepid solution until saturated.

Implementation
• Check the doctor's order and assess the patient's condition.
• Check the medication Kardex for recent administration of an antipyretic *because this can affect patient response to the bath.*
• Explain the procedure to the patient, provide privacy, and make sure the room is warm and free of drafts. Wash your hands thoroughly and put on gloves, if necessary.
• Place a linen-saver pad under the patient *to catch any spills* and a bath blanket over him *for privacy.* Then remove his pajamas. Also remove the top bed linen *to avoid wetting it.*

• Take the patient's temperature, pulse, and respiration *to serve as a baseline.*

• Place the hot water bottle with protective covering on the patient's feet *to reduce the sensation of chilliness.* Place the covered ice bag on his head *to prevent headache and nasal congestion that occur as the rest of the body cools.*

• Wring out each washcloth before sponging the patient *so they don't drip and cause discomfort.*

• Place moist washcloths over the major superficial blood vessels in the axillae, groin, and popliteal areas *to accelerate cooling.* Change the washcloths as they warm.

• Bathe each extremity separately for about 5 minutes; then sponge the chest and abdomen for 5 minutes. Turn the patient, and bathe his back and buttocks for 5 to 10 minutes. Keep the patient covered except for the body part you're sponging.

• Add warm water to the basin as necessary *to maintain the desired water temperature.*

• Check the patient's temperature, pulse, and respirations every 10 minutes. Notify the doctor if the patient's temperature doesn't fall within 30 minutes. Stop the bath when the patient's temperature reaches 1° to 2° F above the desired level *because his temperature will continue to fall naturally.* Continue to monitor his temperature until it stabilizes.

• Observe the patient for chills, shivering, pallor, mottling, cyanosis of the lips or nail beds, and changes in vital signs — especially a rapid, weak, or irregular pulse — *because such signs may indicate an emergency.* If any of these signs occur, discontinue the bath, cover the patient lightly, and notify the doctor.

• If no adverse effects occur, bathe the patient for at least 30 minutes *to reduce temperature.*

• Pat each area dry after sponging but avoid rubbing with the towel *because rubbing increases cell metabolism and produces heat.*

• After finishing the bath, make sure the patient is dry and comfortable. Dress him in a fresh gown and cover him lightly.

• Dispose of liquids and soiled materials properly. If the treatment will be repeated, clean and store the equipment in the patient's room, out of his reach; otherwise, return the items to storage.

• Take temperature, pulse, and respirations 30 minutes after the bath *to determine the treatment's effectiveness.*

Special considerations

If ordered, administer an antipyretic 15 to 20 minutes before the sponge bath *to achieve more rapid fever reduction.* If you're giving an alcohol sponge bath, observe the patient's skin for excessive dryness. Also, keep the emesis basin readily available *because alcohol vapors may cause nausea and vomiting.*

Consider covering the patient's trunk with a wet towel for 15 minutes to speed cooling. Resaturate the towel as necessary.

Refrain from bathing the breasts of a postpartum patient *because they could become overly dry or fissures could develop on the nipples.*

Take a rectal temperature, unless contraindicated, *for accuracy.* Axillary temperatures are unreliable *because the cool compresses applied to these areas alter the readings.* If you must take an oral temperature, do so cautiously *because chills may cause the patient to bite down and shatter the thermometer.* If possible, use an electronic thermometer to take an oral temperature *because it gives the temperature reading more quickly and because it isn't covered with glass, which could break in the patient's mouth.*

Home care

Sponge baths to reduce fever are used most commonly in nonhospital settings; febrile hospitalized patients usually receive antibiotics or antipyretics and, if needed, treatment with hypothermia blankets, which lower and maintain body temperature more effectively than sponge baths.

Complications

Accelerated temperature reduction can provoke seizure activity.

Documentation

Record the date, time, and duration of the bath; the type and temperature of the solution; the patient's temperature, pulse, and respirations before, during, and after the procedure; any complications that arise; and the patient's tolerance for treatment.

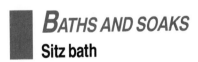

BATHS AND SOAKS
Sitz bath

Also known as a hip bath, a sitz bath involves immersion of the pelvic area in warm or hot water. It is used to relieve discomfort, especially after surgery or childbirth. The bath promotes wound healing by cleaning the perineum and anus, increasing circulation, and reducing inflammation. It also helps relax local muscles.

To be performed correctly, the sitz bath requires frequent checks of water temperature to ensure therapeutic effects, and correct draping of the patient during the bath and prompt dressing after it to prevent vasoconstriction.

Equipment

Sitz tub, portable sitz bath, or regular bathtub ■ bath mat ■ rubber mat ■ bath (utility) thermometer ■ two bath blankets ■ towels ■ hospital gown ■ gloves, if the patient has an open lesion or has been incontinent ■ optional: rubber ring, footstool, overbed table, I.V. pole (to hold irrigation bag), wheelchair or cart, dressings.

A disposable sitz bath kit is available for single-patient use. It includes a plastic basin that fits over a commode and an irrigation bag with tubing and clamp.

Preparation of equipment

Make sure the sitz tub, portable sitz bath, or regular bathtub is clean and disinfected. Or, obtain a disposable sitz bath kit from the central supply department.

Position the bath mat next to the bathtub, sitz tub, or commode. If you're using a tub, place the rubber mat on its surface *to prevent falls.* Place the rubber ring on the bottom of the tub *to serve as a seat for the patient,* and cover the ring with a towel *for comfort. Keeping the patient elevated improves water flow over the wound site and avoids unnecessary pressure on tender tissues.*

If you're using a commercial kit, open the package and familiarize yourself with the equipment.

Fill the sitz tub or bathtub one-third to one-half full, so that the water will reach the seated patient's umbilicus. Use warm water (94° to 98° F [34° to 37° C]) for relaxation or wound cleaning and healing, hot water (110° to 115° F [43° to 46° C]) for heat application. Run the water slightly warmer than desired *because it will cool while the patient prepares for the bath.* Measure the temperature of the water using the bath thermometer.

If you're using a commercial kit, fill the basin to the specified line with water at the prescribed temperature. Place the basin under the commode seat, clamp the irrigation tubing to block water flow, and fill the irrigation bag with water of the same temperature as that in the basin. To create flow pressure, hang the bag above the patient's head on a hook, towel rack, or I.V. pole.

Implementation

• Check the doctor's order and assess the patient's condition.
• Explain the procedure to the patient. Wash your hands thoroughly and put on gloves, if necessary.
• Have the patient void.
• Assist the patient to the bath area, provide privacy, and make sure the area is warm and free of drafts. Help the patient undress, as needed.
• Remove and dispose of any soiled dressings. If a dressing adheres to a wound, allow it to soak off in the tub.
• Assist the patient into the tub or onto the commode, as needed. Instruct him to use the safety rail for balance.

Explain that initially the sensation may be unpleasant *because the wound area is already tender.* Assure him that this discomfort will soon be relieved by the warm water.
• For any apparatus except a regular bathtub, if the patient's feet do not reach the floor and the weight of his legs presses against the edge of the equipment, place a small stool under the patient's feet. *This decreases pressure on local blood vessels.* Also place a folded towel against the patient's lower back *to prevent discomfort and promote correct body alignment.*
• Drape the patient's shoulders and knees with bath blankets *to avoid chills that cause vasoconstriction.*
• If you're using the sitz bath kit, open the clamp on the irrigation tubing *to allow a stream of water to flow continuously over the wound site.* Refill the bag with water of the correct temperature as needed, and encourage the patient to regulate the flow himself. Place the patient's overbed table in front of him *to provide support and comfort.*
• If you're using a tub, check the water temperature frequently with the bath thermometer. If the temperature drops significantly, add warm water. For maximum safety, first help the patient stand up slowly *to prevent dizziness and loss of balance.* Then, with the patient holding the safety rail *for support,* run warm water into the tub. Check water temperature. When the water reaches the correct temperature, help the patient sit down again to resume the bath.
• If necessary, stay with the patient during the bath. If you must leave, show him how to use the call button, and ensure his privacy.
• Check the patient's color and general condition frequently. If he complains of feeling weak, faint, or nauseated or shows signs of cardiovascular distress, discontinue the bath, check the patient's pulse and blood pressure, and assist him back to bed. Use a wheelchair or cart to transport the patient to his room if necessary. Notify the doctor.
• When the prescribed bath time has elapsed—usually 15 to 20 minutes—tell the patient to use the safety rail *for balance* and help him to a standing position slowly *to prevent dizziness and to allow him to regain his equilibrium.*
• If necessary, help the patient to dry himself. Re-dress the wound as needed, and assist the patient to dress and to return to bed or back to his room.
• Dispose of soiled materials properly. Empty, clean, and disinfect the sitz tub, bathtub, or portable sitz bath. Return the commercial kit to the patient's bedside for later use.

Special considerations

Use a regular bathtub only if a special sitz tub, portable sitz bath, or commercial sitz bath kit is unavailable. *Because the application of heat to the extremities causes va-*

sodilation and draws blood away from the perineal area, a regular bathtub is less effective for local treatment than a sitz device.

If the patient will be sitting in a bathtub with his extremities immersed in the hot water, check his pulse before, during, and after the bath *to help detect vasodilation that could make him feel faint when he stands up.*

Tell the patient never to touch an open wound *because of the risk of infection.*

Home care
Instruct the patient to adhere to the manufacturer's guidelines for disposable equipment.

Complications
Weakness or faintness can result from heat or the exertion of changing position. Irregular or accelerated pulse may indicate cardiovascular distress.

Documentation
Record the date, time, duration, and temperature of the bath; wound condition before and after treatment, including color, odor, and amount of drainage; any complications; and the patient's response to treatment.

 # Therapeutic bath

Also referred to as balneotherapy, the therapeutic bath combines water and additives to soothe and relax the patient, clean the skin, relieve inflammation and pruritus, and soften and remove crusts, scales, debris, and old medications. Used primarily for their antipruritic and emollient actions, these baths coat irritated skin with a soothing, protective film. Because they constrict surface blood vessels, they also have an anti-inflammatory effect.

Addition of oatmeal powder, soluble cornstarch, or soybean complex to water creates a colloid bath, which has a soothing effect and is used to treat generalized itching. Oil baths are useful for lubricating dry skin and easing eczematous eruptions. Sodium bicarbonate added to water produces an alkaline bath that has a cooling effect and also helps relieve pruritus. A medicated tar bath may be used to treat psoriasis. The film of tar left on the skin works in combination with ultraviolet light to inhibit the rapid cell turnover characteristic of psoriasis. (See *Comparing therapeutic baths,* page 178.)

A bedridden patient may benefit from a local soak with the therapeutic additive instead of a therapeutic tub bath.

Equipment
Bathtub ▪ bath mat ▪ rubber mat ▪ bath (utility) thermometer ▪ therapeutic additive ▪ measuring device ▪ colander or sieve for oatmeal powder ▪ two washcloths ▪ two towels ▪ hospital gown or loose-fitting cotton pajamas ▪ lubricating cream or ointment, if ordered.

Preparation of equipment
Assemble supplies and draw the bath before bringing the patient to the bath area *to prevent chilling him.* Make sure the tub is clean and disinfected *because a patient with skin breakdown is particularly vulnerable to infection.* Place the bath mat next to the tub and the rubber mat on the bottom of the tub *to prevent falls; the therapeutic additive may make the tub exceptionally slippery.* Fill the tub with 6″ to 8″ (15.2 to 20.3 cm) of water at 95° to 100° F (35° to 37.8° C).

The treatment's purpose and the type of additive used will determine the water temperature. Cool to lukewarm water is used for relieving pruritus and when adding tar or starch. Warm baths are soothing, but water warmer than 100° F causes vasodilation, *which could aggravate pruritus.*

Measure the correct amount of therapeutic additive, according to the doctor's order or package instructions. As the tub is filling, thoroughly mix the additive in the water. Add most substances directly to the water, but place oatmeal powder in a sieve or colander under the tub faucet *to help it dissolve.* Begin with two tablespoons of oatmeal powder; then add more powder or water as needed to regulate the thickness of the oatmeal bath.

When giving a tar bath, wear a plastic apron or protective gown *because tar preparations stain clothing.*

Implementation
● Check the doctor's order, and assess the patient's condition.
● Explain the procedure to the patient and have him void. Wash your hands thoroughly and then escort the patient to the bath area. Close the door *to provide privacy and eliminate drafts.*
● Check the water temperature. Assist the patient to undress, and help him into the tub, if necessary. Advise him to use the safety rails *to prevent falls.*
● Tell him the bath may feel unpleasant at first *because his skin is irritated,* but assure him that the medication will soon coat and soothe his skin.
● Ask the patient to stretch out in the tub and submerge his body up to the chin. If he's capable, give him a washcloth to apply the bath solution gently to his face and other body areas not immersed.

Comparing therapeutic baths

TYPE	AGENTS	PURPOSE
Antibacterial	• Acetic acid • Potassium permanganate • Povidone-iodine	Used to treat infected eczema, dirty ulcerations, furunculosis, and pemphigus
Colloidal	• Aveeno colloidal oatmeal • Aveeno colloidal oatmeal, oilated • Starch and baking soda	Used to relieve pruritus and to soothe irritated skin; indicated for any irritated or oozing condition, such as atopic eczema
Emollient	• Bath oils • Mineral oil	Used to clean and hydrate the skin; indicated for any dry skin condition
Tar	• Bath oils with tar • Coal tar concentrate	Used to treat scaly dermatoses, sometimes in combination with ultraviolet light therapy; loosens scales and relieves pruritus

♦ *Nursing alert.* If the patient is taking a tar bath, tell him not to get the bath solution in his eyes *because tar is an eye irritant.* ♦

• Warn the patient against scrubbing his skin *to prevent further irritation.*

• Add warm water to the bath as needed *to maintain a comfortable temperature.*

• Allow the patient to soak for 15 to 30 minutes. If you must stay with him, pull the bath curtain; *this gives him some privacy and protects him from drafts.* If you must leave the room, show the patient how to use the call button, and ensure his privacy.

• After the bath, assist the patient from the tub. Have him use the safety rails *to prevent falls.*

• Help the patient pat his skin dry with towels. Don't rub the skin *because rubbing removes some solutes and oils clinging to the skin and produces friction, which increases pruritus.*

• Apply lubricating cream or ointment, if ordered, *to help hold water in the newly hydrated skin.*

• Provide a fresh hospital gown or loose-fitting cotton pajamas. Advise the patient to avoid wearing pajamas, underwear, or other clothing that isn't cotton and loose-fitting. *Tight clothing and scratchy or synthetic materials can aggravate skin conditions by causing friction and increasing perspiration.*

• Escort the patient to his room and make sure he's comfortable.

• Drain the bath water, clean and disinfect the tub, and dispose of soiled materials properly. *If you have given an*

oatmeal powder bath, drain and rinse the tub immediately or the powder will cake, making later removal difficult.

Special considerations

Because pruritus seems worse at night, give a therapeutic bath before bedtime, unless ordered otherwise, *to promote restful sleep. Because the patient with a skin disorder may be self-conscious,* maintain eye contact during conversation and avoid staring at his skin. Also, avoid nonverbal expressions and gestures that show revulsion. If the patient wishes, allow him to talk about his condition and how it affects his self-esteem.

Refrain from using soap during a therapeutic bath *because its drying effect counteracts the bath emollient.*

A patient with skin breakdown chills easily, so protect him from drafts. But after the bath, avoid covering or dressing him too warmly *because perspiration aggravates pruritus.* Instruct the patient not to scratch his skin *to prevent excoriation and infection.*

If the patient is confined to bed, you can place the therapeutic additive in a basin of water at 95° to 100° F (35° to 37.8° C) and apply it with a washcloth, using light, gentle strokes.

Home care

• Instruct the patient to bathe only as often as prescribed. *Excessive bathing can dry the skin.*

• Advise the patient to purchase commercial bath oil. *Salad or cooking oils may give clothes an unpleasant odor, and mineral oil mixes poorly with water.*

• Tell the patient to follow manufacturer's instructions for commercially prepared colloid preparations. Colloid for an oatmeal bath can be made at home by putting one-half cup of raw oatmeal into a blender and blending at medium-high speed until the material has the consistency of flour, then sifting it to remove unground pieces.

Documentation
Record the date, time, and duration of the bath. Note the water temperature, the type and amount of additive, skin appearance before and after the bath, the patient's tolerance of the treatment, and the bath's effectiveness.

Soaks

A soak involves the immersion of a body part in warm water or a medicated solution. This treatment helps to soften exudates, facilitate debridement, enhance suppuration, clean wounds or burns, rehydrate wounds, apply medication to infected areas, and increase local blood supply and circulation.

Most soaks are applied with clean tap water and clean technique. Sterile solution and sterile equipment are required for treating wounds, burns, or other breaks in the skin.

Equipment
Basin, or arm or foot tub ▪ bath (utility) thermometer ▪ hot tap water or prescribed solution ▪ cup ▪ pitcher ▪ linen-saver pad ▪ overbed table ▪ footstool ▪ pillows ▪ towels ▪ gauze pads and other dressing materials ▪ gloves, if necessary.

Preparation of equipment
Clean and disinfect the basin or tub. Run hot tap water into a pitcher, or heat the prescribed solution, as applicable. Measure the water or solution temperature with a bath thermometer. If the temperature is not within the prescribed range (usually 105° to 110° F [40.6° to 43.3° C]), add hot or cold water or reheat or cool the solution, as needed. If you're preparing the soak away from the patient's room, heat the liquid slightly above the correct temperature *to allow for cooling during transport.* If the solution for a medicated soak isn't premixed, prepare the dilution and heat it.

Implementation
• Check the doctor's order and assess the patient's condition.

• Explain the procedure to the patient and, if necessary, check his history for previous allergic reaction to the medicated solution. Provide privacy. Wash your hands thoroughly.
• If the soak basin or tub will be placed in bed, make sure the bed is flat beneath it *to prevent spills.* For an arm soak, have the patient sit erect. For a leg or foot soak, ask him to lie down and bend the appropriate knee. For a foot soak in the sitting position, let him sit on the edge of the bed or transfer him to a chair.
• Place a linen-saver pad under the treatment site and, if necessary, cover the pad with a towel *to absorb spillage.*
• Expose the treatment site. Put on gloves before removing any dressing; dispose of the soiled dressing properly. If the dressing is encrusted and stuck to the wound, leave it in place and proceed with the soak. Remove the dressing several minutes later when it has begun to soak free.
• Position the soak basin under the treatment site on the bed, overbed table, footstool, or floor, as appropriate. Pour the heated liquid into the soak basin or tub. Then lower the arm or leg into the basin gradually *to allow adjustment to the temperature change.* Make sure the soak solution covers the treatment site.
• Support other body parts with pillows or towels as needed *to prevent discomfort and muscle strain.* Make the patient comfortable and ensure proper body alignment.
• Check the temperature of the soak solution with the bath thermometer every 5 minutes. If the temperature drops below the prescribed range, remove some of the cooled solution with a cup. Then lift the patient's arm or leg from the basin *to avoid burns,* and add hot water or solution to the basin. Mix the liquid thoroughly and then check its temperature. If the temperature is within the prescribed range, lower the patient's affected part back into the basin.
• Observe the patient for signs of tissue intolerance: extreme redness at the treatment site, excessive drainage, bleeding, or maceration. If such signs develop or the patient complains of pain, discontinue the treatment and notify the doctor.
• After 15 to 20 minutes, or as ordered, lift the patient's arm or leg from the basin and remove the basin.
• Dry the arm or leg thoroughly with a towel. If the patient has a wound, dry the skin around it without touching the wound.
• While the skin is hydrated from the soak, use gauze pads to remove loose scales or crusts.
• Observe the treatment area for general appearance, degree of swelling, debridement, suppuration, and healing. Re-dress the wound, if appropriate.
• Remove the towel and linen-saver pad and make the patient comfortable in bed.

Using intermittent pneumatic compression stockings

For patients with chronic venous disease and sometimes for others at risk for deep venous disease, intermittent pneumatic compression (IPC) stockings may be used during surgery and the postoperative period. These stockings are actually knee- or thigh-length cuffs connected to a pump and hoses. Wrapped from ankle to knee or thigh on each leg, the cuffs imitate normal leg pumping action by sequentially inflating and deflating a series of air cells from the ankle toward the trunk. This milking action propels blood toward the heart, preventing congestion in venous muscle sinuses and valve pockets, and preventing blood backflow. Cuff pressures range from 35 to 55 mm Hg. The cuffs are foam-lined and adjustable to prevent skin irritation.

To operate IPC stockings

Follow the manufacturer's guidelines when operating the IPC unit. The cuffs are marked for placement and positioning. To avoid securing the cuff too tightly, place two fingers between the patient's leg and the cuff before fastening it. If plastic connectors are used, align them on the side of the leg to keep them from pressing against bony prominences when the cuffs are inflated or from pressure against the bed.

Observe cuff filling for at least the first two cycles (approximately 3 or 4 minutes) to ensure correct operation. Only one cuff should fill at a time, from ankle to knee, then thigh. All air cells should then deflate simultaneously. The second cuff follows the same sequence. If the sequence isn't correct and you're sure the cuffs have been properly applied, remove them and have the system checked for malfunction. Also remove the cuffs and check for malfunction if the pump indicator light turns on at any time.

Precautions

Check for proper application, fit, and connections at regular intervals. Assess the patient's skin color, temperature, sensation, and ability to move. If you notice any significant changes, or if the patient experiences numbness, tingling, or leg pain, remove the cuffs and notify the doctor.

• Discard the soak solution, dispose of soiled materials properly, and clean and disinfect the basin. If the treatment is to be repeated, store the equipment in the patient's room, out of his reach; otherwise, return it to the central supply department.

Special considerations

To treat large areas, particularly burns, a soak may be administered in a whirlpool or Hubbard tank.

Documentation

Record the date, time, and duration of the soak; treatment site; solution and its temperature; skin and wound appearance before, during, and after treatment; and the patient's tolerance for treatment.

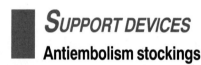

SUPPORT DEVICES
Antiembolism stockings

Elastic antiembolism stockings help prevent deep vein thrombosis (DVT) and pulmonary embolism by compressing superficial leg veins and the soleus muscle. This compression increases venous return by forcing blood into the deep venous system rather than allowing it to pool in the legs and form clots.

Antiembolism stockings can provide equal pressure over the entire leg or a graded pressure that is greatest at the ankle and decreases over the length of the leg. Usually indicated for postoperative, bedridden, elderly, or other patients at risk for DVT, these stockings should not be used on patients with dermatoses or open skin lesions, gangrene, severe arteriosclerosis or other ischemic vascular diseases, pulmonary or any massive edema, recent vein ligation, or vascular or skin grafts. For patients with chronic venous problems, intermittent pneumatic compression stockings may be ordered during surgery and postoperatively. (See *Using intermittent pneumatic compression stockings.*)

Equipment

Tape measure ▪ antiembolism stockings of correct size and length ▪ talcum powder.

Preparation of equipment

Before applying a knee-length stocking: Measure the circumference of the patient's calf at its widest point and leg length from the bottom of the heel to the back of the knee. (See *Measuring for antiembolism stockings.*)

Measuring for antiembolism stockings

Measure the patient carefully to ensure that his antiembolism stockings provide enough compression for adequate venous return.

To choose a *knee-length* stocking of the correct size, measure the circumference of the calf at its widest point (below) and the leg length from the bottom of the heel to the back of the knee (bottom left).

To choose a *thigh-length* stocking, measure the calf as for a knee-length stocking and the thigh at its widest point (below). Then measure leg length from the bottom of the heel to the gluteal fold (bottom right).

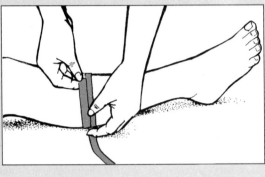

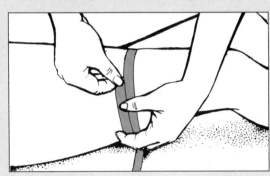

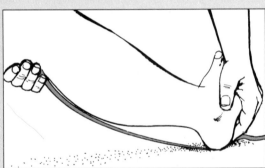

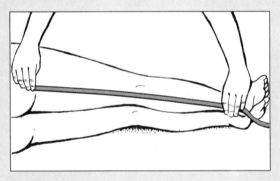

Before applying a thigh-length stocking: Measure the circumference of the calf and thigh at their widest points and the leg length from the bottom of the heel to the gluteal fold.

Before applying a waist-length stocking: Measure the circumference of the calf and thigh at their widest points and the leg length from the bottom of the heel to the waist along the side of the body.

Obtain the correct size stocking according to the manufacturer's specifications. If the patient's measurements are outside the range indicated by the manufacturer, or if his legs are deformed or edematous, ask the doctor if he wants to order custom-made stockings.

Implementation
● Check the doctor's order, and assess the patient's condition. If his legs are cold or cyanotic, notify the doctor before proceeding.
● Explain the procedure to the patient, provide privacy, and wash your hands thoroughly.
● Have the patient lie down. Then dust his ankle with talcum powder *to ease application.*

Applying a knee-length stocking
● Insert your hand into the stocking from the top, and grasp the heel pocket from the inside. Holding the heel, turn the stocking inside out so the foot is inside the

Applying antiembolism stockings: Three key steps

After covering the heel, gather the loose part of the stocking at the toes and pull this portion toward the heel.

Then, gather the loose part of the stocking and bring it over the heel with short, alternating front and back pulls.

Insert index and middle fingers into the gathered part of the stocking at the ankle and ease it upward by rocking it slightly up and down.

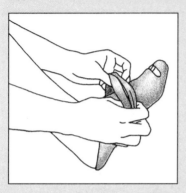

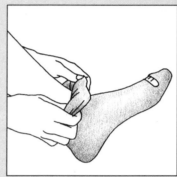

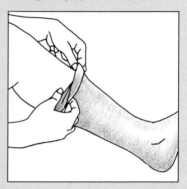

stocking leg. *This method allows easier application than gathering the entire stocking and working it up over the foot and ankle.*

• With the heel pocket down, hook the index and middle fingers of both your hands into the foot section. Facing the patient, ease the stocking over the toes, stretching it sideways as you move it up the foot. Ask the patient to point his toes, if possible, *to ease application.*

• Support the patient's ankle with one hand, and use the other hand to pull the heel pocket under the heel. Then center the heel in the pocket.

• Gather the loose portion of the stocking at the toe, and pull only this section over the heel. Gather the loose material at the ankle, and slide the rest of the stocking up over the heel with short pulls, alternating front and back.

• Insert your index and middle fingers into the gathered stocking at the ankle, and ease the fabric up the leg to the knee.

• Supporting the patient's ankle with one hand, use your other hand to stretch the stocking toward the knee, front and back, *to distribute the material evenly.* The stocking top should be 1″ to 2″ (2.5 to 5 cm) below the bottom of the patella.

• Gently snap the fabric around the ankle *to ensure a tight fit and eliminate gaps that could reduce pressure.*

• Adjust the foot section *for fabric smoothness and toe comfort* by tugging on the toe section. If the stocking has a toe window, make sure it's properly positioned.

• Repeat the procedure for the second stocking, if ordered.

Applying a thigh-length stocking

• Follow the procedure for applying a knee-length stocking, taking care to distribute the fabric evenly below the knee before continuing the procedure.

• With the patient's leg extended, stretch the rest of the stocking over the knee.

• Flex the patient's knee, and pull the stocking over the thigh until the top is 1″ to 3″ (2.5 to 7.6 cm) below the gluteal fold.

• Stretch the stocking from the top, front and back, *to distribute the fabric evenly over the thigh.*

• Gently snap the fabric behind the knee *to eliminate gaps that could reduce pressure.*

Applying a waist-length stocking

• Follow the procedure for applying knee-length and thigh-length stockings, and extend the stocking top to the gluteal fold.

• Fit the patient with the adjustable belt that accompanies the stockings. Make sure that neither the waistband nor the fabric interferes with any incision, drainage tube, catheter, or other external device.

Special considerations

Apply the stockings in the morning, if possible, *before edema develops.* If the patient has been ambulating, ask him to lie down and elevate his legs for 15 to 30 minutes before applying the stockings *to facilitate venous return.*

Don't allow the stockings to roll or turn down at the top or toe *because the excess pressure could cause venous strangulation.* Have the patient wear the stockings in bed and during ambulation *to provide continuous protection against thrombosis.*

Check the patient's toes at least once every 4 hours — more often in the patient with a faint pulse or edema. Note skin color and temperature, sensation, swelling, and ability to move. If complications occur, remove the stockings and notify the doctor immediately.

Be alert for an allergic reaction *because some patients cannot tolerate the sizing in new stockings.* Laundering the stockings before applying them reduces this risk. Remove the stockings at least once daily *to bathe the skin and observe for irritation and breakdown.*

Using warm water and mild soap, wash the stockings when soiled. Keep a second pair of stockings handy *for the patient to wear while the other pair is being laundered.*

Home care

If the patient will require antiembolism stockings after discharge, teach him or a family member how to apply them correctly and explain why it's important that he wear them. (See *Applying antiembolism stockings: Three key steps.*) Instruct the patient or family member to care for the stockings properly and to replace them when they lose their elasticity.

Complications

Obstruction of arterial blood flow — characterized by cold and bluish toes, dusky toenail beds, decreased or absent pedal pulses, and leg pain or cramps — can result from application of antiembolism stockings. Less serious complications, such as an allergic reaction and skin irritation, can also occur.

Documentation

Record the date and time of stocking application and removal, stocking length and size, condition of the leg before and after treatment, condition of the toes during treatment, any complications, and the patient's tolerance of the treatment.

Elastic bandages

Elastic bandages exert gentle, even pressure on a body part. By supporting blood vessels, these rolled bandages promote venous return and prevent pooling of blood in the legs. They're typically used in place of antiembolism stockings to prevent thrombophlebitis and pulmonary embolism in postoperative or otherwise bedridden patients who can't stimulate venous return by muscle activity.

Elastic bandages also minimize joint swelling after trauma to the musculoskeletal system. Used with a splint, they immobilize a fracture during healing. They can provide hemostatic pressure and anchor dressings over a fresh wound or after surgical procedures, such as vein stripping.

Equipment

Elastic bandage of appropriate width ■ tape or pins ■ gauze pads or absorbent cotton.

Bandages usually come in 2″ to 6″ (5 to 15 cm) widths and 4′ and 6′ (1.2 and 1.8 m) lengths. The 3″ (7.6 cm) width is adaptable to most applications. Also available is an elastic bandage with self-closures that eliminate the need for tape or pins.

Preparation of equipment

Select a bandage that wraps the affected body part completely but isn't excessively long. Generally, use a narrower bandage for wrapping the foot, lower leg, hand, or arm and a wider bandage for the thigh or trunk. The bandage should be clean and rolled before application.

Implementation

• Check the doctor's order, and examine the area to be wrapped for evidence of lesions or skin breakdown. If these conditions are present, consult the doctor before applying the elastic bandage.

• Explain the procedure to the patient, provide privacy, and wash your hands thoroughly. Position the patient comfortably, with the body part to be bandaged in normal functioning position *to promote circulation and prevent deformity and discomfort.*

• Avoid applying a bandage to a dependent extremity. If you're wrapping an extremity, elevate it for 15 to 30 minutes before application *to facilitate venous return.*

• Apply the bandage so that two skin surfaces do not remain in contact when wrapped. Place gauze or absorbent cotton as needed between skin surfaces, such as between toes and fingers or under breasts and arms, *to prevent skin irritation.*

• Hold the bandage with the roll facing upward in one hand and the free end of the bandage in the other hand. Hold the bandage roll close to the part being bandaged *to ensure even tension and pressure.*

• Unroll the bandage as you wrap the body part in a spiral or spiral-reverse method. Never unroll the entire bandage before wrapping *because this could produce uneven*

Bandaging techniques

Circular
Each turn encircles the previous one, covering it completely. Use this technique to anchor a bandage.

Spiral
Each turn partially overlaps the previous one. Use this technique to wrap a long, straight body part or one of increasing circumference.

Spiral-reverse
Anchor the bandage and then reverse direction halfway through each spiral turn. Use this technique to accommodate the increasing circumference of a body part.

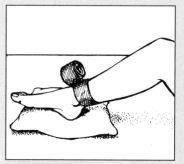 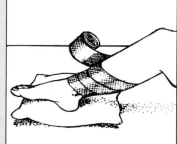 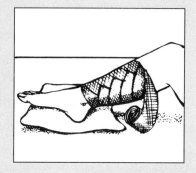

Figure eight
Anchor below the joint, and then use alternating ascending and descending turns to form a figure eight. Use this technique around joints.

Recurrent
This technique includes a combination of recurrent and circular turns. Hold the bandage as you make each recurrent turn and then use the circular turns as a final anchor. Use this technique for a stump, a hand, or the scalp.

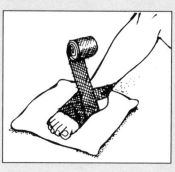 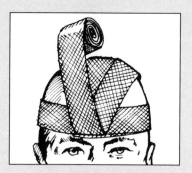 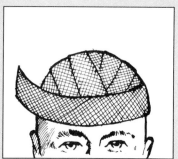

pressure, which interferes with blood circulation and cell nourishment.
• Overlap each layer of bandage by one-half to two-thirds the width of the strip. (See *Bandaging techniques* for specific instructions.)
• Wrap firmly but not too tightly. As you wrap, ask the patient to tell you if the bandage feels comfortable. If he complains of tingling, itching, numbness, or pain, loosen the bandage.

• When wrapping an extremity, anchor the bandage initially by circling the body part twice. *To prevent the bandage from slipping out of place on the foot,* wrap it in a figure eight around the foot, the ankle, and then the foot again before continuing. The same technique works on any joint, such as the knee, wrist, or elbow. Include the heel when wrapping the foot, but never wrap the toes (or fingers) unless absolutely necessary *because the distal extremities are used to detect impaired circulation.*

• When you're finished wrapping, secure the end of the bandage with tape, pins, or self-closures, being careful not to scratch or pinch the patient. Avoid using metal clips *because they typically come loose when the patient moves and may get lost in the bed linens and injure him.*

• Check distal circulation after the bandage is in place *because the elastic may tighten as you wrap.*

• Elevate a wrapped extremity for 15 to 30 minutes *to facilitate venous return.*

• Check distal circulation once or twice every 8 hours *because an elastic bandage that is too tight may result in neurovascular damage.* Lift the distal end of the bandage and assess the skin underneath for color, temperature, and integrity.

• Remove the bandage every 8 hours or whenever it's loose and wrinkled. Roll it up as you unwrap *to ready it for reuse.* Observe the area and provide skin care before rewrapping the bandage.

• Change the bandage at least once daily. Bathe the skin, dry it thoroughly, and observe for irritation and breakdown before applying a fresh bandage.

Special considerations

Wrap an elastic bandage from the distal area to the proximal area *to promote venous return.* Avoid leaving gaps in bandage layers or exposed skin surfaces *because this may result in uneven pressure on the body part.*

Observe the patient for an allergic reaction *because some patients cannot tolerate the sizing in a new bandage.* Laundering it reduces this risk.

Launder the bandage daily or whenever it becomes limp; *laundering restores its elasticity.* Always keep two bandages handy *so one can be applied while the other bandage is being laundered.*

When using an elastic bandage after a surgical procedure on an extremity (such as vein stripping) or with a splint to immobilize a fracture, remove it only as ordered rather than every 8 hours.

Home care

If the patient will be using an elastic bandage at home, teach him or a family member how to apply it correctly and how to assess for restricted circulation. Tell him to keep two bandages available *so he'll always have one to use while the other is being laundered.*

Complications

Arterial obstruction—characterized by a decreased or absent distal pulse, blanching or bluish discoloration of skin, dusky nail beds, numbness and tingling or pain and cramping, and cold skin—can result from elastic bandage application. Edema can occur from obstruction of venous return. Less serious complications include allergic reaction and skin irritation.

Documentation

Record the date and time of bandage application and removal, application site, bandage size, skin condition before application, skin care provided after removal, any complications, the patient's tolerance of the treatment, and any patient teaching.

Binders

Also known as self-closures, binders are lengths of cloth or elasticized material that encircle the chest, abdomen, or groin to provide support, keep dressings in place (especially for patients allergic to tape), reduce tension on wounds and suture lines, and reduce breast engorgement in the non-breast-feeding mother. Typically, cloth binders are fastened with safety pins and elasticized binders are fastened with Velcro. There are no contraindications to their application.

Equipment

Tape measure ■ binder of appropriate size and type ■ safety pins ■ gloves, if necessary.

Commercial elastic binders with Velcro closings are now commonly used instead of standard cotton straight and scultetus binders that require pins. Disposable T-binders are available, and scrotal supports typically replace binders for male patients, except after abdominal-perineal resection. (See *Types of binders,* page 186.) For non-breast-feeding mothers, a snug-fitting support brassiere is usually recommended, but mammary support binders are still available.

Preparation of equipment

Measure the area the binder must fit, and obtain the proper size and type of binder from the central supply department.

Implementation

• Check the doctor's order and assess the patient's condition.

• Explain the procedure to the patient, provide privacy, wash your hands thoroughly, and put on gloves if necessary.

• Raise the patient's bed to its highest position *to avoid muscle strain when applying the binder.*

Types of binders

Breast
Reduces breast engorgement in the non-breast-feeding mother

Scultetus
Keeps suture line intact after abdominal surgery so patient can move more freely, and provides abdominal support after delivery or paracentesis

Straight abdominal
Keeps suture line intact after abdominal surgery so patient can move more freely, and provides abdominal support after delivery or paracentesis

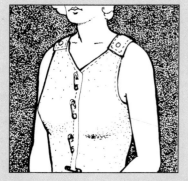

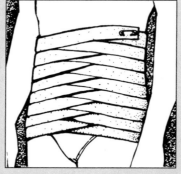

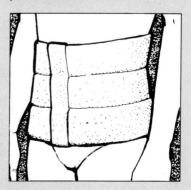

Single T
Keeps perineal dressings in place for the female patient

Double T
Secures perineal dressings for the male patient or for the female patient requiring a bulky dressing

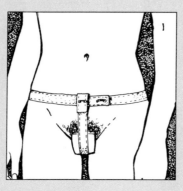

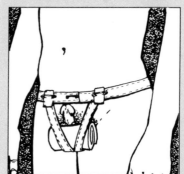

• Change the dressing and inspect the wound or suture line if appropriate.

Applying a straight abdominal binder
• Accordion-fold half of the binder, slip it under the patient, and pull it through from the other side. Make sure the binder is straight, free of wrinkles, and evenly dis-
tributed under the patient. Its lower edge should extend well below the hips.
• Overlap one side snugly onto the other. Then insert one finger under the binder's edge *to ensure a snug fit that's still loose enough to avoid impaired circulation and patient discomfort.*
• Starting at the lower edge, pin the binder together with safety pins spaced about 2″ (5 cm) apart. Place pins well

away from a wound, a pressure point, or a tender and inflamed area *to avoid causing undue and uneven pressure.* Slip your fingers under the binder as you insert the pins *to avoid pricking the patient.* Place the pins horizontally *so they don't interfere with body movement.*
• Make darts in the binder as needed *to provide even snugness.* Avoid making the binder too tight around the diaphragm *because it may interfere with breathing.*

Applying a scultetus binder
• Slide the binder under the patient's hips and buttocks so that its top aligns with the waist and its lowest tail crosses the extreme lower abdomen.
• Adjust the binder so that its solid portion is centered under the patient and its tails are evenly distributed on either side. Spread the tails out flat on the bed *so you can pick them up easily.*
• Beginning at the lower edge of the binder, bring one tail straight across the patient's abdomen. If the tail is too long, fold it over flat at the end. Then hold this tail snugly in place as you bring the opposite tail across on top of it, overlapping the first tail's upper half and continuing with succeeding tail pieces. (See *Applying a scultetus binder.*)
• Secure the top strap, using two safety pins placed horizontally *so they won't interfere with body movement.*

Applying a T-binder
• Slip the T-binder under the patient's waist, with its tails extending below the buttocks. Smooth the waistband and tails *to remove twists, which can chafe and create pressure on the patient's skin.*
• Pull the waistband snugly into position at the patient's waistline or lower across the abdomen. Then fasten it with a safety pin. Next, bring the free tail up between the patient's legs over the dressing or perineal pad.
• For a female patient, bring the single tail up to the center of the waist, loop it behind and over the waistband, and secure it to the waistband by pinning through all layers of material. For a male patient, bring the two tails up on either side of the penis *to provide even support for the testicles.* Loop the ends behind and over the waistband on either side of the midline, and fasten them to the waistband by pinning through all layers of material. *Pinning through multiple layers keeps the straps from slipping sideways as the patient moves.*
• Instruct the patient to call you when he wishes to void or defecate *because the binder must be unfastened and then reapplied.*

Applying a scultetus binder

After centering the binder's solid portion under the patient, with tails distributed evenly on each side, bring the lowest tail straight across the patient's abdomen, hold it snugly, and bring the next higher tail across to overlap it. Alternate tails in this manner, with the next higher tail overlapping the one below it by about half its width.

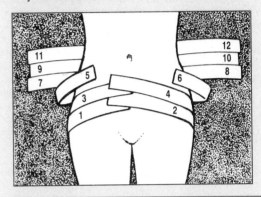

Applying a breast binder
• Slip the binder under the patient's chest so that its lower edge aligns with the waist. Straighten the binder to distribute it evenly on either side of the body.
• Place the binder so that the patient's nipples are centered in the breast tissue. *This ensures proper breast alignment and support and produces faster tissue involution.*
• Pull the binder's edges snugly together and begin pinning upward from the waist. Slip your finger under the binder as you insert the pins *to avoid pricking the patient.* Use at least six pins, and place them horizontally *so they won't interfere with body movement.*
• Make darts in the binder wherever necessary *to provide a snug fit.* Do this by overlapping the material horizontally and pinning it perpendicularly.
• Adjust the shoulder straps to fit properly and secure them with safety pins.

When applying any binder
• Ask the patient if the binder feels comfortable. Tell him that it may feel tight initially but should feel comfortable shortly. Instruct the patient to notify you immediately if the binder feels too tight or too loose or comes apart.
• If the patient can ambulate, ask him to do so *to evaluate the fit of the binder.*

Special considerations

For maximum support, wrap the binder so that it applies even pressure across the body section. Eliminate all wrinkles and avoid placing pressure over bony prominences.

In surgical applications, fasten straight and scultetus binders from the bottom upward *to relieve gravitational pull on the wound.* In obstetric applications, fasten from the top downward *to direct the uterus into the pelvis. Because this places extra pressure on weak abdominal muscles,* observe the patient closely for precipitate delivery. For the obstetric patient, pin the last two straps of the scultetus binder on both sides; for the extremely large patient, pin all straps.

Be careful not to compress any tubes, drains, or catheters and not to position them so that they're working against gravity. Also, don't allow binder placement to interfere with elimination.

Use a double T-binder on a female patient after extensive surgery that requires a large dressing. Use a straight or scultetus binder as a breast binder, if necessary. Pin straps onto the upper front and back for additional support over the shoulders.

Observe the patient and check binder placement every 8 hours. Check the skin for color, palpate it for warmth, check pulses, and assess for tingling or numbness.

Reapply the binder when a dressing needs changing, when the binder becomes loose or too tight, and at other times according to the doctor's orders. When changing the binder, observe the skin for signs of irritation. Provide appropriate skin care before reapplying the binder.

Home care

If the patient will need a binder after discharge from the hospital, teach him and a family member how to remove it, inspect the skin, bathe the area, and reapply it. Tell the patient and family member where binders can be purchased and how to care for them. For a patient with cancer, the American Cancer Society may provide assistance in obtaining binders. If commercially manufactured binders are unavailable, advise the patient and family that a clean towel or discarded sheeting material can be used instead. Periodically reinforce prior teaching and instructions.

Complications

Irritation of the underlying skin can result from perspiration or friction.

Documentation

Record the date and time of binder application, reapplication, and removal; binder type and location; purpose of application; skin condition before and after application; dressing changes or skin care; any complications; and the patient's tolerance of the treatment.

 Pressure dressings

For effective control of capillary or small-vein bleeding, temporary application of pressure directly over a wound may be achieved with a bulk dressing held by a glove-protected hand, bound into place with a pressure bandage, or held under pressure by an inflated air splint. A pressure dressing requires frequent checks for wound drainage to determine its effectiveness in controlling bleeding. Patients who need a pressure dressing may have such diagnoses as fluid volume deficit, impaired skin integrity, impaired tissue integrity, or altered tissue perfusion.

Equipment

Two or more sterile gauze pads ■ roller gauze ■ adhesive tape ■ clean disposable gloves ■ metric ruler.

Preparation of equipment

Obtain the pressure dressing quickly *to avoid excessive blood loss.* Use clean cloth for the dressing if sterile gauze pads are unavailable.

Implementation

• Quickly explain the procedure to the patient *to help decrease his anxiety,* and put on gloves.
• Elevate the injured body part *to help reduce bleeding.*
• Place enough gauze pads over the wound to cover it. Don't clean the wound; *you can do this when the bleeding stops.*
• For an extremity or trunk wound, hold the dressing firmly over the wound and wrap the roller gauze tightly across it and around the body part *to provide pressure on the wound.* Secure the bandage with adhesive tape.
• To apply a dressing to the neck, the shoulder, or another location that can't be tightly wrapped, don't use roller gauze. Instead, apply tape directly over the dressings *to provide the necessary pressure at the wound site.*
• Check pulse, temperature, and skin condition distal to the wound site *because excessive pressure can obstruct normal circulation.*
• Check the dressing frequently *to monitor wound drainage.* Use the metric standard of measurement to determine the amount of drainage, and document these serial measurements for later reference. Do not circle a potentially wet dressing with ink *because this provides no per-*

manent documentation in the medical record and also runs the risk of contaminating the dressing.

• If the dressing becomes saturated, do not remove it *because this will interfere with the pressure.* Instead, apply an additional dressing over the saturated one and continue to monitor and record drainage.

• Obtain additional medical care as soon as possible.

Special considerations
Apply pressure directly to the wound with your gloved hand if sterile gauze pads and clean cloth are unavailable.

Avoid using an elastic bandage to bind the dressing *because it can't be wrapped tightly enough to create pressure on the wound site.*

Complications
Excessively tight application of a pressure dressing can impair circulation.

Documentation
Once the bleeding is controlled, record the date and time of dressing application, the presence or absence of distal pulses, the integrity of distal skin, the amount of wound drainage, and any complications.

WOUND CARE
Management of surgical wounds

Procedures used to manage surgical wounds have several goals. They help prevent infection by barring pathogens from entering the wound. They protect the skin surface from maceration and excoriation caused by contact with irritating drainage. They allow measurement of wound drainage to monitor fluid and electrolyte balance. And they promote patient comfort.

The two principal methods for managing a draining wound are dressing and pouching. Dressing is the best choice when skin integrity is not compromised by caustic or excessive drainage. Lightly seeping wounds with drains, as well as wounds with minimal purulent drainage, usually can be managed with packing and gauze dressings. (See *Choosing a wound dressing.*) In some cases, such as when a wound becomes chronic, it may require an occlusive dressing. (For more information on dressings, see Chapter 13, Skin care.) Copious, excoriating drainage calls for pouching to protect the skin.

Dressing a wound necessitates sterile technique and sterile supplies to prevent contamination. Such dressings

Choosing a wound dressing

For a wound that requires frequent debriding and dressing changes, usually because of drainage or necrosis, most experts would choose a gauze dressing because it allows air to reach the wound and dry it.

Occlusive dressings
However, some experts believe that moisture at the wound surface promotes reepithelialization in some wounds. Thus, they recommend using occlusive or semiocclusive dressings because these dressings maintain moisture better than gauze dressings do. Occlusive dressings are also more comfortable and less painful, probably because they protect exposed cutaneous nerve endings.

For example, chronic leg ulcers have been treated successfully with occlusive, oxygen-impermeable hydrocolloid dressings. Hydrocolloid dressings are compounds of gelatin, pectin, carboxymethylcellulose sodium, and polyisobutylene. The inner part of such dressings interacts with the wound exudate, forming a hydrated gel over the wound. When you remove the dressing, the gel separates and remains on the wound, preventing damage to the new tissue.

Adhesive semipermeable dressings are not as effective as gauze for draining wounds because they "blister" and then leak.

Other dressings
A dressing containing dextranomer beads has been used successfully for wounds that need frequent cleaning. Burns and large pressure ulcers may benefit from biological dressings made from cadaver skin, pigskin, or human amniotic membranes instead of synthetic ones. These dressings reduce fluid loss, minimize local bacterial growth, and help granulation tissue to form. This ensures that the wound will be in the best possible condition for retaining an autograft. A cotton gauze dressing impregnated with crystallized sodium chloride (Mesalt) may help treat infected wounds.

For more on dressings, see the information on burn care and pressure ulcer treatments in Chapter 13, Skin care.

How to put on sterile gloves

Using your nondominant hand, pick up the opposite glove by grasping the exposed inside of the cuff.

Pull the glove onto your dominant hand. Be sure to keep your thumb folded inward to avoid touching the sterile part of the glove. Allow the glove to come uncuffed as you finish inserting your hand, but don't touch the outside of the glove.

Slip the gloved fingers of your dominant hand under the cuff of the loose glove to pick it up.

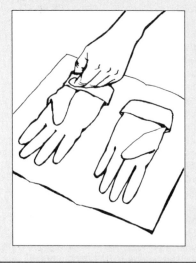
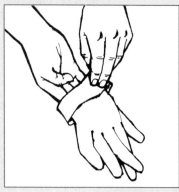
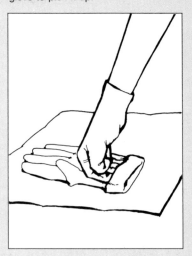

should be changed frequently enough to keep the skin dry.

Equipment
Waterproof trash bag ▪ clean gloves ▪ sterile gloves ▪ gown, if indicated ▪ sterile 4″ × 4″ gauze pads ▪ ABD pads, if needed ▪ sterile cotton-tipped applicators ▪ topical medication, if ordered ▪ adhesive or other tape ▪ soap and water ▪ optional: skin protectant, nonadherent pads, collodion spray, acetone-free adhesive remover or baby oil, normal saline solution, a graduated container, and Montgomery straps, a fish-net tube elasticized dressing support, or a T-binder.

For a wound with a drain: sterile scissors ▪ sterile 4″ × 4″ gauze pads without cotton lining ▪ sump drain ▪ ostomy pouch or other collection bag ▪ precut tracheostomy pads or drain dressings ▪ adhesive tape (paper or silk tape if patient is hypersensitive) ▪ surgical mask.

For pouching a wound: collection pouch with drainage port ▪ sterile gloves ▪ skin protectant ▪ sterile gauze pads.

Several types of prepared equipment are available, including sterile swabs saturated with povidone-iodine, foam dressing for managing open granulating wounds, adhesive gauze, and complete prepackaged, sterile dressing sets, with or without instruments.

Preparation of equipment
Determine the type of dressing being used. Assemble all equipment in the patient's room. Check the expiration date on each sterile package and inspect for tears. Open the waterproof trash bag and place it near the patient's bed. Position the bag *to avoid reaching across the sterile field or the wound when disposing of soiled articles.* Form a cuff by turning down the top of the trash bag *to provide a wide opening and prevent contamination of instruments or gloves by touching the bag's edge.*

Implementation
• Check the doctor's order for specific wound care and medication instructions. Be sure to note the location of surgical drains *to avoid dislodging them during the procedure.* Assess the patient's condition.
• Identify the patient's allergies, especially to adhesive tape and povidone-iodine or other topical solutions or medications.
• Explain the procedure to the patient, provide privacy, and position the patient as necessary. Expose only the wound site *to avoid chilling the patient.*

Slide your nondominant hand into the glove, holding your dominant thumb as far away as possible to avoid brushing against your arm. Allow the glove to come uncuffed as you finish putting it on, but don't touch the skin side of the cuff with your other gloved hand.

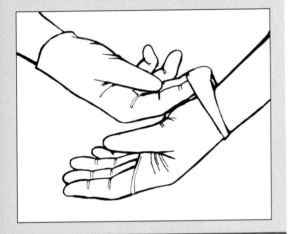

• Wash your hands thoroughly. Put on a gown, if necessary, *to shield your clothing from wound drainage.* Put on clean gloves.

Removing the old dressing
• Loosen the soiled dressing by holding the patient's skin and pulling the tape or dressing toward the wound. *This protects the newly formed tissue and prevents stress on the incision.* Moisten the tape with acetone-free adhesive remover or baby oil, if necessary, *to make removal less painful, particularly from hairy skin.* Don't apply solvents to the incision, *to avoid contaminating the wound.*
• Slowly remove the soiled dressing. If the gauze adheres to the wound, loosen it by moistening with sterile normal saline solution.
• Observe the dressing for the amount, type, color, and odor of drainage.
• Discard the dressing and the gloves in the waterproof trash bag.

Caring for the wound
• Establish a sterile field with all the equipment and supplies you'll need for suture-line care and dressing change, including a sterile dressing set and povidone-iodine swabs. If ointment has been ordered, squeeze the needed amount onto the sterile field. If you're using an antiseptic from an unsterile bottle, pour the antiseptic cleaning agent into a sterile container *so you won't contaminate your gloves.* Then put on sterile gloves. (See *How to put on sterile gloves.*)
• If you won't be using prepackaged sterile povidone-iodine swabs to clean the wound, saturate sterile gauze pads with the prescribed cleaning agent. Avoid using cotton balls *because these may shed particles in the wound, causing irritation, infection, or adhesion.*
• If ordered, obtain a wound culture, then proceed to clean the wound.
• Pick up the moistened gauze pad or swab and squeeze out excess solution.
• Working from the top of the incision, wipe once to the bottom and then discard the gauze pad. With a second moistened pad, wipe from top to bottom in a vertical path next to the incision. (See *Wound-cleaning technique,* page 192.)
• Continue to work outward from the incision in lines running parallel to it. Always wipe from the clean area toward the less clean area, usually top to bottom. Use each gauze pad or swab for only one stroke *to avoid tracking wound exudate and normal body flora from the surrounding skin to the clean areas.* Remember that the suture line is cleaner than the adjacent skin, and the top of the suture line is typically cleaner than the bottom *because more drainage collects at the bottom of the wound.* Avoid cleaning from bottom to top *to prevent further wound contamination.*
• Use sterile cotton-tipped applicators for efficient cleaning of tight-fitting wire sutures, deep and narrow wounds, or wounds with pockets. *Because the cotton on the swab is tightly wrapped, it isn't as likely to leave particles in the wound as a cotton ball.* Remember to wipe only once with each applicator.
• If the patient has a surgical drain, clean the drain's surface last. *Because moist drainage facilitates growth of bacteria,* the drain is considered the most contaminated area. Clean the skin around the drain by wiping in half or full circles from the drain site outward.
• Clean all areas of the wound *to wash away debris, pus, blood, and necrotic material.* Try not to disturb sutures or irritate the incision. Clean to at least 1″ (2.5 cm) beyond the end of the new dressing. If you aren't applying a dressing, clean to at least 2″ (5 cm) beyond the incision.
• Check to see that the incision's edges are lined up properly, and check for signs of infection (heat, redness, swelling, odor), dehiscence, or evisceration. If you observe such signs or the patient reports pain at the wound site, notify the doctor.
• Irrigate the wound, if ordered. (For more information, see "Wound irrigation" in this chapter.)

Wound-cleaning technique

Using a povidone-iodine swab or a sterile gauze pad moistened with the prescribed antiseptic agent, wipe wound areas as shown: Clean a linear wound from top to bottom, and work from the clean area to the less clean area. Use a new swab or pad for each downward stroke. For a puncture wound, wipe the wound area in half or full circles, from the wound site outward, using a new swab or pad for each circular stroke.

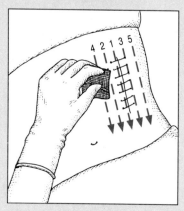 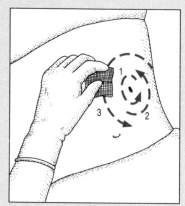

• Wash the skin surrounding the wound with soap and water and pat dry. Avoid oil-based soap *because it may interfere with pouch adherence.* Apply any prescribed topical medication.

• Apply a skin protectant if warranted.

• If ordered, pack the wound with gauze pads or strips folded to fit. Avoid using cotton-lined gauze pads *because cotton fibers can adhere to the wound surface and cause complications.* (See *Packing a wound.*) Pack the wound using the wet-to-damp method. *Soaking the packing material in solution and wringing it out so that it is slightly moist provides a moist wound environment which absorbs debris and drainage. But new tissue won't be disrupted when the packing is removed.*

Applying a fresh gauze dressing

• To apply the new dressing, begin by gently placing sterile 4″ × 4″ gauze pads at the wound center and moving progressively outward to the edges of the wound site. Extend the gauze at least 1″ beyond the incision in each direction, and cover the wound evenly with enough sterile dressings (usually two or three layers) to absorb all drainage until the next dressing change. Use ABD pads to form outer layers, if needed, to provide greater absorbency.

• When the dressing is in place, remove and discard your gloves *because the tape may stick to them, making it difficult to apply.*

• Secure the edges of the dressing to the patient's skin with strips of tape *to maintain the sterility of the wound site.* Or secure the dressing with a T-binder or Montgomery straps *to prevent skin excoriation that may be caused*

by the repeated removal of tape necessitated by frequent dressing changes.

• Make sure the patient is comfortable.

• Properly dispose of solutions and trash bag, and clean or dispose of soiled equipment and supplies according to institutional policy. If the patient's wound has purulent drainage, don't return unopened sterile supplies to the sterile supply cabinet *to prevent cross-contamination of other equipment.*

• For the recently postoperative patient or a patient with complications, check the dressing every 30 minutes or as ordered. For the patient with a properly healing wound, check it at least once every 8 hours.

Dressing a wound with a drain

• Prepare a drain dressing by using sterile scissors to cut a slit in a sterile 4″ × 4″ gauze pad. Fold the pad in half, and cut inward from the center of the folded edge. Don't use a cotton-lined gauze pad *because cutting the gauze opens the lining and releases cotton fibers into the wound.* Prepare a second pad the same way.

• Gently press one folded pad close to the skin around the drain so that the tubing fits into the slit. Press the second folded pad around the drain from the opposite direction so that the two pads encircle the tubing.

• Layer as many uncut sterile 4″ × 4″ gauze pads or ABD pads around the tubing as needed *to absorb expected drainage.* Tape the dressing in place or use a T-binder or Montgomery straps. (See *How to make Montgomery straps,* page 194.)

Pouching a wound

• If the patient's wound is draining heavily or if drainage may damage surrounding skin, you'll need to create a pouch.

• Measure the wound, and cut an opening ⅛″ (0.3 cm) larger than the wound in the collection pouch's facing.

• Apply a skin protectant, as needed. Some protectants are incorporated within the collection pouch and also provide adhesion.

• Make sure the drainage port at the bottom of the pouch is firmly closed *to prevent leaks.* Then gently press the contoured pouch opening around the wound, beginning at its lower edge, *to catch any drainage.*

• To empty the pouch, put on gloves, insert its bottom half into a graduated collection container, and open the drainage port. Note the color, consistency, odor, and amount of fluid. Obtain a culture specimen, if ordered, and send it to the laboratory immediately. Remember to follow isolation precautions when handling infectious drainage.

• Wipe the bottom of the pouch and the drainage port with a gauze pad *to remove any drainage that could irritate the patient's skin or cause an odor.* Then reseal the port. Change the pouch only if it leaks or fails to adhere to the skin. *More frequent changes are unnecessary and only irritate the patient's skin.*

Special considerations

Because many doctors prefer to change the first post-operative dressing themselves *to check the incision,* avoid changing the first dressing unless you have specific instructions to do so. If you have no such order and drainage comes through the dressing, reinforce the dressing with fresh sterile gauze. Request an order to change the dressing, or ask the doctor to change it as soon as possible. A reinforced dressing shouldn't remain in place longer than 24 hours *because it's an excellent medium for bacterial growth.* Replace any dressing that becomes wet from the outside — from spilled drinking water, bath water, or urine, for example — as soon as possible *to prevent wound contamination.*

Consider all dressings and drains infectious.

Use acetone-free adhesive remover to remove any adhesive tape residue. If the doctor wants to avoid debriding the wound, place nonadherent pads directly over the incision before applying gauze pads *because gauze adheres to the wound and debrides it.*

If the patient has two wounds in the same area, cover each separately with layers of sterile 4″ × 4″ gauze pads. Then cover both sites with an ABD pad secured to the patient's skin with tape. Don't eliminate the gauze pads and use only an ABD pad to cover both sites *because*

Packing a wound

Pack the wound cavity carefully with moist gauze pads folded to fit. Make sure that all wound surfaces are covered and kept moist so that complete debridement can take place.

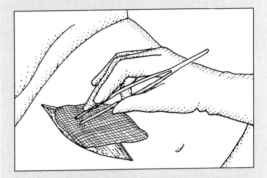

Pack the wound only until all wound surfaces and edges are covered. Packing that overlaps the edge can cause maceration of surrounding tissues.

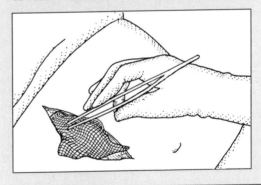

drainage quickly saturates a single pad, promoting cross-contamination.

When packing a wound, don't pack it too tightly *because this may prevent wound edges from contracting and also compresses adjacent capillaries.* Avoid using overly damp packing *because it retards wound closure from within and increases the risk of infection.*

To save time when dressing a wound with a drain, use precut tracheostomy pads or drain dressings instead of custom-cutting gauze pads to fit around the drain. If the patient is sensitive to adhesive tape, use paper or silk tape *because these cause less skin reaction and will peel off*

How to make Montgomery straps

An abdominal dressing requiring frequent changes can be secured with Montgomery straps to promote the patient's comfort. If ready-made straps aren't available, follow these steps to make your own:

• Cut four to six strips of 2" or 3" (5 cm to 7.6 cm) wide nonallergenic tape of sufficient length to allow the tape to extend about 6" (15.2 cm) beyond the wound on each side. (The length of the tape varies, depending on the patient's size and the type and amount of dressing.)

• Fold one end of each strip 2" or 3" back on itself (sticky sides together) to form a nonadhesive tab. Then cut a small hole in the folded tab's center, close to its top edge. Make as many pairs of straps as you'll need to snugly secure the dressing.

• Clean the patient's skin to prevent irritation. After the skin dries, apply a skin protectant. Then apply the sticky side of each tape to a skin barrier sheet composed of opaque hydrocolloidal or nonhydrocolloidal materials, and apply the sheet directly to the skin near the dressing. Next, thread a separate piece of gauze ties, umbilical tape, or twill tape (about 12" [30.5 cm]) through each pair of holes in the straps and fasten each tie as you would a shoelace. Don't stress the surrounding skin by securing the ties too tightly.

• Repeat this procedure according to the number of Montgomery straps needed.

• Replace Montgomery straps whenever they become soiled (every 2 or 3 days). If skin maceration occurs, place new tapes about 1" (2.5 cm) away from any irritation.

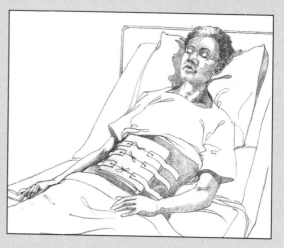

---

more easily than adhesive tape. Use a surgical mask to cradle a chin or jawline dressing; *this provides a secure dressing and avoids the need for shaving the patient's hair.*

If ordered, use a collodion spray or other similar topical protectant instead of a gauze dressing; *this moisture- and contaminant-proof covering dries in a clear impermeable film that leaves the wound visible for observation and avoids the friction caused by a dressing.*

If a sump drain isn't adequately collecting wound secretions, reinforce it with an ostomy pouch or other collection bag. Use waterproof tape to strengthen a spot on the front of the pouch near the adhesive opening; then cut a small "X" in the tape. Feed the drain catheter into the pouch through the "X" cut. Seal the cut around the tubing with more waterproof tape, and then connect the tubing to the suction pump. *This method frees the drainage port at the bottom of the pouch so you don't have to remove the tubing to empty the pouch.* If you use more than one collection pouch for a wound or wounds, be sure to record the volume of drainage separately for each pouch. Avoid using waterproof material over the dressing *because it*

reduces air circulation and predisposes the wound to infection from accumulated heat and moisture.

Home care

Include the patient in all aspects of wound management as early as possible *to allay anxiety and promote self-care.* Teach the importance of aseptic techniques, how to examine the wound for signs of infection and other healing problems, and how to change the dressing. Teach proper positioning, lighting, and use of mirrors so the patient or family members can view the wound clearly. Provide written instructions for all procedures to be performed at home. Urge the patient to call his doctor if he detects signs of infection.

Complications

Allergy to an antiseptic cleaning agent, prescribed topical medication, or adhesive tape may result in skin redness, rash, excoriation, or infection.

Documentation

Record the date, time, and type of wound management procedure; amount of soiled dressing and packing removed; wound appearance (size, condition of margins, presence of necrotic tissue) and odor, if present; type, color, consistency, and amount of drainage for each wound; presence and location of drains; any additional procedures, such as irrigation, packing, or application of a topical medication; type and amount of new dressing or pouch applied; and the patient's tolerance of the procedure.

Record special or detailed wound care instructions and pain management steps on the nursing care plan. Record the color and amount of measurable drainage on the intake and output sheet.

Suture removal

The goal of this procedure is to remove skin sutures from a healed wound without damaging newly formed tissue. The timing of suture removal depends on the shape, size, and location of the sutured incision; the absence of inflammation, drainage, and infection; and the patient's general condition. Usually, for a sufficiently healed wound, sutures are removed 7 to 10 days after insertion. Techniques for removal depend on the method of suturing, but all require sterile procedure to prevent contamination. Although sutures usually are removed by a doctor, in many institutions a nurse may remove them on the doctor's order.

Equipment

Waterproof trash bag ▪ adjustable light ▪ clean gloves, if the wound is dressed ▪ sterile gloves ▪ sterile forceps or sterile hemostat ▪ normal saline solution ▪ sterile gauze pads ▪ antiseptic cleaning agent ▪ sterile curve-tipped suture scissors ▪ povidone-iodine sponges ▪ optional: adhesive butterfly strips or Steri-Strips and compound benzoin tincture or other skin protectant.

Prepackaged, sterile suture-removal trays are available.

Preparation of equipment

Assemble all equipment in the patient's room. Check the expiration date on each sterile package and inspect for tears. Open the waterproof trash bag and place it near the patient's bed. Position the bag properly *to avoid reaching across the sterile field or the suture line when disposing of soiled articles.* Form a cuff by turning down the top of the trash bag *to provide a wide opening and prevent con-*

tamination of instruments or gloves by touching the bag's edge.

Implementation

● If your institution allows you to remove sutures, check the doctor's order *to confirm the exact time and details of this procedure.*
● Check for patient allergies, especially to adhesive tape and povidone-iodine or other topical solutions or medications.
● Tell the patient that you're going to remove the stitches from his wound. Assure him that this procedure typically is painless, but that he may feel a tickling sensation as the stitches come out. Reassure him that because his wound is healing properly, removing the stitches won't weaken the incision.
● Provide privacy, and position the patient so he's comfortable without placing undue tension on the suture line. *Because some patients experience nausea or dizziness during the procedure,* have the patient recline if possible. Adjust the light to have it shine directly on the suture line.
● Wash your hands thoroughly. If the patient's wound has a dressing, put on clean gloves and carefully remove it. Discard the dressing and the gloves in the waterproof trash bag.
● Observe the patient's wound for possible gaping, drainage, inflammation, signs of infection, or embedded sutures. Notify the doctor if the wound has failed to heal properly. The absence of a healing ridge under the suture line 5 to 7 days postinsertion indicates that the line needs continued support and protection during the healing process.
● Establish a sterile work area with all the equipment and supplies you'll need for suture removal and wound care. Put on sterile gloves and open the sterile suture removal tray if you're using one.
● Observing sterile technique, clean the suture line *to decrease the number of microorganisms present and reduce the risk of infection.* The cleaning process should also moisten the sutures sufficiently *to facilitate removal.* You can soften them further, if necessary, with normal saline solution.
● Then proceed according to the type of suture you're removing. (See *Methods for removing sutures,* page 196.) *Because the visible part of a suture is exposed to skin bacteria and is considered contaminated,* be sure to cut sutures at the skin surface on one side of the visible part of the suture. Remove the suture by lifting and pulling the visible end off the skin *to avoid drawing this contaminated portion back through subcutaneous tissue.*
● If ordered, remove only every other suture *to maintain some support for the incision.* Then go back and remove the remaining sutures.

Methods for removing sutures

Removal techniques depend in large part on the type of sutures you must remove. The illustrations below show removal steps for four common suture types. Keep in mind that, for all suture types, it's important to grasp and cut sutures in the correct place to avoid pulling the exposed (thus contaminated) suture material through subcutaneous tissue.

Plain interrupted sutures

Using sterile forceps, grasp the knot of the first suture and raise it off the skin. This will expose a small portion of the suture that was below skin level. Place the rounded tip of sterile curved-tip suture scissors against the skin and cut through the exposed portion of the suture. Then, still holding the knot with the forceps, pull the cut suture up and out of the skin in a smooth continuous motion to avoid causing the patient pain. Discard the suture. Repeat the process for every other suture, initially; if the wound doesn't gape, you can then remove the remaining sutures as ordered.

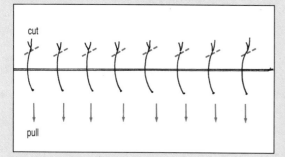

Mattress interrupted sutures

If possible, remove the small visible portion of the suture opposite the knot by cutting it at each visible end and lifting the small piece away from the skin *to prevent pulling it through and contaminating subcutaneous tissue.* Then remove the rest of the suture by pulling it out in the direction of the knot, as shown in the illustration at the top of the next column. If the visible portion is too small to cut twice, cut it once and pull the entire suture out in the opposite direction. Repeat for the remaining sutures and monitor the incision carefully for infection.

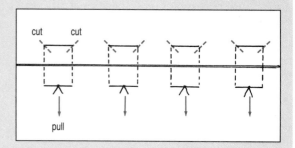

Plain continuous sutures

Cut the first suture on the side opposite the knot. Next, cut the same side of the next suture in line. Then lift the first suture out in the direction of the knot. Proceed along the suture line, grasping each suture where you grasped the knot on the first one.

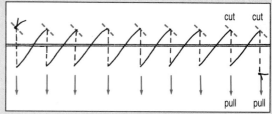

Mattress continuous sutures

Follow the procedure for removing mattress interrupted sutures, first removing the small visible portion of the suture, if possible, *to prevent pulling it through and contaminating subcutaneous tissue.* Then extract the rest of the suture in the direction of the knot.

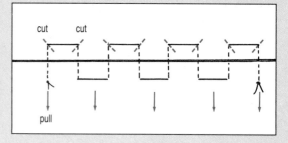

• After removing sutures, wipe the incision gently with gauze pads soaked in an antiseptic cleaning agent or with a povidone-iodine sponge. Apply a light sterile gauze dressing, if needed, *to prevent infection and irritation from clothing*. Then discard your gloves.

• Make sure the patient is comfortable. According to the doctor's preference, inform the patient that he may shower in 1 or 2 days if the incision is dry and heals well.

• Properly dispose of solutions and trash bag, and clean or dispose of soiled equipment and supplies according to institutional policy.

Special considerations

Be sure to check the doctor's order for the time of suture removal. Usually, you'll remove sutures on the head and neck 3 to 5 days after insertion; on the chest and abdomen, 5 to 7 days after insertion; and on the lower extremities, 7 to 10 days after insertion.

However, if the patient has interrupted sutures or an incompletely healed suture line, remove only those sutures specified by the doctor. He may want to leave some sutures in place for an additional day or two *to support the suture line.*

If the patient has both retention and regular sutures in place, check the doctor's order for the sequence in which they are to be removed. *Because retention sutures link underlying fat and muscle tissue and give added support to the obese or slow-healing patient*, these usually remain in place for 14 to 21 days.

Be particularly careful to clean the suture line before attempting to remove mattress sutures. *This decreases the risk of infection when the visible, contaminated part of the stitch is too small to cut twice for sterile removal and must be pulled through the tissue.* After you have removed mattress sutures this way, monitor the suture line carefully *for subsequent infection.*

If the wound dehisces during suture removal, apply butterfly adhesive strips or Steri-Strips to support and approximate the edges and call the doctor immediately to repair the wound.

Apply butterfly adhesive strips or Steri-Strips after any suture removal, if desired, *to give added support to the incision line and prevent lateral tension on the wound from forming a wide scar.* Use a small amount of compound benzoin tincture or other skin protectant *to ensure adherence.* Leave the strips in place for 3 to 5 days, or as ordered.

Home care

If the patient is being discharged, teach him how to remove the dressing and care for the wound. Instruct him to call the doctor immediately if he observes wound discharge or any other abnormal change. Tell him that the redness surrounding the incision should gradually disappear and only a thin line should show after a few weeks.

Documentation

Record the date and time of suture removal, type and number of sutures, appearance of the suture line, any signs of wound complications, any dressings or butterfly strips applied, and the patient's tolerance for the procedure.

 ## Removal of skin staples and clips

Skin staples or clips may be used instead of standard sutures to close lacerations or surgical wounds. Because they can secure a wound more quickly than sutures, they may substitute for surface sutures where cosmetic results are not a prime consideration, such as in abdominal closure. When properly placed, staples and clips distribute tension evenly along the suture line with minimal tissue trauma and compression, facilitating healing and minimizing scarring. Because staples and clips are made from surgical stainless steel, tissue reaction to them is minimal. Usually, doctors remove skin staples and clips, but some institutions permit qualified nurses to perform this procedure.

Skin staples and clips are contraindicated when wound location requires cosmetically superior results or when the incision site makes it impossible to maintain at least a 5 mm distance between the staple and underlying bones, vessels, or internal organs.

Equipment

Waterproof trash bag ▪ adjustable light ▪ clean gloves, if needed ▪ sterile gloves ▪ sterile gauze pads ▪ sterile staple or clip extractor ▪ povidone-iodine solution or other antiseptic cleaning agent ▪ sterile cotton-tipped applicators ▪ optional: butterfly adhesive strips or Steri-Strips, compound benzoin tincture or other skin protectant.

Prepackaged, sterile, disposable staple or clip extractors are available.

Preparation of equipment

Assemble all equipment in the patient's room. Check the expiration date on each sterile package and inspect for tears. Open the waterproof trash bag and place it near the patient's bed. Position the bag *to avoid reaching across the sterile field or the wound when disposing of soiled articles.* Form a cuff by turning down the top of the bag *to provide*

Removing a staple

Position the extractor's lower jaws beneath the span of the first staple, as shown in the first illustration. Squeeze the handles until they're completely closed; then lift the staple away from the skin, as shown in the second illustration. The extractor changes the shape of the staple and pulls the prongs out of the intradermal tissue.

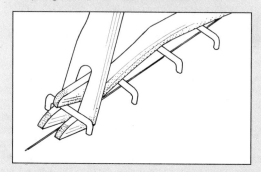

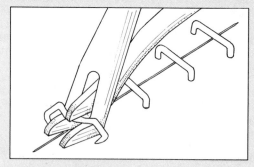

a wide opening and prevent contamination of instruments or gloves by touching the bag's edge.

Implementation
• If your institution allows you to remove skin staples and clips, check the doctor's order *to confirm the exact timing and details of this procedure.*
• Check for patient allergies, especially to adhesive tape and povidone-iodine or other topical solutions or medications.
• Explain the procedure to the patient. Tell him that he may feel a slight pulling or tickling sensation, but little discomfort, during staple removal. Reassure him that because his incision is healing properly, removing the supporting staples or clips won't weaken the incision line.

• Provide privacy, and place the patient in a comfortable position that doesn't place undue tension on the incision. *Because some patients experience nausea or dizziness during the procedure,* have the patient recline if possible. Adjust the light to shine directly on the incision.
• Wash your hands thoroughly.
• If the patient's wound has a dressing, put on clean gloves and carefully remove it. Discard the dressing and the gloves in the waterproof trash bag.
• Assess the patient's incision and notify the doctor of gaping, drainage, inflammation, or other signs of infection.
• Establish a sterile work area with all the equipment and supplies you'll need for removing staples or clips and for cleaning and dressing the incision. Open the package containing the sterile staple or clip extractor, maintaining asepsis. Put on sterile gloves.
• Wipe the incision gently with sterile gauze pads soaked in an antiseptic cleaning agent, or with sterile cotton-tipped applicators, *to remove surface encrustations.*
• Pick up the sterile staple or clip extractor. Then, starting at one end of the incision, remove the first staple or clip. (See *Removing a staple.*) Hold the extractor over the trash bag, and release the handle to discard the staple or clip.
• Repeat the procedure for each staple or clip until all are removed.
• Apply a sterile gauze dressing, if needed, *to prevent infection and irritation from clothing.* Then discard your gloves.
• Make sure the patient is comfortable. According to the doctor's preference, inform the patient that he may shower in 1 or 2 days if the incision is dry and healing well.
• Properly dispose of solutions and the trash bag, and clean or dispose of soiled equipment and supplies according to institutional policy.

Special considerations
Carefully check the doctor's order for the time and extent of staple or clip removal. The doctor may want you to remove only alternate staples or clips initially and to leave the others in place for an additional day or two *to support the incision.*

When removing a staple or clip, place the extractor's jaws carefully between the patient's skin and the staple or clip *to avoid patient discomfort.* If extraction is difficult, notify the doctor; *staples or clips placed too deeply within the skin or left in place too long may resist removal.*

If the wound dehisces after staples or clips are removed, apply butterfly adhesive strips or Steri-Strips to approximate and support the edges, and call the doctor immediately to repair the wound. (See *Types of adhesive skin closures.*)

You may also apply butterfly adhesive strips or Steri-Strips after removing staples or clips even if the wound is healing normally *to give added support to the incision and prevent lateral tension from forming a wide scar.* Use a small amount of compound benzoin tincture or other skin protectant *to ensure adherence.* Leave the strips in place for 3 to 5 days.

Home care
If the patient is being discharged, teach him how to remove the dressing and care for the wound. Instruct him to call the doctor immediately if he observes wound discharge or any other abnormal change. Tell him the redness surrounding the incision should gradually disappear, and that after a few weeks only a thin line should show.

Documentation
Record the date and time of staple or clip removal, the number of staples or clips removed, appearance of the incision, any dressings or butterfly strips applied, any signs of wound complications, and the patient's tolerance for the procedure.

Management of wound dehiscence and evisceration

Although the typical surgical wound heals without incident, occasionally the edges of a wound may fail to join, or may separate even after they seem to be healing normally. This development, called wound dehiscence, may lead to an even more serious complication: evisceraton, where a portion of the viscera (usually a bowel loop) protrudes through the incision. Evisceration, in turn, can lead to peritonitis and septic shock. (See *Recognizing dehiscence and evisceration,* page 200.) Dehiscence and evisceration are most likely to occur 6 or 7 days after surgery. By then, sutures may have been removed and the patient can cough easily and breathe deeply—both of which strain the incision.

Several factors can contribute to these complications. Poor nutrition—whether from inadequate intake or a condition such as diabetes mellitus—may hinder wound healing. Chronic pulmonary or cardiac disease can also slow healing because the injured tissue doesn't get needed nutrients and oxygen. Localized wound infection may limit closure, delay healing, and weaken the incision. And stress on the incision from coughing or vomiting may cause abdominal distention or severe stretching. A

Types of adhesive skin closures

Steri-Strips are used as a primary means of keeping a wound closed after suture removal. They're made of thin strips of sterile, nonwoven, porous fabric tape.

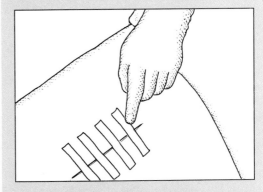

Butterfly closures consist of sterile, waterproof adhesive strips. A narrow, nonadhesive "bridge" connects the two expanded adhesive portions. These strips are used to close small wounds and to assist healing after suture removal.

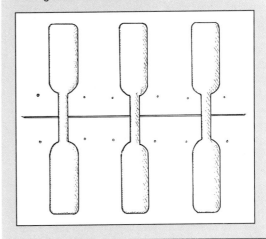

midline abdominal incision, for instance, has a high risk of wound dehiscence.

Equipment
Two sterile towels ■ 1 liter of normal sterile saline solution ■ sterile irrigation set, including a basin, a solution

Recognizing dehiscence and evisceration

In wound dehiscence, the layers of the surgical wound separate. With evisceration, the viscera (in this case, a bowel loop) protrude through the surgical incision.

Wound dehiscence

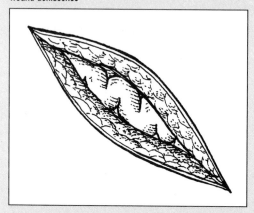

Evisceration of bowel loop

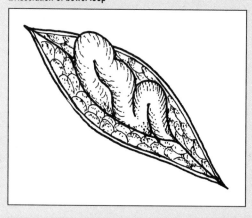

container, and a 50-ml catheter-tip syringe ▪ several large abdominal dressings ▪ sterile, waterproof drape ▪ linen-saver pads ▪ sterile gloves.

If the patient will return to the operating room, make sure you also gather the following equipment: I.V. administration set and I.V. fluids ▪ equipment for nasogastric intubation ▪ sedative, as ordered ▪ suction apparatus.

Implementation

• Provide reassurance and support *to ease the patient's anxiety.* Tell him to stay in bed. If possible, stay with him while someone else notifies the doctor and collects the necessary equipment.

• Place a linen-saver pad under the patient *to keep the sheets dry when you moisten the exposed viscera.*

• Using sterile technique, unfold a sterile towel *to create a sterile field.* Open the package containing the irrigation set, and place the basin, solution container, and 50-ml syringe on the sterile field.

• Open the bottle of normal saline solution and pour about 400 ml into the solution container. Also pour about 200 ml into the sterile basin.

• Open several large abdominal dressings and place them on the sterile field.

• Put on the sterile gloves and place one or two of the large abdominal dressings into the basin *to saturate them with saline solution.*

• Place the moistened dressings over the exposed viscera. Then place a sterile, waterproof drape over the dressings *to prevent the sheets from getting wet.*

• Moisten the dressings every hour by withdrawing saline solution from the container through the syringe and then gently squirting the solution on the dressings.

• When you moisten the dressings, inspect the color of the viscera. If it appears dusky or black, notify a doctor immediately. *With its blood supply interrupted, a protruding organ may become ischemic and necrotic.*

• Keep the patient on absolute bed rest in low Fowler's position (no more than 20 degrees elevation) with his knees flexed. *This prevents injury and reduces stress on an abdominal incision.*

• Monitor the patient's pulse, respirations, blood pressure, and temperature every 15 minutes *to detect shock.*

• If necessary, prepare the patient to return to the operating room. Gather the equipment and start an I.V. infusion, as ordered.

• Insert a nasogastric tube and connect it to continuous or intermittent low suction, as ordered.

• Also administer preoperative medications to the patient as ordered.

• Depending on the circumstances, some of these procedures may not be done at the bedside. For instance, nasogastric intubation may make the patient gag or vomit, causing further evisceration. For this reason, the doctor may choose to have the tube inserted in the operating room with the patient under anesthesia.

• Continue to reassure the patient while you prepare him for surgery. Be sure he has signed a consent form and the operating room staff has been informed about the procedure.

Special considerations

As always, the best treatment is prevention. If you're caring for a postoperative patient who's at risk for poor healing, be sure he gets an adequate supply of protein, vitamins, and calories. Monitor his dietary deficiencies, and discuss any problems with a doctor and a dietitian.

When changing wound dressings, always use sterile technique. Inspect the incision with each dressing change and, if you recognize the early signs of infection, start treatment before dehiscence or evisceration can occur. If local infection develops, clean the wound as necessary to eliminate a buildup of purulent drainage. Always make sure bandages aren't so tight that they limit blood supply to the wound.

After surgery on obese or elderly patients with weak or pendulous abdominal walls, apply an abdominal binder. *You'll do this because large amounts of fatty tissue make approximating the wound edges more difficult and because fatty tissue heals slowly.* A large abdomen can also cause excessive stretching and abdominal wall tension.

Encourage the high-risk patient to splint his abdomen with a pillow during straining, coughing, or sneezing.

If a postoperative patient detects a sudden gush of pinkish serous drainage on his dressing, inspect the incision for dehiscence. If the wound seems to be separating slowly and evisceration hasn't developed, place the patient in the supine position. Apply a butterfly bandage to the wound edges and call the doctor.

Complications

Infection, which can lead to peritonitis and possibly septic shock, is the most severe and most common complication of wound dehiscence and evisceration. Caused by bacterial contamination or by drying of normally moist abdominal contents, infection can impair circulation and lead to necrosis of the affected organ. Immediately covering the wound with sterile, moist dressings reduces the risk of contamination and drying.

Assess for local infection by observing the wound for drainage, purulence, or odor. Inspect the incision for redness, swelling, or local inflammation. Suspect infection with a poorly approximated wound. Also look for signs of systemic infection, such as an increased white blood cell count, fever, and tachycardia.

Documentation

Note when the problem occurred, the patient's activity preceding the problem, his condition, and the time the doctor was notified. Describe the appearance of the wound or eviscerated organ; the amount, color, consistency, and odor of any drainage; and any nursing actions taken. Record the patient's vital signs, his response to the incident, and the doctor's actions.

Finally, be sure you change the patient care plan to reflect nursing actions needed to promote proper healing.

Management of traumatic wounds

Because most traumatic wounds are caused by accidental injury in unsterile conditions, they carry a high risk of local infection that can delay healing, increase scar formation, and lead to a systemic infection such as septicemia. Care of such wounds aims to remove bacteria, prevent infection, promote healing, and minimize scarring.

While caring for a traumatic wound, the nurse can also assess its condition. The type of wound and degree of contamination usually determine which cleaning technique and cleaning agent are most appropriate. Large, deep, or obviously dirty wounds may require analgesic medication and such special procedures as debridement and irrigation.

Equipment

Two sterile basins ■ ordered antiseptic cleaning agent ■ normal saline solution ■ sterile 4″ × 4″ gauze pads ■ sterile gloves and clean gloves ■ sterile cotton-tipped applicators ■ dry sterile dressing, nonadherent pad, or petroleum gauze ■ linen-saver pad ■ optional: scissors, towel, goggles, mask, gown, 50-ml catheter-tip syringe, surgical scrub brush, oral irrigating device, antibiotic ointment, porous tape, sterile forceps, sutures and suture set.

Preparation of equipment

Assemble needed equipment at the patient's bedside. Fill one basin with the ordered cleaning agent and the other with normal saline solution. Make sure the treatment area has enough light to allow careful observation of the wound. Depending on the nature and location of the wound, wear sterile or clean gloves *to avoid spreading infection.*

Implementation

● Wash your hands.
● Explain the procedure to the patient and provide privacy.
● Assess the patient's pain. Administer pain medication, if ordered, except intradermally injected local anesthetics, which are administered by the doctor.
● Place a linen-saver pad under the area to be cleaned.
● If necessary, cut the hair around the wound with scissors *to facilitate cleaning and treatment.*

• Wet a sterile 4″ × 4″ gauze pad with the ordered cleaning agent. Never clean a wound with cotton balls or cotton-filled gauze pads *because cotton fibers may be pulled off and left in the wound, causing contamination.* Clean the wound gently using a circular motion, working outward from the center of the wound to approximately 2″ (5 cm) past its edge. *This motion removes nearby sources of contamination and stimulates circulation to the wound site.* Discard the soiled gauze pad and use fresh ones as necessary.

• Continue cleaning for approximately 5 minutes or until the wound appears clean.

• Wet several 4″ × 4″ gauze pads with the normal saline and rinse the wound with the same circular motion used in cleaning.

• Extremely dirty wounds that require additional cleaning may be scrubbed with a surgical brush or irrigated with jet lavage (such as a 50-ml catheter-tip syringe or an oral irrigating device, such as a Water Pik). Don't use a bulb syringe or I.V. tubing *because these can't provide enough force to remove embedded debris.* Wear goggles, mask, gown, and sterile gloves when you're manually removing embedded debris *to avoid contaminating yourself with aerosolized particles.*

• After the wound has been cleaned, the doctor may debride it *to remove dead tissue and to reduce the risk of infection and scarring.*

• If necessary, the doctor may suture the wound edges using the suture kit provided, or apply sterile strips of porous tape, depending on the wound's depth.

• Apply the ordered antibacterial ointment *to help prevent infection.*

• Apply a dry sterile dressing over the wound *to absorb drainage and to protect the site from bacterial contamination.* Apply a nonadherent pad or petroleum gauze to abrasions *to keep the dressing from sticking to the wound.*

Special considerations

Do not clean a wound with alcohol *because it causes pain and dehydrates tissue.*

The doctor may perform extensive debriding and suturing in the operating room, using the suture kit provided. If this is necessary, pack the wound with gauze pads soaked in normal saline solution before moving the patient to the operating room. Recognize that a wound in an area subjected to repeated traumatic injury may require splinting *to promote complete healing.*

Check the patient's medical history for previous tetanus immunization and, if ordered, arrange for current immunization.

Teach the patient how to care for his wound, and, if necessary, inform him when to return to have his sutures removed.

Complications

The most common complication of traumatic wounds is infection.

Documentation

Record the date and time of the procedure, the size and condition of the wound, the administration of medications, and specific wound care measures.

 # Wound irrigation

Irrigation cleans tissues and flushes cell debris and drainage from an open wound. Irrigation with an antiseptic or antibiotic solution helps the wound heal properly from the inside tissue layers outward to the skin surface; it also helps prevent premature surface healing over an abscess pocket or infected tract. Performed properly, wound irrigation requires strict sterile technique. After irrigation, open wounds usually are packed to absorb additional drainage.

Equipment

Waterproof trash bag ▪ linen-saver pad ▪ emesis basin ▪ clean gloves ▪ sterile gloves ▪ gown, if indicated ▪ prescribed irrigant, such as sterile normal saline solution, hydrogen peroxide, or antibiotic solutions ▪ sterile water or normal saline solution ▪ soft rubber catheter ▪ 50- to 60-ml piston syringe ▪ sterile container ▪ antiseptic cleaning agent ▪ materials as needed for wound care ▪ sterile irrigation and dressing set ▪ povidone-iodine sponges ▪ sterile petroleum jelly.

Preparation of equipment

Assemble all equipment in the patient's room. Check the expiration date on each sterile package and inspect for tears. Check the sterilization date and the date that each bottle of irrigating solution was opened; don't use any solution that's been open longer than 24 hours.

Using aseptic technique, dilute the prescribed irrigant to the correct proportions with sterile water or normal saline solution, if necessary. Let the solution stand until it reaches room temperature, or warm it to 90° to 95° F (32.2° to 35° C).

Open the waterproof trash bag and place it near the patient's bed *to avoid reaching across the sterile field or the wound when disposing of soiled articles.* Form a cuff by turning down the top of the trash bag *to provide a wide opening and prevent contamination by touching the bag's edge.*

Implementation

• Check the doctor's order, and assess the patient's condition. Identify the patient's allergies, especially to povidone-iodine or other topical solutions or medications.
• Explain the procedure to the patient, provide privacy, and position the patient correctly for the procedure. Place the linen-saver pad under the patient *to catch any spills and avoid linen changes.* Place the emesis basin below the wound *so the irrigating solution flows from the wound into the basin.*
• Wash your hands thoroughly. If necessary, put on a gown *to protect your clothing from wound drainage and contamination.* Put on clean gloves.
• Remove the soiled dressing; then discard the dressing and gloves in the trash bag.
• Establish a sterile field with all the equipment and supplies you'll need for irrigation and wound care. Pour the prescribed amount of irrigating solution into a sterile container *so you won't contaminate your sterile gloves later by picking up unsterile containers.* Put on sterile gloves.
• Fill the syringe with the irrigating solution; then connect the rubber catheter to the syringe. Gently instill a slow, steady stream of irrigating solution into the wound until the syringe empties. (See *Irrigating a deep wound.*) Make sure the solution flows from the clean to the dirty area of the wound *to prevent contamination of clean tissue by exudate.* Be sure the solution reaches all areas of the wound.
• Pinch the catheter closed before you withdraw the syringe *to prevent aspirating drainage and contaminating the equipment.*
• Refill the syringe, reconnect it to the catheter, and repeat the irrigation.
• Continue to irrigate the wound until you've administered the prescribed amount of solution or until the solution returns clear. Note the amount of solution administered. Then remove and discard the catheter and syringe in the waterproof trash bag.
• Keep the patient positioned *to allow further wound drainage into the basin.*
• Clean the area around the wound with povidone-iodine sponges or an antiseptic cleaning agent *to help prevent skin breakdown and infection.*
• Pack the wound, if ordered, and apply a sterile dressing. Remove and discard your gloves and gown.
• Make sure the patient is comfortable.
• Properly dispose of drainage, solutions, and trash bag, and clean or dispose of soiled equipment and supplies according to institutional policy. *To prevent contamination of other equipment,* don't return unopened sterile supplies to the sterile supply cabinet.

Irrigating a deep wound

When preparing to irrigate a deep wound, attach a soft rubber catheter to a piston-type syringe. Soft rubber minimizes tissue trauma, irritation, and bleeding. Then gently insert the catheter into the recesses of the wound until you feel resistance. Avoid forcing the catheter into the wound to prevent tissue damage or, in an abdominal wound, intestinal perforation.

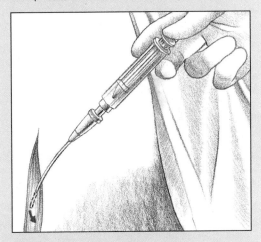

Irrigate the wound with gentle pressure until the solution returns clean. Then position the emesis basin under the wound to collect any remaining drainage.

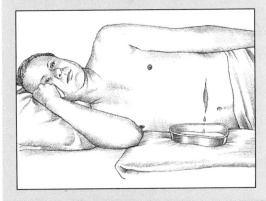

Special considerations

Try to coordinate wound irrigation with the doctor's visit *so he can inspect the wound.* Use only the irrigant specified by the doctor *because others may be erosive or otherwise harmful.* When using an irritating irrigant, such as Dakin's solution, spread sterile petroleum jelly around the wound site *to protect the patient's skin.* Remember to follow your institution's policy concerning wound and skin precautions when appropriate. Irrigate with a bulb syringe only if a piston syringe is unavailable; *the piston syringe reduces the risk of aspirating drainage.* If the wound is small or not particularly deep, you may want to use just the syringe for irrigation.

Home care

If the wound must be irrigated at home, teach the patient or a family member how to perform it using strict aseptic technique. Ask for a return demonstration of the proper technique. Provide written instructions. Arrange for home health supplies and nursing visits, as appropriate. Urge the patient to call his doctor if he detects signs of infection.

Complications

Wound irrigation increases the risk of infection. Excoriation and increased pain may also occur.

Documentation

Record the date and time of irrigation, amount and type of irrigant, appearance of the wound, any sloughing tissue or exudate, amount of solution returned, any skin care performed around the wound, any dressings applied, and the patient's tolerance of the treatment.

 # Closed-wound drain management

Typically inserted during surgery in anticipation of substantial postoperative drainage, a closed-wound drain promotes healing and prevents swelling by suctioning the serosanguineous fluid that accumulates at the wound site. By removing this fluid, the closed-wound drain helps reduce the risk of infection and skin breakdown as well as the number of dressing changes. Hemovac and Jackson-Pratt closed drainage systems are used most commonly.

A closed-wound drain consists of perforated tubing connected to a portable vacuum unit. The distal end of the tubing lies within the wound and usually leaves the body from a site other than the primary suture line to preserve the integrity of the surgical wound. The tubing exit site is treated as an additional surgical wound; the drain is usually sutured to the skin.

If the wound produces heavy drainage, the closed-wound drain may be left in place for longer than 1 week. Drainage must be emptied and measured frequently to maintain maximum suction and prevent strain on the suture line.

Equipment

Graduated cylinder ■ sterile laboratory container, if needed ■ alcohol sponges ■ gloves ■ trash bag ■ sterile gauze pads ■ antiseptic cleaning agent ■ prepackaged povidone-iodine swabs.

Implementation

● Check the doctor's order and assess the patient's condition.
● Explain the procedure to the patient, provide privacy, and wash your hands.
● Unclip the vacuum unit from the patient's bed or gown.
● Using aseptic technique, release the vacuum by removing the spout plug on the collection chamber. The container expands completely as it draws in air.
● Empty the unit's contents into a graduated cylinder, and note the amount and appearance of the drainage. If diagnostic tests will be performed on the fluid specimen, pour the drainage directly into a sterile laboratory container, note the amount and appearance, and send it to the laboratory.
● Maintaining aseptic technique, use an alcohol sponge to clean the unit's spout and plug.
● *To reestablish the vacuum that creates the drain's suction power,* fully compress the vacuum unit. With one hand holding the unit compressed *to maintain the vacuum,* replace the spout plug with your other hand. (See *Using a closed-wound drainage system.)*
● Check the patency of the equipment. Make sure the tubing is free of twists, kinks, and leaks *because the drainage system must be airtight to work properly.* The vacuum unit should remain compressed when you release manual pressure; rapid reinflation indicates an air leak. If this occurs, recompress the unit and make sure the spout plug is secure.
● Secure the vacuum unit to the patient's bedding or, if he is ambulatory, to his gown. Fasten it below wound level *to promote drainage.* Do not apply tension on drainage tubing when fastening the unit *to prevent possible dislodgement.* Remove and discard your gloves and wash your hands thoroughly.
● Observe the sutures that secure the drain to the patient's skin; look for signs of pulling or tearing, and for swelling or infection of surrounding skin. Gently clean

Using a closed-wound drainage system

The portable closed-wound drainage system draws drainage from a wound site, such as the chest wall post-mastectomy shown at left, by means of a Y tube. To empty the drainage, remove the plug and empty it into a graduated cylinder. To reestablish suction, compress the drainage unit against a firm surface to expel air and, while holding it down, replace the plug with your other hand, as shown at right.

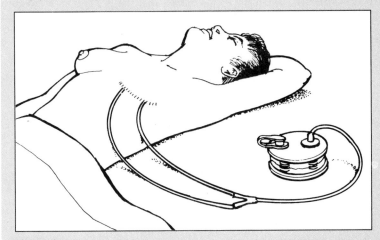
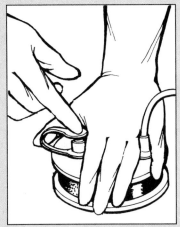

the sutures with sterile gauze pads soaked in an anti-septic cleaning agent or with a povidone-iodine swab.
• Properly dispose of drainage, solutions, and trash bag, and clean or dispose of soiled equipment and supplies according to institutional policy.

Special considerations
Empty the system and measure its contents once during each shift if drainage has accumulated, more often if drainage is excessive. *Removing excess drainage maintains maximum suction and avoids straining the drain's suture line.*

If the patient has more than one closed drain, number the drains *so you can record drainage from each site.*
◆ *Nursing alert.* Be careful not to mistake chest tubes for closed-wound drains *because the vacuum of a chest tube should never be released.* ◆

Complications
Occlusion of the tubing by fibrin, clots, or other particles can reduce or obstruct drainage.

Documentation
Record the date and time you empty the system, the appearance of the drain site and presence of swelling or signs of infection, any equipment malfunction and consequent nursing action, and the patient's tolerance of the treatment. On the intake and output sheet, record drainage color, consistency, type, and amount. If the patient has more than one closed-wound drain, number the drains and record the above information separately for each drainage site.

*R*ADIATION THERAPY
External radiation therapy

About 60% of all cancer patients are treated with some form of external radiation therapy. Also called radiotherapy, this treatment delivers radiation—X-rays or gamma rays—directly to the cancer site. Its effects are local, since only the area being treated experiences direct effects.

Radiation doses are based on the type, stage, and location of the tumor, as well as on the patient's size, condition, and overall treatment goals. Doses are given in increments, usually 3 to 5 times a week, until the total dose is reached.

The goals of radiation therapy include *cure*, in which the cancer is completely destroyed and not expected to recur; *control*, in which the cancer does not progress or regress, but is expected to progress at some later time; or *palliation*, in which radiation is given to relieve symptoms (such as bone pain, seizures, bleeding, headache) caused by the cancer.

Radiation therapy may be augmented by chemotherapy, brachytherapy (radiation implant therapy), or surgery, as needed. (For information on chemotherapy, see Chapter 5, Drug Administration.)

External beam radiation therapy is delivered by machines that aim a concentrated beam of high-energy particles (photons and gamma rays) at the target site. Two types of machines are commonly used: units containing cobalt or cesium as radioactive sources for gamma rays, and linear accelerators that use electricity to produce X-rays. Linear accelerators produce high energy with great penetrating ability. Some (known as orthovoltage machines) produce less powerful electron beams that may be used for superficial tumors.

Equipment
Radiation therapy machine ■ film badge or pocket dosimeter.

Implementation
• Explain the treatment to the patient and his family. Review the treatment goals, and discuss the range of potential adverse effects and interventions to minimize them. Also discuss possible long-term complications and treatment issues. Educate the patient and his family about local cancer services.
• Check to see that the radiation oncology department has obtained informed consent.
• Review the patient's clinical record for recent laboratory and imaging results, and alert the radiation oncology staff to any abnormalities or pertinent results (such as myelosuppression, paraneoplastic syndromes, oncologic emergencies, and tumor progression).
• Transport the patient to the radiology department.
• The patient begins by undergoing simulation (treatment planning), in which the target area is mapped out on his body using a machine similar to the radiotherapy machine. Then the target area is tattooed or marked in ink on his body *to ensure accurate treatments.*
• The doctor and radiation oncologist determine the duration and frequency of treatments, depending on the patient's body size, size of portal, extent and location of cancer, and treatment goals.

• The patient is positioned on the treatment table beneath the machine. Treatments last from a few seconds to a few minutes. Reassure the patient that he won't feel anything and that he will not be radioactive. After treatment is complete, the patient may return home or to his room.

Special considerations
Explain to the patient that the full benefit of radiation treatments may not occur until several weeks or months after treatments begin. Instruct him to report any long-term adverse effects.

Emphasize the importance of keeping follow-up appointments with the doctor.

Refer the patient to a support group, such as a local chapter of the American Cancer Society.

Home care
Instruct the patient and his family on proper skin care and management of the adverse effects of treatment.

Complications
Adverse effects arise gradually and diminish gradually after treatments. They may be acute, subacute (accumulating as treatment progresses), chronic (following treatment), and long-term (arising months to years after treatment). Adverse effects are localized to the area of treatment, and their severity depends on the total radiation dosage, underlying organ sensitivity, and the patient's overall condition.

Common acute and subacute adverse effects can include altered skin integrity, altered GI and genitourinary function, altered fertility and sexual function, altered bone marrow production, fatigue, and alopecia.

Long-term complications or adverse effects may include radiation pneumonitis, neuropathy, skin and muscle atrophy, telangiectasia, fistulas, altered endocrine function, and secondary malignancies.

Other complications of treatment include headache, alopecia, xerostomia, dysphagia, stomatitis, altered skin integrity (wet or dry desquamation), nausea, vomiting, heartburn, diarrhea, cystitis, and fatigue.

Documentation
Record radiation precautions taken during treatment; interventions used, and evaluation of the interventions; grading of adverse effects; teaching given to the patient and family and their responses to it; the patient's tolerance of isolation procedures and the family's compliance with procedures; discharge plans and teaching; and referrals to local cancer services, if any.

Radiation implant therapy

In this treatment, also called brachytherapy, the doctor uses implants of radioactive isotopes (encapsulated in seeds, needles, or sutures) to deliver ionizing radiation within a body cavity or interstitially to a tumor site. Implants can deliver a continuous radiation dose over several hours or days to a specific site while minimizing exposure to adjacent tissues. The implants may be permanent or temporary. Isotopes such as cesium 137 (^{137}Cs), gold 198 (^{198}Au), iodine 125 (^{125}I), iridium 192 (^{192}Ir), palladium 103 (^{103}Pd), and phosphorus 32 (^{32}P) are used to treat cancers. (See *Radioisotopes and their uses,* page 208.)

Common implant sites include the brain, breast, cervix, endometrium, lung, neck, oral cavity, prostate, and vagina.

Brachytherapy is commonly combined with external radiation therapy (teletherapy) for increased effectiveness.

For treatment, the patient is usually placed in a private room (with its own bathroom) located as far away from high-traffic areas as practical. If monitoring shows an increased radiation hazard, adjacent rooms and hallways may also need to be restricted. Consult your hospital's radiation safety policy for specific guidelines.

Equipment
Film badge or pocket dosimeter ▪ RADIATION PRECAUTION sign for door ▪ radiation precaution warning labels ▪ masking tape ▪ lead-lined container ▪ long-handled forceps ▪ male T-binder and two sanitary napkins with safety pin (if Burnett applicator is being used) ▪ optional: lead shield and lead strip.

Preparation of equipment
Place the lead-lined container and long-handled forceps in a corner of the patient's room. Mark a "safe line" on the floor with masking tape 6 feet (180 cm) from the patient's bed *to warn visitors to keep clear of the patient to minimize their radiation exposure.* If desired, place a portable lead shield in the back of the room *to use when providing care.*

Place an emergency tracheotomy tray in the room if an implant will be inserted in the oral cavity or neck.

Implementation
• Explain the treatment and its goals to the patient. Before treatment begins, review radiation safety procedures, visitation policies, potential adverse effects, and interventions for those effects. Also review long-term concerns and home care issues.

• Place the RADIATION PRECAUTION sign on the door.

• Check to see that informed consent has been obtained.

• Ensure that all laboratory tests are performed before beginning treatment. If laboratory work is required during treatment, the badged technician obtains the specimen, labels the collection tube with a radioactive precaution label, and alerts the laboratory personnel before bringing it. If urine tests are needed for ^{32}P therapy, ask the radiation oncology department or laboratory technician how to transport these specimens safely.

• Affix a radiation precaution warning label to the patient's identification wristband.

• Affix warning labels to the patient's chart and Kardex *to ensure staff awareness of the patient's radioactive status.*

• Wear a film badge or dosimeter at waist level during the entire shift. Turn in the radiation badge monthly or according to your hospital's protocol. Pocket dosimeters measure immediate exposures. In many centers, these measurements aren't part of the permanent exposure record but are used to ensure that nurses receive the lowest possible exposure.

• Each nurse must have a personal, nontransferable film badge or ring badge. *Badges document each person's cumulative lifetime radiation exposure.* Only primary caregivers are badged and allowed into the patient's room.

• To minimize exposure to radiation, use the three principles of time, distance, and shielding: Time—plan to give care in the shortest time possible. *Less time equals less exposure.* Distance—work as far away from the radiation source as possible. Give care from the side opposite the implant or from a position allowing the greatest working distance possible. *The intensity of radiation exposure varies inversely as the square of the distance from the source.* Shielding—use a portable shield, if needed and desired.

• Give essential nursing care only; omit bed baths. If ordered, provide perineal care, making sure that wipes, sanitary pads, and similar items are bagged correctly and monitored. (Refer to your hospital's radiation policy.)

• Dressing changes over an implanted area must be supervised by the radiation technician or another designated caregiver.

• Before discharge, a patient's temporary implant must be removed and properly stored by the radiation oncology department. A patient with a permanent implant may not be released until his radioactivity level is less than 5 millirems (mrem) per hour at one meter's distance.

Special considerations
Nurses and visitors who are pregnant or trying to conceive or father a child must not attend patients receiving

Radioisotopes and their uses

Unstable elements, radioisotopes emit three kinds of energy particles as they "decay" to a stable state. These particles are ranked by their penetrating power. *Alpha particles* possess the lowest energy level and are easily stopped by a sheet of paper. More powerful *beta parti-* *cles* can be stopped by the skin's surface. *Gamma rays*, the most powerful, can only be stopped by dense shielding, such as lead. Some isotopes commonly used in cancer treatments are listed below.

ISOTOPE AND INDICATIONS	DESCRIPTION	NURSING CONSIDERATIONS
Cesium 137 (^{137}Cs) Gynecologic cancers	• 30-year half-life • Emits gamma particles • Encased in steel capsules which are placed temporarily in the patient in the operating room	• Elevate the head of the bed no more than 45 degrees. • Encourage fluids and implement a low-residue diet. • Encourage quiet activities; enforce strict bed rest, as ordered.
Iodine 125 (^{125}I) Localized or unresectable tumors; slow-growing tumors; recurrent disease	• 60-day half-life • Emits gamma particles • Permanently implanted as tiny seeds or sutures directly into the tumor or tumor bed	• Because seeds may become dislodged, no linens, body fluids, instruments, or utensils may leave the patient's room until they're monitored. • If a seed is dislodged and found, call the radiation department; use long-handled forceps to put it in a lead-lined container in the room. • Monitor body fluids to detect displaced seeds. Give the patient a 24-hour urine container that can be closed.
Iridium 192 (^{192}Ir) Localized or unresectable tumors	• 74-day half-life • Emits gamma particles • Temporarily implanted as seeds strung inside special catheters that are implanted around the tumor	• If a catheter is dislodged, call the radiation department; use long-handled forceps to put the implant in a lead-lined container in the room.
Palladium 103 (^{103}Pd) Superficial, localized or unresectable intrathoracic or intra-abdominal tumors	• 17-day half-life • Emits gamma particles • Permanently implanted as seeds in the tumor or tumor bed	• See Iodine 125.
Phosphorus 32 (^{32}P) Polycythemia, leukemia, bone metastasis, and malignant ascites	• 14-day half-life • Emits beta particles • Used as an I.V. solution rather than an implant because of its low energy level	• No shielding is required other than a lucite syringe shield. • Patients receiving ^{32}P are placed in a private room with a separate bathroom.
Gold 198 (^{198}Au) Localized male genitourinary tumors	• 3-day half-life • Emits gamma particles • Permanently implanted as tiny seeds directly into the tumor or tumor bed	• If a seed is dislodged and found, call the radiation oncology department for disposal.

radiation implant therapy *because the gonads and developing embryo and fetus are highly susceptible to the damaging effects of ionizing radiation.*

If the patient must be moved out of his room, notify the appropriate department of the patient's status *to give receiving personnel time to make appropriate preparations to receive the patient.* When moving the patient, ensure that the route is clear of equipment and other persons, and that the elevator, if there is one, is keyed and ready to receive the patient. Move the patient in a bed or wheelchair, accompanied by two badged caregivers. If the patient is delayed along the way, stand as far away from the bed as possible until you can continue.

The patient's room must be monitored daily by the radiation oncology department, and disposables must be monitored and removed according to hospital guidelines.

If a code is called on a patient with an implant, follow your hospital's code procedures as well as these steps: Notify the code team of the patient's radioactive status *to exclude any team member who is pregnant or trying to conceive or father a child.* Also notify the radiation oncology department. Cover the implant site with a strip of lead shielding if possible. Don't allow anything to leave the patient's room until it's monitored for radiation. The primary care nurse must remain in the room (as far away from the patient as possible) *to act as a resource person for the patient and to provide film badges or dosimeters to code team members.*

If an implant becomes dislodged, notify the radiation oncology department staff and follow their instructions. Typically, the dislodged implant is collected with long-handled forceps and placed in a lead-shielded canister.

Tell the patient who has had a cervical implant to expect slight to moderate vaginal bleeding after being discharged from the hospital. This flow normally changes color from pink to brown to white. Instruct her to notify the doctor if bleeding increases, persists for more than 48 hours, or has a foul odor. Explain to the patient that she may resume most normal activities but should avoid sexual intercourse and the use of tampons until after her follow-up visit to the doctor (about 6 weeks after discharge). Instruct her to take showers rather than baths for 2 weeks, to avoid douching unless allowed by the doctor, and to avoid activities that cause abdominal strain for 6 weeks.

Refer the patient for sexual or psychological counseling if needed.

If a patient with an implant dies on the unit, notify the radiation oncology department *so they can remove a temporary implant and store it properly.* If the implant was permanent, radiation oncology staff members will determine which precautions to follow before postmortem

care can be provided and before the body can be moved to the morgue.

Complications

Depending on the implant site and total radiation dosage, complications of implant therapy may include dislodgment of the radiation source or applicator, tissue fibrosis, xerostomia, radiation pneumonitis, muscle atrophy, sterility, vaginal dryness or stenosis, fistulas, hypothyroidism, altered bowel habits, infection, airway obstruction, diarrhea, cystitis, myelosuppression, neurotoxicity, and secondary cancers. Encourage the patient and family members to keep in contact with the radiation oncology department and to call them if concerns or physical changes occur.

Documentation

Record radiation precautions taken during treatment; adverse effects of therapy; teaching given to the patient and family and their responses to it; the patient's tolerance of isolation procedures and the family's compliance with procedures; and referrals to local cancer services.

 # Radioactive iodine therapy

Because the thyroid gland concentrates iodine, radioactive iodine 131 (^{131}I) can be used to treat thyroid cancer. This isotope emits beta and gamma radiation, and its half-life (the time required for it to decay to 50% of its original activity) is 8 days. Usually administered orally, ^{131}I is used to treat postoperative residual cancer, recurrent disease, inoperable primary thyroid tumors, invasion of the thyroid capsule, or thyroid ablation as well as cancers that have metastasized to cervical or mediastinal lymph nodes or other distant sites.

Because ^{131}I is absorbed systemically, all body secretions, especially urine, must be considered radioactive. For ^{131}I treatments, the patient usually is placed in a private room (with its own bathroom) located as far away from high-traffic areas as practical. If monitoring shows increased radiation hazard, adjacent rooms and hallways may also need to be restricted. Consult your hospital's radiation safety policy for specific guidelines.

In lower doses, radioactive ^{131}I also may be used to treat hyperthyroidism. Most patients receive this treatment on an outpatient basis and are sent home with appropriate home care instructions.

What to do after ¹³¹I treatment

- Instruct the patient to report any long-term adverse reactions. In particular, review signs and symptoms of hypothyroidism and hyperthyroidism. Also ask him to report any signs and symptoms of thyroid cancer, such as enlarged lymph nodes, dyspnea, bone pain, nausea, vomiting, and abdominal discomfort.
- Although the patient's radiation level at discharge will be safe, suggest that he take extra precautions during the first week, such as using separate eating utensils, sleeping in a separate bedroom, and avoiding bodily contact.
- Sexual intercourse may be resumed 1 week after ¹³¹I treatment. However, urge a female patient to avoid pregnancy for 6 months after treatment, and tell a male patient to avoid impregnating his partner for 3 months after treatment.

Equipment

Film badges, pocket dosimeters, or ring badges ■ RADIATION PRECAUTION sign for door ■ radiation precaution warning labels ■ waterproof gowns ■ clear and red plastic bags for contaminated articles ■ plastic wrap ■ absorbent plastic-lined pads ■ masking tape ■ radioresistant gloves ■ trash cans ■ optional: portable lead shield.

Preparation of equipment

Assemble all necessary equipment in the patient's room. Keep an emergency tracheotomy tray just outside the room or in a handy place at the nurses' station. Place the RADIATION PRECAUTION sign on the door. Affix warning labels to the patient's chart and Kardex *to ensure staff awareness of the patient's radioactive status.*

Place an absorbent plastic back pad on the bathroom floor and under the sink; if the patient's room is carpeted, cover it with such a pad as well. Place an additional pad over the bedside table. Secure plastic wrap over the telephone, television controls, bed controls, mattress, call button, and toilet. *These measures prevent radioactive contamination of working surfaces.*

Keep large trash cans in the room lined with plastic bags (two clear bags inserted inside an outer red bag). Monitor all objects before they leave the room.

Notify the dietitian to supply foods and beverages only in disposable containers and with disposable utensils.

Implementation

- Explain the procedure and review treatment goals with the patient and his family. Before treatment begins, review radiation safety procedures, visitation policies, potential adverse effects, interventions, and home care procedures. (See *What to do after ¹³¹I treatment.*)
- Verify that the doctor has obtained informed consent.
- Check for allergies to iodine-containing substances such as contrast media or shellfish. Review the medication history for thyroid-containing or thyroid-altering drugs and for lithium carbonate, *which may increase ¹³¹I uptake.*
- Review the patient's health history for vomiting, diarrhea, productive cough, and sinus drainage, *which could increase the risk of radioactive secretions.*
- If necessary, remove the patient's dentures *to avoid contaminating them and to reduce radioactive secretions.* Tell him they'll be replaced 48 hours after treatment.
- Affix a RADIATION PRECAUTION label to the patient's identification wristband.
- Encourage the patient to use the toilet rather than a bedpan or urinal, and to flush it three times after each use *to reduce radiation levels.*
- Instruct the patient to remain in his room except for tests or other special reasons. Allow him to ambulate.
- Unless contraindicated, instruct the patient to increase his fluid intake to 3 quarts daily.
- Encourage the patient to chew or suck on hard candy *to keep salivary glands stimulated and to prevent them from becoming inflamed (which may develop in the first 24 hours.)*
- Ensure that all laboratory tests are performed before beginning treatment. If laboratory work is required, the badged laboratory technician obtains the specimen, labels the collection tube with a RADIOACTIVE PRECAUTION label, and alerts the laboratory personnel before transporting it. If urine tests are needed, ask the radiation oncology department or laboratory technician how to transport these specimens safely.
- Wear a film badge or dosimeter at waist level during the entire shift. Turn in the radiation badge monthly or according to your hospital's protocol, and be sure to record your exposures accurately. *Pocket dosimeters measure immediate exposures. These measurements may not be part of the permanent exposure record but help to ensure that nurses receive the lowest possible exposure.*
- Each nurse must have a personal, nontransferable film badge or ring badge. *Badges document each person's cumulative lifetime radiation exposure.* Only primary caregivers are badged and allowed into the patient's room.
- Wear gloves to touch the patient or objects in his room.
- Allow visitors to spend no more than 30 minutes every 24 hours with the patient. Stress that no visitors will be allowed who are under age 18 or who are pregnant or trying to conceive or father a child.

• Restrict direct contact to no more than 30 minutes or 20 millirems (mrem) per day. If the patient is receiving 200 millicuries (mCi) of ^{131}I, remain with him only 2 to 4 minutes and stand no closer than 1' (30 cm) away. If standing 3' (1 m) away, the time limit is 20 minutes; if standing 5' (1.5 m) away, the limit is 30 minutes.
• Give essential nursing care only; omit bed baths. If ordered, provide perineal care, making sure that wipes, sanitary pads, and similar items are bagged correctly and monitored.
• If the patient vomits or urinates on the floor, notify the nuclear medicine department and use nondisposable radioresistant gloves when cleaning the spill. After cleanup, wash your gloved hands, remove the gloves and leave them in the room, then rewash your hands.
• If the patient must be moved from his room, notify the appropriate department of the patient's status *so that receiving personnel can make appropriate arrangements to receive him.* When moving the patient, ensure that the route is clear of equipment and other persons and that the elevator, if there is one, is keyed and ready to receive the patient. Move the patient in a bed or wheelchair, accompanied by two badged caregivers. If the patient is delayed along the way, stand as far away from him as possible until you can continue.
• The patient's room must be cleaned by the radiation oncology department, not by housekeeping. The room must be monitored daily, and disposables must be monitored and removed according to hospital guidelines.
• At discharge, schedule the patient for a follow-up examination. Also arrange for a whole-body scan approximately 7 to 10 days after ^{131}I treatment.
• Inform the patient and his family of community support services for cancer patients.

Special considerations

Nurses and visitors who are pregnant or trying to conceive or father a child must not attend or visit patients receiving ^{131}I therapy *because the gonads and developing embryo and fetus are highly susceptible to the damaging effects of ionizing radiation.*

If a code is called on a patient undergoing ^{131}I therapy, follow your hospital's code procedures as well as these steps. Notify the code team of the patient's radioactive status *to exclude any team member who is pregnant or trying to conceive or father a child.* Also notify the radiation oncology department. Don't allow anything out of the patient's room until it's monitored. The primary care nurse must remain in the room (as far as possible from the patient) *to act as a resource person for the patient and to provide film badges or dosimeters to code team members.*

If the patient dies on the unit, notify the radiology safety officer who will determine which precautions to follow before postmortem care is provided and before the body can be moved to the morgue.

Complications

Myelosuppression is common in patients who have extensive disease or who undergo repeated ^{131}I treatments.

Radiation pulmonary fibrosis may develop if extensive lung metastasis was present when ^{131}I was administered.

Other complications may include nausea, vomiting, headache, radiation thyroiditis, fever, sialadenitis, or pain and swelling at metastatic sites.

Documentation

Record radiation precautions taken during treatment, teaching given to the patient and family and their responses to it, the patient's tolerance of isolation procedures and the family's compliance with procedures, and referrals to local cancer counseling services.

Selected references

Bucholtz, J. "Radiation Therapy," in *Core Curriculum for Oncology Nursing.* Philadelphia: W.B. Saunders Co., 1987.

Campbell, A.D. "Pneumatic Compression Stockings: Preventing Deep Vein Thrombosis and Pulmonary Embolus," *Today's O.R. Nurse* 12(7):4-9, July 1990.

Cooper, D.M. "Optimizing Wound Healing: A Practice Within Nursing's Domain," *Nursing Clinics of North America* 25(1):165-80, March 1990.

Eriksson, J.H. *Oncologic Nursing: A Study and Learning Tool.* Springhouse Notes. Springhouse, Pa.: Springhouse Corp., 1989.

Fahey, V. "An In-depth Look at Deep Vein Thrombosis," *Nursing89* 19(1):86-93, January 1989.

Greenfield, L. "Thyroid Tumors," in *Principles and Practice of Radiation Oncology.* Edited by Perez, C., and Brady, L. Philadelphia: J.B. Lippincott Co., 1987.

Hassey, K.M. "Principles of Radiation Safety and Protection," *Seminars in Oncology Nursing* 3(1):23-29, February 1987.

Jones, P., and Millman, A. "Wound Healing and the Aged Patient," *Nursing Clinics of North America* 25(1):263-77, March 1990.

McCaffery, M., and Beebe, A. *Pain: Clinical Manual for Nursing Practice.* St. Louis: Mosby-Year Book, Inc., 1989.

Porteous, M.J., et al. "Thigh-length Versus Knee-length Stockings in the Prevention of Deep Vein Thrombosis," *British Journal of Surgery* 76(3):296-97, March 1989.

Scurr, J.H., et al. "Regimen for Improved Effectiveness of Intermittent Pneumatic Compression in Deep Venous Thrombosis Prophylaxis," *Surgery* 102(5):816-20, November 1987.

Taylor, C., et al. *Fundamentals of Nursing: The Art and Science of Nursing Care.* Philadelphia: J.B. Lippincott Co., 1989.

Timby, B.K., et al. *Clinical Nursing Procedures.* Philadelphia: J.B. Lippincott Co., 1989.

CHAPTER **5**

Drug Administration

SUSAN J. HART, RN,C, MSN, CCRN

Introduction

Administering drugs is one of your most crucial nursing responsibilities. To ensure safe and effective drug therapy for your patients, you need to be familiar with the indications, customary dosages, and intended effects of prescribed drugs. And you need to assess each patient before administering a drug, delaying or withholding it if necessary. Just as important, you need the skills to be able to administer a drug capably, minimizing your patient's anxiety and maximizing the drug's effectiveness. This chapter will help you perform this task by providing the information you need to give drugs by injection, instillation, inhalation, topical application, and intravascular route. You'll also learn how to add drugs to an I.V. solution, give I.V. bolus injections, and prepare and administer chemotherapeutic drugs.

Selecting the appropriate route

Drugs may be administered by many routes. The *topical,* or dermatomucosal, route includes aural, ocular, nasal, and vaginal administration, oropharyngeal inhalation, and transdermal absorption. The *enteral* route, the most commonly used one, involves drug absorption through the GI tract. The *parenteral* route includes intradermal, subcutaneous, intramuscular, I.V., intrathecal, and intraosseous infusions or injections. The *epidural* route involves giving a drug (usually an anesthetic or narcotic analgesic) through a catheter inserted near the spinal cord by a lumbar puncture.

More than any other factor, the administration route determines the onset of drug effect. For example, drugs administered I.V. act almost instantly because they're immediately available in the bloodstream. Antibiotics, for instance, are commonly given I.V. to provoke a quick, continuous response. Other drugs must be given I.V. because they're ineffective or even dangerous when given by other routes.

Conversely, some drugs—such as NPH insulin or penicillin G procaine—can't be given I.V. because they obstruct blood flow. Drugs administered intrathecally, such as spinal anesthetics, also act rapidly. However, drugs administered orally must be absorbed into the bloodstream before they can take effect. Because their peak effects are therefore delayed, oral drugs are used most often when the patient's condition doesn't require an immediate drug effect.

Avoiding medication errors

Before you administer any medication, always compare the doctor's order with the order on the patient's medication record. Then mentally check off the first five "rights" of drug administration: *right patient, right drug, right dose, right route, and right time.* If the doctor's order and the patient's medication record match, then compare the label on the medication to the medication record. If you find any discrepancies, withhold the drug and verify the order with the doctor or the pharmacist. If a patient questions any of his drugs, always double-check the orders and the dose before administration. Also check the drug's expiration date.

Before giving any drug, you need to be aware of two more "rights": the patient's *right to know why he's getting the drug and what adverse effects to expect, if any;* and his *right to refuse medication.*

Some drugs—such as narcotics, barbiturates, and other controlled substances—have automatic stop dates, mandated by law. Other medications, such as antibiotics, have stop dates set by hospital policy. Check your hospital's policy on how to handle outdated orders, and check drug expiration dates. Also learn your hospital's policies on acceptance and documentation of verbal orders and correct use of p.r.n. (as needed) orders.

Understanding patient response and drug interactions

Assessing a patient's response to medication requires a thorough understanding of his condition and the drug's desired or expected effect. If a patient is receiving an antiarrhythmic, for example, but continues to have premature ventricular contractions, you should tell the doctor that the drug isn't producing the desired effect.

When assessing the patient's response to therapy, also consider the results of laboratory tests, which can indicate a therapeutic effect, adverse effect, or toxic level. For example, prothrombin times help to evaluate the therapeutic effect of warfarin sodium, and low serum potassium levels may signal an adverse effect of certain diuretics. Be aware that some drugs may affect diagnostic test results, causing "false positives." (For example, codeine may elevate cerebrospinal fluid pressure.)

Monitor the patient's condition carefully; such changes as weight loss or gain can affect the action of some drugs. Other factors—such as the patient's age, body build, sex, and emotional state—also may affect the patient's response to drug therapy.

Because many patients receive more than one drug, you should also understand drug *interactions.* A drug interaction is a change in drug absorption, distribution, metabolism, and excretion that may occur with or shortly after administration of another drug. A desirable interaction is the basis for combination therapy, which may be used for additive effect, for helping to maintain an effective blood level, and for minimizing or preventing adverse effects. Some interactions, however, can have undesirable results, such as weakening a drug's desired effects or exaggerating its toxic ones. For example, patients who smoke require larger doses of theophylline than nonsmokers because cigarette smoke activates oxidative enzymes in the liver, increasing drug metabolism.

Watching for adverse effects

When you administer drugs, you also need to recognize and identify adverse effects, toxic reactions, and drug allergies. Some *adverse effects* are transient and subside as the patient develops a tolerance for the drug. Other adverse effects may require a change in therapy.

Toxic reactions to a drug can be acute, resulting from excessive doses, as in acetaminophen overdose, or chronic, resulting from progressive accumulation of the drug in the body. Toxic reactions can also result from impaired metabolism or excretion that can cause elevated blood levels of a drug.

Drug allergy (hypersensitivity) results from an antigen-antibody reaction in susceptible patients. Such a reaction can range from mild urticaria to potentially fatal anaphylaxis. Therefore, always be sure to check for allergies before administering medications. In some instances, sensitivity tests may be done before giving the first dose. Be aware that a negative history does not rule out a future allergic reaction.

Other undesirable effects to watch for when administering drugs include idiosyncratic reactions and dependence.

Document carefully

Documentation aims to preserve an accurate record of patient assessment and interventions as well as your reasons for giving the care specified. Documenting a patient's medications provides a legal record of drugs he received during his hospital stay. Medication administration involves documenting on a medication administration record as well as in the nurses' notes. Many hospitals also require documentation of narcotic administration in a central record.

After administering a drug, document the following on the patient's Kardex or computer file: drug name, dosage, route and time of administration, and your signature and title. In the nurses' notes, include any assessment data that refer to the patient's response to the medication or any adverse effects of the medication.

If your hospital documents medications by computer, be sure to enter each drug immediately after you give it. This gives all health care team members access to current medication information and is especially important if the system has no hard-copy backup. If a patient refuses or is unable to take medication, or if — in your judgment — the patient shouldn't receive the medication, document this on the medication administration record and in the nurses' notes.

Many hospitals use a medication administration record to document medication orders and administration. Usually contained in a Kardex file, the medication administration record serves as the central source for recording the doctor's medication orders and documenting administration. It becomes part of the patient's permanent medical record. When using the medication administration record, know and follow your hospital's policy and procedure for recording medication orders and charting medication administration. Make sure medication orders include the patient's full name, date ordered, drug dose, administration route or method, frequency, and time ordered for the first dose. Some drugs may be ordered with a specific number of doses or a stop date. If that's so, be sure to note this on the medication administration record. Always write legibly. Use only acceptable abbreviations and use them correctly. When in doubt as to how to abbreviate a term, spell it out. When documenting parenteral medications, be sure to include the injection site and the route you used. After administering the first dose, sign your full name, licensure status, and identifying initials in the appropriate place on the medication administration record.

If all medications have been given according to the care plan, no further documentation is needed. However, if your hospital's medication administration record does not include a place to document parenteral administration sites, patient's response to p.r.n. medications, or any deviation from the medication order, further narrative documentation is necessary. Document any patient teaching given, as well as the patient's response and knowledge level.

TOPICAL ADMINISTRATION
Application of topical skin medications

Topical drugs are applied directly to the skin surface. They include lotions, pastes, ointments, creams, powders, shampoos, and aerosol sprays. The medication is absorbed through the epidermal layer into the dermis. The extent of absorption depends on the vascularity of the region. Except for nitroglycerin and certain supplemental hormone replacements, topical medications are commonly used for local, rather than systemic, effects. Ointments have a fatty base, which is an ideal vehicle for such drugs as antimicrobials and antiseptics. Typically, topical medications should be applied two or three times a day to achieve their therapeutic effect.

Equipment

Patient's medication record and chart ■ prescribed medication ■ sterile tongue blades ■ gloves ■ 4″ × 4″ sterile gauze pads ■ transparent semipermeable dressing ■ adhesive tape ■ solvent (such as cottonseed oil).

Implementation

• Verify the order on the patient's medication record by checking it against the doctor's order on the chart.
• Make sure the label on the medication agrees with the medication order. Read the label again before you open the container and as you remove the medication from the container.
• Confirm the patient's identity by asking his name and checking the name, room number, and bed number on his wristband.
• Provide privacy.
• Explain the procedure thoroughly to the patient *because, after discharge, he may have to apply the medication by himself.*
• Wash your hands *to prevent cross-contamination,* and glove your dominant hand.
• Help the patient assume a comfortable position that provides access to the area to be treated.
• Expose the area to be treated. Make sure the skin or mucous membrane is intact (unless the medication has been ordered to treat a skin lesion, such as an ulcer). *Application of medication to broken or abraded skin may cause unwanted systemic absorption and result in further irritation.*
• If necessary, clean the skin of debris, including crusts, epidermal scales, and old medication. You may have to change the glove if it becomes soiled.

Applying a paste, a cream, or an ointment

• Open the container. Place the lid or cap upside down *to prevent contamination of the inside surface.*
• Remove a tongue blade from its sterile wrapper and cover one end with medication from the tube or jar. Then, transfer the medication from the tongue blade to your gloved hand.
• Apply the medication to the affected area with long, smooth strokes that follow the direction of hair growth. *This technique avoids forcing medication into hair follicles, which can cause irritation and lead to folliculitis.* Avoid excessive pressure when applying the medication *because it could abrade the skin.*

• *To prevent contamination of the medication,* use a new tongue blade each time you remove medication from the container.

Removing an ointment

• To remove ointment, wash your hands; then rub solvent on them and apply it liberally to the treated area in the direction of hair growth. Alternatively, saturate a sterile gauze pad with the solvent and use this pad to gently remove the ointment. Remove excess oil by gently wiping the area with the sterile gauze pad. Don't rub too hard to remove the medication *because you could irritate the skin.*

Applying other topical medications

• To apply *shampoos,* follow package directions. (See *Using medicated shampoos,* page 216.)
• To apply *aerosol sprays,* shake the container, if indicated, *to completely mix the medication.* Hold the container 6″ to 12″ (15 to 30 cm) from the skin or follow the manufacturer's recommendation. Spray the medication evenly over the treatment area *to apply a thin film.*
• To apply *powders,* dry the skin surface, making sure to spread skin folds where moisture collects. Then apply a thin layer of powder over the treatment area.
• *To protect applied medications and prevent them from soiling the patient's clothes,* tape an appropriate amount of sterile gauze pad or a transparent semipermeable dressing over the treated area. If you're applying topical medication to the patient's hands or feet, cover the site with white cotton gloves for the hands or terry cloth scuffs for the feet.
• Assess the patient's skin for signs of irritation, allergic reaction, or breakdown.

Special considerations

Never apply medication without first removing previous applications *to prevent skin irritation from an accumulation of medication.*

Be sure to wear gloves *to prevent absorption by your own skin.* If the patient has an infectious skin condition, use sterile gloves and dispose of old dressings according to your hospital's policy.

Don't apply ointments to mucous membranes as liberally as you would to skin *because mucous membranes are usually moist and absorb ointment more quickly than skin does.* Also, don't apply too much ointment to any skin area. *It may cause irritation and discomfort, stain clothing and bedding, and make removal difficult.*

Never apply ointment to the eyelids or ear canal unless ordered. *The ointment may congeal and occlude the tear duct or ear canal.*

Using medicated shampoos

Medicated shampoos include keratolytic and cytostatic agents, coal tar preparations, and lindane (gamma benzene hexachloride) solutions. They can be used to treat such conditions as dandruff, psoriasis, and head lice. However, they're contraindicated in patients with broken or abraded skin.

Since application instructions may vary among brands, check the label on the shampoo before starting the procedure *to ensure use of the correct amount.* Keep the shampoo away from the patient's eyes. If any shampoo should accidentally get in his eyes, irrigate promptly with water. Selenium sulfide, used in cytostatic agents, is extremely toxic if ingested.

To apply a medicated shampoo, follow these steps:
• Prepare the patient for shampoo treatment. (See "Hair care" in Chapter 1.)
• Shake the bottle of shampoo well *to mix the solution evenly.*
• Wet the patient's hair thoroughly and wring out excess water.
• Apply the proper amount of shampoo, as directed on the label.
• Work the shampoo into a lather, adding water as necessary. Part the hair and work the shampoo into the scalp, taking care not to use your fingernails.
• Leave the shampoo on the scalp and hair for as long as instructed (usually 5 to 10 minutes). Then rinse the hair thoroughly.
• Towel-dry the patient's hair.
• After the hair is dry, comb or brush it. Use a fine-tooth comb to remove nits if necessary.

Inspect the treated area frequently for adverse effects, such as signs of an allergic reaction.

Complications
Skin irritation, a rash, or an allergic reaction may occur.

Documentation
Record the medication applied, the time, date and site of application, and the condition of the patient's skin at the time of application. Note subsequent effects of the medication, if any.

 Transdermal drug administration

Through an adhesive disk or measured dose of ointment applied to the skin, transdermal drugs deliver constant, controlled medication directly into the bloodstream for prolonged systemic effect. Medications currently available in transdermal form include nitroglycerin, used to control angina; scopolamine, used to treat motion sickness; estradiol for postmenopausal hormone replacement; clonidine, used to treat hypertension; and fentanyl, a narcotic analgesic used to control chronic pain. Nitroglycerin ointment dilates coronary vessels for up to 4 hours; a nitroglycerin disk can produce the same effect for as long as 24 hours. The scopolamine disk can relieve motion sickness for as long as 72 hours; transdermal estradiol lasts for up to 1 week; clonidine lasts for 24 hours; and fentanyl lasts up to 72 hours.

Contraindications for transdermal application include skin allergies or skin reactions to the drug. Transdermal drugs should not be applied to broken or irritated skin because they would increase irritation, or to scarred or calloused skin, which may impair absorption.

Equipment
Patient's medication record and chart ▪ prescribed medication (disk or ointment) ▪ application strip or measuring paper (for nitroglycerin ointment) ▪ adhesive tape ▪ plastic wrap (optional for nitroglycerin ointment) or semipermeable dressing ▪ optional: gloves.

Implementation
• Verify the order on the patient's medication record by checking it against the doctor's order.
• Wash your hands and, if necessary, don gloves.
• Check the label on the medication *to make sure you'll be administering the correct drug in the correct dose.*
• Confirm the patient's identity by asking his name and checking the name, room number, and bed number on his wristband.
• Explain the procedure to the patient and provide privacy.

Applying transdermal ointment
• Place the prescribed amount of ointment on the application strip or measuring paper, taking care not to get any on your skin. (See *Applying nitroglycerin ointment.)*
• Apply the strip to any dry, hairless area of the body. Don't rub the ointment into the skin.
• Tape the application strip and ointment to the skin.
• If desired, cover the application strip with the plastic wrap, and tape the wrap in place.

Applying nitroglycerin ointment

Unlike most topical medications, nitroglycerin ointment is used for its transdermal *systemic* effect. It's used to dilate the veins and arteries, thus improving cardiac perfusion in a patient with cardiac ischemia or angina pectoris.

To apply nitroglycerin ointment, start by taking the patient's baseline blood pressure *so that you can compare it with later readings.* Gather your equipment. Nitroglycerin ointment, which is prescribed by the inch, comes with a rectangular piece of ruled paper, to be used in applying the medication. Squeeze the prescribed amount of ointment onto the ruled paper, as shown below. Put on gloves, if desired, *to avoid contact with the medication.*

shown below. (Some hospitals require you to use the paper to apply the medication to the patient's skin, usually on the chest or arm. Spread a thin layer of the ointment over a 3″ [7.6 cm] area.) For increased absorption, the doctor may request that you cover the site with plastic wrap or a transparent semipermeable dressing.

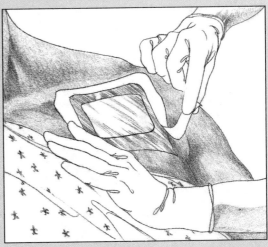

After 5 minutes, record the patient's blood pressure. If it has dropped significantly and he has a headache (from vasodilation of blood vessels in his head), notify the doctor immediately. He may reduce the dose. If the patient's blood pressure has dropped, but he has no symptoms, instruct him to lie still until it returns to normal.

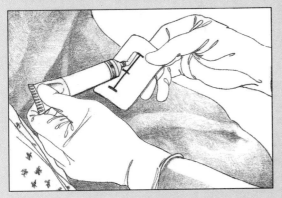

After measuring the correct amount of ointment, tape the paper—drug side down—directly to the skin, as

Applying a transdermal disk

• Open the package and remove the disk.
• Without touching the adhesive surface, remove the clear plastic backing.
• Apply the disk to a dry, hairless area—behind the ear, for example, as with scopolamine. (See *Applying a transdermal medication disk,* page 218.)

After applying transdermal medications

• Store the medication as ordered.
• Instruct the patient to keep the area around the disk or ointment as dry as possible.
• If you didn't wear gloves, wash your hands immediately after applying the disk or ointment *to avoid absorbing the drug yourself.*

Special considerations

Reapply daily transdermal medications at the same time every day *to ensure a continuous effect,* but alternate the application sites *to avoid skin irritation.* Before reapplying nitroglycerin ointment, remove the plastic wrap, application strip, and any remaining ointment from the patient's skin at the previous site.

When applying a scopolamine disk, instruct the patient not to drive or operate machinery until his response to the drug has been determined.

Warn a patient using clonidine disks to check with his doctor before using any over-the-counter cough preparations *because these may counteract the effects of the drug.*

Applying a transdermal medication disk

If the patient will be receiving medication by transdermal disk, instruct him in its proper use, as described below:
• Explain to the patient that the disk consists of several layers. The layer closest to his skin contains a small amount of the drug and allows prompt introduction of the drug into the bloodstream (as indicated by the dots). The next layer controls release of the drug from the main portion of the patch. The third layer contains the main dose of the drug. The outermost layer comprises an aluminized polyester barrier.
• Teach the patient to apply the disk to appropriate skin areas, such as on the upper arm or chest, or behind the ear. Warn him to avoid touching the gel or surrounding tape. Tell him to use a different site for each application to avoid skin irritation. If necessary, he can shave the site. Tell him to avoid any area that may cause uneven absorption, such as skin folds, scars, and calluses, or any irritated or damaged skin areas. Also, tell him not to apply the disk below the elbow or knee.
• Instruct the patient to wash his hands after application to remove any medication that may have rubbed off.
• Warn the patient not to get the disk wet. Tell him to discard the disk if it leaks or falls off, and then to clean the site and apply a new disk at a different site.
• Instruct the patient to apply the disk at the same time at the prescribed interval to ensure continuous drug delivery. Bedtime application is ideal because body movement is reduced during the night. Finally, tell him to apply a new disk about 30 minutes before removing the old one.

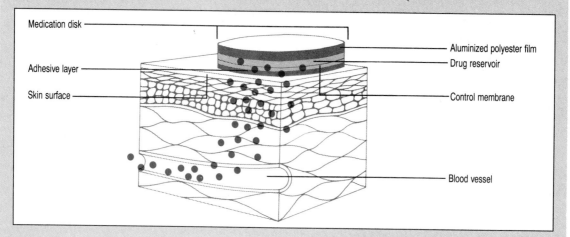

Complications

Skin irritation, such as pruritus or a rash, may occur. The patient may also suffer adverse effects of the drug administered. For example, transdermal nitroglycerin medications may cause headaches and, in elderly patients, postural hypotension. Scopolamine has various adverse effects; dry mouth and drowsiness are the most common. Transdermal estradiol carries an increased risk of endometrial cancer, thromboembolic disease, and birth defects. Clonidine may cause severe rebound hypertension, especially if withdrawn suddenly.

Documentation

Record the type of medication, the date, time, and site of application, and the dose. Also note any adverse effects and the patient's response.

 Application of eye medications

Eye medications—drops, ointments, and disks—serve diagnostic and therapeutic purposes. During an eye examination, eyedrops can be used to anesthetize the eye, dilate the pupil to facilitate examination, and stain the cornea to identify corneal abrasions, scars, or other anomalies. Eye medications can also be used to lubricate the eye, treat certain eye conditions (such as glaucoma and infections), protect the vision of neonates, and lubricate the eye socket for insertion of a prosthetic eye.

Understanding the ocular effects of medications is important because certain drugs may cause eye disorders or have serious ocular effects. For example, anticholinergics, which are often used during eye examinations, can precipitate acute glaucoma in patients with a predisposition to the disorder.

Equipment

Prescribed eye medication ■ patient's medication record and chart ■ sterile cotton balls ■ gloves ■ warm water or normal saline solution ■ sterile gauze pads ■ facial tissues ■ optional: ocular dressing.

Preparation of equipment

Make sure the medication is labeled for ophthalmic use. Then check the expiration date. Remember to date the container the first time you use the medication. After it's opened, an eye medication may be used for a maximum of 2 weeks *to avoid contamination.*

Inspect ocular solutions for cloudiness, discoloration, and precipitation, but remember that some eye medications are suspensions and normally appear cloudy. Don't use any solution that appears abnormal. If the tip of an eye ointment tube has crusted, turn the tip on a sterile gauze pad *to remove the crust.*

Implementation

• Verify the order on the patient's medication record by checking it against the doctor's order on his chart.
• Wash your hands.
• Check the medication label against the medication record.
• Make sure you know which eye to treat *because different medications or doses may be ordered for each eye.*
• Confirm the patient's identity by asking his name and checking the name, room number, and bed number on his wristband.
• Explain the procedure to the patient and provide privacy. Don gloves.
• If the patient is wearing an eye dressing, remove it by gently pulling it down and away from his forehead. Take care not to contaminate your hands.
• Remove any discharge by cleaning around the eye with sterile cotton balls or sterile gauze pads moistened with warm water or normal saline solution. With the patient's eye closed, clean from the inner canthus to the outer canthus, using a fresh sterile cotton ball or sterile gauze pad for each stroke.

• *To remove crusted secretions around the eye,* moisten a gauze pad with warm water or normal saline solution. Ask the patient to close the eye, and then place the gauze pad over it for a minute or two. Remove the pad, and then reapply moist sterile gauze pads, as necessary, until the secretions are soft enough to be removed without traumatizing the mucosa.
• Have the patient sit or lie in the supine position. Instruct him to tilt his head back and toward the side of the affected eye *so excess medication can flow away from the tear duct, minimizing systemic absorption through the nasal mucosa.*
• Remove the dropper cap from the medication container, if necessary, and draw the medication into it. Be careful to avoid contaminating the dropper tip or bottle top.
• Before instilling the eyedrops, instruct the patient to look up and away. *This moves the cornea away from the lower lid and minimizes the risk of touching the cornea with the dropper if the patient blinks.*

Instilling eyedrops

• You may steady the hand in which you're holding the dropper by resting it against the patient's forehead. Then, with your other hand, gently pull down the lower lid of the affected eye and instill the drops in the conjunctival sac. Try to avoid placing the drops directly on the eyeball. (See *Instilling eye medications,* page 220.)

Applying eye ointment

• Squeeze a small ribbon of medication on the edge of the conjunctival sac from the inner to the outer canthus. Cut off the ribbon by turning the tube. If you wish, you can steady the hand holding the medication tube by bracing it against the patient's forehead or cheek.

Using a medication disk

• A medication disk can release medication in the eye for up to 1 week. Pilocarpine, for example, can be administered this way to treat glaucoma. (For specific instructions, refer to *How to insert and remove an eye medication disk,* page 221.)

After instilling eyedrops or eye ointment

• Instruct the patient to close his eyes gently, without squeezing the lids shut. If you instilled drops, tell the patient to blink. If you applied ointment, tell him to roll his eyes behind closed lids *to help distribute the medication over the surface of the eyeball.*
• Use a clean tissue to remove any excess solution or ointment leaking from the eye. Use a fresh tissue for each eye *to prevent cross-contamination.*
• Apply a new eye dressing if necessary. (See "Hot and cold eye compresses" in Chapter 14.)

Instilling eye medications

To instill eyedrops, pull the lower lid down to expose the conjunctival sac. Have the patient look up and away, and squeeze the prescribed number of drops into the sac. Release the patient's eyelid and have him blink to distribute the medication.

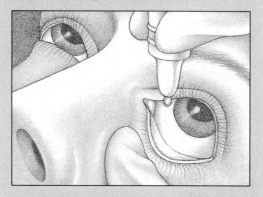

To apply an ointment, gently lay a thin strip of the medication along the conjunctival sac from the inner canthus to the outer canthus. Avoid touching the tip of the tube to the patient's eye. Then, release the eyelid and have the patient roll his eye behind closed lids to distribute the medication.

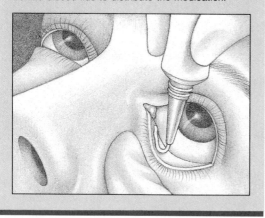

• Return the medication to the storage area. Make sure you store it according to the label's instructions.
• Wash your hands.

Special considerations
When administering an eye medication that may be absorbed systemically (such as atropine), gently press your thumb on the inner canthus for 1 to 2 minutes after instilling drops while the patient closes his eyes. *This helps prevent medication from flowing into the tear duct.*

To maintain the drug container's sterility, never touch the tip of the bottle or dropper to the patient's eyeball, lids, or lashes. Discard any solution remaining in the dropper before returning the dropper to the bottle. If the dropper or bottle tip has become contaminated, discard it and obtain another sterile dropper. *To avoid cross-contamination,* never use a container of eye medication for more than one patient.

Teach the patient to instill eye medications *so that he can continue treatment at home, if necessary.* Review the procedure and ask for a return demonstration.

Complications
Instillation of some eye medications may cause transient burning, itching, and redness. Rarely, systemic effects may also occur.

Documentation
Record the medication instilled or applied, the eye or eyes treated, and the date, time, and dose. Note any adverse effects and the patient's response.

 ## Instillation of eardrops

Eardrops may be instilled to treat infection and inflammation, to soften cerumen for later removal, to produce local anesthesia, or to facilitate removal of an insect trapped in the ear by immobilizing and smothering it. Instillation of ear drops is usually contraindicated if the patient has a perforated eardrum; however, it may be permitted with certain medications and adherence to sterile technique. Other conditions may also prohibit instillation of certain medications into the ear. For instance, instillation of drops containing hydrocortisone is contraindicated if the patient has herpes, another viral infection, or a fungal infection.

Equipment
Prescribed eardrops ▪ patient's medication record and chart ▪ light source ▪ facial tissue or cotton-tipped applicator ▪ optional: cotton ball, bowl of warm water.

How to insert and remove an eye medication disk

Small and flexible, the oval eye medication disk consists of three layers: two soft outer layers and a middle layer containing the medication. Floating between the eyelids and the sclera, the disk stays in the eye while the patient sleeps and even during swimming and athletic activities. The disk frees the patient from having to remember to instill his eyedrops. Once the disk is in place, ocular fluid moistens it, releasing the medication. Eye moisture or contact lenses don't adversely affect the disk. The disk can release medication for up to 1 week before needing replacement. Pilocarpine, for example, can be administered this way to treat glaucoma.

Contraindications include conjunctivitis, keratitis, retinal detachment, and any condition where constriction of the pupil should be avoided.

To insert an eye medication disk
Arrange to insert the disk before the patient goes to bed. *This minimizes the blurring that usually occurs immediately after disk insertion.*
• Wash your hands and don gloves.
• Press your fingertip against the oval disk so it lies lengthwise across your fingertip. It should stick to your finger. Lift the disk out of its packet.
• Gently pull the patient's lower eyelid away from the eye and place the disk in the conjunctival sac. It should lie horizontally, not vertically. The disk will adhere to the eye naturally.

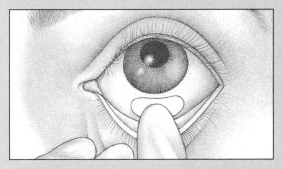

• Pull the lower eyelid out, up, and over the disk. Tell the patient to blink several times. If the disk is still visible, pull the lower lid out and over the disk again. Tell the patient that once the disk is in place, he can adjust its position by *gently* pressing his finger against his closed

lid. Caution him against rubbing his eye or moving the disk across the cornea.
• If the disk falls out, wash your hands, rinse the disk in cool water, and reinsert it. If the disk appears bent, replace it.
• If both of the patient's eyes are being treated with medication disks, replace both disks at the same time *so that both eyes receive medication at the same rate.*
• If the disk repeatedly slips out of position, reinsert it under the upper eyelid. To do this, gently lift and evert the upper eyelid and insert the disk in the conjunctival sac. Then, gently pull the lid back into position and tell the patient to blink several times. Again, the patient may press gently on the closed eyelid to reposition the disk. The more the patient uses the disk, the easier it should be for him to retain it. If he can't, notify the doctor.
• If the patient will continue therapy with an eye medication disk after discharge, teach him to insert and remove it himself. To check his mastery of these skills, have him demonstrate insertion and removal techniques for you.
• Also, teach the patient about possible adverse reactions. Foreign-body sensation in the eye, mild tearing or redness, increased mucous discharge, eyelid redness, and itchiness can occur with the use of disks. Blurred vision, stinging, swelling, and headaches can occur with pilocarpine, specifically. Mild symptoms are common but should subside within the first 6 weeks of use. Tell the patient to report persistent or severe symptoms to his doctor.

To remove an eye medication disk
• You can remove an eye medication disk with one or two fingers. To use one finger, put on gloves and evert the lower eyelid to expose the disk. Then use the forefinger of your other hand to slide the disk onto the lid and out of the patient's eye. To use two fingers, evert the lower lid with one hand to expose the disk. Then pinch the disk with the thumb and forefinger of your other hand and remove it from the eye.
• If the disk is located in the upper eyelid, apply long circular strokes to the patient's closed eyelid with your finger until you can see the disk in the corner of the patient's eye. Once the disk is visible, you can place your finger directly on the disk and move it to the lower sclera. Then remove it as you would a disk located in the lower lid.

Positioning the patient for eardrop instillation

Before instilling eardrops, have the patient lie on his side. Then straighten the patient's ear canal to help the medication reach the eardrum. In an adult, gently pull the auricle *up and back;* in an infant or young child, gently pull *down and back,* as shown here.

Adult

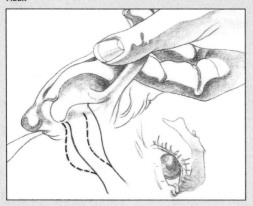

Child

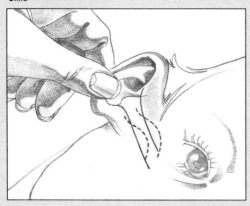

Preparation of equipment

Verify the order on the patient's medication record by checking it against the doctor's order.

To avoid adverse effects (such as vertigo, nausea, and pain) resulting from instillation of eardrops that are too cold, warm the medication to body temperature in the bowl of warm water or carry it in your pocket for 30 minutes before administration. If necessary, test the temperature of the medication by placing a drop on your wrist. *(If the medication is too hot, it may burn the patient's eardrum.)* Before using a glass dropper, make sure it's not chipped *to avoid injuring the ear canal.*

Implementation

• Wash your hands.
• Confirm the patient's identity by asking his name and checking the name, room number, and bed number on his wristband.
• Provide privacy if possible. Explain the procedure to the patient.
• Have the patient lie on the side opposite the affected ear.
• Straighten the patient's ear canal. For an adult, pull the auricle of the ear up and back. For an infant or child under age 3, gently pull the auricle down and back *because the ear canal is straighter at this age.* (See *Positioning the patient for eardrop instillation.)*
• Using a light source, examine the ear canal for drainage. If you find any, clean the canal with the tissue or cotton-tipped applicator *because drainage can reduce the medication's effectiveness.*
• Compare the label on the eardrops to the order on the patient's medication record. Check the label again while drawing the medication into the dropper. Check the label for the final time before returning the eardrops to the shelf or drawer.
• *To avoid damaging the ear canal with the dropper,* gently support the hand holding the dropper against the patient's head. Straighten the patient's ear canal once again and instill the ordered number of drops. *To avoid patient discomfort,* aim the dropper so that the drops fall against the sides of the ear canal, not on the eardrum. Hold the ear canal in position until you see the medication disappear down the canal. Then release the ear.
• Instruct the patient to remain on his side for 5 to 10 minutes *to allow the medication to run down into the ear canal.*
• If ordered, tuck the cotton ball loosely into the opening of the ear canal *to prevent the medication from leaking out.* Be careful not to insert it too deeply into the canal *because this would prevent drainage of secretions and increase pressure on the eardrum.*
• Clean and dry the outer ear.
• If ordered, repeat the procedure in the other ear after 5 to 10 minutes.
• Assist the patient into a comfortable position.
• Wash your hands.

Special considerations

Remember that some conditions make the normally tender ear canal even more sensitive, so be especially gentle when performing this procedure. Wash your hands before and after caring for the patient's ear and between caring for each ear.

To prevent injury to the eardrum, never insert a cotton-tipped applicator into the ear canal past the point where you can see the tip. After applying eardrops to soften cerumen, irrigate the ear as ordered *to facilitate its removal.*

If the patient has vertigo, keep the side rails of his bed up and assist him during the procedure, as necessary. Also, move slowly and unhurriedly *to avoid exacerbating his vertigo.*

Teach the patient to instill the eardrops correctly so that he can continue treatment at home, if necessary. Review the procedure and let the patient try it himself while you observe.

Documentation

Record the medication, the ear treated, and the date, time, and number of eardrops instilled. Also note any signs or symptoms that arise during the procedure, such as drainage, redness, vertigo, nausea, or pain.

Hand-held oropharyngeal inhalers

Hand-held inhalers include the metered-dose inhaler or nebulizer, the turbo-inhaler, and the nasal inhaler. These devices deliver topical medications to the respiratory tract, producing local and systemic effects. The mucosal lining of the respiratory tract absorbs the inhalant almost immediately. Examples of common inhalants are bronchodilators, used to improve airway patency and facilitate mucous drainage, and mucolytics, which attain a high local concentration to liquefy tenacious bronchial secretions.

These inhalers may be contraindicated in patients who can't form an airtight seal around the device, and in patients who lack the coordination or clear vision necessary to assemble a turbo-inhaler. Contraindications for specific inhalant drugs are also possible. For example, bronchodilators are contraindicated if the patient has tachycardia or a history of cardiac arrhythmias associated with tachycardia.

Equipment

Patient's medication record and chart ▪ metered-dose inhaler, turbo-inhaler, or nasal inhaler (see *Types of hand-held inhalers,* page 224) ▪ prescribed medication ▪ normal saline solution (or another appropriate solution) for gargling ▪ optional: emesis basin.

Implementation

● Verify the order on the patient's medication record by checking it against the doctor's order.
● Wash your hands.
● Check the label on the inhaler against the order on the medication record.
● Confirm the patient's identity by asking his name and by checking his name, room number, and bed number on his wristband.
● Explain the procedure to the patient.

Using a metered-dose inhaler

● Shake the inhaler bottle *to mix the medication and aerosol propellant.*
● Remove the mouthpiece and cap from the bottle.
● Insert the metal stem on the bottle into the small hole on the flattened portion of the mouthpiece. Then turn the bottle upside down.
● Have the patient exhale; then place the mouthpiece in his mouth and close his lips around it.
● As you firmly push the bottle down against the mouthpiece, instruct the patient to inhale slowly and to continue inhaling until his lungs feel full. *This action draws the medication into his lungs.* Compress the bottle against the mouthpiece only once.
● Remove the mouthpiece from the patient's mouth, and tell him to hold his breath for several seconds *to allow the medication to reach the alveoli.* Then instruct him to exhale slowly through pursed lips *to keep the distal bronchioles open, allowing increased absorption and diffusion of the drug and better gas exchange.*
● Have the patient gargle with normal saline solution, if desired, *to remove medication from the mouth and back of the throat.* (The lungs retain only about 10% of the inhalant; most of the remainder is exhaled, but substantial amounts may remain in the oropharynx.)
● Rinse the mouthpiece thoroughly with warm water *to prevent accumulation of residue.*

Using a turbo-inhaler

● Hold the mouthpiece in one hand, and with the other hand, slide the sleeve away from the mouthpiece as far as possible.
● Unscrew the tip of the mouthpiece by turning it counterclockwise.
● Firmly press the colored portion of the medication capsule into the propeller stem of the mouthpiece.
● Screw the inhaler together again securely.

Types of hand-held inhalers

These devices use air under pressure to produce a mist containing tiny droplets of medication. Drugs delivered in this form (such as mucolytics or bronchodilators) can travel deep into the lungs.

Nasal inhaler

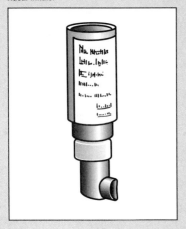

Metered-dose inhaler

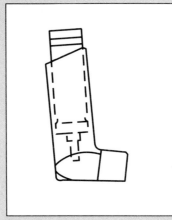

Turbo-inhaler with capsules

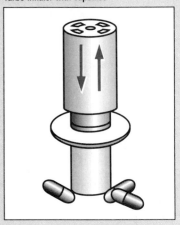

• Holding the inhaler with the mouthpiece at the bottom, slide the sleeve all the way down and then up again *to puncture the capsule and release the medication.* Do this only once.

• Have the patient exhale completely and tilt his head back. Then instruct him to place the mouthpiece in his mouth, close his lips around it, and inhale once — quickly and deeply — through the mouthpiece.

• Tell the patient to hold his breath for several seconds *to allow the medication to reach the alveoli.* (Instruct him not to exhale through the mouthpiece.)

• Remove the inhaler from the patient's mouth, and tell him to exhale as much air as possible.

• Repeat the procedure until all the medication in the device is inhaled.

• Have the patient gargle with normal saline solution, if desired, *to remove medication from the mouth and back of the throat.* Be sure to provide an emesis basin if the patient needs one.

• Discard the empty medication capsule, put the inhaler in its can, and secure the lid. Rinse the inhaler with warm water at least once a week.

Using a nasal inhaler
• Have the patient blow his nose *to clear his nostrils.*

• Shake the medication cartridge and then insert it in the adapter. (When inserting a refill cartridge, first remove the protective cap from the stem.)

• Remove the protective cap from the adapter tip.

• Hold the inhaler with your index finger on top of the cartridge and your thumb under the nasal adapter. The adapter tip should be pointing toward the patient.

• Have the patient tilt his head back. Then tell him to place the adapter tip into one nostril while occluding the other nostril with his finger.

• Instruct the patient to inhale gently as he presses the adapter and the cartridge together firmly *to release a measured dose of medication.* Be sure to follow the manufacturer's instructions. With some medications, such as dexamethasone sodium phosphate (Turbinaire), inhaling during administration is not desirable.

• Tell the patient to remove the inhaler from his nostril and to exhale through his mouth.

• Shake the inhaler, and have the patient repeat the procedure in the other nostril.

• Have the patient gargle with normal saline solution *to remove medication from the mouth and throat.*

• Remove the medication cartridge from the nasal inhaler, and wash the nasal adapter in lukewarm water.

Let the adapter dry thoroughly before reinserting the cartridge.

Special considerations

When using a turbo-inhaler or a nasal inhaler, make sure the pressurized cartridge isn't punctured or incinerated. Store the medication cartridge below 120° F (48.9° C).

Spacer inhalers may be recommended to provide greater therapeutic benefit for children or patients who have difficulty with coordination. A spacer attachment is an extension to the inhaler's mouthpiece that provides more dead-air space for mixing the medication. Some inhalers have built-in spacers.

If you're using a turbo-inhaler, keep the medication capsules wrapped until needed *to keep them from deteriorating.*

Teach the patient how to use the inhaler *so that he can continue treatments himself after discharge,* if necessary. Explain that overdosage — which is common — can cause the medication to lose its effectiveness. Tell him to record the date and time of each inhalation and his response *to prevent overdosage and to help the doctor determine the drug's effectiveness.* Also, note if the patient uses an unusual amount of medication — for example, more than one cartridge for a metered-dose nebulizer every 3 weeks. Inform the patient of possible adverse reactions.

Documentation

Record the inhalant administered, the dose, and the time. Note any significant change in the patient's heart rate after bronchodilation, and any other adverse reactions.

 Instillation of nasal medications

Nasal medications may be instilled by means of drops, a spray (using an atomizer), or an aerosol (using a nebulizer). Most drugs instilled by these methods produce local rather than systemic effects. Drops can be directed at a specific area; sprays and aerosols diffuse medication throughout the nasal passages.

Most nasal medications, such as phenylephrine, are vasoconstrictors, which relieve nasal congestion by coating and shrinking swollen mucous membranes. Because vasoconstrictors may be absorbed systemically, they are usually contraindicated in hypertensive patients. Other types of nasal medications include antiseptics, anesthetics, and corticosteroids. Local anesthetics may be administered to promote patient comfort during rhinolaryngologic examination, laryngoscopy, bronchoscopy, and endotracheal intubation. Corticosteroids reduce inflammation in allergic or inflammatory conditions and in nasal polyps.

Equipment

Prescribed medication ▪ patient's medication record and chart ▪ emesis basin (with nose drops only) ▪ facial tissues ▪ optional: pillow, small piece of soft rubber or plastic tubing, gloves.

Implementation

• Verify the order on the patient's medication record by checking it against the doctor's order. Note the concentration of the medication. Phenylephrine, for example, is available in various concentrations from 0.125% to 1%.
• Confirm the patient's identity by asking his name and checking the name, room number, and bed number on his wristband.
• Explain the procedure to the patient and provide privacy.
• Wash your hands. Don gloves if you notice any drainage from the nares.

Instilling nose drops

• When possible, position the patient so the drops flow back into the nostrils, toward the affected area. (See *Positioning the patient for nose drop instillation,* page 226.)
• Draw up some medication into the dropper.
• Push up the tip of the patient's nose slightly. Position the dropper just above the nostril, and direct its tip toward the midline of the nose *so the drops flow toward the back of the nasal cavity rather than down the throat.*
• Insert the dropper about ⅜" (1 cm) into the nostril. Make sure the dropper doesn't touch the sides of the nostril because *this would contaminate the dropper or could cause the patient to sneeze.*
• Instill the prescribed number of drops, observing the patient carefully for any signs of discomfort.
• *To prevent the drops from leaking out of the nostrils,* ask the patient to keep his head tilted back for at least 5 minutes and to breathe through his mouth. *This also allows sufficient time for the medication to constrict mucous membranes.*
• Keep an emesis basin handy *so the patient can expectorate any medication that flows into the oropharynx and mouth.* Use a facial tissue to wipe any excess medication from the patient's nostrils and face.
• Clean the dropper by separating the plunger and pipette and flushing them with warm water. Allow them to air-dry.

Using a nasal spray

• Have the patient sit upright with his head tilted back slightly. If this position is uncomfortable, have the patient

Positioning the patient for nose drop instillation

To reach the ethmoidal and sphenoidal sinuses, have the patient lie on his back with his neck hyperextended and his head tilted back over the edge of the bed. Support his head with one hand to prevent neck strain.

To reach the maxillary and frontal sinuses, have the patient lie on his back with his head toward the affected side and hanging slightly over the edge of the bed. Ask him to rotate his head laterally after hyperextension, and support his head with one hand to prevent neck strain.

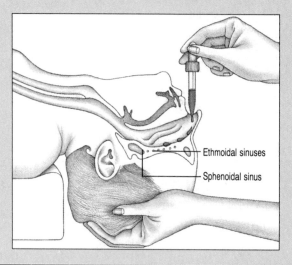

Ethmoidal sinuses

Sphenoidal sinus

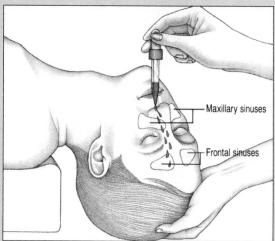

Maxillary sinuses

Frontal sinuses

lie on his back with his shoulders elevated, neck hyperextended, and head tilted back over the edge of the bed. Support his head with one hand *to prevent neck strain.*
• Remove the protective cap from the atomizer.
• *To prevent air from entering the nasal cavity and to allow the medication to flow in properly,* occlude one of the patient's nostrils with your finger. Insert the atomizer tip into the open nostril.
• Instruct the patient to inhale, and as he does so, squeeze the atomizer once, quickly and firmly. Use just enough force to coat the inside of the patient's nose with medication. Then tell the patient to exhale through his mouth.
• If ordered, spray the nostril again. Then repeat the procedure in the other nostril.
• Instruct the patient to keep his head tilted back for several minutes and to breathe slowly through his nose *so the medication has time to work.* Tell him not to blow his nose for several minutes.

Using a nasal aerosol
• Instruct the patient to blow his nose gently *to clear his nostrils.*

• Insert the medication cartridge according to the manufacturer's directions. With some models, you'll fit the medication cartridge over a small hole in the adapter. When inserting a refill cartridge, first remove the protective cap from the stem. Spacer inhalers may be recommended. (See "Hand-held oropharyngeal inhalers" in this chapter.)
• Shake the aerosol well immediately before each use, and remove the protective cap from the adapter tip.
• Hold the aerosol between your thumb and index finger with your index finger positioned on top of the medication cartridge.
• Tilt the patient's head back, and carefully insert the adapter tip in one nostril while sealing the other nostril with your finger.
• Press the adapter and cartridge together firmly *to release one measured dose of medication.*
• Shake the aerosol and repeat the procedure to instill medication into the other nostril.
• Remove the medication cartridge and wash the nasal adapter in lukewarm water daily. Allow the adapter to dry thoroughly before reinserting the cartridge.

To administer drops to relieve ordinary nasal congestion, help the patient to a reclining or supine position with his head tilted slightly toward the affected side. Aim the dropper upward, toward the patient's eye, rather than downward, toward his ear.

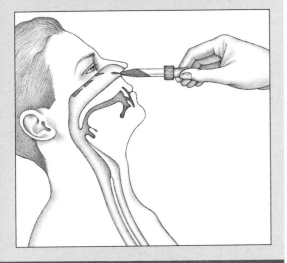

Special considerations

Before instilling nose drops in a young child or an uncooperative patient, attach a small piece of tubing to the end of the dropper *to avoid damaging mucous membranes.*

When using an aerosol, be careful not to puncture or incinerate the pressurized cartridge. Store it at temperatures below 120° F (48.9° C).

To prevent the spread of infection, label the medication bottle so that it will be used only for that patient.

Ideally, a nasal spray should be self-administered by the patient. Teach the patient how to instill nasal medications correctly *so he can continue treatment after discharge,* if necessary. Caution him against using nasal medications longer than prescribed *because they may cause a rebound effect that worsens the condition.* A rebound effect occurs when the medication loses its effectiveness and relaxes the vessels in the nasal turbinates, producing a stuffiness that can be relieved only by discontinuing the medication.

Inform the patient of possible adverse reactions. For example, explain that when receiving corticosteroids by aerosol therapy, therapeutic effects may not appear for 2 days to 2 weeks.

Complications

Some nasal medications may cause restlessness, palpitations, nervousness, and other systemic effects. For example, excessive use of corticosteroid aerosols may cause hyperadrenocorticism and adrenal suppression.

Documentation

Record the medication instilled and its concentration, the number of drops or instillations administered, and whether the medication was instilled in one or both nostrils. Also note the time, date, and any resulting adverse effects.

Insertion of vaginal medications

Vaginal medications include suppositories, creams, gels, and ointments. These medications can be inserted as topical treatment for infection (particularly *Trichomonas vaginalis* and monilial vaginitis) or inflammation, or as a contraceptive. Suppositories melt when they contact the vaginal mucosa, and their medication diffuses topically — as effectively as creams, gels, and ointments.

Vaginal medications usually come with a disposable applicator that enables placement of medication in the anterior and posterior fornices. Vaginal administration is most effective when the patient can remain lying down afterward to retain the medication.

Equipment

Patient's medication record and chart ■ prescribed medication and applicator, if necessary ■ gloves ■ water-soluble lubricant ■ small sanitary pad.

Implementation

• If possible, plan to give vaginal medications at bedtime, when the patient is recumbent.
• Verify the order on the patient's medication record by checking it against the doctor's order.
• Confirm the patient's identity by asking her name and checking the name, room number, and bed number on her wristband.
• Wash your hands, explain the procedure to the patient, and provide privacy.
• Ask the patient to void.
• Ask the patient if she would rather insert the medication herself. If so, provide appropriate instructions. If not, proceed with the following steps.
• Help her into the lithotomy position.
• Expose only the perineum.

How to insert a vaginal suppository

If the suppository is small, place it in the tip of an applicator. Then, lubricate the applicator, hold it by the cylinder, and insert it into the vagina. To ensure the patient's comfort, direct the applicator down initially (toward the spine), and then up and back (toward the cervix), as shown here. When the suppository reaches the distal end of the vagina, depress the plunger.

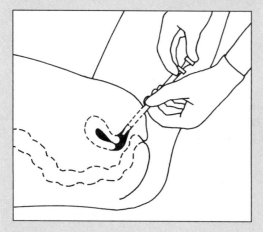

Remove the applicator while the plunger is still depressed.

Inserting a suppository
• Remove the suppository from the wrapper and lubricate it with water-soluble lubricant.
• Put on gloves and expose the vagina.
• With an applicator or the forefinger of your free hand, insert the suppository about 2″ (5 cm) into the vagina. (See *How to insert a vaginal suppository.*)

Inserting ointments, creams, or gels
• Insert the plunger into the applicator. Then fit the applicator to the tube of medication.
• Gently squeeze the tube to fill the applicator with the prescribed amount of medication. Lubricate the applicator.
• Put on gloves and expose the vagina.
• Insert the applicator as you would a small suppository and administer the medication by depressing the plunger on the applicator.

After vaginal insertion
• Remove and discard your gloves.
• Wash the applicator with soap and warm water and store it, unless it is disposable. If the applicator can be used again, label it *so it will be used only for the same patient.*
• *To prevent the medication from soiling the patient's clothing and bedding,* provide a sanitary pad.
• Help the patient return to a comfortable position, and advise her to remain in bed as much as possible for the next several hours.
• Wash your hands thoroughly.

Special considerations
Refrigerate vaginal suppositories that melt at room temperature. If possible, teach the patient how to insert vaginal medication. *She may have to administer it herself after discharge.* Give her a patient-teaching sheet if one is available. Instruct the patient not to wear a tampon after inserting vaginal medication *because it would absorb the medication and decrease its effectiveness.*

Complications
Vaginal medications may cause local irritation.

Documentation
Record the medication administered, the time, and the date. Note adverse effects and any other pertinent information.

 # *ENTERAL ADMINISTRATION*
Oral drug administration

Because oral administration of drugs is usually safest, most convenient, and least expensive, most drugs are commonly administered by this route. Drugs for oral administration are available in many forms: tablets, enteric-coated tablets, capsules, syrups, elixirs, oils, liquids, suspensions, powders, and granules. Some require special preparation before administration, such as mixing with juice to make them more palatable; oils, powders, and granules most often require such preparation.

Oral drugs are sometimes prescribed in higher dosages than their parenteral equivalents because, after absorption through the GI system, they are immediately broken down by the liver before they reach the systemic circulation. Oral administration is contraindicated for unconscious patients; it may also be contraindicated in patients with nausea and vomiting, and in those unable to swallow.

Equipment
Patient's medication record and chart ■ prescribed medication ■ medication cup ■ optional: appropriate vehicle, such as jelly or applesauce, for crushed pills commonly used with children or elderly patients and juice, water, or milk for liquid medications; drinking straw; mortar and pestle for crushing pills.

Implementation
• Verify the order on the patient's medication record by checking it against the doctor's order.
• Wash your hands.
• Check the label on the medication three times before administering it *to make sure you'll be giving the prescribed medication.* Check when you take the container from the shelf or drawer, again before you pour the medication into the medication cup, and again before returning the container to the shelf or drawer. If you're administering a unit-dose medication, check the label for the final time at the patient's bedside immediately after pouring the medication and before discarding the wrapper.
• Confirm the patient's identity by asking his name and checking the name, room number, and bed number on his wristband.
• Assess the patient's condition, including level of consciousness and vital signs, as needed. *Changes in the patient's condition may warrant withholding medication.* For example, you may need to withhold a medication that will slow the patient's heart rate if his apical pulse rate is below 60.
• Give the patient his medication and, as needed, an appropriate vehicle or liquid *to aid swallowing, minimize adverse effects, or promote absorption.* For example, cyclophosphamide is given with fluids to minimize adverse effects; antitussive cough syrup is given without a fluid to avoid diluting its soothing effect on the throat. If appropriate, crush the medication *to facilitate swallowing.*
• Stay with the patient until he has swallowed the drug. If he seems confused or disoriented, check his mouth *to make sure he has swallowed it.* Return and reassess the patient's response within 1 hour after giving the medication.

Special considerations
Make sure you have a written order for every medication given. Verbal orders should be signed by the doctor within the specified time period. (Hospitals usually require a signature within 24 hours; long-term care facilities, within 48 hours.)

Measuring liquid medications

To pour liquids, hold the medication cup at eye level. Use your thumb to mark off the correct level on the cup.

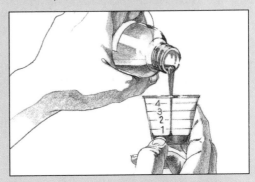

Then set the cup down and read the bottom of the meniscus at eye level *to ensure accuracy.* If you've poured too much medication into the cup, discard the excess. Don't return it to the bottle. Here are a few additional tips:
• Hold the container so that the medication flows from the side opposite the label *so it won't run down the container and stain or obscure the label.* Remove drips from the lip of the bottle first, then from the sides, using a clean, damp paper towel.
• For a liquid measured in drops, use only the dropper supplied with the medication.

Use care in measuring out the prescribed dose of liquid oral medication. (See *Measuring liquid medications.*)

Don't give medication from a poorly labeled or unlabeled container. Don't attempt to label or reinforce drug labels yourself. *This must be done by a pharmacist.*

Never give a medication poured by someone else. Never allow your medication cart or tray out of your sight. *This prevents anyone from rearranging the medications or taking one without your knowledge.* Never return unwrapped or prepared medications to stock containers. Instead, dispose of them and notify the pharmacy. Keep in mind that the disposal of any narcotic drug must be cosigned by another nurse, as mandated by law.

If the patient questions you about his medication or the dosage, check his medication record again. If the medication is correct, reassure him. Make sure you tell him about any changes in his medication or dosage. Instruct him, as appropriate, about possible adverse effects. Ask him to report anything that he feels may be an adverse effect.

To avoid damaging or staining the patient's teeth, give acid or iron preparations through a straw. An unpleasant-tasting liquid can usually be made more palatable if taken through a straw *because the liquid contacts fewer taste buds.*

Oral medications are relatively easy to give to infants *because of their natural sucking instinct and, in infants under 4 months, their undeveloped sense of taste.*

If the patient can't swallow a whole tablet or capsule, ask the pharmacist if the drug is available in liquid form or if it can be administered by another route. If not, ask him if you can crush the tablet or open the capsule and mix it with food. Keep in mind that many enteric-coated or time-release medications and gelatin capsules should not be crushed. Remember to contact the doctor for an order to change the route of administration when necessary.

Documentation

Note the drug administered, the dose, the date and time, and the patient's reaction, if any. If the patient refuses a drug, document the refusal and notify the charge nurse and the patient's doctor, as needed. Also note if a drug was omitted or withheld for other reasons, such as radiology or laboratory tests, or if, in your judgment, the drug was contraindicated at the ordered time. Sign out all narcotics given on the appropriate narcotics central record.

Instillation of drugs through a nasogastric tube

Besides providing an alternate means of nourishment, the nasogastric (NG) tube allows direct instillation of medication into the GI system of patients who can't ingest it orally. Before instillation, the patency and positioning of the tube must be carefully checked because this procedure is contraindicated if the tube is obstructed or improperly positioned or if the patient is vomiting around the tube or his bowel sounds are absent.

Oily medications and enteric-coated or sustained-release tablets are contraindicated for instillation through an NG tube. Oily medications cling to the sides of the tube and resist mixing with the irrigating solution. And crushing enteric-coated or sustained-release tablets to facilitate transport through the tube destroys their intended effect.

Equipment

Patient's medication record and chart ■ prescribed medication ■ towel or linen-saver pad ■ 50- or 60-ml piston type catheter-tip syringe ■ feeding tubing ■ two 4″×4″ gauze pads ■ stethoscope ■ gloves ■ diluent ■ cup for mixing medication and fluid ■ spoon ■ 50 ml of water ■ rubber band ■ gastrostomy tube and funnel, if needed ■ optional: pill-crushing equipment (mortar and pestle, for example), clamp (if not already attached to tube).

For maximum control of suction, use a piston syringe instead of a bulb syringe. The liquid for diluting the medication can be juice, water, or a nutritional supplement.

Preparation of equipment

Gather necessary equipment for use at the patient's bedside. Liquids should be at room temperature. *Administering cold liquid through the NG tube can cause abdominal cramping.* Although this is not a sterile procedure, make sure the cup, syringe, spoon, and gauze are clean.

Implementation

• Verify the order on the patient's medication record by checking it against the doctor's order.

• Wash your hands and don gloves.

• Check the label on the medication three times before preparing it for administration *to make sure you'll be giving the medication correctly.*

• If the prescribed medication is in tablet form, crush the tablets *to ready them for mixing in a cup with the diluting liquid.* Bring the medication and equipment to the patient's bedside.

• Explain the procedure to the patient, if necessary, and provide privacy.

• Confirm the patient's identity by asking his name and checking the name, room number, and bed number on his wristband.

• Unpin the tube from the patient's gown. *To avoid soiling the sheets during the procedure,* fold back the bed linens to the patient's waist and drape his chest with a towel or linen-saver pad.

• Elevate the head of the bed so the patient is in Fowler's position, as tolerated.

• After unclamping the tube, take the 50- or 60-ml syringe and create a 10-cc air space in its chamber. Then attach the syringe to the end of the tube.

• Auscultate the patient's abdomen about 3″ (7.6 cm) below the sternum with the stethoscope. Then, gently insert the 10 cc of air into the tube. You should hear the air bubble entering the stomach. If you hear this sound, gently draw back on the piston of the syringe. *The appearance of gastric contents implies that the tube is patent and in the stomach.* (However, only an X-ray positively confirms the tube's position.) If no gastric contents appear when you draw back on the piston of the syringe, the tube may have risen into the patient's esophagus, in which case you'll have to advance it before proceeding.

• If you meet resistance when aspirating for stomach contents, stop the procedure. *Resistance may indicate a nonpatent tube or improper tube placement.* (Keep in mind that some smaller NG tubes may collapse when aspiration is tried.) If the tube seems to be in the stomach, resistance probably means the tube is lying against the stomach wall. *To relieve resistance,* withdraw the tube slightly or turn the patient.

• After you have established that the tube is patent and in the correct position, clamp the tube, detach the syringe, and lay the end of the tube on the 4″ × 4″ gauze pad.

• Mix the crushed tablets with the diluent. If the medication is in capsule form, open the capsules and empty their contents into the liquid. Pour liquid medications directly into the diluting liquid. Stir well with the spoon. (If the medication was in tablet form, make sure the particles are small enough to pass through the eyes at the distal end of the tube.)

• Reattach the syringe, without the piston, to the end of the tube and open the clamp.

• Deliver the medication slowly and steadily. (See *Giving medications through an NG tube.*)

• If the medication flows smoothly, slowly add more until the entire dose has been given. If the medication doesn't flow properly, don't force it. It may be too thick to flow through the tube. If so, dilute it with water. If you suspect tube placement is inhibiting flow, stop the procedure and reevaluate the placement.

• Watch the patient's reaction throughout the instillation. If he shows any sign of discomfort, stop the procedure immediately.

• As the last of the medication flows out of the syringe, start to irrigate the tube by adding 30 to 50 ml of water. (If your patient is a child, use only 15 to 30 ml of water.) *Irrigation clears medication from the sides of the tube and from the distal end, reducing the risk of clogging.*

• When the water stops flowing, quickly clamp the tube. Detach the syringe and dispose of it properly.

• Fasten the NG tube to the patient's gown.

• Remove the towel or linen-saver pad and replace bed linens.

• Leave the patient in Fowler's position, or have him lie on his right side with the head of the bed partially elevated. Have him maintain this position for at least 30 minutes after the procedure *to facilitate the downward flow of medication into his stomach and prevent esophageal reflux.*

Giving medications through an NG tube

Holding the nasogastric (NG) tube at a level somewhat above the patient's nose, pour up to 30 ml of diluted medication into the syringe barrel. *To prevent air from entering the patient's stomach,* hold the tube at a slight angle and add more medication before the syringe empties. If necessary, raise the tube slightly higher to increase the flow rate.

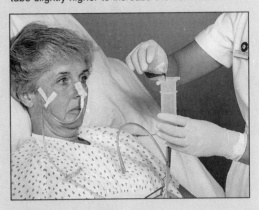

After you've delivered the whole dose, position the patient on her right side, head slightly elevated, *to minimize esophageal reflux.*

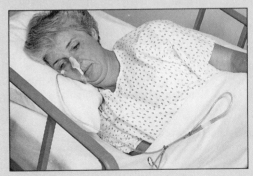

• You may be asked to deliver medications through a gastrostomy tube. (See *Giving medications through a gastrostomy tube,* page 232.) If medication is prescribed for a patient with a gastrostomy feeding button, ask the doctor to order the liquid form of the drug, if possible. If not, you may administer a tablet or capsule if it is dissolved in 30 to 50 ml of warm water (15 to 30 ml for children). To administer medication this way, use the

Giving medications through a gastrostomy tube

Surgically inserted into the stomach, a gastrostomy tube reduces the risk of fluid aspiration into the lungs, a constant danger with a nasogastric (NG) tube.

To administer medication by this route, prepare the patient and medication as you would for an NG tube. Then, gently lift the dressing around the tube *to assess the skin for irritation caused by gastric secretions.* Report any redness or irritation to the doctor. If no irritation appears, follow these steps:

• Remove the dressing that covers the tube. Then remove the dressing or plug at the tip of the tube and attach the syringe or funnel to the tip.

• Release the clamp and instill about 10 ml of water into the tube through the syringe *to check for patency.* If the water flows in easily, the tube is patent. If it flows in slowly, raise the funnel to increase pressure. If the water still doesn't flow properly, stop the procedure and notify the doctor.

• Pour up to 30 ml of medication into the syringe or funnel. Tilt the tube *to allow air to escape as the fluid flows downward.* Just before the syringe empties, add medication as needed.

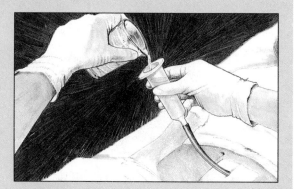

• After giving the medication, pour in about 30 ml of water *to irrigate the tube.*

• Tighten the clamp, place a 4″ × 4″ gauze pad on the end of the tube, and secure it with a rubber band.

• Cover the tube with two more 4″ × 4″ gauze pads, and secure them firmly with tape.

• Keep the head of the bed elevated for at least 30 minutes after the procedure *to aid digestion.*

---

same procedure as for feeding the patient through the button (see Chapter 10, Gastrointestinal care). Then draw up the dissolved medication into a syringe and inject it into the feeding tube.

• Next, withdraw the medication syringe and flush the tube with 50 ml of warm water. (For children, flush the tube with 30 ml.)

• Then replace the safety plug, and keep the patient upright at a 30-degree angle for 30 minutes after giving the medication.

Special considerations

To prevent instillation of too much fluid (more than 400 ml of liquid at one time for an adult), plan the drug instillation so that it doesn't coincide with the patient's regular tube feeding, if possible.

When you must schedule a tube feeding and medication instillation simultaneously, administer the medication first *to ensure that the patient receives the prescribed drug therapy even if he can't tolerate an entire feeding.* Remember to avoid giving the patient foods that interact adversely with the medication.

If the patient receives continuous tube feedings, stop the feeding and check the quantity of residual stomach

contents. If it's greater than 150 ml, withhold the medication and feeding and notify the doctor. *An excessive amount of residual contents may indicate intestinal obstruction or paralytic ileus.*

If the NG tube is attached to suction, be sure to turn off the suction for 20 to 30 minutes after administering medication.

If possible, teach the patient who requires long-term treatment to instill his medication himself through the NG tube. Have him observe you as you perform the procedure several times before you allow him to try it himself.

Be sure to remain with the patient when he performs the procedure for the first few times *so you can provide assistance and answer any questions.* As the patient performs the procedure, give him positive reinforcement and correct any errors in his technique, as necessary.

Documentation

Record the instillation of medication, the date and time of instillation, the dose, and the patient's tolerance of the procedure. On his intake and output sheet, note the amount of fluid instilled.

Buccal and sublingual drug administration

Certain drugs are given buccally or sublingually to prevent their destruction or transformation in the stomach or small intestine. These drugs act quickly because the oral mucosa's thin epithelium and abundant vasculature allow direct absorption into the bloodstream. Drugs given buccally include erythrityl tetranitrate and methyltestosterone; drugs given sublingually include ergotamine tartrate, erythrityl tetranitrate, isoproterenol hydrochloride, isosorbide dinitrate, and nitroglycerin. With this method, the patient must be observed carefully to ensure he doesn't swallow the drug or suffer mucosal irritation.

Equipment
Patient's medication record and chart ▪ prescribed medication ▪ medication cup.

Implementation
• Verify the order on the patient's medication record by checking it against the doctor's order on his chart.
• Wash your hands with warm water and soap. Explain the procedure to the patient if he's never taken a drug buccally or sublingually before.
• Check the label on the medication three times before administering it *to make sure you'll be giving the prescribed medication.* Check when you take the container from the shelf or drawer, right before pouring the medication into the medication cup, and before returning the container to the shelf or drawer. If you're administering a unit-dose medication, check the label for the third time immediately after pouring the medication and again before discarding the wrapper. (Remember: Don't open a unit-dose medication until you're at the patient's bedside.)
• Confirm the patient's identity by asking his name and checking the name and room and bed number on his wristband.
• For buccal administration, place the tablet in the buccal pouch, between the cheek and gum. For sublingual administration, place the tablet under the patient's tongue. (See *Placing drugs in the oral mucosa.*)
• Instruct the patient to keep the medication in place until it dissolves completely *to ensure absorption.*
• Caution him against chewing the tablet or touching it with his tongue *to prevent accidental swallowing.*
• Tell him not to smoke before the drug has dissolved *because nicotine's vasoconstrictive effects slow absorption.*

Placing drugs in the oral mucosa

Buccal and sublingual administration routes allow some drugs, such as nitroglycerin or methyltestosterone, to enter the bloodstream rapidly without being degraded in the GI tract. To give a drug sublingually, place it under the patient's tongue, as shown below, and ask him to leave it there until it's dissolved.

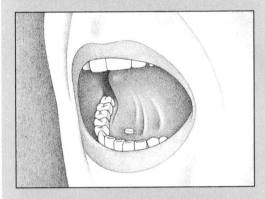

To give a drug buccally, insert it between the patient's cheek and teeth, as shown below. Ask him to close his mouth and hold the tablet against his cheek until the tablet is absorbed.

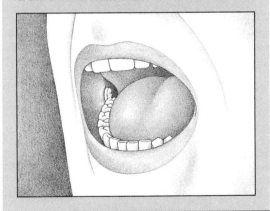

Special considerations
Don't give liquids *because some buccal tablets may take up to 1 hour to be absorbed.* In that case, the patient should rinse his mouth with water *between* doses. Tell the angina patient to wet the nitroglycerin tablet with saliva and keep it under the tongue until fully absorbed.

Complications

Some buccal medications may irritate the mucosa. Alternate sides of the mouth for repeat doses *to prevent continuous irritation of the same site.* Sublingual medications—erythrityl tetranitrate, for example—may cause a tingling sensation under the tongue. If the patient finds this annoying, try placing the drug in the buccal pouch instead.

Documentation

Record the medication administered, the dose, the date and time, and the patient's reaction, if any.

Administration of rectal suppositories or ointments

A rectal suppository is a small, solid, medicated mass, usually cone-shaped, with a cocoa butter or glycerin base. It may be inserted to stimulate peristalsis and defecation or to relieve pain, vomiting, and local irritation. Rectal suppositories commonly contain drugs that reduce fever, induce relaxation, interact poorly with digestive enzymes, or have a taste too offensive for oral use. Rectal suppositories melt at body temperature and are absorbed slowly.

Because insertion of a rectal suppository may stimulate the vagus nerve, this procedure is contraindicated in patients with potential cardiac arrhythmias. It may have to be avoided in patients with recent rectal or prostate surgery because of the risk of local trauma or discomfort during insertion.

An ointment is a semisolid medication used to produce local effects. It may be applied externally to the anus or internally to the rectum. Rectal ointments commonly contain drugs that reduce inflammation or relieve pain and itching.

Equipment

Rectal suppository or tube of ointment and ointment applicator ▪ patient's medication record and chart ▪ 4″ × 4″ gauze pads ▪ gloves ▪ water-soluble lubricant ▪ optional: bedpan.

Preparation of equipment

Store rectal suppositories in the refrigerator until needed *to prevent softening and possible decreased effectiveness of the medication.* A softened suppository is also difficult to handle and insert. To harden it again, hold the suppository (in its wrapper) under cold running water.

Implementation

● Verify the order on the patient's medication record by checking it against the doctor's order.
● Wash your hands with warm soap and water.
● Confirm the patient's identity by asking his name and checking the name, room number, and bed number on his wristband.
● Explain the procedure and the purpose of the medication to the patient.
● Provide privacy.

Inserting a rectal suppository

● Place the patient on his left side in Sims' position. Drape him with the bedcovers *to expose only the buttocks.*
● Put on gloves. Remove the suppository from its wrapper, and lubricate it with water-soluble lubricant.
● Lift the patient's upper buttock with your nondominant hand *to expose the anus.*
● Instruct the patient to take several deep breaths through his mouth *to help relax the anal sphincters and reduce anxiety or discomfort during insertion.*
● Using the index finger of your dominant hand, insert the suppository—tapered end first—about 3″ (7.6 cm), until you feel it pass the internal anal sphincter. Try to direct the tapered end toward the side of the rectum *so it contacts the membranes.* (See *How to administer a rectal suppository or ointment.)*
● Ensure the patient's comfort. Encourage him to lie quietly and, if applicable, to retain the suppository for the appropriate length of time. A suppository administered to relieve constipation should be retained as long as possible (at least 20 minutes) to be effective. Press on the anus with a gauze pad if necessary until the urge to defecate passes.
● Discard the used equipment.

Applying an ointment

● *To apply externally,* wear gloves or use a gauze pad to spread medication over the anal area.
● *To apply internally,* attach the applicator to the tube of ointment and coat the applicator with water-soluble lubricant.
● Expect to use approximately 1″ (2.5 cm) of ointment. *To gauge how much pressure to use during application,* try squeezing a small amount from the tube before you attach the applicator.
● Lift the patient's upper buttock with your nondominant hand *to expose the anus.*
● Instruct the patient to take several deep breaths through his mouth *to relax the anal sphincters and reduce anxiety or discomfort during insertion.*
● Gently insert the applicator, directing it toward the umbilicus.

• Slowly squeeze the tube *to eject the medication.*
• Remove the applicator and place a folded 4″ × 4″ gauze pad between the patient's buttocks to absorb excess ointment.
• Disassemble the tube and applicator. Recap the tube, and clean the applicator thoroughly with soap and warm water.

Special considerations

Because the intake of food and fluid stimulates peristalsis, a suppository for relieving constipation should be inserted about 30 minutes before mealtime *to help soften the feces in the rectum and facilitate defecation.* A medicated retention suppository should be inserted between meals.

Instruct the patient to avoid expelling the suppository. However, if he has difficulty retaining it, place him on a bedpan.

Make sure the patient's call button is handy and watch for his signal *because he may be unable to suppress the urge to defecate.* For example, a patient with proctitis has a highly sensitive rectum and may not be able to retain a suppository for long.

Be sure to inform the patient that the suppository may discolor his next bowel movement. Anusol suppositories, for example, can give feces a silver-gray pasty appearance.

Documentation

Record the administration time, the dose, and the patient's response.

*P*ARENTERAL ADMINISTRATION
Cartridge-injection system

A cartridge-injection system, such as the Tubex or Carpuject, is a convenient, easy-to-use method of injection that facilitates accuracy and sterility. The device consists of a plastic cartridge-holder syringe and a prefilled medication cartridge with needle attached.

The medication is premixed and premeasured, which saves time and helps ensure an exact dose. The medication remains sealed in the cartridge and sterile until the injection is administered

The disadvantage of this system is that not all drugs are available in cartridge form. However, compatible drugs can be added to partially filled cartridges.

How to administer a rectal suppository or ointment

When applying a suppository, direct its tapered end toward the side of the rectum so it contacts the membranes, encouraging absorption of the medication.

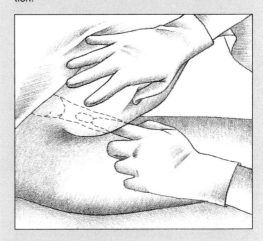

When applying an ointment, be sure to lubricate the applicator to minimize pain on insertion. Direct the applicator tip toward the patient's umbilicus.

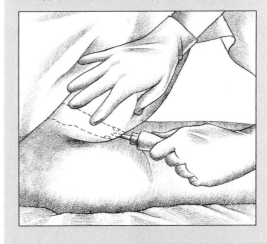

Equipment

Patient's medication record and chart ▪ plastic cartridge-holder syringe ▪ medication-filled cartridge-needle unit ▪ alcohol sponge ▪ additional medication, if prescribed.

The 2-ml Carpuject-type syringe can be adapted to fit a 1-ml cartridge. Plastic syringes can be used with cartridges of any size.

Implementation

• Verify the order on the patient's medication record by checking it against the doctor's order.
• Wash your hands.

Using a Tubex system

• Hold the base of the unit and pull the plunger back. Place the medication cartridge inside the barrel of the unit. Then secure the cartridge by turning the plunger clockwise while holding the barrel. Finally, lock the barrel in place by turning it clockwise.
• Explain the procedure to the patient and provide privacy.
• Remove the needle guard just before the injection. A popping sound indicates that the seal was secure. Expel any air bubbles from the syringe cartridge and administer the medication, as prescribed.
• After the injection, don't resheath the needle *to avoid needle-stick injuries.* Remove the medication cartridge by unscrewing the plunger and barrel and removing the cartridge from the barrel. Discard the cartridge in an appropriate sharps container.

Using a plastic syringe (Carpuject)

• Make sure the medication and dose are correct before loading the syringe.
• Grasp the barrel of the syringe with the open side facing you and pull back the plunger as far as possible.
• Disengage the locking screw by turning it counterclockwise.
• Insert the cartridge-needle unit — needle end first — into the open side of the syringe. Advance and engage the locking screw, and turn it clockwise beyond its initial resistance until it will no longer rotate.
• Advance the plunger rod and screw it clockwise onto the threaded insert in the rubber plunger.
• Remove the needle guard, expel excess air from the cartridge, and administer the injection.
• After the injection, don't resheath the needle *to avoid needle-stick injuries.* Disengage the plunger rod from the plunger by rotating it counterclockwise and pulling it back as far as possible, taking care not to touch the needle.
• Disengage the locking screw by rotating it counterclockwise. Turn the syringe over, and allow the cartridge

to drop out of the holder. Discard the unit in an appropriate sharps container.

Adding a compatible medication to a partially filled cartridge

• Hold the cartridge with the needle end up. Remove the sheath and pull back the plunger rod so the surface of the rubber piston in contact with the medication is set at the mark equal to the combined medication volume.
• Wipe the diaphragm of the vial containing the compatible medication with an alcohol sponge.
• Insert the needle into the single-dose vial. Depress the plunger rod to inject into the vial an amount of air equal to the prescribed amount of medication to be withdrawn from the vial. Pull the rod back *to withdraw the medication.*
• Remove the needle from the vial, expel excess air, and replace the needle guard.
• Proceed to the patient's room to give the injection. Discard the equipment in an appropriate sharps container.

Special considerations

To use a 2-ml syringe holder with a 1-ml cartridge-needle unit, insert a 1-ml cartridge-needle unit into the syringe, engage it in the usual manner, and proceed with the injection. Disengage the cartridge-needle unit and discard it.

Before combining drugs in a cartridge, check appropriate sources for incompatibilities and contraindications. After mixing the drugs, check again for signs of incompatibility, such as discoloration and precipitation. If combining drugs involves the use of a multidose vial, you may want to use a separate needle and syringe to inject air *to prevent contaminating the vial with the cartridge medication.* If combining drugs involves the use of an ampule, you don't have to inject air into it *because an ampule doesn't contain a vacuum.*

Empty cartridges can be obtained and used for medications not readily available in the prefilled cartridge form.

Never use a cartridge-needle unit for successive injections or as a multidose container. Discard the unit after one injection.

To maintain sterility, keep the rubber sheath or needle guard in place until just before the injection.

For patients in isolation, disposable syringes are recommended instead of the cartridge-injection system. If the cartridge-injection system is used under such circumstances, the syringe holder should be kept in the patient's room and must be cleaned properly before it's removed from the room. Once removed from the room, it should be sterilized before being used for other patients or discarded.

Documentation

Record the medications administered, the injection site, and the time of administration. Describe any subsequent effects of the medications.

 Admixture of drugs in a syringe

Combining two drugs in one syringe avoids the discomfort of two separate injections. Usually, drugs can be mixed in a syringe in one of four ways. They may be combined from two multidose vials (as, for example, regular and long-acting insulin), from one multidose vial and one ampule, from two ampules, or from a cartridge-injection system combined with either a multidose vial or ampule.

Such combinations are contraindicated when the drugs aren't compatible, and when the combined doses exceed the amount of solution that can be absorbed from a single injection site.

Equipment

Prescribed medications ■ patient's medication record and chart ■ alcohol sponges ■ syringe and needle ■ optional: cartridge-injection system and filter needle.

The type and size of the syringe and needle depend on the prescribed medications, the patient's body build, and the route of administration.

Medications that come in prefilled cartridges require a cartridge-injection system. (See "Cartridge-injection system" in this chapter.)

Implementation

• Verify that the drugs to be administered agree with the patient's medication record and the doctor's orders.
• Calculate the dose to be given.
• Wash your hands.

To mix drugs from two multidose vials

• Using an alcohol sponge, wipe the rubber stopper on the first vial. *This decreases the risk of contaminating the medication as you insert the needle into the vial.*
• Pull back the syringe plunger until the volume of air drawn into the syringe equals the volume to be withdrawn from the drug vial.
• Without inverting the vial, insert the needle into the top of the vial, making sure that the needle's bevel tip doesn't touch the solution. Inject the air into the vial and withdraw the needle. *This replaces air in the vial to prevent creation of a partial vacuum when the drug is withdrawn.*

• Repeat the above steps for the second vial. Then, after injecting the air into the second vial, invert the vial, withdraw the prescribed dose, and then withdraw the needle.
• Wipe the rubber stopper of the first vial again and insert the needle, taking care not to depress the plunger. Invert the vial, withdraw the prescribed dose, and then withdraw the needle.

To mix drugs from a multidose vial and an ampule

• Using an alcohol sponge, clean the vial's rubber stopper.
• Pull back on the syringe plunger until the volume of air drawn into the syringe equals the volume to be withdrawn from the drug vial.
• Insert the needle into the top of the vial and inject the air. Then invert the vial and withdraw the prescribed dose. Put the sterile needle cover over the needle.
• Wrap the ampule's neck with a piece of sterile gauze or an alcohol sponge *to protect yourself from injury in case the glass splinters.* Break open the ampule, directing the force away from you.
• If desired, switch to the filter needle at this point *to filter out any glass splinters.*
• Insert the needle into the ampule. Be careful not to touch the outside of the ampule with the needle. Draw the correct dose into the syringe.
• If you switched to the filter needle, change back to a regular needle to administer the injection.

To mix drugs from two ampules

• An opened ampule doesn't contain a vacuum. To mix drugs from two ampules in a syringe, calculate the prescribed doses and open both ampules, using aseptic technique. If desired, use a filter needle to draw up the drugs. Then change to a regular needle to administer them.

Special considerations

Insert a needle through the vial's rubber stopper at a slight angle, bevel up, and exert slight lateral pressure. *This way you won't cut a piece of rubber out of the stopper, which can then be pushed into the vial.*

When mixing drugs from multidose vials, be careful not to contaminate one drug with the other. Ideally, the needle should be changed after drawing the first medication into the syringe. This isn't always possible *because many disposable syringes do not have removable needles.*

♦ *Nursing alert.* Never combine drugs if you are unsure of their compatibility, and never combine more than two drugs. (See *Combining drugs in a syringe: A compatibility guide,* page 238.) Although drug incompatibility usually causes a visible reaction, such as clouding, bubbling, or precipitation, some incompatible combinations produce no visible reaction even though they alter the chemical na-

Combining drugs in a syringe: A compatibility guide

	atropine	butorphanol	chlorpromazine	codeine	diazepam	glycopyrrolate	hydromorphone	hydroxyzine	meperidine	morphine	nalbuphine	pentobarbital	phenobarbital	promethazine	scopolamine	secobarbital	sodium bicarbonate	thiopental	
atropine	■	Y	Y		N	Y	Y	Y	Y	P	Y	P		P	P				atropine
butorphanol	Y	■	Y		N			Y	P	Y		N		Y	Y				butorphanol
chlorpromazine	Y	Y	■		N	Y	Y	P	P	P		N		P	P			N	chlorpromazine
codeine				■	N	Y		Y											codeine
diazepam	N	N	N	N	■	N	N	N	N	N	N	N	N	N	N	N	N	N	diazepam
glycopyrrolate	Y		Y	Y	N	■	Y	Y	Y	Y		N		Y	Y	N	N	N	glycopyrrolate
hydromorphone	Y		Y		N	Y	■	Y				Y		Y	Y				hydromorphone
hydroxyzine	Y	Y	P	Y	N	Y	Y	■	P	Y	Y	N		P	Y				hydroxyzine
meperidine	Y	P	P		N	Y		P	■	N		N		Y	P			N	meperidine
morphine	P	Y	P		N	Y		Y	N	■		N?		P?	P			N	morphine
nalbuphine	Y				N			Y			■	N		Y	Y				nalbuphine
pentobarbital	P	N	N		N	N	Y	N	N	N?	N	■		N	Y	Y		Y	pentobarbital
phenobarbital					N								■						phenobarbital
promethazine	P	Y	P		N	Y	Y	P	Y	P?	Y	N		■	P			N	promethazine
scopolamine	P	Y	P		N	Y	Y	Y	P	P	Y	Y		P	■			Y	scopolamine
secobarbital					N	N										■			secobarbital
sodium bicarbonate					N	N					Y						■	N	sodium bicarbonate
thiopental			N		N	N			N	N		Y		N	Y		N	■	thiopental

KEY

Y Compatible

N Not compatible

P Provisionally compatible: use within 15 minutes of preparation

? Conflicting reports on compatibility; mixing not recommended

(A blank space indicates no available data on compatibility.)

ture and action of the drugs. Check appropriate references and a pharmacist when you are unsure about specific compatibility. When in doubt, administer two separate injections. ◆

Some medications are compatible for only a brief time after being combined and should be administered within 10 minutes after mixing. After this time, environmental factors — such as temperature, exposure to light, and humidity — may alter compatibility.

To reduce the risk of contamination, most hospitals dispense parenteral medications in single-dose vials. Insulin is one of the few drugs still packaged in multidose vials. Be careful when mixing regular and long-acting insulin. Draw up the regular insulin first *to avoid contamination by the long-acting suspension. (If a minute amount of the regular insulin is accidentally mixed with the long-acting insulin, it won't appreciably change the effect of the long-acting insulin.)* Check your hospital's policy before mixing insulins.

When you combine a cartridge-injection system and a multidose vial, use a separate needle and syringe to inject air into the multidose vial. *This prevents possible contamination of the multidose vial by the cartridge-injection system.*

Documentation

Record the drugs administered, the injection site, and the time of administration. Document adverse drug effects or other pertinent information.

 Subcutaneous injection

When injected into the adipose (fatty) tissues beneath the skin, a drug moves into the bloodstream more rapidly than if given by mouth. Subcutaneous injection allows slower, more sustained drug administration than intramuscular injection; it also causes minimal tissue trauma and carries little risk of striking large blood vessels and nerves.

Absorbed mainly through the capillaries, drugs recommended for subcutaneous injection include nonirritating aqueous solutions and suspensions contained in 0.5 to 2.0 ml of fluid. Heparin and insulin, for example, are usually administered subcutaneously.

Drugs and solutions for subcutaneous injection are injected through a relatively short needle, using meticulous sterile technique. The most common subcutaneous injection sites are the outer aspect of the upper arm, anterior thigh, loose tissue of the lower abdomen, buttocks, and upper back. Injection is contraindicated in sites that are inflamed, edematous, scarred, or covered by a mole, birthmark, or other lesion. It may also be contraindicated in patients with impaired coagulation mechanisms.

Equipment

Prescribed medication ■ patient's medication record and chart ■ needle of appropriate gauge and length ■ gloves ■ 1- to 3-ml syringe ■ alcohol sponges ■ optional: antiseptic cleaning agent, filter needle, insulin syringe, insulin pump.

Preparation of equipment

Verify the order on the patient's medication record by checking it against the doctor's order.

Inspect the medication *to make sure it's not abnormally discolored or cloudy and that it doesn't contain precipitates.*

Wash your hands. Select a needle of the proper gauge and length. An average adult patient requires a 25G ⅝″ needle; an infant, a child, or an elderly or thin patient, a 25G to 27G ½″ needle.

Remember to check the label on the medication against the medication record. Read the label again as you draw up the medication for injection.

For single-dose ampules: Wrap the ampule's neck in an alcohol sponge and snap off the top, directing the force away from your body. If desired, attach a filter needle to the needle and withdraw the medication. Tap the syringe *to clear air from it.* Cover the needle with the needle sheath.

Before discarding the ampule, check the label against the patient's medication record.

Discard the filter needle and the ampule. Attach the appropriate needle to the syringe.

For single-dose or multidose vials: Reconstitute powdered drugs according to the label's instructions. Make sure that all crystals have dissolved in the solution. Warming the vial by holding it and rolling it between your palms may help to dissolve the drug more quickly.

Clean the vial's rubber stopper with an alcohol sponge. Pull the syringe plunger back until the volume of air in the syringe equals the volume of drug to be withdrawn from the vial.

Insert the needle into the vial. Inject the air, invert the vial, and keep the needle's bevel tip below the level of the solution as you withdraw the prescribed amount of medication. Cover the needle with the needle sheath. Tap the syringe *to clear any air from it.*

Check the drug label against the patient's medication record before returning the multidose vial to the shelf or drawer or before discarding the single-dose vial.

Locating subcutaneous injection sites

Subcutaneous injection sites (shown by dotted areas) include the fat pads on the abdomen, upper hips, upper back, and lateral upper arms and thighs. For subcutaneous injections administered repeatedly, such as insulin, rotate sites. Choose one injection site in one area, move to a corresponding injection site in the next area, and so on. When returning to an area, choose a new site in that area. Preferred injection sites for insulin are the arms, abdomen, thighs and buttocks. Preferred injection sites for heparin injections are in the lower abdominal fat pad just below the umbilicus.

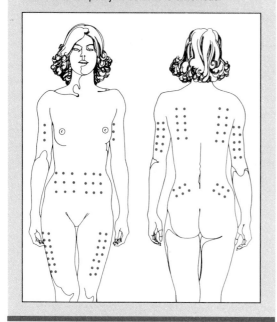

Implementation
• Confirm the patient's identity by asking his name and checking the name, room number, and bed number on his wristband.
• Explain the procedure to the patient and provide privacy.
• Select an appropriate injection site. (See *Locating subcutaneous injection sites.*) Rotate sites according to a schedule for patients who require repeated injections. Use different areas of the body unless contraindicated by the specific drug. (Heparin, for example, should be injected only in certain sites.)

• Put on gloves.
• Position and drape the patient if necessary.
• Clean the injection site with an alcohol sponge, beginning at the center of the site and moving outward in a circular motion. Allow the skin to dry before injecting the drug *to avoid a stinging sensation from introducing alcohol into subcutaneous tissues.*
• Loosen the protective needle sheath.
• With your nondominant hand, grasp the skin around the injection site firmly to elevate the subcutaneous tissue, forming a 1″ (2.5-cm) fat fold.
• Holding the syringe in your dominant hand, insert the loosened needle sheath between the fourth and fifth fingers of your other hand while still pinching the skin around the injection site. Pull back the syringe with your dominant hand *to uncover the needle by grasping the syringe like a pencil.* Don't touch the needle.
• Position the needle with its bevel up.
• Tell the patient he'll feel a prick as the needle is inserted.
• Insert the needle quickly in one motion. (See *Technique for subcutaneous injections.*) Release the patient's skin *to avoid injecting the drug into compressed tissue and irritating nerve fibers.*
• Pull back the plunger slightly *to check for blood return.* If none appears, begin injecting the drug slowly. If blood appears upon aspiration, withdraw the needle, prepare another syringe, and repeat the procedure.
• Don't aspirate for blood return when giving insulin or heparin. *It's not necessary with insulin and may cause a hematoma with heparin.*
• After injection, remove the needle gently but quickly at the same angle used for insertion.
• Cover the site with an alcohol sponge, and massage the site gently (unless you have injected a drug that contraindicates massage, such as heparin or insulin) *to distribute the drug and facilitate absorption.*
• Remove the alcohol sponge and check the injection site for bleeding or bruising.
• Dispose of injection equipment according to hospital policy. *To avoid needle-stick injuries,* don't resheath the needle.

Special considerations
If the medication is available in prefilled syringes, adjust the angle and depth of insertion according to needle length.

For insulin injections
To establish more consistent blood insulin levels, rotate insulin injection sites within anatomic regions. Absorption varies from one region to another. Preferred insulin

injection sites are the arms, abdomen, thighs, and buttocks.

Make sure the type of insulin, unit dosage, and syringe are correct.

When combining insulins in a syringe, make sure they are compatible. Regular insulin can be mixed with all other types. Prompt insulin zinc suspension (Semilente insulin) cannot be mixed with NPH insulin. Follow hospital policy regarding which insulin to draw up first.

Before drawing up insulin suspension, gently roll and invert the bottle to ensure even drug particle distribution. Don't shake the bottle *because this can cause foam or bubbles to develop in the syringe.*

Some patients may benefit from an insulin infusion pump. (See *Types of insulin infusion pumps,* page 242.)

For heparin injections
The preferred site for heparin injection is the lower abdominal fat pad, 2″ (5 cm) beneath the umbilicus, between the right and the left iliac crests. *Injecting heparin into this area, which isn't involved in muscular activity, reduces the risk of local capillary bleeding.* Always rotate the sites from one side to the other.

Don't administer any injections within 2″ of a scar, a bruise, or the umbilicus.

Don't aspirate to check for blood return *because this may cause bleeding into the tissues at the site.*

Don't rub or massage the site after the injection. *Rubbing can cause localized minute hemorrhages or bruises.*

If the patient bruises easily, apply ice to the site for the first 5 minutes after the injection *to minimize local hemorrhage,* then apply pressure.

Complications
Concentrated or irritating solutions may cause formation of sterile abscesses. Repeated injections in the same site can cause lipodystrophy. A natural immune response, this complication can be minimized by rotating injection sites.

Documentation
Record the time and date of the injection, the medication administered and the dose, the injection site and route, and the patient's reaction to the medication.

Intradermal injection

Used primarily for diagnostic purposes, as in allergy or tuberculin testing, intradermal injections are administered in small amounts, usually 0.5 ml or less, into the

Technique for subcutaneous injections

Before giving the injection, elevate the subcutaneous tissue at the site by grasping it firmly.

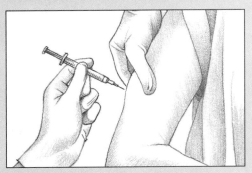

Insert the needle at a 45- or 90-degree angle to the skin surface, depending upon needle length and the amount of subcutaneous tissue at the site. Some medications, such as heparin, should always be injected at a 90-degree angle.

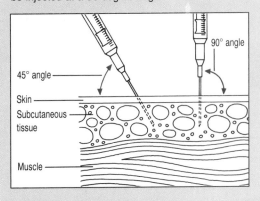

outer layers of the skin. Because little systemic absorption of intradermally injected agents takes place, this type of injection is used primarily to produce a local effect.

The ventral forearm is the most commonly used site for intradermal injection because of its easy accessibility and lack of hair. In extensive allergy testing, the outer aspect of the upper arms may be used, as well as the area of the back located between the scapulae (see *Intradermal injection sites,* page 243.)

Types of insulin infusion pumps

A continuous subcutaneous insulin infusion pump provides long-term insulin therapy for patients with insulin-dependent diabetes mellitus. Complications include infection at the injection site, catheter clogging, and insulin loss from loose reservoir-catheter connections. Insulin pumps work on either a closed-loop or an open-loop system.

Open-loop system
The open-loop pump is used most commonly. It infuses insulin but can't respond to blood glucose changes. These portable, self-contained, programmable insulin pumps are smaller and less obtrusive than ever — about the size of a credit card — and have fewer buttons.

The pump delivers insulin in small (basal) doses every few minutes and large (bolus) doses that the patient sets manually. The system consists of a reservoir containing the insulin syringe, a small pump, an infusion-rate selector that allows insulin release adjustments, a battery, and a plastic catheter with an attached needle leading from the syringe to the subcutaneous injection site. The needle is typically held in place with waterproof tape. The patient can wear the pump on his belt or in his pocket — practically anywhere as long as the infusion line has a clear path to the injection site.

The infusion-rate selector automatically releases about half the total daily insulin requirement. The patient releases the remainder in bolus amounts before meals and snacks. The patient must change the syringe daily; he must change the needle, catheter, and injection site every other day.

Closed-loop system
The self-contained closed-loop system detects and responds to changing blood glucose levels. The typical closed-loop system includes a glucose sensor, a programmable computer, a power supply, a pump, and an insulin reservoir. The computer triggers continuous insulin delivery in appropriate amounts from the reservoir.

Nonneedle catheter system
In an alternate, nonneedle delivery system, a tiny plastic catheter is inserted into the skin over a needle. The needle is then withdrawn, leaving the catheter in place. This pump can be placed in the abdomen, thigh, or flank and should be changed every 2 or 3 days.

Open-loop infusion pump

Close-up of the pump

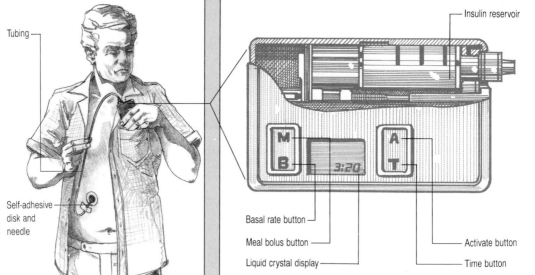

Tubing

Self-adhesive disk and needle

Insulin reservoir

Basal rate button

Meal bolus button

Liquid crystal display

Activate button

Time button

Equipment

Patient's medication record and chart ▪ tuberculin syringe with a 26G or 27G ½″ to ⅝″ needle ▪ prescribed medication ▪ gloves ▪ alcohol sponges.

Implementation

- Verify the patient's identity by checking his name, room number, and bed number on his wristband against his medical record.
- Tell him where you will be giving the injection.
- Instruct the patient to sit up and to extend his arm and support it on a flat surface, with the ventral forearm exposed.
- Put on gloves.
- With an alcohol sponge, clean the surface of the ventral forearm about two or three fingerbreadths distal to the antecubital space. Be sure the test site you have chosen is free of hair or blemishes. Allow the skin to dry completely before administering the injection.
- While holding the patient's forearm in your hand, stretch the skin taut with your thumb.
- With your free hand, hold the needle at a 15-degree angle to the patient's arm, with its bevel up.
- Insert the needle about ⅛″ below the epidermis at sites 2″ (5 cm) apart. Stop when the needle's bevel tip is under the skin, and inject the antigen slowly. You should feel some resistance as you do this, and a wheal should form as you inject the antigen. (See *Giving an intradermal injection,* page 244.) If no wheal forms, you have injected the antigen too deeply; withdraw the needle and administer another test dose at least 2″ (5 cm) from the first site.
- Withdraw the needle at the same angle at which it was inserted. Do not rub the site. *This could irritate the underlying tissue, which may affect test results.*
- Circle each test site with a marking pen, and label each site according to the recall antigen given. Instruct the patient to refrain from washing off the circles until the test is completed.
- Dispose of needles and syringes according to hospital policy.
- Remove and discard your gloves.
- Assess the patient's response to the skin testing in 24 to 48 hours.

Special considerations

In patients hypersensitive to the test antigens, a severe anaphylactic response can result. This requires immediate epinephrine injection and other emergency resuscitation procedures. Be especially alert after giving a test dose of penicillin or tetanus antitoxin.

Intradermal injection sites

The most common intradermal injection site is the ventral forearm. Other sites (indicated by dotted areas) include the upper chest, upper arm, and shoulder blades. Skin in these areas is usually lightly pigmented, thinly keratinized, and relatively hairless, facilitating detection of adverse reactions.

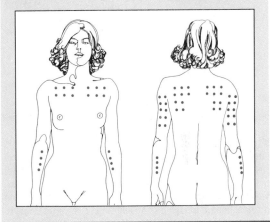

Documentation

Record the type and amount of medication given on the patient's medication record. Also record the time given and the location of the injection site. Note any skin reactions as well as any other adverse reactions.

 Intramuscular injection

Intramuscular (I.M.) injections deposit medication deep into muscle tissue, which is well-vascularized and can absorb it quickly. This route of administration provides rapid systemic action and absorption of relatively large doses (up to 5 ml in appropriate sites). I.M. injections are recommended for patients who are uncooperative or can't take medication orally and for drugs that are altered by digestive juices. Because muscle tissue has few sensory nerves, I.M. injection allows less painful administration of irritating drugs.

The site for an I.M. injection must be chosen carefully, taking into account the patient's general physical status and the purpose of the injection. I.M. injections should not be administered at inflamed, edematous, or irritated

Giving an intradermal injection

Secure the forearm. Insert the needle at a 10- to 15-degree angle so it just punctures skin surface. When injected, the drug should raise a small wheal.

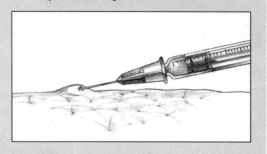

sites or at those containing moles, birthmarks, scar tissue, or other lesions. I.M. injections may also be contraindicated in patients with impaired coagulation mechanisms, and in patients with occlusive peripheral vascular disease, edema, and shock, because these conditions impair peripheral absorption. I.M. injections require sterile technique to maintain the integrity of muscle tissue.

Oral or I.V. routes are preferred for administration of drugs that are poorly absorbed by muscle tissue, such as phenytoin, digoxin, chlordiazepoxide, diazepam, and haloperidol.

Equipment

Patient's medication record and chart ▪ prescribed medication ▪ diluent or filter needle, if needed ▪ 3- to 5-ml syringe ▪ 20G to 25G 1″ to 3″ needle ▪ gloves ▪ alcohol sponges.

The prescribed medication must be sterile. The needle may be packaged separately or already attached to the syringe. Needles used for I.M. injections are longer than subcutaneous needles *because they must reach deep into the muscle.* Needle length also depends on the injection site, the patient's size, and the amount of subcutaneous fat covering the muscle. The needle gauge for I.M. injections should be larger to accommodate viscous solutions and suspensions.

Preparation of equipment

Verify the order on the patient's medication record by checking it against the doctor's order. Also note if the patient has any allergies, especially before the first dose.

Check the prescribed medication for color and clarity. Also note the expiration date. Never use medication that is cloudy or discolored or that contains a precipitate unless the manufacturer's instructions allow it. Remember also that for some drugs (such as suspensions) the presence of drug particles is normal. Observe for any abnormal changes. If in doubt, check with the pharmacist.

Choose equipment appropriate to the prescribed medication and injection site and make sure it works properly. The needle should be straight, smooth, and free of burrs.

Wipe the stopper of the medication vial with an alcohol sponge, and then draw up the prescribed amount of medication using the three-label check system — read the label as you select the medication, as you draw up the medication, and after you have completed drawing up the medication *to verify the correct dosage.*

Then draw about 0.2 cc of air into the syringe according to hospital policy. When the syringe is inverted during the injection, the air bubble rises to the plunger end of the syringe and follows the medication into the injection site. *The air clears the needle of medication and helps prevent leakage into the subcutaneous tissue following injection by creating an air block that reduces reflux (tracking) along the needle path.*

Gather all necessary equipment and proceed to the patient's room.

Implementation

• Confirm the patient's identity by asking his name and checking his wristband for name, room number, and bed number.

• Provide privacy and explain the procedure to the patient.

• Wash your hands.

• Select an appropriate injection site. The gluteal muscles (gluteus medius and minimus and the upper outer corner of the gluteus maximus) are used most commonly for healthy adults, although the deltoid muscle may be used for a small-volume injection (2 ml or less). For infants and children, the vastus lateralis muscle of the thigh is used most often *because it's usually the best developed and contains no large nerves or blood vessels, minimizing the risk of serious injury.* The rectus femoris muscle may also be used in infants but is usually contraindicated in adults. Remember to always rotate injection sites for patients who require repeated injections.

• Position and drape the patient appropriately, making sure the site is well-exposed and that lighting is adequate.

• Loosen the protective needle sheath, but don't remove it.

• After selecting the injection site, gently tap it *to stimulate nerve endings and minimize pain when the needle is inserted.* (See *Locating I.M. injection sites,* page 246.) Then clean the skin at the site with an alcohol sponge. Move the sponge outward in a circular motion to a circumference of about 2″ (5 cm) from the injection site. Then allow the skin to dry *to avoid introducing alcohol into the needle puncture, which causes pain.* Keep the alcohol sponge for later use.

• Don gloves. With the thumb and index finger of your nondominant hand, gently stretch the skin of the injection site taut.

• Holding the syringe in your dominant hand, remove the needle sheath by slipping it between the free fingers of your nondominant hand and then drawing back the syringe.

• Position the syringe at a 90-degree angle to the skin surface, with the needle a couple of inches from the skin. Tell the patient that he will feel a prick as you insert the needle. Then quickly and firmly thrust the needle through the skin and subcutaneous tissue, deep into the muscle.

• Support the syringe with your nondominant hand, if desired. Pull back slightly on the plunger with your dominant hand to aspirate for blood. If no blood appears, place your thumb on the plunger rod and *slowly* inject the medication into the muscle. *A slow, steady injection rate allows the muscle to distend gradually and accept the medication under minimal pressure.* You should feel little or no resistance against the force of the injection. The air bubble in the syringe should follow the medication into the injection site.

♦ *Nursing alert.* If blood appears in the syringe on aspiration, the needle is in a blood vessel. If this occurs, stop the injection, withdraw the needle, prepare another injection with new equipment, and inject another site. Don't inject the bloody solution. ♦

• After the injection, gently but quickly remove the needle at a 90-degree angle.

• Using a gloved hand, cover the injection site immediately with the used alcohol sponge, apply gentle pressure, and unless contraindicated, massage the relaxed muscle *to help distribute the drug and promote absorption.*

• Remove the alcohol sponge and inspect the injection site for signs of active bleeding or bruising. If bleeding continues, apply pressure to the site; if bruising occurs, you may apply ice.

• Watch for adverse reactions at the site for 30 minutes after the injection.

• Discard all equipment according to universal precautions and your hospital's policy. Don't attempt to recap needles; dispose of them in an appropriate sharps container *to avoid needle-stick injuries.*

Special considerations

To slow absorption, some drugs for I.M. administration are dissolved in oil or other special solutions. Mix these preparations well before drawing them into the syringe.

Never use the gluteal muscles (which develop from repeated walking) as the injection site for a child under age 3 or who has been walking for less than a year. Never inject into sensitive muscles, especially those that twitch or tremble when you assess site landmarks and tissue depth with your fingertips. *Injections in these trigger areas may cause sharp or referred pain, such as the pain caused by nerve trauma.*

Keep a rotation record that lists all available injection sites, divided into various body areas, for patients who require repeated injections. Rotate from a site in the first area to a site in each of the other areas. Then return to a site in the first area that is at least 1″ (2.5 cm) away from the previous injection site in that area.

If the patient has experienced pain or emotional trauma from repeated injections, consider numbing the area before cleaning it by holding ice on it for several seconds. If you must inject more than 5 ml of solution, divide the solution and inject it at two separate sites.

Always encourage the patient to relax the muscle you'll be injecting *because injections into tense muscles are more painful than usual and may bleed more readily.*

I.M. injections can damage local muscle cells, causing elevated serum enzyme levels (creatine phosphokinase, [CPK]) that can be confused with the elevated enzymes resulting from damage to cardiac muscle, as in myocardial infarction. To distinguish between skeletal and cardiac muscle damage, diagnostic tests for suspected myocardial infarction must identify the isoenzyme of CPK specific to cardiac muscle (CPK-MB [CPK_2]) and include tests for lactate dehydrogenase (LDH) and aspartate aminotransferase (AST), formerly SGOT. If it's important to measure these enzyme levels, suggest that the doctor switch to I.V. administration, with dosages adjusted accordingly.

Complications

Accidental injection of concentrated or irritating medications into subcutaneous tissue, or into other areas where it can't be fully absorbed, can cause sterile abscesses to develop. Such abscesses result from a natural immune response in which phagocytes attempt to remove the foreign matter.

Failure to rotate sites in patients who require repeated injections can lead to deposits of unabsorbed medications. Such deposits can reduce the desired pharmacologic effect and may lead to abscess formation or tissue fibrosis.

Locating I.M. injection sites

Deltoid

First find the lower edge of the acromial process and the point on the lateral arm in line with the axilla. Insert the needle 1" to 2" (2.5 to 5 cm) below the acromial process, usually two to three fingerbreadths, at a 90-degree angle or angled slightly toward the process. Typical injection: 0.5 ml (range: 0.5 to 2 ml).

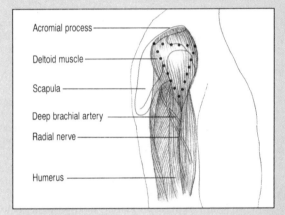

Dorsogluteal

Inject above and outside a line drawn from the posterior superior iliac spine to the greater trochanter of the femur. Or divide the buttock into quadrants and inject in the upper outer quadrant, about 2" to 3" (5 to 7.6 cm) below the iliac crest. Insert the needle at a 90-degree angle. Typical injection: 1 to 4 ml (range: 1 to 5 ml).

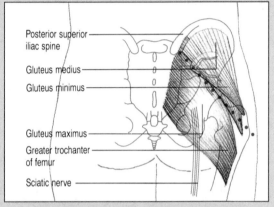

Ventrogluteal

First, locate the greater trochanter of the femur with the heel of your hand. Then, spread your index and middle fingers from the anterior superior iliac spine to as far along the iliac crest as you can reach. Insert the needle between the two fingers at a 90-degree angle to the muscle. (Remove your hand before inserting the needle.) Typical injection: 1 to 4 ml (range: 1 to 5 ml).

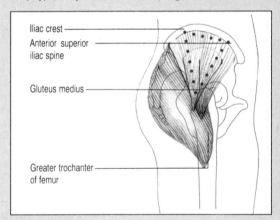

Vastus lateralis

Use the lateral muscle of the quadriceps group, from a handbreadth below the greater trochanter to a handbreadth above the knee. Insert the needle into the middle third of the muscle parallel to the surface on which the patient is lying. You may have to bunch the muscle before insertion. Typical injection: 1 to 4 ml (range: 1 to 5 ml; 1 to 3 ml for infants).

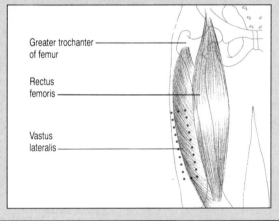

Documentation
Chart the drug administered, dose, date, time, route of administration, and injection site. Also, note the patient's tolerance of injection and its effects, including any adverse effects.

Z-track injection

This method of intramuscular injection prevents leakage, or tracking, into the subcutaneous tissue. Typically, it's used to administer drugs that irritate and discolor subcutaneous tissue, primarily iron preparations, such as iron dextran. It may also be used in elderly patients who have decreased muscle mass. Lateral displacement of the skin during the injection helps to seal the drug in the muscle.

This procedure requires careful attention to technique because leakage into subcutaneous tissue can cause patient discomfort and may permanently stain some tissues.

Equipment
Patient's medication record and chart ▪ two 20G 1¼" to 2" needles ▪ prescribed medication ▪ gloves ▪ 3- to 5-ml syringe ▪ two alcohol sponges.

Preparation of equipment
Verify the order on the patient's medication record by checking it against the doctor's order. Wash your hands. Make sure the needle you're using is long enough to reach the muscle. As a rule of thumb, a 200-pound patient requires a 2" needle; a 100-pound patient, a 1¼" to 1½" needle. Attach one needle to the syringe and draw up the prescribed medication. Then draw 0.2 to 0.5 cc of air (depending on hospital policy) into the syringe. Remove the first needle and attach the second *to prevent tracking the medication through the subcutaneous tissue as the needle is inserted.*

Implementation
• Confirm the patient's identity, explain the procedure, and provide privacy.
• Place the patient in the lateral position, exposing the gluteal muscle to be used as the injection site. The patient may also be placed in the prone position.
• Clean an area on the upper outer quadrant of the patient's buttock with an alcohol sponge.
• Don gloves. Then displace the skin laterally by pulling it away from the injection site. (See *Displacing the skin for Z-track injection*, page 248.)

• Insert the needle into the muscle at a 90-degree angle.
• Aspirate for blood return; if none appears, inject the drug slowly, followed by the air. *Injecting air after the drug helps clear the needle and prevents tracking the medication through subcutaneous tissues as the needle is withdrawn.*
• Wait 10 seconds before withdrawing the needle *to ensure dispersion of the medication.*
• Withdraw the needle slowly. Then release the displaced skin and subcutaneous tissue *to seal the needle track.* Don't massage the injection site or allow the patient to wear a tight-fitting garment over the site *because it could force the medication into subcutaneous tissue.*
• Encourage the patient to walk or to move about in bed *to facilitate absorption of the drug from the injection site.*
• Discard the needles and syringe in an appropriate sharps container. Do not recap needles *to avoid needlestick injuries.*
• Remove and discard your gloves.

Special considerations
Never inject more than 5 ml of solution into a single site using the Z-track method. Alternate gluteal sites for repeat injections.

If the patient is on bed rest, encourage active range-of-motion (ROM) exercises or perform passive ROM exercises *to facilitate absorption from the injection site.*

Complications
Discomfort and tissue irritation may result from drug leakage into subcutaneous tissue.

Documentation
Record the medication, dosage, date, time, and site of injection on the patient's medication record. Include the patient's response to the injected drug.

Intraosseous infusion

When rapid venous infusion is difficult or impossible, intraosseous infusion allows delivery of fluids, medications, or whole blood into the bone marrow. Performed on infants and children, this technique is used in such emergencies as cardiopulmonary arrest or circulatory collapse, hypokalemia from traumatic injury or dehydration, status epilepticus, status asthmaticus, burns, near-drowning, and overwhelming sepsis.

Any drug that can be given I.V. can be given by intraosseous infusion; drug absorption and effectiveness are comparable to the I.V. route. Intraosseous infusion

Displacing the skin for Z-track injection

By blocking the needle pathway after injection, this technique allows I.M. injection while minimizing the risk of subcutaneous irritation and staining from such drugs as iron dextran. The illustrations below show how to perform a Z-track injection.

Before the procedure begins, the skin, subcutaneous fat, and muscle lie in their normal positions.

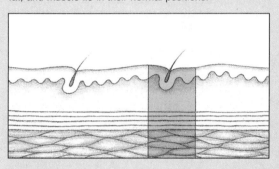

To begin, place your finger on the skin surface, and pull the skin and subcutaneous layers out of alignment with the underlying muscle. You should move the skin about ½" (1 cm).

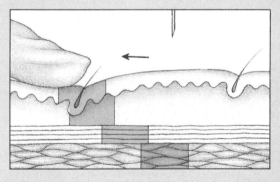

Insert the needle at a 90-degree angle in the site where you initially placed your finger. Inject the drug and withdraw the needle.

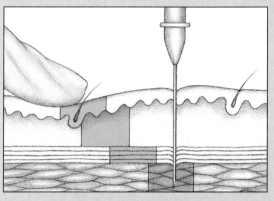

Finally, remove your finger from the skin surface, allowing the layers to return to their normal positions. The needle track (shown by the dotted line) is now broken at the junction of each tissue layer, trapping the drug in the muscle.

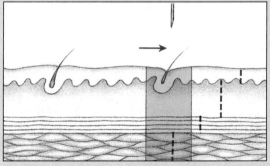

has been used as an acceptable alternative for infants and children.

Intraosseous infusion is commonly undertaken at the anterior surface of the tibia. Alternate sites include the iliac crest, spinous process, or (rarely) the upper anterior portion of the sternum. Only personnel trained in this procedure should perform it. Usually, a nurse will assist. (See *Understanding intraosseous infusion.*)

This procedure is contraindicated in osteogenesis imperfecta, osteopetrosis, and ipsilateral fracture, because of the potential for subcutaneous extravasation. Infusion through an area with cellulitis or an infected burn increases the risk of infection.

Equipment
Bone marrow biopsy needle or specially designed intraosseous infusion needle (cannula and obturator) ■ povidone-iodine sponges ■ sterile gauze pads ■ sterile gloves ■ sterile drape ■ bone marrow set ■ heparinized saline

flush solution ▪ I.V. fluids and tubing ▪ 1% lidocaine ▪ 3- to 5-ml syringe.

Preparation of equipment
Prepare I.V. fluids and tubing, as ordered.

Implementation
• If the patient is conscious, explain the procedure *to allay his fears and promote his cooperation.* Ensure that the patient or a responsible family member understands the procedure and signs a consent form.
• Check the patient's history for hypersensitivity to the local anesthetic. If the patient isn't an infant, tell him which bone site will be infused. Inform him that he will receive a local anesthetic and will feel pressure from needle insertion.
• Provide a sedative, if ordered, before the procedure.
• Position the patient based on the selected puncture site.
• Using sterile technique, clean the puncture site with a povidone-iodine sponge and allow it to dry. Then cover the area with a sterile drape.
• Using sterile technique, hand the doctor the 3- to 5-ml syringe with 1% lidocaine *so that he may anesthetize the infusion site.*
• The doctor inserts the cannula and obturator through the skin and into the bone at an angle of 10 to 15 degrees from vertical. He advances it with a to-and-fro rotary motion through the periosteum until the needle penetrates the marrow cavity. The needle should "give" suddenly as it enters the marrow and should stand erect when released.
• Then the doctor removes the obturator from the needle and attaches a 5-ml syringe. He aspirates some bone marrow *to confirm needle placement.*
• The doctor replaces this syringe with a syringe containing 5 ml of heparinized saline flush solution and flushes the cannula *to confirm needle placement and clear the cannula of clots or bone particles.*
• Next, the doctor removes the syringe of flush solution and attaches I.V. tubing to the cannula *to allow infusion of medications and I.V. fluids.*
• Put on sterile gloves.
• Clean the infusion site with povidone-iodine sponges, and then secure the site with tape and a sterile gauze dressing.
• Monitor vital signs and check the infusion site for bleeding, extravasation, and postinfusion infection.

Special considerations
Intraosseous infusion should be discontinued as soon as conventional vascular access is established (within 2 to 4 hours, if possible). *Prolonged infusion significantly increases the risk of infection.*

Understanding intraosseous infusion

During intraosseous infusion, the bone marrow serves as a noncollapsible vein; thus, fluid infused into the marrow cavity rapidly enters the circulation via an extensive network of venous sinusoids. Here, the needle is shown positioned in the patient's tibia.

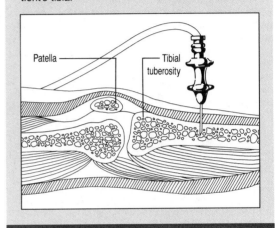

After needle removal, place a sterile dressing over the injection site, and apply firm pressure to the site for 5 minutes.

Intraosseous flow rates are determined by needle size and flow through the bone marrow. Fluids should flow freely if needle placement is correct. Normal saline solution has been administered intraosseously at a rate of 600 ml/minute and up to 2,500 ml/hour when delivered under pressure of 300 mm Hg through a 13G needle.

Complications
Common complications of intraosseous infusion include extravasation of fluid into subcutaneous tissue, resulting from incorrect needle placement; subperiosteal effusion, resulting from failure of fluid to enter the marrow space; and clotting in the needle, resulting from delayed infusion or failure to flush the needle after placement. Other complications include subcutaneous abscess, osteomyelitis, and epiphyseal injury.

Documentation
Record the time, date, location, and the patient's tolerance of the procedure. Document the amount of fluid infused on the input and output record.

Intra-articular injection

An intra-articular injection delivers drugs directly to the synovial cavity of a joint to relieve pain, help preserve function, prevent contractures, and delay muscle atrophy. Drugs commonly administered intra-articularly include corticosteroids, anesthetics, and lubricants. Rarely, antiseptics, analgesics, and counterirritants may be injected by this route. Before intra-articular injection, synovial fluid may be withdrawn to relieve pressure or to be tested in the laboratory.

Usually performed by a doctor with a nurse assisting, intra-articular injection requires sterile technique. It's contraindicated in patients with joint infection, joint instability or fracture, or systemic fungal infection.

Equipment

Patient's medication record and chart ▪ 3-ml and 5- or 10-ml syringes ▪ labels ▪ prescribed medication ▪ sterile towel, gloves, cotton balls, and gauze pads ▪ pillows ▪ sterile emesis basin ▪ antiseptic cleaning agent ▪ sterile fenestrated drape ▪ local anesthetic ▪ 25G ⅝″ needle ▪ 18G 1½″ needle ▪ adhesive bandage ▪ optional: sterile test tubes for synovial fluid aspiration, with appropriate additives and specimen labels, and 10- or 20-ml syringe for aspirating synovial fluid specimen.

Sterile povidone-iodine sponges may be used instead of the antiseptic cleaning agent and the sterile cotton balls or gauze pads.

Preparation of equipment

Verify the order on the patient's medication record by checking it against the doctor's order. Wash your hands. Draw the prescribed amount of medication into the 5- or 10-ml syringe before entering the patient's room. Label the syringe with the name of the medication and the amount. Take the container from which you drew the medication with you *so the doctor can verify the syringe contents.*

Implementation

• Confirm the patient's identity, explain the procedure to him, and provide privacy.
• Position the patient comfortably. The joint to be injected should be stabilized, supported (with pillows, if necessary), and fully exposed. (See *Locating intra-articular injection sites.)*
• Using aseptic technique, open the sterile towel and place it on the bedside stand *to create a sterile field.*
• Using aseptic technique, open the syringes, needles, and cotton balls or gauze pads and drop them onto the sterile field.
• After putting on sterile gloves, the doctor picks up sterile cotton balls or gauze pads and holds them over the emesis basin.
• Pour the antiseptic cleaning agent over the cotton balls or gauze pads.
• The doctor cleans the injection site with the saturated cotton balls or gauze pads. After draping the site, he checks the label on the local anesthetic as you hold the bottle. Then turn it upside down so the doctor can fill the 3-ml syringe.
• The doctor anesthetizes the skin and subcutaneous tissue at the injection site using the 25G ⅝″ needle.

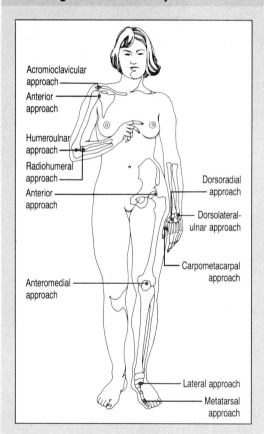

Locating intra-articular injection sites

Acromioclavicular approach

Anterior approach

Humeroulnar approach

Radiohumeral approach

Anterior approach

Anteromedial approach

Dorsoradial approach

Dorsolateral-ulnar approach

Carpometacarpal approach

Lateral approach

Metatarsal approach

To aspirate synovial fluid

• Position the sterile test tubes in the correct order.
• The doctor withdraws synovial fluid with the 18G 1½″ needle using the 10-ml syringe. He leaves the needle in the joint *for the subsequent injection of medication*. The syringe containing the specimen can be set aside until after the procedure.
• After completing the intra-articular injection, the doctor will attach a needle to the specimen syringe and insert appropriate specimens into the test tubes. Label the test tubes appropriately and send them to the laboratory.

To perform intra-articular injection

• Hand the 5- or 10-ml medication syringe — with an 18G 1½″ needle attached — to the doctor, who then injects the medication into the synovial cavity. (If synovial fluid was aspirated, remove the needle and hand the doctor the medication syringe. He attaches the syringe to the needle already in the joint and injects the medication.)
• After the injection, apply pressure to the site and (if appropriate) massage the area gently for 1 or 2 minutes *to facilitate absorption*.
• Apply an adhesive bandage to the site.

Special considerations

Advise the patient to avoid excessive use of the affected joint *because the injected medications may mask pain*.

Complications

Because the medication may infiltrate and initially irritate surrounding tissue, local joint pain may actually increase for 24 to 48 hours after an intra-articular injection. However, fever, persistent increased pain, redness, and swelling may indicate septic arthritis, a serious complication caused by contamination.

Documentation

Record the injected medication, dose, date, time and site of injection, and the doctor's name in your notes. Also note the amount of synovial fluid aspirated, any laboratory studies requested, and the patient's tolerance of the injection.

 # Addition of drugs to an I.V. solution

Various transfer devices can be used to add drugs to an I.V. solution. The common syringe and needle are used to draw up medications, reconstitute powdered drugs, and make transfers. A single- or double-headed needle is used to transfer dissolved medication in a vial to an I.V. bottle while keeping the vacuum intact. A syringe with a filter needle or filter straw can be used to transfer medication from an ampule to a bottle or bag.

Before adding any drug to an I.V. solution, it's necessary to verify the compatibility of the solution with the drug. Adding drugs to blood is contraindicated because it complicates identifying the source of an adverse reaction.

Equipment

Patient's medication record and chart ▪ compatibility and stability guide ▪ drug to be added ▪ I.V. solution ▪ diluent, if necessary ▪ I.V. administration set or sterile I.V. cap ▪ syringe with filter needle ▪ double-headed needle ▪ medication-added labels ▪ alcohol sponges ▪ optional: ampule transfer device, 100-, 250-, or 500-ml container.

You'll also need a needle when using a syringe with a filter needle or filter straw and an ampule transfer device. A 4″ × 4″ gauze pad helps prevent cuts when you break open an ampule. Always use a small, thin needle (such as a 25G 1″) for multiple punctures of a vial or bag. *A small puncture reseals better.*

Preparation of equipment

Verify the order on the patient's medication record by checking it against the doctor's order. Check hospital policy *to see if you're permitted to add the drug to the I.V. solution.* If so, find out how the drug to be added is packaged, and then obtain the appropriate transfer device and any necessary diluent. Inspect the I.V. container for cracks or leaks. Check the compatibility and dosage of the drug, diluent, and I.V. solution. If the drug's stability is limited, mix it in a 100-, 250-, or 500-ml container *to avoid waste and loss of potency.*

Implementation

• Wash your hands.
• Confirm the patient's identity by asking his name and checking the name, room number, and bed number on his wristband.
• Verify that you have the correct drug by comparing its label with the order on the medication record. Read the label as you prepare the drug additive and again after you've added it to the solution.

To use a syringe and needle

• Remove the protective cap from the drug vial and wipe the top of the vial with a sterile alcohol sponge.
• If the drug to be added is a powder, aspirate the correct amount of diluent into the syringe and inject it into the drug vial. Roll the vial between your hands *to dissolve all particles.*

- Wipe the injection port on the I.V. container with an alcohol sponge.
- Inject the drug and gently rotate the vial or invert or rotate the bag *to mix the solution*.

To use a single-headed needle or pin

- Remove the protective cap from the needle or pin on top of the drug vial.
- Invert the drug vial and insert the pin into the I.V. container's main port *so the vacuum draws the drug into the container*. Remove the vial and gently rotate the container *to mix the solution*.

To use a double-headed needle or pin

- Remove the protective cap from the drug vial and wipe the rubber seal with an alcohol sponge, if desired. If you're adding medication to an I.V. bag, remove the protective outer wrapping.
- If the drug to be added is a powder, add the appropriate diluent with a needle and syringe and roll the vial between your hands *to dissolve all particles*.
- Remove the outside cover of the double-headed needle *to expose the shorter needle*. Insert this needle into the drug vial and remove the other half of the needle cover *to expose the longer needle*.
- Wipe the injection port on the I.V. container with an alcohol sponge. Invert the medication vial, and insert the longer needle into the center hole of the appropriate seal. The vacuum then draws the drug into the I.V. container. Remove the vial and gently rotate the container *to mix the solution*.

To use a syringe with a filter needle or straw

- Place the filter needle or straw on the syringe. Then wipe the ampule's neck with an alcohol sponge, wrap it in a 4″ × 4″ gauze pad, and snap off the top, directing the force away from your body.
- Aspirate the ampule's contents with the syringe. Then replace the filter needle or straw with a 25G 1″ needle.
- Inject the drug into the I.V. container and rotate the container *to mix the solution*.

After preparing the solution

- Recheck the drug dose and I.V. solution *to prevent error*.
- Connect the I.V. administration set or sterile protective cap (provided by the manufacturer) to the I.V. container *to prevent contamination*.
- Fill out the medication-added label and place it on the I.V. container. The label should include the date, drug dose, your initials, time the drug was added to the I.V. container, and patient's name, room number, and bed number.

Special considerations

Maintain sterile technique throughout this procedure.

When making multiple drug transfers, add only one drug at a time. Always add the most concentrated drug first and any colored drugs last. Mix the solution thoroughly and examine it for precipitation, discoloration, or cloudiness after adding each drug.

To add a drug to an I.V. solution that has already been hung, always close the flow clamp *to prevent delivering a bolus of the drug to the patient*. Insert a syringe and needle into the injection port of the I.V. container after wiping it with an alcohol sponge. Always rotate the container gently *to mix the solution*. Then open the flow clamp and adjust the flow rate.

When administering an I.V. solution with drugs or other additives, watch for signs of drug sensitivity or intolerance.

Complications

Excessively high drug concentrations in the I.V. solution can cause complications such as sclerosis, thrombosis, hemolysis, or phlebitis. Extravasation of some drugs into subcutaneous tissues can cause tissue necrosis.

Documentation

Record the date and time of administration, your initials or name, the drug name and dosage, the amount and type of I.V. solution infused, and the duration of infusion.

Drug infusion through a secondary I.V. line

A secondary I.V. line is a complete I.V. set — container, tubing, and microdrip or macrodrip system — connected to the lower Y port (secondary port) of a primary line instead of to the I.V. catheter or needle. It can be used for continuous or intermittent drug infusion. When used continuously, a secondary I.V. line permits drug infusion and titration while the primary line maintains a constant total infusion rate.

When used intermittently, a secondary I.V. line is commonly called a *piggyback set*. In this case, the primary line maintains venous access between drug doses. Typically, a piggyback set includes a small I.V. container, short tubing, and a macrodrip system. This set connects to the primary line's upper Y port, also known as a piggyback port. (See *Needle-free piggyback system* for more information.) Antibiotics and histamine₂ receptor antagonists are most commonly administered by intermittent (piggyback) infusion. To make this set work, the primary I.V. container must be positioned below the piggyback container. (The manufacturer provides an extension hook for that purpose.)

I.V. pumps may be used to maintain constant infusion rates, especially with a drug such as lidocaine. A pump allows more accurate titration of drug dosage and helps maintain venous access because the drug is delivered under sufficient pressure to prevent clot formation in the I.V. cannula.

Equipment

Patient's medication record and chart ▪ prescribed I.V. medication ▪ prescribed I.V. solution ▪ administration set with secondary injection port ▪ 22G 1″ needle ▪ alcohol sponges ▪ 1″ adhesive tape ▪ time tape ▪ labels ▪ infusion pump ▪ extension hook and appropriate solution for intermittent piggyback infusion ▪ optional: normal saline solution for infusion with incompatible solutions.

For intermittent infusion, the primary line typically has a piggyback port with a backcheck valve that stops the flow from the primary line during drug infusion and returns to the primary flow after infusion. A volume-control set can also be used with an intermittent infusion line. (For more information, refer to "Use of a volume-control set" in Chapter 6.)

Preparation of equipment

Verify the order on the patient's medication record by checking it against the doctor's order. Wash your hands. Inspect the I.V. container for cracks, leaks, or contamination, and check drug compatibility with the primary solution. See if the primary line has a secondary injection port. If it doesn't, and the medication will be given regularly, replace the I.V. set with a new one that has a secondary injection port.

If necessary, add the drug to the secondary I.V. solution. To do so, remove any seals from the secondary container and wipe the main port with an alcohol sponge. Inject the prescribed medication and gently agitate the solution *to mix the medication thoroughly.* Properly label the I.V. mixture. Insert the administration set spike and attach the needle. Open the flow clamp and prime the line. Then close the flow clamp.

Some medications now come in vials suitable for hanging directly on an I.V. pole. Instead of preparing medication and injecting it into a container, you can inject diluent directly into the medication vial. Then you can spike the vial, prime the tubing, and hang the set as directed.

Needle-free piggyback system

Some drugs can be piggybacked with a needle-free system, which consists of a blunt-tipped plastic insertion device and a rubber injection port. The port may be part of a special administration set or an adaptor for existing administration sets. This rubber injection port has a preestablished slit that can open and reseal immediately.

The needle-free system aims to reduce the risk of accidental needle-stick injuries.

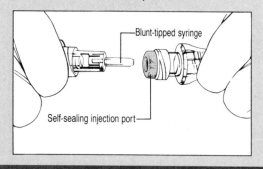

Blunt-tipped syringe

Self-sealing injection port

Implementation

• Confirm the patient's identity by asking his name and checking the name, room number, and bed number on his wristband.

• If the drug is incompatible with the primary I.V. solution, replace the primary solution with a fluid that's compatible with both solutions, such as normal saline, and flush the line before starting the drug infusion. Many hospital protocols require removing the primary I.V. solution and inserting a sterile I.V. plug into the container until you're ready to rehang it. *This will maintain sterility of the solution* and prevent someone else from inadvertently restarting the incompatible solution before the line is flushed with normal saline solution.

• Hang the secondary set's container and wipe the injection port of the primary line with an alcohol sponge.

• Insert the needle from the secondary line into the injection port and tape it securely to the primary line.

• To run the secondary set's container by itself, lower the primary set's container with an extension hook. To run both containers simultaneously, place them at the same height. (See *Assembling a piggyback set,* page 254.)

• Open the clamp and adjust the drip rate. For continuous infusion, set the secondary solution to the desired drip rate; then adjust the primary solution *to achieve the desired total infusion rate.*

Assembling a piggyback set

A piggyback set is useful for intermittent drug infusion. To work properly, its drug container must be positioned higher than the primary set's container.

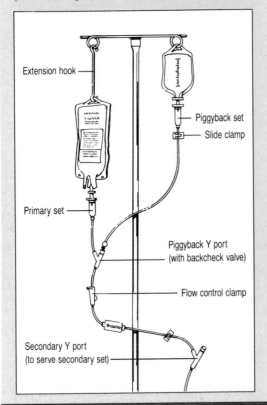

Extension hook

Piggyback set

Slide clamp

Primary set

Piggyback Y port
(with backcheck valve)

Flow control clamp

Secondary Y port
(to serve secondary set)

• For intermittent infusion, adjust the primary drip rate as required upon completion of the secondary solution. If the secondary solution tubing is being reused, close the clamp on the tubing and follow the hospital's policy: Either remove the needle and replace it with a new one, or leave it securely taped in the injection port and label it with the time it was first used. In this case, also leave the empty container in place until you replace it with a new dose of medication at the prescribed time. If the tubing won't be reused, discard it appropriately with the I.V. container.

Special considerations

If hospital policy allows, use a pump for drug infusion. Put a time tape on the secondary container *to help prevent an inaccurate administration rate.*

When reusing secondary tubing, change it according to hospital policy, usually every 48 to 72 hours. Similarly, inspect the injection port for leakage with each use, and change it more often if needed.

Unless you're piggybacking lipids, don't piggyback a secondary I.V. line to a total parenteral nutrition line *because of the risk of contamination.* Check your hospital's policy for possible exceptions.

Complications

Adverse effects and reactions to the infused drug can occur. Repeated punctures of the secondary injection port can damage the seal, possibly allowing leakage or contamination.

Documentation

Record the amount and type of drug and the amount of I.V. solution on the intake and output and medication records. Note the date, duration, and rate of infusion, and the patient's response, where applicable.

Drug administration through a heparin lock

An intermittent infusion injection device — or heparin lock — eliminates the need for multiple venipunctures or for maintaining venous access with a continuous I.V. infusion. This device allows intermittent administration by infusion or by the I.V. bolus or I.V. push injection methods.

Dilute heparin or saline solutions are often injected as the final step in this procedure to prevent clotting in the device. When heparin is used, the device must be flushed with normal saline solution before and after the prescribed medication is administered in case the heparin and the medication are incompatible. The device may then be reflushed with the heparin flush solution.

Equipment

Patient's medication record and chart ■ three 3-ml syringes with 22G or 25G 1″ needles ■ normal saline solution ■ alcohol sponges ■ extra heparin lock ■ prescribed medication in an I.V. container with administration set and needle (for infusion) or in a syringe with needle (for I.V. bolus or push) ■ tourniquet ■ tape ■ gloves ■ optional:

T connector, dilute heparin solution, sterile bacteriostatic water.

The concentration of dilute heparin solution ranges from 10 to 100 units/ml. The solution is available in a cartridge-injection system in doses of 10 to 100 units/ml. If this system is used, substitute its syringe for the 3-ml syringe and the heparin cartridge for the heparin solution. Normal saline solution is available in a similar cartridge system.

Preparation of equipment
Verify the order on the patient's medication record by checking it against the doctor's order. Wash your hands, don gloves, and then wipe the tops of the normal saline solution, heparin flush solution, and medication containers with alcohol sponges. Fill two of the 3-ml syringes (bearing 22G needles) with normal saline solution; if required by hospital policy, draw 1 ml of heparin flush solution into the third syringe. If you'll be infusing medication, insert the administration set spike into the I.V. container, attach the appropriate-sized needle, and prime the line. If you'll be giving an I.V. injection, fill a syringe with the prescribed drug.

Implementation
• Confirm the patient's identity by asking his name and checking the name, room number, and bed number on his wristband. Explain the procedure.
• Don gloves. Wipe the injection port of the intermittent infusion device with an alcohol sponge and insert the needle of a saline-filled syringe.
• Aspirate the syringe and observe for blood *to verify the patency of the device.* If none appears, apply a tourniquet slightly above the site, keep it in place for about 1 minute, and then aspirate again. If blood still doesn't appear, remove the tourniquet and inject the normal saline solution slowly.
♦ *Nursing alert.* Stop the injection immediately if you feel any resistance *because resistance indicates that the device is occluded.* If this occurs, insert a new heparin lock. ♦
• If you feel no resistance, watch for signs of infiltration (puffiness or pain at the site) as you slowly inject the saline solution. If these signs occur, insert a new heparin lock.
• If blood is aspirated, slowly inject the saline and observe for signs of infiltration. *The saline solution flushes out any residual heparin solution that might be incompatible with the medication.*
• Withdraw the saline syringe and needle.

To administer I.V. bolus or push injections
• Insert the needle and syringe with the medication for the I.V. bolus or push injection into the injection port of the device.
• Inject the medication at the required rate. Then remove the needle from the injection port.
• Insert the needle of the remaining saline-filled syringe into the injection port and slowly inject the saline solution *to flush all medication through the device.*
• Remove the needle and syringe, and insert and inject the heparin (or saline) flush solution *to prevent clotting in the device.*

To administer an infusion
• Insert and tape the needle attached to the administration set.
• Open the infusion line and adjust the flow rate as necessary.
• Infuse medication for the prescribed length of time; then flush the device with normal saline solution and heparin flush solution, as you would after a bolus or push injection, according to your hospital's policy.
• To administer fluids and drugs simultaneously or to administer a medication incompatible with the primary I.V. solution, you may want to use a T connector. (See *Using a T connector,* page 256.)

Special considerations
If you're giving a bolus injection of a drug that's incompatible with saline, such as diazepam (Valium), flush the device with bacteriostatic water.

Some hospitals use diluted heparin solution (100 units/ml or 10 units/ml) *to prevent clotting in the cannula.* Other hospitals use 2 to 3 ml of normal saline solution instead. A few hospitals use other solutions or dilutions. Check your hospital's policy.

Intermittent infusion devices should be changed regularly (usually every 48 to 72 hours), according to universal precautions guidelines and hospital policy.

If you're unable to rotate injection sites because the patient has fragile veins, document this fact in your notes.

Complications
Infiltration and a specific reaction to the infused drug are the most common complications.

Documentation
Record the type and amount of drug administered and the times of administration. Include all I.V. solutions used to dilute the medication and flush the line on the intake record. Also document the use of dilute heparin solution.

Using a T connector

The T connector is a piece of small-bore extension tubing 3″ to 6″ (7.6 to 15.2 cm) long. It's fitted with an injection port near the luer-lock connection. This additional injection site allows simultaneous administration of drugs and fluids or of primary I.V. solution and a drug incompatible with it.

To add the T connector, wash your hands and don gloves to minimize exposure to body fluids. Then, explain to the patient what you are about to do, to reduce his anxiety at seeing another piece of I.V. equipment.

Prime the tubing with I.V. fluid, then attach one end of the T connector to the I.V. tubing. Open the slide clamp. Now you're ready to connect the luer-lock tip to the injection cap. Remove the leur-lock tip-protector cap and carefully insert this tip into the injection cap.

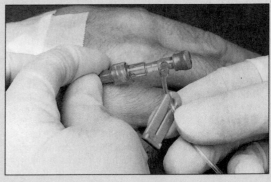

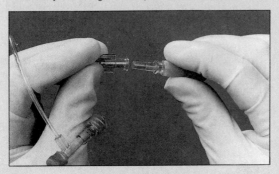

Secure this connector in place with tape. Another I.V. needle can be inserted into the latex injection cap. Finally, document your actions.

I.V. bolus injection

This bolus injection method allows rapid I.V. drug administration. It may be used in an emergency to provide an immediate drug effect. Alternately, it may be used to achieve peak drug levels in the bloodstream or to deliver drugs that can't be diluted, such as diazepam, digoxin, and phenytoin. It may also be used to administer drugs that can't be given I.M. because they're toxic to muscle tissue or because the patient's ability to absorb them is impaired.

The term *bolus* usually refers to the concentration or amount of a drug. I.V. push is a technique for rapid intravenous injection.

Bolus doses of medication may be injected directly into a vein or through an existing I.V. line, or through an implanted vascular access port (VAP). The medication administered by these methods usually takes effect rapidly, so the patient must be monitored for an adverse reaction, such as cardiac arrhythmia. I.V. bolus injections are contraindicated when rapid drug administration could cause life-threatening complications. For certain drugs, the safe rate of injection is specified by the manufacturer.

Some hospital policies specify that only nurses trained in this technique (such as emergency department, critical care, or chemotherapy nurses) can give bolus injections.

Equipment

Patient's medication record and chart ▪ prescribed medication ▪ 20G needle and syringe ▪ diluent, if needed ▪ tourniquet ▪ povidone-iodine sponge ▪ alcohol sponge ▪ sterile 2″ × 2″ gauze pad ▪ gloves ▪ adhesive bandage ▪ tape ▪ optional: winged-tip needle with catheter and second syringe (and needle) filled with normal saline solution; non-coring needle if used with a vascular access port; heparin flush solution.

Winged-tip needles are frequently used for this purpose largely because they can be quickly and easily inserted. This makes them ideal for repeated drug administration, as in weekly or monthly chemotherapy. Another useful dosage form is the ready injectable. (See *Using a ready injectable.*)

Preparation of equipment

Verify the order on the patient's medication record by checking it against the doctor's order. Know the actions, adverse effects, and administration rate of the drug to be injected. Draw up the prescribed medication in the syringe and dilute it if necessary.

Implementation

• Confirm the patient's identity, wash your hands, put on gloves, and explain the procedure.

To give direct injections

• Select the largest vein suitable for an injection. *The larger the vein, the more diluted the drug will become, minimizing vascular irritation.*
• Apply a tourniquet above the injection site *to distend the vein.*
• Clean the injection site with an alcohol sponge or a povidone-iodine sponge, working outward from the puncture site in a circular motion *to prevent recontamination with skin bacteria.*
• If you're using the drug syringe's needle, insert it into the vein at a 30-degree angle with the bevel up. The bevel should reach ¼" (0.6 cm) into the vein. If you're using a winged-tip needle, insert the needle (bevel up), tape the butterfly wings in place when you see blood return in the tubing, and attach the syringe containing the drug.
• Pull back on the plunger of the syringe and check for blood backflow, *which indicates that the needle is in the vein.*
• Remove the tourniquet and inject the drug at the appropriate rate.
• Pull back slightly on the plunger of the syringe and check for blood backflow again. *If blood appears, it indicates that the needle remained in place and all of the injected medication entered the vein.*
• If you're using a winged-tip needle, flush the line with the normal saline solution from the second syringe *to ensure delivery of all the medication into the vein.*
• Withdraw the needle and apply pressure to the injection site with the sterile gauze pad for at least 3 minutes *to prevent hematoma formation.*
• Apply the adhesive bandage to the site after bleeding has stopped.

To give injections through an existing I.V. line

• Check the compatibility of the medication with the I.V. solution.
• Close the flow clamp, wipe the injection port with an alcohol sponge, and inject the drug as you would a direct injection. (Some I.V. lines have a secondary injection port or a T connector; others have a latex cap at the end of the I.V. tubing where the needle is attached.)

Using a ready injectable

A ready injectable—commercially premeasured medication packaged with a syringe and needle—allows for rapid drug administration in an emergency. Usually, preparing a ready injectable takes only 15 to 20 seconds. Other advantages include the reduced risk of breaking sterile technique during administration and the easy identification of medication and dose.

When using a commercially prefilled syringe, make sure to administer precisely the dose prescribed. For example, if a 50 mg/ml cartridge is supplied but the patient's prescribed dose is 25 mg, you must administer only 0.5 ml—half of the volume contained in the cartridge. Be alert for potential medication errors whenever dispensing medications in premeasured dosage forms.

• Open the flow clamp and readjust the flow rate.
• If the drug isn't compatible with the I.V. solution, flush the line with normal saline solution before and after the injection. (For additional information, see "Drug administration through a heparin lock" in this chapter.)

To give a bolus injection through a vascular access port

• Wash your hands, don gloves, and clean the injection site with an alcohol sponge or a povidone-iodine sponge, starting at the center of the port and working outward with a circular motion over a 4" to 5" (10 to 12.7 cm) diameter. Do this three times.
• Palpate the area over the port *to locate the port septum.*
• Anchor the port between your thumb and the first two fingers of your nondominant hand. Then using your dominant hand, insert the needle into the appropriate area of the device and deliver the injection. (See "Implanted vascular access devices" in Chapter 6.)

Special considerations

Because drugs administered by I.V. bolus or push injection are delivered directly into the circulatory system and can produce an immediate effect, signs of an acute allergic reaction or anaphylaxis can develop rapidly. If any signs of anaphylaxis occur (dyspnea, cyanosis, convulsions, or increasing respiratory distress), notify the doctor immediately and begin emergency procedures, as necessary. Also watch for signs of extravasation, such as swelling, the absence of blood backflow, and a sluggish flow rate. If extravasation occurs, stop the injection,

Antidotes for vesicant extravasation

Substances commonly used as antidotes for vesicant extravasation are listed below, along with the extravasated drugs for which they may be given. Antidotes may be instilled through the existing I.V. line or injected subcutaneously with a 1-ml tuberculin syringe in a circle around the infiltrated area. The needle should be changed before each injection of antidote. Some antidotes may be used in combination.

Hyaluronidase (15 units/ml)
This drug may be given as an antidote to aminophylline, calcium solutions, contrast media, dextrose solutions (concentrations of 10% or more), total parenteral nutrition solutions, nafcillin, potassium solutions, vinblastine, vincristine, or vindesine.

Sodium bicarbonate 8.4%
This drug may be given as an antidote to carmustine, daunorubicin, doxorubicin, vinblastine, or vincristine.

Phentolamine
This drug may be given as an antidote to dobutamine, dopamine, epinephrine, metaraminol, or norepinephrine.

Sodium thiosulfate 10%
This drug may be given as an antidote to dactinomycin, mechlorethamine, or mitomycin.

Hydrocortisone sodium succinate (100 mg/ml)
This drug, usually followed by topical application of 1% hydrocortisone cream, may be given as an antidote to doxorubicin or vincristine.

Ascorbic acid
This drug may be injected as an antidote to dactinomycin.

Sodium edetate
This drug may be administered as an antidote to plicamycin.

estimate the amount of infiltration, and notify the doctor. If you're giving diazepam or chlordiazepoxide hydrochloride through a winged-tip needle or I.V. line, flush with bacteriostatic water instead of normal saline solution *to prevent drug precipitation caused by incompatibility.*

Complications
Excessively rapid drug administration may cause adverse effects, depending on the drug administered.

Documentation
Record the amount and type of drug administered, time of injection, appearance of the site, duration of administration, and patient's tolerance of the procedure. Also note the drug's effect and any adverse reactions.

Management of intravenous extravasation

Extravasation is the leakage of infused solution from a vein into surrounding tissue. The result of a needle puncturing the vessel wall or leakage around a venipuncture site, extravasation causes local pain and itching, edema, blanching, and decreased skin temperature in the affected extremity. Extravasation of I.V. solution is often referred to as infiltration, because the fluid infiltrates the tissues.

Extravasation of a small amount of isotonic fluid or a nonirritating drug usually causes only minor discomfort. Treatment involves routine comfort measures, such as the application of warm compresses. However, extravasation of some drugs can severely damage tissue through irritative, sclerotic, vesicant, corrosive, or vasoconstrictive action. (See *Antidotes for vesicant extravasation.*) In these cases, emergency measures must be taken to minimize tissue damage and necrosis, prevent the need for skin grafts or, rarely, avoid possible amputation.

Equipment
Three 25G ⅝" needles ■ antidote for extravasated drug in appropriate syringe ■ 5-ml syringe ■ three tuberculin syringes ■ alcohol sponge or gauze pad soaked in antiseptic cleaning agent ■ 4" × 4" gauze pad ■ cold and warm compresses ■ optional: anti-inflammatory drug ■ 8.4% sodium bicarbonate ■ normal saline solution.

Preparation of equipment
Attach one 25G ⅝" needle to the syringe containing the antidote. Connect the two remaining 25G ⅝" needles to two tuberculin syringes. Then fill the remaining tuberculin syringe with the anti-inflammatory drug, if needed.

Implementation

Opinions differ on the preferred treatment for extravasation; hospital policy will dictate specific actions. They may include some or all of the following steps.
• Stop the infusion immediately and remove the I.V. needle unless you need the route to infiltrate the antidote. Carefully estimate the amount of extravasated solution and notify the doctor.
• Disconnect the tubing from the I.V. needle. Attach the 5-ml syringe to the needle and try to withdraw 3 to 5 ml of blood *to remove any medication or blood in the tubing or needle and provide a path to the infiltrated tissues.*
• Clean the area around the extravasation site with an alcohol sponge or 4″ × 4″ gauze pad soaked in an antiseptic cleaning agent. Then insert the needle of the empty tuberculin syringe into the subcutaneous tissue around the site, and gently aspirate as much of the solution as possible from the tissue.
• Instill the prescribed antidote into the subcutaneous tissue around the site. Then, if ordered, slowly instill an anti-inflammatory drug subcutaneously *to help reduce inflammation and edema.*
• If ordered, instill the prescribed antidote through the I.V. needle.
• Apply cold compresses to the affected area for 24 hours, or apply an ice pack for 20 minutes every 4 hours *to cause vasoconstriction that may localize the drug and slow cell metabolism.* After 24 hours, apply warm compresses and elevate the affected extremity *to reduce discomfort and promote fluid reabsorption.* If the extravasated drug is a vasoconstrictor, such as norepinephrine or metaraminol bitartrate, apply warm compresses only.
• Continuously monitor the I.V. site for signs of abscess or necrosis.

Special considerations

If you're administering a potentially tissue-damaging drug by I.V. bolus or push, first start an I.V. infusion, preferably with normal saline solution. Infuse a small amount of the saline solution, and check for signs of infiltration before injecting the drug.

Know the antidote (if any) for an I.V. drug that can cause tissue necrosis if extravasation occurs. Make sure you're familiar with your hospital's policy regarding the administration of such drugs and their antidotes.

Tell the patient to report any discomfort at the I.V. site. During infusion, frequently check the site for signs of infiltration.

Documentation

Record the site of the extravasation, the patient's symptoms, the estimated amount of infiltrated solution, nursing treatment, the time, and the name of the doctor notified.

Continue to document the appearance of the infiltrated site and any associated symptoms.

Preparation and handling of chemotherapeutic drugs

Administration of chemotherapeutic drugs may cause teratogenic, mutagenic, or carcinogenic effects in patients. However, the risks associated with the caregiver's preparation and handling of these drugs haven't been fully determined. Nor has a preferential technique for handling these drugs been found. Despite these uncertainties, nurses who give chemotherapeutic drugs should follow guidelines from the Occupational Safety and Health Administration (OSHA). What's more, they should keep current with the latest safety guidelines and protocols.

Typically, chemotherapeutic drugs are prepared by a pharmaceutical company or in the hospital pharmacy using a laminar airflow hood and procedures to ensure minimal exposure to potential hazards. Only nurses, doctors, or pharmacists with specialized training should prepare chemotherapeutic drugs.

Equipment

Chemotherapeutic drug ▪ I.V. solution ▪ diluent, if necessary ▪ patient's medication record and chart ▪ compatibility and stability reference source ▪ medication labels ▪ Class II biological safety cabinet (if available) ▪ 18G or 19G needle and hydrophobic filter or dispensing pin ▪ syringes, needles and I.V. tubing with luer-lock fittings ▪ long-sleeved gown ▪ gloves ▪ face shield or goggles ▪ eyewash ▪ plastic absorbent pad ▪ alcohol sponges or sterile gauze pads ▪ impervious containers labeled CAUTION: CHEMOTHERAPY or BIOHAZARD for disposal of unused drug or equipment.

Preparation of equipment

Verify the drug, dosage, and route of administration by checking the medication record against the doctor's order. Check the expiration dates of drugs, solutions, and diluents.

Select syringes, needles, and I.V. tubing with luer-lock fittings *to prevent contamination by leakage.*

Use an 18G or 19G needle and a hydrophobic filter or dispensing pin *to prevent aerosol release from vials.*

Label all syringes, bottles, or bags containing chemotherapeutic drugs with the following information:
• patient's name, identification, and room number
• drug name and dose

• route of administration
• date and time of preparation
• expiration date and time
• vesicant
• storage requirements, if applicable.

Implementation
• Prepare the prescribed drugs in accordance with current product instructions regarding compatibility, stability, and reconstitution technique.

To avoid unnecessary or excessive drug exposure
• Prepare drugs in a Class II biological safety cabinet *for maximum protection.* The blower on the hood should be left on 24 hours a day, 7 days a week. Alternatively, prepare drugs in a quiet work space, away from heating or cooling vents and other personnel.
• Use protective garments (long-sleeved gown, gloves, face shield or goggles) as indicated by institutional policy. Do not wear equipment outside of the preparation area.
• Do not eat, drink, smoke, or apply cosmetics in the drug preparation area.
• Cover the work surface with a clean plastic absorbent pad *to minimize contamination by droplets or spills.* Change the pad when completing each shift or after a spill.
• Consider all equipment used in drug preparation and any unused drug as hazardous waste and dispose according to hospital policy.

To manage accidental exposure
• If skin contact occurs, wash the involved area thoroughly with soap (not a germicidal agent) and water.
• If eye contact occurs, flood the involved eye with water or an isotonic eyewash for at least 5 minutes while holding the eyelid open.
• Obtain a medical evaluation as soon as possible after accidental exposure.

Special considerations
Exercise precautions to avoid skin contact if the medication leaks. Clean all spills immediately according to hospital policy.

Dispose of waste (unused drug and preparation equipment) in impervious containers labeled CAUTION: CHEMOTHERAPY or BIOHAZARD. These must be incinerated or handled as toxic waste.

Complications
Chromosomal damage or liver damage may result from chronic exposure to chemotherapeutic drugs.

Documentation
Document exposure incidents according to established hospital policies.

Administration of chemotherapeutic drugs

Chemotherapeutic drugs may be administered by many routes. These include oral, subcutaneous, I.M., I.V. (using peripheral or central veins), intra-arterial, intracavitary, intrathecal, and intraperitoneal routes. (See *An alternate approach to intraperitoneal chemotherapy.*) The route chosen by the oncologist reflects the drug's pharmacology and the patient's condition. However, most chemotherapeutic drugs are given intravenously.

Chemotherapeutic drugs are hazardous and errors in dosage or administration can cause severe effects or even death. Therefore, these drugs should be reconstituted in a laminar airflow hood by trained personnel. (See "Preparation and handling of chemotherapeutic drugs" in this chapter.) In addition, the patient requires a comprehensive assessment before treatment so that adverse reactions can be prevented or managed effectively.

Equipment
Chemotherapeutic drug ▪ patient's medication record and chart ▪ brown paper bag or aluminum foil if the drug is photosensitive ▪ normal saline solution ▪ syringes and needles ▪ infusion pump or control device (if I.V. infusion is ordered) ▪ gloves ▪ impervious containers labeled CAUTION: CHEMOTHERAPY or BIOHAZARD for disposal of unused drug or equipment.

Preparation of equipment
Verify the drug, dosage, and route of administration by checking the medication record against the doctor's order. Be sure you know the immediate and delayed adverse reactions of the drug being administered. Follow administration guidelines for appropriate procedures in this chapter.

Implementation
• Obtain baseline data, including the patient's history relevant to planned chemotherapy and related medications, the patient's and family's understanding of chemotherapy, and the results of laboratory studies (such as complete blood count, blood urea nitrogen, platelets, creatinine level, and liver function studies).

An alternate approach to intraperitoneal chemotherapy

Administering chemotherapeutic drugs into the peritoneal cavity has several benefits for patients with malignant ascites or ovarian cancer that has spread to the peritoneum. This technique passes drugs directly to the tumor area in the peritoneal cavity, exposing malignant cells to very high concentrations of chemotherapy – up to 1,000 times what could be safely given systemically. What's more, the semipermeable peritoneal membrane permits prolonged exposure of malignant cells to the drug.

Typically, this therapy is performed using a peritoneal dialysis kit, but drugs can also be administered to the peritoneal cavity directly, via the Tenckhoff catheter, shown at right. This method can be performed on an outpatient basis if necessary, and uses equipment that is readily available on most units with oncology patients.

In this technique, the chemotherapy bag is connected directly to the Tenckhoff catheter with a length of I.V. tubing, the solution is infused, and the catheter and I.V. tubing are clamped. Then the patient is asked to change positions every 10 to 15 minutes for 1 hour to move the solution around in the peritoneal cavity. After the prescribed "dwell time," the chemotherapy is al-

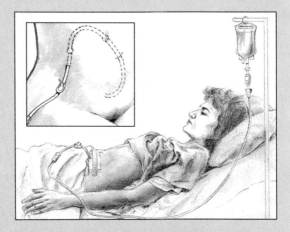

lowed to drain into an I.V. bag. The patient is encouraged to change positions to facilitate drainage. Then the I.V. tubing and catheter are clamped, the I.V. tubing is removed, and a new p.r.n. adapter is fitted to the catheter. Finally, the catheter is flushed with a syringe of heparinized saline.

- Check the patient's chart for the complete chemotherapy protocol order, including the patient's name, the drug's name and dosage, and the route, rate, and frequency of administration. Also check the doctor's order for laboratory values for administration. *The order may specify a reduced drug dosage based on laboratory values.*
- Check to see if antiemetics, fluids, diuretics, or electrolyte supplements have been ordered before, during, or after drug administration.
- Ensure that the patient or a responsible family member has signed the consent form.
- Don gloves when priming I.V. tubing, when purging air bubbles from syringes or I.V. tubing, and when administering chemotherapeutic drugs. *Gloves prevent direct skin contact with drugs.*
- Examine the patient's veins *to determine an administration site,* starting with his hand and proceeding to his forearm. (Remember, the use of veins in the dorsum of the hand or wrist is controversial if you're giving a vesicant drug.)
- Avoid using an existing I.V. line to administer these drugs. Perform a new venipuncture proximal to the old site *to ensure proper needle placement and vein patency.*

Never use a chemotherapeutic drug to test vein patency. Infuse 10 to 20 ml of normal saline solution *to maintain patency.* Administer nonvesicant agents by I.V. push or admixed in a bag of I.V. fluid. Give vesicant agents by I.V. push through a piggyback set connected to a rapidly infusing I.V.
- During administration, watch closely for signs of a hypersensitivity reaction or extravasation. Check for blood return after each 5 ml of medication is injected or according to established guidelines.
- If you suspect extravasation, stop the infusion immediately, leave the needle in place, and notify the doctor. Know the applicable policy for treating extravasation.
- Infuse 20 ml of normal saline solution between all chemotherapeutic medications and before discontinuing the I.V. line.
- Dispose of used needles and syringes carefully. *To prevent aerosol dispersion of chemotherapeutic drugs,* don't clip needles. Place them intact in an impervious container for incineration.
- Dispose of I.V. bags, bottles, gloves, and tubing in a covered trash container. Chemotherapy trash should be incinerated.

• Even though you've used gloves, wash your hands thoroughly with warm soap and water after giving any chemotherapeutic drug.

Special considerations

Evaluate the patient's and family's desire for information and their level of understanding. Instruct them about the chemotherapy, treatment protocol, and schedule of administration. Teach them to recognize the signs and symptoms of extravasation or any other unusual sensations. Instruct them about posttreatment care.

Observe the I.V. administration site frequently for signs of extravasation or allergic reaction (swelling, redness, urticaria). If the patient reports pain, stop the drug immediately and evaluate the site.

During infusion, some drugs need protection from direct sunlight to avoid possible drug breakdown. Cover the vial with a brown paper bag or aluminum foil.

When administering vesicants, avoid sites where damage to underlying tendons or nerves may occur (such as veins in the antecubital fossa, near the wrist, or in the dorsal surface of the hand).

Flush with normal saline solution between drugs *to avoid incompatibility* and after treatment *to clear the line.*

Observe the patient at regular intervals and after treatment for adverse reactions.

If you're unable to remain with the patient during the entire infusion, use a control device or infusion pump *to ensure delivery of the drug within the prescribed time and rate.*

Complications

Adverse effects of chemotherapeutic drugs include extravasation, causing inflammation, ulceration, and possibly necrosis; and loss of vein patency, caused by fibrosis. Other effects include alopecia, anemia, neutropenia, thrombocytopenia, photosensitivity, urticaria, hyperpigmentation, telangiectasis, hyperkeratosis, radiation recall (if drugs are given with or soon after radiotherapy), nausea, vomiting, anorexia, esophagitis, diarrhea, constipation, and stomatitis. Keep in mind that adverse effects vary depending on the drug, dosage, and route of administration.

Anaphylactic reactions may occur with any chemotherapeutic drug. Stop the infusion immediately if the patient displays a local or generalized reaction. Maintain venous access and institute emergency measures as appropriate.

Documentation

Record the location and description of the I.V. site before treatment (and presence of blood return during bolus administration); drugs and dosages administered; sequence of drug administration; needle type and size used; amount and type of flushing solution; and the site's condition after treatment. Also record any adverse reactions, the patient's tolerance of treatment, and the topics you've taught the patient and his family.

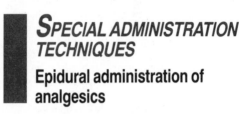

SPECIAL ADMINISTRATION TECHNIQUES
Epidural administration of analgesics

In this procedure, the doctor injects or infuses medication into the epidural space, which lies just outside the subarachnoid space where cerebrospinal fluid (CSF) flows. The drug diffuses slowly into the subarachnoid space of the spinal canal and then into the CSF, which carries it directly into the spinal area—bypassing the blood-brain barrier. In some cases, the doctor injects drugs directly into the subarachnoid space. (See *Understanding intrathecal injections.)*

Epidural analgesia helps manage acute or chronic pain, including moderate to severe postoperative pain. It's especially useful in patients with cancer or degenerative joint disease. This procedure works well because opiate receptors are located along the entire spinal cord. Narcotic drugs act directly on the receptors of the dorsal horn to produce localized analgesia without motor blockade. Narcotics such as morphine, fentanyl, and hydromorphone are administered as either an I.V. bolus dose or by continuous infusion, either alone or in combination with bupivacaine (a local anesthetic). The infusion, given via an epidural catheter, is preferable because it allows a smaller drug dosage to be given continuously. The epidural catheter, inserted near the spinal cord, eliminates the risks of multiple I.M. injections, minimizes adverse cerebral and systemic effects, and eliminates the analgesic peaks and valleys that usually occur with intermittent I.M. injections. (See *Placement of a permanent epidural catheter,* page 264.)

Typically, epidural catheter insertion is performed by an anesthesiologist using aseptic technique. Once the catheter has been inserted, the nurse is responsible for monitoring the infusion and assessing the patient.

Epidural analgesia is contraindicated in patients who have local or systemic infection, neurologic disease, anticoagulant therapy, coagulopathy, spinal arthritis or deformity, hypotension, marked hypertension, or allergy to the prescribed drug.

Equipment

Volume infusion device and epidural infusion tubing (depending on hospital policy) ■ patient's medication record and chart ■ prescribed epidural solutions ■ transparent dressing or sterile gauze pads ■ epidural tray ■ labels for epidural infusion line ■ silk tape ■ optional: monitoring equipment for blood pressure and pulse, apnea monitor.

Have on hand the following drugs and equipment for emergency use: naloxone 0.4 mg I.V.; ephedrine 50 mg I.V.; oxygen; intubation set; hand-held resuscitation bag.

Preparation of equipment

Prepare the infusion device according to the manufacturer's instructions and hospital policy. Obtain an epidural tray. Be sure the pharmacy has been notified ahead of time regarding the medication order *because epidural solutions require special preparation.* Check the medication concentration and infusion rate against the doctor's order.

Implementation

• Explain the procedure and its possible complications to the patient. Tell him he'll feel some pain as the catheter is inserted. Answer any questions he has. Make sure that a consent form has been properly signed and witnessed.
• Position the patient on his side in the knee-chest position, or have him sit on the edge of the bed and lean over a bedside table.
• After the catheter is in place, prime the infusion device, confirm the appropriate medication and infusion rate, and then adjust the device for the correct rate.
• Help the anesthesiologist connect the infusion tubing to the epidural catheter. Then connect the tubing to the infusion pump.
• Bridge-tape all connection sites and label the catheter, infusion tubing, and infusion pump with EPIDURAL INFUSION *to prevent accidental infusion of other drugs into the epidural lines.* Then start the infusion.
• Tell the patient to report immediately any feeling of pain. Instruct him to use a pain scale from 0 to 10, with 0 denoting no pain and 10 denoting the worst pain imaginable. A response of 3 or less typically indicates tolerable pain. If the patient reports a higher pain score, the infusion rate may need to be increased. Call the doctor or change the rate within prescribed limits.
• If ordered, place the patient on an apnea monitor for the first 24 hours after beginning the infusion.
• Change the dressing over the catheter's exit site every 24 to 48 hours, or as needed. The dressing is usually transparent *to allow inspection of drainage* and commonly appears moist or slightly blood-tinged.
• Change the infusion tubing every 48 hours, or as specified by hospital policy.

Understanding intrathecal injections

An intrathecal injection allows the doctor to inject medication into the subarachnoid space of the spinal canal. Certain drugs – such as anti-infectives, or antineoplastics used to treat meningeal leukemia – are administered by this route because they can't readily penetrate the blood-brain barrier through the bloodstream. Intrathecal injection may also be used to deliver anesthetics, such as lidocaine hydrochloride, to achieve regional anesthesia (as in spinal anesthesia or epidural block).

An invasive procedure performed by a doctor under sterile conditions with the nurse assisting, intrathecal injection requires informed patient consent. The injection site is usually between the third and fourth (or fourth and fifth) lumbar vertebrae, well below the spinal cord, to avoid the risk of paralysis. This procedure may be preceded by aspiration of spinal fluid for laboratory analysis.

Contraindications to intrathecal injection include inflammation or infection at the puncture site, septicemia, and spinal deformities (especially when considered as an anesthesia route).

To remove an epidural catheter

• Typically, the anesthesiologist orders analgesics and removes the catheter. However, hospital policy may allow a specially trained nurse to remove the catheter.
• If you feel resistance when removing the catheter, stop and call the doctor for further orders.
• The doctor will want to examine the catheter tip *to rule out any damage during removal,* so be sure to save the catheter.

Special considerations

Assess the patient's respiratory rate and blood pressure every 2 hours for 8 hours, then every 4 hours for 8 hours, during the first 24 hours after starting the infusion. Then assess the patient once per shift, depending on his condition or unless ordered otherwise. Notify the doctor if the patient's respiratory rate is less than 10 breaths/minute or if his systolic blood pressure is less than 90 mm Hg.

Assess the patient's sedation level, mental status, and pain relief status every hour initially, then every 2 to 4 hours, until adequate pain control is achieved. Notify the doctor if the patient appears drowsy or experiences nausea and vomiting, refractory itching, or inability to void,

Placement of a permanent epidural catheter

An epidural catheter is implanted beneath the patient's skin and inserted near the spinal cord at the first lumbar (L1) interspace.

For temporary analgesic therapy (less than 1 week), the catheter may exit directly over the spine and be taped up the patient's back to the shoulder. However, for prolonged therapy, the catheter may be tunneled subcutaneously to an exit site on the patient's side or abdomen, or over his shoulder.

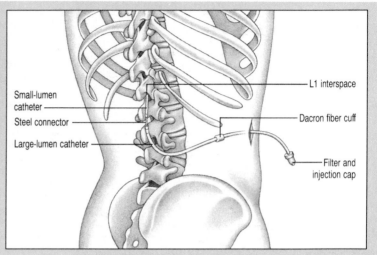

which are adverse effects of certain narcotic analgesics, or if he complains of unrelieved pain.

Assess lower-extremity motor strength every 2 to 4 hours. *If sensory and motor loss occurs, large motor nerve fibers have been affected and dosage may need to be decreased.*

Keep in mind that drugs given epidurally diffuse slowly and may cause adverse effects, including excessive sedation, up to 12 hours after epidural infusion has been discontinued.

The patient should always have a peripheral I.V. line (either continuous infusion or heparin lock) open *to allow immediate administration of emergency drugs.*

If CSF leaks into the dura mater during removal of an epidural catheter, the patient usually experiences headache. This postanalgesia headache worsens with postural changes, such as standing or sitting. The headache can be treated with a " blood patch," in which the patient's own blood (about 10 ml) is withdrawn from a peripheral vein and then injected into the epidural space. When the epidural needle is withdrawn, the patient is instructed to sit up. Because the blood clots seal off the leaking area, the blood patch should relieve the patient's headache immediately. The patient need not restrict his activity after this procedure.

Home care

Home use of epidural analgesia is possible only if the patient or his family is willing and able to learn the care

needed. The patient also must be willing and able to abstain from alcohol and street drugs *because these substances potentiate opiate action.*

Complications

The most common complication of epidural infusion is numbness and leg weakness, which may occur after the first 24 hours and is drug- and concentration-dependent. Identifying the dosage level that provides adequate pain control without causing excessive numbness and weakness requires that the doctor titrate the dosage.

Other complications include respiratory depression, which usually occurs during the first 24 hours (treated with naloxone, 0.2 to 0.4 mg I.V.), pruritus (treated with nalbuphine, 5 mg I.V., or diphenhydramine, 25 mg I.V.), and nausea and vomiting (treated with prochlorperazine, 5 to 10 mg I.V., or metoclopramide, 10 mg I.V.).

Documentation

Record the patient's response to treatment, catheter patency, condition of the dressing and insertion site, vital signs, and assessment results. Also document the labeling of the epidural catheter, changing of the infusion bags, ordered analgesics, if any, and the patient's response.

Drug infusion through an Ommaya reservoir

Also known as the subcutaneous cerebrospinal fluid (CSF) reservoir, the Ommaya reservoir allows delivery of long-term drug therapy to the CSF via the brain's ventricles. The reservoir spares the patient repeated lumbar punctures to administer chemotherapeutic drugs, analgesics, antibiotics, and antifungals. It's most commonly used for chemotherapy and pain management, specifically for treating central nervous system (CNS) leukemia, malignant CNS disease, or meningeal carcinomatosis.

The reservoir is a mushroom-shaped silicone apparatus with an attached catheter. It's surgically implanted beneath the patient's scalp in the nondominant lobe, and the catheter is threaded into the ventricle through a burr hole in the skull. (See *How the Ommaya reservoir works.*) Besides providing convenient, comparatively painless access to CSF, the Ommaya reservoir permits consistent and predictable drug distribution throughout the subarachnoid space and CNS. It also allows measurement of intracranial pressure (ICP).

Before reservoir insertion, the patient may receive a local or general anesthetic, depending on his condition and the doctor's preference. After an X-ray confirms placement of the reservoir, a pressure dressing is applied for 24 hours, followed by a gauze dressing for another day or two. The sutures may be removed in about 10 days. However, the reservoir can be used within 48 hours to deliver drugs, obtain CSF pressure measurements, drain CSF, and withdraw CSF specimens.

The doctor usually injects drugs into the Ommaya reservoir, but a specially trained nurse may perform this procedure if allowed by hospital policy and the state's nurse practice act. This sterile procedure usually takes 15 to 30 minutes.

Equipment
Equipment varies but may include the following: preservative-free prescribed drug ■ gloves ■ povidone-iodine solution ■ sterile towel ■ two 3-ml syringes ■ 25G needle or 22G Huber needle ■ sterile gauze pad ■ collection tubes for CSF, if ordered ■ vial of bacteriostatic normal saline solution.

Preparation of equipment
Using the sterile towel, establish a sterile field near the patient. Prepare a syringe with the preservative-free drug to be instilled and place it, the CSF collection tubes, and the normal saline solution on the sterile field.

How the Ommaya reservoir works

To insert an Ommaya reservoir, the doctor drills a burr hole and inserts the device's catheter through the patient's nondominant frontal lobe into the lateral ventricle. The reservoir, which has a self-sealing silicone injection dome, rests over the burr hole under a scalp flap. This creates a slight, soft bulge on the scalp, approximately the size of a quarter. Usually, drugs are injected into the dome with a syringe.

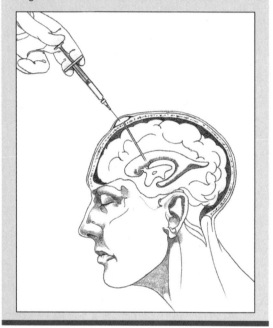

Implementation
• If your patient is scheduled to receive an Ommaya reservoir, explain the procedure before reservoir insertion. Be sure the patient and his family understand the potential complications, and answer any questions they may have. Reassure the patient that any hair shaved for the implant will grow back and that only a coin-sized patch must remain shaved for injections. (Hair regrowth will be slower if the patient is receiving chemotherapy.)

To instill medication
• Obtain baseline vital signs.
• Position the patient so he's either sitting or reclining.

• Put on gloves and prepare the patient's scalp with the povidone-iodine solution, working in a circular motion from the center outward.
• Placing the 25G needle at a 45-degree angle, insert it into the reservoir and aspirate 3 ml of clear CSF into a syringe. (If the aspirate isn't clear, check with the doctor before continuing.)
• Continue to aspirate as many milliliters of CSF as you will instill of the drug. Then detach the syringe from the needle hub, attach the drug syringe, and instill the medication slowly, monitoring for headache, nausea, and dizziness. (Some hospitals use the CSF instead of a pre-servative-free diluent to deliver the drug).
• Instruct the patient to lie quietly for about 15 to 30 minutes after the procedure. *This may prevent meningeal irritation leading to nausea and vomiting.*
• Cover the site with a sterile gauze pad and apply gentle pressure for a moment or two until superficial bleeding stops.
• Monitor the patient for adverse drug reactions and signs of increased ICP, such as nausea, vomiting, pain, or dizziness. Assess for adverse reactions every 30 minutes for 2 hours, then every hour for 2 hours, and finally every 4 hours.

Special considerations

Occasionally, the doctor may wish to prescribe an anti-emetic to be administered 30 minutes before the procedure *to control nausea and vomiting.*

After the reservoir is implanted, the patient may resume normal activities. Instruct him to protect the site from bumps and traumatic injury while the incision heals. Tell him that, unless complications develop, the reservoir may function for years.

Instruct the patient and his family to notify the doctor if any signs of infection develop at the insertion site (for example, redness, swelling, tenderness, or drainage) or if the patient develops headache, neck stiffness, or fever, which may indicate a systemic infection.

Complications

Infection may develop but can usually be treated successfully by injection of antibiotics directly into the reservoir. Persistent infection may require removal of the reservoir.

Catheter migration or blockage may cause symptoms of increased ICP, such as headache and nausea. If the doctor suspects this problem, he may gently push and release the reservoir several times (a technique called *pumping*). With his finger on the patient's scalp, the doctor can feel the reservoir refill. Slow filling suggests catheter migration or blockage, which must be confirmed by computed tomography scan. Surgical correction is required.

Documentation

Record the appearance of the reservoir insertion site before and after access, the patient's tolerance of the procedure, the amount of CSF withdrawn, its appearance, and the name and dose of the drug instilled.

Selected references

Akahoshi, M.P., et al. "Patient Controlled Analgesia via Intrathecal Catheter in Outpatient Oncology Patients," *Journal of Intravenous Nursing* 11(5):289-92, September-October 1988.

Bigelow-Kemp, B., et al. *Fundamentals of Nursing*, 2nd ed. Glenview, Ill.: Scott, Foresman & Co., 1989.

Brown, J.M. "Innovative Antibiotic Therapy at Home," *Journal of Intravenous Nursing* 11(6):397-401, November-December 1988.

Clayton, B., and Stock, Y. *Basic Pharmacology for Nurses*, 9th ed. St. Louis: C.V. Mosby Co., 1989.

Cohen, M.S. "Continuous Epidural Infusions for Acute Postoperative Pain," Part 1. *Current Reviews for Postanesthesia Care Nurses* 11(12):90-96, August 1989.

Cornwell, C.M. "The Ommaya Reservoir: Implications for Pediatric Oncology," *Pediatric Nursing* 16(3):249-51, 256-57, May-June 1990.

Crisis Drugs. Clinical SkillBuilders Series. Springhouse, Pa.: Springhouse Corp., 1991.

Drug Information for the Health Care Professional, 2 vols., 11th ed. Rockville, Md.: United States Pharmacopeial Convention, Inc., 1991.

Drug Information 91—American Hospital Formulary Service. Bethesda, Md.: American Society of Hospital Pharmacists, 1991.

Dunajcik, L. "Controlling the Dangers of Epidural Analgesia," *RN* 51(1):40-45, January 1988.

Earnest, V. *Clinical Skills and Assessment Techniques in Nursing Practice*. Glenview, Ill.: Scott, Foresman & Co., 1989.

Endocrine Problems. NurseReview Series. Springhouse, Pa.: Springhouse Corp., 1991.

Facts and Comparisons. St. Louis, Mo.: Facts and Comparisons, Inc. Updated monthly.

Fiser, D.H. "Intraosseous Infusion," *New England Journal of Medicine* 322(22):1579-81, May 31, 1990.

Fleisher, G. *Textbook of Pediatric Emergency Medicine*, 2nd ed. Baltimore: Williams & Wilkins Co., 1988.

Groenwald, S.L. *Cancer Nursing: Principles and Practice*. Boston: Jones & Bartlett Pubs., Inc., 1987.

Hadaway, L.C. "A Midline Alternative to Central and Peripheral Venous Access," *Caring* 9(5):45-46, 48-50, May 1990.

Hagle, M. "Implantable Devices for Chemotherapy: Access and Delivery," *Seminars in Oncology Nursing* 3(2):96-105, May 1987.

Haight, K. "What You Should Know About Epidural Anesthesia," *Nursing87* 17(9):58-59, September 1987.

Handy, C.M. "Vascular Access Devices: Hospital to Home Care," *Journal of Intravenous Nursing* (Supp.) 12(1):10S-18S, January-February 1989.

Illustrated Manual of Nursing Practice. Springhouse, Pa.: Springhouse Corp., 1991.

I.V. Therapy. Clinical SkillBuilders Series. Springhouse, Pa.: Springhouse Corp., 1991.

Keen, M.F. "Get on the Right Track with Z-track Injections," *Nursing90* 20(8):59, August 1990.

Malloy, Janice. "Administering Intraperitoneal Chemotherapy: A New Approach," *Nursing91* 21(1):58-62, January 1991.

Masoorli, S., and Angeles, T. "PICC Lines: The Latest Home Care Challenge," *RN* 53(1):44-51, January 1990.

Medication Administration and I.V. Therapy Manual: Process and Procedures. Springhouse, Pa.: Springhouse Corp., 1988.

Millam, D. "Avoiding Needle-stick Injuries," *Nursing90* 20(1):61-64, January 1990.

Nurse's Quick Reference. Springhouse, Pa.: Springhouse Corp., 1990.

Nursing92 Drug Handbook. Springhouse, Pa.: Springhouse Corp., 1992.

Oncology Nursing Society. *Cancer Chemotherapy Guidelines: Recommendations for Nursing Practice in the Acute Care Setting.* Pittsburgh, Pa.: Oncology Nursing Society, 1988.

Perry, A.G., and Potter, P.A. *Clinical Nursing Skills and Techniques*, 2nd ed. St. Louis: Mosby-Year Book, Inc., 1990.

Photoguide to Drug Administration. Springhouse, Pa.: Springhouse Corp., 1991.

Physicians' Desk Reference, 46th ed. Oradell, N.J.: Medical Economics Co., Inc., 1992.

Tenenbaum, L. *Cancer Chemotherapy: A Reference Guide.* Philadelphia: W.B. Saunders Co., 1989.

Textbook of Advanced Cardiac Life Support, 2nd ed. Dallas: American Heart Association, 1987.

Timby, B.K. *Clinical Nursing Procedures.* Philadelphia: J.B. Lippincott Co., 1989.

Trissel, L.A. *Handbook on Injectable Drugs*, 5th ed. Bethesda, Md.: American Society of Hospital Pharmacists, 1988.

Wheeler, C.A. "Pediatric Intraosseous Infusion: An Old Technique in Modern Health Care Technology," *Journal of Intravenous Nursing* 12(6):371-76, November-December 1989.

Ziegfeld, C.R. *Core Curriculum for Oncology Nursing.* Philadelphia: W.B. Saunders Co., 1987.

CHAPTER 6

INTRAVASCULAR THERAPY

CHARLES KROZEK, RN, BA, MN

Introduction

Currently, more than 80% of hospitalized patients receive some form of I.V. therapy. Although you may not be called upon to insert all types of I.V. lines, you will be responsible for maintaining these lines and preventing complications throughout therapy. You'll also be responsible for helping the doctor perform minor surgical procedures, such as insertion of central venous (CV) or arterial lines.

This chapter will explain the administration methods and primary uses of I.V. therapy. You'll review how to prepare for I.V. therapy; how to insert, maintain, and remove specific I.V. lines and devices; how to control infection and maintain flow rates; and how to monitor the patient's response to therapy. What's more, you'll find out about patient-teaching responsibilities and home care issues.

I.V. delivery methods

Selection of an I.V. delivery method depends upon the therapy's purpose and duration; the patient's diagnosis, age, and health history; and the condition of his veins. For example, in peripheral I.V. therapy, you'll administer I.V. solutions through a vein in the arm, the hand or, less frequently, the leg or foot. Typically, this method is used for short-term or intermittent therapy.

In CV therapy, you'll administer I.V. solutions through a central vein, such as the right or left subclavian or the internal or external jugular. This method is typically used for patients who need a large volume of fluid or a hypertonic solution, caustic drug, or high-calorie parenteral nutrition solution. Implanted vascular access devices provide a variation on CV infusion. The infused solution enters a central vein through an access device surgically implanted in a subcutaneous pocket. This method of delivery is ordered for patients needing long-term (months to years) I.V. therapy.

Uses of I.V. therapy

The most common uses of I.V. therapy are maintaining and restoring fluid and electrolyte balance, administering drugs, transfusing blood, and delivering parenteral nutrition.

The I.V. route allows rapid, effective drug administration. Commonly infused drugs include antibiotics, thrombolytics, histamine$_2$-receptor antagonists, antineoplastic agents, cardiovascular drugs, anticonvulsants and, most recently, patient-controlled analgesics. Usually, you'll give an I.V drug over a short period — in some cases by direct injection, called I.V. push. (See Chapter 5, Drug administration.)

With blood transfusion, your nursing responsibilities include administering blood and blood components as well as monitoring patients receiving therapy. Transfusion aims to maintain adequate blood volume, prevent cardiogenic shock, increase the blood's oxygen carrying capacity, and maintain hemostasis.

Parenteral nutrition is the administration of nutrients by the I.V. route. Low-concentration parenteral nutrition solutions are administered through a peripheral vein; more highly concentrated ones through a central vein. If you're caring for a patient receiving parenteral nutrition, you'll need to know how to recognize changes in fluid and electrolyte status and in glucose, amino acid, mineral, and vitamin levels. You'll also need to judge your patient's response to the nutrient solution and to detect early signs of complications.

Patient teaching

Many patients are apprehensive about I.V. therapy. To allay their fears, you can provide information that explains and clarifies this therapy. Use pamphlets and videotapes if available. If possible, show the patient the actual equipment and explain how it will be used during therapy.

Allow the patient to express fears and concerns, and convey reassurance by answering his questions fully. You may wish to involve a family member or caregiver in these discussions to further reassure the patient.

Home I.V. therapy

More and more patients are receiving I.V. therapy at home. Home therapy benefits patients by making them feel more comfortable and allowing them to perform many of their normal activities. Its lower cost benefits both patients and hospitals.

Home care patients may receive fluids or such medications as antibiotics, antifungals, chemotherapeutic agents, insulin, chelating agents, or analgesics. More recently, some blood products have been given at home following an initial transfusion in the hospital.

Candidates for home I.V. therapy should be selected carefully. Such patients must be willing and able to administer therapy safely, learn the potential complications and interventions, understand the basics of asepsis, and obtain the necessary supplies. Patients who need help must enlist a home caregiver, such as a family member or friend, to assist them in administering I.V. therapy.

When teaching the home care patient, demonstrate procedures and answer any questions. Have the patient or family members give return demonstrations whenever possible. Teaching should begin in the hospital and should be completed before the patient is discharged. You may wish to include a family member or caregiver in your patient teaching.

Documentation

You need to document I.V. therapy for many reasons. First, an accurate description of your care provides legal protection for you and the hospital. Furthermore, thorough documentation furnishes health care insurers with the records they need of the equipment and supplies used. You may document I.V. therapy on progress notes, a special I.V. therapy sheet or flowchart, or a nursing care plan on the patient's chart. You also must document it on the intake and output sheet.

PERIPHERAL LINES
Preparation for I.V. therapy

Proper selection and preparation of equipment is essential to accurate delivery of an I.V. solution. Selection of an I.V. administration set depends on the rate and type of infusion desired and the type of I.V. solution container used. Two types of drip system are available: the macrodrip and the microdrip set. The macrodrip set can deliver a solution in large quantities and at rapid rates because it delivers a larger amount of solution with each drop than the microdrip set. The microdrip set, used for pediatric and certain adult patients requiring small or closely regulated amounts of I.V. solution, delivers a smaller quantity of solution with each drop.

Administration tubing with a secondary injection port permits separate or simultaneous infusion of two solutions; tubing with a piggyback port and a backcheck valve permits intermittent infusion of a secondary solution and, on its completion, a return to infusion of the primary solution. Vented I.V. tubing is selected for solutions in nonvented bottles; nonvented tubing for solutions in bags or vented bottles. Assembly of I.V. equipment requires aseptic technique to prevent contamination, which can cause local or systemic infection.

Equipment

I.V. solution ■ I.V. administration set ■ in-line filter, if needed ■ I.V. pole ■ alcohol sponges ■ medication and label, if necessary.

Preparation of equipment

Verify the type, volume, and expiration date of the I.V. solution. Discard any outdated solution. If the solution is contained in a glass bottle, inspect for chips or cracks; if it is in a plastic bag, squeeze to detect leaks. Examine the I.V. solution for particles, abnormal discoloration, and cloudiness. If present, discard the solution and notify the pharmacy or dispensing department. If ordered, add medication to the solution, and place a completed medication-added label on the container. (For instructions, see "Addition of drugs to an I.V. solution" in Chapter 5.) Remove the administration set from its box and observe for cracks, holes, and missing clamps.

Implementation

• Wash your hands thoroughly *to prevent introducing contaminants during preparation.*
• Slide the flow clamp of the administration set tubing down to the drip chamber or injection port, and close the clamp.

Preparing a bag

• Place the bag on a flat, stable surface or hang it on an I.V. pole. Then remove the protective cap or tear the tab from the tubing insertion port.
• Remove the protective cap from the administration set spike.
• Holding the port carefully and firmly with one hand, insert the spike with your other hand.

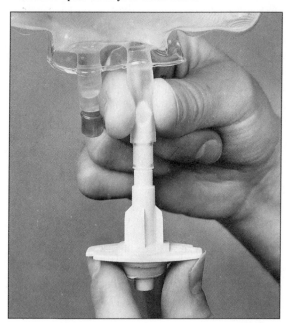

• Hang the bag on the I.V. pole, if you haven't already, and squeeze the drip chamber until it is half full.

Preparing a nonvented bottle
• Remove the bottle's metal cap and inner disk, if present.
• Place the bottle on a stable surface and wipe the rubber stopper with an alcohol sponge.
• Remove the protective cap from the administration set spike, and push the spike through the center of the bottle's rubber stopper. Avoid twisting or angling the spike *to prevent pieces of the stopper from breaking off and falling into the solution.*
• Invert the bottle. If its vacuum is intact, you'll hear a hissing sound and see air bubbles rise (this may not occur if you've already added medication). If the vacuum is not intact, discard the bottle and begin again.
• Hang the bottle on the I.V. pole and squeeze the drip chamber until it is half full.

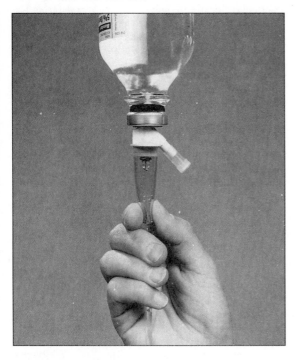

Preparing a vented bottle
• Remove the bottle's metal cap and latex diaphragm *to release the vacuum.* If the vacuum is not intact (except after medication has been added), discard the bottle and begin again.
• Place the bottle on a stable surface and wipe the rubber stopper with an alcohol sponge.
• Remove the protective cap from the administration set

spike, and push the spike through the insertion port next to the air vent tube opening.
• Hang the bottle on the I.V. pole and squeeze the drip chamber until it is half full.

Priming the I.V. tubing
• If necessary, attach a filter to the opposite end of the I.V. tubing, and follow the manufacturer's instructions for filling and priming it. Purge the tubing before attaching the filter *to avoid forcing air into the filter and possibly clogging some filter channels.* Most filters are positioned with the distal end of the tubing facing upward *so that the solution will completely wet the filter membrane and all air bubbles will be eliminated from the line.* (See *When to use an in-line filter,* page 272.)
• If you're not using a filter, aim the distal end of the tubing over a wastebasket or sink and slowly open the flow clamp. (Most distal tube coverings allow the solution to flow without having to remove the protective cover.)
• Leave the clamp open until I.V. solution flows through the entire length of tubing, forcing out all air.
• Invert all Y injection sites and backcheck valves and tap them, if necessary, *to fill them with solution.*

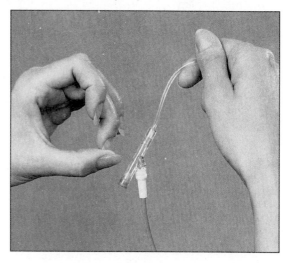

• After priming the tubing, close the clamp. Then loop the tubing over the I.V. pole.
• Label the container with the patient's name and room number, the date and time, the container number, the ordered rate and duration of infusion, and your initials.

Special considerations
Before initiation of I.V. therapy, the patient should be instructed in what to expect. (See *Teaching your patient about I.V. therapy,* page 273.)

When to use an in-line filter

An in-line filter removes pathogens and particles from I.V. solutions, helping to reduce the risk of infusion phlebitis. But because in-line filters are expensive and their installation cumbersome and time-consuming, they're not used routinely. Many institutions require use of a filter only when administering an admixture. If you're unsure of whether to use a filter, check hospital policy or follow this list of do's and don'ts.

Do's
Use an in-line filter:
• when administering solutions to an immunodeficient patient.
• when administering total parenteral nutrition.
• when using additives comprising many separate particles, such as antibiotics requiring reconstitution, or when administering several additives.
• when using rubber injection sites or plastic diaphragms repeatedly.
• when phlebitis is likely to occur.
  Be sure to change the in-line filter according to the manufacturer's recommendations (typically every 24 to 96 hours). *If you don't, bacteria trapped in the filter release endotoxin, a pyrogen small enough to pass through the filter into the bloodstream.*
  Use an add-on filter of larger pore size (1.2 microns) when infusing lipid emulsions and albumin mixed with nutritional solutions.

Don'ts
Don't use an in-line filter:
• when administering solutions with large particles *that will clog a filter and stop I.V. flow,* such as blood and its components, suspensions, lipid emulsions, and high-molecular-volume plasma expanders.
• when administering a drug dose of 5 mg or less *(because the filter may absorb it).*

Always use aseptic technique when preparing I.V. solutions. If you contaminate the administration set or container, replace it with a new one *to prevent introducing contaminants into the system.*

If necessary, you can use vented tubing with a vented bottle. To do this, don't remove the latex diaphragm.

Instead, insert the spike into the larger indentation in the diaphragm.

Change I.V. tubing every 48 or 72 hours according to hospital policy or more frequently if you suspect contamination. Change the filter according to manufacturer's recommendations or sooner if it becomes clogged.

Documentation
Document the type of solution used and any additives to the solution.

Use of a volume-control set

A volume-control set — an I.V. line with a graduated chamber — delivers precise amounts of fluid and shuts off when the fluid is exhausted, preventing air from entering the I.V. line. This device is used as a primary line in children for continuous infusion of fluids or medication. It also may be used as a secondary line in adults for intermittent infusion of medication.

Equipment
Volume-control set ▪ I.V. pole (for setting up a primary I.V. line) ▪ I.V. solution ▪ 20G to 22G 1″ needle ▪ alcohol sponges ▪ medication in labeled syringe and 20G to 22G 1″ needle ▪ tape ▪ label.

Although various models of volume-control sets are available, each one consists of a graduated fluid chamber (120 to 250 ml) with a spike and a filtered air line on top and administration tubing underneath. Floating-valve sets have a valve at the bottom that closes when the chamber empties; membrane-filter sets have a rigid filter at the bottom that, when wet, prevents the passage of air.

Preparation of equipment
Ensure the sterility of all equipment and inspect it carefully *to ensure the absence of flaws.* Take the equipment to the patient's bedside.

Implementation
• Wash your hands, and explain the procedure to the patient. If an I.V. line is already in place, observe its insertion site for signs of infiltration or infection.
• Remove the volume-control set from its box and close all the clamps.
• Remove the protective cap from the volume-control set spike, insert the spike into the I.V. solution container, and hang the container on the I.V. pole.

Teaching your patient about I.V. therapy

Many patients feel apprehensive about peripheral I.V. therapy. So before you begin therapy, teach your patient what to expect before, during, and after the procedure. Thorough patient teaching can reduce anxiety, making therapy easier. Follow these guidelines.

Before insertion
• Describe the procedure. Tell him that "intravenous" means inside the vein and that a plastic catheter or needle will be placed in his vein. Explain that fluids containing certain nutrients or medications will flow from a bag or bottle, through a length of tubing, then through the plastic catheter or needle into his vein.
• Tell him approximately how long the catheter or needle will stay in place. Explain that the doctor will decide how much and what type of fluid the patient needs.
• If the patient will receive a local anesthetic at the insertion site, ask him if he's allergic to lidocaine. If in doubt, use another anesthetic. Tell him this injection will numb the site to reduce the pain of I.V. device insertion.
• If no anesthetic will be used, tell the patient that he may feel transient pain at the insertion site but that the discomfort will stop once the catheter or needle is in place.

• Tell him that I.V. fluid may feel cold at first, but that this sensation should last only a few minutes.

During therapy
• Instruct the patient to report any discomfort after the catheter or needle has been inserted and the fluid has begun to flow.
• Explain any restrictions, as ordered. As appropriate, tell the patient that he may be able to walk while receiving I.V. therapy and, depending on the insertion site and the device, he also may be able to shower or take a tub bath during therapy.
• Teach him how to care for the I.V. line. Tell him not to pull at the insertion site or tubing, not to remove the container from the I.V. pole, and not to kink the tubing or lie on it. Instruct him to call a nurse if the flow rate suddenly slows down or speeds up.

At removal
• Explain that removing a peripheral I.V. line is a simple procedure. Tell the patient that pressure will be applied to the site until the bleeding stops. Reassure him that once the device is out and the bleeding stops, he'll be able to use the affected arm or leg as before therapy.

• Open the air vent clamp and close the upper slide clamp. Then open the lower clamp on the I.V. tubing, slide it upward until it's slightly below the drip chamber, and close the clamp.

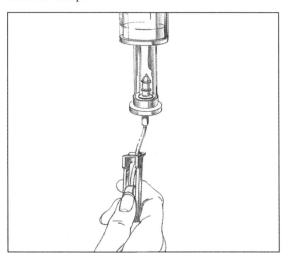

• If you're using a valve set, open the upper clamp until the fluid chamber fills with about 30 ml of solution. Then close the clamp and carefully squeeze the drip chamber until it is half full.
• If you're using a volume-control set with a membrane filter, open the upper clamp until the fluid chamber fills with about 30 ml of solution, and then close the clamp.
• Open the lower clamp and squeeze the drip chamber flat with two fingers of your opposite hand. *If you squeeze the drip chamber with the lower clamp closed, you'll damage the membrane filter.*

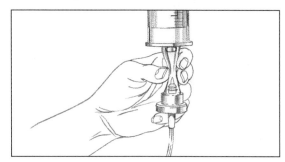

• Keeping the drip chamber flat, close the lower clamp. Now release and reshape the drip chamber so it fills halfway.

• Open the lower clamp, prime the tubing, and close the clamp. To use as a primary line, insert an adapter into the catheter or needle hub. To use as a secondary line, attach a needle to the adapter on the volume-control set. Wipe the Y port of the primary tubing with an alcohol sponge, and insert the needle. Then tape the connection.

• To add medication, wipe the injection port on the volume-control set with an alcohol sponge, and inject the medication. Place a label on the chamber, indicating the drug, the dose, and the date. Don't write directly on the chamber *because the plastic absorbs ink.*

• Open the upper clamp, fill the fluid chamber with the prescribed amount of solution, and close the clamp. Gently rotate the chamber *to mix the medication.*

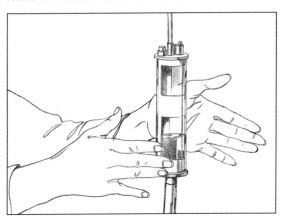

• Turn off the primary solution (if present) or lower the drip rate *to maintain an open line.*

• Open the lower clamp on the volume-control set, and adjust the drip rate as ordered. After completion of the infusion, open the upper clamp and let 10 ml of I.V. solution flow into the chamber and through the tubing *to flush them.*

• If you're using the volume-control set as a secondary I.V. line, close the lower clamp and reset the flow rate of the primary line. If you're using the set as a primary I.V. line, close the lower clamp, refill the chamber to the prescribed amount, and begin the infusion again.

Special considerations

Always check compatibility of the medication and the I.V. solution. If you're using a membrane-filter set, avoid administering suspensions, lipid emulsions, blood, or blood components through it.

If you're using a floating-valve set, the diaphragm may stick after repeated use. If it does, close the air vent and upper clamp, invert the drip chamber, and squeeze it. If the diaphragm opens, reopen the clamp and continue to use the set. If the drip chamber of a floating-valve diaphragm set overfills, immediately close the upper clamp and air vent, invert the chamber, and squeeze the excess fluid from the drip chamber back into the graduated fluid chamber.

Documentation

If you add a drug to the volume-control set, record the amount and type of medication, the amount of fluid used to dilute it, and the date and time of infusion.

Insertion of a peripheral I.V. line

This procedure involves selection of a venipuncture device and insertion site, application of a tourniquet, preparation of the site, and venipuncture. Selection of a venipuncture device and site depends on the type of solution to be used; the frequency and duration of infusion; the patient's age, size, and condition; the patency and location of accessible veins; and, when possible, the patient's preference. Typically, selection focuses on a vein in the nondominant arm or hand. The most favorable venipuncture sites are the cephalic and basilic veins in the lower arm and the veins in the dorsum of the hand; least favorable are the leg and foot veins because of the increased risk of thrombophlebitis.

Antecubital veins can be used if no other venous access is available; to accommodate a large-bore needle; or to administer drugs requiring large volume dilution.

Use of a peripheral line allows administration of fluids, medication, blood, and blood components, and maintains I.V. access to the patient. Insertion is contraindicated in a sclerotic vein, in an edematous or impaired arm or hand, and in the presence of burns or an arteriovenous fistula. Subsequent venipunctures should be performed proximal to a previously used or injured vein.

Equipment

Alcohol sponges ▪ povidone-iodine sponges ▪ antimicrobial ointment, according to hospital policy ▪ gloves ▪ tourniquet (rubber tubing or a blood pressure cuff) ▪ two I.V. needles or I.V. catheter devices ▪ sterile 2″ × 2″ gauze pads or a transparent semipermeable dressing ▪ 1″ nonallergenic tape ▪ I.V. solution with attached and primed administration set ▪ I.V. pole ▪ sharps container ▪ optional: armboard, roller gauze, tube gauze, warm packs,

Comparing venipuncture devices

Most I.V. infusions are delivered through one of three basic types of venipuncture devices: an over-the-needle catheter, a through-the-needle catheter, or a winged infusion set.

Over-the-needle catheter
Purpose: long-term therapy for the active or agitated patient.
Advantages: accidental puncture of the vein is less likely than with a needle; more comfortable for the patient once it's in place; contains radiopaque thread for easy location; some units come with a syringe attached that permits easy check of blood return; some units are equipped with wings.
Disadvantage: more difficult to insert than other devices.

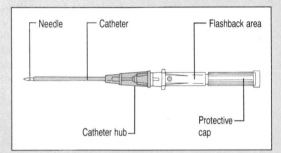

Through-the-needle catheter
Purpose: long-term therapy for the active or agitated patient.
Advantages: accidental puncture of the vein is less likely than with a needle; more comfortable for the patient once it's in place; available in many lengths; most plastic catheters contain radiopaque thread, permitting easy location; one variant, the peripherally inserted central catheter, is inserted in the antecubital vein by

a specially prepared nurse.
Disadvantages: leaking at the site may occur, especially in an elderly patient; if a needle guard isn't used, the catheter may be severed.

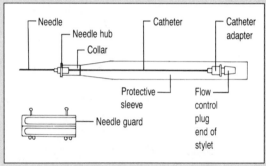

Winged infusion set
Purpose: short-term therapy for any cooperative adult patient; therapy of any duration for an infant or child or for an elderly patient with fragile or sclerotic veins.
Advantages: easiest intravascular device to insert; ideal for I.V. push drugs.
Disadvantage: may easily cause infiltration if a rigid-needle winged infusion device is used.

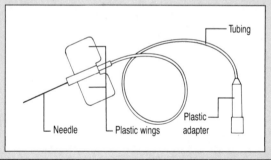

antimicrobial solution (such as 70% alcohol, tincture of iodine, povidone-iodine, or chlorhexidine), local anesthetic (such as 1% lidocaine without epinephrine), U-100 insulin syringe with a 27G needle.

Commercial venipuncture kits are available with or without an I.V. needle or I.V. catheter device (see *Comparing venipuncture devices*). In many hospitals, venipuncture equipment is kept on a tray or cart, allowing choice of the correct needle or catheter and easy replacement of contaminated items.

Preparation of equipment
Check the information on the label of the I.V. solution container, including the patient's name and room number, the type of solution, the time and date of its preparation, the preparer's name, and the ordered infusion rate. Compare the doctor's orders with the solution label *to verify*

Locating hard-to-find veins

You can locate hard-to-find peripheral veins more easily by using a transillumination device such as the Landry Vein Light. This device uses bright light from a pair of adjustable fiber-optic arms to reveal the blood vessels. Secure the light to the patient's limb with tape. Dim the room lights. With the device on its brightest setting, scan the limb below the tourniquet for a vein. The vein appears as a dark line between the fiber-optic arms.

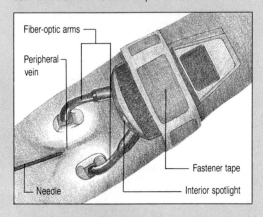

Fiber-optic arms

Peripheral vein

Fastener tape

Needle

Interior spotlight

that the infusion is the correct one. Then select the smallest gauge needle or catheter device available for the infusion unless subsequent therapy will require a larger one. *Smaller gauges cause less trauma to veins, allow greater blood flow around their tips, and reduce the clotting risk.*

If you're using a winged infusion set, connect the adapter to the administration set, and unclamp the line until fluid flows from the open end of the needle cover. Then close the clamp and place the needle on a sterile surface, such as the inside of its packaging.

If you're using a catheter device, open its package *to allow easy access.*

Implementation

● Place the I.V. pole in the proper slot in the patient's bed frame. If you're using a portable I.V. pole, position it close to the patient.
● Hang the I.V. solution with attached primed administration set on the I.V. pole.
● Verify the patient's identity by comparing the information on the solution container with the patient's wristband.

● Wash your hands thoroughly *to avoid spreading microorganisms.* Then explain the procedure to the patient *to ensure his cooperation and reduce anxiety. Anxiety can cause a vasomotor response resulting in venous constriction.*

Selecting the site
● Select the puncture site — preferably a vein in the nondominant arm. For fluid replacement, choose a small vein unless a large vein will be needed for subsequent therapy; *this leaves the large veins available for emergency infusion.* If long-term therapy is anticipated, start with a vein at the most distal site *so you can move proximally as needed for subsequent I.V. insertion sites.* For infusion of an irritating medication, choose a large vein (with plenty of subcutaneous tissue) distal to any nearby joint. Be sure the vein can accommodate the cannula if used.
● Place the patient's arm in a dependent position *to increase capillary fill of the lower arms and hands.* If the patient's skin is cold, warm it by rubbing and stroking the arm, or cover the entire arm with warm packs for 5 to 10 minutes.

Applying the tourniquet
● Apply a tourniquet about 6″ (15.2 cm) above the intended puncture site *to dilate the vein.* Check for a distal pulse. If it is not present, release the tourniquet and reapply it with less tension *to prevent arterial occlusion.*

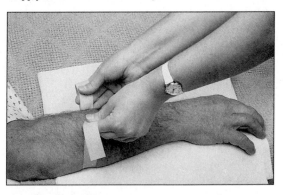

● Lightly palpate the vein with your index and middle fingers, while stretching it to prevent rolling. If the vein feels hard or ropelike, select another.
● If the vein is easily palpable but not sufficiently dilated, one or more of the following techniques may help raise the vein. Flick the skin over the vein with one or two sharp snaps of your finger, place the extremity in a dependent position for several seconds, rub or stroke the skin upward toward the tourniquet or, if you have selected a vein in the arm or hand, tell the patient to open and close his fist several times. If necessary, you may

be able to locate a vein using transillumination. (See *Locating hard-to-find veins.*)

• Leave the tourniquet in place for no more than 2 minutes. If you cannot find a suitable vein and prepare the site in that time, release the tourniquet for a few minutes. Then reapply it and continue the procedure.

Preparing the site

• Put on gloves. Clip the hair around the insertion site, if necessary, and clean the site with one of the following antimicrobials: 70% alcohol solution, povidone-iodine, tincture of iodine, or chlorhexidine. Do not apply alcohol after an iodophor prep *because alcohol negates the effect of the iodophor.* Work in a circular motion outward from the site to a diameter of 2″ to 4″ (5 to 10 cm) *to remove flora that would otherwise be introduced into the vascular system with the venipuncture.* Allow the antimicrobial solution to dry.

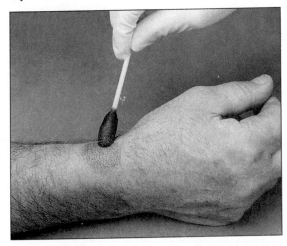

• If ordered, administer a local anesthetic. Make sure the patient is not sensitive to lidocaine. (See *Administering a local anesthetic,* page 278.)

• Hold the skin taut below the site *to stabilize the selected vein.*

• Grasp the needle or catheter. If you're using a *winged infusion set,* hold the short edges of the wings (with the needle's bevel facing upward) between the thumb and forefinger of your dominant hand. Then squeeze the wings together. If you're using an *over-the-needle catheter,* grasp the plastic hub with your dominant hand, remove the cover, and examine the catheter tip. If the edge isn't smooth, discard and replace the device. If you're using a *through-the-needle catheter,* grasp the needle hub with one hand, and unsnap the needle cover. Then rotate the catheter device until the bevel faces upward.

• Using the thumb of your opposite hand, stretch the skin taut below the puncture site *to stabilize the vein.*

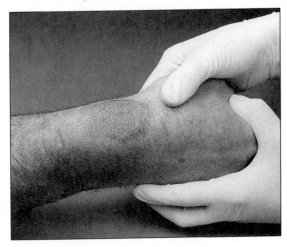

• Lightly press the vein with your thumb about 1½″ (3.8 cm) from the intended insertion site. The vein should feel round, firm, fully engorged, and resilient.

• Tell the patient that you are about to insert the device.

• For the direct approach, hold the needle bevel up and enter the skin directly over the vein at a 30- to 45-degree angle. For the indirect approach, enter the skin slightly adjacent to the vein. Direct the device into the side of the vein wall *to avoid perforating the vein's opposite wall.*

• Advance the device steadily until you meet resistance. Don't penetrate the vein. Lower the needle to a 15- to 20-degree angle, and slowly pierce the vein. You may not always feel a "pop" or a sensation of release when the device enters the vein.

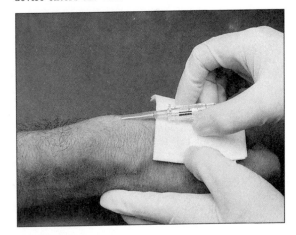

Administering a local anesthetic

Although the procedure isn't recommended by the Intravenous Nurses Society, many doctors order a local anesthetic when starting I.V. therapy to numb the infusion site. If you'll be giving a local anesthetic, follow these guidelines:

• Using a U-100 insulin syringe with a 27G needle, draw up 0.1 ml of 1% lidocaine without epinephrine.
• Clean the venipuncture site.
• Put on gloves. Insert the needle next to the vein, introducing about one-third of it into the skin subcutaneously at a 30-degree angle, as shown here.

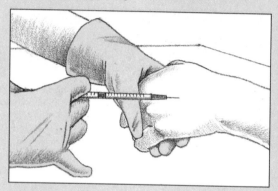

• This lateral approach carries less risk of accidental vein puncture (indicated by blood appearing in the syringe). If the vein is deep, however, inject the lidocaine over the top of it, taking care to avoid injecting the anesthetic into the vein.
• Hold your thumb on the plunger of the syringe during insertion *to avoid unnecessary movement once the needle is under the skin.*
• Without aspirating, quickly inject the lidocaine until a small wheal appears, as shown below. You may not have to administer the entire amount in the syringe.

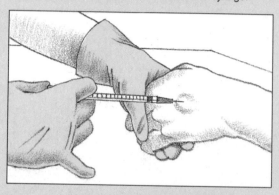

• Quickly withdraw the syringe and massage the wheal with an alcohol sponge. This will make the wheal disappear so the vein won't be hidden. However, you'll see a small pinprick of blood. The skin will be numb for about 30 minutes.
• When numbness occurs, insert the venipuncture device into the skin.

• When you observe blood flashback behind the hub, tilt the needle slightly upward and advance it farther into the vein *to prevent puncture of the posterior vein wall.* (You may not see blood return with a small vein.)
• If you're using a *winged infusion set,* advance the needle fully, if possible, and hold it in place. Release the tourniquet, open the administration set clamp slightly, and check for free flow or infiltration.
• If you're using an *over-the-needle catheter,* advance the device to at least half of its length *to ensure that the catheter itself, not just the introducer needle, has entered the vein.* Then remove the tourniquet.
• Grasp the catheter hub to hold it in place in the vein, and withdraw the needle. As you withdraw it, press lightly on the catheter tip *to prevent bleeding.* (See photograph at right.)
• Advance the catheter up to the hub or until you meet resistance.

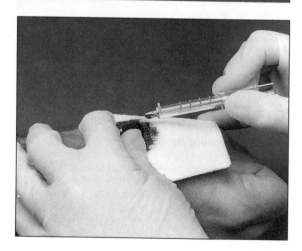

• To advance the catheter while infusing I.V. solution, release the tourniquet and remove the inner needle. Using aseptic technique, attach the I.V. tubing and begin the infusion. While stabilizing the vein with one hand, use the other to advance the catheter into the vein. When the catheter is advanced, decrease the I.V. flow rate. *This method reduces the risk of puncturing the vein's opposite wall because the catheter is advanced without the steel needle and because the rapid flow dilates the vein.*

• To advance the catheter before starting the infusion, first release the tourniquet. While stabilizing the vein with one hand, use the other to advance the catheter up to the hub. Next, remove the inner needle and, using aseptic technique, quickly attach the I.V. tubing. *This method often results in less blood being spilled.*

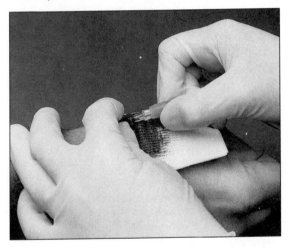

• If you're using a *through-the-needle catheter,* remove the tourniquet, hold the needle in place with one hand and, with your opposite hand, grasp the catheter through the protective sleeve. Then, slowly thread the catheter through the needle until the hub is within the needle collar. Never pull back on the catheter without pulling back on the needle *to avoid severing and releasing the catheter into the circulation, causing an embolus.* If you feel resistance from a valve, withdraw the catheter and needle slightly and reinsert them, rotating the catheter as you pass the valve. Then withdraw the metal needle, and cover it with the protector. Remove the stylet and protective sleeve, and attach the administration set to the catheter hub. Open the administration set clamp slightly, and check for free flow or infiltration.

Dressing the site

• After the venipuncture device has been inserted, clean the skin completely. If necessary, dispose of the inner

How to apply a transparent semipermeable dressing

Instead of using tape to secure the I.V. insertion site, you can apply a transparent semipermeable dressing. Here's how:

• Make sure the insertion site is clean and dry.

• Remove the dressing from the package and, using aseptic technique, remove the protective seal. Avoid touching the sterile surface.

• Place the dressing directly over the insertion site and the hub, as shown. Don't cover the tubing. Also, don't stretch the dressing; doing so *may cause itching.*

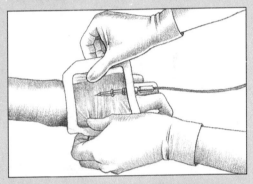

• Tuck the dressing around and under the catheter hub *to make the site impervious to microorganisms.*

• To remove the dressing, grasp one corner, then lift and stretch. If removal is difficult, try loosening the edges with alcohol or water.

needle in a needle receptacle. Then regulate the flow rate.

• You may use a transparent semipermeable dressing to secure the device. (See *How to apply a transparent semipermeable dressing.*)

• If you do not use a transparent dressing, apply antiseptic ointment at the insertion site according to hospital policy; cover with a sterile gauze pad or small adhesive bandage.

• Loop the I.V. tubing on the patient's limb, and secure the tubing with tape. *The loop allows some slack to prevent dislodgment of the catheter from tension on the line.* (See *Methods of taping a venipuncture site,* pages 280 and 281.)

(Text continues on page 282.)

Methods of taping a venipuncture site

If you'll be using tape to secure the venipuncture device to the insertion site, use one of the four basic methods described below.

Chevron method

• Cover the venipuncture site with an adhesive strip or a 2″ × 2″ sterile gauze pad. Then cut a long strip of ½″ (1.3-cm) tape and place it, sticky side up, under the needle and parallel to the short strip of tape (below).

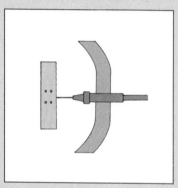

• Cross the ends of the tape over the needle so that the tape sticks to the patient's skin (below).
• Apply a piece of 1″ (2.5-cm) tape across the two wings of the chevron.

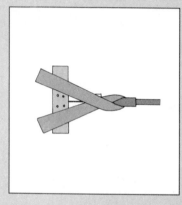

• Loop the tubing and secure it with more tape. Write the date and time of insertion, the type and gauge of the needle, and your initials (below).

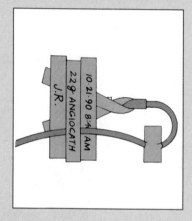

U method

• Cover the venipuncture site with an adhesive strip or a 2″ × 2″ sterile gauze pad. Then place a 2″ (5-cm) strip of ½″ tape, sticky side up, under the tubing (below).

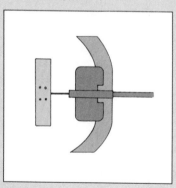

• Bring each side of the tape up, folding it over the wings of the needle. Affix it parallel to the tubing (below).
• Now apply tape as you would with the chevron method.

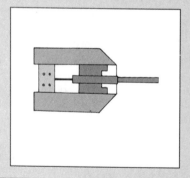

• Write the date and time of insertion, the type and gauge of the needle or catheter, and your initials (below).

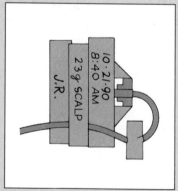

Methods of taping a venipuncture site *(continued)*

Two tape method
• Cover the venipuncture site with an adhesive strip or a 2″ × 2″ gauze pad. Then place a 2″ strip of ½″ tape, sticky side up, under the needle (below).

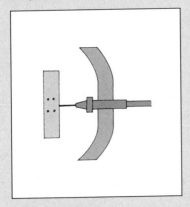

• Fold the tape ends over and affix them to the patient's skin in a U shape (below).
• Place a second strip of ½″ tape, sticky side down, over the needle hub. On the tape, write the date and time of insertion, the type and gauge of the needle or catheter,

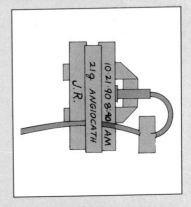

and your initials (below).
   With this method, you can remove the upper strip of tape to check the insertion site while the lower strip anchors the needle.

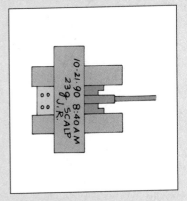

Three tape method
• Cover the venipuncture site with an adhesive strip or a 2″ × 2″ gauze pad (below). Then cut three strips of 1″ tape.
• Place one strip of tape over each wing, keeping the tape parallel to the needle (below).

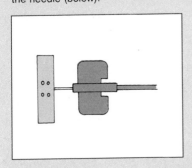

• Now place the other strip of tape perpendicular to the first two. Put it either directly on top of the wings or just below the wings, directly on top of the tubing.

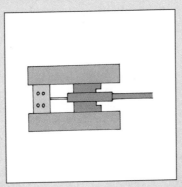

• On the last piece of tape, write the date and time of insertion, the type and gauge of the needle or catheter, and your initials (below).

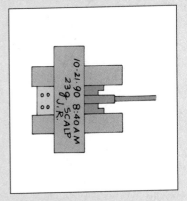

• Label the last piece of tape with the type and gauge of needle or catheter, the date and time of insertion, and your initials. Adjust the flow rate, as ordered.
• If the puncture site is near a movable joint, secure an armboard with roller gauze or tape *to provide stability, because excessive movement can dislodge the needle or catheter and increase the risk of thrombophlebitis and infection.*

Removing a peripheral I.V. line
• Performed upon completion of therapy, for needle or catheter changes, and for suspected infection or infiltration, removal of a peripheral I.V. line usually requires an alcohol sponge, a sterile gauze pad, and an adhesive bandage.
• To remove the I.V. line, first clamp the I.V. tubing *to stop the flow of solution.* Then, gently remove all tape from the skin.
• Using aseptic technique, open the gauze pad and adhesive bandage, and place them within reach. Put on gloves. Hold the sterile gauze pad over the puncture site, and use your other hand to withdraw the needle or catheter slowly and smoothly, keeping it parallel to the skin. (Inspect the catheter tip; if it's not smooth, assess the patient immediately, and notify the doctor.)
• Using the gauze pad, apply firm pressure over the puncture site for 1 to 2 minutes after the device has been removed or until bleeding has stopped.
• Clean the site and apply the adhesive bandage. Or if blood oozes from the site, apply a pressure bandage.
• If drainage appears at the puncture site, send the tip of the device and a sample of the drainage to the laboratory to be cultured according to hospital policy. (A draining site may or may not be infected.) Then clean the area and apply antiseptic ointment and a sterile dressing.
• Instruct the patient to restrict activity for about 10 minutes and to leave the dressing in place for at least 8 hours. If the patient feels lingering tenderness at the site, apply warm packs.

Special considerations
If the patient is elderly, apply the tourniquet carefully *to avoid pinching the skin.* If necessary, apply it over the patient's gown. Make sure skin preparation materials are at room temperature *to avoid vasoconstriction resulting from lower temperatures.* If the patient is allergic to iodine-containing compounds, clean the skin with alcohol.

If you fail to see blood flashback after entering the vein, pull back slightly and rotate the device. If you still fail to see flashback, remove the cannula and try again. If you suspect that the device is in the vein, try these measures to facilitate blood flashback: position the I.V. container below needle level, or insert the needle and syringe into the injection port closest to the puncture site. Then close the clamp on the I.V. tubing and attempt to aspirate. (Keep in mind that, if the device is tightly in place or the patient is extremely dehydrated or hypovolemic, you may not see blood flashback.)

Change a gauze or transparent dressing when you change the administration set (every 48 hours or according to hospital policy).

Be sure to rotate the I.V. site, usually every 48 to 72 hours or according to hospital policy.

When a vein cannot be entered percutaneously, venesection may need to be performed.

Home care
Most patients receiving I.V. therapy at home will have a central venous line. But if you care for a patient going home with a peripheral line, you should teach care of the I.V. site and identify certain complications. If the patient must observe movement restrictions, make sure he understands them.

Teach the patient how to examine the site, and instruct him to notify the doctor if redness, swelling, or discomfort develops; if the dressing becomes moist; or if blood is in the tubing.

Also tell the patient to report any problems with the I.V. line; for instance, if the solution stops infusing or if an alarm goes off on an infusion pump or controller. Explain that the I.V. site will be changed at established intervals by a home care nurse.

If the patient is using an intermittent infusion device, such as a heparin lock, teach him how and when to flush it. Finally, teach the patient to document daily whether the I.V. site is free from pain, swelling, and redness.

Complications
Peripheral line complications can result from the needle or catheter (infection, phlebitis, and embolism) or from the solution (circulatory overload, infiltration, sepsis, and allergic reaction). (See *Risks of peripheral I.V. therapy.*)

Documentation
In your notes or on the appropriate I.V. sheets, record the date and time of venipuncture, the type and gauge of needle or catheter, the location of the insertion site, and the reason the site was changed.

Also document the number of attempts at venipuncture (if you made more than one), the type and flow rate of the I.V. solution, the name and amount of medication in the solution (if any), any adverse reactions and actions taken to correct them, patient teaching and evidence of patient understanding, and your initials.

(Text continues on page 287.)

Risks of peripheral I.V. therapy

COMPLICATION	SIGNS AND SYMPTOMS	POSSIBLE CAUSES	NURSING INTERVENTIONS
Local complications			
Phlebitis	• Tenderness at tip of and proximal to venipuncture device • Redness at tip of catheter and along vein • Puffy area over vein • Vein hard on palpation • Elevated temperature	• Poor blood flow around venipuncture device • Friction from catheter movement in vein • Venipuncture device left in vein too long • Clotting at catheter tip (thrombophlebitis) • Drug or solution with high or low pH or high osmolarity	• Remove venipuncture device. • Apply warm soaks. • Notify doctor if patient has fever. • Document patient's condition and your interventions. ***Prevention*** • Restart infusion using larger vein for irritating solution, or restart with smaller-gauge device *to ensure adequate blood flow.* • Use filter *to reduce risk of phlebitis.* • Tape device securely *to prevent motion.*
Extravasation	• Swelling at and above I.V. site (may extend along entire limb) • Discomfort, burning, or pain at site (but may be painless) • Tight feeling at site • Decreased skin temperature around site • Blanching at site • Continuing fluid infusion even when vein is occluded (although rate may decrease) • Absent backflow of blood	• Venipuncture device dislodged from vein, or perforated vein	• Stop the infusion. Infiltrate the site with an antidote, if appropriate. • Apply ice (early) or warm soaks (later) *to aid absorption.* Elevate limb. • Check for pulse and capillary refill periodically *to assess circulation.* • Restart infusion above infiltration site or in another limb. • Document patient's condition and your interventions. ***Prevention*** • Check I.V. site frequently. • Don't obscure area above site with tape. • Teach patient to observe I.V. site and report pain or swelling.
Catheter dislodgment	• Loose tape • Catheter partly backed out of vein • Solution infiltrating	• Loosened tape, or tubing snagged in bed linens, resulting in partial retraction of catheter; pulled out by confused patient	• If no infiltration occurs, retape without pushing catheter back into vein. If pulled out, apply pressure to I.V. site with sterile dressing. ***Prevention*** • Tape venipuncture securely on insertion.
Occlusion	• No increase in flow rate when I.V. container is raised • Blood backflow in line • Discomfort at insertion site	• I.V. flow interrupted • Heparin lock not flushed • Blood backflow in line when patient walks • Line clamped too long	• Use mild flush injection. Don't force it. If unsuccessful, reinsert I.V. line. ***Prevention*** • Maintain I.V. flow rate. • Flush promptly after intermittent piggyback administration. • Have patient walk with his arm bent at the elbow *to reduce risk of blood backflow.*

(continued)

Risks of peripheral I.V. therapy *(continued)*

COMPLICATION	SIGNS AND SYMPTOMS	POSSIBLE CAUSES	NURSING INTERVENTIONS
Local complications *(continued)*			
Vein irritation or pain at I.V. site	• Pain during infusion • Possible blanching if vasospasm occurs • Red skin over vein during infusion • Rapidly developing signs of phlebitis	• Solution with high or low pH or high osmolarity, such as 40 mEq/liter of potassium chloride, phenytoin, and some antibiotics (vancomycin, erythromycin, and nafcillin)	• Decrease the flow rate. • Try using an electronic flow device *to achieve a steady flow.* ***Prevention*** • Dilute solutions before administration. For example, give antibiotics in 250-ml solution rather than 100 ml. If drug has low pH, ask pharmacist if drug can be buffered with sodium bicarbonate. (Refer to hospital policy.) • If long-term therapy of irritating drug is planned, ask doctor to use central I.V. line.
Severed catheter	• Leakage from catheter shaft	• Catheter inadvertently cut by scissors • Reinsertion of needle into catheter	• If broken part is visible, attempt to retrieve it. If unsuccessful, notify the doctor. • If portion of catheter enters bloodstream, place tourniquet above I.V. site *to prevent progression of broken part.* • Notify doctor and radiology department. • Document patient's condition and your interventions. ***Prevention*** • Don't use scissors around I.V. site. • Never reinsert needle into catheter. • Remove unsuccessfully inserted catheter and needle together.
Hematoma	• Tenderness at venipuncture site • Bruised area around site • Inability to advance or flush I.V. line	• Vein punctured through opposite wall at time of insertion • Leakage of blood from needle displacement • Inadequate pressure applied when catheter discontinued	• Remove venipuncture device. • Apply pressure and warm soaks to affected area. • Recheck for bleeding. • Document patient's condition and your interventions. ***Prevention*** • Choose a vein that can accommodate size of venipuncture device. • Release tourniquet as soon as successful insertion achieved.

Risks of peripheral I.V. therapy *(continued)*

COMPLICATION	SIGNS AND SYMPTOMS	POSSIBLE CAUSES	NURSING INTERVENTIONS
Local complications *(continued)*			
Venous spasm	• Pain along vein • Flow rate sluggish when clamp completely open • Blanched skin over vein	• Severe vein irritation from irritating drugs or fluids • Administration of cold fluids or blood • Very rapid flow rate (with fluids at room temperature)	• Apply warm soaks over vein and surrounding area. • Decrease flow rate. ***Prevention*** • Use a blood warmer for blood or packed red blood cells.
Vasovagal reaction	• Sudden collapse of vein during venipuncture • Sudden pallor, sweating, faintness, dizziness, and nausea • Decreased blood pressure	• Vasospasm from anxiety or pain	• Lower head of bed. • Have patient take deep breaths. • Check vital signs. ***Prevention*** • Prepare patient for therapy *to relieve his anxiety.* • Use local anesthetic *to prevent pain.*
Thrombosis	• Painful, reddened and swollen vein • Sluggish or stopped I.V. flow	• Injury to endothelial cells of vein wall, allowing platelets to adhere and thrombi to form	• Remove venipuncture device; restart infusion in opposite limb if possible. • Apply warm soaks. • Watch for I.V. therapy-related infection; thrombi provide an excellent environment for bacterial growth. ***Prevention*** • Use proper venipuncture techniques *to reduce injury to vein.*
Thrombophlebitis	• Severe discomfort • Reddened, swollen, and hardened vein	• Thrombosis and inflammation	• Same as for thrombosis. ***Prevention*** • Check site frequently. Remove venipuncture device at first sign of redness and tenderness.
Nerve, tendon, or ligament damage	• Extreme pain (similar to electrical shock when nerve is punctured) • Numbness and muscle contraction • Delayed effects, including paralysis, numbness, and deformity	• Improper venipuncture technique, resulting in injury to surrounding nerves, tendons, or ligaments • Tight taping or improper splinting with armboard	• Stop procedure. ***Prevention*** • Don't repeatedly penetrate tissues with venipuncture device. • Don't apply excessive pressure when taping; don't encircle limb with tape. • Pad armboards and tape securing armboards if possible.

(continued)

Risks of peripheral I.V. therapy (continued)

COMPLICATION	SIGNS AND SYMPTOMS	POSSIBLE CAUSES	NURSING INTERVENTIONS
Systemic complications			
Circulatory overload	• Discomfort • Neck vein engorgement • Respiratory distress • Increased blood pressure • Crackles • Increased difference between fluid intake and output	• Roller clamp loosened to allow run-on infusion • Flow rate too rapid • Miscalculation of fluid requirements	• Raise the head of the bed. • Administer oxygen as needed. • Notify the doctor. • Administer medications (probably furosemide) as ordered. ***Prevention*** • Use pump, controller, or rate minder for elderly or compromised patients. • Recheck calculations of fluid requirements. • Monitor infusion frequently.
Systemic infection (septicemia or bacteremia)	• Fever, chills, and malaise for no apparent reason • Contaminated I.V. site, usually with no visible signs of infection at site	• Failure to maintain aseptic technique during insertion or site care • Severe phlebitis, which can set up ideal conditions for organism growth • Poor taping that permits venipuncture device to move, which can introduce organisms into bloodstream • Prolonged indwelling time of device • Weak immune system	• Notify the doctor. • Administer medications as prescribed. • Culture the site and device. • Monitor vital signs. ***Prevention*** • Use scrupulous aseptic technique when handling solutions and tubing, inserting venipuncture device, and discontinuing infusion. • Secure all connections. • Change I.V. solutions, tubing, and venipuncture device at recommended times. • Use I.V. filters.
Air embolism	• Respiratory distress • Unequal breath sounds • Weak pulse • Increased central venous pressure • Decreased blood pressure • Loss of consciousness	• Solution container empty • Solution container empties, and added container pushes air down the line (if line not purged first)	• Discontinue infusion. • Place patient in Trendelenburg's position *to allow air to enter right atrium and disperse via pulmonary artery.* • Administer oxygen. • Notify doctor. • Document patient's condition and your interventions. ***Prevention*** • Purge tubing of air completely before starting infusion. • Use air-detection device on pump or air-eliminating filter proximal to I.V. site. • Secure connections.

Risks of peripheral I.V. therapy *(continued)*

COMPLICATION	SIGNS AND SYMPTOMS	POSSIBLE CAUSES	NURSING INTERVENTIONS
Systemic complications *(continued)*			
Allergic reaction	• Itching • Watery eyes and nose • Bronchospasm • Wheezing • Urticarial rash • Edema at I.V. site • Anaphylactic reaction, which may occur within minutes or up to 1 hour after exposure (flushing, chills, anxiety, agitation, itching, palpitations, paresthesia, throbbing in ears, wheezing, coughing, convulsions, cardiac arrest)	• Allergens, such as medications	• If reaction occurs, stop infusion immediately. • Maintain patent airway. • Notify doctor. • Administer antihistaminic steroid, anti-inflammatory, and antipyretic drugs, as ordered. • Give 0.2 to 0.5 ml of 1:1,000 aqueous epinephrine subcutaneously, as ordered. Repeat at 3-minute intervals and as needed. • Administer cortisone if ordered. ***Prevention*** • Obtain patient's allergy history. Be aware of cross-allergies. • Assist with test dosing. • Monitor patient carefully during first 15 minutes of administration of a new drug.

Insertion of a heparin lock

Also called an intermittent infusion device, a heparin lock consists of either a steel winged-tip needle with tubing that ends in a resealable rubber injection port or a catheter with injection cap attached. Filled with dilute heparin to prevent blood clot formation, the device maintains venous access in patients receiving I.V. medication regularly or intermittently, but not requiring continuous infusion of fluids. A heparin lock proves superior to a keep-vein-open line because it minimizes the risk of fluid overload and electrolyte imbalance. It also cuts costs, reduces the risk of contamination by eliminating I.V. solution containers and administration sets, increases patient comfort and mobility, reduces patient anxiety and, if inserted in a large vein, allows collection of multiple blood samples without repeated venipuncture.

Equipment
Heparin lock ▪ 25G needle ▪ dilute heparin solution in a 1-ml syringe ▪ povidone-iodine sponges ▪ tourniquet ▪ alcohol sponges ▪ venipuncture equipment, sterile dressing, and tape ▪ optional: transparent semipermeable dressing, stretch net protective sleeve.

Some hospitals use a 100 units/ml heparin flush; others, a 10 units/ml flush; and still others, a normal saline solution instead of heparin. Prefilled heparin or saline cartridges are available in both dosages for use in a syringe cartridge holder.

Implementation
• Wash your hands thoroughly *to prevent contamination of the venipuncture site.*
• Explain the procedure to the patient, and describe the purpose of the heparin lock.
• Remove the set from its packaging, wipe the port with an alcohol sponge, and inject a dilute heparin solution or normal saline solution to fill the tubing and 25G needle. *This removes air from the system, preventing formation of an air embolus.*
• Select a venipuncture site, and clean it first with povidone-iodine sponges, wiping outward from the site in a circular motion. Do not wipe off the povidone-iodine with alcohol *because doing so negates its effect.*
• Perform the venipuncture and ensure correct needle placement in the vein. Then release the tourniquet. (See "Venipuncture" in Chapter 3 for complete instructions.)
• Tape the set in place, using the chevron method or an accepted alternative. Loop the tubing, if applicable, so the injection port is free and easily accessible.

Stabilizing a heparin lock

Before inserting or removing a needle from a heparin lock, you must stabilize the device. To do this, grasp the lock just below the injection cap with the thumb and index finger of your nondominant hand, as shown, and hold the device steady during needle insertion and withdrawal.

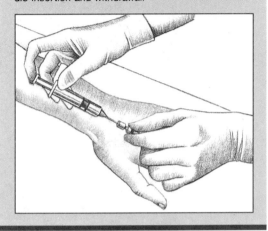

• Apply a sterile dressing. On the last piece of tape used to secure the dressing, write the time, date, and your initials.
• Inject dilute heparin solution or normal saline solution every 6 to 12 hours or according to hospital policy *to maintain the patency of the heparin lock.* Inject the heparin slowly *to prevent stinging.*

Special considerations

Whenever inserting or removing a needle from a heparin lock, be sure to stabilize the device to prevent dislodging it from the vein. (See *Stabilizing a heparin lock.*)

If ordered, obtain a blood sample for activated partial thromboplastin time *before* inserting the intermittent infusion set *because small amounts of heparin can alter the results of this test.*

If the patient has a clotting disorder, use 1 to 2 ml of normal saline solution according to hospital policy, instead of a heparin flush.

If the patient feels a burning sensation during injection of heparin, stop the injection and check needle placement. If the needle is in the vein, inject the heparin at a slower rate *to minimize irritation.* If the needle is not in the vein, remove and discard it. Then select a new

venipuncture site and, using fresh equipment, restart the procedure.

Change the sterile dressing every 24 to 48 hours and the heparin lock every 72 hours according to hospital policy, using a new venipuncture site. Some hospitals use a transparent semipermeable dressing or a stretch net protective sleeve to cover the entire device. *This allows more patient freedom and better observation of the injection site.*

If the doctor orders an I.V. infusion discontinued and a heparin lock inserted in its place, convert the existing line into a heparin lock by disconnecting the I.V. tubing and inserting a male adapter plug into the device. (See *Converting an I.V. line to a heparin lock.*)

Home care

Most patients receiving I.V. therapy at home will have a central venous line. But if you care for a patient who will be going home with a peripheral line, you should teach the patient how to care for the I.V. site and how to identify complications. If the patient must observe movement restrictions, make sure he understands which movements to avoid.

Because the patient may have special drug delivery equipment that differs from the hospital's, be sure to demonstrate the equipment and have the patient give a return demonstration.

Teach the patient to examine the site and to notify the doctor if the dressing becomes moist, if blood appears in the tubing, or if redness, swelling, or discomfort develops.

Also tell the patient to report any problems with the I.V. line — for instance, if the solution stops infusing or if an alarm goes off on the infusion pump controller. Explain that the I.V. site will be changed at established intervals by a home care nurse.

Teach the patient or caregiver how and when to flush the heparin lock. Finally, teach the patient to document daily whether the I.V. site is free from pain, swelling, and redness.

Complications

Use of a heparin lock set has the same potential complications as the use of a peripheral I.V. line. (See "Insertion of a peripheral I.V. line" in this chapter.)

Documentation

Record the date and time of insertion, the type and gauge of needle, and the date and time of each heparin flush.

Maintenance of peripheral I.V. sites and systems

Routine maintenance of I.V. sites and systems includes regular assessment and rotation of the site and periodic changes of the dressing, tubing, and solution. These measures help prevent complications, such as thrombophlebitis and infection. They should be performed according to hospital policy. Typically, I.V. dressings are changed every 48 hours or whenever the dressing becomes wet, soiled, or nonocclusive. I.V. tubing is changed every 48 to 72 hours or according to hospital policy, and I.V. solution is changed every 24 hours or as needed. The site should be assessed every 2 hours if a transparent semipermeable dressing is used, with every dressing change otherwise, and should be rotated every 48 to 72 hours. Sometimes limited venous access will prevent frequent site changes; if so, be sure to assess the site frequently.

Equipment
For dressing changes: sterile gloves ■ povidone-iodine or alcohol sponges ■ povidone-iodine or other antimicrobial ointment, according to hospital policy ■ adhesive bandage, sterile 2″ × 2″ gauze pad, or transparent semipermeable dressing ■ 1″ adhesive tape.

   For solution changes: solution container ■ alcohol sponge.

   For tubing changes: I.V. administration set ■ sterile 2″ × 2″ gauze pad ■ adhesive tape for labeling ■ sterile gloves ■ optional: hemostats.

   For I.V. site change: See "Insertion of a peripheral I.V. line" in this chapter.

   Commercial kits containing the equipment for dressing changes are available.

Preparation of equipment
If your hospital keeps I.V. equipment and dressings in a tray or cart, have it nearby, if possible, *because you may have to select a new venipuncture site, depending on the current site's condition.* If you're changing both the solution and the tubing, attach and prime the I.V. administration set before entering the patient's room.

Implementation
• Wash your hands thoroughly *to prevent the spread of microorganisms.* Remember to wear sterile gloves whenever working near the venipuncture site.

• Explain the procedure to the patient *to allay his fears and ensure cooperation.*

Converting an I.V. line to a heparin lock

Two types of adapter plugs (shown below) allow you to convert an existing I.V. line into a heparin lock. To make the conversion, follow these steps:
• Prime the adapter plug with dilute heparin or normal saline solution, as appropriate.
• Clamp the I.V. tubing and remove the administration set from the catheter or needle hub.
• Insert the male adapter plug.

   Inject the remaining dilute heparin or normal saline solution to fill the line and to prevent clot formation.

Long male adapter
This long adapter plug slides into place.

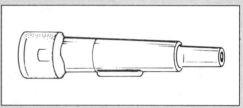

Short male adapter
This short luer-lock adapter plug twists into place.

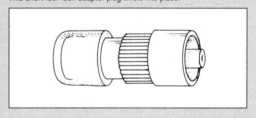

To change the dressing
• Remove the old dressing, open all supply packages, and put on sterile gloves.
• Hold the needle or catheter in place with your nondominant hand *to prevent accidental movement or dislodgment, which could puncture the vein and cause infiltration.*
• Assess the venipuncture site for signs of infection (redness and pain at the puncture site), infiltration (coolness, blanching, and edema at the site), and thrombophlebitis (redness, firmness, pain along the path of the vein, and edema). If any such signs are present, apply pressure to the area with a sterile 2″ × 2″ gauze pad and remove the

catheter or needle. Maintain pressure on the area until the bleeding stops, and apply an adhesive bandage. Then, using fresh equipment and solution, start the I.V. in another appropriate site, preferably on the opposite extremity.

• If the venipuncture site is intact, hold the needle or catheter and carefully clean around the puncture site with a povidone-iodine or alcohol sponge. Work in a circular motion outward from the site *to avoid introducing bacteria into the clean area.* Allow the area to dry completely.

• Apply povidone-iodine or other antimicrobial ointment if hospital policy dictates, and cover with an adhesive bandage or sterile 2″ × 2″ gauze pad. Retape the site, or apply a transparent semipermeable dressing.

• When using a transparent semipermeable dressing, you may omit the povidone-iodine ointment. The transparent dressing allows visualization of the insertion site. It maintains sterility and is placed over the insertion site to halfway up the catheter or needle hub.

To change the solution

• Wash your hands.

• Inspect the new solution container for cracks, leaks, and other damage. Check the solution for discoloration, turbidity, and particulates. Note the date and time the solution was mixed and its expiration date.

• Clamp the tubing when inverting it *to prevent air from entering the tubing.* Keep the drip chamber half full.

• If you're replacing a bag, remove the seal or tab from the new bag and remove the old bag from the pole. Remove the spike, insert it into the new bag, and adjust the flow rate.

• If you're replacing a bottle, remove the cap and seal from the new bottle and wipe the rubber port with an alcohol sponge. Clamp the line, remove the spike from the old bottle, and insert the spike into the new bottle. Then hang the new bottle and adjust the flow rate.

To change tubing

• Reduce the I.V. flow rate, remove the old spike from the container, and hang it on the I.V. pole. Place the cover of the new spike loosely over the old one.

• Keeping the old spike in an upright position above the patient's heart level, insert the new spike into the I.V. container, as shown at the top of the next column.

• Prime the system. Hang the new I.V. container and primed set on the pole, and grasp the new adapter in

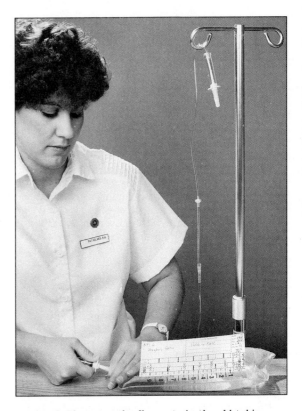

one hand. Then stop the flow rate in the old tubing.

• Put on sterile gloves.

• Place a sterile gauze pad under the needle or catheter hub *to create a sterile field.* Press one of your fingers over the catheter to prevent bleeding.

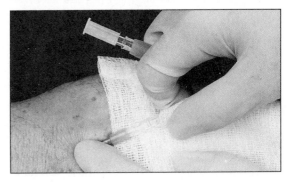

• Gently disconnect the old tubing, being careful not to dislodge or move the I.V. device. (If you have trouble disconnecting the old tubing, use a hemostat to hold the hub securely while twisting the tubing *to remove it.* Or use one hemostat on the venipuncture device and another on the hard plastic end of the tubing. Then pull the hemostats in opposite directions. Don't clamp the hemostats shut; *this may crack the tubing adapter or the venipuncture device.)*

• Remove the protective cap from the new tubing, and connect the new adapter to the needle or catheter. Hold the hub securely *to prevent dislodging the needle or catheter tip.*

• Observe for blood backflow into the new tubing *to verify that the needle or catheter is still in place.* (You may not be able to do this with small-gauge catheters.)

• Adjust the clamp to maintain the appropriate flow rate.

• Retape the needle or catheter hub and I.V. tubing, and recheck the I.V. flow rate *because taping may alter it.*

• Label the new tubing and container with the date and time. Label the solution container with a time strip.

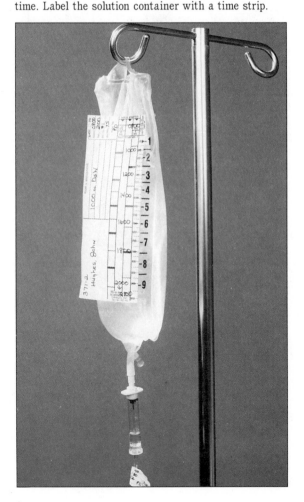

Special considerations

Check the prescribed I.V. flow rate before each solution change *to prevent errors.* If you crack the adapter or hub (or if you accidentally dislodge the needle or catheter from the vein), remove the needle or catheter. Apply pressure and an adhesive bandage to stop any bleeding. Perform a venipuncture at another site and restart the I.V.

Keep in mind that flow rates may change 20% to 40% during an infusion. If you're not using an infusion pump, check the flow rate every hour.

Documentation

Record the time, date, and rate and type of solution (and any additives) on the I.V. flowchart. Also record this information, dressing or tubing changes, and appearance of the site in your notes.

CENTRAL VENOUS AND ARTERIAL LINES
Insertion and removal of a central venous line

A central venous (CV) line is a sterile catheter made of polyurethane, polyvinylchloride (PVC), or silicone rubber (Silastic). It's inserted through a major vein, such as the subclavian vein or, less commonly, the jugular vein. (See *CV catheter pathways,* page 292.)

By giving access to the central veins, CV therapy offers several benefits. It allows monitoring of CV pressure, which indicates blood volume or pump efficiency, and permits aspiration of blood samples for diagnostic tests. It also allows administration of I.V. fluids (in large amounts, if necessary) in emergencies or when decreased peripheral circulation causes peripheral veins to collapse; when prolonged I.V. therapy reduces the number of accessible peripheral veins; when solutions must be diluted (for large fluid volumes or for irritating or hypertonic fluids, such as total parenteral nutrition [TPN] solutions); and when a patient requires long-term venous access. Because repeated blood samples can be drawn through it, the CV line decreases the patient's anxiety and preserves or restores peripheral veins.

A variation of CV therapy, peripheral CV therapy involves the insertion of a catheter into a peripheral vein instead of a central vein, but the catheter tip still lies in the CV circulation. A peripherally inserted central catheter (PICC) usually enters at the basilic vein and

CV catheter pathways

The illustrations below show several common pathways for central venous (CV) catheter insertion. Typically, a CV catheter is inserted into the subclavian vein or the internal jugular vein. The catheter may terminate in the superior vena cava or in the right atrium.

Insertion: Subclavian vein
Termination: Superior vena cava

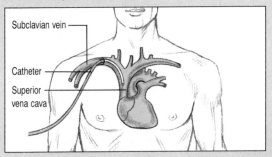

Insertion: Subclavian vein
Termination: Right atrium

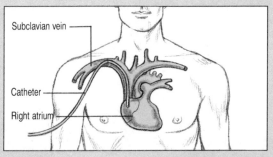

Insertion: Internal jugular vein
Termination: Superior vena cava

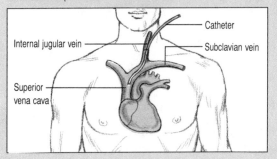

Insertion: Basilic vein (peripheral)
Termination: Superior vena cava

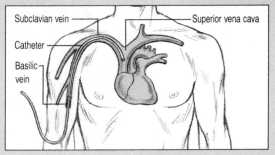

Insertion: Through a subcutaneous tunnel to the subclavian vein
(Dacron cuff helps hold catheter in place)
Termination: Superior vena cava

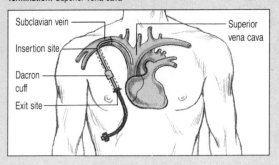

terminates in the subclavian vein, the axillary vein, or the superior vena cava. PICCs may be inserted by a specially prepared nurse. New catheters have longer needles and smaller lumens, facilitating this procedure. PICCs are commonly used in home I.V. therapy, but may also be used with chest injury; chest, neck, or shoulder burns; compromised respiratory function; proximity of a surgical site to the CV line placement site; or if a doctor is not available to insert a CV line.

As with any invasive procedure, however, CV therapy also has its drawbacks. It increases the risk of complications, such as pneumothorax, sepsis, thrombus formation, and vessel and adjacent organ perforation (all life-threatening conditions). Also, the CV line may decrease patient mobility, requires more time and skill to insert than a peripheral I.V. catheter, and costs more than a peripheral I.V. catheter.

Removal of a CV line—a sterile procedure—usually is accomplished by a doctor either at the end of therapy or at the onset of complications. A peripherally inserted central line may be removed by a specially prepared nurse. If the patient may have an infection, the removal procedure includes collection of the catheter tip as a specimen for culture.

Equipment

For insertion of a CV line: shave preparation kit, if necessary ▪ sterile gloves and gowns ▪ blanket ▪ linen-saver pad ▪ sterile towel ▪ sterile drape ▪ masks ▪ povidone-iodine sponges and ointment ▪ alcohol sponges ▪ 70% alcohol solution ▪ hydrogen peroxide ▪ normal saline solution ▪ antibiotic ointment, if necessary ▪ 3-ml syringe with 25G 1″ needle ▪ 1% or 2% injectable lidocaine ▪ dextrose 5% in water ▪ syringes for blood samples ▪ suture material ▪ two 14G or 16G CV catheters ▪ I.V. solution with administration set prepared for use ▪ infusion pump or controller, as needed ▪ sterile 4″ × 4″ gauze pads ▪ 1″ adhesive tape ▪ sterile scissors ▪ heparin or normal saline flushes as needed ▪ portable X-ray machine ▪ optional: transparent semipermeable dressing.

For flushing a catheter: normal saline solution or heparinized normal saline flush solution ▪ alcohol sponge ▪ 70% alcohol solution.

For changing an injection cap: alcohol sponge or povidone-iodine sponge ▪ injection cap ▪ padded clamp.

For removal of a CV line: clean gloves and sterile gloves ▪ sterile suture removal set ▪ sterile drape ▪ alcohol sponges ▪ povidone-iodine ointment ▪ mask ▪ povidone-iodine solution ▪ sterile 4″ × 4″ gauze pads ▪ forceps ▪ tape ▪ sterile, plastic adhesive-backed dressing or transparent semipermeable dressing ▪ sterile culture tube and sterile scissors for a culture, if necessary.

The type of catheter selected depends on the type of therapy to be used. (See *Guide to CV catheters,* pages 294 and 295.)

Some hospitals have prepared trays containing most of the equipment necessary for catheter insertion.

Preparation of equipment

Before insertion of a CV line, confirm catheter type and size with the doctor; usually, a 14G or 16G catheter is selected. Set up the I.V. solution and prime the administration set, using strict aseptic technique. Attach the line to the infusion pump or controller if ordered. Recheck all connections to make sure they're tight. As ordered, notify the radiology department that a portable X-ray machine will be needed.

Implementation

● Wash your hands thoroughly *to prevent the spread of microorganisms.*

To insert a CV line

● Reinforce the doctor's explanation of the procedure, and answer the patient's questions. Ensure that the patient has signed a consent form, if necessary, and check his history for hypersensitivity to iodine or the local anesthetic.

● Place the patient in Trendelenburg's position *to dilate the veins and reduce the risk of air embolism.*

● For subclavian insertion, place a rolled blanket lengthwise between the shoulders *to increase venous distention.* For jugular insertion, place a rolled blanket under the opposite shoulder *to extend the neck, making anatomic landmarks more visible.* Place a linen-saver pad under the appropriate area *to prevent soiling the bed.*

● Turn the patient's head away from the site *to prevent possible contamination from airborne pathogens and to make the site more accessible.* Or, if dictated by hospital policy, place a mask on the patient unless this increases his anxiety or is contraindicated due to his respiratory status.

● Prepare the insertion site. Make sure the skin is free of hair *because hair can harbor microorganisms.* Infection control practitioners recommend clipping the hair close to the skin rather than shaving. *Shaving may cause skin irritation and create multiple small open wounds, increasing the risk of infection.* (If the doctor orders the area to be shaved, try shaving it the evening before catheter insertion; *this allows minor skin irritations to heal partially.*) After you remove the hair, rinse with normal saline solution to remove hair clippings. You may also need to

(Text continues on page 296.)

Guide to CV catheters

TYPE	DESCRIPTION	INDICATIONS	ADVANTAGES AND DISADVANTAGES	NURSING CONSIDERATIONS
Groshong catheter	• Silicone rubber • About 35″ (88.9 cm) long • Closed end with pressure-sensitive two-way valve • Dacron cuff • Single or double lumen • Tunneled	• Long-term central venous (CV) access • Patient with heparin allergy	*Advantages* • Less thrombogenic • Pressure-sensitive two-way valve eliminates frequent heparin flushes • Dacron cuff anchors catheter and prevents bacterial migration *Disadvantages* • Requires surgical insertion • Tears and kinks easily • Blunt end makes it difficult to clear substances from its tip	• Two surgical sites require dressing after insertion. • Handle catheter gently. • Check the external portion frequently for kinks or leaks. • Repair kit is available. • Remember to flush with enough saline solution to clear the catheter, especially after drawing or administering blood.
Short-term, single-lumen catheter	• Polyvinylchloride (PVC) or polyurethane • About 8″ (20.3 cm) long • Lumen gauge varies • Percutaneously placed	• Short-term CV access • Emergency access • Patient who needs only one lumen	*Advantages* • Easily inserted at bedside • Easily removed • Stiffness aids central venous pressure (CVP) monitoring *Disadvantages* • Limited functions • PVC is thrombogenic and irritates inner lumen of vessel • Should be changed every 3 to 7 days (Frequency may depend on hospital's CV line infection rate)	• Minimize patient movement. • Assess frequently for signs of infection and clot formation.
Short-term, multilumen catheter	• PVC or polyurethane • Two, three, or four lumens exiting at ¾″ (2-cm) intervals • Lumen gauges vary • Percutaneously placed	• Short-term CV access • Patient with limited insertion sites who requires multiple infusions	*Advantages* • Same as single-lumen catheter • Allows infusion of multiple (even incompatible) solutions through the same catheter *Disadvantages* • Same as single-lumen catheter	• Know gauge and purpose of each lumen. • Use the same lumen for the same task.

Guide to CV catheters *(continued)*

TYPE	DESCRIPTION	INDICATIONS	ADVANTAGES AND DISADVANTAGES	NURSING CONSIDERATIONS
Hickman catheter	• Silicone rubber • About 35″ long • Open end with clamp • Dacron cuff 11¾″ (29.8 cm) from hub • Single lumen or multilumen • Tunneled	• Long-term CV access • Home therapy	***Advantages*** • Less thrombogenic • Dacron cuff prevents excess motion and migration of bacteria • Clamps eliminate need for Valsalva's maneuver ***Disadvantages*** • Requires surgical insertion • Open end • Requires doctor for removal • Tears and kinks easily	• Two surgical sites require dressing after insertion. • Handle catheter gently. • Observe frequently for kinks and tears. • Repair kit is available. • Clamp catheter with a nonserrated clamp any time it becomes disconnected or opens.
Broviac catheter	• Identical to Hickman except smaller inner lumen	• Long-term CV access • Patient with small central vessels (pediatric or geriatric)	***Advantages*** • Smaller lumen ***Disadvantages*** • Small lumen may limit uses • Single lumen	• Check hospital policy before drawing or administering blood or blood products.
Hickman/ Broviac catheter	• Hickman and Broviac catheters combined • Tunneled	• Long-term CV access • Patient who needs multiple infusions	***Advantages*** • Double-lumen Hickman catheter allows sampling and administration of blood • Broviac lumen delivers I.V. fluids, including total parenteral nutrition ***Disadvantages*** • Same as Hickman catheter	• Know the purpose and function of each lumen. • Label lumens to prevent confusion.
Peripherally inserted central catheter (PICC)	• Silicone rubber • 20″ (50.8 cm) long • Available in 16G, 18G, 20G, and 22G • Can be used as midline catheter • Percutaneously placed	• Long-term CV access • Patient with poor CV access • Patient at risk for fatal complications from CV line insertion • Patient who needs CV access but faces or has had head or neck surgery	***Advantages*** • Peripherally inserted • Easily inserted at bedside with minimal complications • May be inserted by trained registered nurse in some states ***Disadvantages*** • Catheter may occlude smaller peripheral vessels • May be difficult to keep immobile • Single lumen • Long path to CV circulation	• Check frequently for signs of phlebitis and thrombus formation. • Insert catheter above the antecubital fossa. • Basilic vein is preferable to cephalic vein. • Use armboard if necessary. • Catheter may alter CVP measurements.

wash the skin with soap and water before the actual skin preparation *to remove surface dirt and body oils.*

• Establish a sterile field on a table, using a sterile towel or the wrapping from the instrument tray.

• Put on a mask and sterile gloves and gown, and clean the area around the insertion site with sponges soaked in povidone-iodine ointment, working in a circular motion outward from the site to avoid reintroducing contaminants. If the patient is sensitive to iodine, use a solution of 70% alcohol.

• After the doctor puts on a sterile mask, gown, and gloves and drapes the area to create a sterile field, open the packaging of the 3-ml syringe and 25G needle and present it to the doctor, using sterile technique.

• Wipe the top of the lidocaine vial with an alcohol sponge and invert it. The doctor then fills the 3-ml syringe and injects the anesthetic into the site.

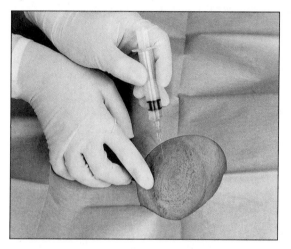

• Open the packaging of the catheter and give it to the doctor using sterile technique. The doctor then inserts the catheter.

• During this time, prepare the I.V. administration set for immediate attachment to the catheter hub. Ask the patient to perform Valsalva's maneuver while the doctor attaches the I.V. line to the catheter hub. *This increases intrathoracic pressure, reducing the possibility of an air embolus.* (See *Teaching Valsalva's maneuver.*)

• After the doctor attaches the I.V. line to the catheter hub, set the flow rate at a keep-vein-open rate to maintain venous access. The doctor then sutures the catheter in place. (See photograph at the top of the next column.)

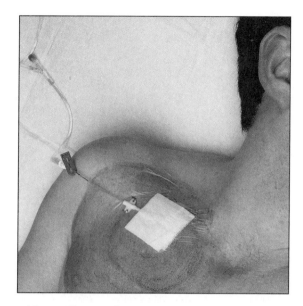

• After an X-ray confirms correct catheter placement, set the flow rate as ordered.

• Use normal saline solution *to remove dried blood that could harbor microorganisms,* and apply povidone-iodine ointment over the site. Place antibiotic ointment at the site if hospital policy directs, secure the catheter with adhesive tape, and apply an occlusive, sterile 4″ × 4″ gauze pad. You may also use a transparent semipermeable dressing, either alone or placed over the gauze pad. Expect some serosanguineous drainage during the first 24 hours. Label the dressing with the time and date of catheter insertion and catheter length (if not imprinted on the catheter).

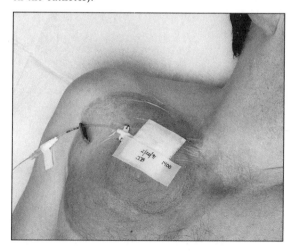

• Place the patient in a comfortable position and reassess his status.

To flush the catheter

• *To maintain patency,* flush the catheter routinely according to your hospital's policy. If the system is being maintained as a heparin lock and the infusions are intermittent, the flushing procedure will vary according to the hospital's policy, the medication administration schedule, and the type of catheter.

• Typically, a CV catheter with a two-way valve (Groshong catheter) must be flushed with normal saline solution weekly. All lumens of a multilumen catheter (except the Groshong) must be flushed regularly. (No flushing is needed with a continuous infusion through a single-lumen catheter.) Most hospitals use a heparinized saline flush solution available in premixed 10-ml multidose vials. Recommended concentrations vary from 10 units of heparin/ml to 1,000 units of heparin/ml. Some hospitals use normal saline solution instead of heparinized saline solution to flush catheters because research suggests that heparin isn't always necessary to keep the line open.

• The recommended frequency for flushing CV catheters varies from once every 12 hours to once weekly. Most clinicians agree that flushing should be done twice daily for 3 to 4 days after insertion, and from once daily to three times a week thereafter.

• The recommended amount of flushing solution also varies. Most hospitals recommend using 3 to 5 ml of solution to flush the catheter, although some hospital policies call for as much as 10 ml of solution. Different catheters require different amounts of solution, and the volume capacity will be altered if the catheter has been cut to fit the patient.

• To perform the flushing procedure, start by cleaning the cap with an alcohol sponge (using a 70% alcohol solution). Allow it to dry.

• Inject the recommended type and amount of flush solution.

• After flushing the catheter, maintain positive pressure by keeping your thumb on the plunger of the syringe while withdrawing the needle. *This prevents blood backflow and potential clotting in the line.*

• CV catheters used for intermittent infusions have injection caps (short luer-lock devices similar to the heparin lock adapters used for peripheral I.V. infusion therapy). Unlike heparin lock adapters, however, these caps contain a small amount of empty space, so you don't have to preflush the cap before connecting it.

To change the injection cap

• The frequency of cap changes varies according to hospital policy and the number of times that the cap is used.

Teaching Valsalva's maneuver

Increased intrathoracic pressure reduces the risk of air embolus during insertion and removal of a central venous catheter. A simple way to achieve this is to ask the patient to perform Valsalva's maneuver: forced exhalation against a closed airway. Instruct the patient to take a deep breath and hold it, and then to bear down for 10 seconds. Then tell the patient to exhale and breathe quietly.

Valsalva's maneuver raises intrathoracic pressure from its normal level of 3 to 4 mm Hg to levels of 60 mm Hg or higher. It also slows the pulse rate, decreases the return of blood to the heart, and increases venous pressure.

This maneuver is contraindicated in patients with increased intracranial pressure. It should not be taught to patients who are not alert or cooperative.

Use strict aseptic technique when changing the cap. Repeated punctures of the injection port increase the risk of infection. Also, pieces of the rubber stopper may break off after repeated punctures, placing the patient at risk for embolism.

• Clean the connection site with an alcohol sponge or a povidone-iodine sponge.

• Instruct the patient to perform Valsalva's maneuver while you quickly disconnect the old cap and connect the new cap, using aseptic technique. If the patient can't perform Valsalva's maneuver, use a padded clamp to prevent air from entering the catheter.

To remove a CV line

• If you'll be removing the CV catheter, first check the patient's record for the most recent placement (confirmed by an X-ray) *to trace the catheter's path as it exits the body.* Make sure that assistance is available if a complication, such as uncontrolled bleeding, occurs during catheter removal. *(Some vessels, such as the subclavian vein, can be difficult to compress.)* Before you remove the catheter, explain the procedure to the patient.

• Place the patient in a supine position *to prevent emboli.*

• Wash your hands and put on clean gloves and a mask.

• Turn off all infusions and prepare a sterile field, using a sterile drape.

• Remove and discard the old dressing and change to sterile gloves.

• Clean the site with an alcohol sponge or with a gauze pad soaked in povidone-iodine solution. Inspect the site for signs of drainage or inflammation.

Key steps in changing a CV dressing

Expect to change your patient's central venous (CV) dressing at least once a week. Many hospitals specify dressing changes two or three times weekly as well as whenever it becomes soiled, moist, or loose. The following illustrations show the key steps you'll perform.

First, don clean gloves and remove the old dressing by pulling it toward the exit site of a long-term catheter or toward the insertion site of a short-term catheter. (This technique helps you avoid pulling out the line.) Remove and discard your gloves.

Next, don sterile gloves and clean the skin around the site three times, using a new alcohol sponge each time. Start at the center and move outward, using a circular motion. Allow the skin to dry and repeat the same cleaning procedure using three swabs soaked in povidone-iodine solution.

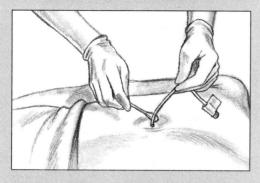

After the solution has dried, cover the site with a dressing, such as the transparent semipermeable dressing shown here. Write the time and date on the dressing.

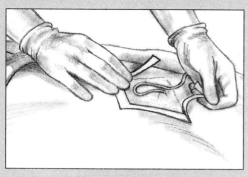

• Clip the sutures and, using forceps, remove the catheter in a slow, even motion. Have the patient perform Valsalva's maneuver as the catheter is withdrawn *to prevent air emboli.*

• Apply povidone-iodine ointment to the insertion site *to seal it.* Then cover the site with a gauze pad, and tape a transparent semipermeable dressing over the gauze. Label the dressing with the date and time of the removal and your initials. Keep the site covered for 48 hours.

• Inspect the catheter *to see if any portions have broken off during removal.* If so, notify the doctor immediately and monitor the patient closely for signs of distress. If a culture is necessary, use sterile scissors to clip approximately 1″ (2.5 cm) off the distal end of the catheter, letting it drop into the sterile culture tube.

• Dispose of the I.V. tubing and equipment properly.

Special considerations

When catheter placement is in doubt, infuse an I.V. solution such as dextrose 5% in water or normal saline solution until correct placement is assured. Or use a heparin lock and flush the line. *Infusing an isotonic solution avoids the risk of vessel wall thrombosis.*

Be alert for such signs of air embolism as sudden onset of pallor, cyanosis, dyspnea, coughing, and tachycardia, progressing to syncope and shock. If any of these signs occur, place the patient on his left side in Trendelenburg's position, and notify the doctor.

After insertion, also watch for signs of pneumothorax, such as shortness of breath, uneven chest movement, tachycardia, and chest pain. Notify the doctor immediately if such signs appear.

Change the dressing at least once a week, according to hospital policy, or whenever it becomes moist, soiled, or nonocclusive. Change the tubing and solution every 24 to 48 hours or according to hospital policy while the CV line is in place. Dressing, tubing, and solution changes for a CV line should be performed using sterile technique. (See *Key steps in changing a CV dressing.*) Assess the site for signs of infection, such as discharge, inflammation, and tenderness.

To prevent air embolism, have the patient perform Valsalva's maneuver each time the catheter hub is open to air. Or close the clamp if the catheter has one. (A Groshong catheter does not require clamping *because it has an internal valve.)*

Home care

Long-term CV catheters allow patients to receive caustic fluids and blood infusions at home. These catheters have a much longer life because they are less thrombogenic and less prone to infection than short-term devices.

A candidate for home therapy must have a family member or friend who can safely and competently administer the I.V. fluids, a backup helper, a suitable home environment, a telephone, transportation, adequate reading skills, and the ability to prepare, handle, store, and dispose of the equipment. The care procedures used in the home are the same as those used in the hospital, except that the home therapy patient uses clean instead of sterile technique.

The overall goal of home therapy is patient safety, so your patient teaching must begin well before discharge. After discharge, a home-therapy coordinator will provide follow-up care until the patient or someone close to him can independently provide catheter care and infusion therapy. Many home therapy patients learn to care for the catheter themselves and to infuse their own medications and solutions.

Complications
Complications can occur at any time during the infusion therapy. Traumatic complications, such as pneumothorax, typically occur upon catheter insertion but may not be noticed until after the procedure is completed. Systemic complications, such as sepsis, typically occur later during infusion therapy. Other complications include phlebitis (especially in peripheral CV therapy) and thrombus formation. (See *Risks of CV therapy*, pages 300 and 301.)

Documentation
Record the time and date of insertion, the length and location of the catheter, the solution infused, the doctor's name, and the patient's response to the procedure. Also document the time of the X-ray, its results, and your notification of the doctor.

After removing a CV line, record the time and date of removal and the type of antimicrobial ointment and dressing applied. Note the condition of the catheter insertion site and collection of a culture specimen.

Insertion and removal of an arterial line

Insertion of an arterial line is a sterile procedure performed by a doctor with the nurse's help. During insertion, the doctor introduces a catheter into the brachial, the radial or — occasionally — the femoral or ulnar artery.

The *brachial* site, which is easily observed and maintained, may provide more accurate blood pressure readings than the radial site because it's closer to the heart. However, using this site necessitates splinting the elbow to stabilize the catheter. The *radial* site, also easily observed and located, may entail difficult and painful catheter insertion because of the artery's small lumen. Catheter insertion into the *femoral* artery, the easiest to locate and puncture in an emergency, carries a risk of severe hemorrhage if the catheter is dislodged.

Once in place at any of these sites, an arterial line allows frequent monitoring of blood pressure and arterial blood gases. The patency of the line is maintained by a continuous flush of heparinized saline solution administered under pressure to reduce the risk of clot formation. Because an arterial line carries the risk of bleeding and thrombosis, its insertion is contraindicated in patients with severe coagulopathy unless the potential benefits outweigh the risks.

Removal of an arterial line (a sterile procedure) may be performed by a doctor or nurse either on completion of therapy or onset of complications.

Equipment
For insertion of an arterial line: I.V. pole ▪ 500-ml bag of 0.9% normal saline solution ▪ heparin, 1 to 2 units/ml in normal saline solution ▪ pressure bag ▪ medication-added label ▪ two 3-ml syringes (one with a 21G to 25G 1″ needle for heparin insertion into normal saline solution, one with a 25G 1″ needle for injection of local anesthetic) ▪ alcohol sponges ▪ nonvented I.V. administration set with microdrip chamber ▪ 6″ extension pressure tubing ▪ continuous flush device ▪ three-way stopcock ▪ dead-end stopcock caps ▪ povidone-iodine sponges and ointment ▪ sterile gloves and mask ▪ 1% or 2% injectable lidocaine ▪ linen-saver pad ▪ sterile towel ▪ 16G to 20G catheter (type and length depend on site, patient's size, and other possible uses of the line) ▪ sterile adhesive bandage ▪ 4″ × 4″ gauze pads ▪ 1″ adhesive tape ▪ optional: suture material, splint or armboard.

For removal of an arterial line: two sterile 4″ × 4″ gauze pads ▪ povidone-iodine ointment ▪ adhesive bandage ▪ sterile gloves and mask ▪ sterile suture removal set ▪ washcloth or pillowcase ▪ small sandbag (for removal from a femoral artery) ▪ alcohol sponges ▪ optional: sterile container and sterile scissors.

Most hospitals use prepackaged arterial line sets containing dead-end caps, connected extension pressure tubing, continuous flush device, and stopcock.

Preparation of equipment
Before insertion of an arterial line, wash your hands thoroughly, and maintain asepsis when setting up the equipment. Inflate the pressure bag to 300 mm Hg, check for air leaks, and release the pressure. Then squeeze the

(Text continues on page 302.)

Risks of CV therapy

PROBLEM	SIGNS AND SYMPTOMS	POSSIBLE CAUSES	NURSING INTERVENTIONS
Pneumothorax, hemothorax, chylothorax, hydrothorax	• Chest pain • Dyspnea • Cyanosis • Decreased breath sounds on affected side • With hemothorax, decreased hemoglobin because of blood pooling • Abnormal chest X-ray	• Lung puncture by catheter during insertion or exchange over a guidewire • Large blood vessel puncture with bleeding inside or outside the lung • Lymph node puncture with leakage of lymph fluid • Infusion of solution into chest area through infiltrated catheter	• Notify doctor. • Remove catheter or assist with removal. • Administer oxygen as ordered. • Set up and assist with chest tube insertion. • Document interventions. ***Prevention*** • Position patient head down with a rolled towel between his scapulae to dilate and expose the internal jugular or subclavian vein as much as possible during catheter insertion. • Assess for early signs of fluid infiltration (swelling in the shoulder, neck, chest, and arm). • Ensure that the patient's immobilized and prepared for insertion. Active patients may need to be sedated or taken to the operating room. • Minimize patient activity after insertion, especially with a peripheral catheter.
Air embolism	• Respiratory distress • Unequal breath sounds • Weak pulse • Increased central venous pressure • Decreased blood pressure • Churning murmur over precordium • Alteration or loss of consciousness	• Intake of air into central venous (CV) system during catheter insertion or tubing changes, or inadvertent opening, cutting, or breaking of catheter	• Clamp catheter immediately. • Turn patient on his left side, head down, so air can enter the right atrium and pulmonary artery. Maintain this position for 20 to 30 minutes. • Don't recommend Valsalva's maneuver because a large air intake worsens the condition. • Administer oxygen. • Notify the doctor. • Document interventions. ***Prevention*** • Purge all air from tubing before hookup. • Teach patient to perform Valsalva's maneuver during catheter insertion and tubing changes. • Use air-eliminating filters. • Use infusion device with air detection capability. • Use luer-lock tubing, tape the connections, or use locking devices for all connections.
Thrombosis	• Edema at puncture site • Erythema • Ipsilateral swelling of arm, neck, and face • Pain along vein • Fever, malaise	• Sluggish flow rate • Composition of catheter material (polyvinylchloride catheters are more thrombogenic) • Hematopoietic status of patient • Preexisting limb edema	• Notify doctor. • Possibly remove catheter. • Possibly infuse anticoagulant doses of heparin. • Verify thrombosis with diagnostic studies. • Apply warm, wet compresses locally. • Don't use limb on affected side for subsequent venipuncture. • Document interventions.

Risks of CV therapy *(continued)*

PROBLEM	SIGNS AND SYMPTOMS	POSSIBLE CAUSES	NURSING INTERVENTIONS
Thrombosis *(continued)*		• Infusion of irritating solutions • Repeated or long-term use of same vein • Preexisting cardiovascular disease	**Prevention** • Maintain steady flow rate with infusion pump, or flush catheter at regular intervals. • Use catheters made of less thrombogenic materials or catheters coated to prevent thrombosis. • Dilute irritating solutions. • Use 0.22-micron filter for infusions.
Infection	• Redness, warmth, tenderness, swelling at insertion or exit site • Possible exudate of purulent material • Local rash or pustules • Fever, chills, malaise • Leukocytosis • Nausea and vomiting • Elevated urine glucose level	• Failure to maintain aseptic technique during catheter insertion or care • Failure to comply with dressing change protocol • Wet or soiled dressing remaining on site • Immunosuppression • Irritated suture line • Contaminated catheter or solution • Frequent opening of catheter or long-term use of single I.V. access site	• Monitor temperature frequently. • Monitor vital signs closely. • Culture the site. • Re-dress aseptically. • Possibly use antibiotic ointment locally. • Treat systemically with antibiotics or antifungals, depending on culture results and doctor's order. • Catheter may be removed. • Draw central and peripheral blood cultures; if the same organism appears in both, then catheter is primary source and should be removed. • If cultures don't match but are positive, the catheter may be removed, or the infection may be treated through the catheter. • Treat patients with antibiotics, as ordered. • If the catheter is removed, culture its tip. • Document interventions. **Prevention** • Maintain sterile technique. Use sterile gloves, masks, and gowns when appropriate. • Observe dressing-change protocols. • Teach about restrictions on swimming, bathing, and so on. (With adequate white blood cell count, the doctor may allow these activities.) • Change wet or soiled dressing immediately. • Change dressing more frequently if catheter is located in femoral area or near tracheostomy. Perform tracheostomy care after catheter care. • Examine solution for cloudiness and turbidity before infusing; check fluid container for leaks. • Monitor urine glucose level in patients receiving total parenteral nutrition (TPN); if greater than 2 +, suspect early sepsis. • Use a 0.22-micron filter (or a 1.2-micron filter for 3-in-1 TPN solutions). • Catheter may be changed frequently. • Keep the system closed as much as possible.

bag of normal saline solution and check for leaks; if none are present, wipe the injection port with an alcohol sponge. Using a 3-ml syringe with a 21G or 25G 1″ needle, inject the prescribed amount of heparin, and gently rotate the bag to mix the solution. Label the bag with the amount of heparin added. Wipe the main port with an alcohol sponge and insert the administration set spike. Invert the bag, open the flow clamp, and squeeze the air from the bag *to reduce the risk of introducing air into the line.* Then close the clamp, place the pressure bag on the I.V. bag, and hang it on the I.V. pole.

Connect the administration set tubing to the continuous flush device's tubing. Secure a three-way stopcock to the patient's side of the device, and attach the pressure tubing to the opposite side of the stopcock. (The transducer is connected to the other port of the continuous flush device.) Then replace the open cap on the transducer port with a dead-end cap *to prevent leakage of arterial blood.* Gently squeeze the drip chamber until it is about one-fourth full of solution. When the bag is pressurized, the chamber will fill further. Remove the cover from the end of the pressure tubing, set the stopcock to the upright (middle) position, and raise the end of the tubing *to expel residual air.* Then open the flow clamp and activate the fast-flush release; the saline solution should run through the system, flushing all air. Tap the continuous flush device to release any air bubbles. Replace the cover, remove the dead-end cap from the stopcock port that vents to air, and open the stopcock to air and the saline solution. Hold this stopcock port upright until solution flows from it, replace the dead-end cap, and close the stopcock port.

Remove the cover from the end of the transducer port, turn the stopcock so the saline solution enters the transducer port, and activate the continuous flush device to remove all air. Replace the dead-end cap. Set the stopcock in the upright position. Close the flow clamp. Inflate the pressure bag to 300 mm Hg, but avoid overfilling the drip chamber. If it does overfill, release the pressure bag, invert the drip chamber, squeeze some solution into the I.V. bag, and repressurize the pressure bag.

Implementation
• Reinforce the doctor's explanation of the procedure, as needed. Check the patient's history for hypersensitivity to the local anesthetic or iodine.
• Confirm the insertion site with the doctor, and position the patient so the site is well lit and accessible. Before the radial site is chosen, Allen's test may be performed to assess blood supply to the hand. (See "Arterial puncture for blood gas analysis" in Chapter 3.)

To insert an arterial line
• Place a linen-saver pad and sterile towel under the arm or leg *to create a sterile field and to prevent blood from soiling the area.*
• After the doctor puts on sterile gloves and mask, open the wrappers of a povidone-iodine sponge and an alcohol sponge. Using sterile technique, the doctor takes the sponges and cleans the insertion site.
• Open the syringe package. Maintaining sterile technique, give the 3-ml syringe with the 25G 1″ needle to the doctor. Then, wipe the rubber stopper of the lidocaine bottle with alcohol and invert the bottle *to allow the doctor to withdraw the anesthetic.* He then injects the local anesthetic into the site.
• Open the catheter packaging. Using sterile technique, the doctor grasps the catheter, inserts it into the artery, and attaches the administration set.
• Open the flow clamp and activate the fast-flush release *to flush blood from the catheter.*
• Temporarily tape the I.V. tubing to the patient's arm to keep it in place during suturing.
• Put on gloves.
• Apply povidone-iodine ointment to the site and cover it with a sterile dressing.
• If necessary, apply an armboard or splint *to immobilize the insertion site.*
• Tape the I.V. tubing to the patient's arm.

To remove an arterial line
• Wash your hands and explain the procedure to the patient. After putting on gloves and a mask, gently remove the dressing *to avoid dislodging the catheter,* and remove any sutures, using the sterile suture removal set.
• Turn off the flow clamp *to prevent fluid leakage.* Withdraw the catheter with a gentle, steady motion, keeping it parallel to the artery *to reduce the risk of traumatic injury.* Immediately apply pressure with a sterile gauze pad for at least 7 minutes to a brachial site, 5 minutes to a radial site, and 10 minutes to a femoral site, or until bleeding ceases.
• Apply povidone-iodine ointment to the site, fold a gauze pad in half, place it over the site, and cover it with an adhesive bandage *to apply pressure.* Check the distal pulse *to detect arterial obstruction from an overly tight bandage.*
• Periodically check the site for bleeding or a hematoma. Place a small sandbag, covered with a washcloth or pillowcase, over a femoral site *to prevent delayed bleeding.* Check for bleeding under the sandbag at least every 15 minutes for the first hour, every 30 minutes for the second hour, and then every hour for 6 hours.
• Watch for changes in pulse intensity, skin color, and temperature of the arm or leg *because they can indicate thrombus formation.* Notify the doctor immediately if you

TROUBLESHOOTING

Managing arterial line problems

MECHANICAL PROBLEM	INTERVENTION	PREVENTION
Air bubbles in the line	• Check for leaks and loose connections in the line. • Flush air through an open stopcock port.	• Flush all air from the line when setting up the equipment. • Avoid rapid, repeated pulling of the pigtail on the fast-flush valve.
Blood clot in the catheter or stopcock	• Flush the catheter, using the fast-flush valve. Never flush an arterial line with a syringe. Systolic back pressure may cause leakage. • Notify the doctor and prepare to replace the line.	• Maintain the flow rate of the heparinized flush solution at 3 to 4 ml/hour. • Flush the catheter, using the fast-flush valve, after aspirating blood samples.
Catheter displacement	• Attempt to aspirate blood. If you can't, notify the doctor and prepare to replace the line. Bloody drainage at the insertion site may indicate displacement.	• Tape the catheter securely. • Splint the arm or leg to stabilize the insertion site.
Blood backflow into the line	• Check the position of all stopcocks. • Check for loose connections. • Flush the catheter, using the fast-flush valve. • Replace the dome if blood backs up into it.	• Always maintain 300 mm Hg of pressure.
Inability to flush the line	• Check the position of all stopcocks, the bag pressure, and the condition of the tubing. Check the catheter for kinks. • If the line still can't be flushed, notify the doctor and prepare to replace it.	• Always maintain 300 mm Hg of pressure.

observe any of these signs, or signs of pulmonary embolus, such as dyspnea, chest pain, tachycardia, coughing, or blood-tinged sputum. (See *Managing arterial line problems.*)

• Change the pressure dressing to an adhesive bandage after 2 hours for a brachial or radial site and after 8 hours for a femoral site, or as ordered by the doctor.

Special considerations

After any insertion, ensure that all connections are tight *because a patient with normal cardiac output can lose 300 to 500 ml of blood per minute from an 18G catheter.*

Avoid obscuring the catheter hub connection with the dressing; the connection must be visible and accessible at all times. Flush the line every hour or according to hospital policy. Check the pressure bag *to ensure a con-*

stant reading of 300 mm Hg. Also check pulses distal to the insertion site every 2 hours *to detect circulatory impairment.* Change the dressing every 72 hours or when it becomes moist, soiled, or nonocclusive, and change the tubing, continuous flush device, and I.V. bag every 24 hours according to hospital policy.

If you suspect infection, clean the insertion site before catheter removal. After the catheter is removed, cut off its tip, using sterile scissors, place it in a sterile container, and send it to the laboratory for culture. Apply antimicrobial ointment to the site according to hospital policy, and apply a sterile dressing.

Complications

For information on complications, see *Risks of using arterial lines,* page 304.

Risks of using arterial lines

COMPLICATION	POSSIBLE CAUSES	SIGNS AND SYMPTOMS	NURSING INTERVENTIONS	PREVENTION
Thrombosis	• Arterial damage • Sluggish rate of flush solution • Inadequately heparinized flush solution • Failure to flush catheter when necessary • Irrigation of clotted catheter with syringe	• Loss or weakening of pulse below site • Loss of warmth, sensation, and mobility below site	• Notify the doctor. He may remove the line or the clot by arteriotomy and Fogarty catheterization.	• Check distal pulse rate and flow rate hourly. • Tape catheter securely; splint limb. • Heparinize the flush solution; flush hourly and after collecting blood. • Never irrigate the catheter with a syringe.
Bleeding and hematoma	• Dislodged catheter • Disconnected line • Blood leakage around catheter	• Bloody dressing; blood flowing from disconnected line • Ecchymosis at the insertion site or of the limb	• Notify the doctor. • If catheter dislodges, put direct pressure on site. • If the line is disconnected, replace contaminated equipment.	• Frequently check the line connections and insertion site. • Tape the catheter securely, and splint the limb.
Air embolism	• Empty I.V. container • Air in the tubing • Loose connections	• Decreased blood pressure • Weak, rapid pulse • Cyanosis • Loss of consciousness	• Turn the patient to his left side so air entering the heart can be absorbed in the pulmonary artery. • Check the line for leaks. • Notify the doctor, and check vital signs. • Administer oxygen if ordered.	• Expel all air from the line before starting the infusion. • Secure all connections and check them routinely. • Change the I.V. container before it runs out.
Systemic infection	• Poor aseptic technique • Contaminated equipment, solution, or medication	• Sudden rise in temperature and pulse rate • Chills • Changes in blood pressure	• Evaluate for other sources of infection. Collect blood sample and specimens of urine, sputum, and I.V. solution for cultures, as ordered. • Notify the doctor.	• Use aseptic technique. • Avoid contaminating the site when bathing the patient. • If the line is disconnected, replace contaminated equipment.
Arterial spasm	• Traumatic catheter insertion • Arterial irritation after catheter insertion	• Intermittent loss or weakening of pulse below the insertion site	• Notify the doctor. • Prepare lidocaine for the doctor to inject into the catheter. Make sure it contains no epinephrine.	• Tape the catheter securely and splint the limb.

Understanding VAPs

Typically, a vascular access port (VAP) is used to deliver intermittent infusion of medication, chemotherapy, or blood products. Because the device is completely covered by the patient's skin, it reduces the risk of extrinsic contamination. Patients may prefer this type of central line because it doesn't alter the body image and requires less routine catheter care.

The VAP consists of a catheter connected to a small reservoir. A septum designed to withstand multiple punctures seals the reservoir.

VAPs come in two basic designs: top entry and side entry. In a top-entry port, the needle is inserted perpendicular to the reservoir. In a side-entry port, the needle is inserted into the septum nearly parallel to the reservoir. (A needle stop prevents the needle from coming out the other side.)

Top-entry VAP

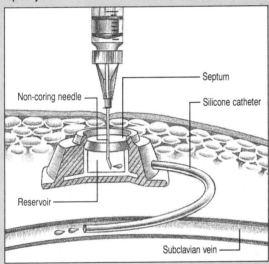

Side-entry VAP

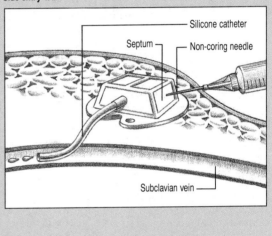

Documentation
At insertion, record the time, date, doctor's name, insertion site, and the type, gauge, and length of the catheter. At removal, record the time, date, doctor's name, condition of the insertion site, and any catheter specimens sent for culture.

Implanted vascular access devices

An implanted vascular access device is surgically implanted under local anesthesia by a doctor. The device consists of a silicone catheter attached to a reservoir, which is covered with a self-sealing silicone rubber septum. Such a device is used most commonly when an external central venous (CV) catheter is not desirable for long term I.V. therapy. The most common type of vascular access device is a vascular access port (VAP). One- and two-piece units with single or double lumens are available. (See *Understanding VAPs*.)

VAPs come in two basic types: top entry (such as Med-i-Port, Port-A-Cath, and Infuse-A-Port) and side entry (such as S.E.A. Port). The VAP reservoir can be made of titanium (such as Port-A-Cath), stainless steel (such as Q-Port), or molded plastic (such as Infuse-A-Port). The type and lumen size selected depend on the patient's therapeutic needs.

Implanted in a pocket under the skin, a VAP functions much like a long-term CV catheter, except that it has no external parts. The attached indwelling catheter tunnels through the subcutaneous tissue so the catheter tip lies in a central vein (the subclavian vein, for example). A

Characteristics of non-coring needles

Unlike a conventional hypodermic needle, a non-coring needle has a deflected point, which slices the port's septum instead of coring it.

When the needle is withdrawn, the septum reseals itself. Non-coring needles come in two types: straight and right angle.

Generally, you can expect to use a right-angle needle with a top-entry port, and a straight needle with a side-entry port. When administering a bolus injection or continuous infusion, you'll use a non-coring needle attached to an extension set, which may also have a side port for drug injections and blood sampling.

Conventional hypodermic needle

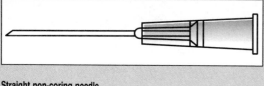

Right-angle non-coring needle

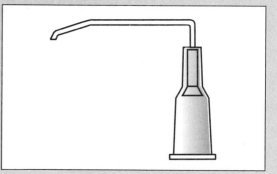

Straight non-coring needle

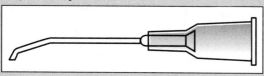

VAP can also be used for arterial access or can be implanted into the epidural space, peritoneum, or pericardial or pleural cavity.

Typically, VAPs deliver intermittent infusions. Most often used for chemotherapy, a VAP can also deliver I.V. fluids, medications, or blood products. You can also use a VAP to obtain blood samples.

VAPs offer several advantages, including minimal activity restrictions, few self-care measures for the patient to learn and perform, and few dressing changes (except when used to maintain continuous infusions or heparin locks). Implanted devices are easier to maintain than external devices. For instance, they require heparinization only once after each use (or periodically if not in use). They also pose less risk of infection because they have no exit site to serve as an entry for microorganisms.

Because VAPs create only a slight protrusion under the skin, many patients find them easier to accept than external infusion devices. Because the device is implanted, however, it may be more difficult for the patient to manage, particularly if the patient will be administering medication or fluids on a daily or frequent basis. And because accessing the device requires inserting a needle through subcutaneous tissue, patients who fear or dislike needle punctures may be uncomfortable using it and may require a local anesthetic. In addition, im-

plantation and removal of the device requires surgery and hospitalization. The comparatively high cost of VAPs makes them worthwhile only for patients who require infusion therapy for at least 6 months.

Implanted VAPs are contraindicated in patients who have been unable to tolerate other implanted devices and in those who may develop an allergic reaction.

Equipment

To implant a VAP: non-coring needles of appropriate type and gauge (see *Characteristics of non-coring needles*) ▪ VAP ▪ sterile gloves ▪ alcohol sponges ▪ extension set tubing, if needed ▪ povidone-iodine swabs ▪ local anesthetic (lidocaine without epinephrine) ▪ ice pack ▪ 5-, 10-, and 20-ml syringes ▪ normal saline and heparin flush solutions ▪ I.V. solution ▪ sterile dressings ▪ luer-lock injection cap ▪ clamp ▪ adhesive skin closures ▪ suture removal set.

To administer a bolus injection: extension set ▪ 10-ml syringe filled with normal saline solution ▪ clamp ▪ syringe containing the prescribed medication ▪ optional: sterile needle filled with heparin flush solution.

To administer a continuous infusion: prescribed I.V. solution or medication ▪ I.V. administration set ▪ filter, if ordered ▪ extension set ▪ clamp ▪ 10-ml syringe filled with normal saline solution ▪ antimicrobial ointment (such as povidone-iodine ointment) ▪ adhesive tape ▪ sterile 2″ × 2″ gauze pad ∎ sterile tape ∎ transparent semi-permeable dressing.

Some hospitals use an implantable port access kit.

Preparation of equipment
Confirm the size and type of the device and the insertion site with the doctor. Attach the tubing to the solution container, prime the tubing with fluid, fill the syringes with saline or heparin flush solution, and prime the non-coring needle and extension set. All priming must be done using strict aseptic technique, and all tubing must be free of air. After you've primed the tubing, recheck all connections for tightness. Make sure that all open ends are covered with sealed caps.

Implementation
• Wash your hands *to prevent spread of microorganisms.*

Assisting with implantation of a VAP
• Reinforce to the patient the doctor's explanation of the procedure, its benefit to the patient, and what's expected of him during and after implantation.
• Although the doctor is responsible for obtaining consent for the procedure, be sure the written document is signed, witnessed, and on the chart.
• Allay the patient's fears and answer questions about movement restrictions, cosmetic concerns, and management regimens.
• Check the patient's history for hypersensitivity to local anesthetic or iodine.
• The doctor will surgically implant the VAP, most likely using a local anesthetic (similar to insertion of a central venous catheter). Occasionally, a patient may receive a general anesthetic for VAP implantation.
• During the implantation procedure, you may be responsible for handing equipment and supplies to the doctor. First, the doctor makes a small incision and introduces the catheter, typically into the superior vena cava through the subclavian, jugular, or cephalic vein. After fluoroscopy verifies the placement of the catheter tip, the doctor creates a subcutaneous pocket over a bony prominence in the chest wall. Then, he tunnels the catheter to the pocket. Next, he connects the catheter to the reservoir, places the reservoir in the pocket, and flushes it with heparin solution. Finally, he sutures the reservoir to the underlying fascia and closes the incision.

Preparing to access the port
• The device can be used immediately after placement, although some edema and tenderness may persist for about 72 hours. This makes the device initially difficult to palpate and slightly uncomfortable for the patient.

• Prepare to access the port, following the specific steps for top-entry or side-entry ports.
• Using aseptic technique, inspect the area around the port for signs of infection or skin breakdown.
• Place an ice pack over the area for several minutes *to alleviate possible discomfort from the needle puncture.* Alternatively, give a local anesthetic after cleaning the area.
• Wash your hands thoroughly and put on sterile gloves. Remember to keep these gloves on throughout the procedure.
• Clean the area with an alcohol sponge, starting at the center of the port and working outward with a firm circular motion over a 4″ to 5″ (10 to 12.7 cm) diameter. Repeat this procedure twice.
• If hospital policy calls for a local anesthetic, check the patient's record for possible allergies. As indicated, anesthetize the insertion site by injecting 0.1 ml of lidocaine (without epinephrine).

Accessing a top-entry port
• Palpate the area over the port to locate the port septum.
• Anchor the port with your nondominant hand. (See *Stabilizing a top-entry VAP*, page 308.) Then, using your dominant hand, aim the needle at the center of the device.
• Insert the needle perpendicular to the port septum. Push the needle through the skin and septum until you reach the bottom of the reservoir.
• Check needle placement by aspirating for blood return.
• If you're unable to obtain blood, remove the needle and repeat the procedure. Inability to obtain blood might indicate that the catheter is lodged against the vessel's wall. Ask the patient to raise his arms, perform Valsalva's maneuver, or change position to free the catheter. If you still don't get a blood return, notify the doctor; a fibrin sleeve on the distal end of the catheter may be occluding the opening.
• Flush the device with normal saline solution. If you detect swelling or if the patient reports pain at the site, remove the needle and notify the doctor.

Accessing a side-entry port
• To gain access to a side-entry port, you'll follow the same procedure as with a top-entry port; however, you'll insert the needle parallel to the reservoir instead of perpendicular to it.

Administering a bolus injection
• Attach the 10-ml syringe filled with saline solution to the end of the extension set and remove all the air. Now attach the extension set to the non-coring needle. Check for a blood return. Then flush the port with normal saline solution, according to your hospital's policy. (Some hos-

Stabilizing a top-entry VAP

This illustration shows the correct way to secure a top-entry vascular access port (VAP). Hold the device between your thumb and first two fingers while inserting a needle into the septum.

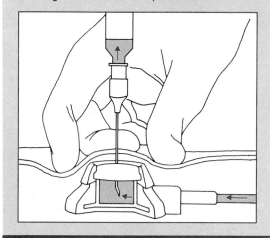

pitals require flushing the port with a sterile needle of heparin solution first.)
• Clamp the extension set and remove the saline syringe.
• Connect the medication syringe to the extension set. Open the clamp and inject the drug, as ordered.
• Examine the skin surrounding the needle for signs of infiltration, such as swelling or tenderness. If you note these signs, stop the injection and intervene appropriately.
• When the injection is complete, clamp the extension set and remove the medication syringe.
• Open the clamp and flush with 5 ml of normal saline solution after each drug injection to minimize drug incompatibility reactions.
• Flush with heparin solution, as hospital policy directs.

Administering a continuous infusion
• Remove all air from the extension set by priming it with an attached syringe of normal saline solution. Now attach the extension set to the non-coring needle.
• Flush the port system with normal saline solution. Clamp the extension set and remove the syringe.
• Connect the administration set, and secure the connections with sterile tape if necessary.
• Unclamp the extension set and begin the infusion.

• Apply a small amount of antimicrobial ointment to the insertion site.
• Affix the needle to the skin. (See *Continuous infusion: Securing the needle.*) Then apply a transparent semipermeable dressing.
• Examine the site carefully for infiltration. If the patient complains of stinging, burning, or pain at the site, discontinue the infusion and intervene appropriately.
• When the solution container is empty, obtain a new I.V. solution container, as ordered.
• Flush with heparin solution as hospital policy directs.

Special considerations
After implantation, monitor the site for signs of hematoma and bleeding. Edema and tenderness may persist for about 72 hours. The incision site requires routine postoperative care for 7 to 10 days. You'll also need to assess the implantation site for signs of infection, device rotation, or skin erosion. You don't need to apply a dressing to the wound site except during infusions or to maintain a heparin lock.

While the patient is hospitalized, a luer-lock injection cap may be attached to the end of the extension set to provide ready access for intermittent infusions. Besides saving nursing time, a luer-lock cap will reduce the discomfort of accessing the port, as well as prolong the life of the port septum by decreasing the number of needle punctures.

If your patient is receiving a continuous or prolonged infusion, you'll need to change the dressing and needle every 5 to 7 days. You'll also need to change the tubing and solution, as you would for a long-term CV infusion. If your patient is receiving an intermittent infusion, you'll need to flush the port periodically with heparin solution. When the VAP isn't being used, flush it every 4 weeks. During the course of therapy, you may have to clear a clotted VAP, as ordered.

If clotting threatens to occlude the VAP, the doctor may order a fibrinolytic agent, such as urokinase, to clear the catheter. The usual dose is 1 ml (5,000 IU/ml of sterile water) of urokinase. *Because such agents increase the risk of bleeding,* urokinase may be contraindicated in patients who have had surgery within the previous 10 days; who have active internal bleeding, such as GI bleeding; or who have experienced central nervous system damage, such as infarction, hemorrhage, traumatic injury, surgery, or primary or metastatic disease within the past 2 months.

Besides performing routine care measures, you must be prepared to handle several common problems that may arise during an infusion with a VAP. These common problems include an inability to flush the VAP, withdraw blood from it, or palpate it. (See *Managing common VAP problems,* page 310.)

Home care

A home care patient needs thorough teaching about procedures and follow-up visits from a home care nurse to ensure safety and successful treatment. If the patient will be accessing the port himself, explain that the most uncomfortable part of the procedure is the actual insertion of the needle into the skin.

Once the needle has penetrated the skin, the patient will feel mostly pressure. Eventually, the skin over the port will become desensitized from frequent needle punctures. Until then, the patient may want to use a topical anesthetic.

Stress the importance of pushing the needle into the port until the patient feels the needle bevel touch the back of the port. Many patients tend to stop short of the back of the port, leaving the needle bevel in the rubber septum.

Also stress the importance of monthly flushes when no more infusions are scheduled. If possible, instruct a family member in all aspects of care.

Complications

A patient who has a VAP faces risks similar to those associated with CV catheters. These include complications such as infection and infiltration. (See *Risks of VAP therapy,* page 311.)

Documentation

Record your assessment findings and interventions according to hospital policy. Include the following information: the type, the amount, the rate, and the duration of the infusion; the appearance of the site; the development of problems, if any, and the steps taken to resolve them.

Also keep a record of all needle and dressing changes for continuous infusions; blood samples obtained, including the type and amount; and patient-teaching topics covered.

Finally, document the removal of the infusion needle, the status of the site, the use of the heparin flush, and any problems you encountered and resolved.

Continuous infusion: Securing the needle

When starting a continuous infusion, you must secure the right-angle non-coring needle to the skin. If the needle hub isn't flush with the skin, place a folded sterile dressing under the hub, as shown. Then apply adhesive skin closures across it.

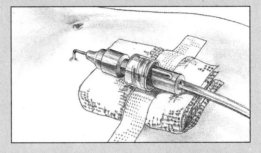

Secure the needle and tubing, using the chevron-taping technique.

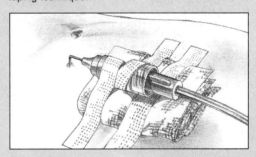

Apply a transparent semipermeable dressing over the entire site.

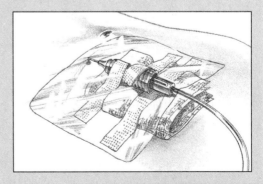

Managing common VAP problems

PROBLEMS AND POSSIBLE CAUSES	NURSING INTERVENTIONS
Inability to flush the device or draw blood	
Kinked tubing or closed clamp	• Check tubing or clamp.
Catheter lodged against vessel wall	• Reposition the patient. • Teach the patient to change his position to free the catheter from the vessel wall. • Raise the arm that's on the same side as the catheter. • Roll the patient to his opposite side. • Have the patient cough, sit up, or take a deep breath. • Infuse 10 ml of normal saline solution into the catheter. • Regain access to the catheter or vascular access port (VAP) using a new needle.
Incorrect needle placement or needle not advanced through septum	• Regain access to the device. • Teach the home care patient to push down firmly on the non-coring needle device in the septum and to verify needle placement by aspirating for a blood return.
Clot formation	• Assess patency by trying to flush the VAP while the patient changes position. • Notify the doctor; obtain an order for urokinase instillation. • Teach the patient to recognize clot formation, to notify the doctor if it occurs, and to avoid forcibly flushing the VAP.
Kinked catheter, catheter migration, or port rotation	• Notify the doctor immediately. • Tell the patient to notify the doctor if he has trouble using the VAP.
Inability to palpate the device	
Deeply implanted port	• Note portal chamber scar. • Use deep palpation technique. • Ask another nurse to try locating the VAP. • Use a 1½″ or 2″ (3.8- or 5-cm) non-coring needle to gain access to the VAP.

 # *F*LOW RATE MANAGEMENT

Flow rate calculation and manual control

Calculated from a doctor's orders, flow rate is usually expressed as the total volume of I.V. solution infused over a prescribed interval or as the total volume given in milliliters per hour (ml/hr). Many devices can regulate the flow of I.V. solution, including clamps, controllers, the flow regulator (or rate minder), and the volumetric pump. (See *Using I.V. clamps,* page 312.)

When regulated by a clamp or controller, flow rate is usually measured in drops per minute; by a volumetric pump, in ml/hr. The flow regulator can be set to deliver the desired amount of solution, also in ml/hr. Less accurate than infusion pumps or controllers, flow regulators are most reliable when used with inactive adult

Risks of VAP therapy

COMPLICATION	SIGNS AND SYMPTOMS	POSSIBLE CAUSES	NURSING INTERVENTIONS
Site infection or skin breakdown	• Erythema and warmth at the port site • Oozing or purulent drainage at vascular access port (VAP) site or pocket • Fever	• Infected incision or VAP pocket • Poor postoperative healing	• Assess site daily for redness; note any drainage. • Notify the doctor. • Administer antibiotics as ordered. • Apply warm soaks for 20 minutes four times a day. *Prevention* • Teach the patient to inspect for and report any redness, swelling, drainage, or skin breakdown at the port site.
Extravasation	• Burning sensation or swelling in subcutaneous tissue	• Needle dislodged into subcutaneous tissue • Needle incorrectly placed in VAP • Needle position not confirmed; needle pulled out of septum	• Stop the infusion. • Notify the doctor; prepare to administer antidote if ordered. • Follow hospital protocol for removing the needle. *Prevention* • Teach the patient how to gain access to the device, verify its placement, and secure the needle before initiating infusion.
Thrombosis	• Inability to flush port or administer infusion	• Frequent blood sampling • Infusion of packed red blood cells (PRBCs)	• Notify the doctor; obtain an order to administer urokinase. *Prevention* • Flush VAP thoroughly right after obtaining blood sample. • Administer PRBCs as a piggyback with normal saline solution and use an infusion pump; flush with saline solution between units.
Fibrin sheath formation	• Blocked port and catheter lumen • Inability to flush port or administer infusion • Possible swelling, tenderness and erythema in neck, chest, and shoulder	• Adherence of platelets to catheter	• Notify the doctor; add heparin (1,000 to 2,000 units) to continuous infusions as ordered. *Prevention* • Use port only to infuse fluids and medications; don't use to obtain blood samples. • Administer only compatible substances through port.

Using I.V. clamps

With a roller clamp or screw clamp, you can increase or decrease flow through the I.V. line by turning a wheel or screw.

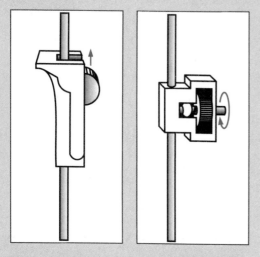

With a slide clamp, you can open or close the line by moving the clamp horizontally. However, you can't make fine adjustments to flow rate.

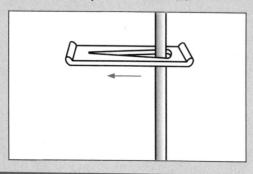

patients. With any device, flow rate can be easily monitored by using a time tape, which indicates the prescribed solution level at hourly intervals.

Equipment

I.V. administration set with clamp ■ 1″ paper or adhesive tape (or premarked time tape) ■ infusion pump and controller (if infusing drugs) ■ watch with second hand ■ drip rate chart, as necessary ■ pen.

Standard macrodrip sets deliver 10 to 20 drops/ml, depending on the manufacturer; microdrip sets, 60 drops/ml; and blood transfusion sets, 10 drops/ml. A commercially available adapter can convert a macrodrip set to a microdrip system.

Implementation

• Flow rate requires close monitoring and correction because such factors as venous spasm, venous pressure changes, patient movement or manipulation of the clamp, and bent or kinked tubing can cause the rate to vary markedly.

To calculate and set the drip rate

• Follow the steps in *Calculating flow rates* to determine the proper drip rate, or use your unit's drip rate chart.
• After calculating the desired drip rate, remove your watch and hold it next to the drip chamber of the I.V. administration set *to allow simultaneous observation of the watch and the drops.*
• Release the clamp to the approximate drip rate. Then count drops for 1 minute *to account for flow irregularities.*
• Adjust the clamp, as necessary, and count drops for 1 minute. Continue to adjust the clamp and count drops until the correct rate is achieved.

To make a time tape

• Calculate the number of milliliters to be infused per hour. Place a piece of tape vertically on the container alongside the volume-increment markers.
• Starting at the current solution level, move down the number of milliliters to be infused in 1 hour, and mark the appropriate time and a horizontal line on the tape at this level. Then continue to mark 1-hour intervals until you reach the bottom of the container.
• Check the flow rate every 15 minutes until it is stable. Then recheck it every hour or according to hospital policy, and adjust as necessary.
• With each check, inspect the I.V. site for complications and assess the patient's response to therapy.

Special considerations

If the infusion rate slows significantly, a slight rate increase may be necessary. If the rate must be increased by more than 30%, consult the doctor. When infusing drugs, use an I.V. pump or controller, if possible, *to avoid flow rate inaccuracies.* Always use a pump or controller when infusing solutions via a central line.

Large-volume solution containers have approximately 10% more fluid than the amount indicated on the bag, to allow for tubing purges. Thus, a 1,000-ml bag or bottle will contain an additional 100 ml; similarly, a 500-ml

Calculating flow rates

When calculating the flow rate of I.V. solutions, remember that the number of drops required to deliver 1 ml varies with the type and manufacturer of the administration set used. The illustration on the left shows a standard (macrodrip) set, which delivers from 10 to 20 drops/ml. The illustration in the center shows a pediatric (microdrip) set, which delivers about 60 drops/ml. The illustration on the right shows a blood transfusion set, which delivers about 10 drops/ml.

To calculate the flow rate, you must know the calibration of the drip rate for each manufacturer's product. As a quick guide, refer to the chart below. Use this formula to calculate specific drop rates:

$$\frac{\text{Volume of infusion (in ml)}}{\text{time of infusion (in minutes)}} \times \text{drip factor (in drops/ml)} = \text{drops/minute}$$

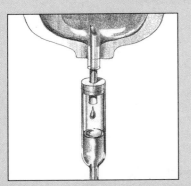 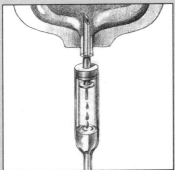 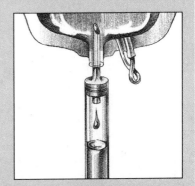

ADMINISTRATION SET	DRIP FACTOR	ORDERED VOLUME					
		500 ml/ 24 hr or 21 ml/hr	1,000 ml/ 24 hr or 42 ml/hr	1,000 ml/ 20 hr or 50 ml/hr	1,000 ml/ 10 hr or 100 ml/hr	1,000 ml/ 8 hr or 125 ml/hr	1,000 ml/ 6 hr or 166 ml/hr
		DROPS/MINUTE TO INFUSE					
Macrodrip							
Abbott	15	5	10	12	25	31	42
Baxter Healthcare	10	3	7	8	17	21	28
Cutter	20	7	14	17	34	42	56
IVAC	20	7	14	17	34	42	56
McGaw	15	5	10	12	25	31	42
Microdrip							
Various manufacturers	60	21	42	50	100	125	166

container will hold an extra 50 ml; and a 250-ml container, 25 ml.

Complications
An excessively slow flow rate may cause insufficient intake of fluids, drugs, and nutrients; an excessively rapid rate of fluid or drug infusion may cause circulatory overload—possibly leading to congestive heart failure and pulmonary edema, as well as drug side effects. (See *Managing I.V. flow rate deviations.*)

Documentation
Record the original flow rate when setting up a peripheral line. If you adjust the rate, record the change, the date and time, and your initials.

 ## Use of I.V. controllers and pumps

Various types of controllers and pumps electronically regulate the flow of I.V. solutions or drugs with extreme accuracy. (See *Regulating flow rate electronically,* page 316.) Controllers regulate gravity flow by counting drops and achieve the desired infusion rate by compressing the I.V. tubing. However, because controllers simply count drops, which aren't always of equal size, these devices fail to achieve the accuracy of volumetric pumps, which measure flow rate in milliliters per hour.

Volumetric pumps, used for high-pressure infusion of drugs or for highly accurate delivery of fluids or drugs, have mechanisms to propel the solution at the desired rate under pressure. (Pressure is brought to bear only when gravity flow rates are insufficient to maintain preset infusion rates.) The peristaltic pump applies pressure to the I.V. tubing to force the solution through it. (Not every peristaltic pump is volumetric; some count drops.) The piston-cylinder pump pushes the solution through special disposable cassettes; most of these pumps operate at high pressures (up to 45 psi) and can deliver 1 to 999 ml/hour with a 97% to 98% accuracy. (Some newer pumps operate at 10 to 25 psi.) The portable syringe pump, another type of volumetric pump, delivers very small amounts of fluid over a long duration. It's used for administering fluids to infants and for delivering intra-arterial drugs. Other special devices include the controlled release infusion system, secondary syringe converter, and patient-controlled analgesia device. (See *Devices for intermittent infusion,* page 317, and *Understanding patient-controlled analgesia,* page 318.)

Controllers and pumps have various detectors and alarms that automatically signal or respond to the completion of an infusion, air in the line, low battery power, and occlusion or inability to deliver at the set rate. Depending on the problem, these devices may sound or flash an alarm, shut off, or switch to a keep-vein-open rate.

Equipment
Controller or peristaltic pump ▪ I.V. pole ▪ I.V. solution ▪ sterile administration set ▪ sterile peristaltic tubing or cassette, if needed ▪ alcohol sponges ▪ adhesive tape.

Tubing and cassette vary with each manufacturer.

Preparation of equipment
To set up a controller: First, attach the controller to the I.V. pole. Then clean the port on the I.V. solution container with an alcohol sponge, insert the administration set spike, and fill the drip chamber no more than halfway *to avoid miscounting the drops.* Rotate the chamber so the fluid touches all sides *to remove any vapor that could interfere with correct drop counting.* Now, prime the tubing and close the clamp. Position the drop sensor above the fluid level in the drip chamber and below the drop port *to ensure correct drop counting.* Insert the peristaltic tubing into the controller, close the door, and open the flow clamp completely.

To set up a volumetric pump: First, attach the pump to the I.V. pole. Then, swab the port on the I.V. container with alcohol, insert the administration set spike, and completely fill the drip chamber *to prevent air bubbles from entering the tubing.* Next, prime the tubing and close the clamp. Now, follow the manufacturer's instructions for placement of tubing.

Implementation
• Position the controller or pump on the same side of the bed as the I.V. or anticipated venipuncture site *to avoid crisscrossing I.V. lines over the patient.* If necessary, perform the venipuncture.
• Plug in the machine and attach its tubing to the needle or catheter hub. If you're using a controller, position the drip chamber 30″ (76.2 cm) above the infusion site *to ensure accurate gravity flow.*
• Depending on the machine, turn it on and press the start button. Set the appropriate dials on the front panel to the desired infusion rate and volume. Always set the volume dial at 50 ml less than the prescribed volume or 50 ml less than the volume in the container *so that you can hang a new container before the old one empties completely.*
• Check the patency of the I.V. line and watch for infiltration. If you're using a controller, monitor the accuracy of the infusion rate.
• Tape all connections and recheck the controller's drip rate *because taping may alter it.*

Managing I.V. flow rate deviations

PROBLEM	CAUSE	INTERVENTION
Flow rate too fast	• Patient or visitor manipulates the clamp	• Instruct the patient not to touch the clamp, and place tape over it. Restrain the patient or administer the I.V. with an infusion pump or a controller, if necessary.
	• Tubing disconnected from the catheter	• Wipe the distal end of the tubing with alcohol, reinsert firmly into the catheter hub, and tape at the connection site. Consider using tubing with luer connections.
	• Change in patient position	• Administer the I.V. with an infusion pump or a controller to ensure the correct flow rate.
	• Bevel against vein wall (positional cannulation)	• Manipulate the cannula, and place a 2″ × 2″ gauze pad under or over the catheter hub to change the angle. Reset the flow clamp at the desired rate. If necessary, remove the cannula and reinsert.
	• Flow clamp drifting as a result of patient movement	• Place tape below the clamp.
Flow rate too slow	• Venous spasm after insertion	• Apply warm soaks over site.
	• Venous obstruction from bending arm	• Secure with an armboard if necessary.
	• Pressure change (decreasing fluid in bottle causes solution to run slower due to decreasing pressure)	• Readjust the flow rate.
	• Elevated blood pressure	• Readjust the flow rate. Use an infusion pump or a controller to ensure correct flow rate.
	• Cold solution	• Allow the solution to warm to room temperature before hanging.
	• Change in solution viscosity from medication added	• Readjust the flow rate.
	• I.V. container too low or patient's arm or leg too high	• Hang the container higher or remind the patient to keep his arm below heart level.
	• Bevel against vein wall (positional cannulation)	• Withdraw the needle slightly, or place a folded 2″ × 2″ gauze pad over or under the catheter hub to change the angle.
	• Excess tubing dangling below insertion site	• Replace the tubing with a shorter piece, or tape the excess tubing to the I.V. pole, below the flow clamp (make sure the tubing is not kinked).
	• Cannula too small	• Remove the cannula in use and insert a larger-bore cannula, or use an infusion pump.
	• Infiltration or clotted cannula	• Remove the cannula in use and reinsert a new cannula.
	• Kinked tubing	• Check the tubing over its entire length and unkink it.
	• Clogged filter	• Remove the filter and replace with a new one.
	• Tubing memory (tubing compressed at area clamped)	• Massage or milk the tubing by pinching and wrapping it around a pencil four or five times. Quickly pull the pencil out of the coiled tubing.

Regulating flow rate electronically

Controllers and infusion pumps, such as the two shown below, electronically regulate the flow of I.V. solutions and drugs. You'll use them when a precise flow rate is required—for instance, when administering total parenteral nutrition solutions and chemotherapeutic or cardiovascular agents.

Controller

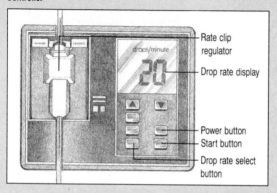

- Rate clip regulator
- Drop rate display
- Power button
- Start button
- Drop rate select button

Infusion pump

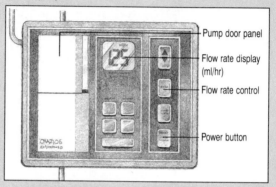

- Pump door panel
- Flow rate display (ml/hr)
- Flow rate control
- Power button

• Turn on the alarm switches. Then explain the alarm system to the patient *to prevent anxiety when a change in the infusion activates the alarm.*

Special considerations

Monitor the pump or controller and the patient frequently *to ensure the device's correct operation and flow rate, and to detect infiltration and such complications as infection and air embolism.*

If electrical power fails, the pumps will automatically switch to battery power.

Check the manufacturer's recommendations before administering opaque fluids, such as blood, because some pumps fail to detect opaque fluids and others may cause hemolysis of infused blood.

Move the tubing in controllers every few hours *to prevent permanent compression or tubing damage.* Change the tubing and cassette every 48 hours or according to hospital policy.

Remove I.V. solutions from the refrigerator 1 hour before infusing them to help release small gas bubbles from the solutions. *Small bubbles in the solution can join to form larger bubbles, which can activate the pump's air-in-line alarm.*

Home care

Be sure the patient and his family understand the purpose of using the pump or controller. If necessary, dem-

onstrate how the device works. Also demonstrate how to maintain the system (tubing, solution, and site assessment and care) until you're confident that the patient and family can proceed safely. As time permits, have the patient repeat the demonstration. Discuss which complications to watch for, such as infiltration, and review what measures to take if complications occur. Schedule a teaching session with the patient or family so you can answer questions they may have about the procedure before the patient's discharge.

Complications

Complications associated with I.V. controllers and pumps are the same as those associated with peripheral lines. (See "Insertion of a peripheral I.V. line" in this chapter.) Keep in mind that infiltration can develop rapidly with infusion by a volumetric pump because the increased subcutaneous pressure won't slow the infusion rate until significant edema occurs.

Documentation

In addition to routine documentation of the I.V. infusion, record the use of a controller or pump on the I.V. record and in your notes.

Devices for intermittent infusion

The devices shown below allow you to deliver precise drug amounts over a prescribed time period from a vial or a syringe.

Controlled release infusion system
Place this device between the I.V. container and the tubing, then attach the drug vial to its side, as shown. The I.V. fluid passes into the device where it mixes with the drug from the vial to deliver a controlled amount of medication to the patient.

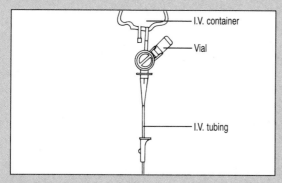

Secondary syringe converter
This special administration set converts any syringe into a piggyback container. The tubing connects to the syringe instead of to a bag or bottle. Follow the same procedure as you would with a minibag, substituting the syringe for the minibag.

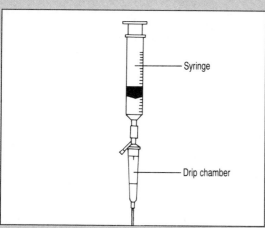

Syringe pump
Battery-operated mini-infusion syringe pumps can be used to infuse small volumes intermittently or continuously. You'll find them especially useful for pediatric patients. The syringe and microbore tubing replace the minibag and piggyback tubing to deliver a precise volume over the prescribed time.

The major disadvantage of the syringe pump is that you need tubing to connect it to the venipuncture device. So when you give a small-volume dose, a portion of the drug remains in the tubing. You can help to limit the amount of drug remaining by using small-volume tubing. (Standard I.V. tubing holds 1.9 ml/foot; small-volume tubing has a smaller lumen and holds only 0.06 ml/foot.)

Also, remember that syringe pumps don't have air detectors. So be sure to eliminate all air from the syringe, tubing, and needle. Use luer-locks and tape all connections. This helps prevent partial disconnections that could cause an air infusion and drug leaks.

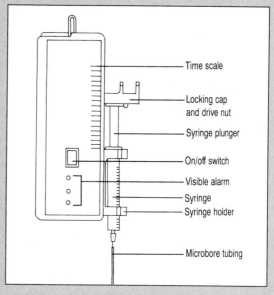

Understanding patient-controlled analgesia

In patient-controlled analgesia (PCA), the patient controls I.V. delivery of an analgesic (usually morphine) by pressing the button on a delivery device. The patient therefore receives analgesia at the level he needs and at the time he needs it. The device prevents the patient from accidentally overdosing by imposing a lock-out time between doses — usually 6 to 10 minutes. During this interval, the patient will not receive any analgesic, even if he pushes the button. The accompanying illustrations show two of the more commonly used PCA devices.

The first device, shown below, is a reusable, battery-operated pump that delivers a drug dose when the patient presses a call button at the end of a cord.

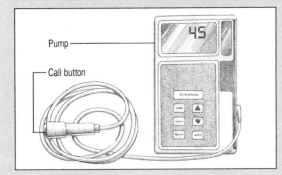

The other device, shown below, is disposable and mechanically operated. It contains an infusor and a unit that's worn like a wristwatch. The patient pushes a button on the device to receive the analgesic from a collapsible chamber.

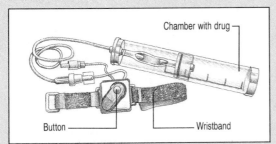

Indications and advantages
Indicated for patients who need parenteral analgesia, PCA therapy is typically given to trauma patients post-operatively and to terminal cancer patients and others with chronic diseases. To receive PCA therapy, a patient must be mentally alert, able to understand and comply with instructions and procedures, and have no history of allergy to the analgesic. Patients ineligible for therapy include those with limited respiratory reserve, a history of drug abuse or chronic sedative or tranquilizer use, or a psychiatric disorder. PCA therapy's advantages include:
• no need for I.M. analgesics
• pain relief tailored to each patient's size and pain tolerance
• a sense of control over pain
• ability to sleep at night with minimal daytime drowsiness
• lower narcotic use compared with patients not on PCA
• improved postoperative deep-breathing, coughing, and ambulation.

PCA setup
To set up a PCA system, the doctor should order:
• a loading dose, given by I.V. push at the start of PCA therapy (typically 25 mg meperidine [Demerol] or 2 mg morphine)
• the appropriate lock-out interval
• the maintenance dose (also called the basal dose)
• the amount the patient will receive when he activates the device
• the maximum amount the patient can receive within a specified time (if an adjustable device is used).

Nursing considerations
Because the primary adverse effect of analgesics is respiratory depression, you must monitor your patient's respiratory rate routinely. Also, check for infiltration into the subcutaneous tissues and for catheter occlusion, which may cause the drug to back up in the primary I.V. tubing. If the analgesic nauseates your patient, you may need to administer an antiemetic drug.

Before your patient starts using the PCA device, teach him how it works. Then have the patient practice with a sample device. Explain that he should take enough analgesic to relieve acute pain but not enough to induce drowsiness.

During therapy, monitor and record the amount of analgesic infused, the patient's respiratory rate, and the patient's assessment of pain relief. If the patient reports insufficient pain relief, notify the doctor.

PARENTERAL NUTRITION
Equipment preparation and site care for total parenteral nutrition

Total parenteral nutrition (TPN) is the parenteral administration of a solution of dextrose, proteins, electrolytes, vitamins, and trace elements in amounts that exceed the patient's energy expenditure and thereby achieve anabolism. Because this solution has about six times the solute concentration of blood, it requires dilution by delivery into a high-flow central vein to avoid injury to the peripheral vasculature. Typically, the solution is delivered to the superior vena cava through an indwelling subclavian vein catheter inserted by the infraclavicular approach or, less commonly, by the supraclavicular, internal jugular, or antecubital fossa approach.

A patient may receive TPN for any of the following reasons:
• debilitating illness lasting longer than 2 weeks
• limited or no oral intake for longer than 7 days, such as in cases of multiple traumatic injuries, severe burns, or anorexia nervosa
• loss of 10% or more of pre-illness weight
• serum albumin level below 3.5 g/dl
• poor tolerance of long-term enteral feedings
• chronic vomiting or diarrhea
• continued weight loss despite adequate oral intake
• GI disorders that prevent or severely reduce absorption, such as bowel obstruction, Crohn's disease, ulcerative colitis, short bowel sydrome, cancer malabsorption syndrome, and bowel fistulas
• inflammatory GI disorders, such as pancreatitis and peritonitis
• excessive nitrogen loss resulting from wound infection, fistulas, or abscesses
• renal or hepatic failure.

TPN also promotes normal growth and development in infants with congenital anomalies, such as tracheoesophageal fistula, gastroschisis, duodenal atresia, cystic fibrosis, meconium ileus, diaphragmatic hernia, volvulus, malrotation of the gut, and annular pancreas.

Because TPN solution supports bacterial growth and the central venous (CV) line gives systemic access, contamination and sepsis are always a risk. Strict surgical asepsis is required during solution, dressing, tubing, and filter changes. Site care and dressing changes should be performed according to hospital policy, usually at least three times weekly (once weekly for transparent dressings), and whenever the dressing becomes wet, soiled, or nonocclusive. Tubing and filter changes are performed every 24 to 48 hours according to hospital policy.

Equipment
Infusion pump and sterile tubing ▪ extension tubing ▪ two pairs of sterile gloves ▪ organic solvent (such as 70% alcohol) ▪ alcohol sponges ▪ antimicrobial solution (such as povidone-iodine) ▪ povidone-iodine ointment (or substitute) ▪ bags or bottles of TPN solution ▪ sterile 4″ × 4″ gauze pads ▪ cotton-tipped applicators ▪ transparent semipermeable dressing ▪ antiseptic adhesive balsam ▪ nonallergenic tape ▪ time tape ▪ optional: two face masks, sterile scissors, sterile drape, precut drain dressing, dextrose 10% in water, 0.22-micron cellulose membrane filter (1.2 microns if solution contains lipid emulsions or albumin), and luer-lock connections.

Some administration sets include single tubing with an in-line filter incorporated into the tubing. Prepackaged dressing kits are available commercially.

Preparation of equipment
Remove the 1-liter, 2-liter, or 3-liter bags or bottles of TPN solution from the refrigerator at least 1 hour before use *because delivery of a chilled solution can cause pain, hypothermia, venous spasm, and venous constriction.*

Double-check the contents of the solution and the doctor's orders. Then observe the solution for cloudiness, turbidity, and particles and the container for cracks; if any of these are present, return the solution to the pharmacy. (See *Types of parenteral nutrition,* pages 320 and 321, to compare solutions.)

Always maintain strict aseptic technique when preparing and handling equipment. Connect, in sequence, the pump tubing, cellulose membrane filter (if applicable), and extension tubing. Tape the tubing connections or use the luer-lock connections, if available, *to prevent accidental separation, which can lead to air embolism, exsanguination, and sepsis.* Squeeze the drip chamber of the tubing before spiking the bag or bottle, turn it upright and, using strict aseptic technique, insert the tubing spike into the port of the TPN container and release the drip chamber. *This prevents accidental dripping of TPN solution from a bottle (bags won't drip).* Start the flow of solution *to prime the tubing and remove air.* Gently tap the tubing *to dislodge air bubbles trapped in the Y ports.* If necessary, attach a time tape to the TPN container *to allow approximate measurement of fluid intake.* Attach the set-up to the infusion pump and prepare it according to the manufacturer's instructions.

Implementation
• Explain the procedure, make sure the bedside area is clean, and open the equipment.
• If required, put on a mask (especially if the patient is immunodeficient), and position the patient supine, with

(Text continues on page 322.)

Types of parenteral nutrition

TYPE	SOLUTION COMPONENTS/LITER	USES	SPECIAL CONSIDERATIONS
Standard I.V. therapy	• Dextrose, water, electrolytes in varying amounts. For example: D_5W = 170 calories/liter, $D_{10}W$ = 340 calories/liter, 0.9% sodium chloride = 0 calories • Vitamins as ordered	• Less than 1 week as nutrition source • Maintains hydration (main function) • Facilitates and maintains normal metabolic function	• Nutritionally incomplete; does not provide sufficient calories to maintain adequate nutritional status
Total parenteral nutrition (TPN) via central venous (CV) line	• Dextrose 20% to 25% in water (1 liter dextrose 25% = 850 nonprotein calories) • Crystalline amino acids 2.5% to 8.5% • Electrolytes, vitamins, trace elements, insulin, and heparin, as ordered • Lipid emulsion 10% to 20% (usually infused as a separate solution, but an infusion system is available in which dextrose, protein, and lipids are mixed in the same container)	• 3 weeks or more • For patients with large caloric and nutrient needs • Provides calories, restores nitrogen balance, and replaces essential vitamins, electrolytes, minerals, and trace elements • Promotes tissue synthesis, wound healing, and normal metabolic function • Allows bowel rest and healing; reduces activity in the gallbladder, pancreas, and small intestine • Improves tolerance of surgery	***Basic solution*** • Nutritionally complete • Requires minor surgical procedure for CV line insertion (can be done at bedside by the doctor) • Highly hypertonic solution • May cause metabolic complications (glucose intolerance, electrolyte imbalance, essential fatty acid deficiency) ***I.V. lipid emulsion*** • May not be used effectively in severely stressed patients (especially burn patients) • May interfere with immune mechanisms • Given via CV line; irritates peripheral vein in long-term use
Total nutrient admixture	• One day's nutrients are contained in a single, 3-liter bag (also called 3:1 solution) • Combines lipids with other parenteral solution components	• 3 weeks or more • For relatively stable patients because solution components can be adjusted just once daily • For other uses, see TPN (above)	• See TPN (above) • Reduces need to handle bag, cutting risk of contamination • Decreases nursing time and reduces need for infusion sets and electronic devices, lowering hospital costs, increasing patient mobility, and allowing easier adjustment to home care • Precludes use of certain infusion pumps because they can't accurately deliver large volumes of solution; precludes use of standard I.V. tubing filters because a 0.22-micron filter blocks lipid and albumin molecules

Types of parenteral nutrition *(continued)*

TYPE	SOLUTION COMPONENTS/LITER	USES	SPECIAL CONSIDERATIONS
Peripheral parenteral nutrition (PPN)	• Dextrose 5% to 12.5% • Crystalline amino acids 2.75% to 4.25% • Electrolytes, trace elements, and vitamins as ordered • Lipid emulsion 10% or 20% (1 liter dextrose 10% and amino acids 3.5% infused at the same time as 1 liter lipid emulsion = 1,440 nonprotein calories [340 from dextrose and 1,100 from lipid emulsion]) • Heparin or hydrocortisone, as ordered	• 3 weeks or less • Maintains nutritional state in patients who can tolerate relatively high fluid volume, in those who usually resume bowel function and oral feedings after a few days, and in those who are susceptible to infections of the CV catheter	***Basic solution*** • Nutritionally complete for a short time • Cannot be used in nutritionally depleted patients • Can't be used in volume-restricted patients because PPN exceeds CV line volume • Doesn't cause weight gain • Avoids insertion and care of CV line, but requires adequate venous access; site must be changed every 48 hours • Delivers less hypertonic solutions than CV line TPN • May cause phlebitis • Less chance of metabolic complications than with central line TPN ***I.V. lipid emulsion*** • As effective as dextrose for caloric source • Diminishes phlebitis if infused at the same time as basic nutrient solution • Irritates vein in long-term use • Reduces carbon dioxide buildup when pulmonary compromise is present
Protein-sparing therapy	• Crystalline amino acids in same amounts as TPN • Electrolytes, vitamins, and minerals as ordered	• 2 weeks or less • May preserve body protein in a stable patient • Augments oral or tube feedings	• Nutritionally complete • Requires little mixing • May be started or stopped any time during the hospital stay • Other I.V. fluids, medications, and blood by-products may be administered through the same I.V. line • Not as likely to cause phlebitis as PPN • Adds a major expense; has limited benefits

his head turned away from the catheter insertion site. If hospital policy dictates and the patient can tolerate it, place a mask over his nose and mouth. Place a sterile drape over the patient if he's being mechanically ventilated.

● Put on gloves.

● Remove the dressing carefully, pulling the tape gently from the skin *to minimize traumatic injury.* Then inspect the skin for signs of infection and the catheter for leaks or other mechanical problems. Remove your gloves.

● Wash your hands, put on sterile gloves, and clean the catheter insertion site three times with alcohol sponges or cotton-tipped applicators soaked in an organic solvent, such as 70% alcohol. Work in a circular motion, moving from the insertion site outward to the edge of the adhesive border *to avoid introducing contaminants from the unclean area.*

● Working in a circular motion, as before, clean the insertion site and the catheter three times with the povidone-iodine solution.

● Instruct the patient to perform Valsalva's maneuver or to hold his breath on deep inspiration as you change the I.V. tubing. If the patient is being mechanically ventilated, change the I.V. tubing immediately after the machine delivers a breath at peak inspiration. *These measures increase intrathoracic pressure and prevent air embolism.*

● Set the infusion pump at the ordered flow rate and start the infusion.

● Ensure that the junction of the catheter tubing is secure (you may use luer-lock connections), remove the contaminated gloves, and put on a sterile pair.

● Following your hospital's policy, use a sterile cotton-tipped applicator or pad to apply povidone-iodine ointment to the skin at the insertion site and to the hub of the catheter at the catheter-tubing junction, being careful not to loosen the connections.

● Do not remove the povidone-iodine solution from the skin *because its antimicrobial effects are long-lasting and continue after drying.*

● Arrange the sterile dressing pads *to shield the catheter and skin from airborne contaminants.* A precut drain dressing may be used around the catheter.

● Apply adhesive balsam to the skin at the perimeter of the drain dressings.

● Tape the dressing securely to the skin.

● You may use a transparent semipermeable dressing instead of the gauze drain dressings and tape. *These allow visualization of the insertion site.* When using these dressings, do not use povidone-iodine ointment at the insertion site.

● Write the catheter insertion date, the date of the dressing change, and your initials on a strip of tape and apply this to the dressing.

● Loop and tape the administration tubing (but not the filter) over the intact dressing *to prevent tension on the catheter and its inadvertent removal if the tubing is pulled.*

Special considerations

If the patient is sensitive or allergic to iodine, use 70% alcohol as the antimicrobial agent. Scrub for 30 seconds or until the applicator comes away visibly clean.

When using a CV line for TPN, the following are contraindicated: infusion of blood or blood products, bolus injection of drugs, simultaneous administration of I.V. solutions, measurement of CV pressure, aspiration of blood for routine laboratory tests, addition of medication to a TPN solution container, and use of three-way stopcocks.

If the patient develops a fever, discontinue the TPN solution and replace it with dextrose 10% in water, infusing it at the same rate as the TPN solution. Change the I.V. tubing and dressing and notify the doctor, who may order bacterial and fungal cultures of the TPN solution, tubing, and blood. Reduction of fever within 4 to 6 hours after withdrawal implicates the solution or the delivery apparatus. If the fever persists, suspect catheter-related sepsis and again notify the doctor, who may then order blood and urine cultures to help determine the cause of infection. If necessary, the doctor will remove the catheter and order fungal and bacterial cultures. Fever usually subsides within 12 to 24 hours after catheter removal.

Observe the patient for signs of thrombosis or thrombophlebitis, such as erythema and edema at the catheter insertion site; ipsilateral swelling of the arm, neck, or face; pain along the course of the vein; and other systemic manifestations. If such signs occur, notify the doctor immediately; he may remove the catheter and start heparin infusion at a peripheral site.

Be alert for swelling at the catheter insertion site *because it indicates extravasation of the TPN solution, which can cause necrosis.* Check the catheter tubing for leaks from mechanical or chemical disruption.

Watch for signs and symptoms of air embolism: dyspnea, apprehension, chest pain, tachycardia, hypotension, cyanosis, seizures, loss of consciousness, and cardiopulmonary arrest. If you suspect air embolism, position the patient in left Trendelenburg's position *to allow air to pass from the pulmonary artery,* and administer supplemental oxygen. It may take several minutes for the air to dissipate.

Observe for catheter retraction from the vein, which may result from loosening of the sutures at the insertion site. Measure catheter length from the insertion site to the hub during dressing changes for verification.

Complications

Catheter-related sepsis is the most serious complication of TPN. Although uncommon, subclavian or jugular vein thrombosis can result from a malpositioned catheter and can precede septicemia. Air embolism, a potentially fatal complication, can occur during tubing replacement, from inadvertent disconnection of tubing and from undetected hairline cracks in the tubing. Extravasation of TPN solution can cause necrosis, with sequential sloughing of the epidermis and dermis.

Documentation

Record the times of dressing, filter, and solution changes; the condition of the catheter insertion site; your observations on the patient's condition; and any complications and resulting treatments.

Patient monitoring during total parenteral nutrition

Total parenteral nutrition (TPN) requires careful monitoring to assess the patient's response to the nutrient solution and to detect early signs of complications. Because the typical patient is in a protein-wasting state, TPN therapy causes marked changes in fluid and electrolyte status and in glucose, amino acid, mineral, and vitamin levels. If the patient displays an adverse reaction or signs of complications, the TPN regimen can be changed as needed.

Assessment of the patient's nutritional status includes physical examination, anthropometric measurements, biochemical determinations, and tests of cell-mediated immunity. Assessment of the patient's condition to detect complications requires recognition of the signs and symptoms of possible complications, understanding of laboratory test results, and careful record keeping.

Because the TPN solution is high in glucose, the infusion must start slowly to allow the patient's pancreatic beta cells to adapt to it by increasing insulin output. Usually, if the adult patient tolerates the TPN solution the first day, the doctor increases the intake to 1 liter every 12 hours for at least 2 days. Within the first 3 to 5 days of TPN, the typical adult patient can tolerate 3 liters of solution daily without adverse reactions. Lipid emulsions also require monitoring. (See *Precautions for giving lipid emulsions*, page 324.)

Equipment

Test kits for blood and urine glucose and urine ketones ■ stethoscope ■ sphygmomanometer ■ watch with second hand ■ scale ■ input and output chart ■ time tape ■ additional equipment for nutritional assessment, as ordered ■ optional: 10% dextrose in water.

If the patient is receiving cephalosporins, methyldopa, aspirin, or large doses of ascorbic acid, Tes-Tape should be used in place of Clinitest reagent tablets *to avoid false positive results in urine glucose and ketone determinations.*

Preparation of equipment

For preparation of the infusion pump and TPN solution, see appropriate sections of this chapter. Attach a time tape to the TPN container to allow approximate measurement of fluid intake. Make sure each bag or bottle has a label listing the expiration date, glucose concentration, and total volume of solution. (If the bag or bottle is damaged and you don't have an immediate replacement, hang a bag of dextrose 10% in water until the new container is ready.)

Implementation

● Explain the procedure to the patient *to diminish his anxiety and encourage cooperation.* Instruct the patient to inform you if he experiences any unusual sensations during the infusion. Begin the infusion at a slow rate (usually 40 ml/hour), as ordered, *to reduce the risk of hyperglycemia.* Then, as ordered, increase the adult patient's infusion rate (usually in 25 ml/hour increments) *to allow the pancreatic beta cells to increase endogenous insulin production, and to establish carbohydrate and water tolerances.*

● Record vital signs every 4 hours, or more often if necessary, *because increased temperature is one of the earliest signs of catheter-related sepsis.*

● Watch for swelling at the catheter site, *which may indicate extravasation of the TPN solution, possibly leading to tissue necrosis.*

● Check blood or urine for glucose and notify the doctor as appropriate.

● Perform I.V. site care and dressing changes at least three times a week (once a week for transparent semipermeable dressings), or whenever the dressing becomes wet, soiled, or nonocclusive. Use strict aseptic technique.

● Expect to change the tubing and filter every 24 to 48 hours, using strict aseptic technique. Make sure all tubing junctions are secure.

● Maintain flow rates, as prescribed, even if the flow falls behind schedule.

● Record daily fluid intake and output accurately. Specify the volume and type of each fluid, and calculate the daily caloric intake. *This record is a diagnostic tool for prompt, precise replacement of fluid and electrolyte deficits.*

Precautions for giving lipid emulsions

You may administer lipid emulsions as part of a total parenteral nutrition (TPN) solution along with a peripheral parenteral nutrition (PPN) solution, or separately through either a central venous line or a peripheral I.V. line. No matter which of these methods you use, be sure to observe these precautions.

Before the infusion
• Use a particulate filter according to the manufacturer's recommendations (usually a 1.2-micron filter). Standard 0.22-micron filters are insufficient because lipid particles clog the filter and disturb the emulsion.
• Aways check the lipid emulsion for separation or an oily appearance. If either condition exists, the emulsion may have been disturbed and should not be used. Never shake the lipid container excessively or use the emulsion if you see any inconsistency in texture or color.
• Never add anything to the lipid emulsion; doing so could cause instability. Also, protect the emulsion from freezing.

During the infusion
• Monitor the patient's vital signs. The flow rate should not exceed 1 ml/minute for the first 30 minutes.

• Check for signs and symptoms of an adverse reaction. Indications of an immediate adverse reaction, which can occur within 2½ hours, include increased temperature, flushing, sweating, pressure sensations over the eyes, nausea, vomiting, headache, chest and back pain, dyspnea, and cyanosis. Indications of a delayed reaction, which occurs up to 10 days after the infusion, include hepatomegaly, splenomegaly, thrombocytopenia, focal seizures, hyperlipidemia, hepatic damage, jaundice, hemorrhagic diathesis, and gastroduodenal ulcer.

After the infusion
• Be aware of the biochemical and clinical signs and symptoms of essential fatty acid disease that may be associated with impaired wound healing, adverse effects on red blood cells, and ineffective prostaglandin synthesis. Check for dry or scaly skin, thinning hair, liver function abnormalities, and thrombocytopenia.
• Discard any unused emulsion; if contaminated, it can support microbial growth. The Centers for Disease Control guidelines recommend allowing lipid emulsions to hang no longer than 12 hours. Follow the manufacturer's recommendations.

• Physically assess the patient daily. If ordered, measure arm circumference and skinfold thickness over the triceps. Weigh the patient at the same time each morning (after voiding), in similar clothing, and on the same scale. Suspect fluid imbalance if the patient gains more than 1.1 lb (0.5 kg) daily.
• Monitor the results of routine laboratory tests and report abnormal findings to the doctor *to allow appropriate changes in the TPN solution.* Laboratory tests usually include serum electrolytes, blood urea nitrogen, and blood glucose at least three times weekly; and liver function studies, complete blood count and differential, and serum albumin, phosphorus, calcium, magnesium, and creatinine once weekly. Studies ordered less frequently include serum transferrin, prothrombin time, creatinine-height index, nitrogen balance, total lymphocyte count, and skin tests.
• Monitor the patient for signs and symptoms of glucose metabolism disturbance, fluid and electrolyte imbalances, and nutritional aberrations. Remember that some patients may require supplementary insulin for the duration of TPN; the pharmacy usually adds insulin directly to the TPN solution.

• Provide emotional support. Keep in mind that patients often associate eating with positive feelings and become disturbed when eating is prohibited.
• Provide frequent mouth care.
• Keep the patient active *to enable him to utilize nutrients more fully.*
• When discontinuing TPN, decrease the infusion rate slowly, depending on the patient's current glucose intake, *to minimize the risk of hyperinsulinemia and resulting hypoglycemia.* Weaning usually takes place over 24 to 48 hours but can be completed in 4 to 6 hours if the patient receives sufficient oral or I.V. carbohydrates. You may use a cyclic administration schedule, as ordered, to wean the patient from TPN to enteral feedings.

Special considerations
Always maintain strict aseptic technique when handling the equipment used to administer therapy. *Because the TPN solution serves as a medium for bacterial growth and the central venous (CV) line provides systemic access, the patient risks infection and sepsis.*

When using a filter, position it as close to the access site as possible. Check the filter's porosity and psi capacity to make sure it exceeds the psi exerted by the infusion pump.

Don't allow TPN solutions to hang for more than 24 hours.

Be careful when using the TPN line for other functions. If using a single-lumen CV catheter, do not use the line to infuse blood or blood products, to give a bolus injection, to administer simultaneous I.V. solutions, to measure CV pressure, or to draw blood for laboratory tests. Never add medication to a TPN solution container. Also, do not use a three-way stopcock, if possible, *because add-on devices increase the risk of infection.*

Complications

Catheter-related, metabolic, and mechanical complications can occur during TPN administration. (See *Dealing with TPN hazards*, pages 326 and 327.)

Documentation

Record serial monitoring indices on the appropriate flow-chart to determine the patient's progress and response. Note any abnormal, adverse, or altered responses.

Peripheral parenteral nutrition

Using a solution that combines amino acids, dextrose (5% to 12.5%) in water, and a lipid emulsion, peripheral parenteral nutrition (PPN) can supply full caloric needs without the risks associated with a central venous (CV) line. Because this combined solution has a lower tonicity than a total parenteral nutrition solution, the success of PPN depends on the patient's tolerance for the large volumes of fluid necessary to supply full nutritional needs. PPN that includes a lipid emulsion is associated with a lower incidence of phlebitis than a solution that contains only amino acids and dextrose.

Patients who don't need to gain weight yet need nutritional support may receive PPN for as long as 2 to 3 weeks. It's used to maintain or restore fluid and electrolyte balance, to maintain homeostasis before and after surgery, and to help a patient meet minimum calorie and protein requirements.

This therapy may also be used as an adjunct to oral or enteral feedings for a patient who needs to supplement his low-calorie intake. Or PPN may be given to a patient who's unable to absorb enteral therapy.

PPN should be used cautiously in patients with severe hepatic damage, coagulation disorders, anemia, and pulmonary disease, and in those at increased risk for fat embolism. It should not be used for patients with mal-nutrition or metabolic disorders, such as pathologic hyperlipidemia, lipid nephrosis, and acute pancreatitis accompanied by hyperlipidemia.

Equipment

Amino acid-dextrose solution at room temperature (dextrose should not exceed 12.5%) ▪ lipid emulsion ▪ two controllers or pumps ▪ Y-type nonphthalate administration set ▪ alcohol sponges ▪ adhesive tape ▪ I.V. pole and venipuncture equipment, if necessary ▪ sterile gloves.

The only additive allowed to the lipid emulsion is sodium heparin (in a small dose), which activates lipase, the enzyme needed to oxidize fatty acids and enhance clearance of fat from the blood. An excessive amount of sodium heparin can deplete the body's stores of lipase.

A nonphthalate administration set, designed especially for simultaneous infusion of lipid emulsion and amino acid-dextrose solution, consists of two lines in a Y configuration. (See *Giving lipids and amino acids together*, page 328.) The vented line is used for the lipid emulsion; the nonvented line, containing a filter, for the amino acid-dextrose solution. This special nonphthalate tubing is necessary because lipids can extract small amounts of phthalates from phthalate-plasticized poly-vinylchloride tubing.

Controllers that can accommodate the special tubing are needed to ensure the correct infusion rate *because the risk of phlebitis is smaller when two components are administered at approximately the same rate.*

Preparation of equipment

Inspect the lipid emulsion for opacity and consistency of color and texture. If the emulsion looks frothy, oily, or contains particles, or if its stability or sterility is questionable, return the bottle to the pharmacy. Avoid shaking the bottle excessively *to prevent aggregation of fat globules.*

Similarly, inspect the amino acid-dextrose solution for cloudiness, turbidity, and particles and the bottle for cracks; if any of these are present, return the bottle to the pharmacy.

Wash your hands and, using aseptic technique, take the nonphthalate tubing from its package. Close the flow clamp *to equalize pressure in the tubing.* Remove the protective cap from the lipid emulsion bottle, and wipe the rubber stopper with an alcohol sponge. Hold the bottle upright, and insert the vented spike through the inner circle of the rubber stopper. Invert the bottle, and squeeze the drip chamber until it fills to the level indicated in the tubing package instructions. Open the flow clamp, allow fat emulsion to flow through to the Y connector, and then close the clamp.

Dealing with TPN hazards

COMPLICATIONS	SIGNS AND SYMPTOMS	INTERVENTIONS
Metabolic hazards		
Hyperglycemia	Fatigue, restlessness, confusion, anxiety, weakness, and (in severe cases) delirium or coma; polyuria; dehydration; elevated glucose levels	• Start insulin therapy or adjust total parenteral nutrition (TPN) flow rate.
Hypoglycemia	Sweating, shaking, irritability when infusion is stopped	• Infuse dextrose 10% in water.
Hyperosmolar nonketotic syndrome	Confusion, lethargy, seizures, coma, hyperglycemia, dehydration, glycosuria	• Stop the dextrose infusion. • Give insulin and 0.45% sodium chloride to rehydrate.
Hypokalemia	Muscle weakness, paralysis, paresthesia, arrhythmias	• Increase potassium supplementation.
Hypomagnesemia	Tingling around mouth, paresthesia in fingers, mental changes, hyperreflexia	• Increase magnesium supplementation.
Hypophosphatemia	Irritability, weakness, paresthesia, coma, respiratory arrest	• Increase phosphate supplementation.
Hypocalcemia	Polyuria, dehydration, elevated blood and urine glucose levels	• Increase calcium supplementation.
Metabolic acidosis	Increased serum chloride level, decreased serum bicarbonate level	• Use acetate or lactate salts of sodium or hydrogen.
Hepatic dysfunction	Increased serum transaminase, lactate dehydrogenase, and bilirubin levels	• Use special hepatic formulations. • Decrease carbohydrates and add I.V. lipids.
Mechanical hazards		
Clotted catheter	Interrupted flow rate, hypoglycemia	• Reposition the catheter. Attempt to aspirate clot. • If unsuccessful, instill urokinase to clear catheter lumen, as ordered.
Dislodged catheter	Catheter out of the vein	• Place a sterile gauze pad on the site and apply pressure.
Air embolism	Apprehension, chest pain, tachycardia, hypotension, cyanosis, seizures, loss of consciousness, cardiac arrest	• Clamp the catheter. • Place patient in Trendelenburg's position on left side. Give oxygen as ordered. • If cardiac arrest occurs, begin cardiopulmonary resuscitation.

Dealing with TPN hazards *(continued)*

COMPLICATIONS	SIGNS AND SYMPTOMS	INTERVENTIONS
Mechanical hazards *(continued)*		
Thrombosis	Erythema and edema at insertion site; ipsilateral swelling of arm, neck, and face; pain at the insertion site and along vein; malaise; fever; tachycardia	• Remove the catheter promptly. • Administer heparin if ordered. • Venous flow studies may be done.
Too-rapid infusion	Nausea, headache, lethargy	• Check the infusion rate. • Check the infusion pump if you're using one.
Extravasation	Swelling of tissue around the insertion site; pain	• Stop the I.V. infusion. • Assess the patient for cardiopulmonary abnormalities. • Chest X-ray may be performed.
Phlebitis	Pain, tenderness, redness, and warmth	• Apply gentle heat to the insertion site. • Elevate the insertion site if possible.
Cracked or broken tubing	Fluid leaking from the tubing	• Apply a padded hemostat above the break to prevent air from entering the line.
Pneumothorax and hydrothorax	Dyspnea, chest pain, cyanosis, decreased breath sounds	• Apply suction. • Chest tube will be inserted.
Sepsis	Fever, chills, leukocytosis, erythema or pus at the insertion site	• Remove the catheter and culture the tip. • Give appropriate antibiotics.

Remove the protective cap from the container of amino acid-dextrose solution, and wipe the rubber stopper with an alcohol sponge. Hold the bottle upright and insert the nonvented spike. Squeeze the drip chamber to eliminate dripping of solution, invert the bottle, and squeeze the drip chamber until the fluid reaches the desired level. Hold the filter with the Y connector facing upward and the air vent downward, and open the clamp. Start the solution flow *to remove air from the filter and line.* Then close the clamp.

If your administration set contains a second Y injection site, insert it and tap gently *to remove all air from the tubing* before closing the clamp.

If you're initiating the infusion, hang the containers on the I.V. pole after inserting the spikes. Always hang the lipid emulsion container higher than the amino acid-dextrose container *so that the lipid emulsion doesn't backflow into the amino acid set.* Then attach the controllers to the I.V. pole, and prepare them according to manufacturer's instructions.

Implementation
• Explain the procedure to the patient *to ease his anxiety and promote his cooperation.*
• Obtain baseline vital signs, as ordered. If necessary, perform a venipuncture. Select the patient's largest available vein as the insertion site *to ensure hemodilution of the irritating PPN solution.* When using a short-term catheter that requires 48- to 72-hour site rotation, try applying heat to the site to facilitate insertion.

To start the infusion
• Connect the administration set to the I.V. needle or catheter hub. Then turn on the controllers and set them to the desired flow rate (start the infusion slowly and increase gradually to ensure tolerance to the hypertonic

Giving lipids and amino acids together

The illustration below shows the setup you'll use to administer lipid emulsions with amino acids. Note that the lipid emulsion container is higher than the amino acid container.

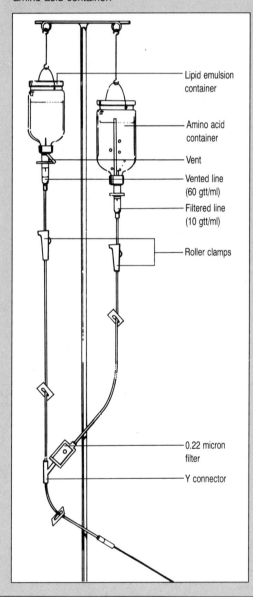

Lipid emulsion container

Amino acid container

Vent

Vented line (60 gtt/ml)

Filtered line (10 gtt/ml)

Roller clamps

0.22 micron filter

Y connector

solution). Next, completely open the flow clamps *to allow the controllers to regulate the flow rate.*
• Monitor vital signs every 10 minutes for the first 30 minutes and every hour thereafter.

To change the solutions
• Remove the protective caps, and wipe the stoppers of the solution containers with alcohol sponges.
• Turn off the controllers, and close the flow clamps. Using strict aseptic technique, remove each spike and insert it in the new container.
• Hang the containers, turn on the controllers, and set the flow rate. Open the flow clamps completely.

To change the solutions and tubing
• Hang the new solution container and tubing alongside the old ones.
• Put on sterile gloves. Examine the skin above the insertion site for signs of phlebitis, such as redness, warmth, and pain. If such signs are present, remove the existing I.V. line and start a line in a different vein, using venipuncture equipment.
• Turn off the controllers, and close the flow clamps on the old tubing. Disconnect the tubing from the needle or catheter hub, and connect the new tubing.
• Open the flow clamps on the new containers to equal, slow flow rates *to prevent clot formation in the needle or catheter while you're inserting the tubing into the controllers.*
• Remove the old tubing from the controllers, and insert the new tubing according to the manufacturer's instructions.
• Turn on the controllers, set them to the desired flow rate, and open the flow clamps completely.
• Remove the old equipment and dispose of it properly.

To change a dressing and needle or catheter
• Change the dressing at intervals specified by hospital policy (usually every 24 to 48 hours), and inspect the insertion site for signs of phlebitis.
• Change the needle or catheter according to hospital policy or at the onset of signs of phlebitis.
• Loop and tape the tubing *to prevent its dislodging from the needle or catheter hub.*

Special considerations
Always use strict aseptic technique when handling equipment, and never reuse a partially empty bottle of lipid emulsion *because it is an excellent medium for bacterial growth.* All bottles, bags, tubing, and filters should be changed every 24 hours. Be alert for signs of sepsis,

such as elevated temperature, chills, malaise, leukocytosis, and altered level of consciousness.

Observe the patient's reaction to the lipid emulsion; usually, the patient experiences a feeling of satiety but occasionally reports an unpleasant metallic taste in his mouth. Monitor the patient's lipid tolerance rate closely. Cloudy plasma in a centrifuged sample of citrated blood indicates that the fat hasn't been cleared from the bloodstream. Lipid emulsion may clear from the blood at an accelerated rate in a patient with full-thickness burns, multiple traumatic injuries, and metabolic imbalance *because catecholamines, adrenocortical hormones, thyroxine, and growth hormone enhance lipolysis and mobilization of fatty acids.*

Check serum triglyceride levels; these should return to normal within 18 hours after infusion of a bottle of lipid emulsion. As ordered, obtain blood samples for laboratory analysis; typically, aspartate aminotransferase (formerly SGOT), alanine aminotransferase (formerly SGPT), alkaline phosphatase, cholesterol, triglyceride, plasma free fatty acid, and coagulation tests are performed weekly *to monitor the patient's response.*

Because lipase synthesis increases insulin requirements, increase the insulin dosage of the patient with diabetes, as ordered. For the patient with hypothyroidism, administer thyroid-stimulating hormone — which affects lipase activity — as ordered, *to prevent intravascular accumulations of triglycerides.*

Monitor for signs and symptoms of adverse reactions to lipid emulsion therapy.

Complications
Immediate or early adverse reactions to lipid emulsion therapy, which reportedly occur in fewer than 1% of patients, include fever, dyspnea, cyanosis, nausea, vomiting, headache, flushing, diaphoresis, lethargy, syncope, chest and back pain, slight pressure over the eyes, irritation at the infusion site, hyperlipemia, hypercoagulability, and thrombocytopenia. Thrombocytopenia has been reported in infants receiving 20% I.V. lipid emulsion.

Delayed but uncommon complications associated with prolonged administration of lipid emulsion include hepatomegaly, splenomegaly, jaundice secondary to central lobular cholestasis, and blood dyscrasias (thrombocytopenia, leukopenia, and transient increases in liver function studies). For unknown reasons, a few patients receiving 20% I.V. lipid emulsion have developed brown pigmentation (I.V. fat pigment) in the reticuloendothelial system.

In a premature or low-birth-weight infant, PPN with lipid emulsion may cause lipid accumulation in the lungs.

Documentation
Record the dates and times of all dressing and cannula changes, the duration and amount of each infusion, and the patient's condition and response to therapy.

Preparation for home parenteral nutrition

Home parenteral nutrition (HPN) makes possible prolonged or indefinite I.V. total parenteral nutrition (TPN). This technique has dramatically improved the health of patients with such chronic conditions as Crohn's disease and malabsorption syndrome, and with such acute conditions as incomplete bowel obstruction and antineoplastic therapy. It has also decreased the duration of hospitalization. Although peripheral parenteral nutrition may be administered at home, long-term TPN is the primary home care therapy.

To prepare for HPN, a barium-impregnated silicone rubber catheter with a Dacron cuff is implanted, usually in the superior vena cava. Its entrance site is on the anterior abdomen to allow the patient to care for the catheter. About 2 to 3 weeks after implantation, firm tissue covers the catheter cuff to provide a physical barrier to microbial contamination.

Preparation for HPN usually necessitates extensive patient teaching and, when possible, instructions for the patient's family.

Typically, patients receiving HPN can ingest part of their caloric requirements during the day and require about 10 to 14 hours of infusion nightly to supply the remaining nutrients. If all the patient's nutrition must be received I.V., a continuous infusion may be necessary. For intermittent and continuous infusion, patient teaching must include techniques for proper care. (See *Teaching topics for home parenteral nutrition,* page 330.)

Equipment
Teaching aids (including audiovisual teaching aids and mannequins) as available ■ I.V. infusion apparatus ■ dressings ■ TPN solution ■ volumetric infusion pump ■ portable I.V. pole or ambulatory TPN vest ■ HPN supplies (including tubing, dressings, TPN solution).

Implementation
• Assess the patient's ability to perform the care routines necessary for HPN, and determine if family members or friends can assist with or perform them. Consider the patient's motivation, mental aptitude, job or other daily

Teaching topics for home parenteral nutrition

Techniques
- ☐ Catheter heparinization
- ☐ How to destroy contaminated needles and syringes
- ☐ Dressing changes
- ☐ Drug administration
- ☐ Hand washing
- ☐ Lipid emulsion administration
- ☐ Tubing changes
- ☐ Pump operation
- ☐ Self-monitoring of intake and output, weight, temperature, diet
- ☐ Solution preparation
- ☐ Use of sterile equipment

Related topics
- ☐ How to detect complications, such as air embolism, thrombosis, clotted or fractured catheter, pump malfunction, metabolic disturbance, solution contamination
- ☐ Financial support, home referral, medical alert, and networking services
- ☐ Follow-up appointments
- ☐ How to maintain procedures when traveling
- ☐ How to find, buy, and store supplies
- ☐ How to schedule infusions
- ☐ Weaning

activities, home environment, and the accessibility of hospitals, home nursing services, and other health care support systems.

• Formulate a teaching plan based on this assessment and on the patient's expectations. Be sure the plan incorporates goals, specifies criteria for meeting them, and proceeds from simple to complex tasks *to allow the patient to develop confidence.* Avoid placing time limits on goals *because learning ability and mastery of tasks requiring manual dexterity vary from patient to patient.*

• If desired, develop a written contract between you and the patient that specifies the goals of HPN and the means to achieve them. Revise the contract as necessary *to reflect changes in the patient's needs and performance. Use of the contractual relationship enhances the patient's independence, minimizes conflict and frustration between patient and nurse, encourages open communication, and promotes a cooperative patient-nurse relationship.*

• Conduct teaching sessions in a quiet area and, if possible, arrange to have a family member present. *When the family member understands the patient's pathophysiology, medical management, and progress, he tends to be less anxious, more satisfied with the quality of health care, and more able to acknowledge the limitations and constraints of HPN.*

• Use a variety of teaching aids *to accommodate differences in the patient's ability.* When teaching the mature patient, use an extensively illustrated manual (if available) that includes goals, equipment, procedures with rationales, suggested learning activities, and evaluations of HPN equipment. Give demonstrations with mannequins (if available) and real equipment *to involve the patient actively and reduce anxiety about performing the HPN tasks.* Stimulate the patient's interest with audiovisual teaching aids.

• Offer positive feedback during all teaching phases.

• Before discharge, critically evaluate the patient's ability to perform HPN tasks and ensure that all essential learning goals have been met.

• Remind the patient to change the catheter site dressing as ordered (usually every 2 to 3 days) or whenever it becomes soiled or nonocclusive and to change administration tubing as scheduled. Tell the patient to wash gently around the site and to take only sponge baths. Tell him he may be allowed to remove his dressing and bathe or shower after the implanted catheter has been in place for 1 month or longer.

• Also remind the patient to prevent contact between the catheter and granular or lint-producing surfaces *to avoid local tissue reaction from airborne particles and surface contaminants.*

• Discuss a suitable TPN schedule with the patient, considering his nutritional needs as well as his life-style. Emphasize his adherence to the prescribed schedule and volume *to prevent glucose imbalance.*

• Arrange for a home care agency to help the patient adjust to HPN and resolve any difficulties (including how to obtain supplies), or notify the hospital's discharge planner *so the appropriate referrals can be made.*

Special considerations
Suggest that the patient wear a medical identification bracelet or subscribe to a medical alert service. Tell the patient that a nurse from the home health care team will always be available in case of emergency.

To preserve as much patient mobility as possible, equipment such as the ambulatory TPN vest is available. This vest is made from lightweight materials and is adjustable to individual specifications. Breast pockets accommodate bags of nutrient solution, which are attached to the front of each shoulder. The pockets vary with the size of the nutrient bags. Y tubing connects these bags to a portable volumetric pump, located in a zippered pocket. To provide balance and enhance patient comfort, the pump empties both bags at the same rate. When the patient is wearing the vest, the administration tubing is coiled in one of the pockets. When the patient is not wearing the vest, the nutrient bags can hang from a clothes hanger.

Because the financial burden of long-term or permanent HPN can be devastating — even for the patient with health insurance — make a social service referral. Inform the elderly patient that Medicare may assume the cost of supplies and pharmaceuticals if he meets eligibility requirements.

Documentation
Record your patient teaching measures and the patient's learning progress in your notes.

BLOOD AND BLOOD COMPONENTS

Transfusion of whole blood and packed cells

Whole-blood transfusion replenishes both the volume and the oxygen-carrying capacity of the circulatory system. Transfusion of packed red blood cells (RBCs), from which 80% of the plasma has been removed, restores only the oxygen-carrying capacity. Both types of transfusion treat decreased hemoglobin and hematocrit levels. Whole blood is usually transfused only when decreased levels result from hemorrhage; packed RBCs are transfused when such depressed levels accompany normal blood volume, avoiding possible fluid and circulatory overload. Both whole blood and packed RBCs contain cellular debris, necessitating in-line filtration during administration. (Washed packed RBCs — commonly used for patients previously sensitized by transfusions — are rinsed with a special solution that removes white blood cells and platelets, thus decreasing the chance of transfusion reaction.)

Depending on hospital policy, two nurses may have to identify the patient and blood product before administering a transfusion to prevent errors and a potentially fatal reaction. The procedure also usually requires a signed patient consent form. If the patient is a Jehovah's Witness, transfusion requires special written permission.

Equipment
Blood recipient set (filter and tubing with drip chamber for blood, or combined set) ■ I.V. pole ■ gloves ■ multiple-lead tubing ■ whole blood or packed RBCs ■ 250 ml of normal saline solution ■ venipuncture equipment, if necessary (should include 18G catheter or 19G needle) ■ optional: ice bag, warm compresses.

Straight-line and Y-type blood administration sets are commonly used. Although filters come in mesh and microaggregate types, the latter type is preferred, especially when transfusing multiple units of blood. New, highly effective leukocyte removal filters are available for use when transfusing blood and packed RBCs. Use of these filters delays a patient from becoming sensitive to transfusion therapy.

For some patients, you may need to use a blood warmer. (See *Using a dry-heat blood warmer*, page 332.)

Administer packed RBCs with a Y-type set. Using a straight-line set forces you to piggyback the tubing *so you can stop the transfusion if necessary but still keep the vein open.* Piggybacking increases the chance of harmful microorganisms entering the tubing as you're connecting the blood line to the established line.

Multiple-lead tubing minimizes the risk of contamination, especially when transfusing multiple units of blood (a straight-line set would require multiple piggybacking). A Y-type set gives you the option of adding normal saline solution to packed cells — decreasing their viscosity — if the patient can tolerate the added fluid volume.

Preparation of equipment
Avoid obtaining either whole blood or packed RBCs until you're ready to begin the transfusion *because RBCs deteriorate after 2 hours when stored at room temperature.* Prepare equipment when you're ready to start the infusion.

Implementation
• Explain the procedure to the patient. Ascertain that he has signed an informed consent form before transfusion therapy.
• Record the patient's vital signs *to serve as baseline values.*
• Obtain whole blood or packed RBCs from the blood bank within 30 minutes of the transfusion start time. Check the expiration date on the blood bag, and observe for abnormal color, RBC clumping, gas bubbles, and extraneous material. Return outdated or abnormal blood to the blood bank.
• Compare the name and number on the patient's wristband with those on the blood bag label. Check the blood bag identification number and ABO blood group and Rh compatibility. Also, compare the patient's blood bank

Using a dry-heat blood warmer

Rapid transfusion of cold blood can lead to hypothermia and may cause arrhythmias. Depending on hospital policy, you may use a dry-heat blood warmer for massive, rapid transfusions and for exchange transfusions in neonates. You can also use this device for transfusions in patients with increased cold agglutinin titers. The warmer maintains a constant temperature of 98.6° F (37° C). To use the blood warmer, follow these steps:

• Attach the blood warmer to an I.V. pole at mattress height. Plug in the device. Prepare and hang a Y-set with a blood bag and normal saline solution.

• Insert the warming bag into the blood warmer. The lead at the bottom of the warming bag is attached to the Y-set. The lead at the top of the warming bag is connected to the patient. Match these leads to the corresponding openings and mount the warming bag on the support pins, keeping the bag flat against the back panel. Then secure the pins.

• Close the blood warmer door and secure the latch. Turn the machine on, and allow it to operate for at least 2 minutes to warm up. (Avoid opening the door at any time during the transfusion. Otherwise, you'll break the vacuum and will have to replace the warming bag.)

• While the blood warmer is heating up, connect the blood-line adapter to the female adapter on the bottom lead. When the desired temperature is indicated on the machine, open the saline line to fill the bag with normal saline solution. Squeeze the outlet chamber until it's flat; continue to hold the chamber. When saline solution appears in the chamber, close the main flow clamp and release the chamber. The chamber then automatically fills halfway with saline solution.

• Remove the adapter cover on the top lead and open the clamp. Expel residual air from the line. Proceed as you would when administering blood with a Y-type set.

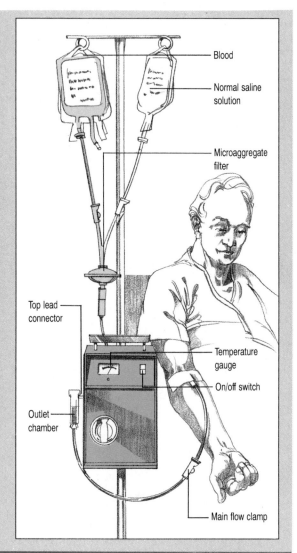

identification number, if present, with the number on the blood bag. Identification of blood and blood products is performed at the patient's bedside by two licensed professionals according to hospital policy.

• Put on gloves. Using a Y-type set, close all the clamps on the set. Then insert the spike of the line you're using for the normal saline solution into the bag of saline so-

lution. Next, open the port on the blood bag and insert the spike of the line you're using to administer the blood or cellular component into the port. Hang the normal saline solution and blood or cellular component on the I.V. pole, open the clamp on the line of saline solution, and squeeze the drip chamber until it's half full of saline solution. Then remove the adapter cover at the tip of the blood administration set, open the main flow clamp, and prime the tubing with saline solution.

• If you're administering packed RBCs with a Y-type set, you can add saline solution to the bag *to dilute the cells* by closing the clamp between the patient and the drip chamber and opening the clamp from the blood. Then lower the blood bag below the saline container and let 30 to 50 ml of saline flow into the packed cells. Finally, close the clamp to the blood bag, rehang the bag, rotate it gently *to mix the cells and saline solution,* and close the clamp to the saline container.

• If the patient doesn't have an I.V. line in place, perform venipuncture, preferably using an 18G catheter or 19G needle. Avoid using an existing line if the needle or catheter lumen is smaller than 20G. Central venous access devices also may be used for transfusion therapy.

• If you're administering whole blood, gently invert the bag several times *to mix the cells.*

• Attach the prepared blood administration set to the venipuncture device and flush it with normal saline solution.

• Then close the clamp to the saline solution and open the clamp between the blood bag and the patient. Adjust the flow clamp closest to the patient to deliver 25 to 30 drops/minute; the patient then receives about 50 ml of blood over 30 minutes *to minimize any transfusion reaction, which usually occurs within this period.*

• Remain with the patient, and watch for signs of transfusion reaction. If such signs develop, record vital signs, stop the transfusion, infuse the saline solution at a keep-vein-open rate, and notify the doctor immediately. If no signs of a reaction appear within 15 minutes, adjust the flow clamp to the ordered infusion rate. Raising and lowering the blood bag *to adjust the rate reduces the risk of hemolysis from pressure on the tubing.* A unit of RBCs may be given over a period of 1 to 4 hours, as ordered.

• After completing the transfusion, put on gloves and flush the filter and tubing with normal saline solution, if recommended by the manufacturer. Then reconnect the original I.V. fluid or discontinue the I.V.

• Return the empty blood bag to the blood bank, and discard the tubing and filter.

• Record the patient's vital signs.

Special considerations

Although some microaggregate filters can be used for up to 10 units of blood, always replace the filter and tubing if more than 1 hour elapses between transfusions. When administering multiple units of blood under pressure, use a blood warmer *to avoid hypothermia.*

For rapid blood replacement, you may need to use a pressure bag. Be aware, however, that excessive pressure may develop, leading to broken blood vessels and ex-travasation, with hematoma and hemolysis of the infusing RBCs. (See *Transfusing blood under pressure,* page 334.)

If the transfusion stops, take the following steps as needed:

• Check that the I.V. container is at least 3' (1 m) above the level of the I.V. site.

• Make sure that the flow clamp is open and that the blood completely covers the filter. If it doesn't, squeeze the drip chamber until it does.

• Gently rock the bag back and forth, agitating any blood cells that may have settled on the bottom.

• Untape the dressing over the I.V. site to check needle placement. Reposition the needle if necessary.

• Flush the line with saline solution and restart the transfusion. Using a Y-type set, close the flow clamp to the patient and lower the blood bag. Next, open the saline clamp and allow some saline solution to flow into the blood bag. Rehang the blood bag, open the flow clamp to the patient, and reset the flow rate.

If a hematoma develops at the I.V. site, immediately stop the infusion. Remove the needle or catheter. Notify the doctor and expect to place ice intermittently on the site for 8 hours; then apply warm compresses. Promote reabsorption of the hematoma by having the patient gently exercise the affected limb. Document your observations and actions.

If the blood bag empties before the next one arrives, administer normal saline solution slowly. If you're using a Y-type set, close the blood-line clamp, open the saline-line clamp, and let the saline solution run slowly until the new blood arrives. Decrease the flow rate or clamp the line before attaching the new unit of blood.

Home care

Standards established by the American Association of Blood Banks, in accordance with federal, state, and local regulations, allow a doctor to order transfusions of blood products (not whole blood) for home care patients. To qualify, a patient must be unable to leave his home without assistance and must have received previous transfusions without difficulties. (See *Administering transfusions in the home,* page 335.)

Complications

Despite increasingly accurate crossmatching precautions, transfusion reactions can occur. (See *Understanding autotransfusion,* page 336.)

Unlike a transfusion reaction, an infectious disease transmitted during a transfusion may go undetected until days, weeks, or even months later, when it produces signs and symptoms. Measures to prevent disease transmission include laboratory testing of blood products and careful

Transfusing blood under pressure

Transfuse blood under pressure only when rapid replacement is necessary. Begin this procedure by selecting the proper equipment—a pressure cuff or a positive-pressure set. The *pressure cuff*, which resembles a sleeve, is placed over the blood bag and inflated; a pressure gauge, attached to the cuff, is calibrated in millimeters of mercury (mm Hg). The *positive-pressure set* is a gravity administration set containing a built-in pressure chamber that increases the flow rate when manual pressure is applied externally to the chamber.

Prepare the patient and set up the equipment just as you would a standard administration set. Connect the tubing to the needle or catheter hub. Throughout the transfusion, watch the patient closely for complications, such as infiltration or extravasation, which can occur quite rapidly.

To use a pressure cuff
• Insert your hand into the pressure-cuff sleeve and pull the blood bag upward through the center opening. Then grasp one loop of the sleeve, slip it through the blood bag loop, and pull the other sleeve loop through it.
• Hang the blood bag on the I.V. pole. Open the flow clamp on the tubing.
• To set the flow rate, turn the screw clamp on the pressure cuff counterclockwise, as shown at upper right.
• Compress the pressure bulb of the cuff to inflate the bag until you achieve the desired flow rate. Then turn the screw clamp clockwise *to maintain this constant flow rate. Note:* As the blood bag empties, the pressure decreases, so check the flow rate regularly and adjust the pressure in the pressure cuff as necessary *to maintain a constant flow rate.* Don't allow the cuff needle to exceed 300 mm Hg *because excessively high pressure may cause hemolysis of red blood cells or even rupture the blood bag.*

To use a positive-pressure set
• Open the upper and lower flow clamps on the administration set. Manually compress and release the pump chamber *to force the blood down the tubing and into the patient,* as shown at right. Allow the pump chamber to refill completely before compressing it again.
• Continue to compress and release the chamber until the blood bag empties or until rapid administration is no longer necessary. *To discontinue transfusion under pressure,* stop compressing the chamber and adjust the flow rate as for standard administration.

Pressure cuff

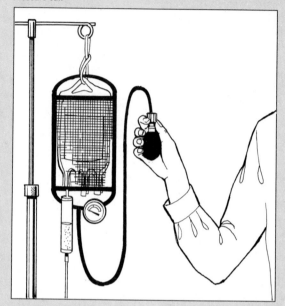

Positive-pressure set

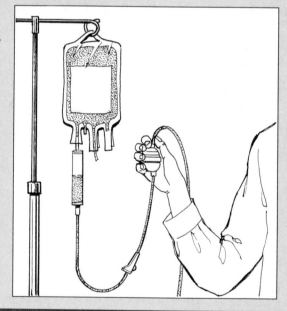

screening of potential donors, neither of which is guaranteed.

Hepatitis C (non-A, non-B) accounts for the majority of posttransfusion hepatitis cases. The tests that detect hepatitis B and hepatitis C can produce false-negative results and may allow some hepatitis cases to go undetected.

When testing for antibodies to human immunodeficiency virus (HIV), keep in mind that antibodies do not appear until about 6 to 12 weeks after exposure. Consequently, blood from a donor exposed to HIV but who has not yet developed antibodies could infect the recipient. The estimated risk of acquiring HIV from blood products varies from 1 in 40,000 to 1 in 153,000, depending on the source.

Many blood banks screen blood for cytomegalovirus (CMV). Blood with CMV is especially dangerous for an immunosuppressed, seronegative patient. Blood banks also test blood for syphilis, although the routine practice of refrigerating blood kills the syphilis organism and virtually eliminates the risk of transfusion-related syphilis.

Circulatory overload and hemolytic, allergic, febrile, and pyogenic reactions can result from any transfusion. Coagulation disturbances, citrate intoxication, hyperkalemia, acid-base imbalance, loss of 2,3-diphosphoglycerate, ammonia intoxication, and hypothermia can result from massive transfusion.

Documentation
Record the date and time of transfusion, the type and amount of transfusion product, the patient's vital signs, and your check of all identification data, and the patient's response. (See *Reviewing transfusion products,* pages 337 and 338.) Document any transfusion reaction and treatment.

Management of transfusion reactions

A transfusion reaction typically stems from a major antigen-antibody reaction and can result from a single or massive transfusion of blood or blood products. Although many reactions occur during transfusion or within 96 hours afterward, infectious diseases transmitted during a transfusion may go undetected until days, weeks, or months later, when signs and symptoms appear.

Transfusion reaction requires immediate recognition and prompt nursing action to prevent further complica-

HOME CARE

Administering transfusions in the home

To administer transfusions to patients at home, follow this procedure:
• Transport blood products in a container with the appropriate coolant for the product. The proper temperature for transporting blood is between 33.8° and 50° F (1° and 10° C); for platelets, between 68° and 75° F (20° and 24° C).
• Encourage the patient to void before beginning the procedure *because the transfusion may take up to 2 hours.*
• Set up and transfuse the product according to your agency's or institution's policy.
• After stopping the infusion, keep the I.V. line open and remain with the patient for at least 30 minutes *to watch for delayed reaction to the procedure.* Take a final set of vital signs, and complete all charting.
• If no reactions occur after 30 minutes, remove the I.V. and give the patient or a caretaker posttransfusion instructions. Place all equipment, including the containers and infusion devices, in a biohazard bag and then into the transport container. Return the container to the blood bank for proper disposal.
• If a transfusion reaction occurs, notify the transfusion service and the patient's doctor immediately.

tions and possible death — particularly if the patient is unconscious or so heavily sedated that he can't report the common symptoms.

Equipment
Normal saline solution ■ I.V. administration set ■ sterile urine specimen container ■ needle, syringe, and tubes for blood samples ■ transfusion reaction report form ■ optional: oxygen, epinephrine, hypothermia blanket, leukocyte removal filter.

Implementation
• As soon as you suspect an adverse reaction, stop the transfusion and start the saline infusion at a keep-vein-open rate *to maintain venous access.* Don't discard the blood bag or administration set.
• Notify the doctor.
• Monitor vital signs every 15 minutes or as indicated by the severity and type of reaction.

Understanding autotransfusion

Autotransfusion is the collection, filtration, and reinfusion of the patient's own blood. The procedure has several advantages over transfusion of bank blood. Autotransfusion uses blood that is warm, safe, and readily available. Most important, because autotransfused blood is autologous, it eliminates disease transmission, transfusion reactions, isoimmunization and, postoperatively, the addition of anticoagulants. Autotransfusion can overcome the objections of certain religious groups who oppose transfusions of donor blood. Unlike bank blood, autologous blood contains normal levels of 2,3-diphosphoglycerate advantageous for tissue oxygenation, potassium, ammonia, and clotting factors (except for fibrinogen); has a normal pH; and appears to have viable platelets. Occasionally, autologous blood causes transient hemoglobinuria because of traumatic injury to red blood cells (RBCs) during collection.

Indications and use
Autotransfusion techniques are used after traumatic injury and before, during, and after surgery. The trauma technique, most commonly used for hemothorax, can also be used in primary injuries of the lungs, liver, chest wall, heart, pulmonary vessels, spleen, kidneys, inferior vena cava, and iliac, portal, and subclavian veins. In this technique, the collection system uses citrated phosphate dextrose to prevent clotting of the collected blood.

The preoperative technique, also called autologous blood donation, is performed primarily for the patient with a rare blood type before major surgery or the patient for whom isoimmunization may complicate future transfusion needs. This technique follows standard blood-bank donation and transfusion procedures.

The intraoperative technique, used most often for thoracic and cardiovascular surgery, can also be used in hip and knee resection, spinal fusion, liver resection, and ruptured ectopic pregnancy. In this technique, a commercial cell washer-processor reduces anticoagulated collected whole blood to washed, packed RBCs for later reinfusion. The postoperative technique is used solely to collect shed mediastinal blood after cardiac surgery.

Autotransfusion is contraindicated in patients with malignant neoplasms, intrathoracic or systemic infections and infestations, coagulopathies, enteric contamination, excessive hemolysis, and when using an antibiotic at a site unsuitable for I.V. administration.

Nursing interventions
• Monitor vital signs, particularly the cardiovascular and respiratory signs.
• Maintain equipment sterility. Monitor and correct problems in the system.
• Monitor controlled suction.
• If an anticoagulant is ordered, ensure the proper ratio of anticoagulant to shed blood. (Consult the manufacturer's guidelines or doctor's order.)
• Monitor laboratory data during and after autotransfusion, particularly the coagulation profile, hemoglobin and hematocrit, arterial blood gas, and calcium levels.
• Document the amount of blood retrieved and reinfused in intake and output records.
• Infuse collected blood within 4 hours of collection.
• Follow the manufacturer's recommendations for proper use of the autotransfusion device.

• Compare the labels on all blood containers to corresponding patient identification forms *to verify that the transfusion was the correct blood or blood product.*
• Notify the blood bank of a possible transfusion reaction and collect blood samples, as ordered. Immediately send these samples, all transfusion containers (even if empty), and the administration set to the blood bank. The blood bank will test these materials to further evaluate the reaction.
• Collect the first posttransfusion urine specimen, mark the collection slip "Possible transfusion reaction," and send it to the laboratory immediately. *The laboratory tests this urine specimen for the presence of hemoglobin, which indicates a hemolytic reaction.*

• Closely monitor intake and output. Note evidence of oliguria or anuria *because hemoglobin deposition in the renal tubules can cause renal damage.*
• If ordered, administer oxygen, epinephrine, or other drugs. If ordered, apply a hypothermia blanket *to reduce fever.*
• Make the patient as comfortable as possible and provide reassurance as necessary. (For specific steps, see *Managing transfusion reactions*, pages 339 to 341.)

Special considerations
Treat all transfusion reactions as serious until proven otherwise. If the doctor anticipates a transfusion reaction, such as one that may occur in a leukemia patient,

(Text continues on page 341.)

Reviewing transfusion products

PRODUCT	DESCRIPTION	NURSING CONSIDERATIONS
Whole blood	500-ml unit contains about 200 ml of red blood cells (RBCs) and about 300 ml of plasma.	• Indicated for massive blood loss and exchange transfusion in neonates. • Multiple-lead tubing (preferably a Y-type set) is recommended over piggybacking on a straight-line set. • Monitor vital signs frequently throughout transfusion. • Administer ABO group- and Rh type-specific product.
RBCs (packed)	350- to 400-ml unit contains about 200 to 250 ml of RBCs (with same amount of hemoglobin as whole blood) and 150 ml of plasma and additive solution (normal saline, adenine, glucose, and mannitol).	• Indicated for inadequate oxygen-carrying capacity. • A filter with larger surface area may be used to increase transfusion rate. • Administer ABO group- and Rh type-specific product, if possible. If not, group- and type-compatible product can be transfused safely.
RBCs (deglycerolized or leukocyte-poor)	200-ml unit contains RBCs suspended in 50 ml of normal saline, with virtually all leukocytes and plasma proteins removed. Deglycerolized RBCs, taken from donors with rare blood types, are first frozen (with glycerol added to preserve RBCs), then thawed and deglycerolized before transfusion. Leukocyte-poor RBCs aren't frozen.	• Same indications as for packed RBCs. Also used to prevent febrile reactions from leukocyte antibodies and to treat immunosuppressed patients. • All tubing should be rubber-free to prevent platelets from sticking. • Transfuse more rapidly than whole blood to prevent platelets from clumping and sticking to side of bag. • Administer ABO group- and Rh type-compatible product if possible. • Inspect unit for color. It should have a yellow tinge. • Agitate bag more often than other blood products because platelets tend to clump. • Adverse reactions are usually slight. • American Red Cross recommends that units of platelet concentrates be pooled in blood bank into transfer packs, rather than administered as single-donor units. Expiration date is usually 2 to 5 days from date of collection, depending on method of storage.
Platelets	30- to 60-ml unit contains about half the number of platelets originally found in 1 unit of whole blood.	• Indicated to treat thrombocytopenia, acute leukemia and marrow aplasia, and to restore platelet count preoperatively in a patient with a count of 100,000/mm³ or less. • ABO compatibility not necessary but recommended for repeated platelet transfusions. • Use a component drip administration set; infuse 100 ml over 15 minutes. • Patients with a history of platelet reaction require premedication with antipyretics and antihistamines. • Avoid administering when the patient has a fever.
Fresh frozen plasma	200- to 250-ml unit contains all coagulation factors and 250 mg of fibrinogen.	• Indicated to expand plasma volume, treat postoperative hemorrhage or shock, and correct coagulation factor deficiencies. • ABO compatibility not necessary. • Use a straight-line set and administer rapidly. • Large volume transfusions may require correction for hypocalcemia.

(continued)

Reviewing transfusion products *(continued)*

PRODUCT	DESCRIPTION	NURSING CONSIDERATIONS
Cryoprecipitated antihemophilic factor	Frozen 20-ml unit contains mostly coagulation Factor VIII, plus 250 mg of fibrinogen.	• Indicated for hemophilia A, von Willebrand's disease, hypofibrinogenemia, and "fibrin glue." • Smaller needle or catheter size (22G or 23G for adults) may be used because product is not viscous. • Use component Y-type set if available. Tubing doesn't have to be rubber-free because product won't stick. • Transfuse more rapidly than whole blood because coagulation factors become unstable after thawing. • Administer ABO group-compatible product. • Patient usually receives multiple units. American Red Cross recommends that they be pooled into transfer packs. Administer all units within 6 hours. • Because product has short half-life, transfusions may need to be repeated frequently, depending on the patient's clinical status.
Granulocytes	Unit volume varies (200-500 ml), but units contain mostly granulocytes (exact number depends on method of salvage) and RBCs, plasma, and platelets.	• Indicated in severe gram-negative infection or severe neutropenia unresponsive to routine forms of therapy in immunosuppressed patient. Also indicated in severe granulocyte dysfunction. • Microaggregate filter is contraindicated because it traps granulocytes. • Administer ABO group-compatible and, when possible, Rh type-compatible and human leukocyte antigen-compatible products. • For best results, administer as soon as possible after salvage. • Procedure must be repeated daily for 4 days or longer to be effective. • Because product consists of white blood cells, watch for chills and fever. Other adverse reactions include coughing and shortness of breath. Continue transfusion if possible but, if severe dyspnea develops, stop transfusion, keep vein open, and notify the doctor.
Serum albumin (5% and 25%) and plasma protein fraction (PPF)	25% albumin comes in 50-ml and 100-ml units. 5% albumin and PPF (essentially the same product) come in 250-ml units.	• Indicated in hypovolemia and hypoproteinemia (in burns, for example). • Because product comes in glass bottle, use administration set supplied with it. The set will have a filtered air inlet. Normal saline solution is not needed as a starter. Product needs no blood filter. • 25% albumin is not usually given at more than 1 ml/minute because of the danger of fluid overload. PPF given at over 10 ml/minute may produce hypotension. • Compatibility testing isn't required because product contains no RBCs or plasma antibodies. • Product is free from HIV and hepatitis viruses. • 25% albumin is used for patient with depleted vascular volume but extravascular fluid accumulation. • Because 25% albumin rapidly mobilizes large volumes of fluid into circulation, watch for pulmonary edema and other signs and symptoms of fluid overload. • Product is stored at room temperature and has an extremely long shelf life. Always check expiration date before administering.

Managing transfusion reactions

REACTION AND CAUSE	SIGNS AND SYMPTOMS	NURSING INTERVENTIONS
Reactions from single transfusion		
Hemolytic ABO or Rh incompatibility, intradonor incompatibility, or improper blood storage	• Shaking, chills, fever, nausea, vomiting, chest pain, dyspnea, hypotension, oliguria, hemoglobinuria, flank pain, abnormal bleeding • May progress to shock and renal failure	• Monitor blood pressure. • Treat shock as indicated by the patient's condition, using I.V. fluids, oxygen, epinephrine, a diuretic, and a vasopressor. • Obtain posttransfusion reaction blood sample and urine specimen for evaluation. • Observe for signs of hemorrhage resulting from disseminated intravascular coagulation. ***Prevention*** • Before transfusion, check donor and recipient blood types to ensure blood compatibility; identify patient with another nurse or doctor present. • Transfuse blood slowly for first 15 to 20 minutes while observing the patient closely.
Febrile Bacterial lipopolysaccharides	• Fever, chills, headache, flank pain	• Relieve symptoms with an antipyretic, antihistamine, or analgesic, as ordered. ***Prevention*** • Premedicate with an antipyretic, antihistamine and, possibly a steroid. • Use leukocyte-poor or washed red blood cells (RBCs).
Allergic Allergen in donor's blood	• Pruritus, urticaria, fever, chills, nausea, vomiting, facial swelling, wheezing, laryngeal edema • May progress to anaphylaxis	• Administer antihistamines. • Monitor for anaphylactic reaction and administer epinephrine and steroids, if indicated. ***Prevention*** • Premedicate with antihistamine if patient has a history of allergic reactions. • Observe the patient closely for the first 20 minutes of the transfusion.
Bacterial contamination Cold-growing, gram-negative organisms, such as species of *Pseudomonas*	• Chills, fever, vomiting, abdominal cramping, diarrhea, shock, signs of renal failure	• Treat with broad-spectrum antibiotic and steroid. ***Prevention*** • Observe blood before transfusion for gas, clots, and dark purple color. • Use air-free, touch-free method to draw and deliver blood. • Maintain strict storage control. • Change blood tubing and filter every 4 hours. • Infuse each unit of blood over 2 to 4 hours; terminate the infusion if time exceeds 4 hours. • Maintain aseptic technique during administration.

(continued)

Managing transfusion reactions *(continued)*

REACTION AND CAUSE	SIGNS AND SYMPTOMS	NURSING INTERVENTIONS
Reactions from single transfusion *(continued)*		
Plasma protein incompatibility Immunoglobulin A (IgA) incompatibility	• Flushing, abdominal pain, diarrhea, chills, fever, dyspnea, hypotension	• Treat for shock by administering oxygen, fluids, epinephrine and, possibly, a steroid, as ordered. *Prevention* • Transfuse only IgA-deficient blood or well-washed RBCs.
Reactions from multiple transfusions		
Hemosiderosis Increased hemosiderin (iron-containing pigment) from RBC destruction, especially after receiving chronic transfusions	• Plasma iron level greater than 200 mg/dl	• Perform a phlebotomy to remove excess iron. *Prevention* • Administer blood only when absolutely necessary.
Bleeding tendencies Low platelet count in stored blood, causing dilutional thrombocytopenia	• Abnormal bleeding and oozing from cut or break in skin surface	• Administer platelets. • Monitor platelet count. *Prevention* • Use only fresh blood (less than 7 days old) when possible.
Elevated blood ammonia level Increased level of ammonia in stored blood	• Forgetfulness, confusion	• Monitor ammonia level. • Decrease the amount of protein in diet. • If indicated, give neomycin sulfate. *Prevention* • Use only RBCs, fresh frozen plasma, or fresh blood, especially if patient has hepatic disease.
Increased oxygen affinity for hemoglobin Decreased level of 2,3-diphosphoglycerate in stored blood. When oxygen's affinity for hemoglobin rises, oxygen stays in the bloodstream and isn't released into tissues.	• Depressed respiratory rate, especially in patients with chronic lung disease	• Monitor arterial blood gas levels and give respiratory support as needed. *Prevention* • Use only RBCs or fresh blood if possible.

Managing transfusion reactions *(continued)*

REACTION AND CAUSE	SIGNS AND SYMPTOMS	NURSING INTERVENTIONS
Reactions from multiple transfusions *(continued)*		
Hypothermia Rapid infusion of large amounts of cold blood, which decreases myocardial temperature	• Shaking, chills, hypotension, ventricular fibrillation • Cardiac arrest if core temperature falls below 86° F (30° C)	• Stop transfusion. • Warm the patient with blankets. • Obtain an ECG. *Prevention* • Warm blood to 95° to 98.6° F (35° to 37° C), especially before massive transfusions.
Hypocalcemia Citrate toxicity occurs when citrate-treated blood is infused rapidly. Citrate binds with calcium, causing a calcium deficiency, or normal citrate metabolism becomes hindered by hepatic disease.	• Tingling in fingers, muscle cramps, nausea, vomiting, hypotension, cardiac arrhythmias, convulsions	• Slow or stop transfusion, depending on reaction. Expect a worse reaction in hypothermic patients or in patients with elevated potassium levels. • Slowly administer calcium gluconate I.V. *Prevention* • Infuse blood slowly. • Monitor potassium and calcium levels. • Use blood less than 2 days old if administering multiple units.
Hyperkalemia An abnormally high level of potassium in stored plasma caused by RBC lysis	• Intestinal colic, diarrhea, muscle twitching, oliguria, renal failure, ECG changes with tall peaked T waves, bradycardia proceeding to cardiac standstill	• Obtain an ECG. • Administer sodium polystyrene sulfonate (Kayexalate) orally or by enema. *Prevention* • Use fresh blood when administering massive transfusions.

he may order prophylactic treatment with antihistamines or antipyretics to precede blood administration.

To avoid a possible febrile reaction, the doctor may order the blood washed *to remove as many leukocytes as possible,* or a leukocyte removal filter may be used during the transfusion.

Documentation

Record the time and date of the transfusion reaction, the type and amount of infused blood or blood products, the clinical signs of the transfusion reaction in order of occurrence, the patient's vital signs, any specimens sent to the laboratory for analysis, any treatment given, and the patient's response to treatment. If required by hospital policy, complete the transfusion reaction form.

 Therapeutic plasma exchange

In therapeutic plasma exchange (TPE), also known as plasmapheresis, blood drawn from a patient's vein (usually in the antecubital fossa or via a large-bore double lumen central venous [CV] access device) flows to a cell separator, where it is divided into plasma and formed elements (red cells, white cells, and platelets) by centrifugation or by microporous membrane filtration. The plasma is then collected in a container for disposal, and the formed elements are mixed with a plasma replacement fluid (proteins, fluid, and electrolytes) and returned to the patient through another vein or CV access device. In another method of TPE, the plasma is separated, filtered to remove the disease mediator, then returned to the patient. In both methods, the extracorporeal circuit contains 150 to 400 ml of blood during plasma exchange, which means that the patient must be able to tolerate decreased blood volume.

TPE may benefit patients with immune-related disorders (such as multiple myeloma, rapidly progressive glomerulonephritis, systemic lupus erythematosus, and rheumatoid arthritis) or with a neuromuscular disorder, such as myasthenia gravis. It is commonly combined with steroid immunosuppressant therapy to suppress pathologic immune responses, thereby preventing further organ or system destruction. The procedure can be performed at the bedside or in a special unit and requires a specially prepared technician or nurse to operate the cell separator, another nurse to monitor and maintain the patient, and a specialized doctor to be in the facility.

Equipment

Vascular access needles, if not in place ■ gloves ■ sterile gauze pads ■ normal saline solution ■ anticoagulant ■ nonallergenic tape ■ aids to help maintain blood flow, such as a rolled ABD pad, tourniquet, blood pressure cuff, or heating pad ■ optional: heparin, 2% lidocaine, immune globulin.

The technician or nurse usually provides all equipment necessary to operate the cell separator.

Preparation of equipment

Using sterile technique, the technician or nurse assembles all necessary equipment and primes the extracorporeal circuit with normal saline solution *to remove air bubbles, preventing formation of an air embolus.* Then she adds an anticoagulant, usually anticoagulant-citrate-dextrose (ACD), *which prevents clotting by citrate binding to the blood's ionized (free) calcium.* ACD only works in the extracorporeal circuit and is neutralized on return to the patient. The doctor may order the addition of calcium gluconate to the plasma replacement solution *to prevent hypocalcemic reactions because albumin in this solution can also bind the returned blood's ionized calcium.*

Implementation

• Explain the procedure to the patient, and verify that he has signed a consent form. Tell him the procedure usually takes 1 to 2 hours but may take longer, depending on the volume of plasma exchanged. Advise him to eat lightly before the procedure.

• Instruct the patient to urinate before the procedure and during the procedure, as necessary. *A full bladder may cause mild hypotension because of fluid shift or vasovagal reaction.*

• Tell the patient to report any symptoms of hypocalcemic paresthesias, such as tingling of mouth, chin, or fingers, during treatment.

• Take vital signs *to serve as baseline values.* Observe universal precautions.

• If an I.V. line is not in place, perform venipunctures *to establish vascular access routes.* Use large-bore vascular access needles *to minimize resistance and prevent damage to blood cells.* Large-bore CV access catheters or dialysis catheters are frequently inserted by a surgeon specifically for plasmapheresis. Obtain blood samples if ordered.

• If ordered, administer 2,000 to 3,000 units of heparin I.V. just before TPE *to prevent clot formation in the vascular access sites.*

• The technician or nurse then connects the patient to the cell separator and starts it. While the machine is operating, observe all solutions *to avoid an air embolus from an empty container.*

• Monitor the patient for signs of hypotension, hypocalcemia, or allergic reaction, which may result from the replacement solution. Temporary reduction of blood flow rate relieves paresthesias from hypocalcemia.

• Take one or more of the following measures *to optimize blood flow,* as necessary. Place the patient in an elevated, semi-Fowler's position *to promote gravity drainage,* and hyperextend the arm on a firm surface, with the wrist supported *to make large veins accessible.* Instruct the patient to squeeze a small, rolled ABD pad *to promote venous blood flow and prevent vessel collapse.* Apply a tourniquet or blood pressure cuff above the peripheral vascular sites *to provide pressure and increase blood pooling.* Place heating pads over the access sites *to dilate the vessels,* but observe for reddened skin, especially in the elderly patient with diminished heat sensitivity. Slightly withdraw or shift the needle *to augment blood flow.*

• After plasma exchange is completed, remove the needles (while wearing gloves) and elevate the affected extremities slightly.

• Firmly hold sterile gauze pads over the puncture sites until bleeding stops. Then apply sterile pressure dressings and secure with nonallergenic tape. Avoid bending the extremities *to prevent vessel scarring and to allow use of the veins for subsequent treatment.* If necessary, note on the patient's chart that the veins shouldn't be used for other purposes between TPE treatments.

• Mark all disposable equipment and plasma bags as contaminated, and discard according to hospital policy.

Special considerations

If possible, withhold drugs until completion of the procedure *to prevent their removal from the blood.* If the unstable patient with myasthenia gravis is undergoing TPE, have emergency equipment available. Monitor the patient's blood pressure and pulse rate at least every 30 minutes. As ordered, give pyridostigmine bromide only if the patient experiences dysphagia or respiratory difficulty.

If the patient is receiving TPE treatments frequently, he may require transfusions of fresh frozen plasma *to replace the normal clotting factors removed from his plasma.* As ordered, give deep I.M. injections of immune globulin in divided doses for 3 days after the procedure *to replace normal immunoglobulins needed to resist infection that also were removed in the plasma.* If permitted by hospital policy, mix 2 ml of 2% lidocaine with 10 ml of immune globulin *to promote patient comfort during injection.*

After TPE, the patient may experience fatigue for 1 or 2 days as a result of decreased plasma protein levels. Advise him to rest frequently during this period and to avoid strenuous activities, if possible.

Unless contraindicated, tell the patient to maintain a high-protein diet to replace lost proteins and to take multivitamins with iron daily. If the patient is receiving steroids and requires a low-sodium diet, emphasize the importance of observing the diet.

Because plasmapheresis and concurrent therapy can cause immunosuppression, advise the patient to avoid people who have colds and other illnesses. Tell him to notify the doctor if any symptoms of an infection develop—even a scratchy throat—so that the schedule for TPE and other therapy can be altered, if necessary. Also advise the patient to notify the doctor of any muscle weakness or cramping.

If the patient is receiving immunosuppressant or steroid therapy, watch for signs of infection and an abnormally low white blood cell count.

Complications
Hypotension can result from fluid shifts without protein replacement or from decreased blood volume. In the elderly patient, diminished cardiac output may cause hypotension after the procedure. Hypocalcemia can result from the binding of ionized calcium by citrate; hypomagnesemia can follow repeated TPE, producing severe, prolonged muscle cramping and tetany. Allergic reaction can result from the protein replacement solution, particularly from the plasma protein fraction. In a patient with myasthenia gravis, cholinergic crisis is possible. In a patient being mechanically ventilated, respiratory secretions may increase for 1 to 2 days after treatment.

Documentation
Record the time of the procedure, the patient's vital signs, tolerance to the procedure, vascular access sites, volume of exchanged plasma, replacement solution, any adverse reactions, and any administration of drugs. Refer to the plasmapheresis flowchart for intake and output measurements, and record them on the intake and output sheet.

Selected references

American Association of Blood Banks. "Blood Transfusion Outside the Hospital," *AJN* 89(4):486-89, April 1989.

Bartlett, K., and Burgoon, D. "Venous Access Devices: Appropriate for Home Use," *Home Healthcare Nurse* 8(2):38-41, March-April 1990.

Brown, J.M. "Evaluation of Surecath Access Devices," *Journal of Intravenous Nursing* 12(5):298-301, September-October 1989.

Delaney, C.W., and Lauer, M.L. *Intravenous Therapy: A Guide to Quality Care.* Philadelphia: J.B. Lippincott Co., 1988.

Freedman, S., et al. "Nursing Considerations in the Administration of Blood Component Therapy," *Seminars in Oncology Nursing* 6(2):155-62, May 1990.

Hadaway, L.C. "Evaluation and Use of Advance I.V. Technology: Central Venous Access Devices," Part I. *Journal of Intravenous Nursing* 12(2):73-82, March-April 1989.

Handy, C.M. "Vascular Access Devices: Hospital to Home Care," *Journal of Intravenous Nursing* 12(Supp.):S10-S18, January-February 1989.

Intravenous Nurses Society. "Intravenous Nursing Standards of Practice," *Journal of Intravenous Nursing* 13(Supp.):S1-S98, April 1990.

Lichtor, J.L. "Transfusion Reactions," Part 2. *Current Reviews for Nurse Anesthetists* 12(4):27-32, July 27, 1989.

Millam, D.A. "Mastering Arterial Punctures," *AJN* 88(9):1213-24, September 1988.

Newman, L.N. "A Side-by-Side Look at Two Venous Access Devices," *AJN* 89(6):826-35, June 1989.

Physicians' Desk Reference (PDR), 44th ed. Oradell, N.J.: Medical Economics Company, 1990.

Plumer, A.L. *Principles and Practice of Intravenous Therapy*, 4th ed. Boston: Little, Brown & Co., 1987.

Viall, C.D. "Your Complete Guide to Central Venous Catheters," *Nursing90* 20(2):34-42, February 1990.

Wheeler, C.A. "Pediatric Intraosseous Infusion: An Old Technique in Modern Healthcare Technology," *Journal of Intravenous Nursing* 12(6):371-76, November-December 1989.

CARDIOVASCULAR CARE

CHERYL MILFORD, RN, MS, CCRN

Introduction

Cardiovascular disorders, the leading cause of death in the United States, affects millions of Americans each year. The responsibility of caring for patients with these disorders pervades nearly every area of nursing practice. As a result, cardiovascular care ranks as one of the most rapidly growing areas of nursing. What's more, it's one of the most rapidly changing fields, with the continuing proliferation of new diagnostic tests, new drug and other treatments, and sophisticated monitoring equipment. Consequently, nurses face a constant challenge to keep up with the latest developments.

Patient teaching

Today, nurses assume much of the responsibility for preparing patients physically and psychologically for their hospitalization and ongoing care. Specifically, they play a pivotal role in teaching patients and their families about test and procedure preparation and follow-up care, drug and other treatments, disease prevention, and life-style modification. Through patient teaching, nurses can help patients reduce stress and comply with prescribed therapy.

Monitoring

Cardiac and hemodynamic monitoring represent critical cardiovascular care responsibilities. Cardiac monitoring involves either hardwire or telemetric systems that continuously record the patient's cardiac activity. This makes monitoring useful not only for assessing cardiac rhythm, but also for gauging a patient's response to drug therapy and for preventing complications associated with diagnostic and therapeutic procedures. Once used only in critical care areas, cardiac monitoring is now performed in high-risk obstetric, general medical, pediatric, and transplantation departments.

Similarly, hemodynamic monitoring has become more widely used since its inception in the 1970s. It uses invasive techniques to measure pressure, flow, and resistance within the cardiovascular system. Made with a pulmonary artery catheter, these measurements are used to guide therapy. Hemodynamic monitoring includes pulmonary artery pressure monitoring, cardiac output measurement, right ventricular ejection fraction and volume measurement, temporary pacing through the pulmonary

artery catheter, and continuous evaluation of mixed venous oxygen saturation.

Treatment

In cardiovascular emergencies, nurses may perform or assist with cardiopulmonary resuscitation, defibrillation, cardioversion, and temporary pacing. Carrying out these life-saving procedures calls for in-depth knowledge of cardiovascular anatomy, physiology, and equipment, as well as sound assessment and intervention techniques. Only nurses with up-to-date information and sharpened skills can provide safe, effective patient care.

MONITORING
Electrocardiography

One of the most valuable and frequently used diagnostic tools, electrocardiography (ECG) measures the heart's electrical activity as waveforms. Impulses moving through the heart's conduction system create electric currents that can be monitored on the body's surface. Electrodes attached to the skin can detect these electric currents and transmit them to an instrument that produces a record (the electrocardiogram) of cardiac activity.

ECG can be used to identify myocardial ischemia and infarction, rhythm and conduction disturbances, chamber enlargement, electrolyte imbalances, and drug toxicity.

The standard 12-lead ECG uses a series of electrodes placed on the extremities and the chest wall to assess the heart from 12 different views (leads). The 12 leads consist of 3 standard bipolar limb leads (designated I, II, III), 3 unipolar augmented leads (aV_R, aV_L, aV_F), and 6 unipolar precordial leads (V_1 to V_6). The limb leads and augmented leads show the heart from the frontal plane. The precordial leads show the heart from the horizontal plane.

The ECG device measures and averages the differences between the electrical potential of the electrode sites for each lead and graphs them over time. This creates the standard ECG complex, called P-QRS-T. The P wave represents atrial depolarization; the QRS complex, ventricular depolarization; and the T wave, ventricular repolarization. (See *Reviewing ECG waveform components*, page 346.)

Variations of standard ECG include exercise ECG (stress ECG) and ambulatory ECG (Holter monitoring). Exercise electrocardiography monitors heart rate, blood

Reviewing ECG waveform components

An electrocardiogram (ECG) waveform has three basic components: P wave, QRS complex, and T wave. These elements can be further divided into a PR interval, J point, ST segment, U wave, and QT interval.

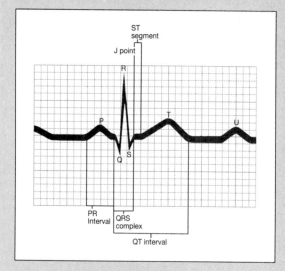

P wave and PR interval
The P wave represents atrial depolarization. The PR interval represents the time it takes an impulse to travel from the atria through the AV node and bundle of His. The PR interval measures from the beginning of the P wave to the beginning of the QRS complex.

QRS complex
The QRS complex represents ventricular depolarization (the time it takes for the impulse to travel through the bundle branches to the Purkinje fibers).

   The Q wave appears as the first negative deflection in the QRS complex; the R wave, as the first positive deflection. The S wave appears as the second negative deflection or the first negative deflection after the R wave.

J point and ST segment
Marking the end of the QRS complex, the J point also indicates the beginning of the ST segment. The ST segment represents part of ventricular repolarization.

T wave and U wave
Usually following the same deflection pattern as the P wave, the T wave represents ventricular repolarization. The U wave follows the T wave, but is not always seen.

QT interval
The QT interval represents ventricular depolarization and repolarization. It extends from the beginning of the QRS complex to the end of the T wave.

---

pressure, and ECG waveforms as the patient walks on a treadmill or pedals a stationary bicycle. For ambulatory ECG, the patient wears a portable Holter monitor to record heart activity continuously over 24 hours.

   ECG may be accomplished using a multichannel or a single-channel method. For the multichannel method, all electrodes are attached to the patient at once and the machine prints a simultaneous view of all leads. The single-channel method requires systematic attachment and removal of selected electrodes and stopping and starting the tracing each time.

Equipment
ECG machine ■ recording paper ■ pre-gelled disposable electrodes or reusable electrodes with suction bulbs, electrode gel, and rubber straps ■ 4″ × 4″ gauze pads ■ moist cloth towel ■ sterile drape ■ optional: shaving supplies, marking pen.

Preparation of equipment
Before using the ECG machine, check the date of its last inspection by the hospital's engineering department. If the period for authorized use has elapsed, avoid using the machine *because even a miniscule leakage of electric current (10 microamperes) may put the patient at risk for life-threatening arrhythmias.*

Implementation
● Explain the procedure to the patient *to allay his fears and promote cooperation.* Inform him that no special preparation is required and that the procedure takes no longer than 15 minutes. Instruct him to relax, lie still, and breathe normally. Advise him not to talk during the procedure *because the movement of his muscles may distort the ECG tracing.*
● Check the patient's history for cardiac medications, and note any current therapy on the test request form.

• Place the patient in the supine position. If he can't tolerate lying flat, help him to assume a semi-Fowler's position.
• Instruct the patient to expose his chest, both ankles, and both wrists for electrode placement. Drape the female patient's chest until chest leads are applied.
• Turn on the machine *to warm up the stylus mechanism*. Check the paper supply.

Multichannel ECG
• Place electrodes on the inner aspect of the wrists, the medial aspect of the lower legs, and the chest. (See *Positioning chest electrodes*.) If using disposable electrodes, remove the paper backing before positioning. Then connect the lead wires after all electrodes are in place. For reusable electrodes, apply electrode gel and affix the electrodes with suction bulbs. Secure the limb electrodes with rubber straps, but avoid tightening them *to prevent circulatory impairment and distortion on the recording.*
• If frequent ECGs will be necessary, use a marking pen to indicate lead positions on the patient's chest *to ensure consistent placement.*
• Set the paper speed to 25 mm/second or as ordered. Calibrate the machine by adjusting the sensitivity to normal and checking the quality and baseline position of the tracing.
• Press the start button and the machine will produce a printout showing all 12 leads simultaneously on thermal or pressure-sensitive recording paper.
• As the machine records the ECG, check to be sure that all leads are represented in the tracing. If not, determine which one has come loose, reattach it, and restart the tracing. Check for artifact in the tracing.
• Also observe to be sure that the wave doesn't peak beyond the top edge of the recording grid. If it does, adjust the machine to bring the wave inside the boundaries.
• When the machine finishes the tracing, remove the electrodes and reposition the patient's gown and bed covers.

Single-channel ECG
• Apply either disposable or standard electrodes to the inner aspects of the wrists and medial aspects of the lower legs.
• Connect each lead wire to the corresponding electrode by inserting the wire prong into the terminal post and tightening the screw.
• Set the paper speed to 25 mm/second or as ordered. Calibrate the machine by adjusting the sensitivity to normal and checking the quality and baseline position of the tracing. Recalibrate the machine after running each lead *to provide a consistent test standard.*

Positioning chest electrodes

To ensure accurate test results, position chest electrodes as follows:

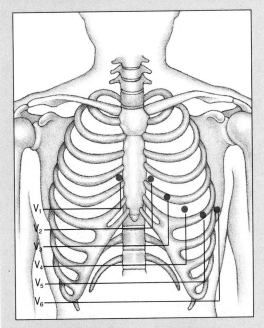

V_1: Fourth intercostal space at right border of sternum
V_2: Fourth intercostal space at left border of sternum
V_3: Halfway between V_2 and V_4
V_4: Fifth intercostal space at midclavicular line
V_5: Fifth intercostal space at anterior axillary line (halfway between V_4 and V_6)
V_6: Fifth intercostal space at midaxillary line, level with V_4

• Turn the lead selector to I. Then mark the lead by writing "I" on the paper strip or by depressing the marking button on the machine (some machines do this automatically). Record for 3 to 6 seconds and then return the machine to the standby mode. Repeat this procedure for leads II, III, aV_R, aV_L, and aV_F.
• Determine proper placement for the chest electrodes. If frequent ECGs are necessary, use a marking pen to indicate lead positions on the patient's chest *to ensure consistent placement.*

• Connect the chest lead wire to the suction bulb in the same manner as you connected the limb electrodes. Apply gel to each of the six chest positions, then firmly press the suction bulb to attach the chest lead to the V_1 position. Mark the strips as before. Then turn the lead selector to V and record V_1 for 3 to 6 seconds. Return the lead selector to standby. Reposition the electrode and repeat the procedure for V_2 to V_6.
• After completing V_6, run a rhythm strip on lead II for at least 6 seconds.
• Assess the quality of the tracings and repeat any that are unclear.
• Disconnect the equipment, remove the electrodes, and wipe the gel from the patient with a moist cloth towel. Wash the gel from the electrodes and dry them thoroughly.

Special considerations
In place of the electrodes and straps on the extremities, suction bulbs may be used *to enhance baseline stability.*

Small areas of hair on the patient's chest or extremities may be shaved, but this usually isn't necessary.

If the patient's skin is exceptionally oily, scaly, or diaphoretic, rub the electrode site with a dry $4'' \times 4''$ gauze pad before applying the electrode *to help reduce interference in the tracing.* During the procedure, ask the patient to breathe normally. If his respirations distort the recording, ask him to hold his breath briefly *to reduce baseline wander in the tracing.*

If the patient has a pacemaker, you can perform ECG with or without a magnet. Be sure to note the presence of a pacemaker and the use of the magnet (to turn off the pacemaker) on the strip.

Documentation
Label the ECG recording with the patient's name, room number, and hospital identification number. If you're sending the ECG to another department for interpretation and mounting, complete all information on the request form. Document in your notes the test's date and time and significant responses by the patient as well.

Cardiac monitoring

Because it allows continuous observation of the heart's electrical activity, cardiac monitoring is used in patients with conduction disturbances or in those at risk for life-threatening arrhythmias. It's also used to evaluate the effects of therapy.

Like other forms of electrocardiography (ECG), cardiac monitoring uses electrodes placed on the patient's chest to transmit electrical signals that are converted into a tracing of cardiac rhythm on an oscilloscope.

Two types of monitoring may be performed: hardwire or telemetry. In *hardwire* monitoring, the patient is connected to a monitor at bedside. The rhythm display appears at bedside, but it may also be transmitted to a console at a remote location. *Telemetry* uses a small transmitter connected to the ambulatory patient to send electrical signals to another location where they are displayed on a monitor screen. (See *Setting up for telemetry.*)

Regardless of the type, cardiac monitors can display the patient's rhythm and heart rate; produce a printed record of cardiac rhythm; and sound an alarm if the patient's heart rate rises above or falls below specified limits. Some monitors can also recognize and count abnormal heartbeats and trigger an alarm if the heartbeats exceed a set limit.

Equipment
Cardiac monitor ■ lead wires ■ patient cable ■ disposable pre-gelled electrodes (the number of electrodes varies from three to five, depending on the manufacturer) ■ alcohol sponges ■ $4'' \times 4''$ gauze pads ■ optional: shaving supplies, washcloth.

Preparation of equipment
Plug the monitor into an electrical outlet and turn it on *to warm up the unit while you prepare the equipment and the patient.* Insert the cable into the appropriate socket in the monitor.

Connect the lead wires to the cable. In some systems, the lead wires are permanently secured to the cable. Each lead wire should indicate the location for attachment to the patient: right arm (RA), left arm (LA), right leg (RL), left leg (LL), and ground (C or V). This should appear on the lead wire—if it's permanently connected—or at the connection of the lead wires and cable to the patient. Then connect an electrode to each of the lead wires, carefully checking that each lead wire is in its correct outlet.

Implementation
• Explain the procedure to the patient, provide privacy, and ask the patient to expose his chest. Wash your hands.
• Determine electrode positions on the patient's chest, based on the system and lead you're using. (See *Understanding lead placement,* pages 350 and 351.)
• If the lead wires and patient cable aren't permanently attached, verify that the electrode placement corresponds to the label on the patient cable.

• If necessary, shave an area about 4″ (10 cm) in diameter around each electrode site. Clean the area with an alcohol sponge and dry it completely *to remove skin secretions that may interfere with electrode function.* Gently abrade the dried area by rubbing it briskly until it reddens *to remove dead skin cells and to promote better electrical contact with living cells.* (Some electrodes have a small, rough patch for abrading the skin; otherwise, use a dry washcloth or a dry gauze pad.)

• Remove the backing from the pre-gelled electrode. Check the gel for moistness. If the gel is dry, discard it and replace it with a fresh electrode.

• Apply the electrode to the site and press firmly *to ensure a tight seal.* Repeat with the remaining electrodes.

• When all the electrodes are in place, check for a tracing on the cardiac monitor. Assess the quality of the ECG. (See *Identifying cardiac monitor problems,* page 352.) To verify that each beat is being detected by the monitor, compare the digital heart rate display with your count of the patient's heart rate.

• If necessary, use the gain control to adjust the size of the rhythm tracing, and the position control to adjust the waveform position on the recording paper.

• Set the upper and lower limits of the heart rate alarm, based on unit policy. Turn the alarm on.

Special considerations
Make sure that all electrical equipment and outlets are grounded *to avoid electric shock and interference (artifacts).* Also ensure that the patient is clean and dry *to prevent electric shock.*

Avoid opening the electrode packages until just before using *to prevent the gel from drying out.*

Avoid placing the electrodes on bony prominences, hairy areas, areas where defibrillator pads will be placed, or areas for chest compression.

If the patient's skin is exceptionally oily, scaly, or diaphoretic, rub the electrode site with a dry 4″ × 4″ gauze pad before applying the electrode *to help reduce interference in the tracing.* During the procedure, ask the patient to breathe normally. If his respirations distort the recording, ask him to hold his breath briefly *to reduce baseline wander in the tracing.*

Assess skin integrity, and reposition the electrodes every 24 hours or as necessary.

Documentation
Record the date and time that monitoring begins and the monitoring lead in your notes. Document a rhythm strip at least every 8 hours with any changes in the patient's condition (or as stated by hospital policy). Label the rhythm strip with the patient's name, room number, the date, and time.

Setting up for telemetry

Telemetry detects arrhythmias that occur during sleep, or when the patient is resting, performing mild exercise, or undergoing stress. It's especially useful for the ambulatory patient because it permits greater freedom than hardwire monitoring and avoids electrical hazards by isolating the monitor system from leakage and accidental shock. To set up a telemetry monitor:

• Insert a battery in the telemetry transmitter, matching the polarity markings on the transmitter case with those on the battery.

• Test the battery's charge by observing the oscilloscope screen, which registers no cardiac activity if the battery is low. In some models, check the battery by pushing the test-light button on the back of the transmitter. If the test light fails to go on, replace the battery. Make sure the lead wire cable is securely attached to the transmitter.

• Show the transmitter to the patient and explain how it works. Before proceeding, answer any questions he may have.

• Apply electrodes to the patient's chest and attach the lead wires to them.

• Place the transmitter in the pouch provided by the manufacturer or hospital. Tie the pouch strings around the patient's neck and waist. Make sure the pouch fits snugly without making the patient uncomfortable. If no pouch is available, place the transmitter in the patient's bathrobe pocket.

• After locating the patient's telemetry monitor in the central console, calibrate it and adjust the heart-rate alarms as you would a hardwire monitor.

• Some units have a button that can be pushed if the patient has symptoms. This causes the central console to print a rhythm strip. Tell the patient how and when to use this button.

• Tell the patient to remove the transmitter if he takes a shower or bath.

If cardiac monitoring will continue after the patient's discharge, ensure that all caregivers have some knowledge of rhythm interpretation and cardiopulmonary resuscitation. Also discuss troubleshooting techniques to use if the monitor malfunctions. As needed, contact the monitor supplier to help in discharge planning.

Understanding lead placement

You'll have several leads and electrodes to place depending on the cardiac monitoring system you're using. The most typical system is the three-electrode system, which uses standard limb leads and a modified version of standard chest leads. To increase monitoring capability, you may need to use the four- or five-electrode system. Review the manufacturer's instructions for your particular system and use the following guidelines to place the leads precisely.

Three-electrode system

In this system, the most commonly used limb lead is lead II, and typically used modified chest leads are MCL₁ and MCL₆ (modified versions of V₁ and V₆). In general, a three-electrode monitoring system has one positive lead and one negative lead. A third lead serves as a ground.

Lead II

For lead II, you'll place the negative electrode at the first intercostal space on the right sternal border, the positive electrode at the fourth intercostal space on the left midclavicular line, and the ground electrode at the fourth intercostal space at the right sternal border.

Lead II measures the electrical flow from the RA (−) to the LL (+), producing good QRS complexes, which reflect ventricular activity, and positive P waves, which show atrial activity.

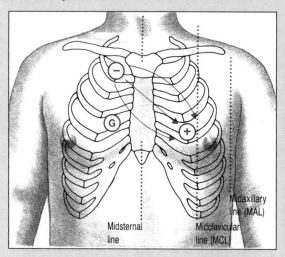

Lead MCL₁

Using MCL₁, the negative electrode would be positioned on the left side of the patient's chest just below the clavicle. The positive electrode would be positioned on the right sternal border at the fourth intercostal space, and the ground electrode would be positioned on the right side of the chest just below the clavicle.

Lead MCL₁ records the sequence of ventricular depolarization better, so it's used to differentiate between right or left bundle-branch block and ectopy. Note that in MCL₁, the positive electrode should be positioned directly over the right ventricle.

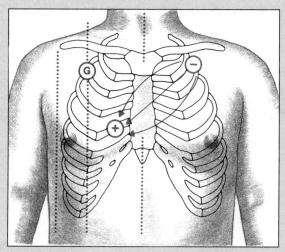

Lead MCL₆

With lead MCL₆, the negative electrode would be positioned just below the left clavicle on the midclavicular line. The positive electrode would be positioned at the left fifth intercostal space on the midaxillary line, and the ground electrode would be positioned just below the right clavicle on the midclavicular line.

Lead MCL₆ allows you to easily see tall QRS complexes so that you can identify right bundle-branch block and ST segment and T wave changes. In MCL₆, the positive electrode lies over the apex of the left ventricle.

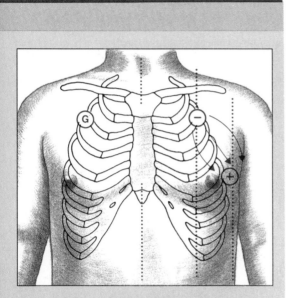

Four- and five-electrode systems

In a four-electrode system, a right leg (RL) electrode is added to provide a permanent ground for all leads used in the three-electrode system. Place this electrode on the 4th or 5th intercostal space, right midclavicular line.

A five-electrode system uses an additional exploratory chest electrode. This lets the examiner obtain any of the six modified chest leads and the standard limb leads as well. Place this lead (marked C or V) on the 3rd or 4th intercostal space, left sternal border.

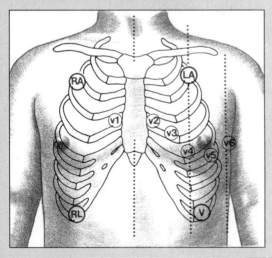

Arterial pressure monitoring

An invasive technique, arterial pressure monitoring provides continuous and accurate arterial pressure readings through a transducer that converts blood pressure into electrical impulses. These impulses are displayed on a monitor screen and recorded on paper tape. A visible and audible alarm sounds when the pressure exceeds preset limits.

The information obtained from arterial pressure monitoring is used to evaluate and guide therapies related to tissue perfusion and oxygenation. This technique also allows procurement of arterial blood samples.

Arterial pressure monitoring requires insertion of an arterial catheter through a large artery, usually the radial or femoral artery. (See *Arterial pressure monitoring setup,* page 353.)

Equipment

Preassembled arterial pressure tubing with flush device and disposable transducer ▪ monitoring equipment ▪ pressure cardule, if necessary ▪ patient cable ▪ heparin flush solution (typically 500 or 1,000 units/500 ml normal saline solution as ordered or according to hospital policy) ▪ pressure bag ▪ I.V. pole ▪ sterile gloves ▪ nonallergenic tape ▪ antimicrobial ointment ▪ dry, sterile dressing ▪ labels.

If you'll need to obtain a blood sample from an arterial line, also assemble: 5-ml syringe ▪ 5- to 10-ml syringe (depending on the amount of blood to be drawn) ▪ two sterile 4″ × 4″ gauze pads ▪ optional: blood collection tubes.

Preparation of equipment

Wash your hands. Maintain sterile technique as you prepare the equipment. If necessary, turn on the monitor to warm it up (be sure that the pressure cardule is in the monitor if one isn't built in). Insert the arterial line tubing spike into the bag of heparinized solution. Make sure that the roller clamp is closed.

To remove air from the bag, invert it. Squeeze the air out through the tubing, or insert a needle into the injection port and squeeze air out through the needle.

If necessary, place the transducer in the pole mount on the I.V. pole. (Some transducers don't need to be mounted; they can be laid on the bed.)

Squeeze the drip chamber until it's about half full. Open the roller clamp. Prime the tubing by activating the flush device. (Follow the manufacturer's directions for flushing the transducer. Many transducers need to be inverted during flushing *so that no air becomes trapped.*)

Identifying cardiac monitor problems

PROBLEM	POSSIBLE CAUSES	SOLUTIONS
False-high-rate alarm	• Monitor interpreting large T waves as QRS complexes, which doubles the rate • Skeletal muscle activity	• Reposition electrodes to lead where QRS complexes are taller than T waves. • Place electrodes away from major muscle masses.
False-low-rate alarm	• Shift in electrical axis from patient movement, making QRS complexes too small to register • Low amplitude of QRS • Poor contact between electrode and skin	• Reapply electrodes. Set gain so height of complex is greater than 1 millivolt. • Increase gain. • Reapply electrodes.
Low amplitude	• Gain dial set too low • Poor contact between skin and electrodes; dried gel; broken or loose lead wires; poor connection between patient and monitor; malfunctioning monitor; physiologic loss of QRS amplitude	• Increase gain. • Check connections on all lead wires and monitoring cable. Replace electrode as necessary. Reapply electrodes, if required.
Wandering baseline	• Poor position or contact between electrodes and skin • Thoracic movement with respirations	• Reposition or replace electrodes. • Reposition electrodes.
Artifact (waveform interference)	• Patient having seizures, chills, or anxiety • Patient movement • Electrodes applied improperly • Static electricity • Electrical short circuit in lead wires or cable • Interference from decreased room humidity	• Notify doctor and treat patient as ordered. Keep patient warm and reassure him. • Help patient relax. • Check electrodes and reapply, if necessary. • Make sure cables don't have exposed connectors. Change static-causing bedclothes. • Replace broken equipment. Use stress loops when applying lead wires. • Regulate humidity to 40%.
Broken lead wires or cable	• Stress loops not used on lead wires • Cables and lead wires cleaned with alcohol or acetone, causing brittleness	• Replace lead wires and retape them, using stress loops. • Clean cable and lead wires with soapy water. *Do not allow cable ends to become wet.* Replace cable as necessary.
60-cycle interference (fuzzy baseline)	• Electrical interference from other equipment in room • Patient's bed improperly grounded	• Attach all electrical equipment to common ground. Check plugs to make sure prongs aren't loose. • Attach bed ground to the room's common ground.
Skin excoriation under electrode	• Patient allergic to electrode adhesive • Electrode on skin too long	• Remove electrodes and apply nonallergenic electrodes and nonallergenic tape. • Remove electrode, clean site, and reapply electrode at new site.

As you flush each vented stopcock, replace it with a sterile dead-end cap. Verify that no air remains in the tubing. Then, insert the heparin flush bag into the pressure bag and inflate the pressure bag to 300 mm Hg, which will create a flow rate between 2 and 5 ml/hour. (Some hospitals recommend inflating the bag with less pressure before insertion, believing that the transducer may be damaged if it's pressurized before insertion.) Connect the monitor cable to the transducer.

If you have a reusable transducer and transducer dome, follow the manufacturer's directions for attaching the dome to the transducer and to the preassembled pressure tubing and flush system. (You may need to place several drops of sterile saline solution or bacteriostatic water on the transducer's surface before attaching the dome.)

Follow the manufacturer's directions to calibrate and zero the equipment if the machine doesn't automatically calibrate. Label the tubing with the date, time, and your initials.

Implementation
• Describe the procedure to the patient and explain its purpose.

Inserting an arterial line
• Prepare the tubing as explained previously. Wash your hands and put on sterile gloves.
• After the doctor positions the arterial catheter, attach the tubing to it, securing the tubing to the catheter with a slight twisting motion. (See "Insertion and removal of an arterial line," Chapter 6.) Secure the catheter with nonallergenic tape or, alternatively, the doctor may suture the catheter in place. Apply antimicrobial ointment and a dry, sterile dressing to the site, according to hospital protocol. Label the dressing with the date, time, and your initials.
• Level the transducer to the phlebostatic axis, located at the fifth intercostal space in the midaxillary line at the level of the right atrium. (See *Locating the phlebostatic axis,* page 354.) Zero the equipment according to the manufacturer's directions.
• Obtain pressure readings. Set alarms between 10 and 20 mm Hg above and below the patient's blood pressure.

Changing arterial line tubing
• Prepare the tubing as explained previously. Wash your hands and put on sterile gloves.
• Determine the length of tubing to be changed. (The tubing to the catheter, to the hub, or to the stopcock closest to the patient may be changed.)
• Turn the alarms off.

Arterial pressure monitoring setup

After insertion of an arterial catheter through a large artery, the catheter is connected to a flush device and a transducer. These are attached to a monitoring system that transforms electrical impulses into an arterial pressure waveform.

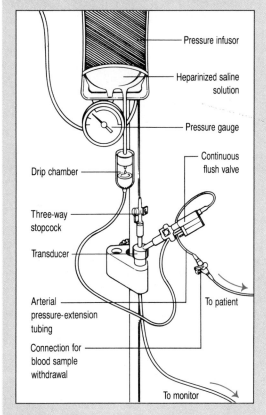

Pressure infusor

Heparinized saline solution

Pressure gauge

Continuous flush valve

Drip chamber

Three-way stopcock

Transducer

Arterial pressure-extension tubing

Connection for blood sample withdrawal

To patient

To monitor

• Clamp the tubing before disconnecting it as needed, depending on the tubing being changed. Disconnect the old segment of tubing, and immediately replace it with new tubing.
• Activate the flush device to clear blood from the line and catheter. Clean any blood from the tubing or catheter, and apply a dry, sterile dressing if the tubing to the catheter was changed.
• Level the transducer, zero the equipment, and set the alarms (as described before).

Locating the phlebostatic axis

The intersection of two imaginary lines approximates the location of the phlebostatic axis, the point where the right atrium and vena cava meet. The tip of the monitoring catheter should rest within the body at this point.

The anterior view shows the vertical line passing from the fourth intercostal space at the right side of the sternum. The lateral view shows the horizontal line passing through the fourth intercostal space, midway between the outermost part of the chest's anterior and posterior surfaces.

Anterior view

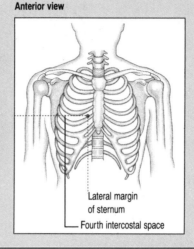

Lateral margin of sternum

Fourth intercostal space

Lateral view

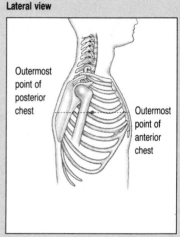

Outermost point of posterior chest

Outermost point of anterior chest

Obtaining a blood sample from an arterial line
• Assemble the equipment, wash your hands, and put on sterile gloves.
• Turn off the alarms.
• Open one package of sterile 4″ × 4″ gauze pads, and position it near the arterial line. Remove the dead-end cap from the stopcock closest to the patient and place it on a sterile 4″ × 4″ gauze pad *to keep the dead-end cap clean.*
• Insert the 5-ml syringe into the stopcock. Turn off the stopcock to the flush solution. Slowly withdraw between 3 and 5 ml of blood from the line; this will be discarded. Turn the stopcock halfway back to the open position, *which closes the system in all directions.* Remove the discard syringe, and replace it with the 5- to 10-ml specimen syringe.
• Turn off the stopcock to the flush solution. Using the specimen syringe, slowly withdraw the required amount of blood from the line. Turn the stopcock to the original position. Remove the syringe.
• Activate the flush device *to clear blood from the tubing.* Turn off the stopcock to the patient, and flush the stopcock port until the solution runs clear. Return the stopcock to the original position. *This opens the flush system to the catheter.* Turn on the alarms. Transfer the blood to the appropriate tubes, and send the specimens to the laboratory.

Special considerations

Always use sterile technique and maintain electrical safety when working with arterial lines. Note that many factors can alter pressure readings and waveforms, including air in the tubing, the transducer, or both; an inappropriate transducer level; loose connections; cracks or leaks in the system; a clot in the catheter; and the catheter tip resting against the vessel wall.

Level and zero the system at the beginning of each shift and after any manipulation of the patient or system. Check the patient's cuff blood pressure for comparison every 4 to 8 hours, depending on hospital policy. Change the dressing and tubing every 24 to 72 hours.

Monitor the patient frequently. Considerable blood can be lost quickly if the system becomes disconnected. (See *What to do if a patient removes his arterial line.*) Keep alarms on at all times, except when replacing tubing, as noted.

Bear in mind that pressure tubing is made of stiff, nondistensible plastic. Inaccurate arterial pressure measurements will result if you use conventional I.V. tubing below the level of the transducer.

Documentation

Document the date and time of the insertion and the dressing and tubing changes. Record the patient's blood pressure as indicated. Observe the shape of the arterial waveform, and note any changes.

Pulmonary artery and capillary wedge pressure monitoring

This procedure uses a pulmonary artery catheter (such as a Swan-Ganz) or a similar catheter, connected to a transducer and a monitor, to measure pulmonary artery pressure (PAP) and pulmonary capillary wedge pressure (PCWP). These measurements allow assessment of the heart's pumping ability and filling pressures, provide information about vascular volume status and the effect of drug therapy, and aid in detecting complications of acute myocardial infarction and other disorders.

Both PAP and PCWP measurements require insertion of a multilumen, balloon-tipped, flow-directed catheter. This type of catheter has evolved from a simple double-lumen monitoring device to the latest six-lumen catheter. (See *A look at the pulmonary artery catheter*, page 356.)

The catheter is inserted by the doctor either percutaneously into the subclavian, jugular, or femoral vein or through a venous cutdown in the antecubital fossa and threaded to the junction of the superior vena cava and right atrium.

Once the catheter lies in the right atrium, the balloon is inflated. Venous circulation carries the catheter tip through the right atrium and ventricle to a small branch of the pulmonary artery where the balloon will be wedged. When the balloon is deflated, the catheter drifts out of this position and into the pulmonary artery, its normal resting place. Catheter progress is usually evaluated by observing waveform changes on a cardiac monitor, but progress can also be tracked fluoroscopically. (See *Monitoring pressure tracings*, page 357.)

Once the catheter is in place, PAP can be monitored continuously and PCWP observed as required. Many hospitals also monitor central venous pressure (CVP) with the pulmonary artery catheter.

Equipment
Pressure cuff ■ balloon-tipped, flow-directed pulmonary artery catheter ■ bag of heparinized normal saline solution (usually 500 ml normal saline solution with 500 or 1,000 units heparin) ■ alcohol sponges ■ medication-added label ■ preassembled disposable pressure tubing with flush device and disposable transducer ■ monitor and monitor cable ■ I.V. pole with transducer mount ■ emergency resuscitation equipment ■ electrocardiogram (ECG) monitor ■ ECG electrodes ■ armboard (for antecubital insertion) ■ lead aprons (if fluoroscope is used during insertion) ■ sutures ■ sterile 4" × 4" gauze pads or other dry occlusive dressing material ■ prepackaged

What to do if a patient removes his arterial line

If the patient removes his arterial line, he's in danger of hypovolemic shock from blood loss. Here's what to do.

What to do first
• Immediately apply direct pressure at the insertion site, and send someone to call the doctor. Because arterial blood flows under high intravascular pressure, be certain to maintain firm, direct pressure for 5 to 10 minutes *to encourage clot formation at the insertion site.*
• Check the patient's I.V. line and, if ordered, increase the flow rate temporarily *to compensate for blood loss.*

When the bleeding stops
• Apply a sterile pressure dressing.
• Reassess the patient's level of consciousness (LOC) and orientation and offer reassurance.
• Estimate the amount of blood loss from your observations of the blood and from changes in the patient's blood pressure and heart rate.
• Assist the doctor as he reinserts the catheter. Ensure that the arm is immobilized and that the tubing and catheter are secured.
• Withdraw blood for a complete blood count and arterial blood gas analysis, as ordered.

Ongoing care
• Frequently assess the patient's vital signs, LOC, skin color and temperature, and circulation to the extremity.
• Watch for further bleeding or hematoma at the insertion site.
• Once the patient has stabilized, diminish the I.V. flow rate to the previous keep-vein-open level.

introducer kit ■ optional: dextrose 5% in water, shaving materials (if a femoral insertion site is used).

If a prepackaged introducer kit is unavailable, obtain the following: an introducer (one size larger than the catheter) ■ sterile tray containing instruments for procedure ■ masks ■ sterile gowns ■ sterile gloves ■ povidone-iodine ointment ■ sutures ■ two 10-ml syringes ■ local anesthetic (1% to 2% lidocaine) ■ one 5-ml syringe ■ 25G ½" needle ■ 1" and 3" tape.

A look at the pulmonary artery catheter

The pulmonary artery catheter is made of pliable radiopaque polyvinylchloride and may contain two to six lumens.

The distal lumen measures pulmonary artery pressure when connected to a transducer and measures pulmonary capillary wedge pressure (PCWP) during balloon inflation. It also permits drawing of mixed venous blood samples.

The proximal lumen measures central venous pressure. The balloon inflation lumen inflates the balloon at the distal tip of the catheter for PCWP measurement.

Other lumens may provide a port for pacemaker electrodes or measurement of mixed venous oxygen saturation with an Opticath catheter.

The latest six-lumen (right ventricular ejection fraction-volumetric oximetry TD) catheter is shown below. It incorporates intracardiac electrodes, which can be used with the thermistor to determine the right ventricular ejection fraction and systolic and end-diastolic right ventricular volumes.

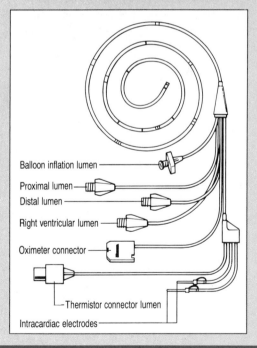

Balloon inflation lumen

Proximal lumen

Distal lumen

Right ventricular lumen

Oximeter connector

Thermistor connector lumen

Intracardiac electrodes

Preparation of equipment

You'll need to obtain at least one single-channel transducer and flush system for PAP and PCWP readings. The number of other systems needed will depend on the catheter inserted and specific monitoring requirements.

Turn on the monitor to allow it to warm up. Be sure the pressure cardule is in the monitor if one isn't built in. Wash your hands and maintain sterile technique as you prepare the equipment.

Insert a tubing spike into the bag of heparinized normal saline solution. Withdraw air from the bag by inserting a large-gauge needle into the bag's injection port and squeezing the bag gently until no air remains. Make sure the roller clamp is closed.

If necessary, place the transducer in the pole mount on the I.V. pole. (Some transducers don't need to be mounted; they can be laid on the bed.)

Squeeze the drip chamber until it's half full. Open the roller clamp and prime the tubing by activating the flush device. (Follow the manufacturer's directions for flushing the transducer and tubing. Many transducers need to be inverted so that air isn't trapped during flushing.) As you flush, replace each vented stopcock with a sterile dead-end cap.

Verify that no air remains in the tubing. Then insert the heparin flush bag into the pressure bag and inflate it to 300 mm Hg. This will create a flow rate between 2 and 5 ml/hour. (Some hospitals recommend inflating the bag with less pressure before insertion, believing that the transducer may be damaged if it's pressurized before insertion.) Connect the monitor cable to the transducer.

If you have a reusable transducer and transducer dome, follow the manufacturer's directions for attaching the dome to the transducer and to the presassembled pressure tubing and flush system. (You may need to place several drops of sterile saline solution or bacteriostatic water on the transducer's surface before attaching the dome.)

Implementation

• Explain the procedure to the patient *to allay his fears and promote cooperation*. Make sure he understands and has signed a consent form.

• Place the ECG electrodes on the patient, if they're not already in place, and connect them to the cardiac monitor. For subclavian catheter insertion, keep the chest electrodes on the side opposite the insertion site.

• Bring the equipment to the same side of the patient as the insertion site. Connect the monitor cable to the transducer, and plug it into the monitor.

Monitoring pressure tracings

Characteristic waveforms appear on the cardiac monitor as the pulmonary artery catheter is passed through the heart.

Right atrial pressure
When the catheter tip reaches the right atrium from the superior vena cava, the waveform looks like the one shown below. The doctor then inflates the balloon. This carries the tip through the tricuspid valve and into the right ventricle.

Normal range
Mean: 3 to 6 mm Hg

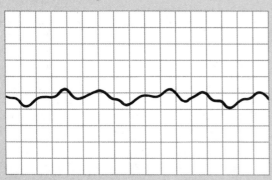

Right ventricular pressure
When the catheter tip reaches the right ventricle, the waveform looks like the one shown below.

Normal range
Systolic: 17 to 22 mm Hg
Diastolic: 1 to 7 mm Hg

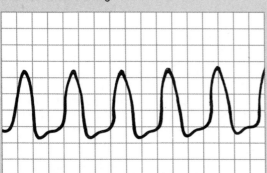

Pulmonary artery pressure
The waveform below appears when the catheter tip has moved through the pulmonic valve and into the pulmonary artery.

Normal range
Systolic: 17 to 32 mm Hg
Diastolic: 4 to 13 mm Hg
Mean: 9 to 19 mm Hg

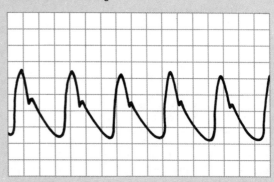

Pulmonary artery wedge pressure
The waveform below appears once the pulmonary artery catheter's balloon, carried by the circulation, becomes wedged in a small vessel. At this point the doctor will deflate the balloon, which causes the catheter tip to slip back into the main branch of the pulmonary artery. The pulmonary artery pressure waveform then reappears.

Normal range
Mean: 8 to 12 mm Hg

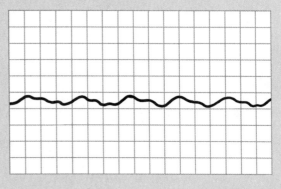

To zero and calibrate the system

• Position the transducer level with the right atrium by locating the fourth intercostal space at the midaxillary line, the phlebostatic axis. Adjust the transducer to the proper level.

• Remove the dead-end cap, and open the stopcock closest to the transducer (or follow the manufacturer's guidelines) *to open the transducer to air.*

• Zero and calibrate it according to the manufacturer's directions. (Some monitors calibrate automatically.) Then replace the dead-end cap, and close the stopcock to this port.

To assist with catheter insertion

• Make sure you have emergency resuscitation equipment available.

• Maintaining sterile technique, open the tray containing the equipment for insertion.

• Position the patient supine or in a slight Trendelenburg's position with the insertion site exposed.

• Put on a mask, and help the doctor to put on a sterile gown, mask, and gloves. If catheter placement will be guided by fluoroscopy, the doctor must wear a lead apron under the sterile gown. You should also put one on. Place a mask over the patient's nose and mouth, if desired.

• Open the supplies as ordered, or assist with the opening of the prepackaged introducer material, maintaining sterile technique.

• Clean the top of the local anesthetic bottle with an alcohol sponge, and invert it *so the doctor can insert the syringe and withdraw the drug.*

• Connect the pressure tubing to the proximal and distal catheter lumens, as ordered. Using the pressure tubing fast-flush device, flush each lumen. The doctor will inflate the balloon and verify its integrity before catheter insertion.

• Once all lines are prepared, the doctor will insert the catheter via the introducer. The balloon is inflated intermittently *to allow normal blood flow and to aid catheter insertion.*

• As the doctor advances the catheter, monitor pressure and ECG tracings *to help locate the catheter if it accidentally moves backward from the pulmonary artery (especially into the right ventricle, which may cause arrhythmias).*

• After the doctor sutures the catheter, put on sterile gloves and apply povidone-iodine ointment to the insertion site *to reduce the risk of infection.*

• Apply a dry, occlusive dressing — either sterile gauze or a transparent dressing — to the site. Then use tape to secure the catheter to the dressing *to prevent accidental dislodgment.*

• If the line was inserted into the antecubital fossa, apply a padded armboard *to keep the arm from bending.*

• Write the date, time, and your initials on a piece of tape and place it on the dressing.

• Remove all used or unnecessary equipment from the room, and properly discard all disposable equipment. Send reusable equipment for sterilization.

• If ordered, arrange for a chest X-ray at the patient's bedside *to verify correct catheter placement.*

To take a PAP reading

• Make sure all the stopcocks are set properly.

• Observe the monitor for pulmonary artery systolic and diastolic waveforms, and obtain waveform strips *for documentation and baseline reference.*

• Record the systolic and diastolic waveform and mean values. Some monitors record these continuously; some require manual setting.

To take a PCWP reading

• Make sure the machine is set to monitor mean pressure.

• To the balloon port, attach a syringe (of the size specified on the catheter shaft) filled with the maximum amount of air (usually 1.0 to 1.5 cc).

• Slowly inject the air from the syringe into the balloon while observing the monitor screen. Inject only until the PAP waveform changes to the PCWP waveform. *The PCWP waveform often occurs before the maximum amount of air is injected — depending on the size of the pulmonary artery.*

• Record the mean pressure.

• Remove the syringe, and leave the port lock in the open position *to allow air to escape and to prevent the balloon from remaining inflated accidentally.*

• Check the waveform on the monitor screen *to verify that the catheter has returned to a pulmonary artery position.*

• According to hospital policy, activate the fast-flush release to flush the catheter, *which helps reposition the catheter tip.*

• Set the high and low alarms as required by hospital policy.

Special considerations

Use aseptic technique throughout the procedure *to avoid infection.* Prevent exsanguination from a disconnection in the system by using luer-locks or other positive locks at all connections, keeping the catheter and all parts of the system unobscured, and making sure the monitor and alarms are on at all times. Always observe electrical-hazard precautions. (For further information, see *Identifying hemodynamic pressure monitoring problems,* pages 360 and 361.)

Activate the fast-flush release at intervals specified by the hospital's policy *to prevent thrombus formation.*

Frequently check the involved extremity, if applicable, for pulse, color, temperature, and sensation. Notify the doctor of any changes.

Change the catheter dressing at each tubing change, when it becomes wet or soiled, or at intervals specified by hospital policy.

Take PAP and PCWP readings at the end of expiration. To do this, assess the patient's chest, noting when he completely exhales because *when he inhales, intrathoracic pressure drops, causing a decline in cardiac pressures. When he exhales, intrathoracic pressure rises causing a slight elevation of cardiac pressures. Because of this, the pressure at the end of expiration is the best indicator of normal cardiac pressures without respiratory interference.*

To prevent infection, change tubing, stopcocks, continuous flush devices, and fluid for infusion every 24 to 72 hours, depending on hospital policy.

Besides monitoring arterial pressures, you can also monitor CVP, if ordered. To do so, set the stopcocks to allow direct communication between the proximal lumen and the transducer; set the monitor to mean; observe the waveform; and record the CVP measurement. Return the stopcocks to their original positions.

Positive pressure ventilation may alter the patient's reading in any direction. Pressures should be recorded with the patient on the ventilator.

Dextrose 5% in water is sometimes used as the I.V. solution *because it's not a plasma expander and doesn't conduct electric current.*

◆ *Nursing alert.* During catheter insertion, alert the doctor immediately if the patient experiences arrhythmias, dyspnea, tachypnea, hemoptysis, stridor, or drastic changes in vital signs or pressure readings. These may indicate cardiac perforation, pulmonary artery rupture, hemorrhage, pneumothorax, or hemothorax. ◆

Note the volume of air needed to achieve a wedge. If the volume of air needed is significantly below that indicated on the catheter, notify the doctor *because the catheter may have migrated distally.* You should feel resistance when inflating the balloon. If you don't, notify the doctor immediately—the balloon may have ruptured.

◆ *Nursing alert.* Never introduce air into a balloon if you suspect it's ruptured; this can cause an air embolus. Prevent balloon rupture by knowing the maximum volume of the balloon, and avoid overinflating the balloon or aspirating from it. Don't leave the balloon wedged for more than 15 to 30 seconds. Air in the flush system can also cause an embolus. ◆

If the waveform won't return to PAP from PCWP, or if it's damping with low numbers and decreased pulmonary artery systolic-diastolic differential, check for equipment problems. Then check the patient's blood pressure and pulse rate. If these aren't changed, the catheter is probably wedged. Because a permanent wedge can cause pulmonary infarct and necrosis, flush the PAP port *to push the catheter tip away from a vessel wall.* (Don't activate the fast-flush release, which could rupture capillaries.) Then check for a slowed drip rate and increased pressure readings—signs that the catheter is still wedged. If it is, turn the patient on his right side, and instruct him to cough as you flush the line. If the waveform doesn't return to the PAP area, turn the patient onto his left side and repeat the procedure. If there's still no change, notify the doctor immediately.

Avoid administering large volumes of fluid and drugs through the distal port *because vessel spasm or rupture may result.*

Complications

Various complications can occur during hemodynamic monitoring. These include infection, air embolism, pulmonary artery perforation, ventricular arrhythmias, tricuspid or pulmonic valve damage, and tension pneumothorax, which may occur during insertion. (See *Risks of using arterial lines,* Chapter 6.)

Documentation

Record the time, size, and type of catheter inserted, insertion site, vital signs, administration of drugs (if any), initial PAP and PCWP readings and tracings, and the patient's tolerance of the procedure. Start a flowchart of PAP· readings and tracings, noting any changes.

 Central venous pressure monitoring

Measurements of central venous pressure (CVP) are monitored with a manometer connected to a catheter that's threaded through the subclavian or jugular vein (or through the basilic, cephalic, or saphenous veins) and placed in or near the right atrium. This procedure accurately determines right atrial pressure, which reflects right ventricular pressure and the pumping ability of the right side of the heart. CVP is also used to assess blood volume and vascular tone.

Because CVP rises only after significant changes have occurred in the left heart or pulmonary venous system, CVP monitoring has been replaced in most hospitals by pulmonary artery catheterization for assessing rapidly changing cardiovascular status. Pulmonary artery catheterization uses pulmonary artery pressure and pulmonary capillary wedge pressure to detect cardiovascular

(Text continues on page 362.)

Identifying hemodynamic pressure monitoring problems

PROBLEM	POSSIBLE CAUSES	INTERVENTIONS
No waveform	• Power supply turned off • Monitor screen pressure range set too low • Loose connection in line • Transducer not connected to amplifier • Stopcock off to patient • Catheter occluded or out of blood vessel	• Check power supply. • Raise monitor screen pressure range, if necessary. • Rebalance and recalibrate equipment. • Tighten loose connections. • Check and tighten connection. • Position stopcock correctly. • Use fast-flush valve to flush line, or try to aspirate blood from catheter. If the line remains blocked, notify the doctor and prepare to replace the line.
Drifting waveforms	• Improper warm-up • Electrical cable kinked or compressed • Temperature change in room air or I.V. flush solution	• Allow monitor and transducer to warm up for 10 to 15 minutes. • Place monitor's cable where it can't be stepped on or compressed. • Routinely zero and calibrate equipment 30 minutes after setting it up. This allows I.V. fluid to warm to room temperature.
Line fails to flush	• Stopcocks positioned incorrectly • Inadequate pressure from pressure bag • Kink in pressure tubing • Blood clot in catheter	• Make sure stopcocks are positioned correctly. • Make sure pressure bag gauge reads 300 mm Hg. • Check pressure tubing for kinks. • Try to aspirate the clot with a syringe. If the line still won't flush, notify the doctor and prepare to replace the line, if necessary. *Important:* Never use a syringe to flush a hemodynamic line.
Artifact (waveform interference)	• Patient movement • Electrical interference • Catheter fling (tip of pulmonary artery catheter moving rapidly in large blood vessel or heart chamber)	• Wait until the patient is quiet before taking a reading. • Make sure electrical equipment is connected and grounded correctly. • Notify the doctor. He may try to reposition the catheter.
False-high readings	• Transducer balancing port positioned below patient's right atrium • Flush solution flow rate is too fast • Air in system • Catheter fling (tip of pulmonary artery catheter moving rapidly in large blood vessel or heart chamber)	• Position balancing port level with the patient's right atrium. • Check flush solution flow rate. Maintain it at 3 to 4 ml/hour. • Remove air from the lines and the transducer. • Notify the doctor, who may try to reposition the catheter.

Identifying hemodynamic pressure monitoring problems *(continued)*

PROBLEM	POSSIBLE CAUSES	INTERVENTIONS
False-low readings	• Transducer balancing port positioned above right atrium • Transducer imbalance • Loose connection	• Position balancing port level with the patient's right atrium. • Make sure the transducer's flow system isn't kinked or occluded and rebalance and recalibrate the equipment. • Tighten loose connections.
Damped waveform	• Air bubbles • Blood clot in catheter • Blood flashback in line • Transducer position • Arterial catheter out of blood vessel or pressed against vessel wall	• Secure all connections. • Remove air from lines and transducer. • Check for and replace cracked equipment. • Refer to "Line fails to flush" (this chart). • Make sure stopcock positions are correct; tighten loose connections and replace cracked equipment; flush line with fast-flush valve; replace the transducer dome if blood backs up into it. • Make sure the transducer is kept at the level of the right atrium at all times. Improper levels give false-high or false-low pressure readings. • Reposition if the catheter is against vessel wall. • Try to aspirate blood to confirm proper placement in the vessel. If you can't aspirate blood, notify the doctor and prepare to replace the line. *Note:* Bloody drainage at the insertion site may indicate catheter displacement. Notify the doctor immediately.
Pulmonary artery wedge pressure tracing unobtainable	• Ruptured balloon • Incorrect amount of air in balloon • Catheter malpositioned	• If you feel no resistance when injecting air, or if you see blood leaking from the balloon inflation lumen, stop injecting air and notify the doctor. If the catheter is left in, label the inflation lumen with a warning not to inflate. • Deflate the balloon. Check label on catheter for correct volume. Reinflate slowly with correct amount. To avoid rupturing the balloon, never use more than the stated volume. • Notify the doctor. Obtain chest X-ray.

Interpreting CVP findings

To interpret pressure readings correctly, establish a normal central venous pressure (CVP) for the patient. The average CVP may range between 3 and 15 cm H_2O or mm Hg, but it varies from patient to patient. To establish a normal range, measure CVP at 15-, 30-, and 60-minute intervals.

What to do if readings vary

If a reading differs from the established range by more than 2 cm H_2O, double-check it by taking vital signs and assessing the patient's cardiopulmonary status.

If these appear stable, check the I.V. line for patency and review the measurement procedure. Remember, a blocked line can cause a false-low reading. Notify the doctor if you're sure the abnormal reading reflects actual CVP and if CVP deviates from the range set for the patient.

Importance of CVP measurements

Don't rely on vital signs to reflect stable cardiovascular states; regular CVP measurements can detect disorders before changes in vital signs are apparent. For example, a high CVP reading may signal congestive heart failure, hypervolemia, vasoconstriction, or early stage cardiac tamponade; a low reading may signal peripheral blood pooling, hypovolemia, vasoconstriction, or vasodilation.

If the CVP changes significantly, the doctor will probably order a chest X-ray to detect possible disorders or to detect possible migration of the catheter tip.

changes. CVP measurements can be obtained directly from the pulmonary artery catheter.

CVP is measured in millimeters of mercury or centimeters of water. The normal range varies with the patient's size, position, and hydration state. (See *Interpreting CVP findings*.)

Equipment

Disposable CVP manometer set with stopcock, extension tubing, and leveling rod or yardstick ▪ I.V. pole ▪ I.V. solution, as ordered ▪ I.V. tubing ▪ tape.

Preparation of equipment

Gather the appropriate equipment and wash your hands. Clamp the manometer to the I.V. pole, spike the I.V. container, and hang it 30″ to 36″ (76.2 to 91.4 cm) above the insertion site *to prevent blood from backing up in the catheter.*

Now examine the stopcock *to learn the proper operating positions.* (See *Stopcock positioning and operation.*)

Next, insert the distal end of the tubing into the left side of the stopcock. Turn the stopcock to the container-to-patient position, open the flow clamp, and flush the tubing. Then turn the stopcock to the container-to-manometer position. Make sure the tubing doesn't contain an in-line filter, which can distort pressure readings. Fill the manometer column with I.V. solution (about 20 to 25 cm H_2O or about 10 cm H_2O higher than the expected CVP value). Then close the flow clamp on the tubing. Avoid overfilling the manometer *to prevent inactivation of the filter and increased risk of contamination; also, if a small plastic ball is used to indicate fluid level in the manometer, it may be forced from the tube and rendered useless.*

Implementation

● Explain the procedure to the patient *to allay his fears and promote cooperation.*
● Loosen the protective cover on the distal end of the extension tubing (from the stopcock to the patient), and ask the patient to perform the Valsalva's maneuver *to avoid formation of an air embolus.* Quickly disconnect the existing I.V. tubing, remove the protective covering from the new tubing, and connect it to the patient's catheter.
● If the patient is unconscious, wait until he inhales fully, and then quickly connect the tubing. Lowering the head of the bed also helps prevent an air embolus in a patient unable to cooperate. If the patient is intubated, maintain full inflation as you connect the tubing. Finally, adjust the flow clamp to the desired infusion rate.
● Place the patient in a supine position (his head can be slightly raised). He doesn't need to be kept flat. *Studies show this to be unnecessary for accurate monitoring as long as the zero mark on the manometer remains at the zero reference point and the patient's position stays the same for each reading.*
● Adjust the position of the manometer so that the stopcock aligns horizontally with the right atrium.
● *To find the position of the right atrium,* locate the fourth intercostal space at the midaxillary line (phlebostatic axis). This site becomes the zero reference point—the location for all subsequent readings.
● If the manometer has a leveling rod, extend it between the zero reference point and the zero mark at the bottom of the manometer scale. If the rod has a small viewing window, a bubble will appear between two lines in the

Stopcock positioning and operation

To ensure accurate central venous pressure readings, the base of the manometer must be aligned with the right atrium. For this reason, the manometer set usually contains a leveling rod to allow you to determine quickly that the base of the manometer is level with the previously determined zero reference point.

After adjusting the manometer's position, examine the typical three-way stopcock. By turning it to any position shown, you can control the direction of fluid flow. Four-way stopcocks are also available; the fourth position blocks all openings.

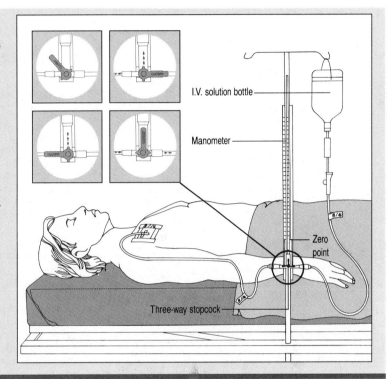

window when the rod is horizontal. If a leveling rod isn't available, use a yardstick with a level attached. With this, you can also watch the bubble for the level.

• When the stopcock of the manometer is level with the right atrium, tape the manometer set to the I.V. pole *to secure its position.* Recheck the level before each pressure reading. If an adjustment is required, first raise or lower the bed and then readjust the manometer on the I.V. pole as necessary *to maintain alignment with the atrium.*

• Check the patency of the line by briefly increasing the infusion rate. If the line is not patent, notify the doctor. Never irrigate a clogged CVP line. *This avoids possible release of a thrombus.* If the line is patent, proceed.

• Turn the stopcock to the container-to-manometer position *to slowly fill the manometer with I.V. solution, as before.*

• Turn the stopcock to the manometer-to-patient position; the fluid level then falls with inspiration, as intrathoracic pressure decreases, and rises slightly with expiration.

• When the fluid column stabilizes, tap the manometer lightly *to dislodge air bubbles that may distort pressure readings.* Then position yourself so that the top of the fluid column is at eye level. Expect the column to rise and fall slightly during breathing. Note the *lowest* level the fluid reaches, and take your reading from the base of the meniscus. If the manometer has a small ball floating on the fluid surface, take the reading from the ball's midline. If the fluid fails to fluctuate during breathing, *the end of the catheter may be pressed against the vein wall.* Ask the patient to cough *to change the catheter's position slightly.*

• Maintain catheter patency by returning the stopcock to the container-to-patient position as soon as you take the reading. Then check for blood backflow.

• Readjust the infusion rate and be sure that all connections are secure *to minimize the risk of hemorrhage or an air embolus.* (Some hospital policies recommend taping all connections for these reasons.)

• Return the patient to a comfortable position.

Other methods for measuring cardiac output

In the *Fick method,* the blood's oxygen content is measured before and after it passes through the lungs. First, blood is removed from the pulmonary and the brachial arteries and analyzed for oxygen content. Then, a spirometer measures oxygen consumption — the amount of air entering the lungs each minute. Next, cardiac output (CO) is calculated using this formula:

$$CO \ (liter/minute) = \frac{oxygen\ consumption\ (ml/min)}{arterial\ oxygen\ content - venous\ oxygen\ content\ (ml/min)}$$

The Fick method is especially useful in detecting low cardiac output levels.

In the *dye dilution test,* a known volume and concentration of dye is injected into the pulmonary artery and measured by simultaneously sampling the amount of dye in the brachial artery. To calculate cardiac output, these values are entered into a formula or plotted into a time and dilution-concentration curve. A computer, similar to the one used for the thermodilution test, performs the computation. Dye dilution measurements are particularly helpful in detecting intracardiac shunts and valvular regurgitation.

Special considerations

If the patient is connected to a ventilator and is receiving positive end-expiratory pressure, you may obtain variable CVP readings. *To detect significant changes,* record all pressure readings while the patient is connected to the ventilator, and take readings at end-expiration before the next inspiration begins. However, if the patient's condition permits, some hospitals allow you to disconnect the ventilator for all CVP readings and reconnect it immediately after the procedure.

Report any deviations from the prescribed CVP range to the doctor. Avoid making pressure observations when the patient is sitting up *because this position causes false-low measurements if the patient has been put in a sitting position within 3 minutes of your manometer reading.* Remember that the patient with chronic obstructive pulmonary disease usually has a high CVP.

Documentation

Record the time, date, and pressure reading. If the patient was placed in a special position, note this on the nursing Kardex to ensure consistent readings.

 # Cardiac output measurement

Measuring cardiac output — the amount of blood ejected from the heart — helps evaluate cardiac function. Normal output is 4 to 8 liters/minute. Low cardiac output can be caused by decreased myocardial contractility from myocardial infarction, drug effects, acidosis, or hypoxia. Other possible causes include decreased left ventricular filling pressure from fluid depletion or increased systemic vascular resistance related to arteriosclerosis or hypertension. Output can also fall below normal as a result of decreased blood flow from the ventricles in valvular heart disease.

High cardiac output can occur with some arteriovenous shunts and from decreased vascular resistance (for example, in septic shock), or it can be unusually high but still normal (for example, in well-conditioned athletes).

Cardiac output is measured indirectly by the thermodilution method. Other methods include the Fick method and the dye dilution test, although these are usually confined to research projects or the cardiac catheterization laboratory. (See *Other methods for measuring cardiac output.*)

In the thermodilution method, a balloon-tipped, flow-directed catheter is inserted into a large vein, advanced to the right side of the heart, and positioned in the pulmonary artery. A solution is injected into the proximal or right atrium port of the pulmonary artery catheter. A computer then calculates the cardiac output from temperature changes in the injected solution in the proximal lumen and the temperature of the pulmonary artery. (See *Closed cardiac output systems.*)

Equipment

Cardiac output machine (portable or within the monitoring system) ▪ bag of 500 ml dextrose 5% in water ▪ closed injection system ▪ 10-ml syringe ▪ stopcocks ▪ optional: equipment for icing injectant.

Preparation of equipment

Gather all the equipment and bring it to the patient's bedside.

Closed cardiac output systems

This illustration shows the equipment needed to measure cardiac output, using a closed injectant delivery system. First, an iced or room-temperature solution is injected into the proximal or right atrium port of the pulmonary artery catheter.

A computer then calculates the cardiac output from temperature changes in the injected material in the proximal lumen and the temperature at the pulmonary artery. The thermistor on the catheter tip measures the temperature at the pulmonary artery. The computer displays the cardiac output as a digital readout.

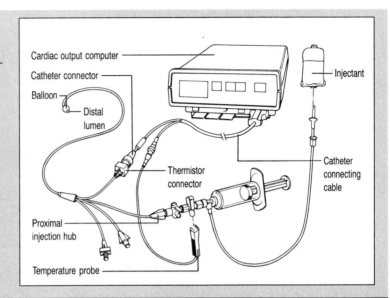

Implementation

• Wash your hands. Explain the procedure to the patient. Tell him that you'll be injecting a solution into the catheter in his heart. Tell him that this will help determine how well his heart is pumping. Assure him that he won't feel any discomfort.
• Place the patient in the supine position (his head can be slightly elevated).
• Attach the thermistor tubing from the cardiac output machine to the thermistor port on the pulmonary artery catheter. *This should accurately measure the patient's core temperature.*
• Attach the temperature probe from the cardiac output machine to the appropriate area on the proximal port *to measure the temperature of the injectant.*
• Before injecting the ordered solution, ensure that the catheter is not in the wedge position *because this position can trigger a false-high reading and damage the pulmonary artery.*
• Remove the stopcock cap and connect the syringe to the stopcock on the proximal lumen so that the syringe and the catheter lumen are in a straight line. Open the stopcock *to instill the injectant as described below.* Using aseptic technique, replace the syringe after each injection.

• If you're using a closed system, spike the 500-ml bag of dextrose 5% in water and prime the system. Connect the leur-lock end of the system to the proximal lumen of the pulmonary artery catheter so that the syringe and the catheter lumen are in a straight line. The closed system should remain in place at all times *to reduce the risk of contamination.* One or more stopcocks may be used between the catheter and the closed system.
• Turn the computer on and calibrate it, if necessary, according to the manufacturer's directions.
• Open the clamp on the closed system and fill the syringe from the bag of dextrose 5% in water.
• Open the stopcock to the patient, and verify that READY appears on the computer. Depress the start button. Inject the solution with one smooth, rapid motion (within 4 seconds). Inject 5 to 10 ml for an adult and 3 ml for a child. Cardiac output values will be displayed on the computer screen. Repeat the procedure two more times, waiting 1 minute between each injection.
• Calculate the average of the three measurements to determine cardiac output.

Understanding pacemaker codes

A permanent pacemaker's three-letter (or sometimes five-letter) code simply refers to how it's programmed.

First letter (chamber that's paced)	**Second letter** (chamber that's sensed)	**Third letter** (how pulse generator responds)
A = atrium	A = atrium	I = inhibited
V = ventricle	V = ventricle	T = triggered
D = dual (both chambers)	D = dual (both chambers)	D = dual (inhibited and triggered)
O = not applicable	O = not applicable	O = not applicable

Examples of two common programming codes:

DDD	VVI
Pace: atrium and ventricle	Pace: ventricle
Sense: atrium and ventricle	Sense: ventricle
Response: inhibited and triggered	Response: inhibited
This is a fully automatic, or universal, pacemaker.	This is a demand pacemaker, inhibited.

• Return all stopcocks to the original positions. With the system closed, verify that the clamp on the injection system is also closed.

Special considerations
If ordered, calculate the cardiac index—divide cardiac output by body surface area. This is a more specific measurement than cardiac output alone. The normal range is 2.5 to 4.2 liters/minute.

You can also use cardiac output data to calculate the systemic vascular resistance and determine the effectiveness of medications.

Although many hospitals ice the injectant before injection, this is usually not necessary if there is a 10° difference between the patient's temperature and that of the room air or the injectant. (The injectant should be at 0° to 4° C to obtain greatest accuracy.) At times, you may need to ice the injectant for a short period to troubleshoot the equipment; refer to the manufacturer's directions.

Documentation
Record the average cardiac output and related calculations. Document the amount and type of injectant used on the intake and output record. Also note the patient's tolerance for the procedure.

TREATMENT
Permanent pacemaker insertion and care

Designed to operate for 3 to 20 years, a permanent pacemaker is self-contained. The surgeon implants the device in a pocket beneath the patient's skin. This is usually done in the operating room or cardiac catheterization laboratory. Nursing responsibilities involve monitoring the electrocardiogram (ECG) and maintaining sterile technique.

Today, permanent pacemakers function in the demand mode, allowing the patient's heart to beat on its own but preventing it from falling below a preset rate. Pacing electrodes can be placed in the atria, in the ventricles, or in both chambers (AV sequential, dual chamber). (See *Understanding pacemaker codes.*)

Candidates for permanent pacemakers include patients with myocardial infarction and persistent bradyarrhythmia and patients with complete heart block or slow ventricular rates stemming from congenital or degenerative heart disease or cardiac surgery. Patients who suffer Stokes-Adams attacks, as well as those with Wolff-Parkinson-White syndrome or "sick sinus syndrome," may also benefit from permanent pacemaker implantation.

Equipment

Sphygmomanometer ■ stethoscope ■ thermometer ■ ECG monitor (with oscilloscope and strip-chart recorder) ■ sterile dressing tray ■ povidone-iodine ointment ■ shaving supplies with razor ■ sterile gauze dressing ■ nonallergenic tape ■ antibiotics ■ analgesics ■ sedatives ■ alcohol sponges ■ emergency resuscitation equipment ■ sterile gown and mask ■ optional: I.V. line for emergency medications.

Implementation

• Explain the procedure to the patient. Provide and review literature from the manufacturer or the American Heart Association so that he can learn about the pacemaker and how it works. Emphasize that the pacemaker merely augments his natural heart rate.
• Ensure that the patient or a responsible family member signs a consent form, and ask the patient if he's allergic to anesthetics or iodine.

Preoperative care

• For transvenous pacemaker insertion, shave the patient's chest from the axilla to the midline and from the clavicle to the nipple line on the side selected by the doctor. If the pacemaker is to be inserted in the axilla, shave that area; for epicardial placement, shave from the nipple line to the umbilicus.
• Establish an I.V. line at a keep-vein-open rate *to administer emergency drugs in case of ventricular arrhythmia.*
• Establish baseline vital signs and a baseline ECG recording.
• Provide sedation, as ordered.

In the operating room

• If you'll be present to monitor arrhythmias during the procedure, put on a gown and mask.
• Help the patient assume a supine position. Have emergency resuscitation equipment on hand.
• Connect the ECG monitor to the patient and run a baseline rhythm strip. Make sure the machine has enough paper to run additional rhythm strips during the procedure. Leave the monitor screen on throughout the procedure.
• During *transvenous* placement, the doctor, guided by a fluoroscope, passes the electrode catheter through the cephalic or external jugular vein and positions it under the trabeculae in the apex of the right ventricle. He then attaches the catheter to the pulse generator, inserts this into a pocket of subcutaneous tissue in the patient's chest wall, and sutures it closed, leaving a small outlet for a drainage tube.
• During *epicardial* placement, the doctor may apply the electrodes directly to the myocardium after he performs

a thoracotomy. In this procedure, the doctor inserts the generator beneath the skin in the subcostal area. If the patient had a temporary pacemaker, the doctor will probably leave it in for 24 hours after the insertion of the permanent implant *in case the new pacemaker doesn't function properly.*

Postoperative care

• Monitor the patient's ECG *to check for arrhythmias and to ensure correct pacemaker functioning.*
• Also monitor the I.V. flow rate; the I.V. line is usually kept in place for 24 to 48 hours postoperatively *to allow for possible emergency treatment of arrhythmias.*
• Check the dressing for signs of bleeding and infection (swelling, redness, or exudate). The doctor may order prophylactic antibiotics for up to 7 days after the implantation.
• Change the dressing and apply povidone-iodine ointment at least once every 24 to 48 hours, or according to doctor's orders and hospital policy. If the dressing becomes soiled or the site is exposed to air, change the dressing immediately, regardless of when you last changed it.
• Check the patient's vital signs and level of consciousness (LOC) every 15 minutes for the first hour, every hour for the next 4 hours, every 4 hours for the next 48 hours, and then once every shift. (Confused, elderly patients with second-degree heart block will not show immediate improvement in LOC.)
◆ *Nursing alert.* Watch for signs and symptoms of a perforated ventricle, with resultant cardiac tamponade: persistent hiccups, distant heart sounds, pulsus paradoxus, hypotension with narrow pulse pressure, increased venous pressure, cyanosis, distended neck veins, decreased urine output, restlessness, or complaints of fullness in the chest. If any of these develop, notify the doctor immediately. ◆
• Relieve patient discomfort with analgesics, as ordered.
• Teach the patient how to take his own pulse rate daily before he's discharged from the hospital. Make sure he understands that he must take a resting pulse rate. Tell him what constitutes an acceptable and unacceptable discrepancy between pulse readings and whom to call if the discrepancy is unacceptable. The lower rate limit is usually 5 beats/minute below the pulse generator setting; the upper limit is usually 90 to 100 beats/minute.

Special considerations

If the patient is a hunter, the doctor usually places the pacemaker battery on the side opposite the one where the gun is held *to avoid damaging it during recoil.* If the patient wears a hearing aid, the pacemaker battery is placed on the opposite side accordingly.

Teaching the patient who has a permanent pacemaker

Teach the patient being discharged with a new, permanent pacemaker about its care and the prevention of complications.

Wound care
Instruct the patient to keep the incision clean and dry and to watch for signs of infection (redness, swelling, draining, warmth, or tenderness). Urge him to follow the doctor's orders about dressing-change procedures. Advise him to wear loose-fitting clothing over the incision until it's healed.

Medications
Tell the patient to take his heart medication exactly as prescribed. Explain that this medication along with his pacemaker ensures a regular heartbeat.

When to call the doctor
Teach the patient to take his pulse daily, at rest, for a full 60 seconds. If he observes a dramatic increase or decrease in his pulse rate, he should contact the doctor. He should also call the doctor if he experiences extreme weakness, chest pain, or shortness of breath.

Precautions
Tell the patient always to carry a card or documents describing the type and rate of his pacemaker. Advise him to avoid strong magnetic fields, such as those produced by magnetic resonance imaging. Electrocautery may also interfere with pacing. To avoid damage from radiation therapy, cover the pacemaker with a lead shield during treatments, and check pacemaker function afterward. Although pacemakers are now adequately shielded from the effects of microwave ovens, advise the patient to avoid standing near the oven while it's operating.

Because the patient's pacemaker may activate airport security devices, advise the patient to alert security personnel that he has a pacemaker. If he has a nuclear pacemaker, he'll need to inform the Nuclear Regulatory Commission (NRC) if he plans to travel abroad.

Provide the patient with an identification card that lists the pacemaker type and manufacturer, serial number, pacemaker rate setting, date implanted, and the doctor's name. (For more information, see *Teaching the patient who has a permanent pacemaker.*)

Watch for signs of pacemaker malfunction.

Complications
After epicardial placement, the patient risks the complications associated with thoracotomy and general anesthesia. Complications of transvenous placement include thrombus and embolus formation and cardiac tamponade, owing to perforation of the ventricular wall.

Both methods of implantation may cause infection or arrhythmia. Other complications involving the pacemaker itself, such as battery failure or a displaced electrode wire, are the same as for a temporary pacemaker.

Documentation
Document the type of pacemaker used, the serial number and the manufacturer's name, the pacing rate, the date of implantation, and the doctor's name. Note whether the pacemaker successfully treated the patient's arrhythmias, and include other pertinent observations, such as the condition of the incision site.

Temporary pacemaker placement and care

Usually performed as an emergency procedure, temporary pacemaker placement may be indicated for symptomatic bradycardia or tachyarrhythmias. A temporary pacemaker consists of a battery-powered pulse generator that the patient wears on his chest, waist, or upper arm. An electrode catheter transmits electrical impulses from the pacemaker to the patient's heart and from the heart back to the pacemaker.

Two types of pacemakers are available. The *fixed-rate pacemaker* fires continuously, regardless of the patient's heart rate, while the more common *demand pacemaker* senses the patient's own rate and fires if that rate drops below a preset limit.

To help place the lead wires, the doctor may use fluoroscopy. In transvenous pacing, the doctor inserts the electrode catheter into the brachial, femoral, subclavian, or jugular vein and advances it into the right ventricle. In transthoracic pacing, he inserts the electrode catheter through the chest wall and into the right ventricle. Transthoracic pacing is usually done in the operating room as part of an open-chest procedure or during cardiac arrest.

Once in the right ventricle, the electrode catheter sends an impulse to the ventricular myocardium, causing ventricular depolarization. If the patient needs atrial pacing alone or in conjunction with ventricular pacing to keep his cardiac output within normal limits, the doctor can place a special temporary electrode in the right atrium.

To maintain normal heart rate until an electrode catheter can be placed transvenously, the doctor or a specially prepared nurse may use transcutaneous (or external) pacing. In this procedure, a pulse generator sends electrical impulses to the heart through two electrode pads placed on the front and back of the patient's chest. Although transcutaneous pacing is quick and noninvasive, it's only used temporarily until pacing can be achieved transvenously.

Equipment
For all temporary pacing: crash cart with emergency drugs and resuscitation equipment ▪ cardiac monitor with strip-chart recorder ▪ equipment for inserting I.V. line and fluids (if patient doesn't have I.V. line in place) ▪ temporary pacemaker generator ▪ electrode catheter ▪ adhesive tape ▪ sterile gloves ▪ sterile dressings ▪ povidone-iodine solution ▪ nonconducting tape or rubber surgical glove ▪ optional: elastic bandage or gauze strips, restraints.

For transvenous pacing: bridging cable ▪ 10-volt battery ▪ shaving kit ▪ guide wire or introducer ▪ sterile gowns ▪ linen-saver pad ▪ alcohol sponges ▪ vial of 1% lidocaine ▪ 5-ml syringe ▪ fluoroscopy equipment, if necessary ▪ fenestrated drape ▪ prepackaged cutdown tray (for antecubital vein placement only) ▪ receptacle for infectious wastes.

For transthoracic pacing: transthoracic needle.

For transcutaneous pacing: transcutaneous pacing generator ▪ transcutaneous pacing electrodes ▪ cardiac monitor ▪ shaving supplies.

Many hospitals use prepackaged trays that contain most, but not all, of the equipment needed.

Preparation of equipment
Set out all appropriate equipment for the specific procedure. For transvenous pacing, connect the bridging cable to the generator, aligning the positive and negative poles. Place a table for sterile supplies and a receptacle for infectious wastes nearby.

Implementation
• If applicable, explain the procedure to the patient. Then follow the steps as outlined below.

For all temporary pacing
• Make sure the patient or a family member signs a consent form before the procedure. (For transvenous pacing, also check the patient's history for hypersensitivity to the local anesthetic.)
• Attach the cardiac monitor to the patient if it's not yet attached.
• Obtain baseline vital signs and an electrocardiogram (ECG) reading.
• Insert an I.V. line if not already present. Begin an I.V. infusion of dextrose 5% water at a keep-vein-open rate.
• Insert a new battery into the pacemaker generator and test it.

For transvenous pacing
• Ensure that the patient lies supine on the table or bed.
• Connect the bridging cable to the generator, and align the positive and negative poles. *This cable allows slack between the electrode catheter and the generator, reducing the risk of accidental catheter displacement.*
• Place a linen-saver pad under the catheter insertion site. If necessary, shave or clip the hair around the insertion site.
• Maintaining a sterile field, open the supply tray.
• Using sterile technique, wipe the skin at the insertion site with alcohol. Use a circular motion, wiping away from the center of the site. Clean a $4'' \times 4''$ area with povidone-iodine. (In some settings the doctor may do this.)
• Cover the insertion site with a fenestrated drape.
• Wipe the rubber stopper of the vial of lidocaine with an alcohol sponge. Then invert the vial *so the doctor can withdraw the anesthetic.*
• After the doctor anesthetizes the insertion site, he'll puncture the vein, insert a guide wire or an introducer, and advance the electrode catheter. As the catheter advances, watch the cardiac monitor. You should see large P waves and small QRS complexes when the electrode catheter reaches the right atrium, then smaller P waves and larger QRS complexes as it reaches the right ventricle. When the catheter touches the right ventricular endocardium, you'll see elevated ST segments and premature ventricular contractions.
• Assess the patient for jaw pain and earache, *which indicate that the electrode catheter has missed the superior vena cava and reached the neck instead.*
• Once the electrode catheter is in place, attach the catheter leads to the bridging cable, lining up the positive and negative poles.
• Set the pacemaker as ordered. (See *Learning about a temporary pacemaker,* page 370.)
• After the doctor sutures the catheter to the insertion site, put on sterile gloves. Cover the insertion site with

Learning about a temporary pacemaker

The three main parameters on a temporary pacemaker are rate, output, and sensitivity. These are set after the pacemaker is inserted. The *rate* is a value representing the number of times the pacemaker paces (or fires) per minute. The rate is based on the reason for pacing, the patient's intrinsic heart rate, and his response to various rates.

The *output* is the amount of charge or electrical stimulation given to the heart chamber each time the pacemaker fires. Expressed in milliamperes (mA), it's determined by testing the patient's ventricular threshold response—the smallest amount of charge needed to stimulate the heart to beat. This amount is also called the *capture level.* With a properly positioned pacemaker wire, the ventricular threshold is usually 0.5 to 1.5 mA. The output is set at two to three times the ventricular threshold because many factors, including the patient's position, can affect the threshold.

The *sensitivity* setting controls how well the pacemaker detects intrinsic electrical activity. It's measured in millivolts and is adjusted to allow either demand pacing (fires only when it senses no intrinsic electrical activity) or asynchronous (fixed) pacing, a rate that's maintained regardless of the intrinsic heartbeat.

The pulse generator should have a transparent removable cover so settings are visible but can't be actually altered. Check and record the threshold and sensitivity at least once daily while the pacemaker is in use, and make adjustments as ordered. If over time fibrous tissue forms around the wire tip, the output setting may need to be increased.

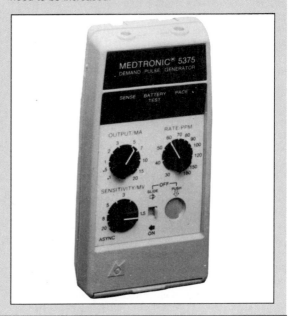

a dry, sterile dressing, and mark the dressing with the date and time.
• Secure the pulse generator to the patient's chest, waist, or upper arm with the fastening tape on the generator or with an elastic bandage or gauze strips.
• Place the cap supplied by the manufacturer over the pacer controls *to avoid an accidental setting change.*
• Assess the patient's vital signs and level of consciousness (LOC) *to determine how well he's tolerating the procedure.* Check the ECG monitor *to make sure the pacemaker is functioning properly.*
• Arrange for a chest X-ray *to check electrode placement.* You'll also need a 12-lead ECG reading as a baseline.
• If the doctor used a femoral or brachial approach, immobilize the patient's limb *to avoid putting stress on the pacing wires.* Tell the patient to wiggle his fingers or toes periodically *to prevent stiffness and to increase circulation.*

For transthoracic pacing
• Put on sterile gloves.
• Clean the skin to the left of the xiphoid process with povidone-iodine solution. Work quickly, *because cardiopulmonary resuscitation (CPR) must be interrupted for this procedure.*
• The doctor will insert a transthoracic needle through the chest wall to the left of the xiphoid process into the right ventricle, then follow it with the electrode catheter as shown on page 371 (top left).
• Connect the electrode catheter to the generator, lining up the positive and negative poles. Then look for signs of ventricular pacing and capture on the ECG monitor.
• The doctor will suture the electrode catheter into place.
• Using sterile technique, cover the insertion site with a sterile 4″ × 4″ dressing and tape. Mark it with the date and time.

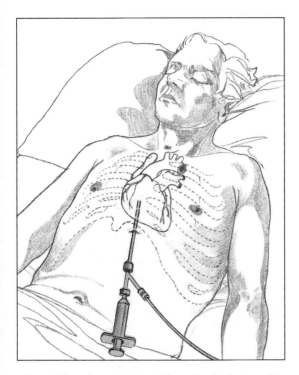

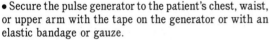

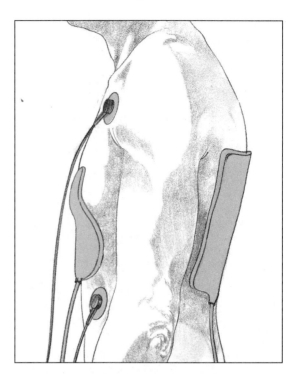

• Secure the pulse generator to the patient's chest, waist, or upper arm with the tape on the generator or with an elastic bandage or gauze.
• Check the patient's peripheral pulses and vital signs to assess his hemodynamic status. If you can't palpate a pulse, continue CPR.
• If you do detect a pulse, continue monitoring the patient.

For transcutaneous pacing
• If you're using a demand pacemaker, attach a lead to the generator.
• If necessary, shave or clip the hair over the areas where you'll place the electrodes.
• Place the electrode marked apex or positive on the left anterior chest at the fourth intercostal space just to the left of the sternum.
• Avoid placing it over the large pectoral muscle *because the resulting muscle stimulation can make the patient uncomfortable.*
• Place the second electrode on the patient's back, in the left subscapular area as shown above (top right).
• Connect the electrodes to the transcutaneous pacing generator.

• Set the output about halfway and turn on the generator.
• Look for pacemaker capture on the cardiac monitor. If you don't see it, increase the output until you do. If you see capture as soon as you turn the generator on, decrease the output until capture disappears and then increase it gradually until capture reappears. Usually, you can adjust the output to 10% above the level where capture was seen. *This keeps the patient from receiving too much stimulation, which could make him uncomfortable.*
• Watch the monitor to check that the pacemaker is working properly. You should see a pacing artifact and a QRS complex greater than 0.14 second followed by a T wave and, if appropriate, no sign of the underlying arrhythmia.
• Check the patient's vital signs, peripheral pulses, and LOC *to assess his response to pacing.*
• Continue monitoring the patient as you prepare him for transvenous pacing.

Special considerations
Make sure all electrical equipment is grounded. Also, insulate the pacemaker by covering all exposed metal parts, such as electrode connections and pacemaker terminals, with nonconducting tape, or place the pacing unit in a dry, rubber surgical glove. Tell the patient not to

Adverse effects of pacemaker placement

Temporary pacemaker placement can cause muscle stimulation, pneumothorax, ectopic beats, ventricular perforation, and perforation of other organs.

Muscle stimulation
If painful muscle stimulation occurs, the electrode may need to be moved away from the pectoral muscle without disturbing cardiac pacing.

Pneumothorax
If pacemaker insertion disrupts the pleural lining, you'll see signs of pneumothorax, such as severe shortness of breath, absent breath sounds on the affected side, and asymmetrical chest movement. If you suspect a pneumothorax, report it immediately. Obtain a chest X-ray, and prepare for chest tube insertion to relieve the pneumothorax, as ordered.

Ectopic beats
If the pacemaker leads irritate the myocardium, you'll see ectopic beats such as premature ventricular contractions (PVCs). If you see frequent PVCs on the cardiac monitor, notify the doctor and prepare emergency medications.

Ventricular perforation
Although a rare complication, perforation of the ventricle can cause life-threatening cardiac tamponade. The classic signs of cardiac tamponade — muffled heart sounds, neck vein distention, restlessness, hypotension, and pulsus paradoxus. The patient may also hiccup as the pacemaker stimulates his diaphragm. Report these signs immediately and anticipate surgery or pericardiocentesis.

Perforation of other organs
During a transthoracic approach, the needle may perforate the stomach, liver, or diaphragm. If it perforates the stomach or liver, the patient will show signs of shock and will need surgical repair of the organ. If the needle perforates the diaphragm, the patient will feel short of breath. A large tear requires surgical repair; smaller tears usually heal without surgery.

use an electric razor or any other nonessential electrical equipment.

If the patient is disoriented or uncooperative, use restraints to prevent accidental removal of pacemaker wires.

If the patient needs emergency defibrillation, make sure the pacemaker can withstand the procedure. If it can't, disconnect it *to avoid damaging the generator.*

Monitor the patient for signs and symptoms of infection, including redness and drainage at the insertion site, malaise, chills, and an increased white blood cell count. If you note such signs and symptoms, tell the doctor, who may order antibiotics. To help prevent infection, maintain sterile technique when changing the dressing.

Complications
The major complication of transcutaneous pacing is painful muscle stimulation. Temporary pacemaker placement can cause more serious complications. (See *Adverse effects of pacemaker placement.*)

Other complications can result from a pacemaker malfunction. A malfunction that causes the pacemaker to fire during the relative refractory phase of repolarization — particularly a failure to sense — can lead to fatal arrhythmias. (See *Identifying pacemaker failure.*)

Documentation
Record the reason for transcutaneous pacing, the time it started, and the locations of the electrodes. For a transvenous or transthoracic pacemaker, note the date, the time, and reason for the temporary pacemaker.

For any temporary pacemaker, record the pacemaker settings. Note the patient's response to the procedure, along with any complications and the interventions taken. If possible, obtain rhythm strips before, during, and after pacemaker placement, and whenever pacemaker settings are changed or when the patient receives treatment for a complication caused by the pacemaker. As you monitor the patient, record his response to temporary pacing and note any changes in his condition.

Code management

Managing a code in a hospital requires knowing the American Heart Association's procedures for basic life support (BLS) and advanced cardiac life support (ACLS). Basic life support includes both cardiopulmonary resuscitation (CPR) and foreign-body removal from an airway. The ACLS procedures treat the effects of a cardiac or respiratory arrest by establishing and maintaining ven-

Identifying pacemaker failure

Life-threatening arrhythmias can result when the patient's pacemaker sends an impulse too weak to stimulate the heart (failure to capture), fails to detect ventricular depolarization (failure to sense), or fails to send an impulse at all (failure to fire). Below are rhythm strips that compare these problems with a normal strip, as well as lists of possible causes and interventions.

Normal
The location of the spike is your first clue that the pacemaker is functioning normally.

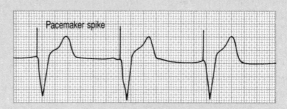

Failure to capture

Causes	Interventions
• Pacemaker output too low	• Increase pacemaker output.
• Catheter dislodged	• Reposition catheter.
• Loose connections	• Secure all connections.

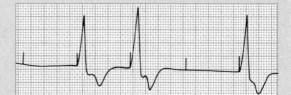

Failure to sense

Cause	Intervention
• Incorrect sensitivity setting	• Adjust sensitivity.

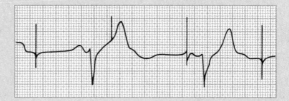

Failure to fire

Causes	Interventions
• Loose lead hookups	• Secure lead hookups.
• Dead battery	• Replace battery.
• Malfunctioning pulse generator	• Replace pulse generator.

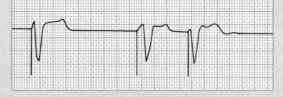

tilation and circulation. ACLS also focuses on recognizing and treating the immediate causes of arrest. It provides step-by-step guidelines for treating different arrhythmias, including such procedures as administering drugs, defibrillating, and establishing a patent airway.

Most hospitals have code teams that respond to respiratory and cardiac emergencies. Members of the code team come from several departments, including anes-thesia, respiratory therapy, electrocardiography, critical care, and I.V. therapy. Each team member has a specific role. Some team members may have standing orders to defibrillate and administer certain drugs.

Although ACLS requires the entire code team, a qualified nurse with standing orders can start several of the ACLS procedures, including defibrillation and drug administration. Once the patient's condition stabilizes, the underlying cause of the cardiac arrest is treated.

Equipment

Crash cart containing: manual resuscitation bag ■ supplemental oxygen supply ■ cardiac monitor ■ I.V. therapy equipment ■ electrodes ■ defibrillator ■ conductive jelly or paste, saline gel pads, or 4″ × 4″ gauze pads and saline solution ■ emergency medications ■ emergency airway equipment ■ laryngoscope ■ needles and syringes ■ dextrose 5% in water ■ cardiac arrest board ■ endotracheal tubes ■ suction equipment ■ nasogastric (NG) tube and water-soluble lubricant.

Preparation of equipment

Good emergency care often depends on the careful stocking of crash carts and a precise knowledge of their contents. Periodically review the equipment on the crash cart *so you don't waste time during a code.* Ensure that the expiration dates for the drugs haven't passed.

Implementation

• As the first nurse to arrive on the scene, you should assess the patient's level of consciousness and his ABCs: airway, breathing, and circulation.

• Call for help. When the second nurse arrives, ask her to call a code and get the crash cart.

• Place a hard surface, such as the headboard from the bed, under the patient and begin CPR. *The hard surface makes chest compressions more effective.* (See "Cardiopulmonary resuscitation" in this chapter.) When the crash cart arrives, replace the headboard with the cardiac arrest board from the cart.

• If you witnessed an arrest or if the cardiac monitor shows an arrest resulting from ventricular tachycardia or ventricular fibrillation, deliver a single precordial thump — a quick, sharp blow to the midsternum — *to try to convert the abnormal rhythm* even before your patient is attached to a cardiac monitor.

• The second nurse is responsible for breathing. She should attach the manual resuscitation bag to a supplemental oxygen source. She ventilates the patient with the bag while you continue chest compressions.

• A third nurse, who's responsible for circulation and cardiac care, should turn on the cardiac monitor. Then she will apply two electrodes, one in the hollow below each clavicle, and a third electrode at the fourth intercostal space at the left sternal border. Exact placement of the remaining electrodes on the abdomen can vary, depending on the specific cardiac monitor being used.

• The nurse should attach a monitor wire to each electrode before placing it on the patient's chest. The electrode seal should be well seated. Avoid placing electrodes on bony prominences or hairy areas, or where defibrillator pads will be placed. Also avoid placing electrodes where chest compressions will be given.

• Assess the patient's cardiac rhythm *to help select the correct treatment.* Follow the ACLS guidelines for the arrhythmia you observe on the monitor. (See *Treating ventricular arrhythmias.*)

• When the code team arrives, allow them to replace you and the other nurses. If necessary, one of you can assist with ACLS procedures, while another documents what happens and who participates in the code. The nurse assigned to the patient should stay in the room during the code *to give the doctor the patient's medical history and describe the events leading to the arrest.*

• Insert a peripheral I.V. line *to administer fluid and emergency drugs.* Choose a large blood vessel, such as the brachial vein, *because smaller peripheral vessels tend to collapse quickly during cardiac arrest.* Use a large-gauge needle *that won't dislodge or injure the vein and cause extravasation and vessel collapse.* (See *Recommendations for code drugs,* pages 378 to 380.)

• Begin an infusion of dextrose 5% in water. Later, other fluids, such as normal saline solution, may be infused *to help prevent circulatory collapse from hypovolemia.*

• Prepare the patient for defibrillation. (See "Defibrillation" in this chapter.)

• Set up portable or wall suction equipment, and suction the patient's oral secretions as necessary *to maintain an open airway.*

• Prepare the equipment for endotracheal tube insertion. Then suction the patient and use the manual resuscitation bag to hyperventilate him with 100% oxygen. Assist the doctor or nurse educated in the procedure to insert the tube. Always assess for bilateral breath sounds immediately after intubation or repositioning. If you hear sounds on only one side, pull the endotracheal tube out slightly. CPR should stop during insertion. If you can't hear bilateral breath sounds, auscultate the epigastric area to rule out gastric intubation.

• Prepare the drugs that may be needed during the code to control heart rate and rhythm. The doctor may order one or more drugs, such as lidocaine, procainamide, bretylium tosylate, atropine sulfate, verapamil, propranolol, or isoproterenol. To improve cardiac output and blood pressure, the doctor may also order epinephrine, norepinephrine, dopamine, dobutamine, amrinone, calcium, digitalis, nitroglycerin, sodium nitroprusside, sodium bicarbonate, or a diuretic — either singly or in combination. You'll give these drugs I.V., although lidocaine, atropine, and epinephrine can also be given endotracheally. Elevate the patient's limb and give him a 50-ml fluid bolus with the I.V. drugs.

Treating ventricular arrhythmias

Advanced cardiac life support (ACLS) guidelines recommend a series of steps for treating sustained ventricular tachycardia (VT), ventricular fibrillation (VF), and asystole. Keep in mind that these steps aren't intended as a strict set of rules. Certain patients will require interventions not covered by these steps.

The following flowcharts show the steps recommended in the ACLS guidelines. Continue following them only if VT, pulseless VT, VF, or asystole persists.

Ventricular tachycardia

If you detect a pulse, you have two possible paths to follow: one for a stable patient, the other for an unstable one. Consider the patient unstable if chest pain, dyspnea, hypotension, congestive heart failure, ischemia, or myocardial infarction develops.

If the patient doesn't have hypotension or pulmonary edema and isn't unconscious, you can use a precordial thump before cardioversion. If cardioversion alone doesn't work, give lidocaine, then procainamide or bretylium.

When VT resolves, infuse the antiarrhythmic that helped resolve the arrhythmia.

No pulse	Pulse present	
Treat as ventricular fibrillation	Stable patient.	Unstable patient.
	Administer oxygen. Establish I.V. access.	Administer oxygen. Consider sedating patient. Establish I.V. access.
	Give lidocaine, 1 mg/kg.	Cardiovert with 50 joules.
	Give lidocaine 0.5 mg/kg every 8 minutes until VT resolves or up to 3 mg/kg.	Cardiovert with 100 joules.
		Cardiovert with 200 joules.
	Give procainamide 20 mg/min until VT resolves or up to 1,000 mg.	Cardiovert with up to 360 joules.
	Cardiovert if patient becomes unstable.	If VT recurs, give lidocaine and cardiovert again starting at the energy level previously successful, then give procainamide or bretylium.

(continued)

Treating ventricular arrhythmias (continued)

Ventricular fibrillation

Treat VF and pulseless VT the same way. After each defibrillation attempt, assess the patient's pulse rate and rhythm. If the arrhythmia recurs after a transient conversion, apply the joule level that produced the conversion.

If possible, intubate the patient earlier than shown on the flowchart—but only if it can be done during the other interventions. If intubation isn't necessary, defibrillate and give epinephrine.

Keep in mind that some doctors prefer administering lidocaine in 0.5 mg/kg boluses every 8 minutes up to a total dose of 3 mg/kg. Also keep in mind that sodium bicarbonate isn't recommended for a routine cardiac arrest.

Witnessed cardiac arrest	Unwitnessed cardiac arrest
Check pulse. If absent, administer precordial thump.	Check pulse.

If pulse is absent, perform cardiopulmonary resuscitation (CPR) until a defibrillator is available.
Check cardiac monitor to detect VF or VT.

Defibrillate with 200 joules.
If unsuccessful, defibrillate with 200 to 300 joules.
If unsuccessful, defibrillate with up to 360 joules.

Check pulse; if absent, perform CPR.
Establish I.V. access.

Give epinephrine 1:10,000, 0.5 to 1.0 mg I.V. push, every 5 minutes.
Intubate when possible.

Defibrillate with up to 360 joules.

Give lidocaine, 1 mg/kg I.V. push.

Defibrillate with up to 360 joules.

Give bretylium, 5 mg/kg I.V. push.
(Consider giving sodium bicarbonate.)

Defibrillate with up to 360 joules.

Give bretylium, 10 mg/kg I.V. push.

Defibrillate with up to 360 joules.

Repeat lidocaine or bretylium.

Defibrillate with up to 360 joules.

Treating ventricular arrhythmias *(continued)*

Asystole

If possible, intubate the patient earlier than shown on the flowchart—but only if it can be done during the other interventions. If he can be ventilated without being intubated, however, CPR and epinephrine administration assume higher initial priorities. The doctor may order epinephrine endotracheally.

When using the guidelines here, keep in mind that sodium bicarbonate isn't recommended for a routine cardiac arrest.

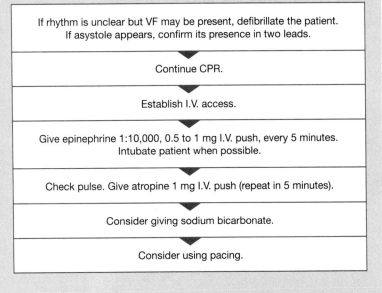

If rhythm is unclear but VF may be present, defibrillate the patient. If asystole appears, confirm its presence in two leads.

Continue CPR.

Establish I.V. access.

Give epinephrine 1:10,000, 0.5 to 1 mg I.V. push, every 5 minutes. Intubate patient when possible.

Check pulse. Give atropine 1 mg I.V. push (repeat in 5 minutes).

Consider giving sodium bicarbonate.

Consider using pacing.

• Assess the patient's cardiac rhythm strip again and, if necessary, defibrillate him.
• Set the defibrillator to 200 joules and deliver the first defibrillation. If that doesn't convert the rhythm, deliver a second defibrillation at between 200 and 300 joules, and, if necessary, a third at not more than 360 joules.
• If the patient's rhythm is converted, but he still has severe bradycardia with reduced cardiac output (from acute heart block, for example), the doctor may order a vasopressor or vagolytic. If that doesn't raise heart rate and cardiac output sufficiently, the doctor may insert a temporary pacemaker.
• Throughout ACLS, take the patient's central pulses—carotid or femoral—frequently. *Remember, the cardiac monitor shows only the heart's electrical activity, not the effectiveness of cardiac compressions.*
• Either during the code (if needed) or after the patient has been stabilized, insert an NG tube *to relieve or prevent gastric distention.*
• After the patient's condition stabilizes, obtain a chest X-ray *to check for complications, such as a fracture or puncture wounds from chest compressions.* The X-ray film will also show whether the endotracheal tube is properly

placed and whether the patient has suffered any other possible complications of intubation.

Special considerations

Because code teams vary among hospitals, you need to know your hospital's specific code team. Make sure you know who should respond to a code, how to notify each team member, what each team member does during the code, and what role you should play.

Besides giving emergency care, you may need to remove the patient's roommate, call for other staff members to help, get more equipment, or call a clergy member to sit with the family.

Complications

Even when performed correctly, CPR can cause fractured ribs, liver laceration, lung puncture, and gastric distention. Defibrillation can cause electric shock, and emergency intubation can result in esophageal or tracheal laceration, subcutaneous emphysema, or accidental right mainstem bronchus intubation. (Decreased or absent breath sounds on the left side of the chest and normal breath sounds on the right may signal accidental right mainstem bronchus intubation.)

(Text continues on page 380.)

Recommendations for code drugs

Use this chart to review medications administered during a code. Note the indications, dosages, and nursing considerations for the following drugs on the crash cart.

DRUG	DOSAGE	NURSING CONSIDERATIONS
Atropine	0.5 mg for bradycardia (1 mg for asystole), I.V. push over 1 to 2 minutes; may be repeated every 5 minutes to a maximum of 2 mg	• Indicated for sinus bradycardia with hemodynamic compromise or with frequent ventricular ectopic beats, and for ventricular asystole • May be given endotracheally if an I.V. line can't be established quickly • May slow heart rate at doses below 0.5 mg • May induce tachycardia
Bretylium	*For resistant ventricular fibrillation:* 5 mg/kg I.V. push followed by defibrillation; if ventricular fibrillation persists, increase to 10 mg/kg and repeat at 15- to 30-minute intervals (maximum dose: 30 mg/kg). *For resistant ventricular tachycardia:* 5 to 10 mg/kg diluted to 50 ml with D₅W and injected I.V. over 8 to 10 minutes. Dose can be repeated in 1 to 2 hours, then every 6 to 8 hours if ventricular tachycardia persists. Or give as a continuous infusion at 2 mg/min.	• Indicated for resistant ventricular fibrillation or tachycardia • Not a first-line drug; use only if ventricular fibrillation isn't converted by lidocaine and defibrillation, if ventricular fibrillation recurs despite lidocaine therapy, or if lidocaine and procainamide fail to control ventricular tachycardia associated with palpable pulse
Calcium chloride	500 mg to 1 gram I.V. (5 to 10 ml of a 10% solution); repeat as ordered.	• Not for routine use in resuscitation efforts, but can be used if patient has hyperkalemia, hypocalcemia, or calcium channel blocker toxicity
Dobutamine	2.5 to 10 mcg/kg/min I.V. infusion; use smallest effective dose, as indicated by hemodynamic parameters	• Indicated for patients with low cardiac output, hypotension, and pulmonary congestion • May induce reflex peripheral vasodilation • Monitor heart rate closely; increase of 10% or more may worsen myocardial ischemia
Dopamine	2 to 5 mcg/kg/min I.V. infusion initially, titrate until the desired response is achieved	• Indicated for hypotension • Drug effects vary with dosage: At 0.5 to 2 mcg/kg/min, it dilates renal and mesenteric vessels without increasing heart rate or blood pressure; at 2 to 10 mcg/kg/min, it increases cardiac output without peripheral vasoconstriction; at over 10 mcg/kg/min, it causes peripheral vasoconstriction
Epinephrine	0.5 to 1 mg I.V. (5 to 10 ml of 1:10,000 solution); repeat every 5 min if necessary	• Indicated for cardiac arrest • May be given endotracheally if I.V. line can't be established quickly • Intracardiac injection indicated only if venous and endotracheal routes unavailable

Recommendations for code drugs *(continued)*

DRUG	DOSAGE	NURSING CONSIDERATIONS
Isoproterenol HCl	Dilute 1 mg (5 ml) in 500 ml of D_5W and infuse 2 to 10 mcg/min; titrate to the heart rate and rhythm.	• Indicated for hemodynamically significant bradycardia unresponsive to atropine in a patient with a palpable pulse • Not indicated for cardiac arrest • Increases cardiac work load, worsening ischemia and arrhythmias in patients with ischemic heart disease • Use until pacemaker therapy begins
Lidocaine	1 mg/kg I.V. bolus (25 to 50 mg/min) as a loading dose, followed by bolus of 0.5 mg/kg every 8 to 10 min for a maximum of 3 mg/kg (300 mg over 1 hr). After a successful resuscitation, set up a continuous I.V. infusion at 2 to 4 mg/min. (Dilute 1 gram of lidocaine in 250 ml of D_5W for a 0.4% solution, or 4 mg/ml.)	• Indicated for ventricular tachycardia, ventricular fibrillation, or premature ventricular contractions that are frequent, close-coupled, multiform in configuration, or arranged in short bursts of two or more in succession • May be used prophylactically when myocardial infarction is suspected but not confirmed to prevent ventricular ectopy • Improves response to defibrillation when patient is in ventricular fibrillation • May be given endotracheally if an I.V. line can't be established quickly
Nitroglycerin	10 mcg/min I.V. initially, increasing by 5 to 10 mcg/min every 3 to 5 min as needed	• Indicated for congestive heart failure, unstable angina • Monitor for hypotension, which could worsen myocardial ischemia • Mean dosage range is 50 to 500 mcg/min; most patients respond to 200 mcg/min or less • Special administration sets (non-PVC plastic tubing) available (with regular tubing, expect reduced drug effect from increased binding to regular plastic; conversely, with special tubing, expect increased drug effect)
Nitroprusside	Dissolve 50 mg in 2 to 3 ml of D_5W, then mix with 250 to 1,000 ml of D_5W, depending on desired concentration. Infuse at 0.5 mcg/kg/min, titrating until the desired effect is achieved. The therapeutic dose ranges from 0.5 to 8 mcg/kg/min.	• Indicated for heart failure and for hypertensive crisis • Wrap container in opaque material to prevent drug deterioration • Monitor blood pressure with intra-arterial line
Norepinephrine	Mix 4 mg of norepinephrine bitartrate per 1,000 ml of D_5W or normal saline solution to yield a 4 mcg/ml solution. Or mix 4 mg per 250 ml to yield a 16 mcg/ml	• Indicated for severe hypotension with low total peripheral resistance • Contraindicated in hypovolemia

(continued)

Recommendations for code drugs *(continued)*

DRUG	DOSAGE	NURSING CONSIDERATIONS
Norepinephrine *(continued)*	solution. (The concentration chosen will depend on the patient's fluid requirements.) Infuse through a central venous catheter at 2 mcg/min; titrate to the desired response.	• Monitor blood pressure with intra-arterial line; false-low blood pressure reading may occur with standard cuff • Cardiac output may increase or decrease, depending on vascular resistance, left ventricle's ability to function, and reflex response • Avoid prolonged use; drug could cause ischemia of vital organs
Procainamide	50 mg I.V. every 5 min, up to 1 gram; maintenance infusion (2 grams in 500 ml) is 1 to 4 mg/min	• Indicated for ventricular arrhythmias, such as premature ventricular contraction or tachycardia, when lidocaine is contraindicated or ineffective • Lower dosage for patients with renal failure • Hypotension from too-rapid infusion • Monitor ECG carefully; if QRS interval widens more than 50% or if PR interval is prolonged, notify doctor and discontinue as ordered
Sodium bicarbonate	1 mEq/kg after acidosis is established, with a maximum of half this dose every 10 min thereafter as needed	• Not recommended for initial resuscitation unless preexisting acidosis is clearly present; hyperventilation should be the primary therapy for controlling acid-base balance
Verapamil	5 mg I.V. initially, followed by 10 mg over 15 to 30 min if paroxysmal supraventricular tachycardia persists and if the patient hasn't had an adverse reaction to the initial dose	• Indicated for atrial arrhythmias, especially paroxysmal supraventricular tachycardia with atrioventricular node conduction • Use cautiously and in lower doses for patients receiving beta-blockers • Monitor for hypotension, severe bradycardia, congestive heart failure, and facilitated accessory conduction in patients with Wolff-Parkinson-White syndrome

Documentation

Many hospitals have code sheets that act as the documentation tool and the doctor's order sheet. Be familiar with any code sheet used at your hospital.

Record the time the patient was found, who found him, whether he suffered from cardiac or respiratory arrest, and who responded to the code. Note when the I.V. line was inserted, where the I.V. site is located, the size of the needle used, and what fluids and drugs the patient received.

If the patient received defibrillation, note the electrocardiogram (ECG) before defibrillation, the number of joules used, and the ECG after defibrillation. Note whether a ventilation mask or an endotracheal tube was used. If the patient was intubated, record who intubated him and what size tube was used. Also note whether you auscultated bilateral breath sounds afterward.

Record any recommended follow-up therapy. If the doctor orders the patient transferred, note where he will be transferred and his condition before transfer. Document any other complications. Also note the interventions to correct them.

Cardiopulmonary resuscitation

An emergency procedure, cardiopulmonary resuscitation (CPR) seeks to restore and maintain the victim's respiration and circulation after his heartbeat and breathing have stopped. The goal is to provide oxygen and blood flow to the heart, brain, and other vital organs until help arrives. CPR is begun as soon as possible after cardiac and respiratory arrest. If the victim's heartbeat and respirations have stopped for less than 4 minutes before intervention, he has a much better chance for complete recovery, as long as the resuscitation is effective.

If the victim's circulation has been stopped for 4 to 6 minutes, brain damage may have occurred. After 6 minutes without circulation, brain damage will almost certainly occur. However, there are exceptions — a drowning victim who's been in cold water or someone who's suffered hypothermia, for instance. If there is any doubt as to how long the victim's pulse and respirations have been absent, CPR should be performed.

The easiest way to remember the basic CPR procedure is to follow the ABC scheme: airway open, breathing restored, then circulation restored. After the airway has been opened and breathing and circulation have been restored, drug therapy, diagnosis by electrocardiogram (ECG), or defibrillation may follow. CPR is contraindicated in "no code" patients.

Equipment
CPR requires no special equipment except a hard surface on which to place the patient.

Implementation
• The following illustrated instructions provide a step-by-step guide for CPR as currently recommended by the American Heart Association.

One-person rescue
• If you're the sole rescuer, expect to open the patient's airway, check for breathing, and assess for circulation before beginning compressions.

Open the airway
• As shown above at right, assess the victim to determine if he's unconscious. Gently shake his shoulders and shout, "Are you okay?" This helps ensure that you don't start CPR on a person who's conscious. Check whether he has an injury, particularly to the head or neck. If you suspect a head or neck injury, move him as little as possible to reduce the risk of paralysis.

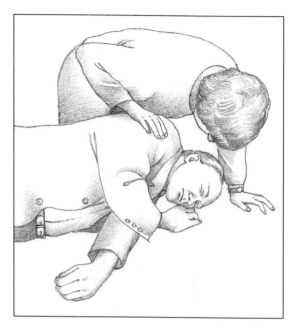

• Call out for help. Send someone to contact the emergency medical service (EMS), if appropriate. Place the victim in a supine position on a hard, flat surface. When moving him, roll his head and torso as a unit. Avoid twisting or pulling his neck, shoulders, or hips.

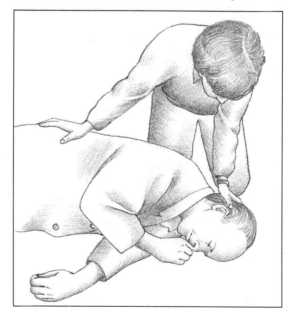

● Kneel near his shoulders. This position will give you easy access to his head and chest.

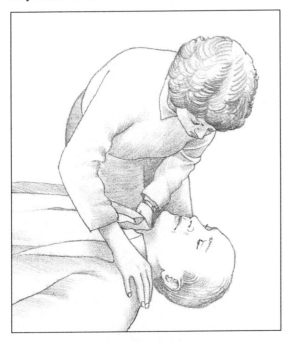

● In many cases, the muscles controlling the victim's tongue will be relaxed, causing the tongue to obstruct the airway. If the victim doesn't appear to have a neck injury, use the *head-tilt/chin-lift maneuver* to open his airway. To accomplish this, first place your hand that's closer to the victim's head on his forehead. Then apply firm pressure. The pressure should be firm enough to tilt the victim's head back. Next place the fingertips of your other hand under the bony part of his lower jaw near the chin. Now lift the victim's chin. At the same time, keep his mouth partially open (as shown above at right).
● Avoid placing your fingertips on the soft tissue under the victim's chin *because this maneuver may inadvertently obstruct the airway you're trying to open.*

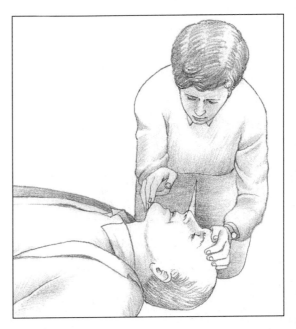

● If you suspect a neck injury, use the *jaw-thrust maneuver* instead of the *head-tilt/chin-lift maneuver.* Kneel at the victim's head with your elbows on the ground. Rest your thumbs on his lower jaw near the corners of the mouth, pointing your thumbs toward his feet. Then place your fingertips around the lower jaw. To open the airway, lift the lower jaw with your fingertips.

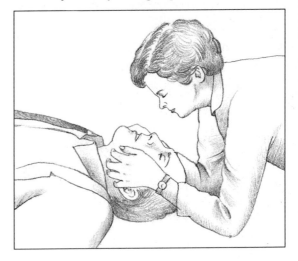

Check for breathing

• While maintaining the open airway, place your ear over the victim's mouth and nose. Now, listen for the sound of air moving, and note whether his chest rises and falls. You may also feel airflow on your cheek. If he starts to breathe, keep the airway open and continue checking his breathing until help arrives.

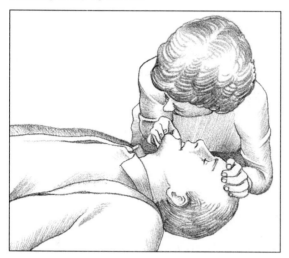

• If the victim doesn't start breathing after you open his airway, begin rescue breathing. Pinch his nostrils shut with the thumb and index finger of the hand you've had on his forehead.

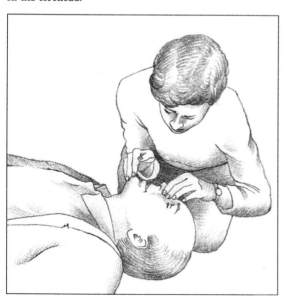

• Take a deep breath and place your mouth over the victim's mouth, creating a tight seal. Give two full ventilations, taking a deep breath after each to allow enough time for his chest to expand and relax and to prevent gastric distention. Each ventilation should last 1 to 1½ seconds.

• If the first ventilation isn't successful, reposition the victim's head and try again. If you're still not successful, he may have a foreign-body airway obstruction. Check for loose dentures. If dentures or any other objects are blocking the airway, follow the procedure for clearing an airway obstruction. (See "Obstructed airway management," Chapter 8.)

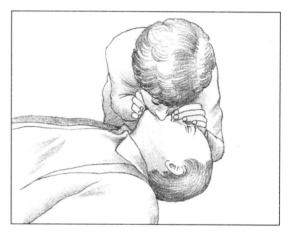

Assess circulation

• Keep one hand on the victim's forehead so his airway remains open. With your other hand, palpate the carotid artery that's closer to you. To do this, place your index and middle fingers in the groove between the trachea and the sternocleidomastoid muscle. Palpate for 5 to 10 seconds.

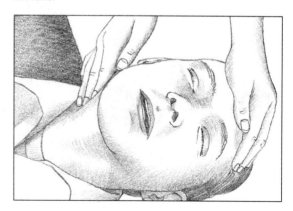

• If you detect a pulse, don't begin chest compressions. Instead, perform rescue breathing by giving the victim 12 ventilations per minute (or one every 5 seconds). After every 12 ventilations, recheck his pulse.

• If there's no pulse and you haven't sent someone for help yet, tell a bystander to call the EMS. Then start giving chest compressions. Make sure your knees are apart for a wide base of support. Using the hand closer to his feet, locate the lower margin of the rib cage. Then move your fingertips along the margin to the notch where the ribs meet the sternum.

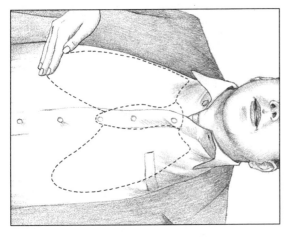

• Place your middle finger on the notch and your index finger next to your middle finger. Your index finger will now be on the bottom of the sternum.

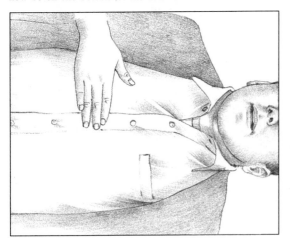

• Put the heel of your other hand on the sternum, next to the index finger. The long axis of the heel of your hand will be aligned with the long axis of the sternum.

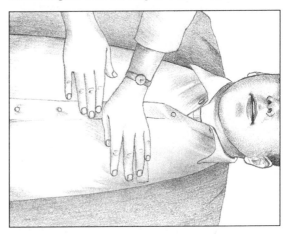

• Take the first hand off the notch and put it on top of the hand on the sternum. Make sure you have one hand directly on top of the other and your fingers aren't on his chest. This position will keep the force of the compression on the sternum and reduce the risk of a rib fracture, lung puncture, or liver laceration.

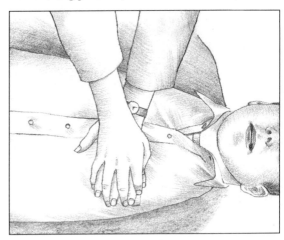

• With your elbows locked, arms straight, and your shoulders directly over your hands, you're ready to give chest compressions. Using the weight of your upper body, compress the victim's sternum 1½" to 2" (3.8 to 5 cm), delivering the pressure through the heels of your hands. After each compression, release the pressure and allow the chest to return to its normal position so that the heart can fill with blood. Don't change your hand position during compressions—you might injure the victim.

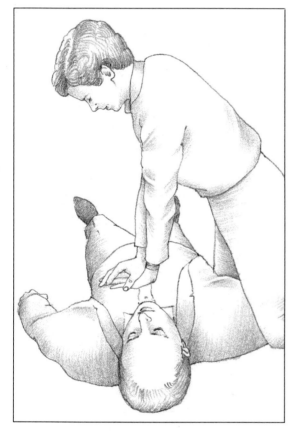

• Give 15 chest compressions at a rate of 80 to 100 per minute. Count, "One and two and three and..." up to 15. Open the airway and give 2 ventilations. Then find the proper hand position again and deliver 15 more compressions. Do four complete cycles of 15 compressions and 2 ventilations.
• Palpate the carotid pulse again. If there's still no pulse, continue performing CPR in cycles of 15 compressions and 2 ventilations. If you're alone, perform CPR for about 1 minute, check the victim's pulse, then try to get help. Return quickly to the victim and continue CPR. Every

few minutes, check for breathing and a pulse. If you detect a pulse but he isn't breathing, give 12 ventilations per minute and monitor his pulse. If he has a pulse and is breathing, monitor his respirations and pulse closely. You should stop performing CPR only when his respirations and pulse return, he's turned over to the EMS, or you're exhausted.

Two-person rescue
If another rescuer arrives while you're giving CPR, follow these steps:
• If you haven't contacted the EMS, tell the second rescuer to do so. He should then return to help with the rescue. If he's not a health care professional, ask him to stand by. Then, if you become fatigued, he can take over one-person CPR.

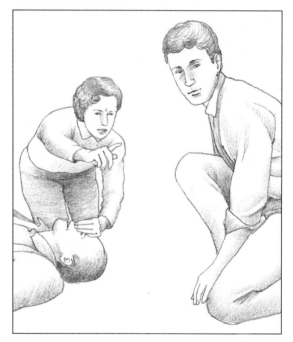

• Have him begin by checking the victim's pulse for 5 seconds after you've given two ventilations. If he doesn't feel a pulse, he should give two ventilations and begin chest compressions.
• If the rescuer is another health care professional, the two of you can perform two-person CPR. He should start assisting after you've finished a cycle of 15 compressions, two ventilations, and a pulse check.

• The second rescuer should get into place opposite you. While you're checking for a pulse, he should be finding the proper hand placement for delivering chest compressions.

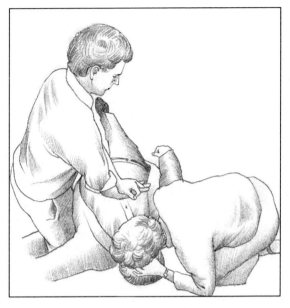

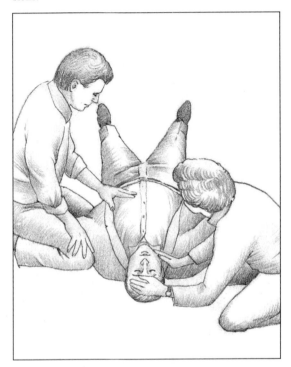

• If you don't detect a pulse, say, "No pulse, continue CPR," and give one ventilation (as shown above at right). Then the second rescuer should begin delivering compressions at a rate of 80 to 100 per minute. Compressions and ventilations should be administered at a ratio of 5 compressions to 1 ventilation. The compressor (at this point, the second rescuer) should count out loud so the ventilator can anticipate when to give ventilations. To ensure that the ventilations are effective, the rescuer performing the chest compressions should stop briefly or at least long enough to observe the victim's chest rise with the air supplied by the rescuer giving ventilations.

• As the ventilator, you must check for breathing and a pulse. Signal the compressor to stop giving compressions for 5 seconds so you can make these assessments.

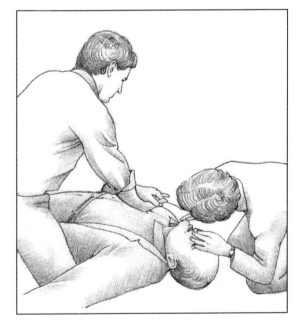

• After a minimum of 10 cycles, the compressor (second rescuer) may call for a switch. This should be done clearly to allow for a smooth transition. The compressor can substitute the word "switch" for the word "one" as he counts compressions. In other words, he'd say, "Switch and two and three and four and five." You'd then give a ventilation and become the compressor by moving down to the victim's chest and placing your hands in the proper position.

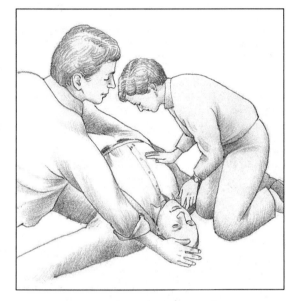

• The second rescuer would become the ventilator and move to the victim's head. He'd check the pulse for 5 seconds. If he found no pulse, he'd say, "No pulse," and give a ventilation. You'd then give compressions at a rate of 80 to 100 per minute — or five compressions for each ventilation. As shown at right above, both of you should continue giving CPR in this manner until the victim's respirations and pulse return, he's turned over to the EMS, or both of you are exhausted.

Special considerations

Although acquired immunodeficiency syndrome (AIDS) isn't known to be transmitted in saliva, some health care professionals may hesitate to give rescue breaths — especially if the victim has AIDS. For this reason, the American Heart Association recommends that all health care professionals learn how to use disposable airway equipment.

A second rescuer may instinctively take the victim's pulse without waiting for the end of a cycle. This is *not*

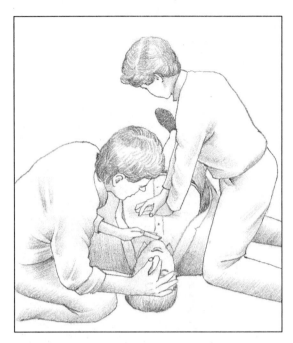

part of the American Heart Association recommendations and may confuse some rescuers. The recommendations aim to have all rescuers act in the same way so that time isn't wasted and all efforts help restore the victim's respirations and heartbeat.

Complications

CPR can cause certain complications — especially if the compressor doesn't place her hands properly on the sternum. These complications include fractured ribs, a lacerated liver, and punctured lungs. Gastric distention, a common complication, results from giving too much air during ventilation. (For more information, see *Managing hazards of CPR,* page 388.)

Documentation

Whenever you perform CPR, document why you initiated it, whether the victim suffered from cardiac or respiratory arrest, when you found the victim and started CPR, and how long the victim received CPR. Note his response and any complications. Also include any interventions taken to correct complications.

If the victim also received advanced cardiac life support, document which interventions were performed, who performed them, when they were performed, and what equipment was used.

Managing hazards of CPR

To prevent complications, make sure to position your hands properly for chest compressions, and check that you're not delivering excessive ventilation. If you suspect the following complications, tell the doctor, but don't stop cardiopulmonary resuscitation (CPR).

Fractured ribs
Once the victim's condition has stabilized, you can detect fractured ribs by palpating for bone displacement and crepitus (a crunching sound). The victim will need rest and pain medication for a fractured rib. If he has a serious fracture, he may need his rib cage splinted.

Liver laceration
Although rare, liver laceration poses a much more serious threat. It usually causes hemorrhage, resulting in shock, decreased blood pressure, increased heart rate, and abdominal distention. You may have trouble distinguishing it from shock caused by respiratory or cardiac arrest. If you suspect liver laceration, tell the doctor. After the victim is stabilized, diagnostic studies, such as peritoneal fluid analysis, may be ordered. Treatment includes fluid resuscitation and surgical repair.

Punctured lung
If the victim has a punctured lung from a broken rib, he may develop a tension pneumothorax. With this complication, air enters – but can't escape – the pleural space, building up positive pressure in the thoracic cavity and collapsing the lung. You may have trouble ventilating a victim with a punctured lung.

Other signs of a tension pneumothorax include asymmetrical chest movement, absent breath sounds on the side where the pneumothorax has developed and, as the condition grows worse, a shift of the trachea away from the affected side. A chest X-ray will be needed to confirm the diagnosis.

The victim will need to have a chest tube or a large-bore needle inserted into the pleural space (at about the second intercostal space) to relieve the pressure caused by trapped air.

Gastric distention
A more common complication of CPR – also signaled by difficulty in giving resuscitative breaths – is gastric distention. Caused by delivering too much air during ventilation, gastric distention can lead to vomiting, which increases the risk of aspiration.

If you notice the victim's stomach becoming distended during CPR, reposition his airway and make sure that his chest, not his stomach, rises and falls during ventilation. If the victim vomits, turn him on his side – preferably away from you. Suction his airway and continue to perform CPR.

Defibrillation

During defibrillation, an electric current passes through the patient's heart via two electrode paddles positioned on his chest. This current depolarizes the myocardium, usually allowing the sinoatrial node to resume control of the heart. This technique is used for ventricular fibrillation and pulseless ventricular tachycardia.

Defibrillation is most effective when initiated as soon as possible following the onset of life-threatening arrhythmia. Specially trained nurses, who are often the first to recognize the need for defibrillation, can perform the procedure in many hospitals.

Patients with a history of ventricular fibrillation may be candidates for an automatic implantable cardioverter defibrillator, a sophisticated device that automatically discharges an electric current when it senses ventricular tachyarrhythmia. (See *Understanding the AICD.*)

Equipment
Defibrillator ■ conductive gel pads ■ crash cart with emergency resuscitation equipment.

Defibrillation paddles are available both in adult size (13 cm in diameter) and in pediatric size (8 cm in diameter), as well as anterolateral and anteroposterior types.

Implementation
• Assess the patient to determine the lack of a pulse. Call for help, and perform cardiopulmonary resuscitation (CPR) until the defibrillator and crash cart arrive.
• Connect the monitoring leads from the defibrillator unit to the patient. Remove any telemetry or bedside monitors *to prevent damage to those units.*
• Assess the patient's cardiac rhythm *for appropriateness for defibrillation.*
• Turn on the defibrillator, and verify that the current indicator lights up. If it doesn't, check the battery or other power source. If the defibrillator can also be used

Understanding the AICD

The automatic implantable cardio-verter defibrillator (AICD) has a pulse generator and lead systems to monitor the heart's activity and deliver shocks as necessary.

The surgeon will position a bipolar lead transvenously in the endocardium of the right ventricle. Or he may place two leads ⅜″ (1 cm) apart on the epicardium of the left ventricle. These leads record the heart rate.

The shocks are delivered by two patch leads sewn onto the heart as shown or by one patch lead and a lead (not shown) placed in the right atrium via the superior vena cava. These leads also detect the amount of time the waveform remains at the baseline—called the probability density function.

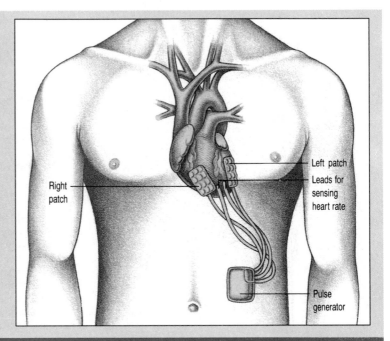

for synchronized cardioversion, make sure it's set on the asynchronous mode. (If it's set on the synchronous mode, the paddles won't discharge during ventricular fibrillation or pulseless ventricular tachycardia.)

• Expose the patient's chest, and apply pads. (See *Paddle placement*, page 390.)

• Apply conductive gel to one paddle, and rub the two paddles together to distribute the gel. Make sure that no excess gel is dripping from the paddles; *excess gel will cause arcing of current.*

• If you are using gel pads, place them where the paddles will be located. Do not cover any of the electrocardiogram (ECG) lead wires or electrodes *to avoid possible electric shock.*

• An alternative defibrillator uses pre-gelled and self-adhesive conductive defibrillator pads in place of gel pads and defibrillator paddles. To use these defibrillator pads, peel the covering off the pads and place them just as you would place the gel pads, either in the regular or anteroposterior position. Then attach the lead wires to the pads, if necessary.

• Set the machine at the energy level for initial defibrillation (200 joules for adults and 2 joules/kg for infants and children).

• Charge the paddles by pressing the charge button on the machine or on the paddles themselves. A blinking light or a constant hissing noise will signal that the paddles are charging. When they're fully charged, the light will stop blinking, the hissing will cease, and the machine may show a digital display of the energy level.

• Apply the paddles over the conductive pads to the chest. Press them firmly against the patient's skin.

• Reassess the patient's cardiac rhythm, pulse, and level of consciousness *to determine the need for defibrillation.*

• Instruct personnel to stand clear of the patient and bed *to avoid the risk of electric shock.*

• Discharge the current by pressing both paddle discharge buttons simultaneously.

• If defibrillation is unsuccessful, repeat the procedure two more times. Increase the energy level as ordered. (For adults, the American Heart Association recommends 200 joules for the first attempt, 200 to 300 joules for the second, and no more than 360 joules for the third.) Perform the three countershocks in rapid succession; it's

Paddle placement

For anterolateral paddle placement, position one paddle to the right of the upper sternum, just below the right clavicle, and the other at the fifth or sixth intercostal space in the left anterior axillary line.

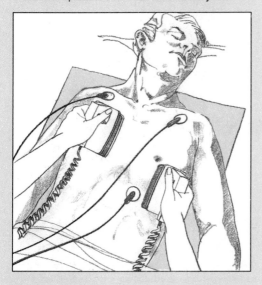

For anteroposterior placement, position the anterior paddle directly over the heart at the precordium, to the left of the lower sternal border. Place the flat posterior paddle under the patient's body beneath the heart and immediately below the scapulae (but not under the vertebral column).

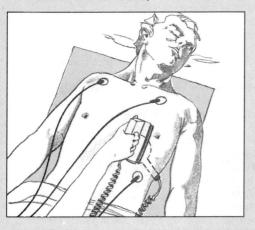

unnecessary to resume CPR between each one. Defibrillation can be done unlimited times, but most hospitals limit the nurse to the three initial countershocks.

• If the patient remains without a pulse after the three initial countershocks, resume CPR and give supplemental oxygen *to ensure maximum oxygenation and perfusion of vital organs.* Begin administering medication.

• If normal rhythm is restored, continue to monitor the patient and provide supplemental oxygen and ventilation as needed.

• If the paddles have been recharged but are not used again, clear the charge by turning the machine off, by adjusting the energy selector dial, or by placing the paddles into their protective housing and discharging them into the machine. *Under no circumstances should the paddles be discharged against each other or into the air.*

• Prepare the defibrillator for immediate reuse by cleaning and restocking any used equipment and medications.

Special considerations

Defibrillators vary from manufacturer to manufacturer, so familiarize yourself with your hospital's equipment. Operation of the defibrillator should be checked at least every 8 hours and after each use.

Defibrillation can be affected by several factors, including paddle size and placement, condition of the patient's myocardium, duration of the arrhythmia, chest resistance, and the number of countershocks.

Complications

Defibrillators can cause electric shock. Also, insufficient conductive medium will cause skin burns and limit the effectiveness of defibrillation.

Documentation

Thorough documentation of the cardiac arrest is essential. This includes the time resuscitation was initiated; the time and energy level of defibrillation; the time, dose, and route of medications administered; the use of CPR; airway maintenance; rhythm strips obtained; and the patient outcome.

 Synchronized cardioversion

Like defibrillation, synchronized cardioversion delivers electric current to the heart to correct an arrhythmia. But these procedures differ in two important ways. With cardioversion, much lower energy levels are used (typically 25 to 100 joules, depending on the arrhythmia being converted), and the burst of electricity is precisely timed to coincide with the peak of the R wave.

You can't use synchronized cardioversion to treat ventricular fibrillation or pulseless ventricular tachycardia because a fibrillating heart doesn't generate an R wave. But the procedure is the treatment of choice for unstable ventricular tachycardia (accompanied by chest pain, dyspnea, and hypotension) and unstable paroxysmal atrial tachycardia that fails to respond to drug therapy.

Synchronized cardioversion may be either an elective or an emergency procedure, during which you may assist a doctor. In an emergency, a qualified nurse may perform the procedure.

Equipment
Defibrillator ■ conductive gel pads ■ sedative ■ crash cart containing emergency resuscitation equipment.

Defibrillation paddles are available in adult (13 cm in diameter) and pediatric (8 cm in diameter) sizes and anterolateral and anteroposterior types as well.

Implementation
• If you have time, explain the procedure to the patient.
• Connect monitoring leads from the defibrillator unit in the crash cart to the patient. Remove telemetry and bedside monitors *to prevent damage to those units.*
• Assess the patient's cardiac rhythm *for appropriateness for cardioversion.*
• Turn the defibrillator on, and verify that the current indicator lights up. If it doesn't, check the battery or other power source.
• Make sure that the defibrillator is set for the synchronous mode *so that the electric current can be delivered with the peak of the R wave.*
• Administer sedation as ordered. The timing of the medication may vary, depending on the medication being administered. If necessary, ask another nurse to ventilate the patient.
• Expose the patient's chest, and apply the conductive pads. If conductive pads aren't available, apply conductive gel to one paddle and rub the two paddles together *to distribute the gel.* Make sure that no excess gel drips off the paddles; *excess gel can cause arcing of current.*
• Position the pads so that one pad is to the right of the sternum, just below the clavicle, and the other pad is at the fifth or sixth intercostal space in the left anterior axillary line.
• Set the machine to the appropriate energy level, usually between 25 and 100 joules. This will vary, depending on the cardiac rhythm.
• If not already done, activate the synchronized mode by depressing the synch button. When the machine is syn-

chronized properly, an indicator should recognize each QRS complex.
• Charge the paddles by pressing the charge button on the machine or on the paddles. A blinking light or a constant hissing noise signals that the paddles are charging. When they're fully charged, the light will remain on, the hissing will cease, and the machine may show a digital display of the energy level.
• Press the paddles firmly to the chest over the conductive pads.
• Reassess the patient's rhythm and pulse *to determine the need for cardioversion.*
• Instruct personnel to stand clear of the patient and bed *to avoid the risk of electric shock.*
• Discharge the current by pushing both paddle discharge buttons simultaneously. Unlike defibrillation, discharge won't occur immediately; you'll notice a slight delay while the defibrillator synchronizes with the R wave.
• If cardioversion is unsuccessful, repeat the procedure two or three more times as ordered, gradually increasing the energy level with each additional countershock. *To prevent complications,* make sure the synchronization indicator remains on each time cardioversion is repeated.
• If normal rhythm is restored, continue to monitor the patient and provide supplemental ventilation as long as needed.
◆ *Nursing alert.* If cardioversion results in ventricular fibrillation or ventricular tachycardia with no pulse, turn the synch switch off, and defibrillate the patient. Have emergency medications available. ◆
• If the paddles have been recharged but are not used again, clear the charge by turning the machine off, adjusting the energy selector dial, or placing the paddles in their protective housing and discharging them into the machine. *The paddles should never be discharged against each other or into the air.*

Special considerations
Defibrillators vary from manufacturer to manufacturer, so familiarize yourself with your hospital's equipment. Operation of the defibrillator should be checked at least every 8 hours and after each use.

Cardioversion can be affected by several factors, including paddle size and placement, condition of the patient's myocardium, duration of the arrhythmia, chest resistance, and the number of countershocks.

Complications
Cardioversion may result in ventricular fibrillation or ventricular tachycardia (with no pulse). Also, insufficient conductive medium will cause skin burns and limit the effectiveness of cardioversion.

Documentation

Thorough documentation of the procedure is essential. Be sure to note the time, dose, and route of medications administered; the energy level used; rhythm strips obtained; and the outcome.

 # Vagal maneuvers

When a patient suffers sinus, atrial, or junctional tachyarrhythmias, vagal maneuvers—Valsalva's maneuver and carotid sinus massage—can slow his heart rate. These maneuvers work by stimulating nerve endings, which respond as they would to an increase in blood pressure. They send this message to the brain stem, which in turn stimulates the autonomic nervous system to increase vagal tone and decrease the heart rate.

In *Valsalva's maneuver,* the patient holds his breath and bears down, raising his intrathoracic pressure. When this pressure increase is transmitted to the heart and great vessels, venous return, stroke volume, and systolic blood pressure decrease. Within seconds, the baroreceptors respond to these changes by increasing the heart rate and causing peripheral vasoconstriction.

When the patient exhales at the end of the maneuver, his blood pressure rises to its previous level. This increase, combined with the peripheral vasoconstriction caused by bearing down, stimulates the vagus nerve, decreasing the heart rate.

In *carotid sinus massage,* manual pressure applied to the left or right carotid sinus slows the heart rate. This method is used both to diagnose and treat tachyarrhythmias.

The patient's response to carotid sinus massage depends on the type of arrhythmia. If he has sinus tachycardia, his heart rate will slow gradually during the procedure and speed up again after it. If he has atrial tachycardia, the arrhythmia may stop and the heart rate may remain slow because the procedure increases atrioventricular (AV) block. With atrial fibrillation or flutter, the ventricular rate may not change; AV block may even worsen. With paroxysmal atrial tachycardia, reversion to sinus rhythm occurs only 20% of the time. Nonparoxysmal tachycardia and ventricular tachycardia won't respond.

Vagal maneuvers are contraindicated for patients with severe coronary artery disease, acute myocardial infarction, or hypovolemia. Carotid sinus massage is contraindicated for patients with cardiac glycoside toxicity or cerebrovascular disease and for patients who have had carotid surgery.

Although usually performed by a doctor, vagal maneuvers may also be done by a specially prepared nurse under a doctor's supervision.

Equipment

Crash cart with emergency medications and airway equipment ■ electrocardiogram (ECG) monitor and electrodes ■ I.V. catheter and tubing ■ tourniquet ■ dextrose 5% in water ■ optional: shaving supplies if needed, cardiotonic drugs.

Implementation

• Explain the procedure to the patient *to ease his fears and promote cooperation.* Ask him to let you know if he feels light-headed.
• Place the patient in a supine position. Insert an I.V. line, if necessary. Then administer dextrose 5% in water at a keep-vein-open rate, as ordered. *This line will be used if emergency drugs become necessary.*
• Prepare the patient's skin, shaving it if necessary, and attach ECG electrodes. Adjust the size of the ECG complexes on the monitor *so that you can see the arrhythmia clearly.*

Valsalva's maneuver

• Ask the patient to take a deep breath and bear down, as if he were trying to defecate. If he doesn't feel light-headed or dizzy, and if no new arrhythmias occur, have him hold his breath and bear down for 10 seconds.

If he does feel dizzy or light-headed, or if you see a new arrhythmia on the monitor—asystole for more than 6 seconds, frequent premature ventricular contractions (PVCs), or ventricular tachycardia or ventricular fibrillation—allow him to exhale and stop bearing down.
• After 10 seconds, ask him to exhale and breathe quietly. If the maneuver was successful, the monitor will show his heart rate slowing before he exhales.

Carotid sinus massage

• Begin by obtaining a rhythm strip, using the lead that shows the strongest P waves.
• Auscultate both carotid sinuses. If you detect bruits, inform the doctor and don't perform carotid sinus massage. If you don't detect bruits, proceed as ordered. (See *Location and technique for carotid sinus massage.*)
• Monitor the ECG throughout the procedure. Stop massaging when the ventricular rate slows sufficiently to permit diagnosis of the rhythm. Or stop as soon as *any* evidence of a rhythm change appears. Have the crash cart handy to give emergency treatment if a dangerous arrhythmia occurs.

Location and technique for carotid sinus massage

Before applying manual pressure to the patient's right carotid sinus, locate the bifurcation of the carotid artery on the right side of the neck. Turn the patient's head slightly to the left and hyperextend the neck. This brings the carotid artery closer to the skin and moves the sternocleidomastoid muscle away from the carotid artery.

Then, using a circular motion, gently massage the right carotid sinus between your fingers and the transverse processes of the spine for 3 to 5 seconds. Don't massage for more than 5 seconds *to avoid risking life-threatening complications.*

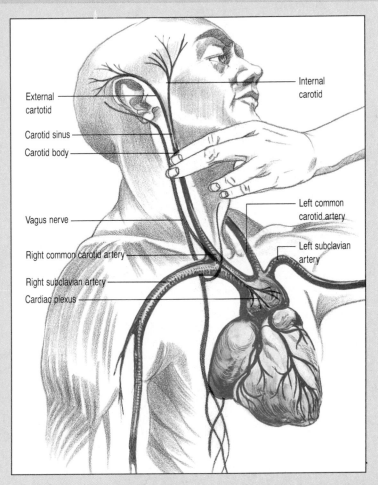

External carotid

Carotid sinus

Carotid body

Vagus nerve

Right common carotid artery

Right subclavian artery

Cardiac plexus

Internal carotid

Left common carotid artery

Left subclavian artery

• If the procedure has no effect within 5 seconds, stop massaging the right carotid sinus and begin to massage the left. If this also fails, administer cardiotonic drugs, as ordered.

Special considerations

Remember that a brief period of asystole—from 3 to 6 seconds—and several PVCs may precede conversion to normal sinus rhythm. If the vagal maneuver succeeded in slowing the patient's heart rate and converting the arrhythmia, continue monitoring him for several hours.

Complications

Use caution when performing carotid sinus massage on elderly patients, patients receiving cardiac glycosides, and patients with heart block, hypertension, coronary artery disease, diabetes mellitus, or hyperkalemia. The procedure may cause arterial pressure to plummet in these patients, although it usually rises quickly afterward. This is particularly true of elderly patients with heart disease. Vagal maneuvers can occasionally cause bradycardia or complete heart block, so monitor the patient's cardiac rhythm closely. (See *Adverse effects of vagal maneuvers,* page 394.)

Adverse effects of vagal maneuvers

Both Valsalva's maneuver and carotid sinus massage are useful for slowing heart rate. However, they can cause complications, some of which are life-threatening.

Valsalva's maneuver
This maneuver can cause bradycardia, accompanied by a decrease in cardiac output, possibly leading to syncope. The bradycardia will usually pass quickly, but if it doesn't or if it advances to complete heart block or asystole, begin basic life support, if necessary, by advanced cardiac life support.

Valsalva's maneuver can mobilize venous thrombi and cause bleeding. Monitor the patient for signs and symptoms of vascular occlusion, including neurologic changes, chest discomfort, and dyspnea. Report such problems at once, and prepare the patient for diagnostic testing or transfer to the intensive care unit (ICU), as ordered.

Carotid sinus massage
Because carotid sinus massage can cause ventricular fibrillation, ventricular tachycardia, and standstill as well as worsening atrioventricular block that leads to junctional or ventricular escape rhythms, you'll need to monitor the patient's electrocardiogram (ECG) closely. If his ECG indicates complete heart block or asystole, start basic life support at once, followed by advanced cardiac life support. If emergency medications don't convert the complete heart block, the patient may need a temporary pacemaker.

Carotid sinus massage can cause cerebral damage from inadequate tissue perfusion, especially in elderly patients. It can also cause a cerebrovascular accident, either from decreased perfusion caused by total carotid artery blockage or from migrating endothelial plaque loosened by carotid sinus compression. Watch the patient carefully during and after the procedure for changes in neurologic status. If you note any, tell the doctor at once and prepare the patient for further diagnostic tests or transfer to the ICU, as ordered.

Documentation
Record the date and time of the procedure, who performed it, and why it was necessary. Note the patient's response, any complications, and the interventions taken. If possible, obtain a rhythm strip before, during, and after the procedure to document changes.

 Pericardiocentesis

This procedure involves needle aspiration of the pericardial sac to remove blood or other fluid that has accumulated in the sac, relieving pressure on the heart. The extracted fluid can then be studied to help diagnose the underlying disease.

Several conditions can lead to fluid accumulation, including pericarditis, malignant neoplasm, and life-threatening cardiac tamponade. Commonly caused by chest trauma or cardiac surgery, cardiac tamponade requires immediate treatment to prevent the rapidly collecting blood from causing cardiac decompensation. If time allows, the doctor may order an echocardiogram to diagnose tamponade before beginning pericardiocentesis, or he'll perform the procedure based on assessment findings alone.

Equipment
Cardiac monitor with strip chart recorder ■ sterile specimen container ■ shaving supplies ■ sterile 4″ × 4″ drain dressings ■ sterile gloves, gowns, and masks ■ povidone-iodine solution ■ vial of 1% or 2% lidocaine ■ adhesive tape ■ sterile 4″ × 4″ gauze pads ■ inside-the-needle I.V. catheter ■ sterile I.V. tubing ■ alcohol sponges ■ sterile drainage container ■ dextrose 5% in water ■ 50-ml syringe ■ three-way stopcock ■ intracardiac needle ■ hemostat ■ optional: sedative.

Many hospitals use prepackaged pericardiocentesis trays that contain most, but not all, of the equipment needed for pericardiocentesis.

Implementation
• Check the patient's history for hypersensitivity to the local anesthetic.
• Obtain baseline vital signs, and administer a sedative, if ordered. Connect a cardiac monitor to the patient. Put on gloves.
• If the patient doesn't have a patent I.V. line for emergency medications, insert a line and administer dextrose 5% in water at a keep-vein-open rate.
• Shave or clip the patient's chest from midsternum to below the xiphoid process. Clean the area, first with

Needle placement in pericardiocentesis

After the doctor anesthetizes the site for needle insertion into the pericardial cavity, he'll connect the 50-ml syringe to a three-way stopcock and attach the intracardiac needle. He'll insert the needle to the left of the xiphoid process and advance it until he obtains a blood or fluid return.

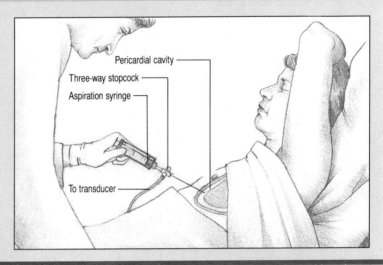

Pericardial cavity

Three-way stopcock

Aspiration syringe

To transducer

alcohol sponges, then with povidone-iodine. Wipe with a circular motion, moving away from the insertion site, *to help prevent infection.* Clean the entire shaved area *in case the myocardium tears during the procedure and the doctor needs to perform a thoracotomy to suture the tear.*
● If the patient's condition allows, elevate his head 60 degrees and support his arms with pillows. *This position makes needle placement easier.*
● Help the doctor put on sterile gloves, gown, and mask. Put on your gown and mask. Open the pericardiocentesis tray, using the outer wrapper to create a sterile field.
● Clean the rubber stopper of the lidocaine vial with an alcohol sponge, and invert it so the doctor can withdraw the anesthetic.
● After the doctor anesthetizes the site, monitor the patient's electrocardiogram (ECG) while the doctor inserts the needle. (See *Needle placement in pericardiocentesis.*) If the ECG pattern changes, notify the doctor *because the needle may have touched or penetrated the ventricle.* The doctor will attach a hemostat to the needle at the chest wall *to keep it from slipping out of position.* Then he will turn the three-way stopcock *to keep air out of the pericardial sac.*
● If the doctor needs a specimen, he'll withdraw the fluid and turn off the stopcock to the patient. Have the sterile specimen container ready for the specimen.
● If the patient has a lot of fluid in the pericardial sac, the doctor may insert a through-the-needle catheter and leave it in place. If so, attach the catheter to sterile

tubing and a sterile drainage container. Don sterile gloves and cover the catheter site with sterile drain dressings. Tape them securely and note the date and time on the dressing.
● Also using sterile technique, cover the intracardiac needle insertion site with sterile 4″ × 4″ gauze pads and tape them securely, noting the date and time on the dressing.
● After the procedure, monitor the patient closely. Report any changes that suggest perforation of the right ventricle or decreasing cardiac output.

Special considerations

Because pericardiocentesis can cause life-threatening complications, the patient should recover in the intensive care unit. (See *Dealing with the hazards of pericardiocentesis,* page 396.)

Despite pericardiocentesis, cardiac tamponade may recur. To relieve the problem, the patient may need pericardiocentesis again or further measures, such as surgery.

Documentation

Record the reason for pericardiocentesis, who performed it, and the outcome. Note the type of fluid aspirated, the presence of clots, and any specimens taken. Record the patient's response during the procedure and his status afterward, noting any complications and interventions taken.

Dealing with the hazards of pericardiocentesis

Needle aspiration of the pericardial sac risks cardiac arrhythmias, hemorrhage, organ puncture, and infection. Here are some guidelines for nursing care if any of these complications develop in your patient.

Cardiac arrhythmias
The most common complication, cardiac arrhythmias, results from the needle touching the myocardium. If you detect arrhythmias, tell the doctor at once, and prepare to administer emergency medications.

Hemorrhage
If the myocardium or a coronary artery is lacerated, the patient will show signs of hemorrhage, increased heart rate, and decreased blood pressure. In a compromised patient, these signs may be masked. To detect lacerations, check the aspirated fluid for clots. If you see any, tell the doctor and prepare for immediate surgical repair and resuscitation efforts.

Organ puncture
If the patient has sudden chest or epigastric pain, dyspnea, or decreasing blood pressure, the needle may have perforated his lung, liver, or stomach. If the needle punctured the lung, the patient will develop a pneumothorax and require immediate chest tube insertion. If the needle punctured the liver or stomach, he'll require surgical repair of the tear to stop the hemorrhaging.

Infection
Assess the patient for signs of infection, including an elevated white blood cell count, fever, chills, and drainage or redness at the insertion site. Notify the doctor if these signs appear. The doctor may order antibiotics along with culture and sensitivity tests.

Ventricular assist device

A temporary life-sustaining treatment for a failing heart, the ventricular assist device (VAD) diverts systemic blood flow from a diseased ventricle into a centrifugal pump. It temporarily reduces ventricular work, allowing the myocardium to rest and contractility to improve. Although used most commonly to assist the left ventricle, this device may also assist the right ventricle or both ventricles. (See *VAD: Help for the failing heart.*)

Candidates for VAD include patients with massive myocardial infarction, irreversible cardiomyopathy, acute myocarditis, an inability to be weaned from cardiopulmonary bypass, valvular disease, bacterial endocarditis, or heart transplant rejection. The device may also be used in those awaiting a heart transplant.

Equipment
Insertion of the ventricular assist device is performed in the operating room.

Implementation
• Before surgery, explain to the patient that food and fluid intake must be restricted and that you will continuously monitor his cardiac function (using an electrocardiogram, a pulmonary artery catheter, and an arterial line). Offer the patient reassurance. Before sending him to the operating room, ensure that he has signed a consent form.
• If time permits, shave the patient's chest and scrub it with an antiseptic solution.
• When the patient returns from surgery, administer analgesics, as ordered.
• Frequently monitor vital signs, intake, and output.
• Keep the patient immobile *to prevent accidental extubation, contamination, or disconnection of the VAD.* Use soft restraints as necessary.
• Monitor pulmonary artery pressures. If you've been prepared to adjust the pump, maintain cardiac output at about 5 to 8 liters/minute, central venous pressure at about 8 to 16 mm Hg, pulmonary capillary wedge pressure at about 10 to 20 mm Hg, mean arterial pressure at greater than 60 mm Hg, and left arterial pressure between 4 and 12 mm Hg.
• Monitor the patient for signs and symptoms of poor perfusion and ineffective pumping, including arrhythmias, hypotension, slow capillary refill, cool skin, oliguria or anuria, confusion, anxiety, and restlessness.
• Administer heparin, as ordered, to prevent clotting in the pump head and thrombus formation. Check for bleeding, especially at the operative sites. Monitor laboratory studies, as ordered, especially complete blood count and coagulation studies.
• Assess the patient's incisions and the cannula insertion sites for signs of infection. Monitor the patient's white blood cell count and differential daily, and take rectal or core temperatures every 4 hours.

VAD: Help for the failing heart

The ventricular assist device (VAD) functions somewhat like an artificial heart. The major difference is that the VAD assists the heart, whereas the artificial heart replaces it. The VAD is designed to aid one or both ventricles. The pumping chambers themselves aren't usually implanted in the patient.

The permanent VAD is implanted in the patient's chest cavity, although it still provides only temporary support. The device receives power through the skin by a belt of electrical transformer coils (worn externally as a portable battery pack). It can also operate off an implanted, rechargeable battery for up to 1 hour at a time.

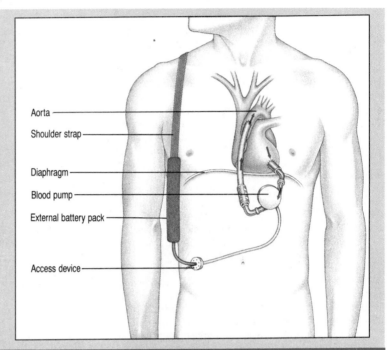

Aorta

Shoulder strap

Diaphragm

Blood pump

External battery pack

Access device

• Change the dressing over the cannula sites daily or according to hospital policy.
• Provide supportive care, including range-of-motion exercises and mouth and skin care.

Special considerations
If ventricular function fails to improve within 4 days, the patient may need a transplant. If so, provide psychological support for the patient and family as they endure referral. You may also initiate the transplant process by contacting the appropriate agency.

The psychological effects of the ventricular assist device can produce stress in the patient, his family, and his close friends. If appropriate, refer them to other support personnel.

Complications
The VAD carries a high risk of complications, including damaged blood cells, which can increase the likelihood of thrombus formation and subsequent pulmonary embolism or cerebrovascular accident.

Documentation
Note the patient's condition following insertion of the VAD. Document any pump adjustments, as well as any complications and interventions.

Intra-aortic balloon counterpulsation

The intra-aortic balloon counterpulsation (IABC) device consists of a single-chamber or multichamber polyurethane balloon attached to an external pump console by a large-lumen catheter. A surgeon advances the balloon catheter up the patient's descending thoracic aorta to a point just distal to the left subclavian artery. The pumping console inflates the balloon with helium or carbon dioxide during diastole and deflates it during systole.

This inflation-deflation cycle, called counterpulsation, is synchronized with the patient's electrocardiogram (ECG), which appears on the console's oscilloscope. IABC increases systemic circulation, improves coronary perfusion, and reduces left ventricular work load. (See *Understanding the balloon pump*.)

The balloon inflates early in diastole, just after the aortic valve closes. Normally, about 70% to 80% of coronary perfusion occurs during diastole. Balloon inflation forces blood toward the aortic valve, which increases pressure in the aortic root and augments diastolic pressure to enhance coronary perfusion. It also forces blood through the brachiocephalic, common carotid, and subclavian arteries arising from the aortic trunk, which improves peripheral circulation.

During systole, blood pressure in the left ventricle must exceed that in the aorta to allow the aortic valve to open and eject blood. The aortic resistance that must be overcome is called afterload. The balloon rapidly deflates just before systole, which reduces aortic volume and decreases aortic pressure and afterload. Because aortic pressure is diminished, the left ventricle doesn't need to work as hard to open the aortic valve. This decreased work load reduces the heart's oxygen requirement and, combined with the more efficient myocardial perfusion provided by the IABC, prevents or reduces myocardial ischemia.

The IABC console can be preset to assist the heart at intervals — for example, it can inflate and deflate every one to four beats, depending on the patient's need and the type of machine used. Inflation and deflation of the balloon is inhibited by certain ventricular arrhythmias.

The balloon catheter can be inserted percutaneously at bedside, in the operating room, or in a cardiac catheterization laboratory. If insertion is performed in the unit, strict aseptic technique must be followed. In some hospitals, technicians help the doctor insert and remove the catheter and troubleshoot problems. The nurse is usually responsible for patient assessment and management.

Before insertion of the balloon catheter, a pulmonary artery catheter, an indwelling urinary catheter, and an arterial line should be inserted. A peripheral I.V. or subclavian line should also be in place for administering fluids and medications as needed. A transducer connected to the IABC console projects a visible arterial pressure waveform on the oscilloscope. A separate monitor and transducer may be required to display pulmonary artery pressures.

Common indications for IABC include left ventricular failure and cardiogenic shock caused by acute myocardial infarction, unstable or preinfarction angina, and high-risk cardiac surgery. IABC may also be used to provide preoperative support to the patient undergoing cardiac catheterization.

Use of IABC is contraindicated by the inability to place the catheter through atherosclerotic vessels and in patients with irreversible brain damage, incompetent aortic valve, dissecting aortic aneurysm, or ventricular fibrillation.

Equipment

IABC console and balloon catheters ■ Dacron graft (for surgically inserted balloon) ■ ECG electrodes ■ I.V. solution and infusion set ■ sedative ■ pain medication ■ arterial line catheter ■ heparin flush solution, transducer, and flush setup ■ pulmonary artery catheter setup ■ temporary pacemaker setup ■ sterile drape ■ sterile gloves ■ suture material ■ povidone-iodine solution and saline or sterile water for irrigation and suction setup ■ oxygen setup and respirator, if necessary ■ defibrillator and emergency drugs ■ ECG monitor ■ fluoroscope ■ indwelling urinary catheter ■ urimeter ■ arterial blood gas (ABG) kits and tubes for laboratory studies ■ povidone-iodine swabs and ointment ■ dressing materials ■ 4″ × 4″ gauze pads ■ shaving supplies ■ optional: atropine, I.V. heparin, low-molecular-weight dextran.

Preparation of equipment

The doctor tests the balloon catheter for leaks before insertion. The pump console's pressure transducer must be balanced, and the oscilloscope monitor on the pump console must be calibrated for accuracy. Depending on hospital policy, balancing and calibration may be performed by the nurse or another specially trained member of the health care team.

IABC setup and operation vary with the manufacturer. Consult the manufacturer's instructions for additional information.

Implementation

• Explain the procedure to the patient. Inform him that the balloon catheter temporarily reduces the heart's work load to promote rapid healing of the ventricular muscle. Tell him that it will be removed after his heart can resume an adequate work load again.

To prepare for intra-aortic balloon insertion

• Make sure the patient or responsible family member understands and signs a consent form. Ensure that the form is on the patient's chart.
• Obtain baseline vital signs, including pulmonary artery pressures if the line is already inserted. Obtain a baseline ECG.
• Apply chest electrodes in a standard lead II position or in whatever position produces the largest R wave on the oscilloscope. *The R wave triggers the inflation-deflation cycle.*
• Assess the patient's respiratory status and administer oxygen as necessary.

Understanding the balloon pump

An intra-aortic balloon pump consists of a multichambered or a single-chambered polyurethane balloon attached to an external pump console by means of a large-lumen catheter.

This external pump works in precise counterpoint to the left ventricle, inflating the balloon with helium or carbon dioxide early in diastole and deflating it just before systole. Balloon inflation forces blood toward the aortic valve, augmenting diastolic pressure and improving cardiac perfusion.

Balloon deflation, which occurs quickly after diastole, reduces aortic volume and pressure and the work load of the left ventricle in opening the aortic valve. This, together with the improved perfusion, helps control myocardial ischemia by lowering the heart's need for oxygen.

Intra-aortic balloon counterpulsation (IABC) can be synchronized with the electrocardiogram (ECG) or the arterial waveform.

In the ECG mode, the R wave triggers balloon deflation (as shown); inflation can occur on the T wave's downslope or after a specific delay following the R wave. (The R wave corresponds to systole; the T wave corresponds to aortic valve closure.)

The arterial wave is a useful alternative when the ECG triggers inconsistent counterpulsation. In the arterial wave mode, deflation is triggered by systolic ejection and inflation is triggered by the dicrotic notch, which corresponds to aortic valve closure and the onset of diastole. For the arterial mode to work, the patient must have a pulse pressure greater than 20 mm Hg and his arterial waveform must have a steep upstroke.

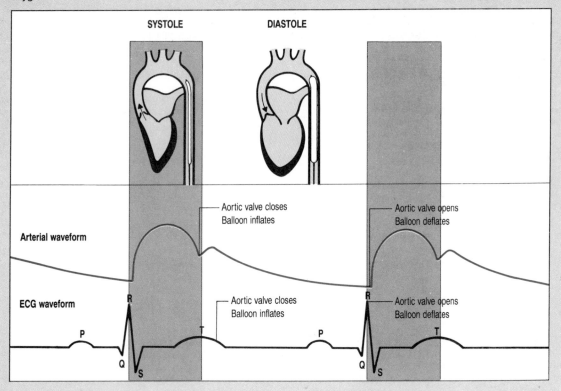

SYSTOLE   DIASTOLE

Aortic valve closes
Balloon inflates

Aortic valve opens
Balloon deflates

Arterial waveform

Aortic valve closes
Balloon inflates

Aortic valve opens
Balloon deflates

ECG waveform

• Prepare and insert a peripheral I.V. line *to deliver medications as ordered.*

• Prepare for and assist with insertion of an arterial line, as indicated, *to allow arterial pressure monitoring. The augmented pressure waveform demonstrates elevated diastolic and lowered systolic pressure and allows you to check proper timing of the inflation-deflation cycle.* (Remember, the balloon should inflate during diastole and deflate during systole.)

• Prepare for and assist with insertion of a pulmonary artery line, as indicated, *to allow measurement of pulmonary artery pressure, to permit aspiration of blood samples, and to perform cardiac output studies.* Increased pressures indicate increased myocardial work load and ineffective balloon pumping. Comparison cardiac output studies may be done on and off the IABC to determine patient progress and potential for weaning.

• If bradycardia occurs, give atropine or prepare the patient for pacemaker insertion, as ordered. The balloon pump is ineffective if the patient has bradycardia.

• Obtain specimens for preoperative laboratory tests, as ordered. These tests usually include blood typing and crossmatching, serum electrolytes, and coagulation studies.

• Insert an indwelling urinary catheter *to allow accurate measurement of urinary output and assessment of fluid balance and renal function.*

• Shave or clip the patient's hair from the lower abdomen to the lower thigh bilaterally, including the pubic area, *to reduce the risk of infection.* Although the catheter is usually inserted in the left side, it may be inserted in the right side if the left artery is diseased.

• Attach another set of ECG monitoring electrodes to the patient unless the ECG pattern is being transmitted from the patient's monitor to the balloon pump monitor.

• Administer a sedative, as ordered.

To insert the intra-aortic balloon

• The surgeon may insert a special intra-aortic balloon catheter percutaneously through the femoral artery into the descending thoracic aorta. This simplified procedure may be performed in the unit or in a cardiac catheterization laboratory.

• If the surgeon chooses not to insert the catheter percutaneously, he inserts the balloon through a femoral arteriotomy. This procedure is best performed in an operating room.

• After making the incision and isolating the artery, the surgeon attaches a Dacron graft to a small opening in the arterial wall, passes the catheter through this graft, and, with optional fluoroscopic guidance, advances it up the descending thoracic aorta and positions the catheter tip between the left subclavian artery and the renal arteries. The surgeon then sews the Dacron graft around the catheter at the insertion point and connects the other end of the catheter to the pumping console.

To monitor the patient after balloon insertion

• Obtain a chest X-ray *to determine correct balloon placement.*

• Observe the arterial pressure pattern every 30 minutes for diastolic augmentation *to verify correctly timed counterpulsation.*

• Measure blood pressure every 15 minutes to 1 hour *to determine the effectiveness of therapy and anticipate the need for vasopressors or vasodilators, such as dopamine or nitroprusside (Nipride).*

• Take apical pulse at least every hour, noting rate and rhythm. *Increased or decreased pulse rate alters the effectiveness of the pump and may require drugs, such as atropine, or pacemaker therapy.*

• Check the patient's temperature every hour. If it's elevated, obtain blood samples for culture, send them to the laboratory immediately, and notify the doctor.

• Measure intake and output hourly.

• Observe for ischemia in the limbs—especially the affected limb—every hour. Be alert for changes in pulse rate, color, temperature, and sensation. Explain to the patient the importance of keeping the affected extremity straight.

♦ *Nursing alert.* Watch for pump interruptions, which may result from loose ECG electrodes or broken wires, static or 60-cycle interference, kinked catheters, and improper body alignment. Elevate the head of the bed no more than 45 degrees, keeping the patient's leg unflexed at the groin *to prevent catheter kinking or forward displacement causing trauma or injury to the aorta.* ♦

• Observe for optimal timing. Balloon inflation should begin when the aortic valve closes or at the dicrotic notch on the arterial waveform. Deflation should occur just before systole. Improper timing includes late inflation, which reduces coronary artery perfusion, and prolonged inflation, which dangerously increases the resistance against which the left ventricle must pump. In both situations, readjust timing according to the manufacturer's guidelines, or notify the person responsible for the balloon pump adjustments.

♦ *Nursing alert.* If the IABC is inadvertently shut off for more than 5 minutes, notify the doctor immediately *to determine the need for heparinization before restarting the balloon. Resumed pumping without adequate anticoagulant precipitates emboli.* ♦

• Check for gas leaks from the catheter or the balloon. Such leaks may be indicated by an alarm on the pump console. If the balloon ruptures, blood will appear in the catheter. If this happens, shut off the pump console and notify the doctor.

◆ *Nursing alert.* If you suspect balloon rupture, promptly place the patient in Trendelenburg's position *to prevent the gas embolus from reaching the brain.* ◆

• If the patient isn't receiving anticoagulants, the doctor may order I.V. heparin or low-molecular-weight dextran *to prevent platelet aggregation on the quiescent balloon.*

• Measure pulmonary artery pressure and pulmonary capillary wedge pressure (PCWP) every 1 to 2 hours, or as ordered. A rising PCWP indicates increased ventricular pressure and work load; notify the doctor if this occurs. Some patients require the administration of I.V. nitroprusside in addition to the IABC *to reduce preload and afterload.*

• Obtain arterial samples for ABG analysis, as ordered. If the patient is connected to a ventilator, perform ventilation checks, suctioning, and respiratory assessment.

• Monitor electrolytes as ordered, especially sodium *to assess fluid balance* and potassium *to prevent cardiac arrhythmias.*

• Monitor hematologic status. Blood products are usually used to maintain the hematocrit at 30%. Platelets may be required if the platelet count drops. Observe for bleeding gums, blood in urine or stool, or petechiae.

• Monitor the results of clotting tests. As ordered, administer heparin through a pressure infusion to maintain the activated partial thromboplastin time at 1½ to 2 times the normal value.

• Turn and position the patient every 2 hours, keeping the affected extremity straight. Provide oral hygiene at least every 4 hours. Give pain medication *for insertion site discomfort,* as ordered.

• Re-dress the balloon site, as ordered, and observe for signs of inflammation or excessive bleeding. Apply pressure *to control bleeding.*

• Prevent constipation *to avoid strain on the patient's heart.*

• If angina occurs, notify the doctor immediately *because the IABC is not effective.*

◆ *Nursing alert.* Watch for signs and symptoms of a dissecting aortic aneurysm, such as a difference in blood pressure between arms; elevated blood pressure; pain in the chest, abdomen, or back; syncope; pallor; diaphoresis; dyspnea; throbbing abdominal mass; and a reduced red blood cell count with an elevated white blood cell count. If you suspect an aortic aneurysm, notify the doctor. ◆

To wean the patient from the intra-aortic balloon

• Assess cardiac index, systemic blood pressure, and PCWP *to evaluate readiness for weaning,* which usually begins about 24 hours after balloon insertion.

• To begin weaning, gradually decrease the frequency of balloon augmentation to 1:2, 1:4, and 1:8 as ordered, and measure the cardiac index at each ratio. (Output is frequently measured both on and off the machine.) Some doctors prefer to wean the patient by diminishing balloon volume; however, this must be done cautiously to avoid reducing volume so much that the balloon can't inflate and deflate forcibly enough to repel platelets. The increased risk of emboli with this method makes it controversial; when using it, some doctors choose to administer I.V. heparin or low-molecular-weight dextran.

• Avoid leaving the patient on a low augmentation setting for more than 2 hours *to skirt the risk of embolus formation.* Check your hospital policy.

To remove the intra-aortic balloon

• The surgeon removes the balloon catheter when augmentation is no longer necessary (for example, when cardiac output improves during weaning). He also removes it if circulation to the limb is seriously compromised; if the patient's condition is considered inoperable during cardiac catheterization; or if the patient's condition deteriorates beyond recovery. Then he closes the Dacron graft and sutures the insertion site. If a percutaneous catheter is in place, the surgeon usually removes it. Pressure must be applied to the site for 15 to 30 minutes or until bleeding stops; in some hospitals, this is the doctor's responsibility.

• After removal of IABC, provide necessary wound care, according to hospital policy.

Complications

Aortic or femoral artery dissection or perforation may occur during balloon insertion. Ischemia or loss of pulses may occur in extremities (especially the legs) from compromised circulation. Thrombi may form on the balloon, predisposing the patient to emboli. Platelets are destroyed during balloon pumping, causing a decrease in circulating platelets (thrombocytopenia). A gas embolus can occur from balloon rupture. Infection may occur at the balloon insertion site.

Documentation

Document all aspects of patient assessment and management. If you're responsible for the IABC device, document all routine checks, problems, and troubleshooting measures. If a technician is responsible for the IABC device, record only when and why the technician was notified, as well as the result of his actions on the patient, if any. Document any teaching of the patient, family, or close friends, as well as responses to therapy and teaching.

Looking at angioplasty

For percutaneous transluminal coronary angioplasty, the doctor must first thread a guide catheter to the occlusion site using fluoroscopic guidance. Once the guide catheter is positioned, the doctor carefully inserts a smaller, double-lumen balloon catheter through the guide catheter to the occlusion and carefully inflates it. The illustration shows balloon inflation and successful arterial dilation.

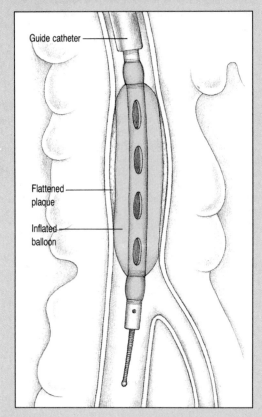

Guide catheter

Flattened plaque

Inflated balloon

Percutaneous transluminal coronary angioplasty

A nonsurgical approach to opening coronary vessels narrowed by arteriosclerosis, percutaneous transluminal coronary angioplasty (PTCA) uses a balloon-tipped catheter that's inserted into a coronary artery. The procedure is performed in the cardiac catheterization laboratory under local anesthesia. Cardiac catheterization usually accompanies PTCA to assess the stenosis and the efficacy of the angioplasty.

Catheterization is used as a visual tool to direct the balloon-tipped catheter through the vessel's area of stenosis. As the balloon is inflated, the plaque is compressed against the vessel wall, allowing coronary blood to flow more freely. (See *Looking at angioplasty.*)

PTCA provides an alternative for patients who are poor surgical risks because of chronic medical problems. It's also useful for patients who have total coronary occlusion, unstable angina, and plaque buildup in several areas, and for those with poor left ventricular function. PTCA is contraindicated in patients with left main coronary artery disease.

Equipment

Povidone-iodine solution ▪ local anesthetic ▪ I.V. solution and tubing ▪ dressing supplies ▪ electrocardiograph (ECG) and electrodes ▪ oxygen ▪ nasal cannula ▪ shaving supplies ▪ sedative ▪ introducer kit ▪ pulmonary artery catheter ▪ contrast medium ▪ emergency medications ▪ heparin for injection ▪ 5-lb (2.3-kg) sandbag ▪ introducer kit for PTCA catheter ▪ sterile gown, gloves, mask, and drapes ▪ optional: nitroglycerin, soft restraints.

Implementation

● Explain the procedure to the patient and his family *to reduce the patient's fears and promote cooperation.*
● Inform the patient that the procedure lasts from 1 to 4 hours and that he'll lie on a hard table during that time.
● Tell him that a catheter will be inserted into an artery or vein in the groin area and that he may feel pressure as the catheter moves along the vessel.
● Mention that he'll be awake during the procedure. He may have to answer questions about how he's feeling and will have to notify the doctor if he experiences any angina.
● Explain that the doctor will inject a contrast medium *to outline the lesion's location.* Warn the patient that during the injection he may feel a hot, flushing sensation or transient nausea.

Before angioplasty

● Check the patient's history for allergies; if he's had allergic reactions to shellfish, iodine, or contrast media, notify the doctor.
● Ensure that the patient has signed a consent form.

- Restrict the patient's food and fluid intake for at least 6 hours before the procedure, or as ordered.
- Ensure that coagulation studies, a complete blood count, serum electrolyte studies, and blood typing and cross-matching have been performed.
- Insert an I.V. line in case emergency medications are needed.

During angioplasty

- Upon arrival at the cardiac catheterization laboratory, apply ECG electrodes and ensure the patency of the I.V.
- Administer oxygen via a nasal cannula, and give the patient a sedative, as ordered.
- Assess the patient's peripheral pulses in all extremities *to use as a baseline.*
- Shave and clean the insertion site with povidone-iodine solution.
- Help the doctor put on a sterile gown and gloves, and help open sterile supplies. The doctor will prepare the site, usually the femoral artery, and inject a local anesthetic *to numb the area.* If the patient doesn't already have a pulmonary artery catheter in place, one may be inserted at this time.
- The doctor inserts a large guide catheter into the femoral artery and sutures it in place. Then he threads an angioplasty catheter through the guide catheter. It's thinner and longer and has a balloon at its tip. Using a thin, flexible guide wire, he then threads the catheter up through the aorta and into the coronary artery to the area of stenosis.
- The doctor injects a contrast medium through the angioplasty catheter and into the obstructed coronary artery *to outline the lesion's location and help assess the blockage.* He'll also inject heparin *to prevent the catheter from clotting.*
- The doctor inflates the catheter's balloon for a gradually increasing amount of time and pressure. The expanding balloon compresses the atherosclerotic plaque against the arterial wall, expanding the arterial lumen. Because balloon inflation deprives the myocardium distal to the inflation area of blood, the patient may experience angina at this time. If balloon inflation fails to decrease the stenosis, a larger balloon may be used.
- After angioplasty, serial angiograms help determine the effectiveness of treatment.
- The doctor removes the angioplasty catheter while leaving the guide catheter in place, *in case the procedure needs to be repeated because of vessel occlusion.* The guide catheter is usually removed 8 to 24 hours after the procedure.

After angioplasty

- When the patient returns to the unit, he may be receiving I.V. heparin or nitroglycerin. He may also have a sandbag on the insertion site *to prevent hematoma formation.*
- Assess the patient's vital signs every 15 minutes for the first hour, then every 30 minutes for 4 hours unless the patient's condition warrants more frequent checking.
- Assess peripheral pulses distal to the catheter insertion site and the color, sensation, temperature, and capillary refill of the extremity.
- Monitor ECG rhythm and arterial pressures.
- Instruct the patient to keep the affected extremity straight; apply soft restraints if necessary. Elevate the head of the bed 15 to 30 degrees.
- Assess the catheter site for hematoma formation, ecchymosis, and hemorrhage. If an area of expanding hematoma formation appears, mark the site and alert the doctor.
- Administer I.V. fluids as ordered, usually 100 ml/hour, *to promote excretion of the contrast medium.* Be sure to assess for signs of fluid overload (distended neck veins, atrial and ventricular gallops, dyspnea, pulmonary congestion, tachycardia, hypertension, and hypoxemia).
- After the doctor removes the catheter, apply direct pressure for at least 10 minutes and monitor the site frequently.

Special considerations

After PTCA, reocclusion may occur. If reocclusion doesn't occur during the first year, the prognosis is usually good if the patient continues his drug regimen and adopts a healthy life-style, including a proper diet and exercise.

Complications

PTCA can cause coronary artery perforation, balloon rupture, reocclusion (necessitating a coronary artery bypass graft), procedure-related myocardial infarction, cardiac tamponade, hematoma formation, and hemorrhage.

Documentation

Note the patient's tolerance for the procedure and his condition after it, including vital signs and the condition of the extremity distal to the insertion site. Document any complications and interventions.

 # Balloon valvuloplasty

Although the treatment of choice for valvular heart disease is surgery, balloon valvuloplasty is an alternative for patients who are poor surgical candidates. It enlarges the orifice of a heart valve that has been narrowed by a congenital defect, calcification, rheumatic fever, or aging.

Balloon valvuloplasty is performed in the cardiac catheterization laboratory under local anesthesia. The doctor inserts a balloon-tipped catheter through the patient's femoral vein or artery, threads it into the heart, and repeatedly inflates it against the leaflets of the diseased valve. This increases the size of the orifice, improving valvular function and helping prevent complications from decreased cardiac output.

Equipment
Povidone-iodine ■ local anesthetic ■ cannula ■ I.V. solution and tubing ■ introducer kit ■ dressing supplies ■ electrocardiograph (ECG) and electrodes ■ pulmonary artery catheter ■ contrast medium ■ oxygen ■ sedative ■ mergency medications ■ shaving supplies ■ heparin for injection ■ introducer kit for balloon catheter ■ sterile gown, gloves, and drapes ■ 5-lb (2.3-kg) sandbag ■ mask and cap ■ optional: nitroglycerin.

Implementation
• Reinforce the doctor's explanation of balloon valvuloplasty to the patient or his parents, including its risks and alternatives.
• Teach the patient what to expect. Inform him that his groin area will be shaved and cleaned with an antiseptic and that he'll feel a brief, stinging sensation when a local anesthetic is injected. Explain that he may feel pressure as the catheter moves along the vessel. Describe the warm, flushed feeling that he's likely to experience from injection of the contrast medium.
• Tell the patient that the procedure may last up to 4 hours and that he may feel discomfort from lying on a hard table for that long.

To prepare for balloon valvuloplasty
• Ensure that the patient has no allergies to shellfish, iodine, or contrast media and that he or his parents have signed a consent form.
• Restrict food and fluid intake for at least 6 hours before valvuloplasty, or as ordered.
• Make sure that the results of routine laboratory studies and blood typing and crossmatching are available.
• Insert an I.V. line to provide access for medications.

To perform balloon valvuloplasty
• Upon the patient's arrival at the cardiac catheterization laboratory, apply ECG electrodes, and ensure the patency of the I.V. line.
• Administer oxygen via a nasal cannula, and give the patient a sedative, as ordered.
• Assess the patient's peripheral pulses in all extremities *to use as a baseline.*
• Shave and clean the insertion site with povidone-iodine.

• Help the doctor put on a sterile gown and gloves, and help open the sterile supplies.
• The doctor will prepare and anesthetize the catheter insertion site (usually at the femoral artery). If it's not already in place, he may insert a pulmonary artery catheter.
• The doctor inserts a large guide catheter into the site. Then he threads a valvuloplasty or balloon-tipped catheter up into the heart.
• The doctor injects a contrast medium to visualize the heart valves and assess the stenosis. Heparin is also injected *to prevent the catheter from clotting.*
• The doctor inflates the balloon on the valvuloplasty catheter at a low pressure for a short time, gradually increasing the time and pressure. If the stenosis isn't reduced, a larger balloon may be used.
• After completion of valvuloplasty, a series of angiograms will be taken to determine the effectiveness of the treatment.
• The doctor sutures the guide catheter in place. It will be removed later after the effects of the heparin have worn off.

To monitor the patient after valvuloplasty
• On return to the unit, the patient may be receiving I.V. heparin or nitroglycerin. He may also have a sandbag on the insertion site *to prevent hematoma formation.*
• Monitor ECG rhythm and arterial pressures.
• Monitor the insertion site frequently for signs of hemorrhage *because exsanguination can occur rapidly.*
• To prevent excessive hip flexion and migration of the catheter, keep the affected leg straight, and elevate the head of the bed no more than 15 degrees.
• For the first hour, monitor vital signs every 15 minutes, then every 30 minutes for 2 hours, and then hourly for the next 5 hours. If vital signs are unstable, notify the doctor and continue to check them every 5 minutes.
• When you take vital signs, assess peripheral pulses distal to the catheter insertion site, and the color, sensation, temperature, and capillary refill time of the extremity.
• Assess the catheter site for hematoma formation, ecchymosis, and hemorrhage. If a hematoma expands, mark the site and alert the doctor.
• As ordered or according to hospital protocol, auscultate regularly for murmurs, which may indicate worsening valvular insufficiency. Notify the doctor if you detect a new or worsening murmur.
• Provide I.V. fluids at a rate of at least 100 ml/hour to help the kidneys excrete the contrast medium. Assess the patient for signs of fluid overload: distended neck veins, atrial and ventricular gallops, dyspnea, pulmonary congestion, tachycardia, hypertension, and hypoxemia.

• After the guide catheter is removed (usually 6 to 12 hours after valvuloplasty), apply direct pressure for at least 10 minutes and monitor the site frequently.

Special considerations
Elderly patients commonly experience restenosis 1 to 2 years after valvuloplasty.

Complications
Severe complications, such as myocardial infarction or calcium emboli, are rare. Other complications include bleeding or hematoma at the insertion site, arrhythmias, circulatory disorders distal to the insertion site, and valvular insufficiency, which can contribute to congestive heart failure and reduced cardiac output.

Documentation
Note the patient's tolerance for the procedure and his condition after it. Document any complications and interventions.

Emergency control of hemorrhage

Hemorrhage results from vascular tissue injury — externally from a laceration, amputation, fracture, crush trauma, or nosebleed; internally from a bleeding ulcer, ruptured spleen, or abdominal or chest trauma. Uncontrolled arterial bleeding can rapidly cause shock, and death can occur. In contrast, venous bleeding, even though heavy at first, is usually controlled quickly by clotting unless the patient is receiving anticoagulant therapy or has a bleeding disorder. However, venous bleeding still requires prompt treatment to prevent heavy blood loss.

Direct pressure over a bleeding vessel is the action of choice for external bleeding. It may help stop blood flow long enough to allow clot formation. If this fails to stop bleeding, applying pressure to the major artery proximal to the injury may slow or stop blood flow and perfusion into the tissues. A tourniquet should be used to control bleeding only if all other measures fail because its use may cause ischemia and necrosis of the affected tissue, possibly necessitating amputation of the limb.

Equipment
In an emergency, equipment consists of whatever is readily available and adaptable for immediate use. External hemorrhage requires thick pads of sterile gauze, sanitary pads, or clean soft cloths, with ties of available materials such as a scarf, stockings, or strips of clothing. Obtain ice bags, if available. If dressings aren't available, use your hands (gloved if possible) to stop excessive bleeding until you can obtain dressings. Tourniquets require a wide fold of cloth or other broad material, such as a belt, blood pressure cuff, scarf, or large handkerchief, and a stick or pencil to tighten the tourniquet.

Implementation
• Explain the procedure to the patient, even if he's comatose, *to help allay his fears and promote cooperation.*

To control external bleeding
• If necessary, cut or tear the patient's clothing *to expose the wound.*
• Elevate an affected extremity above heart level *to stop venous and capillary bleeding.*
• Apply steady, direct pressure on the wound with a clean dressing of sterile gauze, a sanitary pad, or clean, soft cloths. If nothing else is available, use your hands (gloved if possible). Apply ice to the wound, if possible.
• If direct pressure fails to stop bleeding or cannot be applied because of a fracture, apply digital pressure to the arterial pressure point nearest the wound. (See *Locating arterial pressure points,* page 406.) If you're not skilled at locating a pressure point precisely, apply pressure with the heel of your hand to cover the area where the pressure point is located. If you've applied pressure correctly, you'll be unable to detect a pulse below the pressure point, and the patient will feel local tingling or numbness.
• If you've controlled the bleeding, apply a pressure dressing. Using sterile gauze or clean cloths, prepare a compress six to eight layers thick. Tie the dressing in place with any available cloth, such as a scarf, stocking, or strip of clothing. If blood soaks through the dressing, do not remove it; apply additional dressings over the soaked ones and rebandage.
• If bleeding persists — and only as a last resort — apply a tourniquet between the injury site and the heart. Wrap the tourniquet around the extremity, about 2″ (5 cm) above the wound (the tourniquet should not touch the wound edges). Tie it with a half knot, place the stick over the half knot, and tie a square knot over it. Tighten the tourniquet by twisting the stick until bleeding stops. Secure the stick in this position. Leave the tourniquet uncovered, and alert rescuers to its location and time of application. Avoid loosening the tourniquet until the patient reaches the hospital. *Doing so may cause a massive hemorrhage that could be lethal to an already hypovolemic patient, and may release dangerous toxins from injured tissues.*

Locating arterial pressure points

To control hemorrhage, compress the appropriate pressure point—the site at which a large blood vessel can be compressed against bone. Compression of a pressure point controls bleeding in a distinct area (indicated in parentheses after the pressure point).

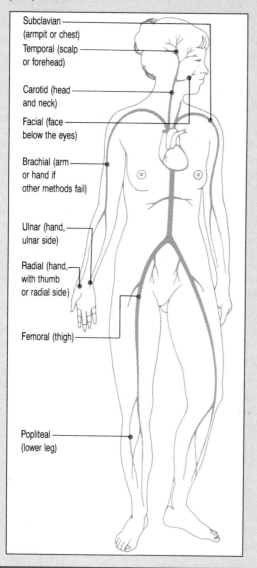

Subclavian (armpit or chest)

Temporal (scalp or forehead)

Carotid (head and neck)

Facial (face below the eyes)

Brachial (arm or hand if other methods fail)

Ulnar (hand, ulnar side)

Radial (hand, with thumb or radial side)

Femoral (thigh)

Popliteal (lower leg)

To control internal bleeding

• If you suspect internal bleeding, keep the patient calm. Don't give liquids unless medical attention will be delayed and there is no GI bleeding. If possible, apply ice bags to the affected area *to reduce swelling*. Place the patient in Trendelenburg's position *to increase cerebral blood flow*. Apply antishock trousers, if indicated.

• After any type of hemorrhage, when bleeding is controlled, take the patient's vital signs and observe for other major injuries. For more information, see *Estimating internal blood loss*.

Special considerations

Be sure not to apply the tourniquet loosely. Loose application may actually increase blood loss *because arterial bleeding continues and the tourniquet prevents venous return.*

Transport the patient to the hospital without delay. If you suspect spinal injury, make sure that the patient is tied to a backboard before movement. Handle a partially severed limb with extreme care *to avoid increasing the extent of injury.* A completely severed limb should accompany the patient on transport. If possible, place the limb in a plastic bag packed in ice. (See *Caring for an amputated body part*, Chapter 12.)

Complications

In hemorrhage, cardiac arrest can result from hypovolemia with secondary anoxia. Even correct application of a tourniquet may cause gangrene and loss of a limb.

Documentation

Be sure to keep a record of the patient's vital signs and an assessment of his condition and injuries (if applicable). Document all nursing interventions. If you used a tourniquet, note the time when you applied it.

 Application and removal of medical antishock trousers

Medical antishock trousers (a MAST suit, also known as a pneumatic antishock garment) are made of inflatable bladders sandwiched between double layers of fabric. When inflated, the suit places external pressure on the lower extremities and abdomen, creating an autotransfusion effect by squeezing blood superiorly and increasing blood volume to the heart, lungs, and brain by up to 30%.

The MAST suit, used to treat shock when systolic blood pressure falls below 80 mm Hg—or below 100 mm Hg when accompanied by signs of shock—can control abdomi-

Estimating internal blood loss

To determine the amount of blood loss from an internal hemorrhage and to pinpoint the probable cause, assess your patient for the signs and symptoms below. (The milliliter amount in parentheses is for a 154-lb [70-kg] patient.)

ESTIMATED BLOOD LOSS	SIGNS AND SYMPTOMS	PROBABLE CAUSES
Less than 10% (500 ml)	• Normal or slightly elevated blood pressure • No orthostatic hypotension • Anxiety	• Fracture • Bleeding ulcer
20% to 25% (1,000 to 1,250 ml)	• Heart rate > 100 beats/minute • Respiratory rate, 20 to 30 breaths/minute • Normal or slightly lowered blood pressure • Narrowed pulse pressure • Normal capillary refill time • Orthostatic hypotension • Reduced urine output (below 30 ml/hour) • Anxiety and restlessness	• Pelvic or long bone fracture • Liver or spleen trauma
30% to 40% (1,500 to 2,000 ml)	• Extremely low urine output • Cool, clammy skin • Tachycardia • Tachypnea • Diminished systolic and elevated diastolic pressures • Narrowed pulse pressure • Cyanosis • Confusion • Decreased level of consciousness	• Multiple trauma with fractures • Spleen rupture • Thoracic injuries • Vascular injuries
40% to 50% (2,000 to 2,500 ml)	• All signs and symptoms in previous category • Weak, thready pulse; may not be palpable • Unresponsiveness	• Ongoing blood loss • Aortic injury • Multiple injuries

nal and lower extremity hemorrhage by creating internal pressure and external tamponade effects. It can also help stabilize and splint pelvic and femoral fractures.

Use of the MAST suit is contraindicated in patients with cardiogenic shock, congestive heart failure, pulmonary edema, tension pneumothorax, and increased intracranial pressure. It should be used cautiously during pregnancy. The MAST suit must be deflated slowly, with continuous blood pressure monitoring, to prevent potentially irreversible shock from hypovolemia. It shouldn't be removed until the patient's blood volume is restored, the patient's condition is stabilized, or the patient is being prepared for surgery. If necessary, the MAST suit can be deflated by stages in the operating room.

Equipment

A MAST suit with foot pump is the only necessary equipment (MAST suits come in a pediatric size for patients 3.5′ to 5′ [1.05 to 1.5 m] tall and an adult size for patients taller than 5′) ■ optional: resuscitation equipment.

Preparation of equipment

Spread open the MAST suit on a smooth surface or blanket *to avoid puncturing it.* Make sure all the stopcock valves are open. Attach the foot pump.

Applying antishock trousers

After taking the patient's baseline vital signs and explaining the treatment, prepare to apply the antishock trousers. On a smooth surface, open the garment with Velcro fasteners down, as shown.

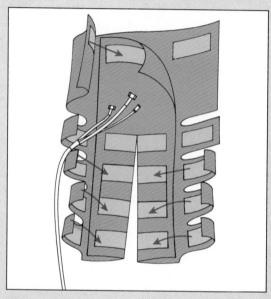

Open all stopcock valves, then attach the foot pump tubing to the valve on the pressure control unit. Can the patient be turned from side to side? If not, slide the garment under him. If he can be turned, place the garment next to him and, with assistance, move him onto it.

Before closing the trousers, remove any sharp objects, such as pieces of glass, stones, keys, or a buckle, that could injure the patient or tear the trousers. As appropriate, pad pressure points and apply lanolin to protect the patient's skin from irritation.

Place the upper edge of the trousers just below the patient's lowest rib. Wrap the right leg compartment around the patient's right leg. Secure the compartment by fastening the Velcro straps from the ankle to the thigh.

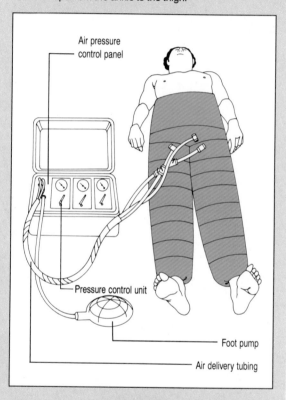

Repeat this procedure for the left leg; then wrap the abdomen. Double-check that all valves are properly positioned.

Implementation

• Explain the procedure to the patient *to allay his fears and ensure his cooperation.*

To apply a MAST suit

• Take vital signs *to establish baseline measurements.* Assess the patient's physical condition *to ensure that there are no contraindications to the use of the suit.*

• Assess the patient's injuries *to determine whether he can be turned from side to side.* If he can't be turned, slide the MAST suit under him. If he can be turned, place the MAST suit next to him and logroll him onto it. You can also set up the MAST suit on a stretcher and place the patient on it in a supine position. (See *Applying antishock trousers.*)

• Examine the patient for sharp objects, such as pieces of glass, *that could injure him or puncture the suit.*

• Double-check the stopcocks to make sure they're all open *so that the MAST suit will inflate uniformly.*
• Inflate the legs of the MAST suit first, then the abdominal segment, to about 20 to 30 mm Hg initially.
• Monitor the patient's blood pressure and pulse rate. Continue to inflate the suit slowly while monitoring vital signs. Stop inflating when the patient's systolic blood pressure reaches the desired level, usually 100 mm Hg.
• Close all stopcocks *to prevent accidental air loss.*
• Monitor the patient's blood pressure, pulse rate, and respirations every 5 minutes *to determine his response to application of the MAST suit.* Check his pedal pulses and temperature periodically. Notify the doctor if the circulation in the patient's feet appears impaired.

To remove a MAST suit
• Before deflation, make sure that I.V. lines are patent, a doctor is in attendance, and emergency resuscitation equipment is immediately available. *Removing a MAST suit may cause the patient's blood pressure to drop rapidly.*
• Open the abdominal stopcock and start releasing small amounts of air. Closely monitor the patient's systolic blood pressure as you do this. If it drops 5 mm Hg, close the stopcock.
♦ **Nursing alert.** Deflating the suit too quickly can allow circulating blood to rush to the abdomen or extremities, causing potentially irreversible shock. ♦
• If you need to stop deflating the MAST suit because of a drop in blood pressure, increase the flow rate of I.V. solutions *to help stabilize blood pressure.*
• If blood pressure is stable, continue to deflate the MAST suit slowly. After deflating the abdominal section, deflate the legs simultaneously.
• When the MAST suit loosens enough, gently pull it off.
• Clean the MAST suit as required, but don't autoclave it or use solvents.

Special considerations
Generally, you should see a therapeutic response to treatment when the MAST suit is inflated to 25 mm Hg. A so-called *morbidity effect,* caused by a change in local circulation, occurs at about 50 mm Hg. Most types of MAST suits have Velcro straps, pop-off valves, or gauges that prevent inflation beyond 104 mm Hg. Normally, the MAST suit shouldn't be left inflated for more than 2 hours, although occasionally it will be used for as long as several days. A range of 25 to 50 mm Hg can usually be maintained for up to 48 hours. For prolonged use, the MAST suit may be inflated at a lower pressure than normal.

A MAST suit is radiolucent, and X-rays can be taken while the patient is wearing it.

Complications
Vomiting can result from compression of the abdomen. Anaerobic metabolism, which can result from the MAST suit's pressure being higher than the patient's systolic pressure, can lead to metabolic acidosis. Skin breakdown may follow prolonged use. When used with severe leg fractures for long periods, tissue sloughing and necrosis caused by increased compartmental pressures have necessitated amputation.

Documentation
Record the time of application and removal and the patient's vital signs before application, during treatment, and after removal.

Selected references

Darovic, F. *Hemodynamic Monitoring: Invasive and Noninvasive Clinical Applications.* Philadelphia: W.B. Saunders Co., 1987.

Hudak, C., et al. *Critical Care Nursing: A Holistic Approach,* 5th ed. Philadelphia: J.B. Lippincott Co., 1990.

Illustrated Manual of Nursing Practice. Springhouse, Pa.: Springhouse Corp., 1991.

Kinkade, S.L., and Lohrman, J. *Critical Care Nursing Procedures: A Team Approach.* Philadelphia: B.C. Decker, Inc., 1990.

Noone, J. "Troubleshooting Thermodilution Pulmonary Artery Catheters," *Critical Care Nurse* 8(2):68, March-April 1988.

Nursing I.V. Drug Handbook, 4th ed. Springhouse, Pa.: Springhouse Corp., 1992.

Schermer, L. "Physiologic and Technical Variables Affecting Hemodynamic Measurements," *Critical Care Nurse* 8(2):33-40, March-April 1988.

Textbook of Advanced Cardiac Support, 2nd ed. Dallas: American Heart Association, 1987.

Vandenbelt, R.J. *Cardiology: A Clinical Approach,* 2nd ed. Chicago: Year-book Medical Publishers, 1987.

RESPIRATORY CARE

VICKI L. BUCHDA, RN, MS

Introduction

No matter where you work, you're sure to encounter patients with respiratory conditions. Such conditions may be acute or chronic, may have developed as a primary disorder, or may result from a cardiac or other disorder.

Caring for the patient with a respiratory condition will challenge your nursing skills. Not only is the patient's oxygenation compromised, but he may develop other problems as well. For instance, the patient may experience ineffective airway clearance and gas exchange, altered cardiac output, altered fluid volume, impaired thermoregulation, and decreased mobility. He may be anxious, cope ineffectively, and have an impaired ability to communicate. In addition, his nutritional status may be compromised. For such a patient, you'll need to develop an individual plan of care to ensure that he achieves optimum gas exchange and physical function.

To meet your care goals, you need to have a working knowledge of the many therapies available to respiratory patients. Although many hospitals have staff who specialize in respiratory procedures, you still need to keep your knowledge up-to-date. That way, you'll understand the rationales behind the patient's treatment, perform or assist with procedures if necessary, recognize complications, and detect the need for additional therapy. You'll also work with other members of the health care team to teach the patient and his family about equipment and procedures necessary for his care.

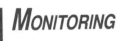

MONITORING
Mixed venous oxygen saturation

This procedure uses a fiber-optic thermodilution pulmonary artery catheter to continuously monitor oxygen delivery to tissues and oxygen consumption by tissues. Monitoring of mixed venous oxygen saturation ($S\bar{v}O_2$) allows rapid detection of impaired oxygen delivery, such as from decreased cardiac output, hemoglobin level, or arterial oxygen saturation. It also helps evaluate a patient's response to drug administration, endotracheal tube suctioning, ventilator setting changes, positive end-expiratory pressure, and fraction of inspired oxygen. $S\bar{v}O_2$

saturation usually ranges from 60% to 80%, with the normal value being 75%.

Equipment

Fiber-optic pulmonary artery (PA) catheter ■ CO-oximeter (monitor) ■ optical module and cable ■ gloves.

Preparation of equipment

Review the manufacturer's instructions for assembly and use of the fiber-optic PA catheter. Connect the optical module and cable to the monitor. Next, peel back the wrapping covering the catheter just enough to uncover the fiber-optic connector. Attach the fiber-optic connector to the optical module, while allowing the rest of the catheter to remain in its sterile wrapping. Calibrate the fiber-optic catheter by following the manufacturer's instructions.

To prepare for the rest of the procedure, follow the instructions for pulmonary catheter insertion, as described in "Pulmonary artery and capillary wedge pressure monitoring," Chapter 7. (See also *$S\bar{v}O_2$ monitoring equipment*, page 412.)

Implementation

- Wash your hands and put on gloves.
- Explain the procedure to the patient *to allay his fears and promote cooperation.*
- Assist with the insertion of the fiber-optic catheter just as you would for a PA catheter.
- Once the catheter is inserted, confirm that the light intensity tracing on the graphic printout is within normal range *to ensure correct positioning and function of the catheter.*
- Observe the digital readout and record the $S\bar{v}O_2$ on graph paper. Repeat readings at least once each hour *to monitor and document trends.*
- Set the machine alarms 10% above and 10% below the patient's current $S\bar{v}O_2$ reading.

To recalibrate the monitor

- Draw a mixed venous blood sample from the distal port of the PA catheter. Send it to the laboratory for analysis *to compare the laboratory's $S\bar{v}O_2$ measurement with the measurement indicated by the fiber-optic catheter.*
- If the catheter values and the laboratory values differ by more than 4%, follow the manufacturer's instructions to enter the $S\bar{v}O_2$ value obtained by the laboratory into the oximeter.
- Recalibrate the monitor every 24 hours, or whenever the catheter has been disconnected from the optical module.

S$\bar{v}$O$_2$ monitoring equipment

The S$\bar{v}$O$_2$ monitoring system consists of a flow-directed pulmonary artery (PA) catheter with fiber-optic filaments, an optical module, and a CO-oximeter. The CO-oximeter displays a continuous digital S$\bar{v}$O$_2$ value; the strip recorder prints a permanent record.

Catheter insertion follows the same technique as with any thermodilution flow-directed PA catheter. The distal lumen connects to an external PA pressure monitoring system; the proximal or central venous pressure (CVP) lumen connects to another monitoring system or to a continuous flow administration unit; and the optical module connects to the CO-oximeter unit.

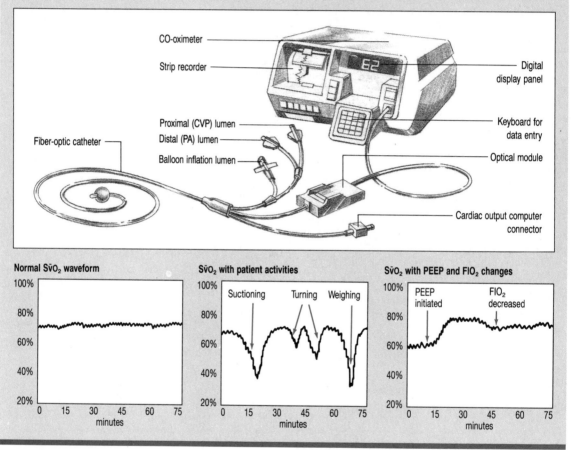

Normal S$\bar{v}$O$_2$ waveform

S$\bar{v}$O$_2$ with patient activities

S$\bar{v}$O$_2$ with PEEP and FIO$_2$ changes

Special considerations

• If the patient's S$\bar{v}$O$_2$ drops below 60%, or if it varies by more than 10% for 3 minutes or longer, reassess the patient. If the S$\bar{v}$O$_2$ does not return to the baseline value after appropriate nursing interventions, notify the doctor. A decreasing S$\bar{v}$O$_2$, or a value less than 60%, indicates impaired oxygen delivery, such as occurs during hemorrhage, hypoxia, shock, arrhythmias, or suctioning. S$\bar{v}$O$_2$ may also decrease as a result of increased oxygen demand from hyperthermia, shivering, or seizures, for example.

• If the intensity of the tracing is low, ensure that all connections between the catheter and oximeter are secure and that the catheter is patent and not kinked.

• If the tracing is damped or erratic, try to aspirate blood from the catheter *to check for patency.* If you can't aspirate blood, notify the patient's doctor *so that he can replace*

How oximetry works

The pulse oximeter allows noninvasive monitoring of a patient's SaO_2 levels by measuring the absorption (amplitude) of light waves as they pass through areas of the body that are highly perfused by arterial blood. Oximetry also monitors pulse rate and amplitude.

Light-emitting diodes in a transducer (photodetector) attached to the patient's body (shown here on the index finger) send red and infrared light beams through tissue. The photodetector records the relative amount of each color absorbed by arterial blood and transmits the data to a monitor, which displays the information with each heartbeat. If the SaO_2 level or pulse rate varies from preset limits, the monitor triggers visual and audible alarms.

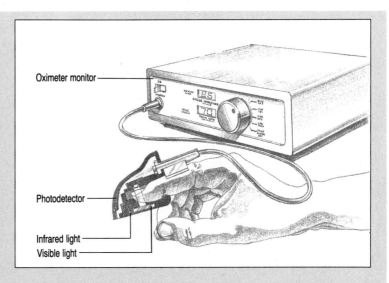

Oximeter monitor

Photodetector

Infrared light

Visible light

the catheter. Also check the PA waveform *to determine whether the catheter has wedged.* If the catheter has wedged, attempt to flush the line. Also turn the patient from side to side and instruct him to cough. If the catheter remains wedged, notify the patient's doctor immediately.
• If the tracing shows a high intensity, the catheter may be pressing against a vessel wall. Flush the line. If the tracing doesn't return to normal, notify the doctor *so he can reposition the catheter.*

Complications
Thrombosis can result from local irritation by the catheter; however, a heparinized flush helps prevent this complication. Thromboembolism also can occur if a thrombus breaks off and lodges in the circulatory system. Monitor the patient for signs and symptoms of infection — such as redness or drainage — at the catheter site.

Documentation
Record the $S\bar{v}O_2$ value on a flowchart and attach a tracing, as ordered. At the same time, note any significant changes in the patient's status and the results of any medical or nursing interventions. For comparison, note the $S\bar{v}O_2$ as measured by the fiber-optic catheter whenever a blood sample is obtained for laboratory analysis of mixed venous oxygen saturation.

Pulse and ear oximetry

Performed intermittently or continuously, oximetry is a relatively simple procedure used to monitor arterial oxygen saturation (SaO_2). Pulse oximetry uses two diodes to send red and infrared light through a pulsating arterial vascular bed, like the one in the fingertip. A photodetector, which is slipped over the finger, measures the transmitted light as it passes through the vascular bed, detects the relative amount of color absorbed by arterial blood, and calculates the exact SaO_2 without interference from surrounding venous blood, skin, connective tissue, or bone. Ear oximetry works by monitoring the transmission of light waves through the vascular bed of a patient's earlobe. However, results will be inaccurate if the patient's earlobe is poorly perfused, as occurs with a low cardiac output. (See *How oximetry works.*)

If the patient has significantly reduced peripheral vascular pulsations, or if he is taking a vasoactive drug, oximetry may be performed through a nasal probe, which detects the pulsations of the septal anterior ethmoidal artery. Capnometry is another procedure used to help assess a patient's cardiovascular and respiratory status

Understanding capnometry

Capnometers monitor carbon dioxide (CO_2) levels, usually by measuring the partial pressure of end-tidal CO_2 in expired air. Most capnometers use infrared absorption spectroscopy to analyze gas samples. Of the common gases in exhaled air, only CO_2 and water vapor absorb infrared light. The capnometer evaporates water vapor by dehumidifying the gas sample, leaving only CO_2 to be measured.

Capnometers display CO_2 values in one of three ways: as a percentage, in millimeters of mercury (mm Hg), or in kilopascals. The monitor also displays CO_2 values graphically as a continuous waveform (capnogram).

Capnometry allows you to measure ventilation, perfusion, and metabolism noninvasively. First used in the operating room by anesthesiologists, capnometry may also be used for patients being mechanically ventilated, weaned from a mechanical ventilator, or resuscitated by cardiopulmonary resuscitation in the intensive care unit or emergency department.

Setting up the capnometer

Begin by calibrating the capnometer according to the manufacturer's instructions. Then attach the power cord to the receptacle on the monitor. After making sure the sample tube assembly is in good condition, connect one end to the sample inlet connector. You'll connect the other end when you're ready to use the monitor.

The capnograph has audible and visual alarms to alert you to a CO_2 value above or below the limits you set. The monitor also has alarms to warn of monitor failure and apnea. Be sure to set these controls as ordered, following the manufacturer's instructions.

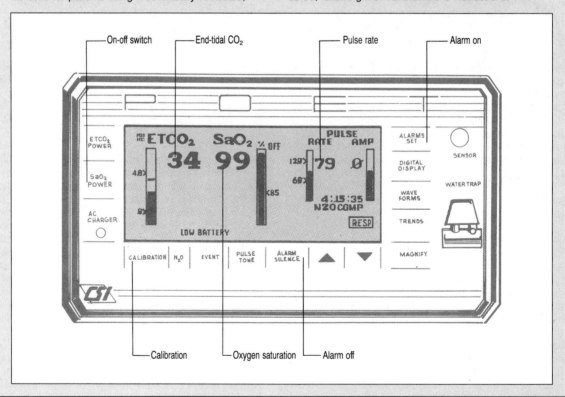

by monitoring carbon dioxide levels. (See *Understanding capnometry.*)

Equipment

Oximeter ■ finger or ear probe ■ alcohol sponges ■ nail polish remover, if necessary.

Preparation of equipment

Review the manufacturer's instructions for assembly of the oximeter.

Implementation

• Explain the procedure to the patient.

To perform pulse oximetry

• Select a finger for the test. Although the index finger is commonly used, a smaller finger may be selected if the patient's fingers are too large for the equipment. Make sure the patient isn't wearing false fingernails, and remove any nail polish from the test finger. Place the transducer (photodetector) probe over the patient's finger so that light beams and sensors oppose each other. If the patient has long fingernails, position the probe perpendicular to the finger if possible, or clip the fingernail.
• If you're testing a neonate or a small infant, wrap the probe around the foot so that light beams and detectors oppose each other. (See "Transcutaneous PO_2 monitoring," Chapter 15.) For a large infant, use a probe that fits on the great toe and secure it to the foot.
• Turn on the power switch. If the device is working properly, a beep will sound, a display will light momentarily, and the pulse searchlight will flash. The SaO_2 and pulse rate displays will show stationary zeros. After four to six heartbeats, the SaO_2 and pulse rate displays will supply information with each beat, and the pulse amplitude indicator will begin tracking the pulse.

To perform ear oximetry

• Using an alcohol sponge, massage the patient's earlobe for 10 to 20 seconds. Mild erythema indicates adequate vascularization. Following the manufacturer's instructions, attach the ear probe to the patient's earlobe or pinna. Use the ear probe stabilizer for prolonged or exercise testing. Be sure to establish good contact on the ear; *an unstable probe may set off the low-perfusion alarm.* After the probe has been attached for a few seconds, a saturation reading and pulse waveform will appear on the oximeter's screen. Leave the ear probe in place for 3 or more minutes until readings stabilize at the highest point, or take three separate readings and average them. Make sure you revascularize the patient's earlobe each time.

• After the procedure, remove the probe, turn off and unplug the unit, and clean the probe by gently rubbing it with an alcohol sponge.

Special considerations

If oximetry has been performed properly, readings are typically accurate. However, certain factors may interfere with accuracy. For example, an elevated bilirubin level may falsely lower SaO_2 readings, while elevated carboxyhemoglobin or methemoglobin levels (such as occur in heavy smokers or urban dwellers) can cause a falsely elevated SaO_2 reading.

Certain intravascular substances — such as lipid emulsions and dyes — can also prevent accurate readings. Other factors that may interfere with accurate results include excessive light (such as from phototherapy, surgical lamps, direct sunlight, and excessive ambient lighting), excessive patient movement, excessive ear pigment, hypothermia, hypotension, and vasoconstriction.

If light is a problem, cover the probes; if patient movement is a problem, move the probe or select a different probe; and if ear pigment is a problem, reposition the probe, revascularize the site, or use a finger probe. (See *Diagnosing pulse oximeter problems,* page 416.)

Normal SaO_2 levels for ear and pulse oximetry are 95% to 100% for adults, and 93.8% to 100% by 1 hour after birth for healthy, full-term neonates. Lower levels may indicate hypoxemia that warrants intervention. For such patients, follow hospital policy or the doctor's orders, which may include increasing oxygen therapy. If SaO_2 levels decrease suddenly, you may need to resuscitate the patient immediately. Notify the doctor of any significant change in the patient's condition.

Documentation

Document the procedure, including the date, time, procedure type, oximetric measurement, and any action taken. Record reading on appropriate flowcharts if indicated.

Bedside spirometry

This procedure measures forced vital capacity (FVC) and forced expiratory volume (FEV), allowing calculation of other pulmonary function indices, such as timed forced expiratory flow rate. Depending on the type of spirometer used, bedside spirometry can also allow direct measurement of vital capacity and tidal volume.

Bedside spirometry aids in diagnosing pulmonary dysfunction before it appears on an X-ray or physical ex-

Diagnosing pulse oximeter problems

To maintain a continuous display of SaO$_2$ levels, you'll need to keep the monitoring site clean and dry. Make sure the skin doesn't become irritated from adhesives used to keep disposable probes in place. You may need to change the site if this happens. Disposable probes that irritate the skin also can be replaced by nondisposable models that don't need tape.

Another common problem with pulse oximeters is the failure of the devices to obtain a signal. Your first reaction if this happens should be to check the patient's vital signs. If they're sufficient to produce a signal, then check for the following problems:

• *Poor connection.* See if the sensors are properly aligned. Make sure that wires are intact and securely fastened and that the pulse oximeter is plugged into a power source.

• *Inadequate or intermittent blood flow to the site.* Check the patient's pulse rate and capillary refill time and take corrective action if blood flow to the site is decreased. This may mean loosening restraints, removing tight-fitting clothes, taking off a blood pressure cuff, or checking arterial and I.V. lines. If none of these interventions works, you may need to find an alternate site. Finding a site with proper circulation may also prove challenging when a patient is receiving vasoconstrictive drugs.

• *Equipment malfunctions.* Remove the pulse oximeter from the patient, put the alarm limits at 85% and 100%, and try the instrument on yourself or another healthy person. This will tell you if the equipment is working correctly.

amination, evaluating its severity, and determining the patient's response to therapy. By allowing assessment of the relationship of flow rate to vital capacity, it helps distinguish between obstructive and restrictive pulmonary disease. It's also useful for evaluating preoperative anesthesia risk. Because the required breathing patterns can aggravate conditions such as bronchospasm, use of the bedside spirometer requires a review of the patient's history and close observation during testing.

Equipment

Spirometer ■ disposable mouthpiece ■ breathing tube, if required ■ spirographic chart, if required ■ chart and pen, if required ■ noseclips ■ optional: vital capacity predicted-values table.

Preparation of equipment

Review the manufacturer's instructions for assembly and use of the spirometer. If necessary, firmly insert the breathing tube *to ensure a tight connection.* If the tube comes preconnected, check the seals for tightness and the tubing for leaks. Check the operation of the recording mechanism, and insert a chart and pen if necessary.

Insert the disposable mouthpiece and make sure it's tightly sealed.

Implementation

• Explain the procedure to the patient. Emphasize that his cooperation is essential *to ensure accurate results.*

• Instruct the patient to remove or loosen any constricting clothing, such as a brassiere, *to prevent alteration of test results from restricted thoracic expansion and abdominal mobility.* Instruct the patient to void *to prevent abdominal discomfort.* Don't perform pulmonary function tests immediately after a large meal *because the patient will experience abdominal discomfort.*

• If the patient wears dentures that fit poorly, remove them *to prevent incomplete closure of his mouth, which could allow air to leak around the mouthpiece.* If his dentures fit well, leave them in place *to promote a tight seal.*

• Plug in the spirometer and set the baseline time.

• If desired, allow the patient to practice the required breathing with the breathing tube unhooked. After practice, replace the tube and check the seal.

• Tell the patient not to breathe through his nose. If the patient has difficulty complying, apply noseclips.

• To measure vital capacity, instruct the patient to inhale as deeply as possible, and then insert the mouthpiece so that his lips are sealed tightly around it *to prevent air leakage and ensure an accurate digital readout or spirogram recording.* (See *Digital bedside spirometer.*)

• Tell him to exhale completely. Then remove the mouthpiece *to prevent recording his next inspiration.*

• Allow the patient to rest and repeat the procedure twice.

• To measure FEV and FVC, repeat this procedure with the chart or timer on, but instruct the patient to exhale as quickly and completely as possible. Tell him when to start, and turn on the recorder or timer at the same time.

• Allow the patient to rest and repeat the procedure twice.

• After completing the procedure, discard the mouthpiece, remove the spirographic chart, and follow the manufacturer's instructions for cleaning and sterilizing.

Special considerations

Encourage the patient during the test; *this may help him to exhale more forcefully, which can be significant.* If the patient coughs during expiration, wait until coughing subsides before repeating the measurement.

Read the vital capacity directly from the readout or spirogram chart. The FVC is the highest volume recorded on the curve. Of the three trials, accept the highest recorded exhalation as the vital capacity result.

To determine the percentage of predicted vital capacity, first determine the patient's predicted value from the vital capacity predicted-values table, then calculate the percentage by using the following formula:

$$\frac{\text{observed vital capacity}}{\text{predicted vital capacity}} \times 100 = \% \text{ predicted vital capacity}$$

To determine the FEV for a specified time, mark the point on the spirogram where it crosses the desired time, and draw a straight line from this point to the side of the chart, which indicates volume in liters. This measurement is usually calculated for 1, 2, and 3 seconds and reported as a percentage of vital capacity. A healthy patient will have exhaled 75%, 85%, and 95% respectively of his FVC. Calculate this percentage by using the following formula:

$$\frac{\text{observed forced}}{\text{observed vital capacity}} \times 100 = \% \text{ vital capacity}$$

Complications

Forced exhalation can cause dizziness or light-headedness, precipitate or worsen bronchospasm, rapidly increase exhaustion (possibly to where the patient will require mechanical support), and increase air trapping in the emphysemic patient.

Documentation

Record the date and time of the procedure; the observed and calculated values, including FEV at 1, 2, and 3 seconds; any complications and the nursing action taken; and the patient's tolerance for the procedure.

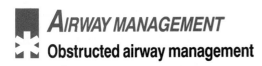

AIRWAY MANAGEMENT
Obstructed airway management

Sudden airway obstruction may occur when a foreign body lodges in the throat or bronchus; when the patient aspirates blood, mucus, or vomitus; when the tongue

Digital bedside spirometer

Various models of bedside spirometers are commercially available. The instrument shown below has a digital readout. Other models display results on an individual chart record or on a roll of chart paper.

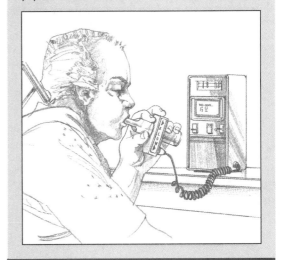

blocks the pharynx; or when the patient experiences traumatic injury, bronchoconstriction, or bronchospasm.

An obstructed airway causes anoxia, which in turn leads to brain damage and death in 4 to 6 minutes. The Heimlich maneuver uses an upper-abdominal thrust to create diaphragmatic pressure in the static lung below the foreign body sufficient to expel the obstruction. The Heimlich maneuver is used in conscious adult patients; if the patient is unconscious, an abdominal thrust should be used. However, the abdominal thrust is contraindicated in pregnant women, markedly obese patients, and patients who have recently undergone abdominal surgery. For such patients, a chest thrust, which forces air out of the lungs to create an artificial cough, should be used. The finger sweep maneuver is then used to manually remove the foreign body from the mouth.

These maneuvers are contraindicated in a patient with incomplete or partial airway obstruction or when the patient can maintain adequate ventilation to dislodge the foreign body by effective coughing. However, the patient's inability to speak, cough. or breathe demands immediate action to dislodge the obstruction. (Also see "Cardiopulmonary resuscitation" in Chapter 7 [for adults] and [for children] in Chapter 16.)

Implementation
• Determine the patient's level of consciousness by tapping his shoulder and asking, "Are you choking?" If he has a complete airway obstruction, he won't be able to answer because airflow to his vocal cords will be blocked. If he makes crowing sounds, his airway is partially obstructed, and you should encourage him to cough. This will either clear the airway or make the obstruction complete. For a complete obstruction, intervene as follows, depending on whether the patient is conscious or unconscious.

Conscious adult
• Tell the patient that you'll try to dislodge the foreign body.
• Standing behind the patient, wrap your arms around her waist. Make a fist with one hand and place the thumb side against her abdomen, slightly above the umbilicus and well below the xiphoid process. Then grasp your fist with the other hand.

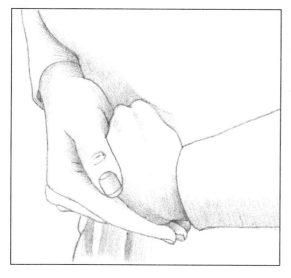

• Squeeze the patient's abdomen 6 to 10 times with quick inward and upward thrusts. Each thrust should be a separate and distinct movement; each should be forceful enough to create an artificial cough that will dislodge an obstruction (top right).

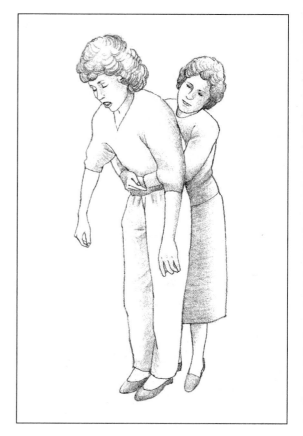

• Make sure you have a firm grasp on the patient because she may lose consciousness and need to be lowered to the floor. Look around the floor for objects that may harm her. Then, if she does lose consciousness, lower her carefully to the floor. Support her head and neck to prevent injury, and continue as described below.

Unconscious adult
• If you come upon an unconscious patient, ask any witnesses what happened. Begin cardiopulmonary resuscitation (CPR) and attempt to ventilate the patient. If you're unable to ventilate her, reposition her head and try again.
• If you still can't ventilate the patient, or if a conscious patient loses consciousness during abdominal thrusts, kneel astride her thighs.
• Place the heel of one hand on top of the other. Then place your hands between her umbilicus and the tip of her xiphoid process at the midline. Push inward and upward with 6 to 10 quick abdominal thrusts (top left, page 419).

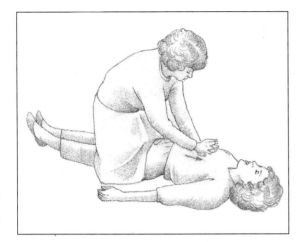

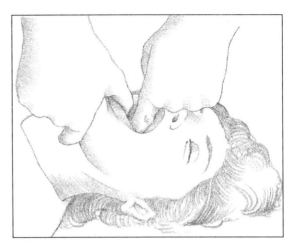

• After delivering the abdominal thrusts, open the patient's airway by grasping the tongue and lower jaw with your thumb and fingers. Lift the jaw *to draw the tongue away from the back of the throat and away from any foreign body.*

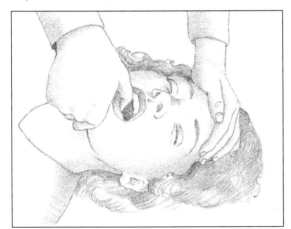

• If you can see the object, remove it by inserting your index finger deep into the throat at the base of her tongue. Using a hooking motion, remove the obstruction. Keep in mind that some clinicians object to a blind finger sweep—using your finger when you can't see the obstruction—*because your finger acts as a second obstruction.* They believe that, in most cases, the tongue-jaw lift described above should be enough to dislodge the obstruction (top right).

• After the object is removed, try to ventilate the patient. Then assess for spontaneous respirations, and check for a pulse. Proceed with CPR if necessary.
• If the object is not removed, try to ventilate the patient. If you can't, repeat the abdominal thrust maneuver described above in sequence until you clear the airway.

Obese or pregnant adult
• If the patient is conscious, stand behind her and place your arms under her armpits and around her chest.
• Place the thumb side of your clenched fist against the middle of the sternum, avoiding the margins of the ribs and the xiphoid process. Grasp your fist with your other hand and perform a chest thrust with enough force to expel the foreign body. Continue until the patient expels the obstruction or loses consciousness.

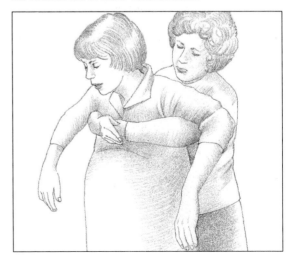

• If the patient loses consciousness, carefully lower her to the floor.
• Kneel close to the patient's side and place the heel of one hand just above the bottom of the patient's sternum. The long axis of the heel of your hand should align with the long axis of the patient's sternum. Place the heel of your other hand on top of that, making sure your fingers don't touch the patient's chest. Deliver each thrust forcefully enough to remove the obstruction.

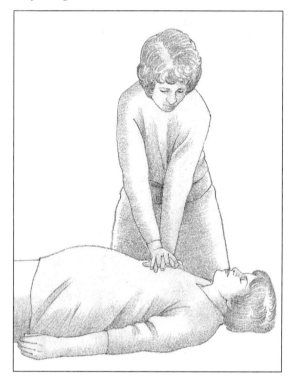

Child
• If the child is conscious and can stand, perform abdominal thrusts using the same technique as you would with an adult, but with less force.
• If he's unconscious or lying down, kneel at his feet; if he's a large child, kneel astride his thighs. If he's lying on a treatment table, stand by his side. Deliver abdominal thrusts as you would for an adult patient, but use less force. (Never perform a blind finger sweep on a child *because you risk pushing the foreign body further back into the airway.*)

Infant
• Whether the infant is conscious or not, place him face down so that he's straddling your arm with his head lower than his trunk. Rest your forearm on your thigh and deliver four back blows with the heel of your hand between the infant's shoulder blades.

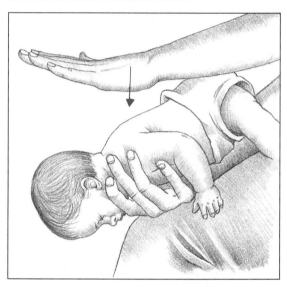

• If you haven't removed the obstruction, place your free hand on the infant's back. Supporting his neck, jaw, and chest with your other hand, turn him over onto your thigh. Keep his head lower than his trunk.
• Position your fingers. To do so, imagine a line between the infant's nipples and place the index finger of your free hand on his sternum, just below this imaginary line. Then place your middle and ring fingers next to your index finger and lift the index finger off his chest. Deliver four chest thrusts as you would for chest compression, but at a slower rate. (As with a child, never perform a blind finger sweep.)

Special considerations
If your patient vomits during abdominal thrusts, quickly wipe out his mouth with your fingers and resume the maneuver as necessary.

Even if your efforts to clear the airway don't seem to be effective, keep trying. As oxygen deprivation increases, smooth and skeletal muscles relax, making your maneuvers more likely to succeed.

Complications
Nausea, regurgitation, and achiness may develop after the patient regains consciousness and can breathe in-

dependently. He may also be injured, possibly from incorrect placement of the rescuer's hands or because of osteoporosis or metastatic lesions that increase the risk of fracture. Examine the patient for injuries, such as ruptured or lacerated abdominal or thoracic viscera.

Documentation

Record the date and time of the procedure, the patient's actions before the obstruction, the approximate length of time it took to clear the airway, and the type and size of the object removed. Also note his vital signs after the procedure, any complications that occurred and nursing actions taken, and his tolerance of the procedure.

⌐⌐ Oropharyngeal airway

An oropharyngeal airway, a curved rubber or plastic device, is inserted into the mouth to the posterior pharynx to establish or maintain a patent airway. In an unconscious patient, the tongue usually obstructs the posterior pharynx. The oropharyngeal airway conforms to the curvature of the palate, removing the obstruction and allowing air to pass around and through the tube. It also facilitates oropharyngeal suctioning. The oropharyngeal airway is intended for short-term use, as in the postanesthesia or postictal stage. It may be left in place longer as an airway adjunct to prevent the orally intubated patient from biting the endotracheal tube.

The oropharyngeal airway is not the airway of choice for the patient with loose or avulsed teeth or recent oral surgery. Inserting this airway in the conscious or semiconscious patient may stimulate vomiting and laryngospasm; therefore, you'll usually insert the airway only in unconscious patients.

Equipment

For inserting: oral airway of appropriate size ■ tongue blade ■ padded tongue blade ■ gloves ■ optional: suction equipment, hand-held resuscitation bag or oxygen-powered breathing device.

For cleaning: hydrogen peroxide ■ water ■ basin ■ optional: pipe cleaner.

For reflex testing: cotton-tipped applicator.

Preparation of equipment

Select an airway of appropriate size for your patient; *an oversized airway can obstruct breathing by depressing the epiglottis into the laryngeal opening.* Usually, you'll select a small size (100 mm, Guedel size 5) for an infant or child, a medium size (90 mm, Guedel size 4) for the average adult, and a large size (80 mm, Guedel size 3) for the large or obese adult. Confirm the correct size by placing the airway flange beside the patient's cheek, parallel to his front teeth. If it's the right size, the airway curve should reach to the angle of the jaw.

Implementation

● Explain the procedure to the patient even though he may not appear to be alert. Provide privacy and put on gloves *to prevent contact with body fluids.* If the patient is wearing dentures, remove them *so they don't cause further airway obstruction.*
● If necessary, suction the patient.
● Place the patient in the supine position with his neck hyperextended, if this is not contraindicated.
● Insert the airway using the cross-finger or the tongue blade technique. (See *Inserting an oral airway,* page 422.)
● Auscultate the lungs to ensure adequate ventilation.
● After the airway is inserted, position the patient on his side *to decrease the risk of aspiration of vomitus.*
● Perform mouth care every 2 to 4 hours, as needed. Begin by holding the patient's jaws open with a padded tongue blade and gently removing the airway. Place the airway in a basin and rinse it with hydrogen peroxide followed by water. If secretions remain, use a pipe cleaner to remove them. Complete standard mouth care and reinsert the airway.
● While the airway is removed for mouth care, observe the mouth's mucous membranes *because tissue irritation or ulceration can result from prolonged airway use.*
● Frequently check the position of the airway *to ensure correct placement.*
● When the patient regains consciousness and is able to swallow, remove the airway by pulling it outward and downward, following the mouth's natural curvature. After the airway is removed, test the patient's cough and gag reflexes *to ensure that removal of the airway wasn't premature, and that the patient can maintain his own airway.*
● To test for gag reflex, use a cotton-tipped applicator to touch both sides of the posterior pharynx. To test for cough reflex, gently touch the posterior oropharynx with the cotton-tipped applicator.

Special considerations

Clear breath sounds on auscultation indicate that the airway is the proper size and that it's in the correct position.

Avoid taping the airway in place *because untaping it could delay airway removal, thus increasing the risk of aspiration.*

Evaluate the patient's behavior *to provide the cue for airway removal.* The patient is likely to gag or cough as

Inserting an oral airway

Unless this position is contraindicated, hyperextend the patient's head as shown below before using either the cross-finger or tongue blade insertion method.

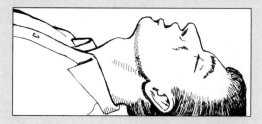

To insert an oral airway using the cross-finger method, place your thumb on the patient's lower teeth and your index finger on his upper teeth. Gently open his mouth by pushing his teeth apart.

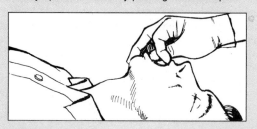

Insert the airway upside down to avoid pushing the tongue towards the pharynx, and slide it over the tongue toward the back of the mouth. Rotate the airway as it approaches the posterior wall of the pharynx so that it points downward, as shown below.

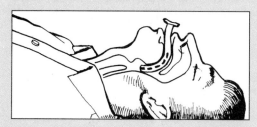

To use the tongue blade technique, open the patient's mouth and depress his tongue with the blade. Guide the airway over the back of the tongue as you did for the cross-finger technique.

he becomes more alert, indicating that he no longer needs the airway.

Complications
Tooth damage or loss, tissue damage, and bleeding may result from insertion.

If the airway is too long, it may press the epiglottis against the entrance of the larynx, producing complete airway obstruction. If the airway is not inserted properly, it may push the tongue posteriorly, aggravating the problem of upper airway obstruction.

To prevent traumatic injury, make sure that the patient's lips and tongue are not between his teeth and the airway.

Immediately after inserting the airway, check for respirations. If respirations are absent or inadequate, initiate artificial positive pressure ventilation by using a mouth-to-mask technique, a hand-held resuscitation bag, or an oxygen-powered breathing device. (See "Manual ventilation" in this chapter.)

Documentation
Record the date and time of the airway's insertion; size of the airway; removal and cleaning of the airway; condition of mucous membranes; any suctioning; any adverse reactions and the nursing action taken; and the patient's tolerance of the procedure.

◼ Nasopharyngeal airway

Insertion of a nasopharyngeal airway — a soft rubber or latex uncuffed catheter — establishes or maintains a patent airway. This airway is the typical choice for patients who've had recent oral surgery or facial trauma, and for patients with loose, cracked, or avulsed teeth. It's also used to protect the nasal mucosa from injury when the patient needs frequent nasotracheal suctioning.

The airway follows the curvature of the nasopharynx, passing through the nose and extending from the nostril to the posterior pharynx. The bevel-shaped pharyngeal end of the airway facilitates insertion, and its funnel-shaped nasal end helps prevent slippage.

Insertion of a nasopharyngeal airway is preferred when an oropharyngeal airway is contraindicated or fails to maintain a patent airway. A nasopharyngeal airway is contraindicated if the patient is receiving anticoagulant therapy or has a hemorrhagic disorder, sepsis, or pathologic nasopharyngeal deformity.

Equipment

For insertion: nasopharyngeal airway of proper size ■ tongue blade ■ water-soluble lubricant ■ gloves ■ optional: suction equipment.

For cleaning: hydrogen peroxide ■ water ■ basin ■ optional: pipe cleaner.

Preparation of equipment

Measure the diameter of the patient's nostril and the distance from the tip of his nose to his earlobe. Select an airway of slightly smaller diameter than the nostril and of slightly longer length (1″ [2.5 cm]) than measured. The sizes for this type of airway are labeled according to their internal diameter.

The recommended size for a large adult is 8 to 9 mm; for a medium adult, 7 to 8 mm; for a small adult, 6 to 7 mm. Lubricate the distal half of the airway's surface with a water-soluble lubricant *to prevent traumatic injury during insertion.*

Implementation

• Put on gloves.
• In nonemergency situations, explain the procedure to the patient.
• Properly insert the airway. (See *Inserting a nasopharyngeal airway.*)
• Once the airway is inserted, check it regularly *to detect dislodgment or obstruction.*
• When the patient's natural airway is patent, remove the airway in one smooth motion. If the airway sticks, apply lubricant around the nasal end of the tube and around the nostril; then gently rotate the airway until it's free.

Special considerations

If the patient coughs or gags, the tube may be too long. If so, remove the airway and insert a shorter one. At least once every 8 hours, remove the airway *to check nasal mucous membranes for irritation or ulceration.* Clean the airway by placing it in a basin and rinsing it with hydrogen peroxide and then with water. If secretions remain, use a pipe cleaner to remove them. Reinsert the clean airway into the other nostril (if it's patent) *to avoid skin breakdown.*

Complications

Sinus infection may result from obstruction of sinus drainage. Insertion of the airway may injure the nasal mucosa and cause bleeding and possible aspiration of blood into the trachea. Suction as necessary to remove secretions or blood. If the tube is too long, it may enter the esophagus and cause gastric distention and hypoventilation during artificial ventilation.

Inserting a nasopharyngeal airway

First, hold the airway beside the patient's face to be sure it's the proper size, as shown here. It should be slightly smaller than the patient's nostril diameter and slightly longer than the distance from the tip of his nose to his earlobe.

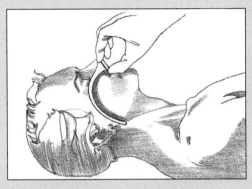

To insert the airway, hyperextend the patient's neck (unless contraindicated). Then, push up the tip of his nose and pass the airway into his nostril, as shown below. Avoid pushing against any resistance *to prevent tissue trauma and airway kinking.*

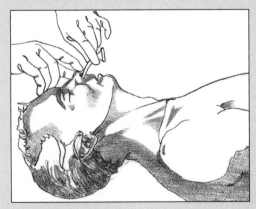

To check for correct airway placement, first close the patient's mouth. Then, place your finger over the tube's opening to detect air exchange. Also depress the patient's tongue with a tongue blade and look for the airway tip behind the uvula.

Semiconscious patients usually tolerate this type of airway better than conscious patients; however, it may still precipitate laryngospasm and vomiting.

When you insert the airway, remember to use a chin-lift or jaw-thrust technique to anteriorly displace the patient's mandible. Immediately after insertion, assess the patient's respirations. If absent or inadequate, initiate artificial positive-pressure ventilation with a mouth-to-mask technique, a hand-held resuscitation bag, or an oxygen-powered breathing device.

Documentation
Record the date and time of the airway's insertion; size of the airway; removal and cleaning of the airway; shifts from one nostril to the other; condition of the mucous membranes; suctioning; complications and nursing action taken; and the patient's reaction to the procedure.

⌐⌐ Esophageal airways

Esophageal airways, such as the esophageal gastric tube airway (EGTA) and the esophageal obturator airway (EOA), are used temporarily (for up to 2 hours) to maintain ventilation in the comatose patient during cardiac or respiratory arrest. These devices avoid tongue obstruction, prevent air from entering the stomach, and keep stomach contents from entering the trachea. They can be inserted only after a patent airway is established.

Although health care providers must have special training to insert an EGTA or EOA, insertion of these airways is much simpler than endotracheal intubation. One reason is that these devices do not require visualization of the trachea or hyperextension of the neck. This makes them useful for treating patients with suspected spinal cord injuries.

Because conscious and semiconscious patients will reject an esophageal airway, one should not be used unless the patient is unconscious and not breathing. These airways are also contraindicated if facial trauma prevents a snug mask fit or if the patient has an absent or weak gag reflex, has recently ingested toxic chemicals, has esophageal disease, or has taken an overdose of narcotics that can be reversed by naloxone. In addition, because pediatric sizes aren't currently available, these airways should not be used in patients under age 16.

Equipment
Esophageal tube ▪ face mask ▪ #16 or #18 French nasogastric (NG) tube (for EGTA) ▪ 35-cc syringe ▪ intermittent gastric suction equipment ▪ oral suction equipment ▪ optional: hand-held resuscitation bag, water-soluble lubricant.

Preparation of equipment
Gather the equipment (see *Types of esophageal airways*). Fill the face mask with air *to check for leaks.* Inflate the esophageal tube's cuff with 35 cc of air *to check for leaks;* then, deflate the cuff. Connect the esophageal tube to the face mask (the lower opening on an EGTA) and listen for the tube to click *to determine proper placement.*

Implementation
• Lubricate the first inch (2.5 cm) of the tube's distal tip with a water-soluble lubricant, I.V. fluid, the patient's saliva, or tap water. With an EGTA, also lubricate the first inch of the NG tube's distal tip.

To insert an esophageal airway
• Assess the patient's condition *to determine if he's a safe candidate for an esophageal airway.*
• If the patient's condition permits, place him in the supine position with his neck in a neutral or semiflexed position. *Hyperextension of the neck may cause the tube to enter the trachea instead of the esophagus.* Remove his dentures, if applicable.
• Insert your thumb deeply into the patient's mouth behind the base of his tongue. Place your index and middle fingers of the same hand under the patient's chin and lift his jaw straight up.
• With your other hand, grasp the esophageal tube just below the mask in the same way you'd grasp a pencil. *This promotes gentle maneuvering of the tube and reduces the risk of pharyngeal trauma.*
• Still elevating the patient's jaw with one hand, insert the tip of the esophageal tube into the patient's mouth. Gently guide the airway over the tongue into the pharynx and then into the esophagus, following the natural pharyngeal curve. No force is required for proper insertion; the tube should easily seat itself. If you encounter resistance, withdraw the tube slightly and readvance it. When the tube is fully advanced, the mask should fit snugly over the patient's mouth and nose. When this is accomplished, the cuff will lie below the level of the carina. If the cuff is above the carina, it may, when inflated, compress the posterior membranous portion of the trachea and cause tracheal obstruction.
• *Because the tube may enter the trachea,* deliver positive-pressure ventilation before inflating the cuff. Watch for chest rise *to confirm that the tube is in the esophagus.*
• Once the tube is properly in place in the esophagus, draw 35 cc of air into the syringe, connect the syringe to the tube's cuff-inflation valve, and inflate the cuff.

Types of esophageal airways

Gastric tube airway

This airway consists of an inflatable mask and an esophageal tube, as shown at right. The transparent face mask has two ports: a lower one for insertion of an esophageal tube and an upper one for ventilation, which can be maintained with a hand-held resuscitation bag. The inside of the mask is soft and pliable; it molds to the patient's face and makes a tight seal, preventing air loss.

The proximal end of the esophageal tube has a one-way, nonrefluxing valve that blocks the esophagus. This valve prevents air from entering the stomach, thus reducing the risk of abdominal distention and aspiration. The distal end of the tube has an inflatable cuff that rests in the esophagus just below the tracheal bifurcation, preventing pressure on the noncartilaginous tracheal wall.

During ventilation, air is directed into the upper port in the mask and, with the esophagus blocked, enters the trachea and lungs.

Obturator airway

This airway consists of an adjustable, inflatable, transparent face mask with a single port, attached by a snap lock to a blind esophageal tube.

When properly inflated, the transparent mask prevents air from escaping through the nose and mouth, as shown at right.

The esophageal tube has 16 holes at its proximal end through which air or oxygen introduced into the port of the mask is transferred to the trachea. The tube's distal end is closed and circled by an inflatable cuff. When the cuff is inflated, it occludes the esophagus, preventing air from entering the stomach and acting as a barrier against vomitus and involuntary aspiration.

Esophageal gastric tube airway

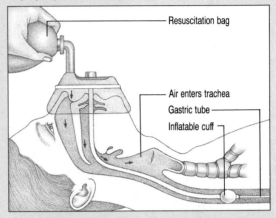

Resuscitation bag

Air enters trachea

Gastric tube

Inflatable cuff

Esophageal obturator airway

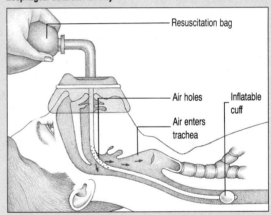

Resuscitation bag

Air holes

Inflatable cuff

Air enters trachea

Avoid overinflation *because this can cause esophageal trauma.*
• If you've inserted an EGTA, insert the NG tube through the lower port on the face mask and into the esophageal tube, and advance it to the second marking so it reaches 6″ (15.2 cm) beyond the distal end of the esophageal tube. Suction stomach contents using intermittent gastric suction *to decompress the stomach.* This is particularly necessary after mouth-to-mouth resuscitation, which introduces air to the stomach. Leave the tube in place during resuscitation.

• For both airways, attach a hand-held resuscitation bag or a mechanical ventilator to the face mask port (upper port) on the EGTA. Up to 100% of the fraction of inspired oxygen can be delivered this way.
• Monitor the patient *to ensure adequate ventilation.* Watch for chest movement, and suction the patient if mucus blocks the EOA tube perforations or in any way interrupts respiration.

To remove an esophageal airway

• Assess the patient's condition *to determine if it's appropriate to remove the airway.* The airway may be removed if respirations are spontaneous and number 16 to 20 breaths/minute. If 2 hours have elapsed since airway insertion and respirations are not spontaneous and at the normal rate, the patient must be switched to an artificial airway that can be used for long-term ventilation, such as an endotracheal tube.

• Detach the mask from the esophageal tube.

• If the patient is conscious, place him on his left side, if possible, *to avoid aspiration during removal of the esophageal tube.* If he's unconscious and requires an endotracheal tube, insert it or assist with its insertion and inflate the cuff of the endotracheal tube before removing the esophageal tube. *With the esophageal tube in place, the endotracheal tube can be guided easily into the trachea, and stomach contents are less likely to be aspirated when the esophageal tube is removed.*

• Deflate the cuff on the esophageal tube by removing air from the inflation valve with a syringe. Don't try to remove the tube with the cuff inflated *because it may perforate the esophagus.*

• Turn the patient's head to the side, if possible, *to avoid aspiration.*

• Remove the EGTA or EOA in one swift, smooth motion, following the natural pharyngeal curve *to avoid esophageal trauma.*

• Perform oropharyngeal suctioning *to remove any residual secretions.*

• Assist the doctor as required in monitoring and maintaining adequate ventilation for the patient.

Special considerations

Keep EGTAs and EOAs stored in the manufacturer's package until use *to preserve their natural curve.*

To ease insertion, you may prefer to direct the airway along the right side of the patient's mouth *because the esophagus is located to the right of and behind the trachea.* Or you may advance the tube tip upward toward the hard palate, then invert the tip and glide it along the tongue surface and into the pharynx. *This keeps the tube centered, avoids snagging it on the sides of the throat, and eases insertion in the patient with clenched jaws.*

Watch the unconscious patient as he regains consciousness. Restrain his hands *if he tries to remove the airway.* Explain the procedure to him, if possible, *to reduce his apprehension.* Observe also for retching and, if it occurs, remove the airway immediately *because the accumulation of vomitus blocked by the airway cuff may perforate the esophagus. To help prevent complications,* do not leave the EOA in place for more than 2 hours.

A mechanical ventilator attached to an endotracheal or tracheostomy tube maintains more exact tidal volume than a mechanical ventilator attached to an esophageal airway.

Complications

EOAs may be inferior to endotracheal intubation in providing adequate oxygenation and ventilation. Esophageal airways may cause esophageal injuries, including rupture, and in semiconscious patients, may cause laryngospasm, vomiting, and aspiration. The EOA does not prevent aspiration of foreign material from the mouth and pharynx into the trachea and bronchi.

Documentation

Record the date and time of the procedure, type of airway inserted, patient's vital signs and level of consciousness, removal of the airway, any alternative airway inserted after extubation, and any complications and the nursing action taken.

 # Oronasopharyngeal suction

Oronasopharyngeal suction removes secretions from the pharynx by means of a suction catheter inserted through the mouth or nostril. Used to maintain a patent airway, this procedure is indicated for the patient who's unable to clear his airway effectively with coughing and expectoration; for example, the unconscious or severely debilitated patient, or the intubated patient who has secretions pooled above the cuff of the artificial airway.

The procedure should be done as often as necessary, depending on the patient's condition.

Because the catheter may inadvertently slip into the lower airway or esophagus, oronasopharyngeal suction is an aseptic procedure that requires sterile equipment. However, clean technique may be used for a tonsil tip suction device. In fact, an alert patient can use a tonsil tip suction device himself to remove secretions.

Nasopharyngeal suctioning should be used with caution in patients who have nasopharyngeal bleeding or spinal fluid leakage into the nasopharyngeal area. Also be alert when performing this procedure on patients receiving anticoagulant therapy or who have blood dyscrasias because these conditions increase the risk for bleeding.

Equipment

Wall suction or portable suction apparatus ▪ collection bottle ▪ connecting tubing ▪ water-soluble lubricant ▪

normal saline solution or sterile water ■ disposable sterile container ■ sterile suction catheter (a #12 or #14 French for an adult, #8 or #10 French for a child, or pediatric feeding tube for an infant) ■ sterile gloves ■ tonsil tip suction device ■ clean gloves ■ nasopharyngeal or oropharyngeal airway (optional for frequent suctioning) ■ overbed table ■ waterproof trash bag ■ soap, water, and 70% alcohol for cleaning catheters.

A sterile catheter, disposable container, and sterile gloves are available in a commercially prepared kit.

Preparation of equipment
Before beginning, check your hospital's policy to determine whether a doctor's order is required for oronasopharyngeal suctioning. Also review the patient's blood gas or oxygen saturation values, and check vital signs. Evaluate the patient's ability to cough and deep breathe *to determine his ability to move secretions up the tracheobronchial tree.* Check the patient's history for a deviated septum, nasal polyps, nasal obstruction, traumatic injury, epistaxis, or mucosal swelling.

If no contraindications exist, gather and place the suction equipment on the patient's overbed table or bedside stand. Position the table or stand on your preferred side of the bed *to facilitate suctioning.* Attach the collection bottle to the suctioning unit, and attach the connecting tubing to it. Date and then open the bottle of normal saline solution or sterile water. Open the waterproof trash bag.

Implementation
• Explain the procedure to the patient, even if he is unresponsive. Inform the patient that suctioning may stimulate transient coughing or gagging, but tell him that coughing helps to mobilize secretions. If the patient has been suctioned previously, simply summarize the reasons for the procedure. Continue to reassure the patient throughout the procedure *to minimize anxiety and fear. Anxiety and fear can increase oxygen consumption.* Also ask the patient which nostril is more patent.
• Wash your hands.
• Place the patient in semi-Fowler's or high Fowler's position, if tolerated, *to promote lung expansion and effective coughing.*
• Turn on the suction from the wall or portable unit and set the pressure according to hospital policy. Usually, the pressure may be set between 80 and 120 mm Hg; higher pressures cause excessive trauma without enhancing secretion removal. Occlude the end of the connecting tubing *to check suction pressure.*
• Using strict aseptic technique, open the suction catheter kit or the sterile catheter, container, and gloves. Put on the gloves and consider your dominant hand sterile

and your nondominant hand nonsterile. Using your nondominant (nonsterile) hand, pour the sterile water or saline into the sterile container.
• With your nondominant hand, place a small amount of water-soluble lubricant on the sterile area. The lubricant is used *to facilitate passage of the catheter during nasopharyngeal suctioning.*
• Pick up the catheter with your dominant (sterile) hand and attach it to the connecting tubing. Use your nondominant hand to control the suction valve while your dominant hand manipulates the catheter.
• Instruct the patient to cough and breathe slowly and deeply several times before beginning suction. *Coughing helps loosen secretions and may decrease the amount of suctioning necessary, while deep breathing helps minimize or prevent hypoxia.* (See *Tips on airway clearance,* page 428.)

For nasal insertion
• Raise the tip of the patient's nose with your nondominant hand *to straighten the passageway and facilitate insertion of the catheter.* Without applying suction, gently insert the suction catheter into the patient's nares. Roll the catheter between your fingers *to help it advance through the turbinates.* Continue to advance the catheter approximately 5″ to 6″ (12.7 to 15 cm) until you reach the pool of secretions or the patient begins to cough.

For oral insertion
• Without applying suction, gently insert the catheter into the patient's mouth. Advance the catheter approximately 3″ to 4″ (7.6 to 10 cm) along the side of the patient's mouth until you reach the pool of secretions or the patient begins to cough. Suction both sides of the patient's mouth and pharyngeal area.
• Using intermittent suction, withdraw the catheter from either the mouth or the nose with a continuous rotating motion *to minimize invagination of the mucosa into the catheter's tip and side ports.* Apply suction for only 10 to 15 seconds at a time *to minimize tissue trauma.*
• Between passes, wrap the catheter around your dominant hand *to prevent contamination.*
• If secretions are thick, clear the lumen of the catheter by dipping it in water and applying suction.
• Repeat the procedure until gurgling or bubbling sounds stop and respirations are quiet.
• After completing suctioning, pull your sterile glove off over the coiled catheter and discard it and the nonsterile glove along with the container of water.
• Flush the connecting tubing with normal saline solution or water.
• Replace the used items *so they're ready for the next suctioning,* and wash your hands.

Tips on airway clearance

Deep breathing and coughing are vital for removing secretions from the lungs. Additional methods to help clear the airway include diaphragmatic breathing and forced expiration. Here's how to teach these methods to your patients.

Diaphragmatic breathing

First, tell the patient to lie supine, with his head elevated 15 to 20 degrees on a pillow. Tell him to place one hand on his abdomen, and then to inhale so that he can feel his abdomen rise. Explain that this is what's known as "breathing with the diaphragm."

Next, instruct the patient to exhale slowly through his nose — or, even better, through pursed lips — while letting his abdomen collapse. Explain that this action decreases his respiratory rate and increases his tidal volume.

Suggest that the patient perform this exercise for 30 minutes several times a day. After he becomes accustomed to the position, and after he's learned to breathe using his diaphragm, he may apply abdominal weights of 4 to 5 kg. The weights enhance the movement of the diaphragm toward the head during expiration.

To enhance the effectiveness of exercise, the patient may also manually compress the lower costal margins, perform straight leg lifts, and coordinate the breathing technique with a physical activity, such as walking.

Forced expiration

Another technique you should teach the patient is forced expiration. First, explain that forced expiration helps clear secretions while causing less traumatic injury than does a cough.

To perform the technique, tell the patient to forcefully expire without closing his glottis, starting with a mid- to low-lung volume. Tell him to follow this expiration with a period of diaphragmatic breathing and relaxation.

Advise the patient that if his secretions are in the central airways, he may have to use a more forceful expiration or a cough to clear them.

Special considerations

If the patient has no history of nasal problems, alternate suctioning between nostrils *to minimize traumatic injury.*

If repeated oronasopharyngeal suctioning is required, the use of a nasopharyngeal or oropharyngeal airway will *help with catheter insertion, reduce traumatic injury, and promote a patent airway. To facilitate catheter insertion for oropharyngeal suctioning,* depress the patient's tongue with a tongue blade, or ask another nurse to do so. *This helps you to visualize the back of the throat and also prevents the patient from biting the catheter.*

If the patient has excessive oral secretions, consider using a tonsil tip catheter *because this allows the patient to remove oral secretions independently, as needed.*

Let the patient rest after suctioning while you continue to observe him. The frequency and duration of suctioning depends on the patient's tolerance for the procedure and on any complications.

Home care

Oronasopharyngeal suctioning may be performed in the home using a portable suction machine. Under these circumstances, suctioning is a clean rather than a sterile procedure. Properly cleaned catheters can be reused, putting less financial strain on patients.

Catheters should be cleaned by first washing them in soapy water and then boiling them for 10 minutes or soaking them in 70% alcohol for 3 to 5 minutes. The catheters should then be rinsed with normal saline solution or tap water.

Whether the patient requires disposable or reusable suction equipment, you should make sure that the patient and his caregivers have received proper teaching and support.

Complications

Increased dyspnea caused by hypoxia and anxiety may result from this procedure. Hypoxia can result because oxygen from the oronasopharynx is removed with the secretions. The amount of oxygen removed varies, depending upon the duration of the suctioning, suction flow and pressure, the size of the catheter in relation to the size of the patient's airway, and the patient's physical condition.

In addition, bloody aspirate can result from prolonged or traumatic suctioning. Water-soluble lubricant can help to minimize traumatic injury.

Documentation

Record the date, time, reason for suctioning, and technique used; amount, color, consistency, and odor (if any) of the secretions; the patient's respiratory status before and after the procedure; any complications and the nursing action taken; and the patient's tolerance for the procedure.

▚ ▚ Endotracheal intubation

This procedure involves the oral or nasal insertion of a flexible tube through the larynx into the trachea for the purposes of controlling the airway and mechanically ventilating the patient. Performed by a doctor, anesthetist, respiratory therapist, or nurse educated in the procedure, endotracheal intubation usually occurs during emergency situations, such as cardiopulmonary arrest, or in diseases, such as epiglottitis. However, intubation may also occur under more controlled circumstances, such as just before surgery. In these instances, endotracheal intubation requires patient teaching and preparation.

Advantages of the procedure are that it establishes and maintains a patent airway, protects against aspiration by sealing off the trachea from the digestive tract, permits removal of tracheobronchial secretions in patients who can't cough effectively, and provides a route for mechanical ventilation. Disadvantages are that it bypasses normal respiratory tract defenses against infection, reduces cough effectiveness, and prevents verbal communication.

Oral endotracheal intubation is contraindicated in patients with acute cervical spinal injury and degenerative spinal disorders, while nasal intubation is contraindicated in patients with apnea, bleeding disorders, chronic sinusitis, or nasal obstructions.

Equipment
Two endotracheal tubes (one spare) in the appropriate size ▪ 10-cc syringe ▪ stethoscope ▪ gloves ▪ lighted laryngoscope with a handle and blades of various sizes, curved and straight ▪ sedative ▪ local anesthetic spray, such as xylocaine (for conscious patients) ▪ mucosal vasoconstricting agent (for nasal intubation) ▪ overbed or other table ▪ water-soluble lubricant ▪ adhesive or other strong tape or Velcro tube holder ▪ compound benzoin tincture ▪ transparent adhesive dressing, if necessary ▪ gloves ▪ oral airway or bite block (for oral intubation) ▪ suction equipment ▪ hand-held resuscitation bag with sterile swivel adapter ▪ humidified oxygen source ▪ optional: prepackaged intubation tray, sterile gauze pad, stylet, Magill forceps, sterile water, and sterile basin.

Preparation of equipment
Quickly gather the individual supplies or use a prepackaged intubation tray, which will contain most of the necessary supplies. Select an endotracheal tube of the appropriate size. Typically, this will be size 2.5 to 5.5 mm, uncuffed, for children. Adult sizes range from 6 to 10 mm and are cuffed. The typical size for oral intubation in women is 7.5 mm and

in men, 9 mm. Select a sightly smaller tube for nasal intubation.

Check the light in the laryngoscope by snapping the appropriate sized blade into place; if the bulb doesn't light, replace the batteries or the laryngoscope (whichever will be quicker).

Using sterile technique, open the package containing the endotracheal tube and, if desired, the other supplies as well, on an overbed table. Pour the sterile water into the basin. Then, *to ease insertion,* lubricate the first inch (2.5 cm) of the distal end of endotracheal tube with the water-soluble lubricant, using aseptic technique. Do this by either placing some of the lubricant on the gauze pad and wiping it on the tube, or by squeezing the lubricant directly onto the tube. Use only water-soluble lubricant *because it can be absorbed by mucous membranes.*

Next, attach the syringe to the port on the tube's exterior pilot cuff. Slowly inflate the cuff, observing for uniform inflation. If desired, submerge the tube in the sterile water and watch for air bubbles, *which would indicate a leak.* Then use the syringe to deflate the cuff.

A stylet may be used on oral intubations *to stiffen the tube.* Lubricate the entire stylet *so that it can be easily removed after intubation.* Insert the stylet into the tube so that its distal tip lies about ½" (1.3 cm) inside the distal end of the tube. Make sure that the stylet does not protrude from the tube *to avoid vocal cord trauma.* Prepare the humidified oxygen source and the suction equipment for immediate use. If the patient is in bed, remove the headboard *to provide easier access.*

Implementation
● Administer medication, as ordered, *to decrease respiratory secretions, induce amnesia or analgesia, and help calm and relax the conscious patient.* Remove dentures and bridgework, if present.
● Administer oxygen until the tube is inserted *to prevent hypoxia.*
● Place the patient supine in the sniffing position so that his mouth, pharynx, and trachea are extended. For a blind intubation, place the patient's head and neck in a neutral position.
● Put on gloves.
● For oral intubation, spray local anesthetic (such as xylocaine) deep into the patient's posterior pharynx *to diminish the gag reflex and reduce patient discomfort.* For nasal intubation, spray a local anesthetic and a mucosal vasoconstricting agent into the patient's nasal passages *to anesthetize and shrink the nasal turbinates and reduce the chance of bleeding.*
● If necessary, suction the patient's pharynx just before tube insertion *to improve visualization of the patient's pharynx and vocal cords.*

• Time each intubation attempt, limiting attempts to less than 30 seconds *to prevent hypoxia.*

Intubation with direct visualization
• Stand at the head of the patient's bed. Using your right hand, hold the patient's mouth open by crossing your index finger over your thumb, placing your thumb on the patient's upper teeth and your index finger on his lower teeth. This technique *provides greater leverage.*
• Grasp the laryngoscope handle in your left hand and gently slide the blade into the right side of the patient's mouth. Center the blade and push the patient's tongue to the left. Hold the patient's lower lip away from his teeth *to prevent the lip from being traumatized.*
• Advance the blade *to expose the epiglottis.* When using a straight blade, insert the tip under the epiglottis; when using a curved blade, insert the tip between the base of the tongue and the epiglottis.
• Lift the laryngoscope handle upward and away from your body at a 45-degree angle *to reveal the vocal cords.* Avoid pivoting the laryngoscope against the patient's teeth *to prevent damaging them.*
• If desired, have an assistant apply pressure to the cricoid ring *to occlude the esophagus and minimize gastric regurgitation.*
• When performing an oral intubation, insert the endotracheal tube into the right side of the patient's mouth. When performing a nasotracheal intubation, insert the endotracheal tube through the nostril and into the pharynx. Then use Magill forceps to guide the tube through the vocal cords.
• Guide the tube into the vertical openings of the larynx between the vocal cords, being careful not to mistake the horizontal opening of the esophagus for the larynx. If the vocal cords are closed because of a spasm, wait a few seconds for them to relax, and then gently guide the tube past them *to avoid traumatic injury.*
• Advance the tube until the cuff disappears beyond the vocal cords. Avoid advancing the tube farther *to avoid occluding a major bronchus and precipitating lung collapse.*
• Holding the endotracheal tube in place, quickly remove the stylet, if present.

Blind nasotracheal intubation
• Pass the endotracheal tube along the floor of the nasal cavity. If necessary, use gentle force to pass the tube through the nasopharynx and into the pharynx.
• Listen and feel for air movement through the tube as it's advanced *to ensure that the tube is properly placed in the airway.*
• Slip the tube between the vocal cords when the patient inhales *because the vocal cords separate on inhalation.*

• Once the tube is past the vocal cords, the breath sounds should become louder. If, at any time during tube advancement, breath sounds disappear, withdraw the tube until they reappear.

After intubation
• Inflate the tube's cuff with 5 to 10 cc of air until you feel resistance. Once the patient is mechanically ventilated, you'll use the minimal-leak technique or the minimal occlusive volume technique to establish correct inflation of the cuff. (For instructions on how to measure tracheal cuff pressure, see "Endotracheal tube care" in this chapter.)
• Remove the laryngoscope. If the patient was intubated orally, insert an oral airway or bite block *to prevent the patient from obstructing airflow or puncturing the tube with his teeth.*
• *To ensure correct tube placement,* observe for chest expansion and auscultate for bilateral breath sounds. If the patient is unconscious or uncooperative, use a hand-held resuscitation bag while observing for upper chest movement and auscultating for breath sounds. Feel the tube's tip for warm exhalations and listen for air movement. Observe for condensation forming inside the tube.
• If you don't hear any breath sounds, auscultate over the stomach while ventilating with the resuscitation bag. Stomach distention, belching, or a gurgling sound indicates esophageal intubation. Immediately deflate the cuff and remove the tube. After reoxygenating the patient *to prevent hypoxia,* repeat insertion using a sterile tube *to prevent contamination of the trachea.*
• Auscultate bilaterally *to exclude the possibility of endobronchial intubation.* If you fail to hear breath sounds on both sides of the chest, you may have inserted the tube into one of the mainstem bronchi (usually the right one because of its wider angle at the bifurcation); such insertion occludes the other bronchus and lung and results in atelectasis on the obstructed side. Or the tube may be resting on the carina, resulting in dry secretions that obstruct both bronchi. (The patient's coughing and fighting the ventilator will alert you to the problem.) To correct these situations, deflate the cuff, withdraw the tube 1 to 2 mm, auscultate for bilateral breath sounds, and reinflate the cuff.
• Once you've confirmed correct tube placement, administer oxygen or initiate mechanical ventilation, and suction if indicated.
• *To secure tube position,* apply compound benzoin tincture to each cheek and let it dry *for enhanced tape adhesion.* Tape the tube firmly with adhesive or other strong tape or use a Velcro tube holder. (See *Three methods to secure an endotracheal tube,* pages 432 and 433.)

• Inflate the cuff with the minimal-leak technique or the minimal occlusive volume technique. For the *minimal-leak technique*, attach a 10-cc syringe to the port on the tube's exterior pilot cuff, and place a stethoscope on the side of the patient's neck. Inject small amounts of air with each breath until you hear no leak. Then aspirate 0.1 cc of air from the cuff *to create a minimal air leak.* Record the amount of air needed to inflate the cuff *for subsequent monitoring of tracheal dilatation or erosion.* For the *minimal occlusive volume technique,* follow the first two steps of the minimal-leak technique, placing your stethoscope over the trachea instead of the side of the neck. Then aspirate until you hear a small leak on inspiration, and add just enough air to stop the leak. Record the amount of air needed to inflate the cuff for subsequent monitoring of tracheal dilatation or erosion.

• Clearly mark the tube's exit point from the mouth or nose with pen or tape. If you can't mark the tube, note the centimeter marking on the tube where the tube exits the mouth or nose. *Periodic monitoring of this mark can reveal tube displacement.*

• Make sure a chest X-ray is taken *to verify tube position.*

• Place a swivel adapter between the tube and the humidified oxygen source *to allow for intermittent suctioning and to reduce tube tension.*

• Place the patient on his side with his head in a comfortable position *to avoid tube kinking and airway obstruction.*

• Auscultate both sides of the chest and watch chest movement as indicated by the patient's condition *to ensure correct tube placement and full lung ventilation.* Give frequent oral care to the orally intubated patient and position the endotracheal tube *to prevent formation of pressure ulcers and to avoid excessive pressure on the sides of the mouth.* Give frequent nasal and oral care to the nasally intubated patient *to prevent formation of pressure ulcers and drying of oral mucous membranes.*

• Suction secretions through the endotracheal tube as the patient's condition indicates *to clear secretions and prevent mucus plugs from obstructing the tube.*

Special considerations

Orotracheal intubation is preferred in emergencies because insertion is easier and faster than with nasotracheal intubation. However, maintaining exact tube placement is more difficult, and the tube must be well secured *to avoid kinking and prevent bronchial obstruction or accidental extubation.* Orotracheal intubation is also poorly tolerated by the conscious patient because it stimulates salivation, coughing, and retching.

Nasotracheal intubation is preferred for elective insertion when the patient is capable of spontaneous ventilation for a short period. Blind intubation is typically used in conscious patients who risk imminent respiratory arrest or who have cervical spinal injury.

Although nasotracheal intubation is more comfortable than oral intubation, it's also more difficult to perform. Because the tube passes blindly through the nasal cavity, the procedure causes greater tissue trauma, increases the risk of infection by nasal bacteria introduced into the trachea, and risks pressure necrosis of the nasal mucosa. However, exact tube placement is easier and the risk of dislodgment is lower. The cuff on the endotracheal tube maintains a closed system that permits positive-pressure ventilation and protects the airway from aspiration of secretions and gastric contents.

Although low-pressure cuffs have significantly reduced the incidence of tracheal erosion and necrosis caused by cuff pressure on the tracheal wall, overinflation of a low-pressure cuff can negate this benefit. Use the minimal-leak technique to avoid these complications. Inflating the cuff a bit more to make a complete seal with the least amount of air is the next most desirable method.

Always record the volume of air needed to inflate the cuff. A gradual increase in this volume indicates tracheal dilatation or erosion. A sudden increase in volume indicates rupture of the cuff and requires immediate reintubation if the patient is being ventilated, or if he requires continuous cuff inflation to maintain a high concentration of delivered oxygen. Once the cuff has been inflated, measure its pressure at least every 8 hours *to avoid overinflation.* Normal cuff pressure is about 18 mm Hg.

Complications

Endotracheal intubation can result in apnea caused by reflex breath-holding or interruption of oxygen delivery; bronchospasm; aspiration of blood, secretions, or gastric contents; tooth damage or loss; and injury to the lips, mouth, pharynx, or vocal cords. It can also result in laryngeal edema and erosion; and tracheal stenosis, erosion, and necrosis. Nasotracheal intubation can result in nasal bleeding, laceration, sinusitis, and otitis media.

Documentation

Record the date and time of the procedure; its indication and success or failure; tube type and size; cuff size, amount of inflation, and inflation technique; administraton of medication; initiation of supplemental oxygen or ventilation therapy; results of chest auscultation and results of the chest X-ray; any complications and the nursing action taken; and the patient's reaction to the procedure.

(Text continues on page 434.)

Three methods to secure an endotracheal tube

Before taping the tube in place, make sure the patient's face is clean, dry, and free of beard stubble. If possible, suction his mouth and dry the tube just before taping. Also check the reference mark on the tube to ensure correct placement. After taping, always check for bilateral breath sounds to ensure that the tube hasn't been displaced by manipulation.

To tape the tube securely, use one of the following three methods.

Method 1

Cut two 2″ (5-cm) strips and two 15″ (38-cm) strips of 1″ (2.5-cm) cloth adhesive tape. Then cut a 13″ (33-cm) slit in one end of each 15″ strip, as shown below.

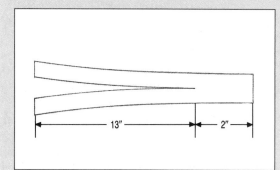

Apply compound benzoin tincture to the patient's cheeks. Place the 2″ strips on his cheeks, creating a new surface on which to anchor the tape securing the tube. *When frequent retaping is necessary, this helps preserve the patient's skin integrity.* If the patient's skin is excoriated or at risk, you can use a transparent semipermeable dressing to protect the skin.

Apply the benzoin tincture to the tape on the patient's face and to the part of the tube where you will be applying the tape.

On the side of the mouth where the tube will be anchored, place the unslit end of the long tape on top of the tape on the patient's cheek.

Wrap the top half of the tape around the tube twice, pulling the tape as tight as possible around the tube. Then, directing the tape over the patient's upper lip, place the end of the tape on the patient's other cheek. Cut off any excess tape. Use the lower half of the tape to secure an oral airway, if necessary, as shown at the top of the next column.

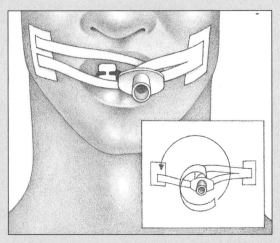

Or twist the lower half of the tape around the tube twice and attach it to the original cheek. *Taping in opposite directions places equal traction on the tube.*

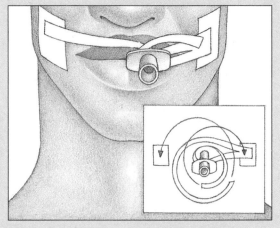

If you've taped in an oral airway or are concerned about the tube's stability, apply the other 15″ strip of tape in the same manner as the first, starting on the other side of the patient's face. If the tape around the tube is too bulky, use only the upper part of the tape and cut off the lower part. If the patient has copious oral secretions, seal the tape by cutting a 1″ piece of paper tape, coating it with benzoin tincture, and placing the paper tape over the adhesive tape.

Three methods to secure an endotracheal tube *(continued)*

Method 2

Cut one piece of 1″ cloth adhesive tape long enough to wrap around the patient's head and overlap in front. Then cut an 8″ (20-cm) piece of tape and center it on the longer piece, sticky sides together. Next, cut a 5″ (12-cm) slit in each end of the longer tape, as shown below.

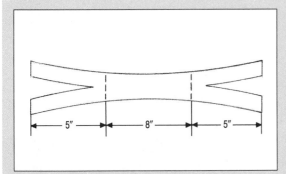

Method 3

Cut a tracheostomy tie in two pieces, one a few inches longer than the other, and cut two 6″ (15.2-cm) pieces of 1″ cloth adhesive tape. Then cut a 2″ slit in one end of both pieces of tape. Fold back the other end of the tape ½″ so the sticky sides are together and cut a small hole in it, as shown below.

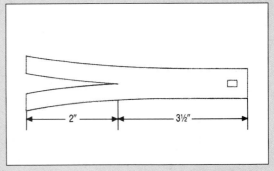

Apply benzoin tincture to the patient's cheeks, under his nose, and lower lip. (Don't spray benzoin directly on the patient's face because the vapors can be irritating if inhaled and can also harm the eyes.)

Place the top half of one end of the tape under the patient's nose and wrap the lower half around the endotracheal tube. Place the lower half of the other end of the tape along the lower lip and wrap the top half around the tube.

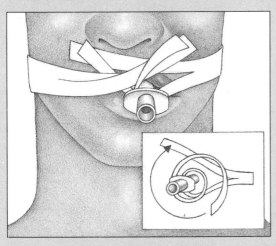

Apply benzoin tincture to the part of the endotracheal tube that will be taped. Wrap the split ends of each piece of tape around the tube, one piece on each side. Overlap the tape to secure it.

Apply the free ends of the tape to both sides of the patient's face. Then insert tracheostomy ties through the holes in the tape and knot the ties.

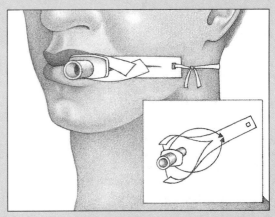

Bring the longer tie behind the patient's neck. *Knotting the ties on the side prevents the patient from lying on the knot and developing a pressure ulcer.*

Endotracheal tube care

The intubated patient requires meticulous care to ensure airway patency and prevent complications until he can maintain independent ventilation. This care includes frequent assessment of airway status, maintenance of proper cuff pressure to prevent tissue ischemia and necrosis, careful repositioning of the tube to avoid traumatic manipulation, and constant monitoring for complications. Endotracheal tube repositioning is done for patient comfort or if a chest X-ray shows improper placement. Move the tube from one side of the mouth to the other to prevent pressure ulcers.

Equipment

For maintaining the airway: stethoscope ▪ suction equipment ▪ gloves.

For repositioning the tube: 10-cc syringe ▪ compound benzoin tincture ▪ stethoscope ▪ adhesive or nonallergenic tape or Velcro tube holder ▪ suction equipment ▪ sedative or 2% lidocaine ▪ gloves ▪ hand-held resuscitation bag with mask in case of accidental extubation ▪ equipment for measuring cuff pressure (listed below).

For measuring cuff pressure: 10-cc syringe ▪ three-way stopcock ▪ cuff pressure manometer or blood pressure manometer with tubing ▪ stethoscope ▪ suction equipment ▪ gloves.

For removing the tube: 10-cc syringe ▪ suction equipment ▪ supplemental oxygen source with mask ▪ cool-mist large-volume nebulizer ▪ hand-held resuscitation bag with mask ▪ gloves ▪ equipment for reintubation.

Preparation of equipment

For repositioning the endotracheal tube: Assemble all equipment at the patient's bedside. Using sterile technique, set up the suction equipment.

For measuring cuff pressure: Assemble all equipment at the patient's bedside. If measuring with a blood pressure manometer, attach the syringe to one stopcock port; then attach the tubing from the manometer to another port of the stopcock. Turn off the stopcock port where you'll be connecting the pilot balloon cuff *so that air can't escape from the cuff.* Use the syringe to instill air into the manometer tubing until the pressure reading reaches 10 mm Hg. *This will prevent sudden cuff deflation when you open the stopcock to the cuff and the manometer.*

For removing the endotracheal tube: Assemble all equipment at the patient's bedside. Set up the suction and supplemental oxygen equipment. Have ready all equipment for emergency reintubation.

Implementation

• Explain the procedure to the patient even if he doesn't appear to be alert. Provide privacy, wash your hands thoroughly, and put on gloves.

To maintain airway patency

• Auscultate the patient's lungs at any sign of respiratory distress. If you detect an obstructed airway, determine the cause and treat accordingly. If secretions are obstructing the lumen of the tube, suction the secretions from the tube. (See "Tracheal suction" in this chapter.)
• If the tube has slipped from the trachea into the right or left mainstem bronchus, breath sounds will be absent over one lung. As ordered, obtain a chest X-ray to verify tube placement and, if necessary, reposition the tube.

To reposition the endotracheal tube

• Get help from a respiratory therapist or another nurse *to prevent accidental extubation during the procedure if the patient coughs.*
• Suction the patient's trachea through the endotracheal tube to remove any secretions, *which can irritate the bronchi and cause the patient to cough during the procedure. Coughing increases the risk of traumatic injury to the vocal cords and the likelihood of dislodging the tube.* Then suction the patient's pharynx *to remove any secretions that may have accumulated above the tube cuff. This helps to prevent aspiration of secretions during cuff deflation.*
• *To prevent traumatic manipulation of the tube,* instruct the assisting nurse to hold it as you carefully untape the tube or unfasten the Velcro tube holder. When freeing the tube, be sure to locate any identifying landmark, such as a number on the tube, or measure the distance from the patient's mouth to the top of the tube *so you have a reference point when moving the tube.*
• Next, deflate the cuff by attaching a 10-cc syringe to the pilot balloon port and aspirating air until you meet resistance and the pilot balloon deflates. Deflate the cuff before moving the tube *because the cuff forms a seal within the trachea and movement of an inflated cuff can damage the tracheal wall and vocal cords.*
• Reposition the tube as necessary, noting new landmarks or measuring the length. Then immediately reinflate the cuff. To do this, instruct the patient to inhale, and slowly inflate the cuff using a 10-cc syringe attached to the pilot balloon port. As you do this, use your stethoscope to listen to the patient's neck *to determine the presence of an air leak.* Once air leakage ceases, stop cuff inflation and, while still listening to the patient's neck with your stethoscope, aspirate a small amount of air until you detect a slight leak. *This creates a minimal air leak, which indicates that the cuff is inflated at the lowest pressure possible to create an adequate seal.* If the patient

is being mechanically ventilated, aspirate to create a minimal air leak during the inspiratory phase of respiration *because the positive pressure of the ventilator during inspiration will create a larger leak around the cuff.* Note the number of cubic centimeters of air required to inflate the cuff to achieve a minimal air leak.

• Measure cuff pressure (as described below) and compare the reading with previous pressure readings *to prevent overinflation.* Then use benzoin and tape to secure the tube in place, or refasten the Velcro tube holder.

• Make sure the patient is comfortable and the airway patent. Properly clean or dispose of equipment.

To measure cuff pressure

• Once the cuff is inflated, measure its pressure at least every 8 hours *to avoid overinflation.* (See *How to measure tracheal cuff pressure,* pages 436 and 437.)

To remove the endotracheal tube

• When you're authorized to remove the tube, obtain another nurse's assistance *to prevent traumatic manipulation of the tube when it's untaped or unfastened.*

• Elevate the head of the patient's bed to approximately 90 degrees.

• Suction the patient's oropharynx and nasopharynx *to remove any secretions that may have accumulated above the cuff and to help prevent aspiration of secretions when the cuff is deflated.*

• Using a hand-held resuscitation bag or the mechanical ventilator, give the patient several deep breaths through the endotracheal tube *to hyperinflate his lungs and increase his oxygen reserve.*

• Attach a 10-cc syringe to the pilot balloon port and aspirate air until you meet resistance and the pilot balloon deflates. If you fail to detect an air leak around the deflated cuff, notify the doctor immediately, and *do not proceed with extubation. Absence of an air leak may indicate marked tracheal edema and can result in total airway obstruction if the endotracheal tube is removed.*

• If you detect the proper air leak, untape or unfasten the endotracheal tube while the assisting nurse stabilizes the tube.

• Insert a sterile suction catheter through the endotracheal tube. Then apply suction and ask the patient to take a deep breath and to open his mouth fully and pretend to cry out. *This causes abduction of the vocal cords and reduces the risk of laryngeal trauma during withdrawal of the tube.*

• Simultaneously remove the endotracheal tube and the suction catheter in one smooth, outward and downward motion, following the natural curve of the patient's mouth. *Suctioning during extubation removes secretions retained at the end of the tube and prevents aspiration.*

• Give the patient supplemental oxygen. For highest humidity, use a cool-mist, large-volume nebulizer *to help decrease airway irritation, patient discomfort, and laryngeal edema.*

• Encourage the patient to cough and deep breathe. Remind him that a sore throat and hoarseness are to be expected and will gradually subside.

• Make sure the patient is comfortable and the airway is patent. Clean or dispose of equipment properly.

• After extubation, auscultate the patient's lungs frequently and watch for signs of respiratory distress. Be especially alert for stridor or other evidence of upper airway obstruction. If ordered, draw an arterial sample for blood gas analysis.

Special considerations

When repositioning a tube, be especially careful in patients with highly sensitive airways. Sedation or direct instillation of 2% lidocaine to numb the airway may be indicated in such patients. *Because the lidocaine is absorbed systemically,* you must have a doctor's order to use it.

After extubation of a patient who's been intubated for an extended time, keep reintubation supplies readily available for at least 12 hours, or until you're sure the patient can tolerate extubation.

Never extubate a patient unless someone skilled at intubation is readily available.

When measuring cuff pressure, keep the connection between the measuring device and the pilot balloon port tight *to avoid an air leak that could compromise cuff pressure.* If you're using a stopcock, do not leave the manometer in the off position *because air will leak from the cuff if the syringe accidentally comes off.* Also note the volume of air needed to inflate the cuff. A gradual increase in this volume indicates tracheal dilatation or erosion. A sudden increase in volume indicates rupture of the cuff and requires immediate reintubation if the patient is being ventilated, or if he requires continuous cuff inflation to maintain a high concentration of delivered oxygen.

If you inadvertently cut the pilot balloon on the cuff, immediately call the person responsible for intubation in your hospital, who will remove the damaged endotracheal tube and replace it with one that's intact. Don't remove the tube yourself before assistance arrives *because a tube with an air leak is better than no airway.*

Complications

Traumatic injury to the larynx or trachea may result from manipulation of the tube, accidental extubation, or slippage of the tube into the right bronchus.

Aspiration of upper airway secretions, underventilation, or coughing spasms may occur if a leak is created during cuff pressure measurement. Ventilatory failure

How to measure tracheal cuff pressure

An endotracheal or tracheostomy cuff provides a closed system for mechanical ventilation so the desired tidal volume can be delivered to the patient's lungs. It also protects the patient's lower respiratory tract from secretions or gastric contents that may accumulate in the pharynx.

To function properly, the cuff must exert enough pressure on the tracheal wall to seal the airway. Excessive pressure, however, can compromise blood flow to the tracheal mucosa. The ideal pressure is the lowest amount needed to seal the airway, known as minimal occlusive volume (MOV). Many authorities recommend maintaining a cuff pressure lower than venous perfusion pressure—usually about 18 mm Hg. Actual cuff pressure will vary with each patient; to keep it within safe limits, measure MOV at least once each shift.

Taking the measurement
Before the procedure, gather a three-way stopcock, a 10-cc syringe partially filled with air, a mercury manometer, and suction equipment. Then suction the endotracheal tube and the patient's oropharynx to remove secretions that have accumulated above the cuff.

Connect the ports of the three-way stopcock to the manometer tubing, the syringe, and the pilot balloon of the cuff. Close the port to the pilot balloon so air can't escape from the cuff.

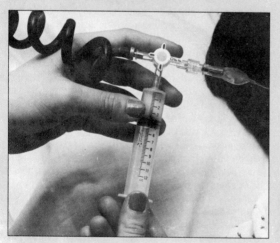

Instill air from the syringe into the manometer tubing until the pressure reading reaches 10 mm Hg. (When

you open the stopcock to the cuff and the manometer, this air will prevent sudden cuff deflation.)

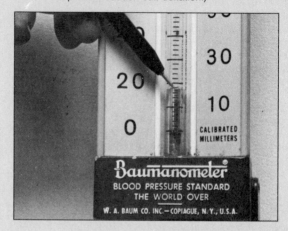

Close the stopcock to the syringe. Then record the manometer reading on expiration; this is the cuff pressure at MOV. (The mercury level will fluctuate as the patient inhales and exhales.) If cuff pressure is less than 25 mm Hg, turn off the stopcock to the pilot balloon.

Rechecking minimal occlusive volume
If cuff pressure exceeds 25 mm Hg, double-check your reading. Turn off the stopcock to the manometer and deflate the cuff completely. Reinflate the cuff until you no longer hear an air leak on inspiration. (Airways become

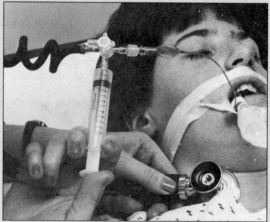

How to measure tracheal cuff pressure *(continued)*

larger on inspiration than on expiration, so if you stop reinflating the cuff when you no longer hear a leak on expiration, a leak may still occur on inspiration.)

Auscultate the patient's trachea. A smooth, hollow sound indicates a sealed airway; a loud, gurgling sound indicates an air leak.

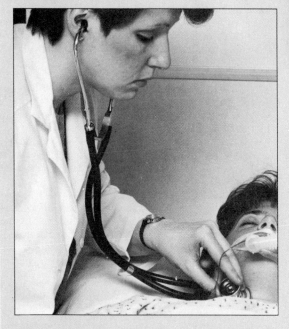

If you hear an air leak on inspiration, add air to the cuff in 0.1-cc increments until you can't hear the leak. Then remove air from the cuff until you auscultate a small leak on inspiration, and add just enough air to stop the leak. Repeat the steps you took above to record the manometer reading on expiration. Then turn off the stop-cock to the pilot balloon and disconnect the stopcock. If the cuff pressure still exceeds 25 mm Hg, notify the doctor. Document your findings.

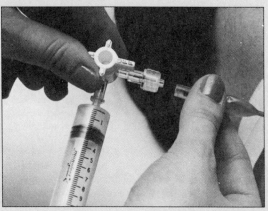

Special considerations

A patient with a high airway pressure or positive end-expiratory pressure may need an extremely high cuff pressure to seal the airway. Ask the doctor if the patient can tolerate such a high cuff pressure or a minimal leak in the cuff, or if he should be reintubated. Then document the decision and the reasons behind it.

If the tube is too small, you may not be able to seal the airway without overinflating the cuff. Report this to the doctor, because the tube may need to be replaced with a larger one.

Record the amount of air needed for reinflation. A gradual increase in the amount needed to reach MOV may indicate tracheal malacia (an abnormal softening of the tracheal tissue). Maintaining cuff pressure at the lowest possible level and inflating it to MOV will keep cuff-related complications to a minimum.

---

and airway obstruction, caused by laryngospasm or marked tracheal edema, are the gravest possible complications of extubation.

Documentation

After tube repositioning, record the date and time of the procedure, reason for repositioning (such as malposition shown by chest X-ray or prevention of pressure ulcers around the mouth), new tube position, total amount of air in the cuff after the procedure, any complications and the nursing action taken, and the patient's tolerance of the procedure.

After cuff pressure measurement, record the date and time of the procedure, cuff pressure, total amount of air in the cuff after the procedure, any complications and the nursing action taken, and the patient's tolerance of the procedure.

After extubation, record the date and time of extubation, presence or absence of stridor or other signs of upper airway edema, type of supplemental oxygen administered, any complications and required subsequent therapy, and the patient's tolerance of the procedure.

Tracheotomy

A tracheotomy involves the surgical creation of an external opening — called a tracheostomy — into the trachea and insertion of an indwelling tube to maintain the airway's patency. If all other attempts to establish an airway have failed, a doctor may perform a tracheotomy at a patient's bedside. This procedure may be necessary when an airway obstruction results from laryngeal edema, foreign body obstruction, or a tumor. An emergency tracheotomy also may be performed when endotracheal intubation is contraindicated.

Use of a cuffed tracheostomy tube provides and maintains a patent airway, prevents the unconscious or paralyzed patient from aspirating food or secretions, allows removal of tracheobronchial secretions from the patient unable to cough, replaces an endotracheal tube, and permits the use of positive-pressure ventilation.

When laryngectomy accompanies a tracheotomy, a laryngectomy tube — a shorter version of a tracheostomy tube — may be inserted by the doctor. In addition, the patient's trachea is sutured to the skin surface. Consequently, with a laryngectomy, accidental tube expulsion doesn't precipitate immediate closure of the tracheal opening. Once healing occurs, the patient has a permanent neck stoma through which respiration takes place.

Although tracheostomy tubes come in plastic and metal, plastic tubes are commonly used in emergencies because they have a universal adapter for respiratory support equipment, such as a mechanical ventilator, and a cuff to allow positive-pressure ventilation.

Equipment

Tracheostomy tube of the proper size (usually #13 to #38 French or #00 to #9 Jackson) with obturator ▪ tracheostomy tape ▪ sterile tracheal dilator ▪ vein retractor ▪ sutures and needles ▪ 4″ × 4″ gauze pads ▪ sterile drapes, gloves, mask, and gown ▪ sterile bowls ▪ stethoscope ▪ sterile tracheostomy dressing ▪ pillow ▪ tracheostomy ties ▪ suction apparatus ▪ alcohol sponge ▪ povidone-iodine solution ▪ sterile water ▪ 5-ml syringe with 22G needle ▪ local anesthetic, such as lidocaine ▪ oxygen therapy device ▪ oxygen source ▪ emergency equipment, including: suctioning equipment, sterile obturator, sterile tracheostomy tube, sterile inner cannula, sterile tracheostomy tube and inner cannula one size

smaller than tubes in use, sterile tracheal dilator or sterile hemostats. Many hospitals use prepackaged sterile trays that contain most of the equipment necessary for a tracheotomy.

Preparation of equipment

Make sure one person stays with the patient while another obtains the necessary equipment. Wash your hands and then, maintaining sterile technique, open the tray and the packages containing the solution containers. Take the tracheostomy tube from its container and place it on the sterile field. If necessary, set up the suction equipment and make sure it works. Once the doctor opens the sterile bowls, pour in the appropriate solution.

Implementation

• Explain the procedure to the patient, even if he's unresponsive.
• Assess his condition and provide privacy. Maintain ventilation until the doctor performs the tracheotomy.
• Wipe the top of the local anesthetic vial with an alcohol sponge. Invert the vial *so the doctor can withdraw the anesthetic,* using the 22G needle attached to the 5-ml syringe.
• Before the doctor begins, place a pillow under the patient's shoulders and neck and hyperextend his neck.
• Assist the doctor as needed with the insertion of the tracheostomy tube. (See *Assisting with a tracheotomy.*)
• When the tube is in position, attach it to the appropriate oxygen therapy device.
• Inject air into the distal cuff port *to inflate the cuff.*
• The doctor will suture the corners of the incision and secure the tracheostomy tube with tape.
• Put on sterile gloves.
• Apply the sterile tracheostomy dressing under the tracheostomy tube flange. Place the tracheostomy ties through the openings of the tube flanges, and tie them on the side of the patient's neck. *This allows easy access and prevents pressure necrosis at the back of the neck.*
• Clean or dispose of the used equipment according to your hospital's policy. Replenish all supplies as needed.
• Make sure that a chest X-ray is ordered *to confirm tube placement.*

Special considerations

Assess the patient's vital signs and respiratory status every 15 minutes for 1 hour, then every 30 minutes for 2 hours, then every 2 hours until his condition is stable.

Monitor the patient carefully for signs of infection. Ideally, the tracheotomy should be performed using sterile technique, as described. But in an emergency, this may not be possible.

Assisting with a tracheotomy

To perform a tracheotomy, the doctor will first clean the area from the chin to the nipples with povidone-iodine solution. Next, he'll place sterile drapes on the patient and locate the area for the incision—usually 1 to 2 cm below the cricoid cartilage. Then he'll inject a local anesthetic.

He'll make a horizontal or vertical incision into the skin. (A vertical incision helps avoid arteries, veins, and nerves on the lateral borders of the trachea.) Then he'll dissect subcutaneous fat and muscle and move the muscle aside with vein retractors to locate the tracheal rings. He'll make an incision between the second and third tracheal rings as shown at top right. He'll use hemostats to control bleeding.

He'll inject a local anesthetic into the tracheal lumen to suppress the cough reflex, and then he'll create a stoma in the trachea. When this is done, carefully apply suction to remove blood and secretions that may obstruct the airway or be aspirated into the lungs. The doctor then will insert the tracheostomy tube and obturator into the stoma, as shown in the next illustration. After inserting the tube, he'll remove the obturator.

Apply a sterile tracheostomy dressing and anchor the tube with tracheostomy ties, as shown in the bottom illustration. Check for air movement through the tube and auscultate the lungs *to ensure proper placement.*

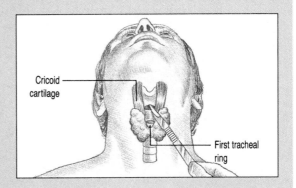

Cricoid cartilage

First tracheal ring

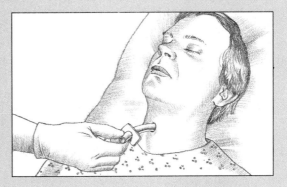

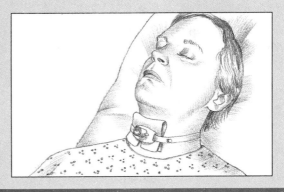

Make sure the following equipment is always at the patient's bedside:
• suctioning equipment *because the patient may need his airway cleared at any time*
• the sterile obturator used to insert the tracheostomy tube *in case the tube is expelled*
• a sterile tracheostomy tube and obturator (the same size as the one used) *in case the tube must be replaced quickly*
• a spare, sterile inner cannula *that can be used if the cannula is expelled*

• a sterile tracheostomy tube and obturator one size smaller than the one used, *which may be needed if the tube is expelled and the trachea begins to close*

• a sterile tracheal dilator or sterile hemostats *to maintain an open airway before inserting a new tracheostomy tube.*

Review emergency first-aid measures and always follow your hospital's policy concerning an expelled or blocked tracheostomy tube. When a blocked tube can't be cleared by suctioning or by withdrawing the inner cannula, hospital policy may require you to stay with the patient while someone else calls the doctor or the appropriate code. You should continue trying to ventilate the patient with whatever method works, such as a hand-held resuscitation bag. Don't remove the tracheostomy tube entirely; doing so may close the airway completely.

Use extreme caution if you try to reinsert an expelled tracheostomy tube because of the risks of tracheal trauma, perforation, compression, and asphyxiation.

Complications

An emergency tracheotomy can cause an airway obstruction (from improper tube placement), hemorrhage, edema, a perforated esophagus, subcutaneous or mediastinal emphysema, aspiration of secretions, tracheal necrosis (from cuff pressure), infection, or lacerations of arteries, veins, or nerves.

Documentation

Record the reason for the procedure, the date and time it took place, and the patient's respiratory status before and after the procedure. Include any complications that occurred during the procedure, the amount of cuff pressure, and the respiratory therapy initiated after the procedure. Also note how the patient responded to the respiratory therapy.

 # Tracheostomy care

Whether a tracheotomy is performed in an emergency situation or after careful preparation, as a permanent measure or as temporary therapy, tracheostomy care has identical goals: to ensure airway patency by keeping the tube free of mucus buildup, to maintain mucous membrane and skin integrity, to prevent infection, and to provide psychological support.

The patient may have one of three types of tracheostomy tube — metal, plastic, or rubber. The metal tube, used mainly for long-term therapy, has three parts — an outer cannula, an inner cannula, and an obturator that guides insertion of the outer cannula. Some plastic tubes have the same three parts. Most, however, consist of the obturator and one single-walled tube that doesn't require removal for cleaning (because encrustations are less likely to form on nonmetal materials), and a cuff. The red rubber James tube, which doesn't have an inner cannula, is used infrequently because its surface may become roughened with use, making sterility difficult to guarantee.

Whichever tube is used, tracheostomy care should be performed using aseptic technique until the stoma has healed to prevent infection. For recently performed tracheotomies, use sterile gloves for all manipulations at the tracheostomy site. Once the stoma has healed, clean gloves may be substituted for sterile ones.

Tracheostomy care may be given at various intervals, depending on the patient's need. It may be necessary as often as every 30 minutes just after tube insertion; it should never be suspended for more than 8 hours. If the patient will be discharged with a tracheostomy, care measures include teaching him home care using clean technique.

Equipment

For aseptic stoma and outer-cannula care: waterproof trash bag ■ two sterile solution containers ■ normal saline solution ■ hydrogen peroxide ■ sterile cotton-tipped applicators ■ sterile 4″ × 4″ gauze pads ■ sterile gloves ■ prepackaged sterile tracheostomy dressing (or 4″ × 4″ gauze pad) ■ equipment and supplies for suctioning and for mouth care ■ water-soluble lubricant or topical antibiotic cream ■ materials as needed for cuff procedures and for changing tracheostomy ties (see below).

For aseptic inner-cannula care: all of the preceding equipment plus a prepackaged commercial tracheostomy-care set, or sterile forceps ■ sterile nylon brush ■ sterile 6″ (15-cm) pipe cleaners ■ clean gloves ■ a third sterile solution container ■ disposable temporary inner cannula (for a patient on a ventilator).

For changing tracheostomy ties: 30″ (76-cm) length of tracheostomy twill tape ■ bandage scissors ■ sterile gloves ■ hemostat.

For emergency tracheostomy tube replacement: sterile tracheal dilator or sterile hemostat ■ sterile obturator that fits the tracheostomy tube in use ■ extra sterile tracheostomy tube and obturator in appropriate size ■ suction equipment and supplies.

Keep these supplies in full view in the patient's room at all times for easy access in case of emergency. Consider taping an emergency sterile tracheostomy tube in a sterile wrapper to the head of the patient's bed for easy access in an emergency.

For cuff procedures: 5- or 10-cc syringe ■ padded hemostat ■ stethoscope.

Preparation of equipment

Wash your hands and assemble all equipment and supplies in the patient's room. Check the expiration date on each sterile package and inspect for tears. Open the waterproof trash bag and place it next to you *so you can avoid reaching across the sterile field or the patient's stoma when discarding soiled items.* Form a cuff by turning down the top of the trash bag *to ensure a wide opening and prevent contamination of instruments or gloves on the bag's edge.*

Establish a sterile field near the patient's bed (usually on the overbed table), and place equipment and supplies on it. Pour normal saline solution, hydrogen peroxide, or a mixture of equal parts of both solutions into one of the sterile solution containers; then pour normal saline solution into the second sterile container for rinsing. For inner-cannula care, you may use a third sterile solution container to hold the gauze pads and cotton-tipped applicators saturated with cleaning solution. If you'll be replacing the disposable inner cannula, open the package containing the new inner cannula while maintaining sterile technique. Obtain or prepare new tracheostomy ties, if indicated.

Implementation

● Assess the patient's condition *to determine his need for care.*
● Explain the procedure to the patient, even if he is unresponsive. Provide privacy.
● Place the patient in semi-Fowler's position (unless it's contraindicated) *to decrease abdominal pressure on the diaphragm, thereby promoting lung expansion.*
● Remove any humidification or ventilation device.
● Using sterile technique, suction the entire length of the tracheostomy tube *to clear the airway of any secretions that may hinder oxygenation.* (See "Tracheal suction" in this chapter.)
● Reconnect the patient to the humidifier or ventilator, if necessary.

To clean a stoma and outer cannula

● Put on sterile gloves if you're not already wearing them.
● With your dominant hand, saturate a sterile gauze pad with the cleaning solution. Squeeze out the excess liquid *to prevent accidental aspiration.* Then wipe the patient's neck under the tracheostomy tube flanges and twill tapes.
● Saturate a second pad and wipe until the skin surrounding the tracheostomy is cleaned. Use additional pads or cotton-tipped applicators to clean the stoma site

and the tube's flanges. Wipe only once with each pad and then discard it *to prevent contamination of a clean area with a soiled pad.*
● Rinse debris and peroxide (if used) with one or more sterile 4″ × 4″ gauze pads dampened in normal saline solution. Dry the area thoroughly with additional sterile gauze pads; then apply a new sterile tracheostomy dressing.
● Remove and discard your gloves.

To clean a nondisposable inner cannula

● Put on sterile gloves.
● Using your nondominant hand, remove and discard the patient's tracheostomy dressing. Then, with the same hand, disconnect the ventilator or humidification device and unlock the tracheostomy tube's inner cannula by rotating it counterclockwise. Place the inner cannula in the container of hydrogen peroxide.
● Working quickly, use your dominant hand to scrub the cannula with the sterile nylon brush. If the brush doesn't slide easily into the cannula, use a sterile pipe cleaner.
● Immerse the cannula in the container of normal saline solution and agitate it for about 10 seconds *to rinse it thoroughly.*
● Inspect the cannula for cleanliness. Repeat the cleaning process if necessary. If the cannula is clean, tap it gently against the inside edge of the sterile container *to remove excess liquid and prevent aspiration.* Don't dry the outer surface *because a thin film of moisture acts as a lubricant during insertion.*
● Reinsert the inner cannula into the patient's tracheostomy tube. Lock it in place and then gently pull on it *to be sure it's positioned securely.* Reconnect the mechanical ventilator. Apply a new sterile tracheostomy dressing.
● If the patient can't tolerate being disconnected from the ventilator for the time it takes to clean the inner cannula, replace the existing inner cannula with a clean one and reattach the mechanical ventilator. Then clean the cannula just removed from the patient and store it in a sterile container until the next time tracheostomy care is performed.

To care for a disposable inner cannula

● Put on clean gloves.
● Using your dominant hand, remove the patient's inner cannula. After evaluating the secretions in the cannula, discard it properly.
● Pick up the new inner cannula, touching only the outer locking portion. Insert the cannula into the tracheostomy and, following the manufacturer's instructions, lock it securely.

To change tracheostomy ties

• Obtain assistance from another nurse or a respiratory therapist *because of the risk of accidental tube expulsion during this procedure.* Patient movement or coughing can dislodge the tube.

• Wash your hands thoroughly and put on sterile gloves, if you're not already wearing them.

• If you're not using commercially packaged tracheostomy ties, prepare new ties from a 30" (76-cm) length of twill tape by folding one end back 1" (2.5 cm) on itself. Then, with the bandage scissors, cut a ½" (1.3-cm) slit down the center of the tape from the folded edge.

• Prepare the other end of the tape in the same way.

• Hold both ends together and, using scissors, cut the resulting circle of tape so that one piece is approximately 10" (25 cm) long, and the other is about 20" (51 cm) long.

• Assist the patient into the semi-Fowler's position, if possible.

• After your assistant puts on gloves, instruct her to hold the tracheostomy tube in place *to prevent its expulsion during replacement of the ties.* However, if you must perform the procedure without assistance, fasten the clean ties in place before removing the old ties *to prevent tube expulsion.*

• With the assistant's gloved fingers holding the tracheostomy tube in place, cut the soiled tracheostomy ties with the bandage scissors or untie them and discard the ties. Be careful not to cut the tube of the pilot balloon.

• Thread the slit end of one new tie a short distance through the eye of one tracheostomy tube flange from the underside; use the hemostat, if necessary, to pull the tie through. Then thread the other end of the tie completely through the slit end, and pull it taut so it loops firmly through the tube's flange. *This avoids knots that can cause discomfort, tissue irritation, pressure, and necrosis at the patient's throat.*

• Fasten the second tie to the opposite flange in the same manner.

• Instruct the patient to flex his neck while you bring the ties around to the side and tie them together with a square knot. *Flexion produces the same neck circumference as coughing and helps prevent an overly tight tie.* Instruct your assistant to place one finger under the tapes as you tie them *to ensure that they're tight enough to avoid slippage but loose enough to prevent choking or jugular vein constriction.* Placing the closure on the side *allows easy access and prevents pressure necrosis at the back of the neck when the patient is recumbent.*

• After securing the ties, cut off the excess tape with the scissors and instruct your assistant to release the tracheostomy tube.

• Make sure the patient is comfortable and can reach the call button easily.

• For the patient with traumatic injury, radical neck dissection, or cardiac failure, check tracheostomy-tie tension frequently *because neck diameter can increase from swelling and cause constriction;* also check frequently for the neonatal or restless patient *because ties can loosen,* possibly predisposing to tube misplacement.

To conclude tracheostomy care

• Replace any humidification device.

• Give oral care, as needed, *because the oral cavity can become dry and malodorous or develop sores from encrusted secretions.*

• Observe soiled dressings and any suctioned secretions for amount, color, consistency, and odor.

• Properly clean or dispose of all equipment, supplies, solutions, and trash, according to hospital policy.

• Take off and discard your gloves.

• Make sure that the patient is comfortable and that he can easily reach the call button.

• Make sure all necessary supplies are readily available at the bedside.

• Repeat the procedure at least once every 8 hours or as needed. Change the dressing as often as necessary, whether or not you also perform the entire cleaning procedure, *because a dressing wet with exudate or secretions predisposes the patient to skin excoriation, breakdown, and infection.*

To deflate and inflate a tracheostomy cuff

• Read the cuff manufacturer's instructions *because cuff types and procedures vary widely.*

• Assess the patient's condition, explain the procedure to him, and reassure him. Wash your hands thoroughly.

• Help the patient into the semi-Fowler's position, if possible, or place him in a supine position *so secretions above the cuff site will be pushed up into the mouth if the patient is receiving positive-pressure ventilation.*

• *Suction the oropharyngeal cavity to prevent any pooled secretions from descending into the trachea after cuff deflation.*

• Release the padded hemostat clamping the cuff inflation tubing, if a hemostat is present.

• Insert a 5- or 10-cc syringe into the cuff pilot balloon and very slowly withdraw all air from the cuff. Leave the syringe attached to the tubing *for later reinflation of the cuff. Slow deflation allows positive lung pressure to push secretions upward from the bronchi. Cuff deflation may also stimulate the patient's cough reflex, producing additional secretions.*

• Remove any ventilation device. Suction the lower airway through any existing tube *to remove all secretions.* Then return the patient to the ventilation device.

• Maintain cuff deflation for the prescribed period of time. Observe the patient for adequate ventilation, and suction as necessary. If the patient has difficulty breathing, reinflate the cuff immediately by depressing the syringe plunger very slowly. Inject the least amount of air necessary to achieve an adequate tracheal seal.

• When inflating the cuff, you may use the minimal-leak technique or the minimal occlusive volume technique *to help gauge the proper inflation point.* (For more information, see "Endotracheal intubation" and "Endotracheal tube care" in this chapter.)

• If you're inflating the cuff using cuff-pressure measurement, be careful not to exceed 25 mm Hg. If the pressure exceeds 25 mm Hg, notify the doctor *because you may need to change to a larger size tube, use higher inflation pressures, or permit a larger air leak.* A cuff pressure of about 18 mm Hg is usually recommended.

• After you've inflated the cuff, if the tubing doesn't have a one-way valve at the end, clamp the inflation line with a padded hemostat (to protect the tubing), and remove the syringe.

• Check for a leak-free cuff seal. Even with minimal cuff inflation, you should feel no air coming from the patient's mouth, nose, or tracheostomy site, and a conscious patient shouldn't be able to speak.

• Be alert for air leaks from the cuff itself. Suspect a leak if injection of air fails to inflate the cuff or increase cuff pressure, if you're unable to inject the amount of air you withdrew, if the patient can speak, if ventilation fails to maintain adequate respiratory movement with pressures or volumes previously considered adequate, or if air escapes during the ventilator's inspiratory cycle.

• Note the exact amount of air used to inflate the cuff *to detect tracheal malacia if more air is consistently needed.*

• Make sure the patient is comfortable and can easily reach the call button and communication aids.

• Properly clean or dispose of all equipment, supplies, and trash, according to hospital policy.

• Replenish any used supplies and make sure all necessary emergency supplies are at the bedside.

Special considerations

Keep appropriate equipment at the patient's bedside for immediate use in an emergency. (For a list, see "Tracheotomy" in this chapter.)

Consult the doctor about first-aid measures you can use for your tracheostomy patient should an emergency occur. Follow hospital policy regarding procedure if a tracheostomy tube is expelled or if the outer cannula becomes blocked. If the patient's breathing is obstructed—for example, when the tube is blocked with mucus that can't be removed by suctioning or by withdrawing the inner cannula—call the appropriate code

and provide manual resuscitation with a hand-held resuscitation bag or reconnect the patient to the ventilator. Don't remove the tracheostomy tube entirely *because this may allow the airway to close completely.* Use extreme caution when attempting to reinsert an expelled tracheostomy tube *because of the risk of tracheal trauma, perforation, compression, and asphyxiation.* Reassure the patient until the doctor arrives (usually a minute or less in this type of code or emergency).

Refrain from changing tracheostomy ties unnecessarily during the immediate postoperative period before the stoma track is well formed (usually 4 days) *to avoid accidental dislodgment and expulsion of the tube.* Unless secretions or drainage is a problem, ties can be changed once a day.

Refrain from changing a single-cannula tracheostomy tube or the outer cannula of a double-cannula tube. Because of the risk of tracheal complications, the doctor usually changes the cannula, with the frequency of change depending on the patient's condition.

If the patient's neck or stoma is excoriated or infected, apply a water-soluble lubricant or topical antibiotic cream as ordered. Remember not to use a powder or an oil-based substance on or around a stoma *because aspiration can cause infection and abscess.*

Replace all equipment, including solutions, regularly according to hospital policy *to reduce the risk of nosocomial infections.*

Home care

If the patient is being discharged with a tracheostomy, start self-care teaching as soon as he's receptive. Teach the patient how to change and clean the tube. If he's being discharged with suction equipment (a few patients are), make sure he and his family feel knowledgeable and comfortable about using this equipment.

Complications

The following complications can occur within the first 48 hours after tracheostomy tube insertion: hemorrhage at the operative site, causing drowning; bleeding or edema within the tracheal tissue, causing airway obstruction; aspiration of secretions; introduction of air into the pleural cavity, causing pneumothorax; hypoxia or acidosis, triggering cardiac arrest; and introduction of air into surrounding tissues, causing subcutaneous emphysema.

Secretions collecting under dressings and twill tape can encourage skin excoriation and infection. Hardened mucus or a slipped cuff can occlude the cannula opening and obstruct the airway. Tube displacement can stimulate the cough reflex if the tip rests on the carina, or can cause blood vessel erosion and hemorrhage. Just the presence of the tube or cuff pressure can produce tracheal erosion and necrosis.

Documentation
Record the date and time of the procedure; type of procedure; the amount, consistency, color, and odor of secretions; stoma and skin condition; the patient's respiratory status; change of the tracheostomy tube by the doctor; the duration of any cuff deflation; the amount of any cuff inflation; and cuff pressure readings and specific body position. Note any complications and the nursing action taken; any patient or family teaching and their comprehension and progress; and the patient's tolerance of the treatment.

 Tracheal suction

This procedure involves the removal of secretions from the trachea or bronchi by means of a catheter inserted through the mouth, nose, tracheal stoma, tracheostomy tube, or endotracheal tube. Besides removing secretions, tracheal suctioning also stimulates the cough reflex. This procedure helps maintain a patent airway to promote optimal exchange of oxygen and carbon dioxide and to prevent pneumonia that results from pooling of secretions. Performed as frequently as the patient's condition warrants, tracheal suction calls for strict aseptic technique.

Equipment
Oxygen source (wall or portable unit, or hand-held resuscitation bag with a mask, 15-mm adapter, or a positive end-expiratory pressure [PEEP] valve, if indicated) ■ wall or portable suction apparatus ■ collection container ■ connecting tube ■ suction catheter kit, or a sterile suction catheter, one sterile glove, one clean glove, and a disposable sterile solution container ■ 1-liter bottle of sterile water or normal saline solution ■ sterile water-soluble lubricant (for nasal insertion) ■ syringe for deflating cuff of endotracheal or tracheostomy tube ■ waterproof trash bag ■ optional: sterile towel.

Preparation of equipment
Choose a suction catheter of appropriate size. The diameter should be no larger than half the inside diameter of the tracheostomy or endotracheal tube *to minimize hypoxia during suctioning.* (A #12 or #14 French catheter

may be used for an 8-mm or larger tube.) Place the suction apparatus on the patient's overbed table or bedside stand. Position the table or stand on your preferred side of the bed *to facilitate suctioning.*

Attach the collection container to the suction unit and the connecting tube to the collection container. Label and date the normal saline solution or sterile water. Open the waterproof trash bag.

Implementation
● Before suctioning, determine whether your hospital requires a doctor's order and obtain one, if necessary.
● Assess the patient's vital signs, breath sounds, and general appearance *to establish a baseline for comparison after suctioning.* Review the patient's arterial blood gas values and oxygen saturation levels if they're available. Evaluate the patient's ability to cough and deep breathe *because this will help move secretions up the tracheobronchial tree.* If you'll be performing nasotracheal suctioning, check the patient's history for a deviated septum, nasal polyps, nasal obstruction, nasal trauma, epistaxis, or mucosal swelling.
● Wash your hands. Explain the procedure to the patient, even if he is unresponsive. Tell him that suctioning usually causes transient coughing or gagging, but that coughing is helpful for removal of secretions. If the patient has been suctioned previously, summarize the reasons for suctioning. Continue to reassure the patient throughout the procedure *to minimize anxiety, promote relaxation, and decrease oxygen demand.*
● Unless contraindicated, place the patient in the semi-Fowler's or high Fowler's position *to promote lung expansion and productive coughing.*
● Remove the top from the normal saline solution or water bottle.
● Open the package containing the sterile solution container.
● Using strictly aseptic technique, open the suction catheter kit and put on the gloves. If using individual supplies, open the suction catheter and the gloves, placing the sterile glove on your dominant hand and the nonsterile glove on your nondominant hand.
● Using your nondominant (nonsterile) hand, pour the normal saline solution or sterile water into the solution container.
● Place a small amount of water-soluble lubricant on the sterile area. *Lubricant may be used to facilitate passage of the catheter during nasotracheal suctioning.*
● Place a sterile towel over the patient's chest, if desired, *to provide an additional sterile area.*

• Using your dominant (sterile) hand, remove the catheter from its wrapper. Keep it coiled *so it can't touch a nonsterile object.* Using your other hand to manipulate the connecting tubing, attach the catheter to the tubing.

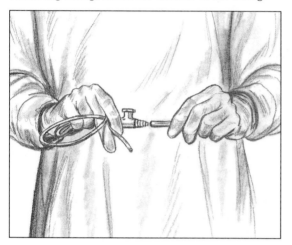

• Occlude the suction port *to assess suction pressure,* as shown below. Set the suction pressure according to hospital policy. Typically, pressure may be set between 80 and 120 mm Hg. *Higher pressures don't enhance secretion removal and may cause traumatic injury.*

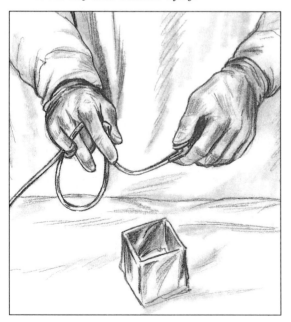

• Dip the catheter tip in the saline solution *to lubricate the outside of the catheter and reduce tissue trauma during insertion.*
• With the catheter tip in the sterile solution, occlude the control valve with the thumb of your nondominant hand. Suction a small amount of solution through the catheter, as shown below, *to lubricate the inside of the catheter to facilitate passage of secretions through it.*

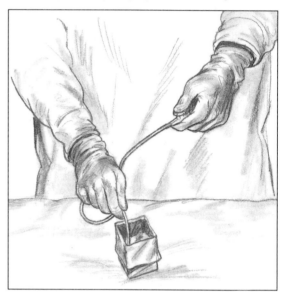

• For nasal insertion of the catheter, lubricate the tip of the catheter with the sterile, water-soluble lubricant *to reduce tissue trauma during insertion.*
• If the patient is not intubated, or is intubated but is not receiving supplemental oxygen or aerosol, instruct him to take three to six deep breaths *to help minimize or prevent hypoxia during suctioning.*
• If the patient is not intubated but is receiving oxygen, evaluate his need for preoxygenation. If indicated, instruct the patient to take three to six deep breaths while using his supplemental oxygen. (If needed, the patient may continue to receive supplemental oxygen during suctioning by leaving his nasal cannula in one nostril or by keeping the oxygen mask over his mouth.)
• If the patient is being mechanically ventilated, preoxygenate him by using either a hand-held resuscitation bag or the sigh mode on the ventilator. To use the resuscitation bag, set the oxygen flow meter at 15 liters/minute, disconnect the patient from the ventilator, and deliver three to six breaths with the resuscitation bag, as shown on page 446.

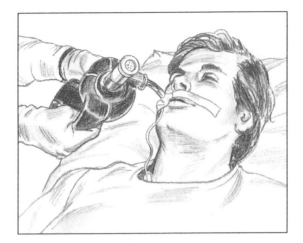

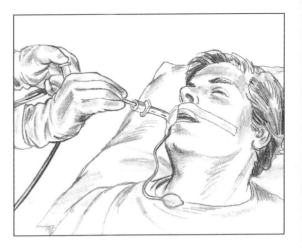

• If the patient is being maintained on PEEP, evaluate the need to use a resuscitation bag with a PEEP valve.
• To preoxygenate using the ventilator, first adjust the fraction of inspired oxygen (FIO_2) and tidal volume according to hospital policy and patient need. Then, either use the sigh mode or manually deliver three to six breaths. If you have an assistant for the procedure, the assistant can manage the patient's oxygen needs while you perform the suctioning.

Nasotracheal insertion in a nonintubated patient
• Disconnect the oxygen from the patient, if applicable.
• Using your nondominant hand, raise the tip of the patient's nose *to straighten the passageway and facilitate insertion of the catheter.*
• Insert the catheter into the patient's nostril while gently rolling it between your fingers *to help it advance through the turbinates.*
• As the patient inhales, quickly advance the catheter as far as possible. Do not apply suction during insertion *to avoid oxygen loss and tissue trauma.*
• If the patient coughs as the catheter passes through the larynx, briefly hold the catheter still and then resume advancement when the patient inhales.

Insertion in an intubated patient
• If you are using a closed system, see *Closed tracheal suctioning.*
• Using your nonsterile hand, disconnect the patient from the ventilator.
• Using your sterile hand, gently insert the suction catheter into the artificial airway, as shown at upper right. Advance the catheter, without applying suction, until you meet resistance. If the patient coughs, pause briefly and then resume advancement.

Suctioning the patient
• After inserting the catheter, apply suction intermittently by removing and replacing the thumb of your nondominant hand over the control valve. Simultaneously use your dominant hand to withdraw the catheter as you roll it between your thumb and forefinger. *This rotating motion prevents the catheter from pulling tissue into the tube as it exits, thus avoiding tissue trauma.* Never suction more than 5 to 10 seconds at a time *to prevent hypoxia.*
• If the patient is intubated, use your nondominant hand to stabilize the tip of the endotracheal tube as you withdraw the catheter *to prevent mucous membrane irritation or accidental extubation.*
• If applicable, resume oxygen delivery by reconnecting the source of oxygen or ventilation, and hyperoxygenating the patient's lungs before continuing *to prevent or relieve hypoxia.*
• Observe the patient and allow him to rest for a few minutes before the next suctioning. The timing of each suctioning and the length of each rest period depend on his tolerance for the procedure and the absence of complications. *To enhance secretion removal*, encourage the patient to cough between suctioning attempts.
• Observe the secretions. If they're thick, clear the catheter periodically by dipping the tip in the saline solution and applying suction. Normally, sputum is watery and tends to be sticky. Tenacious or thick sputum usually indicates dehydration. Watch for color variations. White or translucent color is normal; yellow indicates pus; green indicates retained secretions or *Pseudomonas* infection; brown usually indicates old blood; red indicates fresh blood; and a "red currant jelly" appearance indicates *Klebsiella* infection. When sputum contains blood, note whether it is streaked or well mixed. Also indicate how often blood appeared.

Closed tracheal suctioning

The closed tracheal suction system eliminates the need to disconnect the patient from the mechanical ventilator for suctioning.

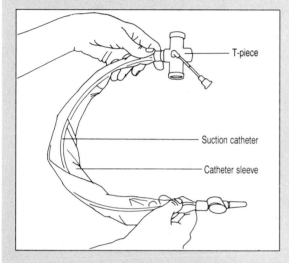

T-piece

Suction catheter

Catheter sleeve

As a result, the patient can maintain the tidal volume, oxygen concentration, and positive-end expiratory pressure delivered by the ventilator while being suctioned. In turn, this reduces the occurrence of suction-induced hypoxemia.

Another advantage of this system is a reduced risk of infection, even when the same catheter is used many times. Because the catheter remains in a protective sleeve, gloves are not required.

To perform the procedure, gather a closed suction control valve, a T-piece to connect the artificial airway to the ventilator breathing circuit, and a catheter sleeve that encloses the catheter and has connections at each end for the control valve and T-piece. Then follow these steps:
• Remove the closed suction system from its wrapping. Attach the control valve to the connecting tubing.
• Depress the thumb suction control valve and keep it depressed while setting the suction pressure to the desired level.
• Connect the T-piece to the ventilator breathing circuit, making sure that the irrigation port is closed; then connect the T-piece to the patient's endotracheal or tracheostomy tube, as shown at upper right.

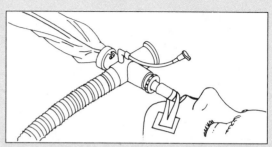

• With one hand keeping the T-piece parallel to the patient's chin, use the thumb and index finger of the other hand to advance the catheter through the tube and into the patient's tracheobronchial tree, as shown below. It may be necessary to gently retract the catheter sleeve as you advance the catheter.

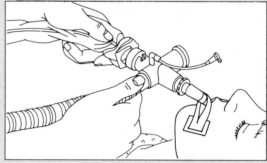

• While continuing to hold the T-piece and control valve, apply intermittent suction and withdraw the catheter until it reaches its fully extended length in the sleeve. Repeat the procedure as necessary.
• To instill normal saline solution into the airway, advance the catheter approximately 6″ (15 cm) into the tube and inject the solution into the irrigation port. Suction as needed.
• After suctioning is complete, flush the catheter by maintaining suction while slowly introducing normal saline or sterile water into the irrigation port.
• Place the thumb control valve in the off position.
• Dispose of and replace the suction equipment and supplies according to hospital policy. Change the closed suction system every 24 hours to minimize the risk of infection.

Tracheal suctioning at home

If a patient can't mobilize secretions effectively by coughing, he may have to perform tracheal suctioning at home using either clean or aseptic technique. Most patients use clean technique; they perform thorough hand washing and may don a clean glove. However, a patient with poor hand-washing technique, recurrent respiratory infections, recent surgery, or a compromised immune system may need to use aseptic technique.

Clean technique
Because the cost of disposable catheters can be prohibitive, many patients reuse disposable catheters, but the practice remains controversial. If the catheter has thick secretions adhering to it, the patient may clean it with Control III, a quaternary compound.

An alternative to disposable catheters is to use nondisposable, red rubber catheters. Consult institutional policy regarding the care and cleaning of suction catheters in the home setting. Some protocols recommend soaking such catheters in soapy water, then placing them in boiling water for 10 minutes; or soaking them in 70% alcohol for 3 to 5 minutes, then rinsing in normal saline solution.

Supplies needed
Obviously, the supplies needed will vary with the technique used. If the patient will be using clean tech-

nique he'll need suction catheter kits (or clean gloves, suction catheters, and a basin), and distilled water. If he'll be using sterile technique, the suction catheters and gloves will need to be sterile, as will the basin and the water (or normal saline).

The type of suction machine necessary will depend upon the patient's needs. You'll need to evaluate the amount of suction the machine provides, how easy it is to clean, the volume of the collection bottles, how much it costs, and whether the machine has an overflow safety device to prevent secretions from entering the compressor. You'll also need to determine whether the patient needs a machine that operates on batteries and, if so, how long the batteries will last, and if and how they can be recharged.

Nursing goals
Before discharge, the patient and his family should demonstrate the suctioning procedure. They also need to recognize the indications for suctioning, the signs and symptoms of infection, the importance of adequate hydration, and when to use adjunct therapy, such as aerosol therapy, chest physiotherapy, oxygen therapy, or a hand-held resuscitation bag. At discharge, arrange for a home health care provider and a durable medical equipment vendor to follow up with the patient.

If the patient's heart rate and rhythm are being monitored, observe for arrhythmias. Should they occur, stop suctioning and ventilate the patient.

After suctioning
• After the procedure, hyperoxygenate the patient being maintained on a ventilator with the hand-held resuscitation bag or by using the ventilator's sigh mode, as described earlier.
• Readjust the FIO₂ and, for ventilated patients, the tidal volume, to the ordered settings.
• After suctioning the lower airway, assess the patient's need for upper airway suctioning. If the cuff of the endoctracheal or tracheostomy tube is inflated, suction the upper airway before deflating the cuff with a syringe. (See "Oronasopharyngeal suction" and "Endotracheal tube care" in this chapter for more information.) Always change the catheter and sterile glove before resuctioning the lower airway *to avoid introducing microorganisms into the lower airway.*

• Discard the gloves and the catheter in the waterproof trash bag. Clear the connecting tubing by aspirating the remaining saline solution or water. Discard and replace suction equipment and supplies according to hospital policy. Wash your hands.
• Auscultate lungs bilaterally and take vital signs, if indicated, *to assess the procedure's effectiveness.*

Special considerations
Raising the patient's nose into the sniffing position helps align the larynx and pharynx and may facilitate passing the catheter during nasotracheal suctioning. If the patient's condition permits, have an assistant extend the patient's head and neck above his shoulders. The patient's lower jaw may need to be moved up and forward. If the patient is responsive, ask him to stick out his tongue *so he will not be able to swallow the catheter during insertion.*

During suctioning, the catheter typically is advanced as far as the mainstem bronchi. However, because of tracheobronchial anatomy, the catheter tends to enter the right mainstem bronchi instead of the left. Using an angled catheter (such as a Coude or Bronchitrac L) may help you guide the catheter into the left mainstem bronchus. Rotating the patient's head to the right seems to have a limited effect.

Studies show that instillation of normal saline solution into the trachea before suctioning may stimulate the patient's cough but does not liquefy the patient's secretions. Keeping the patient adequately hydrated and using bronchial hygiene techniques seems to have a greater effect on mobilizing secretions.

In addition to the closed tracheal method, oxygen insufflation offers a new approach to suctioning. Oxygen insufflation suctioning uses a double lumen catheter that allows oxygen insufflation during the suctioning procedure.

Do not allow the collection container on the suction machine to become more than ¾ full *to keep from damaging the machine.*

Home care
See *Tracheal suctioning at home.*

Complications
Because oxygen is removed along with secretions, the patient may experience hypoxemia and dyspnea. Anxiety may alter respiratory patterns. Cardiac arrhythmias can result from hypoxia and stimulation of the vagus nerve in the tracheobronchial tree. Tracheal or bronchial trauma can result from traumatic or prolonged suctioning.

Patients with compromised cardiovascular or pulmonary status are at risk for hypoxemia, arrhythmias, hypertension, or hypotension. Patients with a history of nasopharyngeal bleeding, who are taking anticoagulants, who have a recent tracheostomy, or who have a blood dyscrasia incur an increased risk of bleeding as a result of suctioning. Use caution when suctioning patients who have increased intracranial pressure because it may increase pressure further.

If the patient experiences laryngospasm or bronchospasm (rare complications) during suctioning, disconnect the suction catheter from the connecting tubing and allow the catheter to act as an airway. Discuss with the patient's doctor the use of bronchodilators or lidocaine to reduce the risk of this complication.

Documentation
Record the date and time of the procedure, the technique used, and the reason for suctioning; amount, color, consistency, and odor (if any) of the secretions; any complications and the nursing action taken; and pertinent data regarding the patient's subjective response to the procedure.

Cricothyrotomy

When endotracheal intubation or a tracheotomy can't be performed quickly to establish an airway, an emergency cricothyrotomy may be necessary. Performed rarely, this procedure involves puncturing the trachea through the cricothyroid membrane.

Usually, your role will be to assist a doctor with this procedure. But if a doctor isn't available and the patient is likely to die before he can be intubated, you may have to perform the procedure yourself. Ideally, cricothyrotomy is performed using sterile technique but, in an emergency, this may not be possible.

Equipment
Have one person stay with the patient while another collects the necessary equipment.

For scalpel or needle cricothyrotomy: sterile gloves ■ povidone-iodine solution ■ sterile 4″ × 4″ gauze pads ■ dilator ■ tape ■ oxygen source.

For scalpel cricothyrotomy: scalpel ■ #6 or smaller tracheostomy tube (if available) ■ hand-held resuscitation bag or T tube and wide-bore oxygen tubing.

For needle cricothyrotomy: 14G (or larger) inside-the-needle or over-the-needle catheter ■ 10-ml syringe ■ tape ■ I.V. extension tubing ■ hand-operated release valve or pressure-regulating adjustment valve.

Implementation
• Hyperextend the patient's neck *to expose the area of the incision site.*
• Have someone hold the patient's head in the correct position while you perform the procedure. (See *Performing an emergency cricothyrotomy,* page 450.)

Special considerations
Immediately after the procedure, check for bleeding at the insertion site, subcutaneous emphysema or inadequate ventilation from an incorrectly placed airway, and tracheal or vocal cord damage.

Complications
Hemorrhage, perforation of the thyroid or esophagus, and subcutaneous or mediastinal emphysema may occur from this procedure. Infection may also occur several days after the procedure — especially if sterile technique wasn't used.

Documentation
Your documentation of the procedure should include the date, time, and circumstances requiring the procedure

Performing an emergency cricothyrotomy

To perform this procedure, first put on sterile gloves and clean the patient's neck with a gauze pad soaked in povidone-iodine solution. To reduce the risk of contamination, use a circular motion, working outward from the incision site.

• Locate the precise insertion site by sliding your thumb and fingers down to the thyroid gland. You'll know you've located its outer borders when the space between your fingers and thumb widens.

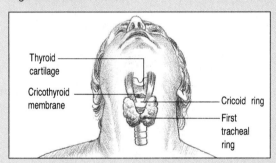

Thyroid cartilage

Cricothyroid membrane

Cricoid ring

First tracheal ring

• Move your finger across the center of the gland, over the anterior edge of the cricoid ring.

Using a scalpel

• Make a horizontal incision, less than ½″ (1.3 cm) long, in the cricothyroid membrane just above the cricoid ring.
• Insert a dilator to prevent tissue from closing around the incision. If a dilator isn't available, insert the handle of the scalpel and rotate it 90 degrees, as shown below.

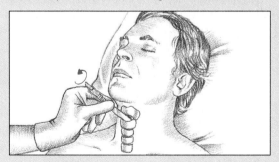

• If a small tracheostomy tube (#6 or smaller) is available, insert it into the opening and secure it to help maintain a patent airway. If a tracheostomy tube isn't available, tape the dilator or scalpel handle in place until a tracheostomy tube is available.

• If the patient can breathe spontaneously, attach a humidified oxygen source to the tracheostomy tube with a T tube; if he can't, attach a hand-held resuscitation bag. You'll need to inflate the cuff of the tracheostomy tube with a syringe to provide positive-pressure ventilation.
• Auscultate bilaterally for breath sounds, and take the patient's vital signs.
• Dispose of the gloves properly and wash your hands.

Using a needle

• Attach a 10-ml syringe to a 14G (or larger) through-the-needle or over-the-needle catheter. Then insert the catheter into the cricothyroid membrane just above the cricoid ring.
• Direct the catheter downward at a 45-degree angle to the trachea to avoid damaging the vocal cords. Maintain negative pressure by pulling back the syringe plunger as you advance the catheter. You'll know the catheter has entered the trachea when air enters the syringe.

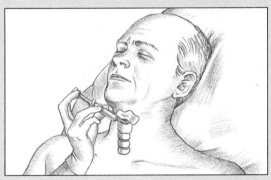

• When the catheter reaches the trachea, advance it and remove the needle and syringe. Tape the catheter in place.
• Attach the catheter hub to one end of the I.V. extension tubing. At the other end, attach a hand-operated release valve or a pressure-regulating adjustment valve. Connect the entire assembly to an oxygen source.
• Press the release valve to introduce oxygen into the trachea and inflate the lungs. When you can see that they're inflated, release the valve to allow passive exhalation. Adjust the pressure-regulating valve to the minimum pressure needed for adequate lung inflation.
• Auscultate bilaterally for breath sounds, and take the patient's vital signs.
• Dispose of the gloves properly and wash your hands.

and the patient's vital signs. Note whether the patient initiated spontaneous respirations after the procedure. Record how much and by what method oxygen was delivered. If any procedures were performed after the airway was established — endotracheal intubation, for example — note them.

OTHER TREATMENTS
Oxygen administration

A patient will need oxygen therapy when hypoxemia results from a respiratory or cardiac emergency or an increase in metabolic function.

In a *respiratory emergency,* oxygen administration enables the patient to reduce his ventilatory effort. When conditions such as atelectasis or adult respiratory distress syndrome impair diffusion, or when lung volumes are decreased from alveolar hypoventilation, this procedure boosts alveolar oxygen levels.

In a *cardiac emergency,* oxygen therapy helps meet the increased myocardial work load as the heart tries to compensate for hypoxemia. Oxygen administration is particularly important for a patient whose myocardium is already compromised — perhaps from a myocardial infarction or cardiac arrhythmia.

When *metabolic demand* is high — in cases of massive trauma, burns, or high fever, for instance — oxygen administration supplies the body with enough oxygen to meet its cellular needs. This procedure also increases oxygenation in the patient with a reduced blood oxygen-carrying capacity, perhaps from carbon monoxide poisoning or sickle cell crisis.

The adequacy of oxygen therapy is determined by arterial blood gas (ABG) analysis, oximetry monitoring, and clinical examinations. The patient's disease, physical condition, and age will help determine the most appropriate method of administration.

Equipment
The equipment needed depends on the type of delivery system ordered (see *Guide to oxygen delivery systems,* pages 453 to 456) and includes selections from the following list: oxygen source (wall unit, cylinder, liquid tank, or concentrator) ▪ flowmeter ▪ adapter, if using a wall unit, or a pressure-reduction gauge, if using a cylinder ▪ sterile humidity bottle and adapters ▪ sterile distilled water ▪ OXYGEN PRECAUTION sign ▪ appropriate oxygen delivery system (a nasal cannula, simple mask, partial rebreather mask, or nonrebreather mask for low-flow and variable oxygen concentrations; a venturi mask, aerosol mask, tracheostomy collar, T tube, tent, or oxyhood for high-flow and specific oxygen concentrations) ▪ small-diameter and large-diameter connection tubing ▪ flashlight (for nasal cannula) ▪ water-soluble lubricant ▪ gauze pads and tape (for oxygen masks) ▪ jet adapter for Venturi mask (if adding humidity) ▪ optional: oxygen analyzer.

Preparation of equipment
Although a respiratory therapist typically is responsible for setting up, maintaining, and managing the equipment, you need a working knowledge of the oxygen system being used.

Check the oxygen outlet port *to verify flow.* Pinch the tubing near the prongs *to ensure that an audible alarm will sound if the oxygen flow stops.*

Implementation
● Assess the patient's condition. In an emergency, verify that he has an open airway before administering oxygen.
● Explain the procedure to the patient and let him know why he needs oxygen *to ensure his cooperation.*
● Check the patient's room *to make sure it's safe for oxygen administration.* Whenever possible, replace electrical devices with nonelectric ones and post a NO SMOKING sign in the patient's room. If the patient is a child and is in an oxygen tent, remove all toys that may produce a spark. *Oxygen supports combustion and the smallest spark can cause a fire.*
● Place an OXYGEN PRECAUTION sign over the patient's bed and on the door to his room.
● Assist in placing the oxygen delivery device on the patient. Make sure it fits properly and is stable.
● Monitor the patient's response to oxygen therapy. Check his ABG values during initial adjustments of oxygen flow. Once the patient is stabilized, pulse oximetry may be used instead. Check the patient frequently for signs of hypoxia, such as decreased level of consciousness, increased heart rate, arrhythmias, restlessness, perspiration, dyspnea, use of accessory muscles, yawning or flared nostrils, cyanosis, and cool, clammy skin.
● Observe the patient's skin integrity *to prevent skin breakdown on pressure points from the oxygen delivery device.* Wipe moisture or perspiration from the patient's face and from the mask as needed.
● If the patient will be receiving oxygen at a concentration above 60% for more than 24 hours, watch carefully for signs of oxygen toxicity. Remind the patient frequently to cough and deep breathe *to prevent atelectasis.* Also, *to prevent the development of serious lung damage,* measure ABG values repeatedly *to determine whether high oxygen concentrations are still necessary.*

Types of home oxygen therapy

Home oxygen therapy can be administered using an oxygen tank, an oxygen concentrator, or liquid oxygen.

Oxygen tank
Commonly used for patients who need oxygen on a standby basis or who need a ventilator at home, the oxygen tank has several disadvantages, including its cumbersome design and the need for frequent refills. Because oxygen is stored under high pressure, the oxygen tank also poses a potential hazard.

Oxygen concentrator
The oxygen concentrator extracts oxygen molecules from room air. It can be used for low oxygen flow (less than 4 liters/minute) and doesn't need to be refilled with oxygen. However, because the oxygen concentrator runs on electricity, it won't function during a power failure.

Liquid oxygen
This option is used commonly by patients who are oxygen-dependent but still mobile. The system includes a large liquid reservoir for home use. When the patient wants to leave the house, he fills a portable unit worn over the shoulder; this supplies oxygen for up to several hours, depending on the liter flow.

Special considerations
Never administer oxygen at more than 2 liters/minute by nasal cannula to a patient with chronic lung disease unless you have a specific order to do so. *This is because some patients with chronic lung disease have become dependent on a state of hypercapnia and hypoxia to stimulate their respirations; therefore, supplemental oxygen could cause them to stop breathing.* However, long-term oxygen therapy of 12 to 17 hours daily may help patients with chronic lung disease to sleep better, survive longer, and experience a reduced incidence of pulmonary hypertension.

When monitoring a patient's response to a change in oxygen flow, check the pulse oximetry monitor or measure ABG values 20 to 30 minutes after adjusting the flow. In the interim, monitor the patient closely for any adverse response to the change in oxygen flow.

Home care
Before discharging a patient who will receive home oxygen therapy, make sure you know the types of oxygen therapy, the kinds of services that are available to him, and the service schedules offered by local home suppliers. Together with the doctor and the patient, choose the device best-suited to the patient. (See *Types of home oxygen therapy.*)

If the patient will be receiving transtracheal oxygen therapy, teach him how to properly clean and care for the catheter. (See *Transtracheal catheter care,* page 457.) Tell the patient to keep the skin surrounding the insertion site clean and dry to prevent infection.

No matter which device the patient uses, you'll need to evaluate his and his family's ability and motivation to administer oxygen therapy at home. Make sure they understand the reason the patient is receiving oxygen and the safety issues for administering oxygen. Teach them how to properly use and clean the equipment and supplies.

If your patient will be discharged with oxygen for the first time, make sure his health insurance covers home oxygen. If it doesn't, find out what criteria he must meet to obtain coverage. Without a third-party payer, the patient may not be able to afford home oxygen therapy.

Documentation
Record the date and time of oxygen administration; the type of delivery device; the oxygen flow rate; the patient's vital signs, skin color, respiratory effort, and lung sounds; subjective patient response before and after initiation of therapy; and any patient or family teaching.

Manual ventilation

A hand-held resuscitation bag is an inflatable device that can be attached to a face mask or directly to an endotracheal or tracheostomy tube to allow manual delivery of oxygen or room air to the lungs of a patient who can't breathe by himself. Usually used in an emergency, manual ventilation also can be performed while the patient is disconnected temporarily from a mechanical ventilator, such as during a tubing change, during transport, or before suctioning. In such instances, use of the hand-held resuscitation bag maintains ventilation. Oxygen administration with a resuscitation bag can help improve a compromised cardiorespiratory system.

(Text continues on page 456.)

Guide to oxygen delivery systems

Patients may receive oxygen through one of several administration systems. Each has its own benefits, drawbacks, and indications for use. Advantages and disadvantages of each system are compared below and on the following pages.

Nasal cannula
Oxygen is delivered through plastic cannulas in the patient's nostrils.

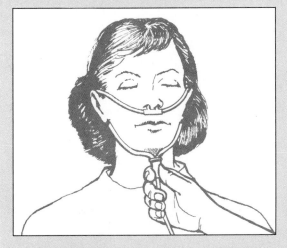

Advantages: safe and simple; comfortable and easily tolerated; nasal prongs can be shaped to fit any face; effective for low oxygen concentrations; allows movement, eating, and talking; inexpensive and disposable.

Disadvantages: can't deliver concentrations higher than 40%; can't be used in complete nasal obstruction; may cause headaches or dry mucous membranes if flow rate exceeds 6 liters/minute; can dislodge easily.

Administration guidelines: Ensure patency of the patient's nostrils with a flashlight. If patent, hook the cannula tubing behind the patient's ears and under the chin. Slide the adjuster upward under the chin to secure the tubing. If using an elastic strap to secure the cannula, position it over the ears and around the back of the head. Avoid applying too tightly, which can result in excess pressure on facial structures and cannula occlusion as well. With a nasal cannula, oral breathers achieve the same oxygen delivery as nasal breathers.

Simple mask
Oxygen flows through an entry port at the bottom of the mask and exits through large holes on the sides of the mask.

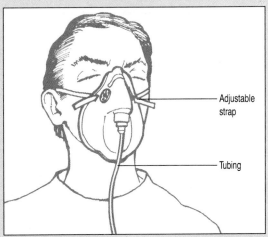

Adjustable strap

Tubing

Advantages: can deliver concentrations of 40% to 60%.

Disadvantages: hot and confining; may irritate patient's skin; tight seal that may cause discomfort is required for higher oxygen concentration; interferes with talking and eating; impractical for long-term therapy because of imprecision.

Administration guidelines: Select the mask size that offers the best fit. Place the mask over the patient's nose, mouth, and chin, and mold the flexible metal edge to the bridge of the nose. Adjust the elastic band around the head to hold the mask firmly but comfortably over the cheeks, chin, and bridge of the nose. For elderly or cachectic patients with sunken cheeks, tape gauze pads to the mask over the cheek area to try to create an airtight seal. Without this seal, room air dilutes the oxygen, preventing delivery of the prescribed concentration. A minimum of 5 liters/minute is required in all masks to flush expired carbon dioxide from the mask so the patient doesn't rebreathe it.

(continued)

Guide to oxygen delivery systems *(continued)*

Partial rebreather mask

The patient inspires oxygen from a reservoir bag along with atmospheric air and oxygen from the mask. The first third of exhaled tidal volume enters the bag; the rest exits the mask. Because air entering the reservoir bag comes from the trachea and bronchi, where no gas exchange occurs, the patient rebreathes the oxygenated air he just exhaled.

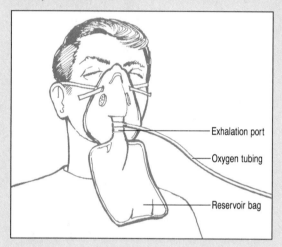

Exhalation port

Oxygen tubing

Reservoir bag

Advantages: effectively delivers concentrations of 40% to 60%; openings in mask allow patient to inhale room air if oxygen source fails.

Disadvantages: tight seal required for accurate oxygen concentration may cause discomfort; interferes with eating and talking; hot and confining; may irritate skin; bag may twist or kink; impractical for long-term therapy.

Administration guidelines: Follow procedures listed for the simple mask. If the reservoir bag collapses more than slightly during inspiration, raise the flow rate until you see only a slight deflation. Marked or complete deflation indicates insufficient oxygen flow; carbon dioxide will accumulate in the mask and bag. Keep the reservoir bag from twisting or kinking. Ensure free expansion by making sure it lies outside the patient's gown and bedcovers.

Nonrebreather mask

On inhalation, a one-way valve opens, directing oxygen from a reservoir bag into the mask. On exhalation, gas exits the mask through the one-way valve and enters the atmosphere. The patient only breathes air from the bag.

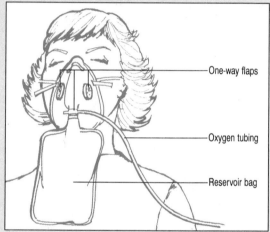

One-way flaps

Oxygen tubing

Reservoir bag

Advantages: delivers the highest possible oxygen concentration (60% to 90%) short of intubation and mechanical ventilation; effective for short-term therapy; doesn't dry mucous membranes; can be converted to a partial rebreather mask, if necessary, by removing the one-way flap.

Disadvantages: requires a tight seal, which may be difficult to maintain and may cause discomfort; may irritate the patient's skin; impractical for long-term therapy.

Administration guidelines: Follow procedures listed for the simple mask. Make sure the mask fits very snugly. Make sure the one-way valves or flaps are secure and functioning. Because the mask excludes room air, valve malfunction can cause carbon dioxide buildup and suffocate an unconscious patient. If the reservoir bag collapses more than slightly during inspiration, raise the flow rate until you see only a slight deflation. Marked or complete deflation indicates an insufficient flow rate. Keep the reservoir bag from twisting or kinking. Ensure free expansion by making sure it lies outside the patient's gown and bedcovers.

Guide to oxygen delivery systems *(continued)*

CPAP mask

This system allows the spontaneously breathing patient to receive continuous positive airway pressure (CPAP) with or without an artificial airway.

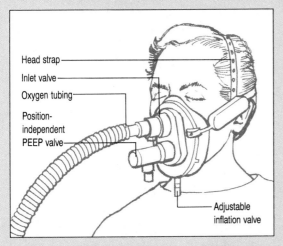

Advantages: noninvasively improves arterial oxygenation by increasing functional residual capacity; allows the patient to avoid intubation; allows the patient to talk and cough without interrupting positive pressure.

Disadvantages: requires a tight fit, which may cause discomfort; heightened risk of aspiration if the patient vomits; increased risk of pneumothorax, diminished cardiac output, and gastric distention; contraindicated in patients with chronic obstructive pulmonary disease, bullous lung disease, low cardiac output, or tension pneumothorax.

Administration guidelines: Place one strap behind the patient's head and the other strap over his head to ensure a snug fit. Attach one latex strap to the connector prong on one side of the mask. Then, use one hand to position the mask on the patient's face while using the other hand to connect the strap to the other side of the mask. After the mask is applied, assess the patient's respiratory, circulatory, and GI function every hour. Watch for signs of pneumothorax, decreased cardiac output, a drop in blood pressure, and gastric distention.

Transtracheal oxygen

The patient receives oxygen through a catheter inserted into the base of his neck in a simple outpatient procedure.

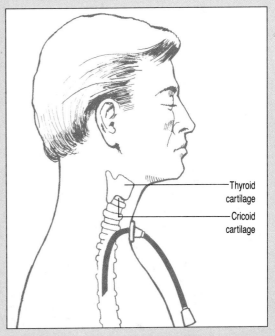

Advantages: supplies oxygen to the lungs throughout the respiratory cycle; provides continuous oxygen without hindering mobility; doesn't interfere with eating or talking; doesn't dry mucous membranes; catheter can easily be concealed by a shirt or scarf.

Disadvantages: not suitable for use in patients at risk for bleeding or those with severe bronchospasm, uncompensated respiratory acidosis, pleural herniation into the base of the neck, or high corticosteroid dosages.

Administration guidelines: After insertion, obtain a chest X-ray to confirm placement. Monitor the patient for bleeding, respiratory distress, pneumothorax, pain, coughing, or hoarseness. Don't use the catheter for about 1 week following insertion to decrease the risk of subcutaneous emphysema.

(continued)

Guide to oxygen delivery systems *(continued)*

Venturi mask

The mask is connected to a Venturi device that mixes a specific volume of air and oxygen.

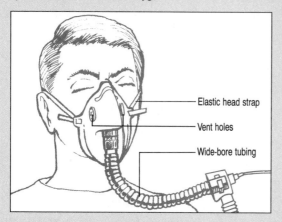

- Elastic head strap
- Vent holes
- Wide-bore tubing

Advantages: delivers highly accurate oxygen concentration despite patient's respiratory pattern because the same amount of air is always entrained; dilute jets can be changed or dial turned to change oxygen concentration; doesn't dry mucous membranes; humidity or aerosol can be added.

Disadvantages: confining and may irritate skin; oxygen concentration may be altered if mask fits loosely, tubing kinks, oxygen intake ports become blocked, flow is insufficient, or patient is hyperpneic; interferes with eating and talking; condensate may collect and drip on the patient if humidification is used.

Administration guidelines: Make sure that the oxygen flow rate is set at the amount specified on each mask and that the Venturi valve is set for the desired fraction of inspired oxygen.

Aerosols

A face mask, hood, tent, or tracheostomy tube or collar is connected to wide-bore tubing that receives aerosolized oxygen from a jet nebulizer. The jet nebulizer, which is attached near the oxygen source, adjusts air entrainment in a manner similar to the Venturi device.

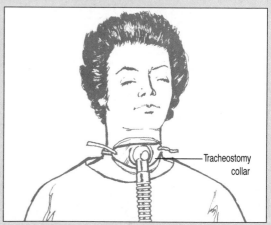

- Tracheostomy collar

Advantages: administers high humidity; gas can be heated (when delivered through artificial airway) or cooled (when delivered through a tent).

Disadvantages: condensate collected in the tracheostomy collar or T tube may drain into the tracheostomy; the weight of the T tube can put stress on the tracheostomy tube.

Administration guidelines: Guidelines vary with the type of nebulizer used, including the ultrasonic, large volume, small volume, and in-line. When using a high-output nebulizer, watch for signs of overhydration, pulmonary edema, crackles, and electrolyte imbalance.

Equipment

Hand-held resuscitation bag ▪ mask ▪ oxygen source (wall unit or tank) ▪ oxygen tubing ▪ nipple adapter attached to oxygen flowmeter ▪ optional: positive end-expiratory pressure (PEEP) valve, oxygen accumulator.

Preparation of equipment

Unless the patient is intubated or has a tracheostomy, select a mask that fits snugly over the mouth and nose. Attach the mask to the resuscitation bag.

If oxygen is readily available, connect the hand-held resuscitation bag to the oxygen. Attach one end of the tubing to the bottom of the bag and the other end to the nipple adapter on the flowmeter of the oxygen source.

Turn on the oxygen and adjust the flow rate according to the patient's condition. For example, if the patient has a low partial pressure of oxygen in arterial blood, he'll need a higher fraction of inspired oxygen (FIO_2). To increase the concentration of inspired oxygen, you can add an oxygen accumulator (also called an oxygen reservoir). This device, which attaches to an adapter on the bottom

Transtracheal catheter care

Teach the patient with a transtracheal catheter how to care for the catheter as well as the skin surrounding the catheter. If the patient has a Heimlich Micro-Trach, tell him to clean around the catheter twice a day using a soapy cotton-tipped applicator and water. He also needs to irrigate the catheter while it's in place, two to three times a day, using normal saline solution. Tell him that this serves to loosen secretions and stimulate coughing. Instruct the patient to change the catheter once a month.

SCOOP catheter
If the patient has a SCOOP catheter, tell him to clean it two to three times a day to keep it free of mucus. Tell him that, before he begins cleaning, he should put on a nasal cannula, disconnect the oxygen tubing from the catheter, and then connect it to the cannula. Instruct the patient to irrigate the catheter by instilling 1½ ml of normal saline solution into the catheter, as shown in the illustration below. Forewarn him that this may make him cough.

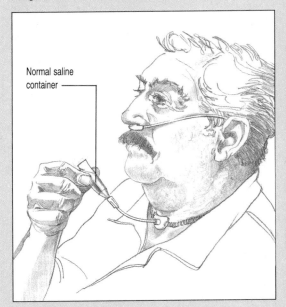

Normal saline container

Next, tell him to insert a cleaning rod (which he's cleaned beforehand) through the catheter as far as possible and then to pull it back.

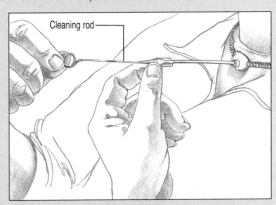

Cleaning rod

After he has removed and reinserted the rod three times, tell him to remove the rod, instill 1½ ml of normal saline solution into the catheter, and then reconnect the oxygen tubing to the catheter. As a final step, instruct him to clean the rod with antimicrobial soap and to store it in a dry place.

In addition to cleaning the catheter while it remains in place, the patient with a SCOOP 1 catheter needs to remove the catheter at least once weekly—the patient with a SCOOP 2 catheter at least once daily—for a more thorough cleaning. (The SCOOP 2 catheter has extra side holes to facilitate oxygen distribution.) After the catheter is removed, tell the patient to use antimicrobial soap, a cleaning rod, and lukewarm tap water to clean the catheter.

Reminders
Remind the patient never to remove or insert a SCOOP catheter while oxygen is flowing through it. Rather, he should put on a nasal cannula, disconnect the catheter from the oxygen source, and then remove the catheter. Next, he should insert a second SCOOP catheter, coated with water-soluble lubricant. Once the second catheter is secured, he can resume oxygen delivery through the catheter.

How to apply a hand-held resuscitation bag and mask

Place the mask over the patient's face so that the apex of the triangle covers the bridge of his nose and the base lies between his lower lip and chin.

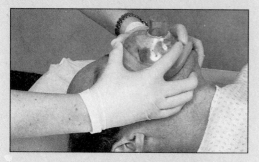

Make sure that the patient's mouth remains open underneath the mask. Attach the bag to the mask and to the tubing leading to the oxygen source.

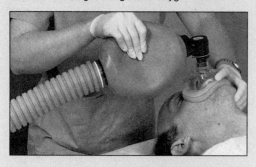

Or, if the patient has a tracheostomy or endotracheal tube in place, remove the mask from the bag and attach the hand-held resuscitation bag directly to the tube.

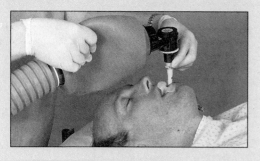

of the bag, permits an FIO_2 of up to 100%. Then, if time allows, set up suction equipment.

Implementation

• Before using the hand-held resuscitation bag, check the patient's upper airway for foreign objects. If present, remove them *because this alone may restore spontaneous respirations in some instances. Also, foreign matter or secretions can obstruct the airway and impede resuscitation efforts.* Suction the patient *to remove any secretions that may obstruct the airway.* If necessary, insert an oropharyngeal or nasopharyngeal airway *to maintain airway patency.* If the patient has a tracheostomy or endotracheal tube in place, suction the tube.

• If appropriate, remove the bed's headboard and stand at the head of the bed *to help keep the patient's neck extended and to free space at the side of the bed for other activities, such as cardiopulmonary resuscitation.*

• Tilt the patient's head backward, if not contraindicated, and pull his jaw forward *to move the tongue away from the base of the pharynx and prevent obstruction of the airway.* (See *How to apply a hand-held resuscitation bag and mask.*)

• Keeping your nondominant hand on the patient's mask, exert downward pressure *to seal the mask against his face.* For the adult patient, use your dominant hand to compress the bag every 5 seconds *to deliver about 1 liter of air.* For a child, deliver 15 breaths/minute, or one compression of the bag every 4 seconds; for the infant, 20 breaths/minute, or one compression every 3 seconds. Infants and children should receive 250 to 500 cc of air with each bag compression.

• Deliver breaths with the patient's own inspiratory effort, if any is present. Don't attempt to deliver a breath as the patient exhales.

• Observe the patient's chest *to ensure that it rises and falls with each compression.* If ventilation fails to occur, check the fit of the mask and the patency of the patient's airway; if necessary, reposition the patient's head and ensure patency with an oral airway.

Special considerations

Avoid neck hyperextension if the patient has a possible cervical injury; instead, use the jaw-thrust technique to open the airway. If you need both hands to keep the patient's mask in place and maintain hyperextension, use the lower part of your arm to compress the bag against your side.

Observe for vomiting through the clear part of the mask. If vomiting occurs, stop the procedure immediately, lift the mask, wipe and suction vomitus, and resume resuscitation.

Underventilation commonly occurs because the hand-held resuscitation bag is difficult to keep positioned tightly on the patient's face while ensuring an open airway. What's more, the volume of air delivered to the patient varies with the type of bag used and the hand size of the person compressing the bag. An adult with a small or medium-sized hand may not consistently deliver 1 liter of air. For these reasons, have someone assist with the procedure, if possible. (See *Using a PEEP valve.*)

Complications
Aspiration of vomitus can result in pneumonia, and gastric distention may result from air forced into the patient's stomach.

Documentation
In an emergency, record the date and time of the procedure; manual ventilation efforts; any complications and the nursing action taken; and the patient's response to treatment, according to your hospital's protocol for respiratory arrest.

In a nonemergency situation, record the date and time of the procedure, reason and length of time the patient was disconnected from mechanical ventilation and received manual ventilation, any complications and the nursing action taken, and the patient's tolerance for the procedure.

Mechanical ventilation

A mechanical ventilator moves air in and out of a patient's lungs. However, although the equipment serves to ventilate a patient, it does not ensure adequate gas exchange. Mechanical ventilators may use either positive or negative pressure to ventilate patients.

Positive pressure ventilators exert a positive pressure on the airway, which causes inspiration and, at the same time, increases the patient's tidal volume. The inspiratory cycles of these ventilators may vary according to volume, pressure, or time. For example, a volume-cycled ventilator—the type used most commonly—delivers a preset volume of air to the patient each time, regardless of the amount of resistance by the patient's lungs. A pressure-cycled ventilator generates flow until the machine reaches a preset pressure, regardless of the volume delivered or the time required to achieve the pressure. A time-cycled ventilator generates flow for a preset amount of time.

Negative pressure ventilators act by creating negative pressure, which pulls the patient's thorax outward and allows air to flow into the patient's lungs. Examples of negative pressure ventilators are the iron lung, the cui-

---

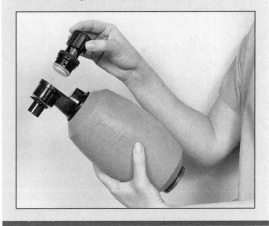

rass (chest shell), and the body wrap (Pneumowrap or Pulmo-wrap). Negative pressure ventilators are used primarily to treat patients with neuromuscular disorders, such as Guillain Barré syndrome, myasthenia gravis, and poliomyelitis.

Other indications for ventilator use include central nervous system disorders, such as cerebral hemorrhage and spinal cord transsection, adult respiratory distress syndrome, pulmonary edema, chronic obstructive pulmonary disease, flail chest, and acute hypoventilation.

Equipment
Oxygen source ■ air source that can supply 50 psi ■ mechanical ventilator ■ humidifier ■ ventilator circuit tubing, connectors, and adapters ■ condensation collection trap ■ spirometer, respirometer, or electronic device to measure flow and volume ■ in-line thermometer ■ probe for gas sampling and measuring airway pressure ■ bacterial filter ■ gloves ■ hand-held resuscitation bag with reservoir ■ suction equipment ■ sterile distilled water ■ equipment for arterial blood gas (ABG) analysis ■ soft restraints, if indicated ■ optional: oximeter.

Preparation of equipment

In most hospitals, respiratory therapists assume responsibility for setting up the ventilator. If necessary, check the manufacturer's instructions for setting it up. In most cases, you'll need to add sterile distilled water to the humidifier and connect the ventilator to the appropriate gas source.

Implementation

• Verify the doctor's order for ventilator support. If the patient is not already intubated, prepare him for intubation. (See "Endotracheal intubation" in this chapter.)
• When possible, explain the procedure to the patient and his family *to help reduce anxiety and fear.* Assure the patient and his family that staff members are nearby to provide care.
• Perform a complete physical assessment and draw blood for ABG analysis *to establish a baseline.*
• Suction the patient if necessary.
• Plug the ventilator into the electrical outlet and turn it on. Adjust the settings on the ventilator as ordered. (See *Mechanical ventilation glossary.*) Make sure that the ventilator's alarms are set, as ordered, and that the humidifier is filled with sterile distilled water.
• Put on gloves if you haven't already. Connect the endotracheal tube to the ventilator. Observe for chest expansion and auscultate for bilateral breath sounds *to verify that the patient is being ventilated.*
• Monitor the patient's ABG values after the initial ventilator setup (usually 20 to 30 minutes), after any changes in ventilator settings, and as the patient's clinical condition indicates *to determine whether the patient is being adequately ventilated and to avoid oxygen toxicity.* Be prepared to adjust ventilator settings depending on ABG analysis.
• Check the ventilator tubing frequently for condensation, *which can cause resistance to airflow and which may also be aspirated by the patient.* As needed, drain the condensate into a collection trap or briefly disconnect the patient from the ventilator (ventilating him with a hand-held resuscitation bag if necessary), and empty the water into a receptacle. Do not drain the condensate into the humidifer *because the condensation may be contaminated with the patient's secretions.*
• Check the in-line thermometer to make sure that the temperature of the air delivered to the patient is close to body temperature.
• When monitoring the patient's vital signs, count spontaneous breaths as well as ventilator-delivered breaths.
• Change, clean, or dispose of the ventilator tubing and equipment in accordance with hospital policy *to reduce the risk of bacterial contamination.* Typically, ventilator tubing should be changed every 24 to 48 hours, sometimes more often.
• When ordered, begin to wean the patient from the ventilator. (See *Weaning the patient from the ventilator,* page 462.)

Special considerations

Be sure that the ventilator alarms are on at all times. *These alarms alert the nursing staff to potentially hazardous conditions and changes in patient status.* If an alarm sounds and the problem can't be identified easily, disconnect the patient from the ventilator and use a hand-held resuscitation bag to ventilate him. (See *Responding to ventilator alarms,* page 463.)

Provide emotional support to the patient during all phases of mechanical ventilation *to reduce anxiety and promote successful treatment.* Even if the patient is unresponsive, continue to explain all procedures and treatments to him.

Unless contraindicated, turn the patient from side to side every 1 to 2 hours *to facilitate lung expansion and removal of secretions.* Perform active or passive range-of-motion exercises for all extremities *to reduce the hazards of immobility.* If the patient's condition permits, position him upright at regular intervals *to increase lung expansion.* When moving the patient or the ventilator tubing, be careful to prevent condensation in the tubing from flowing into the lungs *because aspiration of this contaminated moisture can cause infection.* Provide care for the patient's artificial airway as needed.

Assess the patient's peripheral circulation, and monitor his urine output for signs of decreased cardiac output. Watch for signs and symptoms of fluid volume excess or dehydration.

Place the call light within the patient's reach, and establish a method of communication, such as a communication board, *because intubation and mechanical ventilation impair the patient's ability to speak.* An artificial airway may help the patient to speak *by allowing air to pass through his vocal cords.*

Administer a sedative or neuromuscular blocking agent, as ordered, *to relax the patient or eliminate spontaneous breathing efforts that can interfere with the ventilator's action.* Remember that the patient receiving a neuromuscular blocking drug requires close observation *because of his inability to breathe or communicate.*

If the patient is receiving a neuromuscular blocking agent, make sure that he also receives a sedative. *Neuromuscular blocking agents cause paralysis without altering the patient's level of consciousness.* Reassure the patient and his family that the paralysis is temporary. Also make sure that emergency equipment is readily available in case the ventilator malfunctions or the patient is extu-

Mechanical ventilation glossary

Although a respiratory therapist usually monitors ventilator settings based on the doctor's order, you should understand each of the following terms.

Assist-control mode: The ventilator delivers a preset tidal volume at a preset rate; however, the patient can initiate additional breaths, which trigger the ventilator to deliver the preset tidal volume at positive pressure.

Continuous positive airway pressure (CPAP): A setting that prompts the ventilator to deliver positive pressure to the airway throughout the respiratory cycle. It works only on patients who can breathe spontaneously.

Control mode: The ventilator delivers a preset tidal volume at a fixed rate, regardless of whether the patient is breathing spontaneously or not.

Fraction of inspired oxygen (FIO$_2$): The amount of oxygen delivered to the patient by the ventilator. The dial on the ventilator that sets this percentage is labelled by the term oxygen concentration or oxygen percentage.

I:E ratio: This ratio compares the duration of inspiration to the duration of expiration. The I:E ratio of normal, spontaneous breathing is 1:2, meaning that expiration is twice as long as inspiration.

Inspiratory flow rate (IFR): The IFR denotes the tidal volume delivered within a certain time. Its value can range from 20 to 120 liters/minute.

Minute ventilation or minute volume (V̇E): This measurement results from the multiplication of respiratory rate and tidal volume.

Peak inspiratory pressure (PIP): Measured by the pressure manometer on the ventilator, peak inspiratory pressure reflects the amount of pressure required to deliver a preset tidal volume.

Positive end-expiratory pressure (PEEP): In this mode, the ventilator is triggered to apply positive pressure at the end of each expiration to increase the area for oxygen exchange by helping to inflate and keep open collapsed alveoli.

Pressure support ventilation (PSV): This mode allows the ventilator to apply a preset amount of positive pressure when the patient inspires spontaneously. PSV increases tidal volume while decreasing the patient's breathing work load.

Respiratory rate: Also called frequency, this is the number of breaths per minute delivered by the ventilator.

Sensitivity setting: A setting that determines the amount of effort the patient must exert to trigger the inspiratory cycle.

Sigh volume: A ventilator-delivered breath that is 1½ times as large as the patient's tidal volume.

Synchronized intermittent mandatory ventilation (SIMV): The ventilator delivers a preset number of breaths at a specific tidal volume. The patient may supplement these mechanical ventilations with his own breaths, in which case the tidal volume and rate are determined by his own inspiratory ability.

Tidal volume (VT): Tidal volume refers to the volume of air delivered to the patient with each cycle, usually 12 to 15 cc/kg.

---

bated accidentally. Continue to explain all procedures to the patient, and take extra steps to ensure his safety, such as raising the side rails during turning and covering and lubricating his eyes.

Ensure that the patient gets adequate rest and sleep *because fatigue can delay weaning from the ventilator.* Provide subdued lighting, safely muffle equipment noises, and restrict staff access to the area *to promote quiet during rest periods.*

When weaning the patient, continue to observe for signs of hypoxia. Schedule weaning to fit comfortably and realistically with the patient's daily regimen. Avoid scheduling sessions after meals, baths, or lengthy therapeutic or diagnostic procedures. Have the patient help

you set up the schedule *to give him some sense of control over a frightening procedure.* As the patient's tolerance for weaning increases, help him sit up out of bed *to improve his breathing and sense of well-being.* Suggest diversionary activities *to take his mind off breathing.*

Home care

If the patient will be discharged on a ventilator, evaluate the family's or the caregiver's ability and motivation to provide such care. Well before discharge, develop a teaching plan that will address the patient's needs. For example, teaching should include information about ventilator care and settings, artificial airway care, suctioning, respiratory therapy, communication, nutrition,

Weaning the patient from the ventilator

Successful weaning depends on the patient's ability to breathe on his own. That means he must have a spontaneous respiratory effort that can keep him ventilated, a stable cardiovascular system, and sufficient respiratory muscle strength and level of consciousness to sustain spontaneous breathing. He also should meet some or all of the following criteria.

Criteria
- PaO_2 of 60 mm Hg (50 mm Hg or the ability to maintain baseline levels if he has chronic lung disease) or a fraction of inspired oxygen (FIO_2) at or below 0.4
- $PaCO_2$ of less than 40 mm Hg (or normal for the patient), or an FIO_2 of 0.4 or less if his $PaCO_2$ is 60 mm Hg or more
- Vital capacity of more than 10 ml/kg of body weight
- Maximum inspiratory pressure over −20 cm H_2O
- Minute ventilation under 10 liters/minute with a respiratory frequency of less than 28 to 30 breaths/minute
- Forced expiratory volume in the first second of more than 10 ml/kg of body weight
- Ability to double his spontaneous resting minute ventilation
- Adequate natural airway or a functioning tracheostomy
- Ability to cough and mobilize secretions
- Successful withdrawal of any neuromuscular blocker, such as pancuronium
- Clear or clearing chest X-ray
- Absence of infection, acid-base or electrolyte imbalance, hyperglycemia, arrhythmias, renal failure, anemia, fever, or excessive fatigue

Short-term ventilation
If the patient has received mechanical ventilation for a short time, weaning may be accomplished by progressively decreasing the frequency and tidal volume of the ventilated breaths. Then the patient's endotracheal tube can be converted to a T tube to assess whether his spontaneous respirations are adequate before extubation. If the patient has been mechanically ventilated with 5 cm H_2O or less of PEEP, the adequacy of his spontaneous breathing can be assessed by using a trial of CPAP on the ventilator.

Long-term ventilation
If the patient has received mechanical ventilation for a long time, weaning is usually accomplished by switching the ventilator to pressure support ventilation (PSV), with or without intermittent mandatory ventilation (IMV). This way, each of the patient's spontaneous breaths is augmented by the ventilator. As the patient's own respirations improve, the IMV and the PSV can be decreased.

If the patient doesn't progress satisfactorily using one of these methods, an alternative method of weaning is to disconnect the patient from the ventilator and place him on a T tube or tracheostomy collar for the ordered amount of time before reconnecting him to the ventilator. The patient then alternates between being on and off the ventilator, with the time off the ventilator increasing with each trial. Eventually, the patient will be able to breathe on his own all day. But, even then, he should be reconnected to the ventilator for a few nights so that he can obtain adequate rest and conserve the energy required to breathe on his own the next day.

---

therapeutic exercise, the signs and symptoms of infection, and ways to troubleshoot minor equipment malfunctions.

Also evaluate the patient's need for adaptive equipment, such as a hospital bed, wheelchair or walker with a ventilator tray, patient lift, and bedside commode. Determine whether the patient needs to travel; if so, select appropriate portable and backup equipment.

Before discharge, have the patient's caregiver demonstrate his ability to use the equipment. At discharge, contact a durable medical equipment vendor and a home health nurse to follow up with the patient. Also refer the patient to community resources, if available.

Complications
Mechanical ventilation can cause tension pneumothorax, decreased cardiac output, oxygen toxicity, fluid volume excess caused by humidification, infection, and such GI complications as distention or bleeding from stress ulcers.

Documentation
Document the date and time of initiation of mechanical ventilation. Name the type of ventilator used for the patient, and note its settings. Describe the patient's subjective and objective response to mechanical ventilation (including vital signs, breath sounds, use of accessory muscles, intake and output, and weight). List any complications and nursing actions taken. Record all pertinent

Responding to ventilator alarms

SIGNAL	POSSIBLE CAUSE	INTERVENTIONS
Low-pressure alarm	• Tube disconnected from ventilator	• Reconnect the tube to the ventilator.
	• Endotracheal tube displaced above vocal cords or tracheostomy tube extubated	• Check tube placement and reposition if needed. If extubation or displacement has occurred, ventilate the patient manually and call the doctor immediately.
	• Leaking tidal volume from low cuff pressure (from an underinflated or ruptured cuff or a leak in the cuff or one-way valve)	• Listen for a whooshing sound around the tube, indicating an air leak. If you hear one, check cuff pressure. If you can't maintain pressure, call the doctor; he may need to insert a new tube.
	• Ventilator malfunction	• Disconnect the patient from the ventilator and ventilate him manually if necessary. Obtain another ventilator.
	• Leak in ventilator circuitry (from loose connection or hole in tubing, loss of temperature-sensitive device, or cracked humidification jar)	• Make sure all connections are intact. Check for holes or leaks in the tubing and replace if necessary. Check the humidification jar and replace if cracked.
High-pressure alarm	• Increased airway pressure or decreased lung compliance caused by worsening disease	• Auscultate the lungs for evidence of increasing lung consolidation, barotrauma, or wheezing. Call the doctor if indicated.
	• Patient is biting on oral endotracheal tube	• Insert a bite block if needed.
	• Secretions in airway	• Look for secretions in the airway. To remove them, suction the patient or have him cough.
	• Condensate in large-bore tubing	• Check tubing for condensate and remove any fluid.
	• Intubation of right mainstem bronchus	• Check tube position. If it has slipped, call the doctor; he may need to reposition it.
	• Patient coughing, gagging, or attempting to talk	• If the patient fights the ventilator, the doctor may order a sedative or neuromuscular blocking agent.
	• Chest wall resistance	• Reposition the patient if it improves chest expansion. If repositioning doesn't help, administer the prescribed analgesic.
	• Failure of high-pressure relief valve	• Have the faulty equipment replaced.
	• Bronchospasm	• Assess the patient for the cause. Report to the doctor and treat as ordered.

laboratory data, including ABG analysis results and oxygen saturation levels.

During weaning, record the date and time of each session; the weaning method; and baseline and subsequent vital signs, oxygen saturation levels, and ABG values. Again describe the patient's subjective and objective responses (including level of consciousness, respiratory effort, arrhythmias, skin color, and need for suctioning).

List all complications and nursing actions taken. If the patient was receiving pressure support ventilation (PSV) or using a T-piece or tracheostomy collar, note the duration of spontaneous breathing and the patient's ability to maintain the weaning schedule. If using intermittent mandatory ventilation, with or without PSV, record the control breath rate, the time of each breath reduction, and the rate of spontaneous respirations.

Incentive spirometry

This procedure involves using a breathing device to help the patient achieve maximal ventilation. The device measures respiratory flow or respiratory volume and induces the patient to take a deep breath and hold it for several seconds. This deep breath produces increased lung volume and inflation of alveoli and also facilitates venous return. In addition, this exercise establishes alveolar hyperinflation for a longer time than is possible with a normal deep breath, thus preventing and reversing the alveolar collapse that produces atelectasis and pneumonitis.

Devices used for incentive spirometry are designed to give the patient a visual incentive to breathe deeply. Some are activated when the patient inhales a certain volume of air; afterward, the device estimates the amount of air inhaled. Others contain plastic floats, which are raised according to the amount of air the patient pulls through the device when he inhales.

Incentive spirometry benefits the patient on prolonged bed rest, especially the postoperative patient who may regain his normal respiratory pattern slowly because of such predisposing factors as abdominal or thoracic surgery, advanced age, inactivity, obesity, smoking, and a decreased ability to cough effectively and expel lung secretions.

Equipment
Flow or volume incentive spirometer, as indicated, with sterile disposable tube and mouthpiece ▪ stethoscope ▪ watch ▪ tape.

The tube and mouthpiece are sterile on first use and clean on subsequent uses.

Preparation of equipment
Assemble the ordered equipment at the patient's bedside. Read the manufacturer's instructions for spirometer setup and operation. Remove the sterile flow tube and mouthpiece from the package and attach them to the device. Set the flow rate or volume goal, as determined by the doctor or respiratory therapist and based on the patient's preoperative performance. Turn on the machine if necessary.

Implementation
• Assess the patient's condition.
• Explain the procedure to the patient, making sure he understands the importance of performing this exercise regularly *to maintain alveolar inflation.* Wash your hands.

• Assist the patient to a comfortable sitting or semi-Fowler's position *to promote optimal lung expansion.* If you're using a flow incentive spirometer and the patient is unable to assume or maintain this position, he can perform the procedure in any position as long as the device remains upright. *Tilting a flow incentive spirometer decreases the required patient effort and reduces the exercise's effectiveness.*
• Auscultate the patient's lungs *to provide a baseline for comparison with posttreatment auscultation.*
• Instruct the patient to insert the mouthpiece and close his lips tightly around it *because a weak seal may alter flow or volume readings.*
• Instruct the patient to exhale normally and then inhale as slowly and as deeply as possible. If the patient has difficulty with this step, tell him to suck as he would through a straw, but to do so more slowly. Ask the patient to retain the entire volume of air he inhaled for 3 seconds or, if you're using a device with a light indicator, until the light turns off. This deep breath creates sustained transpulmonary pressure near the end of inspiration and is sometimes called a sustained maximal inspiration.
• Tell the patient to remove the mouthpiece and exhale normally. Allow him to relax and take several normal breaths before attempting another breath with the spirometer. Repeat this sequence 5 to 10 times during every waking hour. Note tidal volumes.
• Evaluate the patient's ability to cough effectively, and encourage him to cough after each effort *because deep lung inflation may loosen secretions and facilitate their removal.* Observe any expectorated secretions.
• Auscultate the patient's lungs and compare findings with the first auscultation.
• Instruct the patient to remove the mouthpiece. Wash the device in warm water and shake it dry. Avoid immersing the spirometer itself *because this enhances bacterial growth and impairs the internal filter's effectiveness in preventing inhalation of extraneous material.*
• Place the mouthpiece in a plastic storage bag between exercises, and label it and the spirometer, if applicable, with the patient's name *to avoid inadvertent use by another patient.*

Special considerations
If the patient is scheduled for surgery, make a preoperative assessment of his respiratory pattern and capability to ensure the development of appropriate postoperative goals. Then teach the patient to use the spirometer before surgery *so that he can concentrate on your instructions and practice the exercise.* A preoperative evaluation will also help in establishing a postoperative therapeutic goal.

Avoid exercising at mealtime *to prevent nausea*. If the patient has difficulty breathing only through his mouth, provide a noseclip *to fully measure each breath*. Provide paper and pencil so the patient can note exercise times. Exercise frequency varies with condition and ability.

Immediately after surgery, monitor the exercise frequently *to ensure compliance and assess achievement*.

Documentation
Record any preoperative teaching and preoperative flow or volume levels; date and time of the procedure; type of spirometer; flow or volume levels achieved; number of breaths taken; patient's condition before and after the procedure; his tolerance of the procedure; and results of both auscultations.

If you've used a flow incentive spirometer, compute *volume* by multiplying the setting by the duration the patient kept the ball (or balls) suspended, as follows. If the patient suspended the ball for 3 seconds at a setting of 500 cc during each of 10 breaths, multiply 500 cc by 3 seconds and then record this total (1,500 cc) and the number of breaths: 1,500 cc × 10 breaths. If you've used a volume incentive spirometer, take the volume reading directly from the spirometer. For example, record 1,000 cc × 5 breaths.

Intermittent positive-pressure breathing

Intermittent positive-pressure breathing (IPPB) delivers room air or oxygen into the lungs at a pressure higher than atmospheric pressure. This delivery ceases when pressure in the mouth or in the breathing circuit tube increases to a predetermined airway pressure.

IPPB was once the mainstay of pulmonary therapy, with its proponents claiming that the device delivered aerosolized medications deeper into the lungs, decreased the work of breathing, and assisted in the mobilization of secretions. Studies now show that IPPB has no clinical benefit over hand-held nebulizers. However, IPPB may be useful in helping asthmatics with hypercapnia and impending respiratory failure avoid intubation and mechanical ventilation. Although IPPB easily inflates healthy alveoli, it may have little effect on alveoli with thickened or obstructed walls—the walls most difficult to inflate.

Typically, personnel from the respiratory therapy department deliver these treatments.

Equipment
IPPB machine ■ breathing circuit tubing ■ other necessary tubing (usually one or two sections) ■ mouthpiece or mask ■ noseclips, if necessary ■ source of pressurized gas at 50 psi, if necessary ■ oxygen, if desired ■ prescribed medication, such as isoetharine hydrochloride (Bronkosol) and normal saline solution ■ 3-ml syringe with needle ■ sphygmomanometer ■ stethoscope ■ facial tissues and waste bag, or specimen cup ■ optional: suction equipment.

Preparation of equipment
Follow the manufacturer's instructions to set up the equipment properly.

Implementation
● Explain the procedure to the patient *to ensure his cooperation*. Tell him to sit erect in a chair, if possible, *to allow for optimal lung expansion*. Otherwise, place him in semi-Fowler's position. Wash your hands.
● Take baseline blood pressure and heart rate, especially if a bronchodilator will be administered, and listen to breath sounds for posttreatment comparisons.
● Instruct the patient to breathe deeply and slowly through his mouth as if sucking on a straw. Encourage the patient to let the machine do the work.
● During treatment, instruct the patient to hold his breath for a few seconds after full inspiration *to allow for greater distribution of gas and medication*. Then instruct him to exhale normally.
● During treatment, take the patient's blood pressure and heart rate. *IPPB treatment increases intrathoracic pressure and may temporarily decrease cardiac output and venous return, resulting in tachycardia, hypotension, or headache. Monitoring also detects reactions to the bronchodilator*. If you find a sudden change in blood pressure or increase in heart rate by 20 or more beats, stop the treatment and notify the doctor.
● If the patient is tolerating the treatment, continue until the medication in the nebulizer is exhausted, usually about 10 minutes.
● After treatment, or as needed, have the patient expectorate into tissues or a specimen cup, or suction him as necessary. Listen to his breath sounds and compare them to the pretreatment assessment.
● Shake excess moisture from the nebulizer and the mouthpiece or mask. After 24 hours of use, either discard the equipment or clean it with warm, soapy water. After washing, rinse with warm water and immerse in glutaraldehyde solution (Control III) for 10 minutes. Then remove the equipment, rinse in warm water, and air dry. Once it's dry, store in a clean plastic bag.

Special considerations

If possible, avoid administering IPPB treatment immediately before or after a meal *because the treatment may induce nausea, and because a full stomach reduces lung expansion.*

Never give IPPB treatment without medication in the nebulizer *because this could dry the patient's airways and make secretions more difficult to mobilize.* If the purpose of treatment is to mobilize secretions, use a specimen cup to measure the secretions obtained.

If the patient wears dentures, leave them in place *to ensure a proper seal,* but remove them if they slide out of position. If the patient has an artificial airway, use a special adapter, such as mechanical ventilation tubing, to give IPPB treatments. When using a mask to administer treatments, allow the patient frequent rest periods and observe for gastric distention *because this is more likely to occur with a mask.*

If the patient's blood pressure is stable during the initial treatment, you may not need to check it during subsequent treatments unless he has a history of cardiovascular disease, hypotension, or sensitivity to any drug delivered in the treatment.

Complications

Gastric insufflation may result from swallowed air and occurs more commonly with a mask than with a mouthpiece. Dizziness can result from hyperventilation. The work of breathing can be increased, especially if the patient is uncomfortable with or frightened by the machine. Decreased blood pressure can result from decreased venous return, especially in the patient with hypovolemia or cardiovascular disease. Increased intracranial pressure can result from impeded venous return from the brain. Spontaneous pneumothorax may result from increased intrathoracic pressure; this complication is rare, but is most likely to occur in patients with emphysematous blebs.

Documentation

Record the date, time, and duration of treatment; medication administered; pressure used; vital signs; breath sounds before and after treatment; amount of sputum produced; any complications and nursing actions taken; and the patient's tolerance of the procedure.

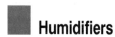 **Humidifiers**

Humidifiers, which deliver a maximum amount of water vapor without producing particulate water, are used to prevent drying and irritation of the upper airway in conditions where the upper airway is inflamed, such as croup, or when secretions are particularly thick and tenacious.

Some humidifiers heat the water vapor, which raises the moisture-carrying capacity of gas and thus increases the amount of humidity delivered to the patient. Room humidifiers add humidity to an entire room, while humidifiers added to gas lines humidify only the air being delivered to the patient. (See *Comparing humidifiers.*)

Equipment

Humidifier ▪ bottled distilled water, or tap water if the unit has a demineralizing capability ▪ container for waste water ▪ bleach ▪ white vinegar.

Preparation of equipment

For a bedside humidifier: Open the reservoir and add sterile distilled water to the fill line; then close the reservoir. Keep all room windows and doors closed tightly to maintain adequate humidification. Then plug the unit into the electrical outlet.

For a heated vaporizer: Remove the top and fill the reservoir to the fill line with tap water. Replace the top securely. Then place the vaporizer about 4 feet from the patient, directing the steam toward but not directly onto the patient. Place the unit in a spot where it can't be overturned *to avoid hot water burns.* This is especially important if children will be in the room.

Plug the unit into an electrical outlet. Steam should soon rise from the unit into the air. Close all windows and doors to maintain adequate humidification.

For a diffusion head humidifier: Unscrew the humidifier reservoir and add sterile distilled water to the appropriate level. (If using a disposable unit, screw the cap with the extension onto the top of the unit.) Then screw the reservoir back onto the humidifier and attach the flowmeter to the oxygen source.

Screw the humidifier onto the flowmeter until the seal is tight. Then set the flowmeter at a rate of 2 liters/minute and check for gentle bubbling.

Next, check the positive-pressure release valve by occluding the end valve on the humidifier. The pressure should back up into the humidifier, signaled by a high-pitched whistle. If this doesn't occur, tighten all connections and try again.

For a cascade bubble diffusion humidifier: Unscrew the cascade reservoir and add sterile distilled water to the fill line. Screw the top back onto the reservoir. Then plug in the heater unit, and set the temperature between 95° F (35° C) and 100.4° F (38° C).

EQUIPMENT

Comparing humidifiers

TYPE	DESCRIPTION AND USES	ADVANTAGES AND DISADVANTAGES
Bedside	• Spinning disc splashes water against baffle, creating small drops and increasing evaporation; motor disperses mist to directly humidify room air	*Advantages* • May be used with all oxygen masks and nasal cannulas • Easy to operate • Inexpensive *Disadvantages* • Produces humidity inefficiently • Can't be used for patient with bypassed upper airway • May harbor bacteria and molds
Heated vaporizer	• Provides direct humidification to room air by heating the water in the reservoir	*Advantages* • May be used with all oxygen masks and nasal cannulas • Easy to operate • Inexpensive *Disadvantages* • Can't guarantee the amount of humidity delivered • Risk of burn injury if the machine is knocked over
Diffusion head	• In-line humidifier most commonly used with low-flow oxygen delivery systems; gas flows through porous diffuser in reservoir to increase gas-liquid interface; provides humidification to patients using a nasal cannula or oxygen mask (except the Venturi mask)	*Advantages* • Easy to use • Inexpensive *Disadvantages* • Provides only 20% to 30% humidity at body temperature • Can't be used for a patient with bypassed upper airway
Cascade bubble diffusion	• Gas is forced through plastic grid in reservoir of warmed water to create fine bubbles; commonly used in patients receiving mechanical ventilation or continuous positive airway pressure therapy	*Advantages* • Delivers 100% humidity at body temperature • The most effective of all evaporative humidifiers *Disadvantages* • If correct water level isn't maintained, mucosa can become irritated

Implementation
• Check to be sure that the humidifier or vaporizer has been prepared properly.

For a bedside humidifier
• Direct the humidifier unit's nozzle away from the patient's face (but toward the patient) for effective treatment. Check for a fine mist emission from the nozzle, which indicates proper operation.
• Check the unit every 4 hours for proper operation, and the water level every 8 hours. When refilling, unplug the unit, discard any old water, wipe with a disinfectant, rinse the reservoir container, and refill with sterile distilled water as necessary.
• Keep the unit cleaned and refilled with sterile water *to reduce the risk of bacterial growth*. Replace the unit every 7 days and send used units for proper decontamination.

For a heated vaporizer
• Check the unit every 4 hours for proper functioning.
• If steam production seems insufficient, unplug the unit, discard the water and refill with half distilled water and half tap water, or clean the unit well.

• Check the water level in the unit every 8 hours. To refill, unplug the unit, discard any old water, wipe with a disinfectant, rinse the reservoir container, and refill with tap water as necessary.

For a diffusion head humidifier
• Attach the oxygen delivery device to the humidifier and then to the patient. Then adjust the flowmeter to the appropriate oxygen flow rate.
• Check the reservoir every 4 hours. If the water level drops too low, empty the remaining water, rinse the jar, and refill it with sterile water. (As the reservoir water level decreases, the evaporation of water in the gas decreases, reducing humidification of the delivered gas.)
• Change the humidification system regularly *to prevent bacterial growth and invasion.*
• Periodically assess the patient's sputum; *if too thick, it can hinder mobilization and expectoration.* If this occurs, the patient requires a device that can provide higher humidity.

For a cascade bubble diffusion humidifier
• Assess the temperature of the inspired gas near the patient's airway every 2 hours when used in critical care and every 4 hours when used in general patient care. If the cascade becomes too hot, drain the water and replace it. *Overheated water vapor can cause respiratory tract burns.*
• Check the reservoir's water level every 2 to 4 hours, and fill as necessary. *If the water level falls below the minimum water level mark, humidification will decrease to that of room air.*
• Be alert for condensation buildup in the tubing, which can result from the very high humidification produced by the cascade.
• Check the tubing frequently and empty the condensate as necessary *so it cannot drain into the patient's respiratory tract, encourage growth of microorganisms, or obstruct dependent sections of tubing.* To do so, disconnect the tubing, drain the condensate into a container, and dispose of it properly. Never drain the condensate into the humidification system.
• Change the cascade regularly according to your hospital's policy.

Special considerations
Because it creates a humidity level comparable to that of ambient air, the diffusion head humidifier is only used for oxygen flow rates greater than 4 liters/minute.

Because the bedside humidifier doesn't deliver a precise amount of humidification, assess the patient regularly *to determine the effectiveness of therapy.* Ask him if he has noticed any improvement and evaluate his sputum.

Like the bedside humidifier, the heated vaporizer doesn't deliver a precise amount of humidification, so assess the patient regularly by asking if he's feeling better and by examining his sputum.

Keep in mind that a humidifier, if not kept clean, can cause or aggravate respiratory problems, especially for people allergic to molds. Refer to your hospital's policy for changing and disposing of humidification equipment.

Home care
Make sure the patient and his family understand the reason for using a humidifier and that they know how to use the equipment. Give the patient specific, written guidelines concerning all aspects of home care.

Instruct a patient using a bedside humidifier at home to fill it with plain tap water and to periodically use sterile distilled water *to prevent mineral buildup.* Also advise him to run white vinegar through the unit *to help clean it, prevent bacterial buildup, and dissolve deposits.*

Tell the patient to rinse a heated vaporizer unit with bleach and water every 5 days. Also run white vinegar through it *to help clean it, prevent bacterial buildup and dissolve any deposits.*

Complicatons
Cascade humidifiers can cause aspiration of tubal condensation and, if the air is heated, can cause pulmonary burns. Humidifiers, if contaminated, can cause infection.

Documentation
Record the date and time when humidification began and was discontinued; the type of humidifier; the flow rate (of a gas system); thermometer readings (if heated); any complications and the nursing action taken; and the patient's reaction to humidification.

 # Nebulizer therapy

An established component of respiratory care, nebulizer therapy aids bronchial hygiene by restoring and maintaining mucous blanket continuity; hydrating dried, retained secretions; promoting expectoration of secretions; humidifying inspired oxygen; and delivering medications. The therapy may be administered through nebulizers that have a large or small volume, are ultrasonic, or are placed inside ventilator tubing.

Ultrasonic nebulizers are electrically driven and use high-frequency vibrations to break up surface water into particles. The resultant dense mist can penetrate the smaller airways and is useful for hydrating secretions and inducing a cough. Large-volume nebulizers are used to provide humidity for an artificial airway, such as a tracheostomy, and small-volume nebulizers are used to deliver medications, such as bronchodilators. In-line nebulizers are used to deliver medications to patients who are being mechanically ventilated. In this instance, the nebulizer is placed in the inspiratory side of the ventilatory circuit, as close to the endotracheal tube as possible.

Many questions still exist regarding aerosol therapy, including what type of fluid to use, the types of medications that can be delivered, and the effectiveness of therapy. (See *Comparing nebulizers,* page 470.)

Equipment

For an ultrasonic nebulizer: ultrasonic gas-delivery device ▪ large-bore oxygen tubing ▪ nebulizer couplet compartment.

For a large-volume nebulizer (such as Venturi jet): pressurized gas source ▪ flowmeter ▪ large-bore oxygen tubing ▪ nebulizer bottle ▪ sterile distilled water ▪ heater (if ordered) ▪ in-line thermometer (if using heater).

For a small-volume nebulizer (such as a mini-nebulizer): pressurized gas source ▪ flowmeter ▪ oxygen tubing ▪ nebulizer cup ▪ mouthpiece or mask ▪ normal saline solution ▪ prescribed medication.

For an in-line nebulizer: pressurized gas source ▪ flowmeter ▪ nebulizer cup ▪ normal saline solution ▪ prescribed medication.

Preparation of equipment

For an ultrasonic nebulizer: Fill the couplet compartment on the nebulizer to the level indicated.

For a large-volume nebulizer: Fill the water chamber to the indicated level with sterile distilled water. Avoid using saline solution *to prevent corrosion.* Add a heating device, if ordered, and place a thermometer in-line between the outlet port and the patient, as close to the patient as possible, *to monitor the actual temperature of the inhaled gas and to avoid burning the patient.* If the unit will supply oxygen, analyze the flow at the patient's end of the tubing *to ensure delivery of the prescribed oxygen percentage.*

For a small-volume nebulizer: Draw up the prescribed medication, inject it into the nebulizer cup, and add the prescribed amount of saline solution or water. Attach the mouthpiece, mask, or other gas-delivery device.

For an in-line nebulizer: Draw up the medication and diluent, remove the nebulizer cup, quickly inject the medication, and then replace the cup. If using an intermittent positive-pressure breathing machine, attach the mouthpiece and mask to the machine. (For more information, see "Intermittent positive-pressure breathing" in this chapter.)

Implementation

● Explain the procedure to the patient and wash your hands.

● Take the patient's vital signs and auscultate his lung fields *to establish a baseline.* If possible, place the patient in a sitting or high Fowler's position to encourage full lung expansion and promote aerosol dispersion. Encourage the patient to take slow, even breaths during the treatment.

Ultrasonic nebulizer

● Before beginning, administer an inhaled bronchodilator (metered dose inhaler or small-volume nebulizer) *to prevent bronchospasm.*

● Turn on the machine and check the outflow port *to ensure proper misting.*

● Check the patient frequently during the procedure *to observe for adverse reactions.* Watch for labored respirations *because ultrasonic nebulizer therapy may hydrate retained secretions and obstruct airways.* Take the patient's vital signs and auscultate his lung fields.

● Encourage the patient to cough and expectorate, or suction as needed.

Large-volume nebulizer

● Attach the delivery device to the patient.

● Encourage the patient to cough and expectorate, or suction as needed.

● Check the water level in the nebulizer at frequent intervals and refill or replace as indicated. When refilling a reusable container, discard the old water *to prevent infection from bacterial or fungal growth,* and refill the container to the indicator line with sterile distilled water.

● Change the nebulizer unit and tubing according to hospital policy *to prevent bacterial contamination.*

● If the nebulizer is heated, tell the patient to report any warmth, discomfort, or hot tubing *because these may indicate a heater malfunction.* Use the in-line thermometer to monitor the temperature of the gas the patient is inhaling. If you turn off the flow for more than 5 minutes, unplug the heater *to avoid overheating the water and burning the patient when the aerosol is resumed.*

Small-volume nebulizer

● After attaching the flowmeter to the gas source, attach the nebulizer to the flowmeter and then adjust the flow to at least 10 liters/minute *to ensure adequate functioning* but not more than 14 liters/minute to prevent excess venting.

● Check the outflow port *to ensure adequate misting.*

● Remain with the patient during the treatment, which lasts 15 to 20 minutes, and take his vital signs *to detect any adverse reaction to the medication.*

Comparing nebulizers

TYPE	DESCRIPTION AND USES	ADVANTAGES AND DISADVANTAGES
Ultrasonic 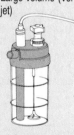	• Uses high-frequency sound waves to create an aerosol mist	**Advantages** • Provides 100% humidity • About 20% of its particles reach the lower airways • Loosens secretions **Disadvantages** • May precipitate bronchospasms in the asthmatic patient • Infants have increased risk of overhydration
Large volume (Venturi jet)	• Supplies cool or heated moisture to a patient whose upper airway has been bypassed by endotracheal intubation or a tracheostomy, or who has recently been extubated	**Advantages** • Provides 100% humidity with cool or heated devices • Provides oxygen and aerosol therapy • Can be used for long-term therapy **Disadvantages** • Nondisposable units increase risk of bacterial growth • Condensate can collect in large-bore tubing • If correct water level isn't maintained in reservoir, mucosal irritation may result from breathing hot, dry air • Infants have increased risk of overhydration from mist
Small volume (mini-nebulizer, Maxi-mist)	• Hand-held device, used to deliver aerosolized medication	**Advantages** • Conforms to patient's physiology, allowing him to inhale and exhale on his own • Can cause less air trapping than medication administered by intermittent positive-pressure breathing • May be used with compressed air, oxygen, or compressor pump • Compact and disposable **Disadvantages** • Procedure takes a long time if patient needs nurse's assistance • Medication distributed unevenly if patient doesn't breathe properly

• Encourage the patient to cough and expectorate, or suction as necessary.
• Change the nebulizer cup and tubing according to hospital policy *to prevent bacterial contamination.*

In-line nebulizer
• Turn on the machine and check the outflow port *to ensure proper misting.*
• Remain with the patient during the treatment, which lasts 15 to 20 minutes, and take his vital signs *to detect any adverse reaction to the medication.*

• Encourage the patient to cough and suction excess secretions as necessary.
• Auscultate the patient's lungs *to evaluate the effectiveness of therapy.*

Special considerations
When using high-output nebulizers, such as an ultrasonic nebulizer, in pediatric patients or in patients with a delicate fluid balance, be alert for signs of overhydration (exhibited by unexplained weight gain occurring over

several days after the beginning of therapy), pulmonary edema, crackles, and electrolyte imbalance.

Also, if oxygen is being delivered concomitantly, the fraction of inspired oxygen (FIO_2) may be diluted if the flow is not adequate. Therefore, if the mist disappears when the patient inhales, increase the gas flow.

Complications

Nebulized particulates can irritate the mucosa in some patients and cause bronchospasm and dyspnea. Other complications include airway burns (when heating elements are used), infection from contaminated equipment (although rare), and adverse reactions from medications.

Documentation

Record the date, time, and duration of therapy; type and amount of medication; FIO_2, or oxygen flow, if administered; baseline and subsequent vital signs and breath sounds; and patient's response to treatment.

Chest physiotherapy

This procedure includes postural drainage, chest percussion and vibration, and coughing and deep breathing exercises. Together, these techniques mobilize and eliminate secretions, reexpand lung tissue, and promote efficient use of respiratory muscles. Of critical importance to the bedridden patient, chest physiotherapy (PT) helps prevent or treat atelectasis and may also help prevent pneumonia — respiratory complications that can seriously impede recovery.

Postural drainage performed in conjunction with percussion and vibration encourages peripheral pulmonary secretions to empty by gravity into the major bronchi or trachea, and is accomplished by sequential repositioning of the patient. Usually, secretions drain best with the patient positioned so the bronchi are perpendicular to the floor. Lower and middle lobe bronchi usually empty best with the patient in the head-down position; upper lobe bronchi, in the head-up position.

Percussing the chest with cupped hands mechanically dislodges thick, tenacious secretions from the bronchial walls. Vibration can be used with percussion or as an alternative to it in a patient who is frail, in pain, or recovering from thoracic surgery or trauma.

Candidates for chest PT include patients who expectorate large amounts of sputum, such as those with bronchiectasis and cystic fibrosis. The procedure has not been proven effective in treating patients with status asthmaticus, lobar pneumonia, or acute exacerbations of chronic bronchitis when the patient has scant secretions and is being mechanically ventilated. Chest PT has little value for treating patients with stable, chronic bronchitis.

Contraindications may include active pulmonary bleeding with hemoptysis and the immediate posthemorrhage stage, fractured ribs or an unstable chest wall, lung contusions, pulmonary tuberculosis, untreated pneumothorax, acute asthma or bronchospasm, lung abscess or tumor, bony metastasis, head injury, and recent myocardial infarction.

Equipment

Stethoscope ▪ pillows ▪ tilt or postural drainage table (if available) or adjustable hospital bed ▪ emesis basin ▪ facial tissues ▪ suction equipment, as needed ▪ equipment for oral care ▪ trash bag ▪ optional: sterile specimen container, mechanical ventilator, supplemental oxygen.

Preparation of equipment

Gather the equipment at the patient's bedside. Set up suction equipment, if needed, and test its function.

Implementation

● Explain the procedure to the patient, provide privacy, and wash your hands.
● Auscultate the patient's lungs *to determine baseline respiratory status.*
● Position the patient as ordered. In generalized disease, drainage usually begins with the lower lobes, continues with the middle lobes, and ends with the upper lobes. In localized disease, drainage begins with the affected lobes and then proceeds to the other lobes *to avoid spreading the disease to uninvolved areas.* (See *Positioning patients for postural drainage,* pages 472 and 473.)
● Instruct the patient to remain in each position for 10 to 15 minutes. During this time, perform percussion and vibration, as ordered. (See *Performing percussion and vibration,* page 474.)
● After postural drainage, percussion, or vibration, instruct the patient to cough *to remove loosened secretions.* First, tell him to inhale deeply through his nose and then exhale in three short huffs. Then have him inhale deeply again and cough through a slightly open mouth. Three consecutive coughs are highly effective. An effective cough sounds deep, low, and hollow; an ineffective one, high-pitched. Have the patient perform exercises for about 1 minute and then rest for 2 minutes. Gradually progress to a 10-minute exercise period four times daily.
● Provide oral hygiene *because secretions may taste foul or have a stale odor.*
● Auscultate the patient's lungs *to evaluate the effectiveness of therapy.*

Positioning patients for postural drainage

The following illustrations show you the various postural drainage positions and the areas of the lungs affected by each.

Lower lobes: Posterior basal segments
Elevate the foot of the bed 30 degrees. Have the patient lie prone with his head lowered. Position pillows under his chest and abdomen. Percuss his lower ribs on both sides of his spine.

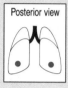

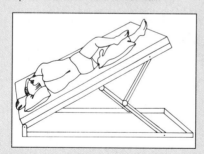

Lower lobes: Lateral basal segments
Elevate the foot of the bed 30 degrees. Instruct the patient to lie on his abdomen with his head lowered and his upper leg flexed over a pillow for support. Then have him rotate a quarter turn upward. Percuss his lower ribs on the uppermost portion of his lateral chest wall.

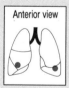

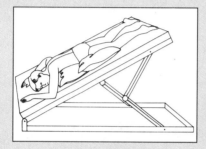

Lower lobes: Anterior basal segments
Elevate the foot of the bed 30 degrees. Instruct the patient to lie on his side with his head lowered. Then place pillows as shown (above, right). Percuss with a slightly

cupped hand over his lower ribs just beneath the axilla. If an acutely ill patient has trouble breathing in this position, adjust the bed to an angle he can tolerate. Then begin percussion.

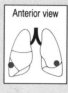

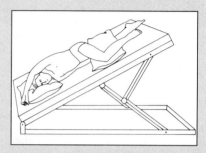

Lower lobes: Superior segments
With the bed flat, have the patient lie on his abdomen. Place two pillows under his hips. Percuss on both sides of his spine at the lower tip of his scapulae.

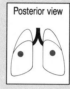

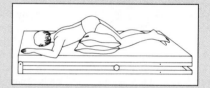

Right middle lobe: Medial and lateral segments
Elevate the foot of the bed 15 degrees. Have the patient lie on his left side with his head down and his knees flexed. Then have him rotate a quarter turn backward. Place a pillow beneath him. Percuss with your hand moderately cupped over the right nipple. For a woman, cup your hand so that its heel is under the armpit and your fingers extend forward beneath the breast.

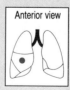

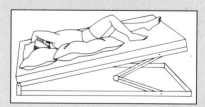

Positioning patients for postural drainage *(continued)*

Left upper lobe: Superior and inferior segments, lingular portion

Elevate the foot of the bed 15 degrees. Have the patient lie on his right side with his head down and knees flexed. Then have him rotate a quarter turn backward. Place a pillow behind him, from shoulders to hips. Percuss with your hand moderately cupped over his left nipple. For a woman, cup your hand so that its heel is beneath the armpit and your fingers extend forward beneath the breast.

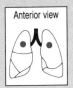
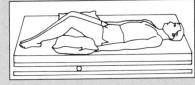

Anterior view

Upper lobes: Anterior segments

Make sure the bed is flat. Have the patient lie on his back with a pillow folded under his knees. Then have him rotate slightly away from the side being drained. Percuss between his clavicle and nipple.

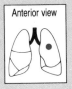
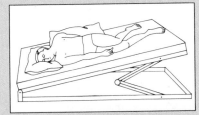

Anterior view

Upper lobes: Apical segments

Keep the bed flat. Have the patient lean back at a 30-degree angle against you and a pillow. Percuss with a cupped hand between his clavicles and the top of each scapula.

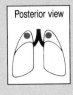
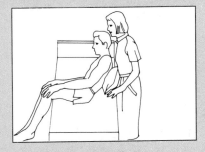

Posterior view

Upper lobes: Posterior segments

Keep the bed flat. Have the patient lean over a pillow at a 30-degree angle. Percuss and clap his upper back on each side.

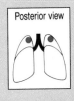
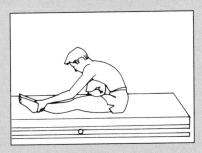

Posterior view

Special considerations

For optimal effectiveness and safety, modify chest PT according to the patient's condition. For example, initiate or increase the flow of supplemental oxygen, if indicated. Also, suction the patient who has an ineffective cough reflex. If the patient tires quickly during therapy, shorten the sessions *because fatigue leads to shallow respirations and increased hypoxia.*

Maintain adequate hydration in the patient receiving chest PT *to prevent mucus dehydration and promote easier mobilization.* Avoid performing postural drainage immediately before or within 1½ hours after meals *to avoid nausea and aspiration of food or vomitus.*

Because chest percussion can induce bronchospasm, any adjunct treatment (for example, intermittent positive-pressure breathing, aerosol, or nebulizer therapy) should precede chest PT.

Refrain from percussing over the spine, liver, kidneys, or spleen *to avoid injury to the spine or internal organs.* Also avoid performing percussion on bare skin or the female patient's breasts. Percuss over soft clothing (but not over buttons, snaps, or zippers) or place a thin towel over the chest wall. Remember to remove jewelry that might scratch or bruise the patient.

Explain coughing and deep breathing exercises pre-operatively, so the patient can practice them when he's pain-free and better able to concentrate. Postoperatively, splint the patient's incision using your hands or, if possible, teach the patient to splint it himself *to minimize pain during coughing.*

Performing percussion and vibration

To perform percussion, instruct the patient to breathe slowly and deeply, using the diaphragm, *to promote relaxation*. Hold your hands in a cupped shape, with fingers flexed and thumbs pressed tightly against your index fingers. Percuss each segment for 1 to 2 minutes by alternating your hands against the patient in a rhythmic manner. Listen for a hollow sound on percussion *to verify correct performance of the technique*.

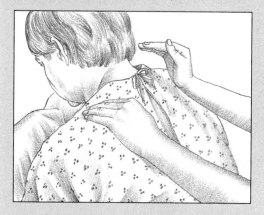

To perform vibration, ask the patient to inhale deeply and then exhale slowly through pursed lips. During exhalation, firmly press your fingers and the palms of your hands against the chest wall. Tense the muscles of your arms and shoulders in an isometric contraction *to send fine vibrations through the chest wall*. Vibrate during five exhalations over each chest segment.

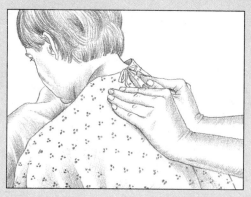

Complications

During postural drainage in head-down positions, pressure on the diaphragm by abdominal contents can impair respiratory excursion and lead to hypoxia or postural hypotension. The head-down position also may lead to increased intracranial pressure, which precludes the use of chest PT in a patient with acute neurologic impairment. Vigorous percussion or vibration can cause rib fracture, especially in the patient with osteoporosis. In an emphysematous patient with blebs, coughing could lead to pneumothorax.

Documentation

Record the date and time of chest PT; positions for secretion drainage and length of time each is maintained; chest segments percussed or vibrated; color, amount, odor, and viscosity of secretions produced, and presence of any blood; any complications and nursing actions taken; and the patient's tolerance of treatment.

 # Thoracentesis

This procedure involves aspiration of fluid or air from the pleural space. It relieves pulmonary compression and respiratory distress by removing accumulated air or fluid that results from injury or such conditions as tuberculosis or cancer. It also provides a specimen of pleural fluid or tissue for analysis, and allows instillation of chemotherapeutic agents or other medications into the pleural space.

Thoracentesis is contraindicated in patients with bleeding disorders.

Equipment

Most hospitals use a prepackaged thoracentesis tray that typically includes the following: sterile gloves ▪ sterile drapes ▪ 70% isopropyl alcohol or povidone-iodine solution ▪ 1% or 2% lidocaine ▪ 5-ml syringe with 21G and 25G needles for anesthetic injection ▪ 17G thoracentesis needle for aspiration ▪ 50-ml syringe ▪ three-way stopcock and tubing ▪ sterile specimen containers ▪ sterile hemostat ▪ sterile 4″ × 4″ gauze pads.

You'll also need the following: adhesive tape ▪ sphygomomanometer ▪ gloves ▪ stethoscope ▪ laboratory request slips ▪ drainage bottles ▪ optional: Teflon catheter, shaving supplies, biopsy needle, prescribed sedative with 3-ml syringe and 21G needle, and drainage bottles, if the doctor expects a large amount of drainage.

Preparation of equipment

Assemble all equipment at the patient's bedside or in the treatment area. Check the expiration date on each sterile package and inspect for tears. Prepare the necessary laboratory request form. Be sure to list current antibiotic therapy on the laboratory forms *because this will be considered in analyzing the specimens.* Make sure the patient has signed an appropriate consent form. Note any drug allergies, especially to the local anesthetic. Have the patient's chest X-rays available.

Implementation

• Explain the procedure to the patient. Inform him that he may feel some discomfort and a sensation of pressure during the needle insertion. Provide privacy and emotional support. Wash your hands.
• Administer the prescribed sedative, as ordered.
• Obtain baseline vital signs and assess respiratory function.
• Position the patient. Make sure he's firmly supported and comfortable. Although the choice of position is variable, you'll usually seat the patient on the edge of the bed with his legs supported and his head and folded arms resting on a pillow on the overbed table. Or have him straddle a chair backward and rest his head and folded arms on the back of the chair. If the patient is unable to sit, turn him on the unaffected side with the arm of the affected side raised above his head. Elevate the head of the bed 30 to 45 degrees if such elevation isn't contraindicated. *Proper positioning stretches the chest or back and allows easier access to the intercostal spaces.*
• Remind the patient not to cough, breathe deeply, or move suddenly during the procedure *to avoid puncture of the visceral pleura or lung.* If the patient coughs, the doctor will briefly halt the procedure and withdraw the needle slightly *to prevent puncture.*
• Expose the patient's entire chest or back, as appropriate.
• Shave the aspiration site, as ordered.
• Wash your hands again before touching the sterile equipment. Then, using sterile technique, open the thoracentesis tray and assist the doctor as necessary in disinfecting the site.
• If an ampule of local anesthetic is not included in the sterile tray and a multidose vial of local anesthetic is to be used, assist the doctor by wiping the rubber stopper with an alcohol sponge and holding the inverted vial while the doctor withdraws the anesthetic solution.
• After draping the patient and injecting the local anesthetic, the doctor attaches a three-way stopcock with tubing to the aspirating needle and turns the stopcock to prevent air from entering the pleural space through the needle.

• Attach the other end of the tubing to the drainage bottle.
• The doctor then inserts the needle into the pleural space and attaches a 50-ml syringe to the needle's stopcock. A hemostat may be used *to hold the needle in place and prevent pleural tear or lung puncture.* As an alternative, the doctor may introduce a Teflon catheter into the needle, remove the needle, and attach a stopcock and syringe or drainage tubing to the catheter *to reduce the risk of pleural puncture by the needle.*
• Support the patient verbally throughout the procedure and keep him informed of each step. Assess him for signs of anxiety and provide reassurance as necessary.
• Check vital signs regularly during the procedure. Continually observe the patient for such signs of distress as pallor, vertigo, faintness, weak and rapid pulse, decreased blood pressure, dyspnea, tachypnea, diaphoresis, chest pain, blood-tinged mucus, and excessive coughing. Alert the doctor if such signs develop *because they may indicate complications such as hypovolemic shock or tension pneumothorax.*
• Put on gloves and assist the doctor as necessary in specimen collection, fluid drainage, and dressing the site.
• After the doctor withdraws the needle or catheter, apply pressure to the puncture site, using a sterile 4″ × 4″ gauze pad. Then apply a new sterile gauze pad and secure it with tape.
• Place the patient in a comfortable position, take his vital signs, and assess his respiratory status.
• Label the specimens properly and send them to the laboratory.
• Discard disposable equipment. Clean nondisposable items and return them for sterilization.
• Check the patient's vital signs and the dressing for drainage every 15 minutes for 1 hour. Then continue to assess the patient's vital signs and respiratory status as indicated by his condition.

Special considerations

To prevent postthoracentesis pulmonary edema and hypovolemic shock, fluid is removed slowly, and no more than 1,000 ml of fluid is removed during the first 30 minutes. *Removing the fluid increases the negative intrapleural pressure, which can lead to edema if the lung doesn't reexpand to fill the space.*

Pleuritic or shoulder pain may indicate pleural irritation by the needle point.

A chest X-ray is usually ordered after the procedure *to detect pneumothorax and evaluate the results of the procedure.*

Complications

Pneumothorax (possibly leading to mediastinal shift and requiring chest tube insertion) can occur if the needle punctures the lung and allows air to enter the pleural cavity. Pyogenic infection can result from contamination during the procedure. Other potential difficulties include pain, cough, anxiety, dry taps, and subcutaneous hematoma.

Documentation

Record the date and time of thoracentesis; location of the puncture site; volume and description (color, viscosity, odor) of the fluid withdrawn; specimens sent to the laboratory; vital signs and respiratory assessment before, during, and after the procedure; any postprocedural tests, such as chest X-ray; any complications and the nursing action taken; and the patient's reaction to the procedure.

▧ Chest tube insertion

The pleural space normally contains a thin layer of lubricating fluid that allows the lungs to move without friction during respiration. An excess of fluid (hemothorax or pleural effusion), air (pneumothorax), or both in this space alters intrapleural pressure and causes partial or complete lung collapse.

Chest tube insertion permits the drainage of air or fluid from the pleural space. Usually performed by a doctor with a nurse assisting, this procedure requires sterile technique. The insertion site varies, depending on the patient's condition and the doctor's judgment. For pneumothorax, the second intercostal space provides the usual site because air rises to the top of the intrapleural space. For hemothorax or pleural effusion, the sixth to the eighth intercostal spaces are common sites because fluid settles to the lower levels of the intrapleural space. For removal of air and fluid, a chest tube is inserted into a high and a low site. Following insertion, one or more chest tubes are connected to a thoracic drainage system that removes air, fluid, or both from the pleural space and prevents backflow into that space, thus promoting lung reexpansion. (See "Thoracic drainage" in this chapter.)

Equipment

Two pairs of sterile gloves ▪ sterile drape ▪ povidone-iodine solution ▪ vial of 1% lidocaine ▪ 10-ml syringe ▪ alcohol sponge ▪ 22G 1″ needle ▪ 25G ⅝″ needle ▪ sterile scalpel (usually with #11 blade) ▪ sterile forceps ▪ two rubber-tipped clamps for each chest tube inserted ▪ sterile

4″ × 4″ gauze pads ▪ two sterile 4″ × 4″ drain dressings (gauze pads with slit) ▪ 3″ or 4″ sturdy, elastic tape ▪ 1″ adhesive tape for connections ▪ chest tube of appropriate size (#16 to #20 French catheter for air or serous fluid; #28 to #40 French catheter for blood, pus, or thick fluid), with or without a trocar ▪ sterile Kelly clamp ▪ suture material (usually 2-0 silk with cutting needle) ▪ thoracic drainage system ▪ sterile drainage tubing, 6′ (1.8 m) long, and connector ▪ sterile Y connector (for two chest tubes on the same side) ▪ optional: antimicrobial ointment, petroleum gauze.

Preparation of equipment

Check the expiration date on the sterile packages and inspect for tears. In a nonemergency situation, make sure that the patient has signed the appropriate consent form. Then assemble all equipment in the patient's room and set up the thoracic drainage system. Place it next to the patient's bed below the chest level *to facilitate drainage.*

Implementation

- Explain the procedure to the patient, provide privacy, and wash your hands.
- Record baseline vital signs and respiratory assessment.
- Position the patient appropriately. (See *Positioning the patient for chest tube insertion.*)
- Place the chest tube tray on the overbed table. Open it using sterile technique.
- The doctor puts on sterile gloves and prepares the insertion site by cleaning the area with povidone-iodine solution.
- Wipe the rubber stopper of the lidocaine vial with an alcohol pad. Then invert the bottle and hold it for the doctor to withdraw the anesthetic.
- After the doctor anesthetizes the site, he makes a small incision and inserts the chest tube. Then he either immediately connects the chest tube to the thoracic drainage system or momentarily clamps the tube close to the patient's chest until he can connect it to the drainage system. He may then secure the tube to the skin with a suture.
- As the doctor is inserting the chest tube, reassure the patient and assist the doctor as necessary.
- Open the packages containing the 4″ × 4″ drain dressings and gauze pads, and put on sterile gloves. If desired, apply antimicrobial ointment to the insertion site. Then place two 4″ × 4″ drain dressings around the insertion site, one from the top and the other from the bottom. Place several 4″ × 4″ gauze pads on top of the drain dressings. Tape the dressings, covering them completely.
- Tape the chest tube to the patient's chest distal to the insertion site *to help prevent accidental dislodgment of the tube.*

Positioning the patient for chest tube insertion

If the patient has a *pneumothorax,* place him in high Fowler's, semi-Fowler's, or the supine position. The doctor will insert the tube in the anterior chest at the midclavicular line in the second to the third intercostal space.

If the patient has a *hemothorax,* have him lean over the overbed table or straddle a chair with his arms dangling over the back. The doctor will insert the tube in the fourth to sixth intercostal space at the midaxillary line.

For either pneumothorax or hemothorax, the patient may lie on his unaffected side with his arms extended over his head.

If the patient has had a *thoracotomy,* the doctor usually will insert one or two chest tubes during surgery (typically a basilar tube and an apical tube). The patient will be positioned on his unaffected side with his arms elevated.

Semi-Fowler's position

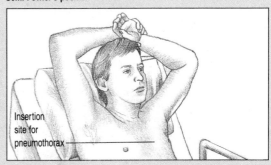

Insertion site for pneumothorax

Leaning forward

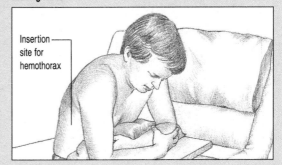

Insertion site for hemothorax

Lying on side

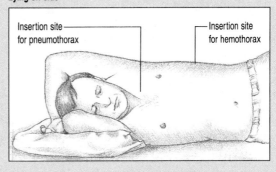

Insertion site for pneumothorax

Insertion site for hemothorax

• Tape the junction of the chest tube and the drainage tube *to prevent their separation.*
• Coil the drainage tubing and secure it to the bed linen with tape and a safety pin, providing enough slack for the patient to move and turn. *These measures prevent the drainage tubing from getting kinked or dropping to the floor,* *which would impair drainage into the bottle, and they help prevent accidental dislodgment of the chest tube.*
• Immediately after the drainage system is connected, instruct the patient to take a deep breath, hold it momentarily, and slowly exhale *to assist drainage of the pleural space and lung reexpansion.*

Performing needle thoracentesis

For a patient with life-threatening tension pneumothorax, a needle thoracentesis temporarily relieves pleural pressure until a doctor can insert a chest tube.

How needle thoracentesis works
A needle attached to a flutter valve is inserted into the affected pleural space. (If no flutter valve is available, one can be made from a perforated finger cot or glove and attached with a rubber band.) Trapped air escapes via the flutter valve when the patient exhales, instead of being retained under pressure. The flutter valve also prevents more air from entering the patient's involved lung during inhalation.

How to perform the procedure
If a doctor isn't available, you may need to perform this procedure. Here's how to proceed.

• Clean the skin around the second intercostal space at the midclavicular line with povidone-iodine solution. Use a circular motion, starting at the center and working outward.
• Insert a sterile 16G (or larger) needle over the superior portion of the rib and through the tissue covering the pleural cavity. The vein, artery, and nerve lie behind the rib's inferior border.
• Listen for a hissing sound. This signals the needle's entry into the pleural cavity.
• If you're using a flutter valve, secure it to the needle. The arrow on the valve indicates the direction of airflow.
• Place a sterile glove on the distal end of the valve to collect the drainage.
• Leave the needle in place until a chest tube can be inserted.

• After the procedure, a portable chest X-ray is done *to check tube position.*
• Take the patient's vital signs every 15 minutes for 1 hour, then as his condition indicates. Auscultate his lungs at least every 4 hours following the procedure *to assess air exchange in the affected lung.* Diminished or absent breath sounds indicate that the lung hasn't reexpanded.

Special considerations
If the patient's chest tube comes out, immediately cover the site with 4″ × 4″ gauze pads and tape them in place. Stay with the patient and monitor his vital signs every 10 minutes. Observe the patient for signs of tension pneumothorax (hypotension, distended neck veins, absent breath sounds, tracheal shift, hypoxemia, weak and rapid pulse, dyspnea, tachypnea, diaphoresis, and chest pain). Instruct another staff member to notify the doctor and gather equipment needed to reinsert the tube. (See also *Performing needle thoracentesis.*)

Place the rubber-tipped clamps at the bedside. If a drainage bottle breaks, a commercial system cracks, or a tube disconnects, clamp the chest tube momentarily as close to the insertion site as possible. *Because no air or liquid can escape from the pleural space while the tube is clamped,* observe the patient closely for signs of tension pneumothorax while the clamp is in place.

A piece of petroleum gauze may be wrapped around the tube at the insertion site *to make an airtight seal.*

The tube may be clamped with large, smooth, rubber-tipped clamps for several hours before removal. *This allows time to observe the patient for signs of respiratory distress, an indication that air or fluid remains trapped in the pleural space.* A chest tube is usually removed within 7 days of insertion *to prevent infection along the tube tract.* (See *Removing a chest tube.*)

Documentation
Record the date and time of chest tube insertion, the insertion site, drainage system used, presence of drainage and bubbling, vital signs and auscultation findings, any complications, and the nursing action taken.

 Thoracic drainage

Because negative pressure in the pleural cavity exerts a suction force that keeps the lungs expanded, any chest trauma that upsets this pressure may cause lung collapse. Consequently, one or more chest tubes may be surgically inserted and then connected to a thoracic drainage system. Thoracic drainage uses gravity and possibly suction to restore negative pressure and remove any material that collects in the pleural cavity. An underwater seal in the drainage system allows air and fluid to escape from the pleural cavity, but doesn't allow air to reenter. The system may include one, two, or three bottles to collect drainage, create a water seal, and control suction. Or it may be a self-contained, disposable system that combines the features of a multibottle system in a compact, one-piece unit. Because you're less likely to use a bottle system, the procedure here details use of a disposable system. (See *Comparing closed drainage systems,* page 480.)

Specifically, thoracic drainage may be ordered to remove accumulated air, fluids (blood, pus, chyle, serous fluids, gastric juices), or solids (blood clots) from the pleural cavity; to restore negative pressure in the pleural cavity; or to reexpand a partially or totally collapsed lung.

Equipment

Thoracic drainage system (Pleur-evac, Argyle, Ohio, or Thora-Klex system, which can function as gravity draining systems or be connected to suction to enhance chest drainage) ■ sterile distilled water (usually 1 liter) ■ adhesive tape ■ sterile clear plastic tubing ■ bottle or system rack ■ two rubber-tipped Kelly clamps ■ sterile 50-ml catheter-tip syringe ■ suction source, if ordered.

Preparation of equipment

Check the doctor's order to determine the type of drainage system to be used and specific procedural details. If appropriate, request the drainage system and suction system from the central supply department. Collect the appropriate equipment and take it to the patient's bedside.

Implementation

• Explain the procedure to the patient, and wash your hands.
• Maintain sterile technique throughout the entire procedure, and whenever you make changes in the system or alter any of the connections *to avoid introducing pathogens into the pleural space.*

To set up a commercially prepared disposable system

• Open the packaged system and place it on the floor in the rack supplied by the manufacturer *to avoid accidentally knocking it over or dislodging the components.* After the system is prepared, it may be hung from the side of the patient's bed.
• Remove the plastic connector from the short tube that's attached to the water-seal chamber. Using a 50-ml catheter-tip syringe, instill sterile distilled water into the water-seal chamber until it reaches the 2-cm mark, or the mark specified by the manufacturer. The Ohio and Thora-Klex systems are ready to use but, with the Thora-

---

Removing a chest tube

Once the patient's lung has reexpanded, you may assist the doctor in removing the chest tube. To do so, first obtain the patient's vital signs and perform a respiratory assessment. Then, after explaining the procedure to the patient, you'll administer an analgesic, as ordered, 30 minutes before tube removal. Then follow the steps listed below:
• Place the patient in semi-Fowler's position or on his unaffected side.
• Place a linen-saver pad under the affected side *to protect the linen from drainage and to provide a place to put the chest tube after removal.*
• Put on clean gloves and remove the chest tube dressings, being careful not to dislodge the chest tube. Discard soiled dressings.
• The doctor puts on sterile gloves, holds the chest tube in place with sterile forceps, and cuts the suture anchoring the tube.
• Make sure the chest tube is securely clamped, and then instruct the patient to perform Valsalva's maneuver by exhaling fully and bearing down. *Valsalva's maneuver effectively increases intrathoracic pressure.*
• The doctor holds an airtight dressing, usually petroleum gauze, *so that he can cover the insertion site with it immediately after removing the tube.* After he removes the tube and covers the insertion site, secure the dressing with tape. Be sure to cover the dressing completely with tape *to make it as airtight as possible.*
• Dispose of the chest tube, soiled gloves, and equipment according to hospital policy.
• Take vital signs, as ordered, and assess the depth and quality of the patient's respirations. Assess the patient carefully for signs and symptoms of pneumothorax, subcutaneous emphysema, or infection.

Klex system, 15-ml of sterile water may be added to help detect air leaks. Replace the plastic connector.
• If suction is ordered, remove the cap (also called the muffler or atmosphere vent cover) on the suction-control chamber *to open the vent.* Next, instill sterile distilled water until it reaches the 20-cm mark or the ordered level, and recap the suction-control chamber.
• Using the long tube, connect the patient's chest tube to the closed drainage collection chamber. Secure the connection with tape.

Comparing closed drainage systems

One-bottle system

The one-bottle system is the easiest drainage system to use. It drains by gravity, combining drainage collection and the water-seal chamber. This system is not recommended for excessive drainage.

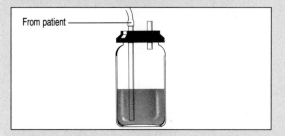

Two-bottle system

The two-bottle system collects drainage in the first bottle and uses the second bottle as the water-seal chamber. This system is not recommended for excessive drainage.

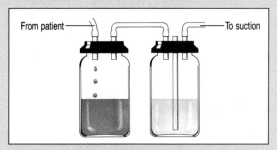

Three-bottle system

In the three-bottle system, the first bottle collects drainage, the second bottle acts as the water-seal chamber, and the third bottle is the suction-control chamber. This system can handle excessive drainage.

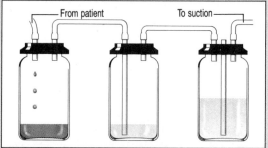

Disposable drainage systems

Commercially prepared disposable systems combine drainage collection, water seal, and suction control in one unit, as shown here. These systems ensure patient safety with positive- and negative-pressure relief valves and have a prominent air-leak indicator. Some systems produce no bubbling sound.

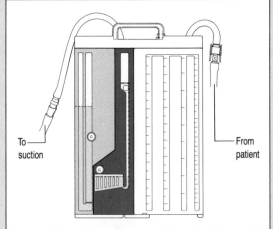

• Connect the short tube on the drainage system to the suction source and turn on the suction. Gentle bubbling should begin in the suction chamber, *indicating that the correct suction level has been reached.*

To manage closed chest underwater seal drainage
• Repeatedly note the character, consistency, and amount of drainage in the drainage collection chamber.
• Mark the drainage level in the drainage collection chamber by noting the time and date at the drainage level on the chamber every 8 hours (or more often) if there is a large amount of drainage.
• Check the water level in the water-seal chamber every 8 hours. If necessary, carefully add sterile distilled water until the level reaches the 2-cm mark indicated on the water-seal chamber of the commercial system.
• Check for fluctuation in the water-seal chamber as the patient breathes. Normal fluctuations of 2″ to 4″ (about 5 to 10 cm) reflect pressure changes in the pleural space during respiration. To check for fluctuation when a suction system is being used, momentarily disconnect the suction system so the air vent is opened, and observe for fluctuation.
• Check for intermittent bubbling in the water-seal chamber. This occurs normally when the system is removing air from the pleural cavity. If bubbling isn't readily apparent during quiet breathing, have the patient take a deep breath or cough. Absence of bubbling indicates that the pleural space has sealed.
• Check the water level in the suction-control chamber. Detach the chamber or bottle from the suction source; when bubbling ceases, observe the water level. If necessary, add sterile distilled water to bring the level to the −20-cm line, or as ordered.
• Check for gentle bubbling in the suction control chamber *because it indicates that the proper suction level has been reached.* Vigorous bubbling in this chamber increases the rate of water evaporation.
• Periodically check that the air vent in the system is working properly. *Occlusion of the air vent results in a buildup of pressure in the system that could cause the patient to develop a tension pneumothorax.*
• Coil the system's tubing and secure it to the edge of the bed with a rubber band or tape and a safety pin. Avoid creating dependent loops, kinks, or pressure on the tubing *because they may interfere with chest drainage.* Avoid lifting the drainage system above the patient's chest *because fluid may flow back into the pleural space.*
• Be sure to keep two rubber-tipped clamps at the bedside. These are used to clamp the chest tube if a bottle breaks or the commercially prepared system cracks, or to locate an air leak in the system.

• Encourage the patient to cough frequently and breathe deeply *to help drain the pleural space and expand the lungs.*
• Instruct him to sit upright *for optimal lung expansion* and to splint the insertion site while coughing *to minimize pain.*
• Check the rate and quality of the patient's respirations and auscultate his lungs periodically *to assess air exchange in the affected lung.* Diminished or absent breath sounds may indicate that the lung has not reexpanded.
• Tell the patient to report any breathing difficulty immediately. Notify the doctor immediately if the patient develops cyanosis, rapid or shallow breathing, subcutaneous emphysema, chest pain, or excessive bleeding.
• When clots are visible, you may be able to strip (or milk) the tubing, depending on your hospital's policy. This is a controversial procedure because it creates high negative pressure that could suck viable lung tissue into the drainage ports of the tube, with subsequent ruptured alveoli and pleural air leak. Strip the tubing only when clots are visible. Use an alcohol sponge or lotion as a lubricant on the tube and pinch it between your thumb and index finger about 2″ (5 cm) from the insertion site. Using the other thumb and index finger, compress the tubing as you slide your fingers down the tube or use a mechanical stripper. After stripping, release the thumb and index finger pinching the tube near the insertion site.
• Check the chest tube dressing at least every 8 hours. Palpate the area surrounding the dressing for crepitus or subcutaneous emphysema, which indicates that air is leaking into the subcutaneous tissue surrounding the insertion site. Change the dressing if necessary or according to hospital policy.
• Encourage active or passive range-of-motion (ROM) exercises for the patient's arm or the affected side if he has been splinting the arm. Usually, the thoracotomy patient will splint his arm to decrease his discomfort.
• Give ordered pain medication as needed *for comfort and to help with deep breathing, coughing, and ROM exercises.*
• Remind the ambulatory patient to keep the drainage system below chest level and to be careful not to disconnect the tubing *to maintain the water seal.* With a suction system, the patient must stay within range of the length of tubing attached to a wall outlet or portable pump.

Special considerations
Instruct staff and visitors to avoid touching the equipment *to prevent complications from separated connections.*

If excessive continuous bubbling is present in the water-seal chamber, especially if suction is being used, rule out a leak in the drainage system. Try to locate the leak by clamping the tube momentarily at various points along its length. Begin clamping at the tube's proximal end and work down toward the drainage system, paying special attention to the seal around the connections. If any connection is loose, push it back together and tape it securely. *The bubbling will stop when a clamp is placed between the air leak and the water seal.* If you clamp along the tube's entire length and the bubbling doesn't stop, the drainage unit may be cracked and need replacement.

If the commercially prepared drainage collection chamber fills, replace it. To do this, double-clamp the tube close to the insertion site (use two clamps facing in opposite directions), exchange the system, remove the clamps, and retape the bottle connection. Never leave the tubes clamped for more than a minute or two *to prevent a tension pneumothorax, which may occur when clamping stops air and fluid from escaping.*

If the commercially prepared system cracks, clamp the chest tube momentarily with the two rubber-tipped clamps at the bedside (placed there at the time of tube insertion). Place the clamps close to each other near the insertion site; they should face in opposite directions *to provide a more complete seal.* Observe the patient for altered respirations while the tube is clamped. Then replace the damaged equipment. (Prepare the new unit before clamping the tube.)

Instead of clamping the tube, you can submerge the distal end of the tube in a container of normal saline solution *to create a temporary water seal while you replace the bottle.* Check your hospital's policy for the proper procedure.

Complications
Tension pneumothorax may result from excessive accumulation of air, drainage, or both, and eventually may exert pressure on the heart and aorta, causing a precipitous fall in cardiac output.

Documentation
Record the date and time thoracic drainage began, type of system used, amount of suction applied to the pleural cavity, presence or absence of bubbling or fluctuation in the water-seal chamber, initial amount and type of drainage, and the patient's respiratory status.

At the end of each shift, record the frequency of system inspection; how frequently chest tubes were milked or stripped; amount, color, and consistency of drainage; presence or absence of bubbling or fluctuation in the water-seal chamber; the patient's respiratory status; condition of the chest dressings; pain medication, if given; and any complications and the nursing action taken.

 # Phrenic pacing

Also known as diaphragm pacing, this procedure induces respiration via a surgically implanted device that stimulates the phrenic nerve. The implanted device prompts the phrenic impulse in response to electrical signals from an external transmitter and antenna. This impulse causes the diaphragm to descend smoothly, drawing air into the lungs.

The phrenic pacemaker is implanted most commonly in patients with chronic dysfunction of the respiratory-control center, or with muscle paralysis caused either by high cervical spinal cord trauma or by innervational or synaptic malfunction. Spinal cord damage is the most common cause of respiratory muscle paralysis. Other innervational causes include amyotrophic lateral sclerosis (Lou Gehrig's disease) and Guillain-Barré syndrome; synaptic malfunction can stem from myasthenia gravis. Depending on the cervical or brain stem area affected, the patient with one of these progressive disorders may need partial or total ventilatory support.

A control dysfunction—stemming from tumor, hemorrhage, cerebrovascular accident, or central alveolar hypoventilation (Ondine's curse)—can affect voluntary or involuntary respiration, depending on the site of the cerebral lesion. Because the spinal cord is divided into two tracts, voluntary respiration can be maintained after loss of involuntary control.

Loss of involuntary respiratory control usually requires implantation of only one pacemaker, which controls breathing during sleep. Loss of both voluntary and involuntary control requires implantation of two pacemakers, one for each phrenic nerve, each operated alternately for 12 hours to prevent diaphragm fatigue. Pacing schedules can range from continuous bilateral diaphragm pacing to unilateral pacing on alternating sides. Some patients may require supplemental mechanical ventilation during the day or at night. Usually, patients need to initiate phrenic pacing gradually.

For phrenic pacing to succeed, the patient's lungs, diaphragm, and phrenic nerves should be normal, and his anterior horn cells intact from the third to the fifth cervical vertebrae. Phrenic nerve pacing is indicated only to correct chronic respiratory malfunction, not an acute disorder.

Equipment
Pacing antenna ■ transmitter ■ 9-volt batteries ■ battery tester ■ adhesive or nonallergenic tape ■ stethoscope ■ watch ■ spirometer ■ 10-ml syringe ■ mechanical venti-

lator, as needed ■ suction equipment ■ sphygmomanometer ■ optional: capnometer, oximeter, abdominal binder.

Preparation of equipment

Check the doctor's order for the transmitter setting and specific pacing schedule. Wash your hands. Using the battery tester, check the transmitter's battery *to ensure an adequate charge.* If necessary, replace the battery. Adjust the transmitter's amplitude dial to the ordered setting, if necessary. *To ensure that each stimulation is effective,* pacing is usually performed at or slightly above the patient's maximum setting (the setting that produces maximum diaphragmatic contraction) instead of at the threshold setting (the lowest setting that produces any stimulation). Tape the dial securely *to prevent accidental movement.* Have a ventilator available and ready to use if the patient is totally dependent on respiratory support.

Implementation

• After the device has been surgically implanted, assess the patient's condition before beginning the pacing trial.
• Make sure the patient is awake *because you'll need his cooperation.* Explain the procedure to him and provide privacy.
• Feel the patient's chest wall to find the surgically implanted receiver. Apply the antenna to the skin directly over the receiver and tape it securely in place.
• Assist the patient into position, as ordered (usually flat or with the head of the bed elevated 30 degrees). If possible, avoid a sitting position *because it inhibits diaphragmatic movement and causes minute volume to drop sharply.* If the patient must sit, try to counteract this effect by applying an abdominal binder *to elevate the diaphragm to its maximum position.*
• Tell the patient you'll activate the pacemaker after his next expiration. Then, after the expiration, turn on the transmitter.
• Observe the patient's abdomen for respiratory movement, and auscultate his lungs bilaterally for breath sounds.
• Tell the patient the pacemaker induces inspiration 10 to 15 times a minute (faster for an infant or small child) and shuts off automatically during expiration.

To monitor initial pacing trials

• Turn the patient frequently from side to side *to prevent atelectasis from diminished respiratory movement on the non-paced side.*
• Using a spirometer, monitor minute and tidal volumes, as ordered. If the patient has a tracheostomy, use the syringe *to inflate the tracheostomy cuff for minute-volume calculations and to deflate it again for the remainder of pacing time.*

• Monitor the patient's oxygenation status using an oximeter and capnometer, as ordered, *to ensure that the patient's oxygenation is within a safe range, and to determine the patient's ability to tolerate decreased pacing.*
• Monitor the patient's blood pressure, pulse, and respirations closely. Observe for signs of diaphragm fatigue, such as patient fatigue, decreased tidal volumes and abdominal (diaphragm) movement. Also observe for signs of hypoxia and hypercapnia, such as tachycardia, hypotension, or cyanosis. If any of these symptoms occur, stop phrenic pacing, resume mechanical ventilation or have the patient resume voluntary respiration, and notify the doctor.
• Keep the patient informed of his progress and reassure him that the pacemaker is operating correctly, especially during the initial pacing trials. Occasionally, tell him how long the trials must continue.

To stop pacing

• Tell the patient that you'll turn off the pacemaker after his next expiration, and that he'll have to breathe voluntarily or with the help of a ventilator. Then, after expiration, turn off the transmitter switch. If necessary, connect the patient to the ventilator.
• Watch the patient closely *to ensure adequate ventilation.* Check for abdominal movement and auscultate bilaterally for breath sounds.
• Untape and remove the antenna. Check the antenna site for redness or irritation.
• Store the pacing equipment and supplies in the patient's room in preparation for the next pacing trial.
• Make sure the patient is comfortable and breathing properly before you leave.

Special considerations

If the pacemaker fails to function properly, first check the battery. If the battery is charged, change the antenna. If the pacemaker still fails to function, switch to a mechanical ventilator, if necessary.

Reduce the dependent patient's fear of pacemaker failure by making sure he has access to an alarm system. For the quadriplegic, this means a system he can activate with his mouth or head in an emergency.

Auscultate the patient's lungs at least several times every 8 hours, and suction as necessary.

Discontinue pacing during times when the patient's intrathoracic pressure changes, such as during vomiting or endotracheal suctioning, *because phrenic stimulation may draw aspirate into the lungs.*

If the patient has trouble swallowing and is being fed through a gastric tube, wait at least 30 minutes after meals before beginning a pacing session. *This reduces the risk of aspiration, which can result from the high intrathoracic pressures generated by pacing.* If the patient is quadriplegic or being paced full-time for some other reason, teach him to swallow food just after the end of inspiration *to prevent aspiration.*

Avoid giving the patient with a phrenic pacemaker tranquilizers, sedatives, or antihistamines *because these may further depress the respiratory drive.*

Caution the patient not to change any of the pacemaker settings *because these are preset by the doctor according to the results of flow studies.* Tell him to keep the transmitter and antenna dry *to prevent minor electric shock and malfunction.* This will restrict the patient being paced full-time to sponge baths. Instruct him to avoid twisting the antenna connection *because it could break off.*

Warn the patient not to lean against any large metal surfaces while pacing *because the conducting surface will direct current from the pacemaker battery, causing the pacemaker to falter or stop.*

Begin patient teaching and discharge planning as early as possible. If possible, involve the patient's family.

Complications

Injury to one or both phrenic nerves prevents the pacemaker from adequately supporting ventilation. Injury may occur during or after surgery, from damage by the pacemaker's electrode cuff, or from reduced blood supply to the nerve. The phrenic nerve can recover spontaneously — completely or partially — but recovery usually takes a year or longer.

Diaphragm fatigue may follow prolonged stimulation of the phrenic nerve. Infection at the implant site may occur, indicated by fever, elevated white blood cell count, and redness, swelling, and discharge around the operative site.

The implanted receiver may fail mechanically because of seepage of body fluids into its electrical components. Receiver failure may follow a period of erratic pacing or sharp pain over the operative site, but the pacer may also fail without warning. Be alert for patient complaints of sharp chest pain, shortness of breath, absence of air exchange, or erratic pacing, *which may signal pacemaker failure.*

Upper airway obstruction may result from or be worsened by pacing in patients with central alveolar hypoventilation.

Early symptoms of airway obstruction include confusion, restlessness, tachycardia, and diaphoresis. Late symptoms include stridor, chest wall retractions, and cyanosis.

Documentation

Record the date and time that phrenic pacing begins for the patient. State the duration of the pacing session, the side paced, the minute and tidal volumes in liters, and the average minute volume. Also record the patient's respiratory rate, the patient's position, and the use of an abdominal binder.

Note the time when the patient resumes spontaneous or ventilator-assisted breathing. Record any complications and the nursing actions taken. Describe the patient's tolerance of the procedure.

Selected references

Bodai, B., et al. "A Clinical Evaluation of an Oxygen Insufflation/ Suction Catheter," *Heart & Lung* 16(1):39-46, January 1987.

Campbell, E.J., et al. "Subjective Effects of Humidification of Oxygen for Delivery by Nasal Cannula: A Prospective Study," *Chest* 93(2):289-93, February 1988.

Carroll, P. "Safe Suctioning," *Nursing89* 19(9):48-51, September 1989.

Chulay, M. "Arterial Blood Gas Changes with Hyperinflation and Hyperoxygenation Suctioning Intervention in Critically Ill Patients," *Heart & Lung* 17(6):654-61, November 1988.

Collins, T.R., and Sahn, S.A. "Thoracocentesis: Clinical Value, Complications, Technical Problems, and Patient Experience," *Chest* 91(6):817-22, June 1987.

Dolan, J.T. *Critical Care Nursing: Clinical Management Through the Nursing Process.* Philadelphia: F.A. Davis Co., 1991.

Erickson, R.S. "Mastering the Ins and Outs of Chest Drainage," Part 1. *Nursing89* 19(5):36-44, May 1989.

Ferland, P. "Are You Ready for Ventilator Patients?" *Nursing91* 21(1):42-47, January 1991.

Geisman, L.K. "Advances in Weaning from Mechanical Ventilation," *Critical Care Nursing Clinics of North America* 1(4):697-705, December 1989.

Gray, J., et al. "The Effects of Bolus Normal-Saline Instillation in Conjunction with Endotracheal Suctioning," *Respiratory Care* 35(8):785-90, August 1990.

Hess, D., et al. "The Effect of Hand Size, Resuscitator Brand, and Use of Two Hands on Volumes Delivered During Adult Bag-Valve Ventilation," *Respiratory Care* 34(9):805-10, September 1989.

Kacmarek, R.M., et al. *The Essentials of Respiratory Care,* 3rd ed. St. Louis: Mosby-Year Book, Inc., 1990.

Kersten, L. *Comprehensive Respiratory Nursing: A Decision-Making Approach.* Philadelphia: W.B. Saunders Co., 1989.

Kim, M.J., et al. *Pocket Guide to Nursing Diagnoses.* St. Louis: C.V. Mosby Co., 1989.

Kozier, B., and Erb, G. *Techniques in Clinical Nursing: A Nursing Process Approach,* 3rd ed. Menlo Park, Calif.: Addison-Wesley Publishing Co., 1989.

Miller, J.I., et al. "Phrenic Nerve Pacing of the Quadriplegic Patient," *Journal of Thoracic Cardiovascular Surgery* 99(1):35-40, January 1990.

Miracle, V., and Allnutt, D. "Using a Manual Resuscitator Correctly," *Nursing90* 20(5):49-51, May 1990.

Pasterkamp, H., et al. "Nomenclature Used by Health Care Professionals to Describe Breath Sounds in Asthma," *Chest* 92(2):346-52, August 1987.

Rogge, J., et al. "Effectiveness of Oxygen Concentrations less than 100% before and after Endotracheal Suction in Patients with Chronic Obstructive Pulmonary Disease," *Heart & Lung* 18(1):64-71, January 1989.

Shapiro, B., et al. *Clinical Applications of Respiratory Care.* St. Louis: Mosby-Year Book, Inc., 1991.

Spearing, C., and Cornell, D.J. "Incentive Spirometry: Inspiring Your Patient to Breathe Deeply," *Nursing87* 17(9):50-51, September 1987.

Stevens, S.A., and Becker, K.L. "How to Perform Picture-Perfect Respiratory Assessment," *Nursing88* 18(1):57-63, January 1988.

Stone, K., and Turner, B. "Endotracheal Suctioning," *Annual Review of Nursing Research* 7:27-49, 1989.

Textbook of Advanced Cardiac Life Support, 2nd ed. Dallas: American Heart Association, 1987.

Timby, B.K., et al. *Clinical Nursing Procedures.* Philadelphia: J.B. Lippincott Co., 1989.

Wilson, E.B., and Malley, N. "Discharge Planning for the Patient with a New Tracheostomy," *Critical Care Nurse* 10(7):73-79, July-August 1990.

Winters, C. "Monitoring Ventilator Patients for Complications," *Nursing88* 18(6):38-41, June 1988.

CHAPTER 9

NEUROLOGIC CARE

DIANE BROADBENT FRIEDMAN, RN, MSN, CS

Introduction

Effective neurologic care aims to preserve and restore optimal nervous system function. And precise nursing skills, meticulously applied, are indispensable to achieving effective care. More and more, these nursing skills require mastery of sophisticated techniques and equipment.

Neurologic assessment

Appropriate supportive care requires that you assess and document neurologic vital signs. At the same time, you also need to assess other systems for complications of neurologic dysfunction.

Be sure to assess neurologic vital signs—especially the patient's orientation level. Many neurologic patients experience changes in perception—ranging from confusion to psychosis—from neurologic dysfunction. Unaddressed, this disorientation further impairs the patient's ability to participate in his recovery. Recognizing this will help you intervene appropriately.

To record and track assessment findings, use special neurologic assessment forms or flowcharts. In common use at most hospitals, these charts separate and grade components of a neurologic assessment, assisting the nurse and other caregivers to quickly recognize changes in neurologic status and to plan subsequent care.

Respiratory assessment constitutes an important part of an overall neurologic assessment. That's because patients with neurologic damage—especially those with traumatic brain or spinal cord injuries—are at considerable risk for respiratory complications. These injuries may depress the respiratory control center and paralyze the muscles used for breathing. As a result, brain tissue, which is especially sensitive to blood oxygen levels, can quickly be damaged by inadequate oxygenation.

Thorough respiratory care goes hand in hand with neurologic care. Frequent position changes, chest physiotherapy, and tracheal suctioning are typical interventions. Additional techniques for preventing complications and promoting comfort include pain management and therapeutic touch.

Rehabilitation

Neurologic rehabilitation begins on admission and touches all aspects of daily care. Because neurologic impairment can alter every area of function, the patient's identity may disintegrate. Consequent rehabilitation procedures must address the psychosocial and physiologic changes associated with the patient's condition—a task that requires enormous time and patience.

The success of rehabilitation efforts may hinge largely on the patient's ability to adapt to significant—even profound—changes. Keep in mind that various factors influence this adaptation: the patient's age, the deficit itself, and available support systems—to name a few. Another ingredient needed for effective rehabilitation is sensitive and skilled nursing care. Such care can dramatically improve the patient's prospects of positive adaptation and recovery.

MONITORING
Neurologic vital signs

Neurologic vital signs supplement the routine measurement of temperature, pulse rate, and respirations by evaluating the patient's level of consciousness (LOC), pupillary activity, and level of orientation to place, time, date, situation, and person. They provide a simple, indispensable tool for quickly checking the patient's neurologic status.

LOC—the degree of response to stimuli—reflects brain stem function and usually provides the first sign of central nervous system deterioration. Changes in *pupillary activity*—pupil size, shape, equality, and response to light—may signal increased intracranial pressure (ICP). *Level of orientation* evaluates higher cerebral functions and processing abilities.

Evaluating muscle strength and tone, reflexes, and posture also may help identify nervous system damage. Finally, ongoing assessment of routine vital signs helps detect neurologic changes or trends. In particular, respiratory rate and pattern can help locate brain lesions and determine their size.

Equipment

Penlight ■ thermometer ■ sterile cotton ball or cotton-tipped applicator ■ stethoscope ■ sphygmomanometer ■ pupil size chart ■ optional: pencil or pen.

Implementation

● Explain the procedure to the patient, even if he's unresponsive. Then wash your hands and provide privacy.

Using the Glasgow coma scale

The Glasgow coma scale provides a standard reference for assessing or monitoring a patient with suspected or confirmed brain injury. You measure three responses to stimuli — eye opening, motor response, and verbal response — and assign a number to each of the possible responses within these categories. A score of 3 is the lowest and 15 is the highest. A score of 7 or less indicates coma. This scale is commonly used in the emergency department, at the scene of an accident, and for periodic evaluation of the hospitalized patient.

CHARACTERISTIC	RESPONSE	SCORE
Eye opening	• Spontaneous	4
	• To verbal command	3
	• To pain	2
	• No response	1
Best motor response	• Obeys commands	6
	• To painful stimuli	
	Localizes pain; pushes stimulus away	5
	Flexes and withdraws	4
	Abnormal flexion	3
	Extension	2
	No response	1
Best verbal response (Arouse patient with painful stimuli, if necessary)	• Oriented and converses	5
	• Disoriented and converses	4
	• Uses inappropriate words	3
	• Makes incomprehensible sounds	2
	• No response	1
	Total:	3 to 15

Assess LOC and orientation

• Assess the patient's LOC by evaluating his responses. Use standard guidelines, such as the Glasgow coma scale. (See *Using the Glasgow coma scale.*) Begin by measuring the patient's response to verbal, light tactile (touch), or painful (nail bed pressure) stimuli. First, ask the patient his full name. If he responds appropriately, assess his orientation to place, time, date, and situation. Ask the patient where he is and then what day, season, and year it is. (Expect disorientation to affect the sense of date first, then time, place, caregivers, and finally self.) When the patient responds verbally, assess the quality of replies. For example, garbled words indicate difficulty with the motor nerves that govern speech muscles. Rambling responses indicate difficulty with thought processing and organization.

• Assess the patient's ability to understand and follow one-step commands that require a motor response. For example, ask him to open and close his eyes or stick out his tongue. Note whether the patient can maintain his LOC. If you must gently shake the patient to keep him focused on your verbal commands, he may sustain neurologic compromise.

• If the patient doesn't respond to commands, apply a painful stimulus. With moderate pressure, squeeze the nail beds on fingers and toes, and note his response. Check motor responses bilaterally *to rule out monoplegia (paralysis of a single area) and hemiplegia (paralysis of one side of the body).*

Examine pupils and eye movement

• Ask the patient to open his eyes. If he doesn't respond, gently lift his upper eyelids. Inspect each pupil for size and shape, and compare the two for equality. To evaluate pupil size more precisely, use a chart showing the various pupil sizes (in increments of 1 mm, with the normal diameter ranging from 2 to 6 mm). Remember, pupil size varies considerably, and some patients have normally unequal pupils (anisocoria). Also see if the pupils are positioned in, or deviated from, the midline.

• Test the patient's direct light response. First, darken the room. Then hold each eyelid open in turn, keeping the other eye covered. Swing the penlight from the patient's ear toward the midline of the face. Shine the light directly into the eye. Normally, the pupil constricts immediately. When you remove the penlight, the pupil should

dilate immediately. Wait about 20 seconds before testing the other pupil *to allow it to recover from reflex stimulation.*
• Now test consensual light response. Hold both eyelids open, but shine the light into one eye only. Watch for constriction in the other pupil, *which indicates proper nerve function at the optic chiasm.*
• Brighten the room and have the conscious patient open his eyes. Observe the eyelids for ptosis or drooping. Then check extraocular movements. Hold up one finger and ask the patient to follow it with his eyes alone. As you move the finger up, down, laterally, and obliquely, see if the patient's eyes track together to follow your finger (conjugate gaze). Watch for involuntary jerking or oscillating eye movements (nystagmus).
• Check accommodation. Hold up one finger midline to the patient's face and several feet away. Have the patient focus on your finger. Then gradually move your finger toward his nose while he still focuses on your finger. This should cause his eyes to converge and both pupils to constrict equally.
• Test the corneal reflex by rapidly moving the palm of your hand toward the patient's open eyes. *This forces a cushion of air against the corneas, which normally causes an immediate blink reflex.* Repeat for the other eye.
• If the patient is unconscious, test the oculocephalic (doll's eye) reflex. Hold the patient's eyelids open. Then quickly, but gently, turn the patient's head to one side, then the other. If the patient's eyes move in the opposite direction from the side to which you turn the head — eyes move right when the head moves left — the reflex is intact.
♦ *Nursing alert.* Never test the doll's eye reflex if you know or suspect that the patient has a cervical spine injury. ♦

Evaluate motor function
• If the patient is conscious, test his grip strength in both hands at the same time. Extend your hands, ask the patient to squeeze your fingers as hard as he can, and compare the strength of each hand. Grip strength is usually slightly stronger in the dominant hand.
• Test arm strength by having the patient close his eyes and hold his arms straight out in front of him with the palms up. See if either arm drifts downward or pronates, *which indicates muscle weakness.*
• Test leg strength by having the patient raise his legs, one at a time, against gentle downward pressure from your hand. Gently push down on each leg at the midpoint of the thigh *to evaluate muscle strength.*
• If the patient is unconscious, estimate the strength of spontaneous and reflex movements. Apply a painful stimulus to elicit movement. Exert pressure on each fingernail bed with a pencil or pen. If the patient withdraws from this stimulus, compare the strength of each limb.

Identifying warning postures

Decorticate and decerebrate posturing are ominous signs of central nervous system deterioration.

Decorticate (abnormal flexion)
In decorticate posturing, the patient's arms are adducted and flexed, with the wrists and fingers flexed on the chest. The legs may be stiffly extended and internally rotated, with plantar flexion of the feet.

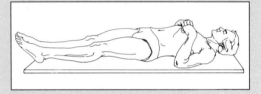

The decorticate posture may indicate a lesion of the frontal lobe, internal capsule, or cerebral peduncles.

Decerebrate (extension)
In decerebrate posturing, the patient's arms are adducted and extended with the wrists pronated and the fingers flexed. One or both of the legs may be stiffly extended, with plantar flexion of the feet.

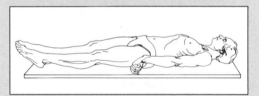

The decerebrate posture may indicate lesions of the upper brain stem.

♦ *Nursing alert.* If decorticate or decerebrate posturing develops in response to painful stimuli, notify the doctor immediately. (See *Identifying warning postures.*) ♦
• Flex and extend the extremities on both sides *to evaluate muscle tone.*
• Test the plantar reflex in all patients. Stroke the lateral aspect of the sole of the patient's foot with your thumbnail or another moderately sharp object. Normally, this elicits flexion of all toes. Watch for a positive Babinski's sign —

Understanding ICP monitoring

Intracranial pressure (ICP) can be monitored using one of four systems.

Intraventricular catheter monitoring

In this procedure, which monitors ICP directly, the doctor inserts a small polyethylene or silicone rubber catheter into the lateral ventricle through a burr hole.

Although this method measures ICP most accurately, it carries the greatest risk of infection. This is the only type of ICP monitoring that allows evaluation of brain compliance and drainage of significant amounts of cerebrospinal fluid (CSF).

Contraindications usually include stenotic cerebral ventricles, cerebral aneurysms in the path of catheter placement, and suspected vascular lesions.

Subarachnoid bolt monitoring

This procedure involves insertion of a special bolt into the subarachnoid space through a twist-drill burr hole that's positioned in the front of the skull behind the hairline.

Placing the bolt is easier than placing an intraventricular catheter, especially if a computerized tomography (CT) scan reveals that the cerebrum has shifted or the ventricles have collapsed. This type of ICP monitoring also carries less risk of infection and parenchymal damage because the bolt doesn't penetrate the cerebrum.

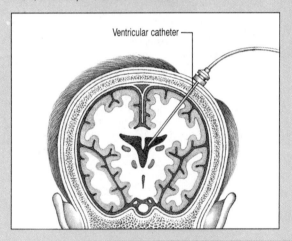

Ventricular catheter

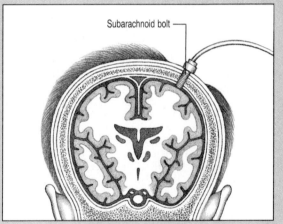

Subarachnoid bolt

dorsiflexion of the great toe with fanning of the other toes—*which indicates an upper motor neuron lesion.*
• Test for Brudzinski's and Kernig's signs in patients suspected of having meningitis.

Complete the neurologic examination

• Take the patient's temperature, pulse rate, respiration rate, and blood pressure. Especially note his pulse pressure—the difference between systolic pressure and diastolic pressure—*because widening pulse pressure can indicate increasing ICP.*

Special considerations

♦ *Nursing alert.* If the previously stable patient suddenly develops a change in neurologic or routine vital signs,

further assess his condition, and notify the doctor immediately.♦

Documentation

Baseline data require detailed documentation; subsequent notes can be brief unless the patient's condition changes. Record the patient's LOC and orientation, pupillary activity, motor function, and routine vital signs, as hospital policy directs. To save time while keeping complete records, the hospital may let you use abbreviations. Use only commonly understood abbreviations and terms to avoid misinterpretation of the patient's status. Examples include the following:
• A + O × 4—alert and oriented to person, place, time, and date

Epidural sensor monitoring
The least invasive with the lowest incidence of infection, this method uses a tiny fiber-optic sensor inserted into the epidural space through a burr hole.

Unlike an intraventricular catheter or a subarachnoid bolt, the sensor can't become occluded with blood or brain tissue. Accuracy is questionable, however, because the epidural sensor doesn't measure ICP directly from a CSF-filled space. Several types of sensors are available; some can be recalibrated repeatedly. Fiber-optic sensors must be calibrated before they're inserted.

Intraparenchymal monitoring
In this procedure, the doctor inserts a catheter through a small subarachnoid bolt and, after puncturing the dura, advances the catheter a few centimeters into the brain's white matter. There's no need to balance or calibrate the equipment after insertion.

Although this method doesn't provide direct access to CSF, measurements are accurate because brain tissue pressures correlate well with ventricular pressures. Intraparenchymal monitoring may be used to obtain ICP measurements in patients with compressed or dislocated ventricles.

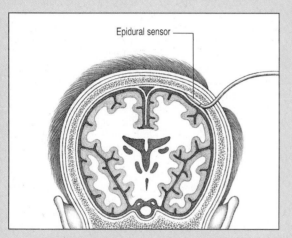

Epidural sensor

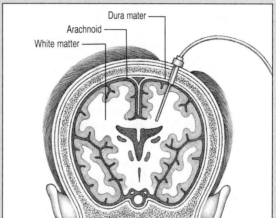

Dura mater
Arachnoid
White matter

- PERRLA — pupils equal, round, reactive to light and accommodation
- PERL — pupils equal, reactive to light
- EOM — extraocular movements

Also describe the patient's behavior — difficult to arouse by gentle shaking, sleepy, unresponsive to painful stimuli.

Intracranial pressure monitoring

This procedure measures pressure exerted by the brain, blood, and cerebrospinal fluid (CSF) against the inside of the skull. Indications for monitoring intracranial pressure (ICP) include head trauma with bleeding or edema, overproduction or insufficient absorption of CSF, cerebral hemorrhage, and space-occupying brain lesions. ICP monitoring can detect elevated ICP early, before clinical danger signs develop. Prompt intervention can then help avert or diminish neurologic damage caused by cerebral hypoxia and shifts of brain mass.

The four basic ICP monitoring systems feature ventricular catheter, subarachnoid bolt, epidural sensor, and intraparenchymal pressure monitoring. (See *Understanding ICP monitoring.*) Regardless of the system used, the procedure is always performed by a neurosurgeon in the operating room, emergency department, or critical care unit. Insertion of an ICP monitoring device requires sterile technique to reduce the risk of central nervous system (CNS) infection. Setting up equipment for the monitoring systems also requires strict asepsis.

Equipment
Monitoring unit and transducers, as ordered ■ 16 to 20 sterile 4″ × 4″ gauze pads ■ linen-saver pads ■ shave preparation tray or hair scissors ■ sterile drapes ■ povidone-iodine solution ■ sterile gown ■ surgical mask ■ two pairs of sterile gloves ■ povidone-iodine ointment ■ head dressing supplies (two rolls of 4″ elastic gauze dressing, one roll of 4″ roller gauze, adhesive tape) ■ optional: suction apparatus, a yardstick.

Preparation of equipment
Monitoring units and setup protocols are varied and complex and differ among hospitals. Check your hospital's guidelines for your particular unit and its preparation.

Various models of preassembled ICP monitoring units are available, each with its own setup protocols. These units are designed to reduce the risk of infection by eliminating the need for multiple stopcocks, manometers, and transducer dome assemblies. Some hospitals use units that have miniaturized transducers rather than transducer domes.

Implementation
• Explain the procedure to the patient or his family. Make sure the patient or a responsible family member has signed a consent form. Determine if the patient is allergic to iodine preparations.
• Provide privacy if the procedure is being done in an open emergency department or intensive care unit.
• Obtain baseline routine and neurologic vital signs *to aid in prompt detection of decompensation during the procedure.*
• Place the patient in the supine position and elevate the head of the bed 30 degrees, or as ordered. Document the number of bed crank rotations, or hang a yardstick on an I.V. pole and mark the exact elevation.
• Place linen-saver pads under the patient's head. Shave or clip his hair at the insertion site, as indicated by the doctor, *to decrease the risk of infection.* Carefully fold and remove the linen-saver pads *to avoid spilling loose hair onto the bed.* Drape the patient with sterile drapes. Scrub the insertion site for 2 minutes with povidone-iodine solution.
• The doctor puts on the sterile gown, mask, and sterile gloves. He then opens the interior wrap of the sterile supply tray and proceeds with insertion of the catheter or bolt.
• *To facilitate placement of the device,* hold the patient's head in your hands or attach a long strip of 4″ roller

gauze to one side rail and bring it across the patient's forehead to the opposite rail. Reassure the conscious patient *to help ease his anxiety.* Talk to him frequently *to assess his level of consciousness (LOC) and detect signs of deterioration.* Watch for cardiac arrhythmias and abnormal respiratory patterns.
• After insertion, apply povidone-iodine ointment and a sterile dressing to the site. The doctor will then connect the catheter to the appropriate monitoring device, depending on the system used.
• If the doctor has set up a drainage system, attach the drip chamber to the headboard or the bedside I.V. pole, as ordered.
♦ *Nursing alert.* Positioning the drip chamber too high may raise ICP; positioning it too low may cause excessive CSF drainage. ♦
• Inspect the insertion site at least every 24 hours or according to hospital policy for redness, swelling, and drainage. Clean the site, reapply povidone-iodine, and apply a fresh sterile dressing.
• Hourly, or as ordered, assess the patient's clinical status, and take routine and neurologic vital signs. Make sure you have obtained orders for waveforms and pressure parameters from the doctor.
• Observe digital ICP readings and waves. Remember, the pattern of readings is more significant than any single reading. (See *Interpreting ICP waveforms.*) If you observe continually elevated ICP readings, note how long they're sustained. If they last several minutes, notify the doctor immediately. Finally, record and describe any CSF drainage.

Special considerations
In infants, ICP monitoring can be performed without penetrating the scalp. In this external method, a photoelectric transducer with a pressure-sensitive membrane is taped to the anterior fontanel. The transducer responds to pressure at the site and transmits readings to a bedside monitor and recording system. The external method is restricted to infants because pressure readings can be obtained only at fontanels, the incompletely ossified areas of the skull.

Osmotic diuretic agents, such as mannitol, reduce cerebral edema by shrinking intracranial contents. Given by I.V. drip or bolus, mannitol draws water from tissues into plasma; it does not cross the blood-brain barrier. Monitor serum electrolyte levels and osmolality readings closely because *the patient may become dehydrated very quickly.* Be aware that a rebound increase in ICP may occur. (See *Nursing management of increased ICP,* page 494.) If your patient has congestive heart failure or severe renal dysfunction, monitor for problems in adapting to the increased intravascular volumes.

Interpreting ICP waveforms

Three waveforms, A, B, and C, are used to monitor intracranial pressure (ICP). *A waves* are an ominous sign of intracranial decompensation and poor compliance. *B waves* correlate with changes in respiration, and *C waves* with changes in arterial pressure.

A normal ICP waveform typically shows a steep upward systolic slope followed by a downward diastolic slope with a dicrotic notch. In most cases, this waveform occurs continuously and indicates an ICP between 0 and 15 mm Hg—normal pressure.

Normal waveform

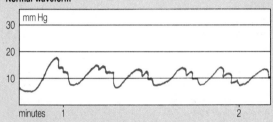

The most clinically significant ICP waveforms are A waves (shown below), which may reach elevations of 50 to 100 mm Hg, persist for 5 to 20 minutes, then drop sharply—signaling exhaustion of the brain's compliance mechanisms. A waves may come and go, spiking from temporary rises in thoracic pressure or from any condition that increases ICP beyond the brain's compliance limits. Activities such as sustained coughing or straining with bowel movements can cause temporary elevations in thoracic pressure.

A waves

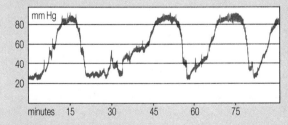

B waves, which appear sharp and rhythmic, with a sawtooth pattern, occur every 1½ to 2 minutes and may reach elevations of 50 mm Hg. The clinical significance of B waves isn't clear, but they correlate with respiratory changes and may occur more frequently with decreas-

ing compensation. Because B waves sometimes precede A waves, notify the doctor if B waves occur frequently.

B waves

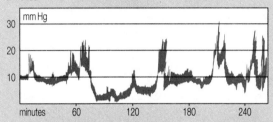

Like B waves, C waves are rapid and rhythmic, but not as sharp. Clinically insignificant, they may fluctuate with respirations or systemic blood pressure changes.

C waves

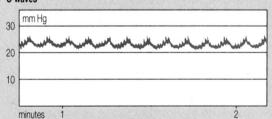

A waveform that looks like the one shown below signals a problem with the transducer or monitor. Check for line obstruction, and determine if the transducer needs rebalancing.

Waveform showing equipment problem

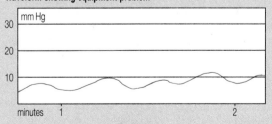

Nursing management of increased ICP

By performing nursing care gently, slowly, and cautiously, you can best help to manage increased ICP rather than possibly compound it. You may even be able to reduce it significantly. If possible, urge your patient to participate in his own care. Here are some steps you can take to manage increased ICP.

• Plan your care to include rest periods between activities. *This allows the patient's ICP to return to baseline, thus avoiding lengthy and cumulative pressure elevations.*

• Try to speak to the patient before attempting any procedures, even if he appears comatose. Touch him on an arm or leg first before touching him in a more personal area, such as the face or chest. This is especially important if the patient doesn't know you, or if he's confused or sedated.

• Suction the patient only when needed *to remove secretions and maintain airway patency.* Avoid depriving him of oxygen for long periods while suctioning; always hyperventilate the patient with oxygen after the procedure. Monitor his heart rate while suctioning. If multiple catheter passes are needed to clear secretions, hyperventilate the patient between them *to bring ICP as close to baseline as possible.*

• Promote venous drainage. Keep the patient's head in the midline position, even when he's positioned on his side. Avoid neck flexion or hip flexion greater than 90 degrees, and keep the head of the bed elevated 30 to 45 degrees.

• *To avoid increasing intrathoracic pressure, which raises ICP,* discourage Valsalva's maneuver and isometric muscle contractions. To avoid isometric contractions, distract the patient when giving him painful injections (by asking him to wiggle his toes and by massaging the area before injection to relax the muscle) and have him concentrate on breathing through difficult procedures such as bed-to-stretcher transfers. Tell the patient to relax as much as possible during position changes, *to keep him from holding his breath when moving around in bed.* If necessary, administer a stool softener *to help prevent constipation and unnecessary straining at stool.*

• If the patient is heavily sedated, monitor respiratory rate and blood gas levels. *Depressed respirations will compromise ventilations and oxygen exchange. Maintaining adequate respiratory rate and volume helps reduce ICP.*

• If you're in a specialty unit, you may be able to routinely hyperventilate the patient to counter sustained ICP elevations. This procedure is one of the best ways to reduce high ICP at bedside for short periods. Consult your hospital's protocol.

Fluid restriction, usually 1,200 ml to 1,500 ml per day, avoids causing or increasing cerebral edema.

Although steroid therapy is controversial, steroids may be used to lower elevated ICP by reducing sodium and water concentration in the brain. *Because they may also produce peptic ulcers,* they're usually given with antacids and cimetidine or ranitidine. Observe for possible GI bleeding. Also monitor urine glucose and acetone levels because *steroids may cause glycosuria in patients with borderline diabetes.*

Barbiturate-induced coma depresses the reticular activating system and reduces the brain's metabolic demand. Reduced demand for oxygen and energy reduces cerebral blood flow, thereby lowering ICP.

Hyperventilation with oxygen from a hand-held resuscitation bag or respirator helps rid the patient of excess carbon dioxide, thereby constricting cerebral vessels and reducing cerebral blood volume and ICP. However, only normal brain tissues respond, because blood vessels in damaged areas have reduced vasoconstrictive ability.

Before tracheal suctioning, hyperventilate the patient with 100% oxygen, as ordered. Apply suction for a maximum of 15 seconds. Avoid inducing hypoxia *because it greatly increases cerebral blood flow.*

Because fever raises brain metabolism, which increases cerebral blood flow, fever-reduction (achieved by administering acetaminophen, alcohol sponge baths, and a hypothermia blanket) also helps to reduce ICP. However, rebound increases in ICP and brain edema may occur if rapid rewarming takes place after hypothermia or if cooling measures induce shivering.

Withdrawal of CSF through the drainage system reduces CSF volume, and thus reduces ICP. Although less commonly used, surgical removal of a skull-bone flap provides room for the swollen brain to expand. If this procedure is performed, keep the site clean and dry *to prevent infection* and maintain sterile technique when changing the dressing.

Complications

CNS infection, the most common hazard of ICP monitoring, can result from contamination of the equipment setup or of the insertion site.

♦ *Nursing alert.* Excessive loss of CSF can result from faulty stopcock placement or a drip chamber that's positioned too low. Such loss can rapidly decompress the cranial contents and damage bridging cortical veins, leading to hematoma formation. Decompression can also lead to rupture of existing hematomas or aneurysms, causing hemorrhage. ♦

Watch for signs of impending or overt decompensation: papilledema; pupillary dilation (unilateral or bilateral); decreased pupillary response to light; decreasing LOC; rising systolic blood pressure and widening pulse pressure; bradycardia; slowed, irregular respirations; and, in late decompensation, decerebrate posturing.

Documentation

Record the time and date of the insertion procedure and the patient's response. Note the insertion site and the type of monitoring system used. Record ICP digital readings and waveforms hourly in your notes, on a flowchart, or directly on readout strips, depending on the hospital's policy. Document any factors that may affect ICP — for example, drug therapy, stressful procedures, or sleep.

Record routine and neurologic vital signs hourly, and describe the patient's clinical status. Note the amount, character, and frequency of any CSF drainage (for example, between 6 p.m. and 7 p.m., 15 ml of blood-tinged CSF).

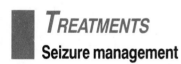

TREATMENTS
Seizure management

When a patient has a generalized seizure, nursing care aims to protect him from injury and prevent serious complications. Appropriate care also includes observation of seizure characteristics to help determine the area of the brain involved.

Seizures are classified as partial or generalized. Partial seizures are usually unilateral, involving a localized or focal area of the brain. A *jacksonian* seizure, for example, has a focal onset and progresses in stepwise fashion, reflecting the spread of seizure activity in the brain. Generalized seizures involve the entire brain and are known as *absence (petit mal)* and *tonic-clonic (grand mal)* seizures. An absence seizure occurs most often in children and usually begins with a brief change in level of consciousness. A tonic-clonic seizure typically begins with a loud cry. Then the patient falls and loses consciousness. Tonic and clonic movements and autonomic nervous system dysfunction follow. Prolonged seizure activity — known as status epilepticus — requires emergency medical intervention.

Patients considered at risk for seizures include those with a history of seizures and those with conditions that may predispose them to seizures. These conditions include hypoglycemia, hypoxia, electrolyte imbalances, drug or alcohol withdrawal, and central nervous system trauma. Patients at risk for seizures need precautionary measures to help prevent injury if a seizure occurs. (See *Precautions for generalized seizures,* page 496.)

Equipment

Oral airway ■ suction equipment ■ equipment for I.V. line insertion ■ 1 liter of normal saline solution ■ anticonvulsant, such as diazepam, phenytoin, or phenobarbital, as ordered ■ emergency resuscitation equipment ■ 50-ml bolus of dextrose 50% in water, as ordered ■ 100-mg bolus of thiamine, as ordered ■ pillows, side rail pads, blankets, or other soft material ■ optional: endotracheal intubation set.

Implementation

● If you're with a patient when he experiences an aura, help him into bed, raise the side rails, and adjust the bed flat. If he's away from his room, lower him to the floor and place a pillow, blanket, or other soft material under his head *to keep it from hitting the floor.*
● Stay with the patient during the seizure, and be ready to intervene if complications, such as airway obstruction, develop. If necessary, have another staff member obtain the appropriate equipment and notify the doctor.
● If the patient is in the beginning of the tonic phase and if according to hospital protocol, you may insert an oral airway into his mouth *so his tongue doesn't block his airway.* If an oral airway isn't available, don't try to hold his mouth open or place your hands inside *because you may be bitten.* Once the patient's jaw becomes rigid, don't try to force the airway into place *because you may break his teeth or cause other injury.* Some clinicians advocate waiting until the seizure subsides before inserting the airway.
● Move sharp or hard objects out of the patient's way, and loosen his clothing.
● Don't forcibly restrain the patient or restrict his movements during the seizure, *because the force of the patient's tonic-clonic movements against restraints may cause muscle strain or even joint dislocation.*

Precautions for generalized seizures

By taking appropriate precautions, you can help protect a patient from injury, aspiration, and airway obstruction should he have a seizure. Plan your precautions using information obtained from the patient's history. What kind of seizure has the patient had before? Is he aware of exacerbating factors? Sleep deprivation, missed doses of anticonvulsants, even upper respiratory infections can increase seizure frequency in some persons who have had seizures. Was his previous seizure an acute episode or did it result from a chronic condition?

Gather the equipment
Based on answers provided in the patient's history, you can tailor your precautions to his needs. Start by gathering the appropriate equipment, including a hospital bed with full-length side rails, commercial side rail pads or six bath blankets (four for a crib), adhesive tape, an oral airway, and oral or nasal suction equipment.

Bedside preparations
Now carry out the precautions you think appropriate for the patient. Remember that a patient with preexisting seizures who's being admitted for a change in medication, treatment of an infection, or detoxification may have an increased risk of seizures.
• Explain the reasons for the precautions to the patient.
• *To protect the patient's limbs, head, and feet from injury if he has a seizure while in bed,* cover the side rails, headboard, and footboard with side rail pads or bath blankets. If you use blankets, keep them in place with adhesive tape. Be sure to keep the side rails raised while the patient is in bed *to prevent falls.* Keep the bed in a low position *to minimize any injuries that may occur if the patient climbs over the rails.*

• Place an airway at the patient's bedside, or tape it to the wall above the bed, according to your hospital's protocol. Keep suction equipment nearby *in case you need to establish a patent airway.* Explain to the patient how the airway will be used.
• If the patient has frequent or prolonged seizures, prepare an I.V. heparin lock *to facilitate administration of emergency medications.*

If a seizure begins
• If the patient experiences a typical seizure warning sign, such as an aura, help him into his bed and raise the side rails. Make sure he knows to put on his call light and immediately get into bed if he experiences an aura when you're not nearby.
• If the patient is confused and walking about after a seizure begins, walk with him and guide him back to his bed; don't try to restrain him.
• If the patient becomes cyanotic, have oxygen available at the bedside *to provide maximum saturation as soon as possible,*
• Never attempt to insert an airway once the seizure itself has started.
• *Alert:* Many clinicians disapprove of using airways, reasoning that seizure onset is commonly so rapid that there's no time to insert such a device before the patient's jaws clench shut. Rather than try to pry the jaws apart, these clinicians advocate waiting until after the seizure passes, then opening the jaws and turning the patient on his side. This also avoids upsetting the patient, who may feel traumatized by an artificial airway. Little research has been done to establish the efficacy of one method over another.

• Continually assess the patient during the seizure. Observe the earliest symptom, such as head or eye deviation, as well as how the seizure progresses, what form it takes, and how long it lasts. *Your description may help determine the seizure's type and cause.*
• After the tonic-clonic phase, maintain a patent airway by turning the patient on his side and applying suction. *He'll be less likely to aspirate vomitus if he's on his side.*
• If ordered, establish an I.V. line and infuse normal saline solution at a keep-vein-open rate.
• If the seizure lasts longer than 10 minutes, administer an anticonvulsant, as ordered. (See *Administering emergency anticonvulsants.*)

• For a patient known to be diabetic, administer 50 ml of dextrose 50% in water by I.V. push, as ordered. For a patient known to be an alcoholic, a 100-mg bolus of thiamine may stop the seizure.
• If the seizure is prolonged and the patient becomes hypoxemic, begin resuscitation measures. Rarely, the patient may require endotracheal intubation.
• If the seizure continues despite medical treatment, you may need to prepare the patient for general anesthesia to stop seizure activity. Electroencephalogram monitoring should be performed in the neurologic intensive care unit *to determine when the seizure activity stops.*

Administering emergency anticonvulsants

A seizure that lasts longer than 10 minutes, or two seizures that occur without the patient's awakening in the interval, signals a condition known as status epilepticus, which requires emergency intervention. After ensuring a patent airway, you'll need to administer an anticonvulsant, such as diazepam or phenytoin, as ordered. If these drugs are ineffective, phenobarbital may be given.

Diazepam
Give an adult 5 to 20 mg of diazepam by slow I.V. push at a rate of 2 to 5 mg/minute, as ordered. You can repeat this dose every 5 to 10 minutes to a maximum dose of 60 mg.

For an elderly or debilitated patient, wait 20 to 30 minutes to repeat the dose. For a child age 5 or older, give 0.5 to 1 mg every 2 to 5 minutes to a total of 10 mg. Repeat this pattern in 2 to 4 hours. For an infant older than 1 month, administer 0.5 mg every 2 to 5 minutes to a total dose of 5 mg. This pattern may be repeated in 2 to 4 hours. Do not give intramuscularly.

Some clinicians prefer to administer lorazepam in children (0.5 mg/kg I.V., repeatable in 15 minutes), because it's less likely to cause respiratory depression than diazepam. However, the manufacturer does not recommend its use for this indication in children under age 18.

Phenytoin
If the doctor orders phenytoin for an adult, administer 150 to 200 mg (or 8 to 18 mg/kg) by direct I.V. injection at a rate of 50 mg/minute. After 30 minutes, you may administer another 100 to 150 mg at the same rate. For a child, give 10 to 15 mg/kg at 0.5 to 1.5 mg/kg/minute. The maximum daily dose is 20 mg/kg. Do not give intramuscularly.

Intravenous diazepam has a rapid onset—less than 1 minute—but its duration of action is only about 30 minutes. Phenytoin's onset is slower (30 minutes to 1 hour) but its duration is 8 to 12 hours. If ordered, both drugs may be given simultaneously—diazepam followed by phenytoin—as long as they're not given in the same syringe.

Phenobarbital
Give an adult 200 to 600 mg by I.V. push. Keep infusion rate below 60 mg/minute. For a child, the usual dose is 15 to 25 mg/kg I.V., given over 10 to 15 minutes.

Special considerations
After the seizure, monitor vital signs and mental status every 15 to 30 minutes for 2 hours. If the patient remains obtunded for more than 2 hours, notify the doctor. When the patient does awaken, reorient and reassure him because he may be anxious, afraid, or embarrassed. Ask him about his aura or activities preceding the seizure. The type of aura (auditory, visual, gustatory, olfactory, or somatic) helps pinpoint the site in the brain where the seizure originated.

Because a seizure commonly indicates an underlying disorder, such as meningitis or a metabolic or electrolyte imbalance, a complete diagnostic workup will be ordered if the cause of the seizure isn't evident.

Complications
The patient may experience an injury, respiratory difficulty, and decreased mental capability.

Common injuries include scrapes and bruises suffered when the patient hits objects during the seizure and traumatic injury to the tongue caused by biting. If you suspect a serious injury, such as a fracture or deep laceration, notify the doctor and arrange for appropriate evaluation and treatment.

Changes in respiratory function may include aspiration, airway obstruction, and hypoxemia. After the seizure, complete a full respiratory assessment, notifying the doctor if you suspect a problem.

Expect most patients to experience a postictal period of decreased mental status lasting 30 minutes to 24 hours. Reassure your patient that this does not indicate incipient brain damage.

Documentation
Note that the patient requires seizure precautions; also record all precautions taken. Record the date and time a seizure began, as well as its duration and any precipitating factors. Identify any sensation that may be considered an aura. Describe any involuntary behavior occurring at onset, such as lip smacking, chewing movements, or hand and eye movements. Record any incontinence occurring during the seizure.

Note the patient's response to the seizure, the medications given, any complications resulting from the medications or the seizure, and any interventions performed. Finally, note the patient's postseizure mental status.

Cerebrospinal fluid drains

Cerebrospinal fluid (CSF) drainage aims to reduce CSF pressure to the desired level and then to maintain it at that level. Fluid can be withdrawn from the lateral ventricle (ventriculostomy) or lumbar subarachnoid space, depending on the indication and the desired outcome. Ventricular drainage is used to reduce increased intracranial pressure (ICP), whereas lumbar drainage is used to aid healing of the dura mater. External CSF drainage is used most commonly to manage increased ICP and to facilitate spinal or cerebral dural healing after traumatic injury or surgery. In either case, CSF is drained by a catheter or a ventriculostomy tube in a sterile, closed drainage collection system.

Other therapeutic uses include ICP monitoring via the ventriculostomy; direct instillation of medications, contrast media, or air for diagnostic radiology; and aspiration of CSF for laboratory analysis.

To place the ventricular drain, the doctor inserts a ventricular catheter through a burr hole in the patient's skull. Usually, this is done in the operating room, with the patient receiving a general anesthetic. To place the lumbar subarachnoid drain, the doctor may administer a local spinal anesthetic at bedside or in the operating room. (See *Methods of CSF drainage.*)

Equipment
Overbed table ▪ sterile gloves ▪ sterile cotton-tipped applicators ▪ povidone-iodine solution ▪ alcohol sponges ▪ sterile fenestrated drape ▪ 3-ml syringe for local anesthetic ▪ 25G ¾″ needle for injecting anesthetic ▪ local anesthetic (usually 1% lidocaine) ▪ 18G or 20G sterile spinal needle or Tuohy needle ▪ #5 French whistle-tip catheter or ventriculostomy tube ▪ external drainage set (includes drainage tubing and sterile collection bag) ▪ suture material ▪ 4″ × 4″ dressings ▪ paper tape ▪ lamp or other light source ▪ I.V. pole ▪ optional: ventriculostomy tray, twist drill, pain medication (such as an analgesic), anti-infective agent (such as an antibiotic).

Preparation of equipment
Open all equipment using sterile technique. Check all packaging for breaks in seals and for expiration dates. After the doctor places the catheter, connect it to the external drainage system tubing. Secure connection points with tape or a connector.

Place the collection system, including drip chamber and collection bag, on an I.V. pole.

Implementation
• Explain the procedure to the patient and family. Consent should be obtained by the doctor from the patient or responsible family member and should be documented according to hospital guidelines.
• Wash your hands thoroughly.
• Perform a baseline neurologic assessment, including vital signs, *to help detect alterations or signs of deterioration.*

Inserting a ventricular drain
• Place the patient in a supine position.
• Place the equipment tray on the overbed table and unwrap the tray.
• Adjust the height of the bed *so that the doctor can perform the procedure comfortably.*
• Illuminate the area of the catheter insertion site.
• The doctor will clean the insertion site and administer a local anesthetic.
• To insert the drain, the doctor will request a ventriculostomy tray with a twist drill. After completing the ventriculostomy, he will connect the drainage system. (*Note:* Although this procedure can be done at bedside under emergency conditions, it's usually done in the operating room.)

Inserting a lumbar subarachnoid drain
• Position the patient in a side-lying position with his chin tucked to his chest and knees drawn up to his abdomen, as for a lumbar puncture. Urge the patient to remain as still as possible during the procedure *to minimize discomfort and traumatic injury.*
• To insert the drain, the doctor attaches a Tuohy needle (or spinal needle) to the whistle-tip catheter. *The needle guides the catheter into the subarachnoid space.* After the doctor removes the needle, he connects the drainage system and sutures or tapes the catheter securely in place.

Monitoring CSF drainage
• Maintain a continuous hourly output of CSF by raising or lowering the drip chamber. To maintain CSF outflow, the drip chamber should be slightly lower than or at the level of the lumbar drain insertion site. Sometimes you may need to carefully raise or lower the drip chamber *to increase or decrease CSF flow.* (For ventricular drains, the drip chamber should be slightly lower than or at the level of the ventricular drain insertion site. However, for treating increased ICP, the chamber should be set higher than the foramen of Monro.)
• Check the dressing frequently for drainage, which could indicate CSF leakage.
• Check the tubing for patency by watching the CSF drops in the drip chamber.

Methods of CSF drainage

Cerebrospinal fluid (CSF) drainage aims to control intracranial pressure (ICP) during treatment for traumatic injury or other conditions that cause a rise in ICP. Two procedures are commonly used, as detailed below.

For a ventricular drain, the doctor makes a burr hole in the patient's skull and inserts the catheter into the ventricle. The distal end of the catheter is connected to a closed drainage system.

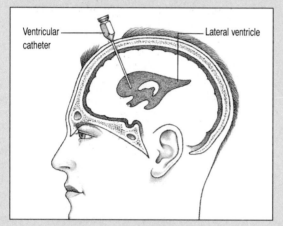

For a lumbar drain, the doctor inserts a catheter beneath the dura into the L3-L4 interspace.

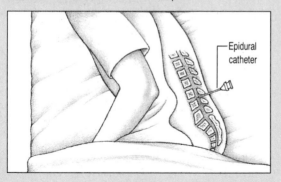

Drainage catheters lead to a sterile, closed collection system affixed securely to the bed or to an I.V. pole. The drip chamber should be set at the level ordered by the doctor.

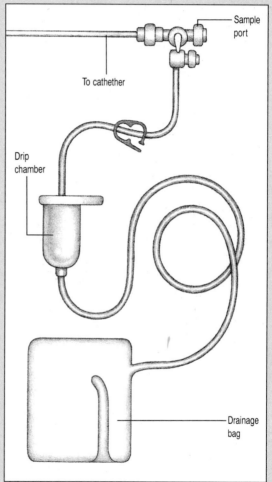

• Observe CSF for color, clarity, amount, blood, and sediment. CSF specimens for laboratory analysis should be obtained from the collection port attached to the tubing, not from the collection bag.
• Change the collection bag when it's full or every 24 hours, according to your hospital policy.

Special considerations

Maintenance of a continual hourly output of CSF is essential *to prevent overdrainage or underdrainage.* Underdrainage or lack of CSF may reflect kinked tubing, catheter displacement, or a drip chamber placed higher than the catheter insertion site. Overdrainage can occur if the drip chamber is placed too far below the catheter insertion site.

Raising or lowering the head of the bed can affect the CSF flow rate. When changing the patient's position, reposition the drip chamber as well.

Patients may experience chronic headache during continuous CSF drainage. Reassure the patient that this is not unusual; administer analgesics as appropriate.

Complications

Signs of excessive CSF drainage include headache, tachycardia, diaphoresis, and nausea. Acute overdrainage may result in collapsed ventricles, tonsillar herniation, and medullary compression. If drainage accumulates too rapidly, clamp the system and notify the doctor immediately. This constitutes a potential neurosurgical emergency.

Cessation of drainage may indicate clot formation. If you can't quickly identify the cause of the obstruction, notify the doctor.

If drainage is blocked, the patient may develop signs of increased ICP. (If the lumbar drain was placed to aid dural wound healing, blockage may cause a CSF leak in the wound area).

Infection may cause meningitis. Administer antibiotics, as ordered, to prevent this.

Documentation

Record the time and date of the insertion procedure and the patient's response. Record routine vital signs and neurologic assessment findings at least every 4 hours.

Document the color, clarity, and amount of CSF at least every 8 hours. Record hourly and 24-hour CSF outputs. Also describe the condition of the dressing.

Halo-vest traction

Halo-vest traction immobilizes the head and neck after traumatic injury to the cervical vertebrae, the most common of all spinal injuries. This procedure, which can prevent further injury to the spinal cord, is performed by an orthopedic surgeon, with nursing assistance, in the emergency department, a specially-equipped room, or in the operating room after surgical reduction of vertebral injuries. The halo-vest traction device consists of a metal ring that fits over the patient's head and metal bars that connect the ring to a plastic vest that distributes the weight of the entire apparatus around the chest. (See *Comparing halo-vest traction devices.*)

Once in place, halo-vest traction allows the patient greater mobility than does traction with skull tongs. It also carries less risk of infection, because it doesn't require skin incisions and drill holes to position skull pins.

Equipment

Halo-vest traction unit ■ halo ring ■ cervical collar or sandbags (if needed) ■ plastic vest ■ board or padded headrest ■ tape measure ■ halo ring conversion chart ■ scissors and razor ■ 4″ × 4″ gauze pads ■ povidone-iodine solution ■ sterile gloves ■ Allen wrench ■ four positioning pins ■ multiple-dose vial of 1% lidocaine (with or without epinephrine) ■ alcohol sponges ■ 3-ml syringe ■ 25G needles ■ five sterile skull pins (one more than needed) ■ torque screwdriver ■ sheepskin liners ■ cotton-tipped applicators ■ ordered cleaning solution ■ medicated powder or cornstarch ■ sterile water or normal saline solution ■ optional: hair dryer, pain medication (such as an analgesic).

Most hospitals supply packaged halo-vest traction units that include software (jacket and sheepskin liners), hardware (halo, head pins, upright bars, and screws), and tools (torque screwdriver, two conventional wrenches, Allen wrench, and screws and bolts). These units don't include sterile gloves, povidone-iodine solution, sterile drapes, cervical collars, or equipment for injection of local anesthetic.

Preparation of equipment

Obtain a halo-vest traction unit with halo rings and plastic vests in several sizes. Check the expiration date of the prepackaged tray, and check the outside covering for damage *to ensure the sterility of the contents.* Then assemble the equipment at the patient's bedside.

Implementation

● Check the support that was applied to the patient's neck on the way to the hospital. If necessary, apply the cervical collar immediately or immobilize the head and neck with sandbags. Keep the cervical collar or sandbags in place until the halo is applied. This support will then be carefully removed *to facilitate application of the vest. Because the patient is likely to be frightened,* try to reassure him.

● Remove the headboard and any furniture at the head of the bed *to provide ample working space.* Then carefully place the patient's head on a board or on a padded headrest that extends beyond the edge of the bed.

◆ *Nursing alert.* Never put the patient's head on a pillow before applying the halo *to avoid further injury to the spinal cord.* ◆

● Elevate the bed to a working level that gives the doctor easy access to the front and back of the halo unit.

Comparing halo-vest traction devices

TYPE	DESCRIPTION	ADVANTAGES
Low profile (standard)	• Traction and compression are produced by threaded support rods on either side of the halo ring. • Flexion and extension are obtained by moving the swivel arm to an anterior or posterior position, depending on the location of the skull pins.	• Immobilizes cervical spine fractures while allowing patient mobility • Facilitates surgery of the cervical spine and permits flexion and extension • Allows airway intubation without losing skeletal traction • Facilitates necessary alignment by an adjustment at the junction of the threaded support rods and horizontal frame
Mark II (type of low profile)	• Traction and compression are produced by threaded support rods on either side of the halo ring. • Flexion and extension are obtained by swivel clamps, which allow the bars to intersect and hold at any angle.	• Enables doctors to assemble the metal framework more quickly • Allows unobstructed access for anteroposterior and lateral X-rays of the cervical spine • Allows patient to wear his usual clothing because uprights are shaped closer to the body
Mark III (update of Mark II)	• Traction and compression are produced by threaded support rods on either side of the halo ring. • Flexion and extension are accommodated by a serrated split articulation coupling attached to the halo ring, which can be adjusted in 4-degree increments.	• Simplifies application while promoting patient comfort • Eliminates shoulder pressure and discomfort by using a flexible padded strap instead of the vest's solid plastic shoulder • Accommodates the tall patient with modified hardware and shorter uprights and allows unobstructed access for medial and lateral X-rays
Trippi-Wells tongs	• Traction is produced by four pins that compress the skull. • Flexion and extension are obtained by adjusting the midline vertical plate.	• Applies tensile force to the neck or spine while allowing patient mobility • Makes it possible to change from mobile to stationary traction without interrupting traction • Adjusts to three planes for mobile and stationary traction • Allows unobstructed access for medial and lateral X-rays

• Stand at the head of the bed and see if the patient's chin lines up with his midsternum, *indicating proper alignment*. If ordered, support the patient's head in your hands and gently rotate the neck into alignment without flexing or extending it.

To assist with application of the halo
• Ask another nurse to help you with the procedure.
• Explain the procedure to the patient, wash your hands, and provide privacy.
• Have the assisting nurse hold the patient's head and neck stable while the doctor removes the cervical collar or sandbags. Maintain this support until the halo is secure, while you assist with pin insertion.
• The doctor first measures the patient's head with a tape measure and refers to the halo ring conversion chart to determine the correct ring size. (The ring should clear the head by 1.5 cm and fit 1 cm above the bridge of the nose.)
• The doctor selects four pin sites: 1 cm above the lateral one-third of each eyebrow and 1 cm above the top of each ear in the occipital area. He also takes into account the degree and type of correction needed to provide proper cervical alignment.
• Trim and shave the hair at the pin sites with scissors or a razor *to facilitate subsequent care and help prevent infection*. Then, use 4″ × 4″ gauze pads soaked in povidone-iodine solution to clean the sites.
• Open the halo-vest unit using sterile technique *to avoid contamination*. The doctor puts on the sterile gloves and removes the halo and the Allen wrench. He then places the halo over the patient's head and inserts the four positioning pins *to hold the halo in place temporarily*.
• Help the doctor prepare the anesthetic. First, clean the injection port of the multiple-dose vial of lidocaine with the alcohol sponge. Then, invert the vial so the doctor can insert a 25G needle attached to the 3-ml syringe and withdraw the anesthetic.
• The doctor injects the anesthetic at the four pin sites. He may change needles on the syringe after each injection.
• The doctor removes four of the five skull pins from the sterile setup and firmly screws in each pin at a 90-degree angle to the skull. When the pins are in place, he removes the positioning pins. He then tightens the skull pins with the torque screwdriver.

To apply the vest
• After the doctor measures the patient's chest and abdomen, he selects a vest of appropriate size.
• Place the sheepskin liners inside the front and back of the vest *to make it more comfortable to wear and to help prevent pressure ulcers*.

• Help the doctor carefully raise the patient while the other nurse supports the head and neck. Slide the back of the vest under the patient and gently lay him down. The doctor then fastens the front of the vest on the patient's chest using Velcro straps.
• The doctor attaches the metal bars to the halo and vest and tightens each bolt in turn, *to avoid tightening any single bolt completely, causing maladjusted tension*. Once halo-vest traction is in place, X-rays should be taken immediately *to check the depth of the skull pins and verify proper alignment*.

To care for the patient
• Take routine and neurologic vital signs at least every 2 hours for 24 hours (preferably every hour for 48 hours) and then every 4 hours until stable. (See *Performing a head-to-toe assessment*, Chapter 1.)
♦ *Nursing alert.* Notify the doctor immediately if you observe any loss of motor function or any decreased sensation, *which could indicate spinal cord trauma.* ♦
• Put on gloves. Gently clean the pin sites every 4 hours with cotton-tipped applicators dipped in cleaning solution. Rinse the sites with sterile water or normal saline solution *to remove any excess cleaning solution*. Then clean the pin sites with povidone-iodine solution or other ordered solution. *Meticulous pin site care prevents infection and removes debris that might block drainage and lead to abscess formation.* Watch for signs of infection—a loose pin, swelling or redness, purulent drainage, pain at the site—and notify the doctor if these signs develop.
• The doctor retightens the skull pins with the torque screwdriver 24 and 48 hours after the halo is applied. If the patient complains of a headache after the pins are tightened, obtain an order for an analgesic. If pain occurs with jaw movement, notify the doctor *because this may indicate that pins have slipped onto the thin temporal plate.*
• Examine the halo-vest unit every shift *to make sure that everything is secure and that the patient's head is centered within the halo*. If the vest fits correctly, you should be able to insert one or two fingers under the jacket at the shoulder and chest when the patient is lying supine.
• Wash the patient's chest and back daily. First, place the patient on his back. Loosen the bottom Velcro straps *so you can get to the chest and back*. Then, reaching under the vest, wash and dry the skin. Check for tender, reddened areas or pressure spots that may develop into ulcers. If necessary, use a hair dryer to dry damp sheepskin *because moisture predisposes the skin to pressure ulcer formation*. Lightly dust the skin with medicated powder or cornstarch *to prevent itching*. If itching persists, check to see if the patient is allergic to sheepskin and if any drug he's taking might cause a skin rash. If the hospital's policy allows, change the vest lining, as necessary.

• Turn the patient on his side (less than 45 degrees) to wash his back. Then close the vest.

• Be careful not to put any stress on the apparatus, *which could knock it out of alignment and lead to subluxation of the cervical spine.*

Special considerations

♦ *Nursing alert.* Keep two conventional wrenches available at all times. In the event of cardiac arrest, use the wrenches to remove the distal anterior bolts. Pull the two upright bars outward. Unfasten the Velcro straps and remove the front of the vest. Use the sturdy back of the vest as a board for cardiopulmonary resuscitation (CPR). *To prevent subluxating the cervical injury,* start CPR with the jaw thrust, which avoids hyperextension of the neck. Pull the patient's mandible forward, while maintaining proper head and neck alignment. *This pulls the tongue forward to open the airway.* ♦

Never lift the patient up by the vertical bars. *This could strain or tear the skin at the pin sites, or misalign the traction.*

To prevent falls, walk with the ambulatory patient. Remember, he'll have trouble seeing objects at or near his feet, and the weight of the halo-vest unit (about 10 pounds) may throw him off balance. If the patient is in a wheelchair, lower the leg rests *to prevent the chair from tipping backward.*

Because the vest limits chest expansion, routinely assess pulmonary function, especially in a patient with pulmonary disease.

Home care

Teach the patient to turn slowly — in small increments — to avoid losing his balance. Remind him to avoid bending forward *because the extra weight of the halo apparatus may cause him to fall.* Teach him to bend at the knees, rather than the waist. Have a physical therapist teach him how to use assistive devices to extend his reach and to help him put on socks and shoes. Suggest wearing shirts or blouses that button in front and that are larger than usual to accommodate the halo-vest.

Most importantly, teach the patient about pin site care and about shampooing and hair care.

Complications

Manipulating the patient's neck during application of halo-vest traction may cause subluxation of the spinal cord, or it could push a bone fragment into the spinal cord, possibly compressing the cord and causing paralysis below the break.

Inaccurate positioning of the skull pins can lead to a puncture of the dura mater, causing a loss of cerebrospinal fluid and a serious central nervous system infec-

tion. Nonsterile technique during application of the halo or inadequate pin site care can also lead to infection at the pin sites. Pressure ulcers can develop if the vest fits poorly or chafes the skin.

Documentation

Record the date and time that the halo-vest traction was applied. Also note the length of the procedure and the patient's response. After application, record routine and neurologic vital signs. Document pin site care and note any signs of infection.

 ## Care of skull tongs

Applying skeletal traction with skull tongs immobilizes the cervical spine after a fracture or dislocation, invasion by tumor or infection, or surgery. Three types of skull tongs are commonly used: Crutchfield, Gardner-Wells, and Vinke. (See *Types of skull tongs,* page 504.) Crutchfield tongs are applied by incising the skin with a scalpel, drilling a hole in the exposed skull, and inserting the pins on the tongs into the hole. Gardner-Wells tongs and Vinke tongs are applied less invasively. Gardner-Wells tongs have spring-loaded pins attached to the tongs. These pins are advanced gently into the scalp. Then the tongs are tightened to secure the apparatus.

Once any tong device is in place, traction is created by extending a rope from the center of the tongs over a pulley and attaching weights to it. With the help of X-ray monitoring, the weights are then adjusted to establish reduction, if necessary, and to maintain alignment. Nursing care of the patient with skull tongs requires meticulous pin site care (three times a day to prevent infection) and frequent observation of the traction apparatus to make sure it's working properly.

Equipment

Three medicine cups ▪ one bottle each of ordered cleaning solution, normal saline solution, and povidone-iodine solution ▪ sterile, cotton-tipped applicators ▪ sandbags or cervical collar (hard or soft) ▪ fine mesh gauze strips ▪ 4″ × 4″ gauze pads ▪ sterile gloves ▪ sterile basin ▪ sterile scissors ▪ hair clippers ▪ optional: turning frame, antibacterial ointment.

Preparation of equipment

Bring the equipment to the patient's room. Place the medicine cups on the bedside table. Fill one cup with a small amount of cleaning solution, one with normal saline solution, and one with povidone-iodine solution. Then set

Types of skull tongs

Skull (or cervical) tongs consist of a stainless steel body with a pin at the end of each arm. Each pin is about ⅛″ (0.3 cm) in diameter with a sharp tip.

On *Crutchfield tongs,* the pins are placed about 5″ (12.7 cm) apart in line with the long axis of the cervical spine.

On *Gardner-Wells tongs,* the pins are farther apart. They are inserted slightly above the patient's ears.

On *Vinke tongs,* the pins are placed at the parietal bones, near the widest transverse diameter of the skull, about 1″ (2.5 cm) above the helix.

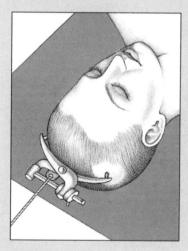 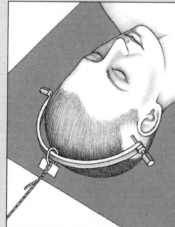 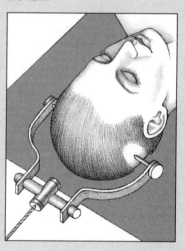

out the cotton-tipped applicators. Keep the sandbags or cervical collar handy for emergency immobilization of the head and neck if the pins in the tongs should slip.

Implementation

• Explain the procedure to the patient. Wash your hands. Inform the patient that pin sites usually feel tender for several days after the tongs are applied. Tell him that he'll also feel some muscular discomfort in the injured area.

• Before providing care, observe each pin site carefully for signs of infection, such as loose pins, swelling or redness, or purulent drainage. Use hair clippers to trim the patient's hair around the pin sites, when necessary, *to facilitate assessment and care.*

• Put on gloves, and gently wipe each pin site with a cotton-tipped applicator dipped in cleaning solution *to loosen and remove crusty drainage.* Repeat with a fresh applicator, as needed, for thorough cleaning. Use a separate applicator for each site *to avoid cross-contamination.*

Next, wipe each site with normal saline solution *to remove excess cleaning solution.* Finally, wipe with povidone-iodine *to provide asepsis at the site and prevent infection.*

• After providing care, discard all pin-site cleaning materials.

• If the pin sites are infected, apply a povidone-iodine wrap, as ordered. First, obtain strips of fine mesh gauze, or cut a 4″ × 4″ gauze pad into strips (using sterile scissors and wearing sterile gloves). Soak the strips in a sterile basin of povidone-iodine solution or normal saline solution, as ordered, and squeeze out the excess solution. Wrap one strip securely around each pin site. Leave the strip in place to dry until you provide care again. *Removing the dried strip aids in debridement and helps clear the infection.*

• Check the traction apparatus—rope, weights, pulleys—at the start of each shift, every 4 hours, and as necessary (for example, after position changes). Make sure the rope hangs freely and that the weights never rest on the floor or become caught under the bed.

Special considerations

Occasionally, the doctor may prefer an antibacterial ointment for pin site care instead of povidone-iodine solution. *To remove old ointment,* wrap a cotton-tipped applicator with a 4″ × 4″ gauze pad, moisten it with cleaning solution, and gently clean each site. Keep a box of sterile gauze pads handy at the patient's bedside.

Watch for signs and symptoms of loose pins, such as persistent pain or tenderness at pin sites, redness, and drainage. The patient may also report feeling or hearing the pins move.

If you suspect a pin has loosened or slipped, don't turn the patient until the doctor examines the skull tongs and fixes them as needed.

If the pins pull out, immobilize the patient's head and neck with sandbags or apply a cervical collar. Then carefully remove the traction weights. Apply manual traction to the patient's head by placing your hands on each side of the mandible and pulling very gently, while maintaining proper alignment. Once you stabilize the alignment, have someone send for the doctor immediately. Remain calm and reassure the patient. Once traction is reestablished, take neurologic vital signs.

♦ *Nursing alert.* Never add or subtract weights to the traction apparatus without an order from the doctor. *This can cause a neurologic impairment.* ♦

Take neurologic vital signs at the beginning of each shift, every 4 hours, and as necessary (for example, after turning or transporting the patient). Carefully assess the function of cranial nerves, *which may be impaired by pin placement.* (See *Performing a head-to-toe assessment,* Chapter 1.) Note any asymmetry, deviation, or atrophy. Review the patient's chart to determine baseline neurologic vital signs on admission to the hospital and immediately after the tongs were applied.

Monitor respirations closely and keep suction equipment handy. Remember, injury to the cervical spine may affect respiration. So be alert for signs of respiratory distress, such as unequal chest expansion and an irregular or altered respiratory rate or pattern.

Patients with skull tongs may be placed on a turning frame *to facilitate turning without disrupting vertebral alignment.* Establish a turning schedule for the patient — usually a supine position for 2 hours and then a prone position for 1 hour — *to help prevent complications of immobility.*

Complications

Infection, excessive tractive force, or osteoporosis can cause the skull pins to slip or pull out. Because this interrupts traction, the patient must receive immediate attention to prevent further injury.

Documentation

Record the date, time, and type of pin site care and the patient's response to the procedure in your notes. Describe any signs of infection. Also, note if any weights were added or subtracted. Record neurologic vital signs, the patient's respiratory status, and the turning schedule on the Kardex.

Pain management

When a patient feels severe pain, he seeks medical help not only because he wants relief but also because he believes the pain signals a serious problem. This perception produces anxiety, which in turn increases the pain. To assess and manage pain properly, the nurse must depend on the patient's subjective description in addition to objective tools.

Several interventions can be used to manage pain. These include analgesics, emotional support, comfort measures, and cognitive techniques to distract the patient. Severe pain usually requires a narcotic analgesic. Invasive measures such as epidural analgesia (see Chapter 5, Drug administration) or patient-controlled analgesia (see Chapter 6, Intravascular therapy) may also be required.

Equipment

Pain assessment tool or scale ▪ oral hygiene supplies ▪ water ▪ nonnarcotic analgesic (such as aspirin or acetaminophen) ▪ optional: patient-controlled analgesia (PCA) device; mild narcotic (such as oxycodone or codeine); strong narcotic (such as methadone, levorphanol, morphine, or hydromorphone).

Implementation

● Explain to the patient how pain medications work together with other pain management therapies to provide relief. Also explain that management aims to keep pain at a low level to permit optimal bodily function.

● Assess the patient's pain by asking key questions and noting his response to the pain. For instance, ask him to describe the duration, severity, and source of his pain. Look for physiologic or behavioral clues to the pain's severity. (See *How to assess pain,* page 506.)

● Develop nursing diagnoses. Appropriate nursing diagnostic categories include pain, anxiety, activity intolerance, fear, potential for injury, knowledge deficit, powerlessness, and self-care deficit.

● Work with the patient to develop a nursing care plan, using interventions appropriate to the patient's life-style.

How to assess pain

To assess pain properly, you'll need to consider the patient's description and your observations of the patient's physical and behavioral responses. Start by asking the following series of key questions (bearing in mind that the patient's responses will be shaped by his prior experiences, self-image, and beliefs about his condition):
• Where is the pain located? How long does it last? How often does it occur?
• What does the pain feel like? (Have the patient describe it.)
• What relieves the pain or makes it worse?
• How do you usually get relief from it?

Ask the patient to rank his pain on a scale of 0 to 10, with 0 denoting lack of pain and 10 denoting the worst pain level. This helps the patient verbally evaluate pain therapies.

Observe the patient's behavioral and physiologic responses to pain. Physiologic responses may be sympathetic or parasympathetic.

Behavioral responses
These include altered body position, moaning, sighing, grimacing, withdrawal, crying, restlessness, muscle twitching, and immobility.

Sympathetic responses
These are commonly associated with mild to moderate pain and include pallor, elevated blood pressure, dilated pupils, skeletal muscle tension, dyspnea, tachycardia, and diaphoresis.

Parasympathetic responses
These are commonly associated with severe, deep pain and include pallor, decreased blood pressure, bradycardia, nausea and vomiting, weakness, dizziness, and loss of consciousness.

Give medications
• If the patient is allowed oral intake, begin with a nonnarcotic analgesic, such as acetaminophen or aspirin every 4 to 6 hours as ordered.
• Then, if the patient needs more relief than a nonnarcotic analgesic provides, you may administer a mild narcotic (such as oxycodone or codeine) as ordered.
• If the patient needs still more pain relief, you may administer a strong narcotic (such as methadone, levorphanol, morphine, or hydromorphone) as prescribed. Administer oral medications if possible. Check the appropriate drug information for each medication you administer.
• If ordered, teach the patient to use a PCA device. *Such a device can help the patient manage his pain and decrease his anxiety.*

Provide emotional support
• Show your concern by spending time talking with the patient. Because of his pain and his inability to manage it, the patient may be anxious and frustrated. Such feelings worsen his pain.

Perform comfort measures
• Periodically reposition the patient *to reduce muscle spasms and tension and to relieve pressure on bony prominences.* Increasing the angle of the bed can reduce the pull on an abdominal incision, diminishing pain. If appropriate, elevate a limb *to reduce swelling, inflammation, and pain.*
• Give the patient a back massage *to help relax tense muscles.*
• Perform passive range-of-motion exercises *to prevent stiffness and further loss of mobility, relax tense muscles, and provide comfort.*
• Provide oral hygiene. Keep a fresh water glass or cup at the bedside. *Many medications tend to dry the mouth.*
• Wash the patient's face and hands.

Use cognitive therapy
• Help the patient enhance the effect of analgesics by using such techniques as distraction, guided imagery, deep breathing, and relaxation. You can easily use these "mind-over-pain" techniques at the bedside. Choose whichever method the patient feels most comfortable with. If possible, start these techniques when the patient feels little or no pain. If he feels persistent pain, begin with short, simple exercises. Before beginning, dim the lights, remove the patient's restrictive clothing, and eliminate noise from the environment.
• For *distraction,* have the patient recall an interesting or pleasant experience or focus his attention on an enjoyable activity. For instance, have him use music as a

These may include prescribed medications, emotional support, comfort measures, cognitive techniques, and education about pain and its management. Emphasize the importance of maintaining good bowel habits, respiratory function, and mobility *because pain may exacerbate any problems in these areas.*
• Implement your care plan. Because individuals respond to pain differently, you'll find that what works for one person may not work for another.

distraction by turning on the radio when the pain begins. Have him close his eyes and concentrate on listening, raising or lowering the volume as his pain increases or subsides. Note, however, that distraction is usually effective only against brief pain episodes lasting less than 5 minutes.

• For *guided imagery,* help the patient concentrate on a peaceful, pleasant image. Encourage him to concentrate on the details of the image he has selected by asking about its sight, sound, smell, taste, and touch. The positive emotions evoked by this exercise minimize pain.

• For *deep breathing,* have the patient stare at an object, then slowly inhale and exhale as he counts aloud to maintain a comfortable rate and rhythm. Have him concentrate on the rise and fall of his abdomen. Encourage him to feel more and more weightless with each breath while he concentrates on the rhythm of his breathing or on any restful image.

• For *muscle relaxation,* have the patient focus on a particular muscle group. Then ask him to tense the muscles and note the sensation. After 5 to 7 seconds, tell him to relax the muscles and concentrate on the relaxed state. Have him note the difference between the tense and relaxed states. After he tenses and relaxes one muscle group, have him proceed to another and another until he's covered his entire body.

Special considerations

Evaluate your patient's response to pain management. If he's still in pain, reassess him and alter your care plan as appropriate.

Remind the patient that results of cognitive therapy techniques improve with practice. Help the patient through the initial sessions.

Remember that patients receiving narcotic analgesics are at risk for developing tolerance, dependence, or addiction. The patient with acute pain may have a smaller risk of dependence or addiction than the patient with chronic pain.

If a patient receiving an opioid analgesic experiences abstinence syndrome when the drug is withdrawn abruptly, suspect physical dependence. The signs and symptoms include anxiety, irritability, chills and hot flashes, excessive salivation and tearing, rhinorrhea, sweating, nausea, vomiting, and seizures. These signs and symptoms are likely to begin in 6 to 12 hours and peak in 24 to 72 hours. To reduce the risk of dependence, discontinue a narcotic by decreasing the dose gradually each day. Also, you may switch to an oral narcotic and decrease its dose gradually.

If a patient becomes addicted, his behavior will be characterized by compulsive drug use and a craving for the drug to experience effects other than pain relief. A patient demonstrating such behavior usually has a preexisting problem that's exacerbated by the narcotic use. Discuss the addicted patient's problem with support personnel, and make appropriate referrals to experts.

During periods of intense pain, the patient's ability to concentrate diminishes. If your patient experiences such pain, help him to select a cognitive technique that's simple to use. Once he selects a particular technique, encourage him to use it consistently.

Complications

The most common adverse effects of analgesics include respiratory depression (the most serious), sedation, constipation, nausea, and vomiting.

Documentation

Document each step of the nursing process. Describe the subjective information you elicited from the patient, using his own words. Note the location, quality, and duration of the pain, as well any precipitating factors.

Record your nursing diagnoses, and include the pain relief method selected. Summarize your actions and the patient's response. If the patient's pain wasn't relieved, note alternate treatments to consider the next time pain occurs. Also record any complications of drug therapy.

Transcutaneous electrical nerve stimulation

Transcutaneous electrical nerve stimulation (TENS) is based on the gate theory of pain, which proposes that painful impulses pass through a "gate" in the brain. TENS is done with a portable, battery-powered device that transmits painless electrical current to peripheral nerves or directly to a painful area over relatively large nerve fibers. This treatment effectively alters the patient's perception of pain by blocking painful stimuli traveling over smaller fibers. Used for patients after surgery and those with chronic pain, a TENS device reduces the need for analgesic drugs and may allow the patient to resume normal activities. (See *Positioning TENS electrodes,* page 508.) Typically, a course of TENS treatments lasts 3 to 5 days. Some conditions, such as phantom limb pain, may require continuous stimulation; other conditions such as a painful arthritic joint require shorter periods (3 to 4 hours).

The TENS device is contraindicated in patients with cardiac pacemakers because it can interfere with pacemaker function. The procedure is also contraindicated

Positioning TENS electrodes

In transcutaneous electrical nerve stimulation (TENS), electrodes placed around peripheral nerves (or an incisional site) transmit mild electrical pulses to the brain. The current is thought to block pain impulses. The patient can influence the level and frequency of his pain relief by adjusting the controls on the device.

Typically, electrode placement varies even though patients may have similar complaints. Electrodes can be placed in several ways:
• to cover the painful area or surround it, as with muscle tenderness or spasm or painful joints

• to "capture" the painful area between electrodes, as with incisional pain

In peripheral nerve injury, electrodes should be placed proximal to the injury (between the brain and the injury site) to avoid increasing pain. Placing electrodes in a hypersensitive area also increases pain. In an area lacking sensation, electrodes should be placed on adjacent dermatomes.

The illustrations show combinations of electrode placement (black squares) and areas of nerve stimulation (shaded red) for low back and leg pain.

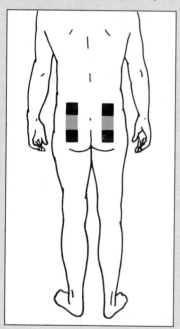
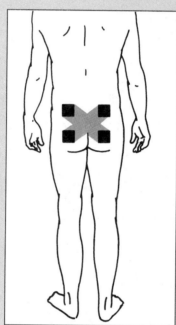
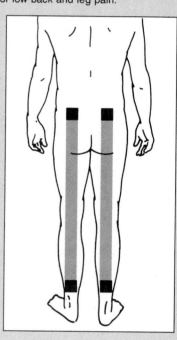

for pregnant patients because its effect on the fetus is unknown. It's also contraindicated in patients who are senile. TENS should be used cautiously in all patients with cardiac disorders. TENS electrodes should not be placed on the head or neck of patients with vascular disorders or seizure disorders. Recent studies have raised questions about the efficacy of TENS treatments.

Equipment
Transcutaneous electrical nerve stimulator ▪ alcohol sponges ▪ electrodes ▪ electrode gel ▪ warm water and

soap ▪ lead wires ▪ charged battery pack ▪ battery recharger ▪ adhesive patch or nonallergenic tape.

Commercial TENS kits are available. They include the stimulator, lead wires, electrodes, spare battery pack, battery recharger, and sometimes the adhesive patch.

Preparation of equipment
Before beginning the procedure, always test the battery pack to make sure it's fully charged.

Implementation

• Wash your hands. Provide privacy. If the patient has never seen a TENS unit before, show him the device and explain the procedure.

Before TENS treatment

• With an alcohol sponge, thoroughly clean the skin where the electrode will be applied. Then dry the skin.
• Apply electrode gel to the bottom of each electrode.
• Place the ordered number of electrodes on the proper skin area, leaving at least 2″ (5 cm) between them. Then secure them with the adhesive patch or nonallergenic tape. Tape all sides evenly *so the electrodes are firmly attached to the skin.*
• Plug the pin connectors into the electrode sockets. *To protect the cords,* hold the connectors — not the cords themselves — during insertion.
• Turn the channel controls to the "off" position or to the position recommended in the operator's manual.
• Plug the lead wires into the jacks in the control box.
• Turn the amplitude and rate dials slowly, as the manual directs. (The patient should feel a tingling sensation.) Then adjust the controls on this device to the prescribed settings or to settings that are most comfortable. Most patients select stimulation frequencies of 60 to 100 Hertz.
• Attach the TENS control box to part of the patient's clothing, such as a belt, pocket, or bra.
• *To make sure the device is working effectively,* monitor the patient for signs of excessive stimulation, such as muscular twitches, or signs of inadequate stimulation, signaled by the patient's inability to feel any mild tingling sensation.

After TENS treatment

• Turn off the controls and unplug the electrode lead wires from the control box.
• If another treatment will be given soon, leave the electrodes in place; if not, remove them.
• Clean the electrodes with soap and water, and clean the patient's skin with alcohol sponges. (Don't soak the electrodes in alcohol *because it will damage the rubber.*)
• Remove the battery pack from the unit and replace it with a charged battery pack.
• Recharge the used battery pack *so it's always ready for use.*

Special considerations

If you must move the electrodes during the procedure, turn off the controls first. Follow the doctor's orders regarding electrode placement and control settings. *Incorrect placement of the electrodes will result in inappropriate pain control. Setting the controls too high can cause pain; setting them too low will fail to relieve pain.* Never place the electrodes near the patient's eyes or over the nerves that innervate the carotid sinus or laryngeal or pharyngeal muscles *to avoid interference with critical nerve function.*

If TENS is used continuously for postoperative pain, remove the electrodes at least daily *to check for skin irritation, and provide skin care.*

If appropriate, let the patient study the operator's manual. Teach him how to place the electrodes properly and how to take care of the TENS unit.

Documentation

On the patient's medical record and the nursing care plan, record the electrode sites and the control settings. Document the patient's tolerance to treatment. Also evaluate pain control.

Selected references

American Association of Neuroscience Nurses. *Neuroscience Nursing: Phenomena and Practice.* Edited by Mitchell, P.H., et al. Norwalk, Conn.: Appleton & Lange, 1988.

Clevenger, V. "Nursing Management of Lumbar Drains," *Journal of Neuroscience Nursing* 22(4):227-31, August 1990.

Friedman, D. "Taking the Scare Out of Caring for Seizure Patients," *Nursing88* 18(2):52-60, February 1988.

Inturrisi, C.E. "Management of Cancer Pain: Pharmacology and Principles of Management," *Cancer* 63(11 Supp.):2308-20, June 1, 1989.

Leppik, I.E. "Status Epilepticus: The Next Decade," *Neurology* 40(5 Supp. 2):4-9, May 1990.

McCaffery, M., and Beebe, A. *Pain: Clinical Manual for Nursing Practice.* St. Louis: C.V. Mosby Co., 1989.

McGuire, L. "Administering Analgesics: Which Drugs Are Right for Your Patient?" *Nursing90* 20(4):34-42, April 1990.

Ropper, A.H., and Kennedy, S.F. *Neurological and Neurosurgical Intensive Care,* 2nd ed. Rockville, Md.: Aspen Pubs., Inc., 1988.

Santilli, N., and Sierzant, T.L. "Advances in the Treatment of Epilepsy," *Journal of Neuroscience Nursing* 19(3):141-57, June 1987.

CHAPTER 10

GASTROINTESTINAL CARE

DANIELE SHOLLENBERGER, RN, MSN

Introduction

Gastrointestinal (GI) conditions affect just about everyone at one time or another. These conditions, so intimately tied to psychological health and stability, range from simple changes in bowel habits to life-threatening disorders requiring major surgery and radical life-style changes.

Just as GI conditions vary widely, so does patient care. For example, the patient with simple constipation may need minimal nursing intervention consisting of brief teaching about diet and exercise. However, the patient with colorectal cancer may need ongoing nursing care ranging from encouragement and support during the diagnostic workup to meticulous colostomy care during recovery.

Your role in GI procedures

Therapeutic GI procedures vary greatly, reflecting the wide spectrum of systemic abnormalities. They may involve feeding a patient through a tube, teaching a patient how to use a gastrostomy feeding button, or minimizing a patient's anxiety before abdominal surgery or his discomfort after it.

To carry out responsibilities like these successfully, you need to address both the emotional and the physical needs of the patient. Where to place an incision or which type of colostomy to use have important emotional implications for the patient. Your knowledge of anatomy and physiology, as well as a familiarity with surgical procedures, influences your plan of care and ultimately how the patient responds.

For some GI procedures, you'll need to provide considerable emotional support, especially if they prove uncomfortable or embarrassing to the patient. Helping the patient undergoing such a procedure to maintain his sense of dignity, while at the same time eliciting his cooperation, requires a skillful blend of compassion and judgment.

For many GI procedures, you'll need to work cooperatively with staff, including the pharmacist, doctors, laboratory personnel, diagnostic technicians, dietitians, and others.

NASAL AND ORAL ACCESS
Nasogastric tube insertion and removal

Usually inserted to decompress the stomach, a nasogastric (NG) tube can prevent vomiting after major surgery. Normally, the patient has the tube for 48 to 72 hours after surgery, by which time peristalsis usually resumes. An NG tube may remain in place for shorter or longer periods, however, depending on its use.

The NG tube has other diagnostic and therapeutic applications, especially in assessing and treating upper GI bleeding, collecting gastric contents for analysis, performing gastric lavage, aspirating gastric secretions, and administering medications and nutrients.

Inserting an NG tube requires close observation of the patient and verification of proper placement. Removing the tube requires careful handling to prevent injury or aspiration. The tube must be inserted with extra care in pregnant patients and in those with an increased risk of complications. For example, the doctor will order an NG tube for a patient with aortic aneurysm, myocardial infarction, gastric hemorrhage, or esophageal varices only if he believes that the benefits outweigh the risks of intubation.

Most NG tubes have a radiopaque marker or strip at the distal end so that the tube's position can be verified by X-ray studies. If the position can't be confirmed, the doctor may order fluoroscopy to verify placement.

The most common NG tubes are the Levin tube, which has one lumen, and the Salem sump tube, which has two lumens, one for suction and drainage and a smaller one for ventilation. Air flows through the vent lumen continuously. This protects the delicate gastric mucosa by preventing a vacuum from forming should the tube adhere to the stomach lining. (See *Types of NG tubes,* page 512.) The Moss tube, which has a triple lumen, is usually inserted during surgery.

Equipment

For inserting an NG tube: tube (usually #14, #16, or #18 French for a normal adult) ■ towel or linen-saver pad ■ facial tissues ■ emesis basin ■ penlight ■ 1″ or 2″ nonallergenic tape ■ gloves ■ water-soluble lubricant ■ cup or glass of water with straw (if appropriate) ■ stethoscope ■ tongue blade ■ catheter-tip or bulb syringe or irrigation set ■ safety pin ■ ordered suction equipment ■ optional: metal clamp, ice, warm water, large basin or plastic container, rubber band.

Types of NG tubes

The doctor will choose the type and diameter of nasogastric (NG) tube that best suits the patient's needs, including lavage, aspiration, enteral therapy, or stomach decompression. Common choices include the Levin, Salem sump, and Moss tubes.

Levin tube

This rubber or plastic tube has a single lumen, a length of 42" to 50" (107 to 127 cm), and holes at the tip and along the side.

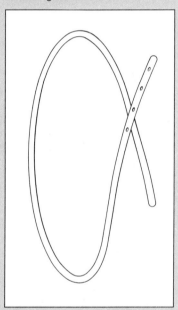

Salem sump tube

This double lumen tube is made of clear plastic and has a blue sump port (pigtail) that allows atmospheric air to enter the patient's stomach. Thus, the tube floats freely and doesn't adhere to or damage gastric mucosa. The larger port of this 48" (122-cm) tube serves as the main suction conduit. The tube has openings at the sides and the tip; markings at 45, 55, 65, and 75 cm; and a radiopaque line to verify placement.

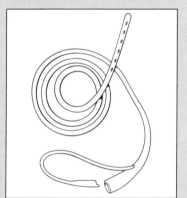

Moss tube

This tube has a radiopaque tip and three lumens. The first, positioned and inflated at the cardia, serves as a balloon inflation port. The second is an esophageal aspiration port. The third is a duodenal feeding port.

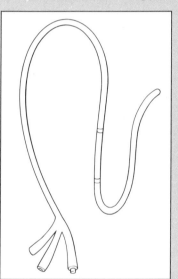

For removing an NG tube: stethoscope ▪ catheter-tip syringe ▪ normal saline solution ▪ towel or linen-saver pad ▪ adhesive remover ▪ optional: clamp.

Preparation of equipment

Inspect the NG tube for defects, such as rough edges or partially closed lumens. Then, check the tube's patency by flushing it with water. *To ease insertion,* increase a stiff tube's flexibility by coiling it around your gloved fingers for a few seconds or by dipping it into warm water. Stiffen a limp tube by briefly chilling it in ice.

Implementation

• Whether you're inserting or removing an NG tube, be sure to provide privacy and wash and glove your hands before inserting the tube.

To insert an NG tube

• Explain the procedure to the patient *to ease anxiety and promote cooperation.* Inform her that she may experience some nasal discomfort, that she may gag, and that her eyes may water. Emphasize that swallowing will ease the tube's advancement.

• Agree on a signal that the patient can use if she wants you to stop briefly during the procedure.

• Gather and prepare all necessary equipment.

• Help the patient into high Fowler's position unless contraindicated.
• Stand at the patient's right side if you're right-handed or at her left side if you're left-handed *to ease insertion.*
• Drape the towel or linen-saver pad over the patient's chest *to protect her gown and bed linens from spills.*
• Have the patient gently blow her nose *to clear her nostrils.*
• Place the facial tissues and emesis basin well within the patient's reach.
• Help the patient face forward with her neck in a neutral position.
• *To determine how long the NG tube must be to reach the stomach,* hold the end of the tube at the tip of the patient's nose. Extend the tube to the patient's earlobe and then down to the xiphoid process.

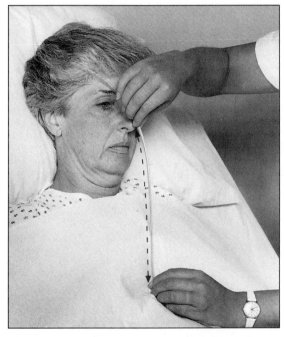

• Mark this distance on the tubing with the tape. (Average measurements for an adult range from 22″ to 26″ [56 to 66 cm].)
• *To determine which nostril will allow easier access,* use a penlight and inspect for a deviated septum or other abnormalities. Ask the patient if she ever had nasal surgery or a nasal injury. Assess airflow in both nostrils by occluding one nostril at a time while the patient breathes through her nose. Choose the nostril with the better airflow.

• Lubricate the first 3″ (7.6 cm) of the tube with a water-soluble gel *to minimize injury to the nasal passages. Using a water-soluble lubricant prevents lipoid pneumonia that may result from aspirating an oil-based lubricant or from accidental slippage of the tube into the trachea.*
• Instruct the patient to hold her head straight and upright.
• Grasp the tube with the end pointing downward, curve it if necessary, and carefully insert it into the more patent nostril.

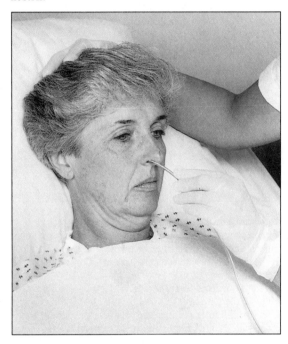

• Aim the tube downward and toward the ear closer to the chosen nostril. Advance it slowly *to avoid pressure on the turbinates and resultant pain and bleeding.*
• When the tube reaches the nasopharynx, you'll feel resistance. Instruct the patient to lower her head slightly *to close the trachea and open the esophagus.* Then, rotate the tube 180 degrees toward the opposite nostril *to redirect it so that the tube won't enter the patient's mouth.*
• Unless contraindicated, offer the patient a cup or glass of water with a straw. Direct her to sip and swallow as you slowly advance the tube (top left, page 514). *This helps the tube pass to the esophagus.* (If you aren't using water, ask the patient to swallow.)

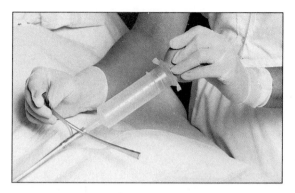

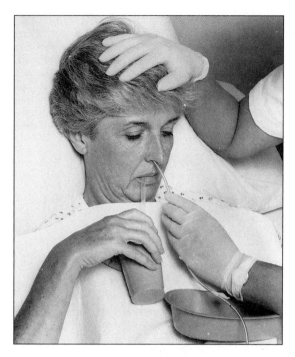

To ensure proper tube placement

• Use a tongue blade and penlight to examine the patient's mouth and throat for signs of a coiled section of tubing (especially in an unconscious patient). Coiling indicates an obstruction.

• Keep an emesis basin and facial tissues readily available for the patient.

• As you carefully advance the tube and the patient swallows, watch for respiratory distress signs, *which may mean the tube is in the bronchus and must be removed immediately.*

• Stop advancing the tube when the tape mark reaches the patient's nostril.

• Attach a catheter-tip or bulb syringe to the tube and try to aspirate stomach contents. If you do not obtain stomach contents, position the patient on her left side *to move the contents into the stomach's greater curvature*, and aspirate again (see illustration above at right).

Note: When confirming tube placement, never place the tube's end in a container of water. *If the tube should be mispositioned in the trachea, the patient may aspirate water.* Besides, water without bubbles does not confirm proper placement. *Instead, the tube may be coiled in the trachea or the esophagus.*

• If you still can't aspirate stomach contents, advance the tube 1″ to 2″ (2.5 to 5 cm). Then inject 10 cc of air into the tube. At the same time, auscultate for air sounds with your stethoscope placed over the epigastric region. *You should hear a whooshing sound if the tube is patent and properly positioned in the stomach.*

• If these tests don't confirm proper tube placement, you'll need X-ray verification.

• Secure the NG tube to the patient's nose with nonallergenic tape (or other designated tube holder). You will need about 4″ (10 cm) of 1″ tape. Split one end of the tape up the center about 1½″ (3.8 cm). Make tabs on the split ends (by folding sticky sides together). Stick the uncut tape end on the patient's nose so that the split in the tape starts about ½″ (1.3 cm) to 1½″ from the tip of her nose. Crisscross the tabbed ends around the tube. Then apply another piece of tape over the bridge of the nose to secure the tube.

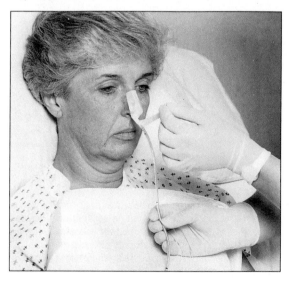

• Alternatively, stabilize the tube with a prepackaged product that secures and cushions it at the nose.

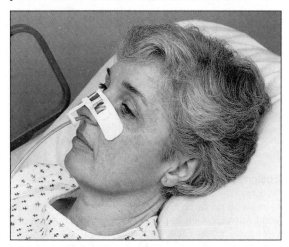

• *To reduce discomfort from the weight of the tube,* tie a slip knot around the tube with a rubber band, and then secure the rubber band to the patient's gown with a safety pin, or wrap another piece of tape around the end of the tube and leave a tab. Then fasten the tape tab to the patient's gown with a safety pin.
• Attach the tube to suction equipment, if ordered, and set the designated suction pressure.

To remove an NG tube
• Explain the procedure to the patient, informing her that it may cause some nasal discomfort and sneezing or gagging.
• Assess bowel function by auscultating for peristalsis or flatus.
• Help the patient into semi-Fowler's position. Then drape a towel or linen-saver pad across her chest *to protect her gown and bed linens from spills.*
• Using a catheter-tip syringe, flush the tube with 10 ml of normal saline solution *to ensure that the tube doesn't contain stomach contents that could irritate tissues during tube removal.*
• Untape the tube from the patient's nose, and then unpin it from her gown.
• Clamp the tube by folding it in your hand.
• Ask the patient to hold her breath *to close the epiglottis.* Then withdraw the tube gently and steadily. (When the distal end of the tube reaches the nasopharynx, you can pull it quickly.)
• When possible, immediately cover and remove the tube *because its sight and odor may nauseate the patient.*

• Assist the patient with thorough mouth care, and clean the tape residue from her nose with adhesive remover.
• For the next 48 hours, monitor the patient for signs of GI dysfunction, including nausea, vomiting, abdominal distention, and food intolerance. GI dysfunction may necessitate reinsertion of the tube.

Special considerations
A helpful device for calculating the correct tube length is Ross-Hanson tape. Place the narrow end of this measuring tape at the tip of the patient's nose. Again, extend the tape to the patient's earlobe and down to the tip of the xiphoid process. Mark this distance on the edge of the tape labeled "nose to ear to xiphoid." The corresponding measurement on the opposite edge of the tape is the proper insertion length.

If the patient has a deviated septum or other nasal condition that prevents nasal insertion, pass the tube orally after removing any dentures, if necessary. Sliding the tube over the tongue, proceed as you would for nasal insertion.

When using the oral route, remember to coil the end of the tube around your hand. *This helps curve and direct the tube downward at the pharynx.*

If your patient lies unconscious, tilt her chin toward her chest *to close the trachea.* Then advance the tube between respirations *to ensure that it doesn't enter the trachea.*

While advancing the tube in an unconscious patient (or in a patient who can't swallow), stroke the patient's neck *to encourage the swallowing reflex and to facilitate passage down the esophagus.*

While advancing the tube, observe for signs that it has entered the trachea, such as choking or breathing difficulties in a conscious patient and cyanosis in an unconscious patient or a patient without a cough reflex. If these signs occur, remove the tube immediately. Allow the patient time to rest; then try to reinsert the tube.

After tube placement, vomiting suggests tubal obstruction or incorrect position. Assess immediately to determine the cause.

Home care
An NG tube may be inserted or removed at home. Indications for insertion include gastric decompression and short-term feeding. A home care nurse or the patient may insert the tube, deliver the feeding, and remove the tube. See *Using an NG tube at home,* page 516.

Complications
Potential complications of prolonged intubation with an NG tube include skin erosion at the nostril, sinusitis, esophagitis, esophagotracheal fistula, gastric ulceration,

Using an NG tube at home

If your patient will need to have a nasogastric (NG) tube in place at home — for short-term feeding or gastric decompression, for example — find out who will insert the tube. If the patient will have a home care nurse, identify her and, if possible, tell the patient when to expect her.

If the patient or a family member will perform the procedure, you'll need to provide additional instruction and supervision. Use this checklist to assemble your teaching topics:

☐ how and where to obtain equipment needed for home intubation
☐ how to insert the tube
☐ verifying tube placement by aspirating stomach contents
☐ correcting tube misplacement
☐ preparing formula for tube feeding
☐ how to store formula, if appropriate
☐ administering formula through the tube
☐ how to remove and dispose of an NG tube
☐ how to clean and store a reusable NG tube
☐ how to use the NG tube for gastric decompression, if appropriate
☐ how to set up and operate suctioning equipment
☐ troubleshooting suctioning equipment
☐ how to perform mouth care and other hygienic procedures.

and pulmonary and oral infection. Additional complications that may result from suction include electrolyte imbalances and dehydration.

Documentation
Record the type and size of the NG tube and the date, time, and route of insertion. Also note the type and amount of suction, if used, and describe the drainage, including the amount, color, character, consistency, and odor. Note the patient's tolerance of the procedure. When you remove the tube, make sure to record the date and time. Describe the color, consistency, and amount of gastric drainage. Again, note the patient's tolerance of the procedure.

Nasogastric tube care

Providing effective nasogastric (NG) tube care requires meticulous monitoring of the patient and the equipment. Monitoring the patient involves checking drainage from the NG tube and assessing GI function. Monitoring the equipment involves verifying correct tube placement and irrigating the tube to ensure patency and to prevent mucosal damage.

Specific care varies only slightly for the most commonly used NG tubes: the single-lumen Levin tube and the double-lumen Salem sump tube.

Equipment
Irrigant (usually normal saline solution) ▪ irrigant container ▪ 60-ml catheter-tip syringe ▪ bulb syringe ▪ suction apparatus ▪ lemon-glycerin swabs or toothbrush and toothpaste ▪ petroleum jelly ▪ 1½″ or 1″ nonallergenic tape ▪ water-soluble lubricant ▪ gloves ▪ stethoscope ▪ linen-saver pad ▪ optional: emesis basin.

Preparation of equipment
Make sure the suction equipment works properly. (See *Common gastric suction devices*.) When using a Salem sump tube with suction, connect the larger, primary lumen (for drainage and suction) to the suction equipment and select the appropriate setting, as ordered (usually low constant suction). If the doctor doesn't specify the setting, follow the manufacturer's directions. A Levin tube usually calls for intermittent low suction.

Implementation
• Explain the procedure to the patient and provide privacy.
• Wash your hands and put on gloves.

To irrigate the NG tube
• Review the irrigation schedule (usually every 4 hours), if the doctor orders this procedure.
• Inject 10 cc of air and auscultate the epigastric area with a stethoscope and aspirate stomach contents *to check correct positioning in the stomach and to prevent the patient from aspirating the irrigant.*
• Measure the amount of irrigant in the bulb syringe or in the 60-ml catheter-tip syringe (usually 30 ml) *to maintain an accurate intake and output record.*
• When using suction with a Salem sump tube or a Levin tube, unclamp and disconnect the tube from the suction equipment while holding it over a linen-saver pad or an emesis basin *to collect any drainage.*

Common gastric suction devices

A variety of portable or wall-mounted suction devices are available for applying negative pressure to nasogastric (NG) and other drainage tubes. Two common types are shown here.

Portable suction machine
In the portable suction machine, a vacuum created intermittently by an electric pump draws gastric contents up the NG tube and into the collecting bottle.

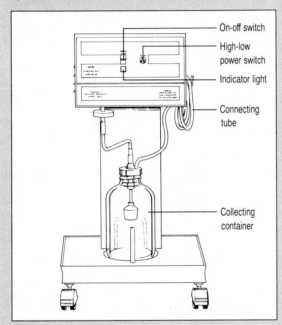

- On-off switch
- High-low power switch
- Indicator light
- Connecting tube
- Collecting container

Stationary suction machine
A stationary wall-unit apparatus can provide intermittent or continuous suction. On-off switches and variable power settings let you set and adjust the suction force on either machine.

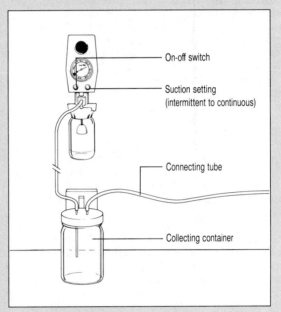

- On-off switch
- Suction setting (intermittent to continuous)
- Connecting tube
- Collecting container

• Slowly instill the irrigant into the NG tube. (When irrigating the Salem sump tube, you may instill small amounts of solution into the vent lumen without interrupting suction; however, you should instill greater amounts into the larger, primary lumen.)
• Gently aspirate the solution with the bulb syringe or 60-ml catheter-tip syringe or connect the tube to the suction equipment, as ordered. *Gentle aspiration prevents excessive pressure on a suture line and on delicate gastric mucosa.*
• Reconnect the tube to suction after completing irrigation.

To instill a solution through the NG tube
• If the doctor orders *instillation,* inject the solution, and do not aspirate it. Note the amount of instilled solution as "intake" on the intake and output record.
• Reattach the tube to suction as ordered.
• After attaching the Salem sump tube's primary lumen to suction, instill 10 to 20 cc of air into the vent lumen *to verify patency.* Listen for a soft hiss in the vent. If you don't hear this sound, suspect a clogged tube; recheck patency by instilling 10 ml of normal saline solution and 10 to 20 cc of air in the vent.

To monitor patient comfort and condition
• Provide mouth care once a shift or as needed. Depending on the patient's condition, use lemon-glycerin swabs

to clean his teeth or assist him to brush them with toothbrush and toothpaste. Coat the patient's lips with petroleum jelly *to prevent dryness from mouth breathing.*

• Change the tape securing the tube as needed or at least daily. Clean the skin, apply fresh tape, and dab water-soluble lubricant on the nostrils as needed.

• Regularly check the tape that secures the tube *because sweat and nasal secretions may loosen the tape.*

• Assess bowel sounds regularly (every 4 to 8 hours) *to verify GI function.*

• Measure the drainage amount and update the intake and output record every 8 hours. Be alert for electrolyte imbalances with excessive gastric output.

• Inspect gastric drainage. Note color, consistency, odor, and amount. Normal gastric secretions have no color or appear yellow-green from bile and have a mucoid consistency. Immediately report any drainage with a coffee-bean color. *This may indicate bleeding.* If you suspect that the drainage contains blood, use a screening test (such as Hematest) for occult blood according to your hospital's protocol.

Special considerations

Irrigate the NG tube with 30 ml of irrigant before and after instilling medication. (See "Instillation of drugs through a nasogastric tube," Chapter 5.) Wait about 30 minutes, or as ordered, after instillation before reconnecting the suction equipment *to allow sufficient time for the medication to be absorbed.*

When no drainage appears, check the suction equipment for proper function. Then, holding the NG tube over a linen-saver pad or an emesis basin, separate the tube and the suction source. Check the suction equipment by placing the suction tubing in an irrigant container. If the apparatus draws the water, check the NG tube for proper function. Be sure to note the amount of water drawn into the suction container on the intake and output record.

A dysfunctional NG tube may be clogged or incorrectly positioned. Attempt to irrigate the tube, reposition the patient, or rotate and reposition the tube. However, if the tube was inserted during surgery, avoid this maneuver *to ensure that the movement doesn't interfere with gastric or esophageal sutures.* Notify the doctor.

If you can ambulate the patient and interrupt suction, disconnect the NG tube from the suction equipment. Clamp the tube *to prevent stomach contents from draining out of the tube.*

If the patient has a Salem sump tube, watch for gastric reflux in the vent lumen when pressure in the stomach exceeds atmospheric pressure. This problem may result from a clogged primary lumen or from a suction system that's set up improperly. Assess the suction equipment for proper functioning. Then, irrigate the NG tube and

instill 30 cc of air into the vent tube *to maintain patency.* Don't attempt to stop reflux by clamping the vent tube. Unless contraindicated, elevate the patient's torso more than 30 degrees, and keep the vent tube above his midline *to prevent a siphoning effect.*

Complications

Epigastric pain and vomiting may result from a clogged or improperly placed tube. Any NG tube — the Levin tube in particular — may move and aggravate esophagitis, ulcers, or esophageal varices, causing hemorrhage. Perforation may result from aggressive intubation. Dehydration and electrolyte imbalances may result from removing body fluids and electrolytes by suctioning. Pain, swelling, and salivary dysfunction may signal parotitis, which occurs in dehydrated, debilitated patients. Intubation can cause nasal skin breakdown and discomfort and increased mucous secretions. Aspiration pneumonia may result from gastric reflux. Vigorous suction may damage the gastric mucosa and cause significant bleeding, possibly interfering with endoscopic assessment and diagnosis.

Documentation

Regularly record tube placement confirmation (usually every 4 to 8 hours). Keep a precise record of fluid intake and output, including the instilled irrigant in fluid input. Track the irrigation schedule and note the actual time of each irrigation. Describe drainage color, consistency, odor, and amount. Also note tape change times and condition of the nares.

Gastric lavage

After poisoning or a drug overdose, especially in patients who have central nervous system depression or an inadequate gag reflex, gastric lavage flushes the stomach and removes ingested substances through a nasogastric (NG) tube. For patients with gastric or esophageal bleeding, lavage with tepid or iced water or normal saline solution may be used to stop bleeding. However, some controversy exists over the effectiveness of iced lavage for this purpose. (See *Is iced lavage effective?*) Typically, this procedure is done in the emergency department or intensive care unit by a doctor, gastroenterologist, or a nurse, although the wide-bore lavage tube is almost always inserted by the gastroenterologist.

Gastric lavage is contraindicated after ingestion of a corrosive substance (such as lye, ammonia, or mineral acids) because the NG tube may perforate the already compromised esophagus.

Correct NG tube placement is essential for patient safety because accidental misplacement (in the lungs, for example) followed by lavage can be fatal. Other complications of gastric lavage include bradyarrhythmias and aspiration of gastric fluids.

Equipment

Lavage setup (two graduated containers for drainage, three pieces of large-lumen rubber tubing, Y connector, and a clamp or hemostat) ■ 2 to 3 liters of normal saline solution or tap water, as ordered ■ I.V. pole ■ basin of ice, if ordered ■ Ewald tube or any large-lumen gastric tube, typically #36 to #40 French (see *Using wide-bore gastric tubes,* page 520) ■ water-soluble lubricant or anesthetic ointment ■ stethoscope ■ ½″ nonallergenic tape ■ 50-ml bulb or catheter-tip syringe ■ gloves ■ linen-saver pad or towel ■ Yankauer or tonsil-tip suction device ■ suction apparatus ■ labeled specimen container ■ laboratory request form ■ norepinephrine ■ optional: patient restraints, charcoal tablets.

A prepackaged, syringe-type irrigation kit may be used for lavage. For poisoning or a drug overdose, however, the lavage setup may be more appropriate to use *because it's a faster and more effective means of diluting and removing the harmful substance.*

Preparation of equipment

Set up the lavage equipment. (See *Preparing for gastric lavage,* page 521.)

If iced lavage is ordered, chill the desired irrigant (water or normal saline solution) in a basin of ice.

Lubricate the end of the NG tube with the water-soluble lubricant or anesthetic ointment.

Implementation

• Explain the procedure to the patient, provide privacy, and wash your hands.
• Put on gloves.
• Drape the towel or linen-saver pad over the patient's chest *to protect him from spills.*
• The doctor inserts the NG tube nasally and advances it slowly and gently *because forceful insertion may injure tissues and cause epistaxis.* He then checks the tube's placement by injecting about 30 cc of air into the tube with the bulb syringe and then auscultating the patient's abdomen with a stethoscope. If the tube is in place, he'll hear the sound of air entering the stomach.
• *Because the patient may vomit when the NG tube reaches the posterior pharynx during insertion,* be prepared to suction the airway immediately with either a Yankauer or a tonsil-tip suction device.

Is iced lavage effective?

Some experts question the effectiveness of using an iced irrigant for gastric lavage to treat GI bleeding. Here's why.

Iced irrigating solutions stimulate the vagus nerve, which triggers increased hydrochloric acid secretion. In turn, this stimulates gastric motility, which can irritate the bleeding site.

Some clinicians prefer using unchilled normal saline solution (which may prevent rapid electrolyte loss) or even water if the patient must avoid sodium. These clinicians point out that no research exists to support the use of iced irrigant to stop acute GI bleeding.

• Once the NG tube passes the posterior pharynx, assist the patient into Trendelenburg's position and turn him toward his left side in a three-quarter prone posture. *This position minimizes passage of gastric contents into the duodenum and may prevent the patient from aspirating vomitus.*
• After securing the NG tube nasally or orally and making sure the irrigant inflow tube on the lavage setup is clamped, connect the unattached end of this tube to the NG tube. Allow the stomach contents to empty into the drainage container before instilling any irrigant. *This confirms proper tube placement and decreases the risk of overfilling the stomach with irrigant and inducing vomiting.* If you're using a syringe irrigation set, aspirate stomach contents with a 50-ml bulb or catheter-tip syringe before instilling the irrigant.
• Once you confirm proper tube placement, begin gastric lavage by instilling about 250 ml of irrigant *to assess the patient's tolerance and prevent vomiting.* If you're using a syringe, instill about 50 ml of solution at a time until you've instilled between 250 and 500 ml.
• Clamp the inflow tube and unclamp the outflow tube *to allow the irrigant to flow out.* If you're using the syringe irrigation kit, aspirate the irrigant with the syringe and empty it into a calibrated container. Measure the outflow amount to be sure that it at least equals the amount of irrigant you instilled. *This prevents accidental stomach distention and vomiting.* If the drainage amount falls significantly short of the instilled amount, reposition the tube until sufficient solution flows out. Gently massage the abdomen over the stomach to promote outflow.
• Repeat the inflow-outflow cycle until returned fluids appear clear. *This signals that the stomach no longer holds harmful substances or that bleeding has stopped.*

Using wide-bore gastric tubes

If you need to deliver a large volume of fluid rapidly through a gastric tube (when irrigating the stomach of a patient with profuse gastric bleeding or poisoning, for example), a wide-bore gastric tube usually serves best. Typically inserted orally, these tubes remain in place only long enough to complete the lavage and evacuate stomach contents.

Ewald tube

In an emergency, using this single-lumen tube with several openings at the distal end allows you to aspirate large amounts of gastric contents quickly.

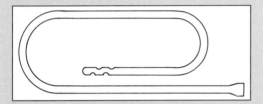

Levacuator tube

This tube has two lumens. Use the larger lumen for evacuating gastric contents; the smaller, for instilling an irrigant.

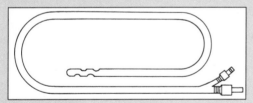

Edlich tube

This single-lumen tube has four openings near the closed distal tip. A funnel or syringe may be connected at the proximal end. Like the Ewald tube, the Edlich tube lets you withdraw large quantities of gastric contents quickly.

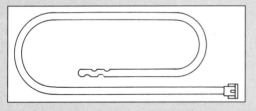

• Assess the patient's vital signs, urine output, and level of consciousness (LOC) every 15 minutes. Notify the doctor of any changes.
• If ordered, remove the NG tube.

Special considerations

To control GI bleeding, the doctor may order continuous irrigation of the stomach with an irrigant and a vasoconstrictor, such as norepinephrine. After the stomach absorbs norepinephrine, the portal system delivers the drug directly to the liver, where it's metabolized. *This prevents the drug from circulating systemically and initiating a hypertensive response.* Or the doctor may use an alternate drug-delivery method, directing you to clamp the outflow tube for a prescribed period after instilling the irrigant and the vasoconstrictive medication and before withdrawing it. *This allows the mucosa time to absorb the drug.*

Never leave a patient alone during gastric lavage. Observe continuously for any changes in his LOC, and monitor vital signs frequently *because the natural vagal response to intubation can depress the patient's heart rate.*

If you need to restrain the patient, secure restraints on the same side of the bed or stretcher *so that you can free them quickly without moving to the other side of the bed.* Avoid restraining the patient in a "spread eagle" position, *which would prevent him from turning and leave him at risk for aspirating vomitus.*

Remember also to keep tracheal suctioning equipment nearby and watch closely for airway obstruction caused by vomiting or excess oral secretions. Throughout gastric lavage, you may need to suction the oral cavity frequently *to ensure an open airway and prevent aspiration.* For the same reasons, and if he doesn't exhibit an adequate gag reflex, the patient may require an endotracheal tube before the procedure.

When aspirating the stomach for ingested poisons or drugs, be sure to save the contents in a labeled container to send to the laboratory for analysis. If ordered, after lavage to remove poisons or drugs, mix charcoal tablets with the irrigant (whether it's water or normal saline solution) and administer the mixture through the NG tube. The charcoal will absorb remaining toxic substances. The tube may be clamped temporarily, allowed to drain via gravity, attached to intermittent suction, or removed.

When performing gastric lavage to stop bleeding, keep precise intake and output records *to determine the amount of bleeding.* When the patient has large volumes of fluid instilled and withdrawn, serum electrolyte or arterial blood gas levels (or both) may be measured during or at the end of lavage.

Complications

Vomiting and subsequent aspiration, the most common complication of gastric lavage, occurs more often in a groggy patient. Bradyarrhythmias also may occur. After iced lavage especially, the patient's body temperature may drop, thereby triggering cardiac arrhythmias.

Documentation

Record the date and time of lavage; the size and type of NG tube used; the volume and type of irrigant; and the amount of drained gastric contents. Record this information on the intake and output record sheet, and include your observations, noting, for example, color and consistency of drainage. Also keep precise records of the patient's vital signs and LOC, any drugs instilled through the tube, the time the tube was removed, and how well the patient tolerated the procedure.

 Feeding tube insertion and removal

Inserting a feeding tube nasally or (sometimes) orally into the stomach or duodenum allows a patient who can't or won't eat to receive nourishment. The feeding tube also permits supplemental feedings in a patient who has exceptionally high nutritional requirements — an unconscious patient or one with extensive burns, for example. Typically, the procedure is done by a nurse, as ordered. The preferred feeding tube route is nasal, but the oral route may be used for patients with such conditions as a deviated septum or a head or nose injury.

The doctor may order duodenal feeding when the patient can't tolerate gastric feeding or when he expects gastric feeding to produce aspiration. Absence of bowel sounds or possible intestinal obstruction contraindicates using a feeding tube.

Feeding tubes differ somewhat from standard nasogastric tubes. Made of silicone, rubber, or polyurethane, feeding tubes have small diameters and great flexibility. This reduces oropharyngeal irritation, necrosis from pressure on the tracheoesophageal wall, distal esophageal irritation, and discomfort from swallowing. To facilitate passage, some feeding tubes are weighted with tungsten, and some need a guide wire to keep them from curling in the back of the throat.

These small-bore tubes usually have radiopaque markings and a water-activated coating, which provides a lubricated surface.

 ## Preparing for gastric lavage

Prepare the lavage setup as follows:
• Connect one of the three pieces of large-lumen tubing to the irrigant container.
• Insert the Y connector stem in the other end of the tubing.
• Connect the remaining two pieces of tubing to the free ends of the Y connector.
• Place the unattached end of one of the tubes into one of the drainage containers. (Later, you'll connect the other piece of tubing to the patient's gastric tube.)
• Clamp the tube leading to the irrigant.
• Suspend the entire setup from the I.V. pole, hanging the irrigant container at the highest level.

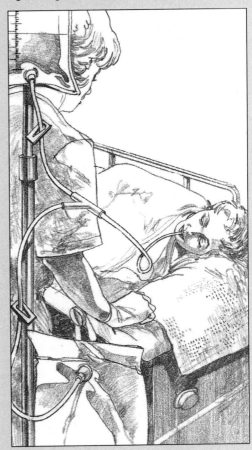

Equipment

For insertion: feeding tube (#6 to #18 French, with or without guide) ■ linen-saver pad ■ gloves ■ nonallergenic tape ■ water-soluble lubricant ■ cotton-tipped applicators ■ skin preparation (such as tincture of benzoin) ■ facial tissues ■ penlight ■ small cup of water with straw, or ice chips ■ emesis basin ■ 60-ml syringe ■ stethoscope.

    During use: mouthwash or saltwater solution ■ toothbrush.

    For removal: linen-saver pad ■ tube clamp ■ bulb syringe.

Preparation of equipment

Have the proper size tube available. Usually, the doctor orders the smallest-bore tube that will allow free passage of the liquid feeding formula. Read the instructions on the tubing package carefully *because tube characteristics vary according to the manufacturer.* (For example, some tubes have marks at the appropriate lengths for gastric, duodenal, and jejunal insertion.)

    Examine the tube *to make sure it's free of defects, such as cracks or rough or sharp edges.* Next, run water through the tube. *This checks for patency, activates the coating, and allows for easier removal of the guide.*

Implementation

● Explain the procedure to the patient and show him the tube *so he knows what to expect and can cooperate more fully.*
● Provide privacy and wash your hands. Put on gloves.
● Assist the patient into semi-Fowler's (or high Fowler's) position.
● Place a linen-saver pad across the patient's chest *to protect him from spills.*
● *To determine the tube length needed to reach the stomach,* first extend the distal end of the tube from the tip of the patient's nose to his earlobe. Coil this portion of the tube around your fingers *so the end will remain curved until you insert it.* Then extend the uncoiled portion from the earlobe to the xiphoid process. Use a small piece of nonallergenic tape to mark the total length of these two portions.

To insert the tube nasally

● Using the penlight, assess nasal patency. Inspect nasal passages for a deviated septum, polyps, or other obstructions. As the patient breathes through his nose, occlude one nostril, then the other, *to determine which has the better airflow.* Assess the patient's history of nasal injury or surgery.
● Lubricate the curved tip of the tube (and the feeding tube guide, if appropriate) with a small amount of water-soluble lubricant *to ease insertion and prevent tissue injury.*

● Ask the patient to hold the emesis basin and facial tissues in case he needs them.
● *To advance the tube,* insert the curved, lubricated tip into the more patent nostril and direct it along the nasal passage toward the ear on the same side. When it passes the nasopharyngeal junction, turn the tube 180 degrees *to aim it downward into the esophagus* and advance it. Then, give him a small cup of water with a straw, or ice chips. Direct him to sip the water or suck on the ice and swallow frequently, without clamping his teeth down on the tube. *This will ease the tube's passage.* Advance the tube as he swallows.

To insert the tube orally

● Have the patient lower his chin *to close his trachea,* and ask him to open his mouth.
● Place the tip of the tube at the back of the patient's tongue, give water, and instruct the patient to swallow, as above.

To position the tube

● Keep passing the tube until the tape marking the appropriate length reaches the patient's nostril or lips.
● *To check tube placement,* attach the syringe filled with 10 cc of air to the end of the tube. Gently inject the air into the tube as you auscultate the patient's abdomen with the stethoscope about 3″ (7.6 cm) below the sternum. Listen for a whooshing sound, *which signals that the tube reached its target in the stomach.* If the tube remains coiled in the esophagus, you'll feel resistance when you inject the air, or the patient may belch.
● If you hear the whooshing sound, gently try to aspirate gastric secretions. Successful aspiration confirms correct tube placement. If no gastric secretions return, the tube may be in the esophagus. You'll need to advance the tube or reinsert it before proceeding.
● After confirming proper tube placement, remove the tape marking the tube length.
● Tape the tube to the patient's nose and remove the guide wire. *Note:* In some cases, X-rays may be ordered to verify tube placement.
● *To advance the tube to the duodenum,* especially a tungsten-weighted tube, position the patient on his right side. *This lets gravity assist tube passage through the pylorus.* Move the tube forward 2″ to 3″ (5 to 7.6 cm) hourly until X-ray studies confirm duodenal placement. (An X-ray film must confirm placement before feeding begins *because duodenal feeding can cause nausea and vomiting if accidentally delivered to the stomach.)*
● Apply skin preparation to the patient's cheek before securing the tube with tape. *This helps the tube adhere to the skin and also prevents irritation.*

• Tape the tube securely to the patient's cheek *to avoid excessive pressure on his nostrils.*

To remove the tube
• Protect the patient's chest with a linen-saver pad.
• Flush the tube with air, clamp or pinch it *to prevent fluid aspiration during withdrawal,* and withdraw it gently but quickly.
• Promptly cover and discard the used tube.

Special considerations
Flush the feeding tube every 8 hours with up to 60 ml of normal saline solution or water *to maintain patency.* Retape the tube at least daily and as needed. Alternate taping the tube toward the inner and outer side of the nose *to avoid constant pressure on the same nasal area.* Inspect the skin for redness and breakdown.

Provide nasal hygiene daily using the cotton-tipped applicators and water-soluble lubricant *to remove crusted secretions.* Assist the patient with oral hygiene at least twice daily. Help him brush his teeth, gums, and tongue with mouthwash or a mild saltwater solution.

If the patient can't swallow the feeding tube, use a guide *to aid insertion.*

Precise feeding-tube placement is especially important *because small-bore feeding tubes may slide into the trachea without causing immediate signs or symptoms of respiratory distress, such as coughing, choking, gasping, or cyanosis.* However, the patient will usually cough if the tube enters the larynx. To be sure that the tube clears the larynx, ask the patient to speak. If he can't, the tube is in the larynx. Withdraw the tube at once and reinsert.

When aspirating gastric contents to check tube placement, pull gently on the syringe plunger *because negative pressure may collapse a small-bore feeding tube or traumatize the stomach lining or bowel.* If you meet resistance during aspiration, stop the procedure *because resistance may result simply from the tube lying against the stomach wall.* If the tube coils above the stomach, you'll be unable to aspirate stomach contents. To rectify this, change the patient's position or withdraw the tube a few inches, readvance it, and try to aspirate again. If the tube was inserted with a guide wire, do not use the guide wire to reposition the tube. The doctor may do so, using fluoroscopic guidance.

Home care
If your patient will use a feeding tube at home, make appropriate home care nursing referrals and teach the patient and caregivers how to use and care for a feeding tube. Help them understand how to obtain equipment, to insert and remove the tube, to prepare and store feeding formula, and to troubleshoot tube position and patency.

Complications
Prolonged intubation may lead to skin erosion at the nostril, sinusitis, esophagitis, esophagotracheal fistula, gastric ulceration, and pulmonary and oral infection.

Documentation
For tube insertion, record the date, time, tube type and size, site of insertion, area of placement, and confirmation of proper placement. Also record the name of the person performing the procedure. For tube removal, record the date and time and describe the patient's tolerance of the procedure.

Tube feedings

This procedure involves delivery of a liquid feeding formula directly to the stomach (known as gastric gavage), duodenum, or jejunum. Gastric gavage typically is indicated for a patient who can't eat normally because of dysphagia or oral or esophageal obstruction or injury. Gastric feedings also may be given to an unconscious or intubated patient or to a patient recovering from GI tract surgery who can't ingest food orally.

Duodenal or jejunal feedings decrease the risk of aspiration because the formula bypasses the pylorus. Jejunal feedings result in reduced pancreatic stimulation; thus, the patient may require an elemental diet.

Usually, patients receive gastric feedings on an intermittent schedule. For duodenal or jejunal feedings, however, most patients seem to better tolerate a continuous slow drip.

Liquid nutrient solutions come in various formulas for administration through a nasogastric tube, small-bore feeding tube, gastrostomy or jejunostomy tube, percutaneous endoscopic gastrostomy or jejunostomy tube, or gastrostomy feeding button. (For more information, see "Transabdominal tube feeding and care" later in this chapter. Also see *Managing tube feeding problems,* page 524.) Tube feeding is contraindicated in patients who have no bowel sounds or suspected intestinal obstruction.

Equipment
For gastric feedings: feeding formula ■ graduated container ■ 120 ml of water ■ gavage bag with tubing and flow regulator clamp ■ towel or linen-saver pad ■ 60-ml syringe ■ stethoscope ■ optional: infusion controller and tubing set (for continuous administration), adapter to connect gavage tubing to feeding tube.

For duodenal or jejunal feedings: feeding formula ■ enteral administration set containing a gavage container,

Managing tube feeding problems

COMPLICATION	INTERVENTIONS
Aspiration of gastric secretions	• Discontinue feeding immediately. • Perform tracheal suction of aspirated contents if possible. • Notify the doctor. Prophylactic antibiotics and chest physiotherapy may be ordered. • Check tube placement before feeding to prevent complication.
Tube obstruction	• Flush the tube with warm water or cranberry juice. If necessary, replace the tube. • Flush the tube with 50 ml of water after each feeding to remove excess sticky formula, which could occlude the tube.
Nasal or pharyngeal irritation or necrosis	• Provide frequent oral hygiene using mouthwash or lemon-glycerin swabs. Use petroleum jelly on cracked lips. • Change the tube's position. If necessary, replace the tube.
Vomiting, bloating, diarrhea, or cramps	• Reduce the flow rate. • Administer metoclopramide to increase GI motility. • Warm the formula. • For 30 minutes after feeding, position the patient on his right side with his head elevated to facilitate gastric emptying. • Notify the doctor. He may want to reduce the amount of formula being given during each feeding.
Constipation	• Provide additional fluids if the patient can tolerate them. • Administer a bulk-forming laxative. • Increase fruit, vegetable, or sugar content of the feeding.
Electrolyte imbalance	• Monitor serum electrolyte levels. • Notify the doctor. He may want to adjust the formula content to correct the deficiency.
Hyperglycemia	• Monitor blood glucose levels. • Notify the doctor of elevated levels. • Administer insulin if ordered. • The doctor may adjust the sugar content of the formula.

drip chamber, roller clamp or flow regulator, and tube connector ■ I.V. pole ■ 60-ml syringe with adapter tip ■ water ■ optional: pump administration set (for an enteral infusion pump), Y connector, antidiarrheal medication (such as paregoric, tincture of opium, or diphenoxylate hydrochloride).

For nasal and oral care: cotton-tipped applicators ■ water-soluble lubricant ■ lemon-glycerin swabs ■ petroleum jelly.

A bulb syringe or large catheter-tip syringe may be substituted for a gavage bag if necessary. The doctor may order an infusion pump *to ensure accurate delivery of prescribed formula.*

Preparation of equipment
Be sure to refrigerate formulas prepared in the dietary department or pharmacy. Refrigerate commercial formulas only after opening them.

Check the date on all formula containers. Discard expired commercial formula. Use powdered formula within 24 hours of mixing. Always shake the container well *to mix the solution thoroughly.*

Allow the formula to warm to room temperature before administration. Never warm it over direct heat *because heat may curdle the formula or change its chemical composition. Also, hot formula may injure the patient.*

Pour 60 ml of water into the graduated container. After closing the flow clamp on the administration set, pour the appropriate amount of formula into the gavage bag. Hang no more than a 4- to 6-hour supply at one time *to prevent bacterial growth.*

Open the flow clamp on the administration set *to remove air from the lines. This keeps air from entering the patient's stomach and causing distention and discomfort.*

Implementation

- Provide privacy and wash your hands.
- Inform the patient that he will receive nourishment through the tube, and explain the procedure to him. If possible, give him a schedule of subsequent feedings.
- If the patient has a nasal or oral tube, cover his chest with a towel or linen-saver pad *to protect him and the bed linens from spills.*
- Assess the patient's abdomen for bowel sounds and distention.

To deliver a gastric feeding

- Elevate the bed to semi-Fowler's or high Fowler's position *to prevent aspiration by gastroesophageal reflux and to promote digestion.*
- Check placement of the feeding tube *to be sure it hasn't slipped out since the last feeding.* Never give a tube feeding until you're sure the tube is properly positioned in the patient's stomach. *Administering a feeding through a misplaced tube can cause formula to enter the patient's lungs.*
- *To check tube patency and position,* remove the cap or plug from the feeding tube, and use the syringe to inject 5 to 10 cc of air through the tube. At the same time, auscultate the patient's stomach with the stethoscope. Listen for a whooshing sound to confirm tube positioning in the stomach. Also aspirate stomach contents to confirm tube patency and placement.
- *To assess gastric emptying,* aspirate and measure residual gastric contents. Reinstill any aspirate obtained.
- Connect the gavage bag tubing to the feeding tube. Depending on the type of tube used, you may need to use an adapter to connect the two.
- If you're using a bulb or catheter-tip syringe, remove the bulb or plunger and attach the syringe to the pinched-off feeding tube *to prevent excess air from entering the patient's stomach, causing distention.* If you're using an infusion controller, thread the tube from the formula container through the controller according to the manufacturer's directions. Purge the tubing of air and attach it to the feeding tube.

- Open the regulator clamp on the gavage bag tubing and adjust the flow rate appropriately. When using a bulb syringe, fill the syringe with formula and release the feeding tube *to allow formula to flow through it.* The height at which you hold the syringe will determine flow rate. When the syringe is three-quarters empty, pour more formula into it.
- To prevent air from entering the tube and the patient's stomach, never allow the syringe to empty completely. If you're using an infusion controller, set the flow rate according to the manufacturer's directions. Always administer a tube feeding slowly — typically 200 to 350 ml over 10 to 15 minutes, depending on the patient's tolerance and the doctor's order — *to prevent sudden stomach distention, which can cause nausea, vomiting, cramps, or diarrhea.*
- After administering the appropriate amount of formula, flush the tubing by adding about 60 ml of water to the gavage bag or bulb syringe. *This maintains the tube's patency by removing excess formula, which could occlude the tube.*
- If you're administering a continuous feeding, flush the feeding tube every 4 hours *to help prevent tube occlusion.* Monitor gastric emptying every 4 hours.
- To discontinue gastric feeding (depending on the equipment you're using), close the regulator clamp on the gavage bag tubing, disconnect the syringe from the feeding tube, or turn off the infusion controller.
- Cover the end of the feeding tube with its plug or cap *to prevent leakage and contamination of the tube.*
- Leave the patient in semi-Fowler's or high Fowler's position for at least 30 minutes.
- Rinse all reusable equipment with warm water. Dry it and store it in a convenient place for the next feeding. Change equipment every 24 hours or according to the hospital's policy.

To deliver a duodenal or jejunal feeding

- Elevate the head of the bed and place the patient in the low Fowler's position.
- Open the enteral administration set and hang the gavage container on the I.V. pole.
- If you're using a nasoduodenal tube, measure its length *to check tube placement.* Remember that you may not get any residual when you aspirate the tube.
- Open the flow clamp and regulate the flow to the desired rate. To regulate the rate using a volumetric infusion pump, follow the manufacturer's directions for setting up the equipment. Most patients receive small amounts initially, with volumes increasing gradually once tolerance is established.
- Flush the tube every 4 hours with water *to maintain patency and provide hydration.* A needle catheter jejunos-

tomy tube may require flushing every 2 hours *to prevent formula buildup inside the tube.* A Y connector may be useful for frequent flushing. Attach the continuous feeding to the main port and use the side port for flushes.

Special considerations

If the feeding solution doesn't initially flow through a bulb syringe, attach the bulb and squeeze it gently to start the flow. Then remove the bulb. Never use the bulb to force the formula through the tube.

If the patient becomes nauseated or vomits, stop the feeding immediately. The patient may vomit if the stomach becomes distended from overfeeding or delayed gastric emptying.

To reduce oropharyngeal discomfort from the tube, allow the patient to brush his teeth or care for his dentures regularly, and encourage frequent gargling. If the patient is unconscious, administer oral care with lemon-glycerin swabs every 4 hours. Use petroleum jelly on dry, cracked lips. (Remember: Dry mucous membranes may indicate dehydration, which requires increased fluid intake.) Clean the patient's nostrils with cotton-tipped applicators, apply lubricant along the mucosa, and assess the skin for signs of breakdown.

During continuous feedings, assess the patient frequently for abdominal distention. Flush the tubing by adding about 50 ml of water to the gavage bag or bulb syringe. *This maintains the tube's patency by removing excess formula, which could occlude the tube.*

If the patient develops diarrhea, administer small, frequent, less concentrated feedings, or administer bolus feedings over a longer time. Also, make sure that the formula isn't cold and that proper storage and sanitation practices have been followed. The loose stools associated with tube feedings make extra perineal and skin care necessary. Giving paregoric, tincture of opium, or diphenoxylate hydrochloride may improve the condition. Changing to a formula with more fiber may eliminate liquid stools.

If the patient becomes constipated, the doctor may increase the fruit, vegetable, or sugar content of the formula. Assess the patient's hydration status *because dehydration may produce constipation.* Increase fluid intake as necessary. If the condition persists, administer an appropriate drug or enema, as ordered.

Drugs can be administered through the feeding tube. Except for enteric-coated drugs or sustained-release medications, crush tablets or open and dilute capsules in water before administering them. Be sure to flush the tubing afterward *to ensure full instillation of medication.* Keep in mind that some drugs may change the osmolarity of the feeding formula and cause diarrhea.

Small-bore feeding tubes may kink, making instillation impossible. If you suspect this problem, try changing the patient's position, or withdraw the tube a few inches and restart. Never use a guide wire to reposition the tube.

Constantly monitor the flow rate of a blended or high-residue formula *to determine if the formula is clogging the tubing as it settles. To prevent such clogging,* squeeze the bag frequently to agitate the solution.

Glycosuria, hyperglycemia, and diuresis can indicate an excessive carbohydrate level, leading to hyperosmotic dehydration, which may be fatal. Collect urine specimens every 4 to 6 hours, and blood specimens, as ordered. Monitor urine and blood glucose levels *to assess glucose tolerance.* (A patient with a serum glucose level of less than 200 mg/100 ml and without glycosuria is considered stable.) Also monitor serum electrolytes, blood urea nitrogen, serum glucose, serum osmolality, and other pertinent findings *to determine the patient's response to therapy and assess his hydration status*.

Check the flow rate hourly to ensure correct infusion. (With an improvised administration set, use a time tape to record the rate *because it's difficult to get precise readings from an irrigation container or enema bag.*)

For duodenal or jejunal feeding, most patients tolerate a continuous drip better than bolus feedings. *Bolus feedings can cause such complications as hyperglycemia, glucosuria, and diarrhea.*

Until the patient acquires a tolerance for the formula, you may need to dilute it to half or three-quarters strength to start, and increase it gradually. Patients under stress or who are receiving steroids may experience a pseudodiabetic state. Assess them frequently to determine the need for insulin.

Home care

Patient education for home tube feeding includes instructions on an infusion control device to maintain accuracy, use of the syringe or bag and tubing, care of the tube and insertion site, and formula-mixing. Formula may be mixed in an electric blender according to package directions. Formula not used within 24 hours must be discarded. If the formula must hang for more than 8 hours, advise the patient to use a gavage or pump administration set with an ice pouch to decrease the incidence of bacterial growth. Tell him to use a new bag daily.

Family members should be instructed in signs and symptoms to report to the doctor or home care nurse, as well as measures to take in an emergency.

Complications

Erosion of esophageal, tracheal, nasal, and oropharyngeal mucosa can result if tubes are left in place for a long time. If possible, use smaller-lumen tubes *to prevent such irritation. Check hospital policy regarding the frequency of changing feeding tubes to prevent complications.*

Using the gastric route, frequent or large-volume feedings can cause bloating and retention. Dehydration, diarrhea, and vomiting can cause metabolic disturbances. Glycosuria, cramping, and abdominal distention usually indicate intolerance.

Using the duodenal or jejunal route, clogging of the feeding tube is common. The patient may experience metabolic, fluid, and electrolyte abnormalities including hyperglycemia, glycosuria, hyperosmolar dehydration, coma, edema, hypernatremia, and essential fatty acid deficiency.

The patient also may experience dumping syndrome, in which a large amount of hyperosmotic solution in the duodenum causes excessive diffusion of fluid through the semipermeable membrane and results in diarrhea. In a patient with low serum albumin levels, these symptoms may result from low oncotic pressure in the duodenal mucosa.

Documentation

On the intake and output sheet, record the date, volume of formula, and volume of water. In your notes, include abdominal assessment (including tube exit site, if appropriate); amount of residuals; verification of tube placement; amount, type, and time of feeding; and tube patency. Discuss the patient's tolerance to the feeding, including nausea, vomiting, cramping, diarrhea, and distention. Note the result of blood and urine tests, hydration status, and any drugs given through the tube. Include the date and time of administration set changes, oral and nasal hygiene, and results of specimen collections.

Nasoenteric-decompression tube insertion and removal

The nasoenteric-decompression tube is inserted nasally and advanced beyond the stomach into the intestinal tract. It's used to aspirate intestinal contents for analysis and to treat intestinal obstruction. The tube may also help to prevent nausea, vomiting, and abdominal distention after GI surgery. A doctor will usually insert or remove a nasoenteric-decompression tube, but sometimes, a nurse will remove it.

A balloon or rubber bag at one end of the tube holds mercury (or air or water) to stimulate peristalsis and facilitate the tube's passage through the pylorus and into the intestinal tract. (See *Common types of nasoenteric-decompression tubes,* page 528.)

Equipment

Sterile 10-cc syringe ■ 21G needle ■ nasoenteric-decompression tube ■ container of water ■ 5 to 10 ml of mercury or water, as ordered ■ suction-decompression equipment ■ gloves ■ towel or linen-saver pad ■ water-soluble lubricant ■ 4″ × 4″ gauze pad ■ ½″ nonallergenic tape ■ bulb syringe or 60-ml catheter-tip syringe ■ stethoscope ■ cotton-tipped applicators ■ rubber band ■ safety pin ■ clamp ■ specimen container ■ optional: basin of ice or warm water, penlight, waterproof marking pen, glass of water with straw, ice chips, local anesthetic.

Preparation of equipment

Stiffen a flaccid tube by chilling it in a basin of ice *to facilitate insertion.* To make a stiff tube flexible, dip it into warm water.

To check the tube's balloon for leaks, inject 10 cc of air into the balloon with a 10-cc syringe and 21G needle. Immerse the balloon in a container of water and watch for air bubbles. Bubble-free water means a leak-free balloon. Then remove the balloon from the water. Mercury, air, or water are then added to the balloon with a syringe, depending on the type of tube used. Follow the manufacturer's recommendations.

Set up suction-decompression equipment, if ordered, and make sure it works properly.

Implementation

• Explain the procedure to the patient, forewarning him that he may experience some discomfort. Provide privacy and adequate lighting. Wash your hands and put on gloves.

• Position the patient as the doctor specifies. The most common positions to facilitate tube insertion are semi-Fowler's or high Fowler's positions. You may also need to help the patient hold his neck in a hyperextended position.

• Protect the patient's chest with a linen-saver pad or towel.

• Agree with the patient on a signal that can be used to stop the insertion briefly if necessary.

To assist with insertion

• The doctor assesses the patency of the patient's nostrils. To evaluate which nostril has better airflow in a conscious patient, he holds one nostril closed and then the other as the patient breathes. In an unconscious patient, he examines each nostril with a penlight *to check for polyps, a deviated septum, or other obstruction.*

Common types of nasoenteric-decompression tubes

The type of nasoenteric-decompression tube chosen for your patient will depend on the size of the patient and his nostrils, the estimated duration of intubation, and the reason for the procedure. For example, to remove viscous material from the patient's intestinal tract, the doctor may select a tube with a wide bore and a single lumen.

Whichever tube you use, you'll need to provide good mouth care and check the patient's nostrils often for signs of irritation. If you see any signs of irritation, re-tape the tube so it doesn't cause tension. Then, lubricate the nostril. Or check with the doctor to see if the tube can be inserted through the other nostril.

Most tubes are impregnated with a radiopaque mark so that placement can be confirmed easily by X-ray or other imaging technique. The following are among the most commonly used types of nasoenteric-decompression tubes.

Cantor tube
This single-lumen, 10′ (3 m) long tube has a balloon that can hold mercury at its distal tip. The Cantor tube may be used to relieve bowel obstructions and to aspirate intestinal contents.

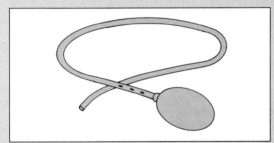

Harris tube
Measuring only 6′ (1.8 m) long, this single-lumen tube (top right) also ends with a balloon that holds mercury. Used chiefly for treating a bowel obstruction, the Harris tube allows lavage of the intestinal tract — usually with a Y tube attached.

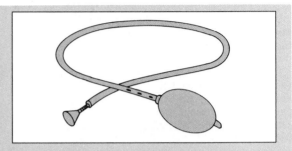

Miller-Abbott tube
This 10′ tube has two lumens: one for inflating the distal balloon with air and one for instilling mercury or water. Also used for bowel obstruction, the tube allows aspiration of intestinal contents.

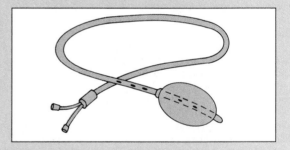

Dennis tube
This three-lumen sump tube is used to decompress the intestinal tract before or after GI surgery. Each lumen is marked to denote its use: irrigation, drainage, and balloon inflation.

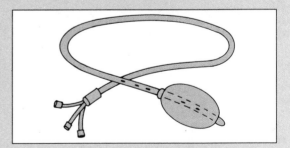

• *To decide how far the tube must be inserted to reach the stomach,* the doctor places the tube's distal end at the tip of the patient's nose and then extends the tube to the earlobe and down to the xiphoid process. He either marks the tube with a waterproof marking pen or holds it at this point.

• The doctor applies water-soluble lubricant to the first few inches of the tube *to reduce friction and tissue trauma and to facilitate insertion.*

• If the balloon already contains mercury or water, the doctor holds it so the fluid runs to the bottom. Then he pinches the balloon closed *to retain the fluid as the insertion begins.*

• Direct the patient to breathe through his mouth or to pant as the balloon enters his nostril. After the balloon begins its descent, the doctor releases his grip on it, *allowing the weight of the fluid to pull the tube into the nasopharynx.* When the tube reaches the nasopharynx, the doctor instructs the patient to lower his chin and to swallow. In some cases, the patient may sip water through a straw *to facilitate swallowing as the tube advances.* After the tube reaches the trachea, however, the patient won't be offered water. *This prevents injury from aspiration.* The doctor continues to advance the tube slowly *to prevent it from curling or kinking in the stomach.*

• *To confirm the tube's passage into the stomach,* the doctor aspirates stomach contents with a bulb syringe.

• When the doctor confirms proper placement of a Miller-Abbott tube, he injects the appropriate amount of mercury (commonly between 2 and 5 ml) into the balloon lumen.

• *To keep the tube out of the patient's eyes and to help avoid undue skin irritation,* fold a 4″ × 4″ gauze pad in half and tape it to the patient's forehead with the fold directed toward the patient's nose. The doctor can slide the tube through this sling, leaving enough slack for the tube to advance.

• Position the patient, as directed, *to help advance the tube.* Commonly, the patient will lie on his right side until the tube clears the pylorus (about 2 hours). The doctor confirms passage by X-ray.

• After the tube clears the pylorus, the doctor may direct you to advance it 2″ to 3″ (5 to 7.6 cm) every hour and to reposition the patient until the premeasured mark reaches the patient's nostril. Gravity and peristalsis will help to advance the tube. (Notify the doctor if you cannot advance the tube.)

• Be sure to keep the remaining premeasured length of tube well lubricated *to ease passage and prevent irritation.*

• Avoid taping the tube while it advances to the premeasured mark, unless the doctor directs you to do so.

• After the tube progresses the necessary distance, the doctor will order an X-ray *to confirm tube positioning.* Once the tube's in place, secure the external tubing with tape *to prevent further progression.*

• Loop a rubber band around the tube and pin the rubber band to the patient's gown with a safety pin.

• If ordered, attach the tube to intermittent suction.

To remove the tube

• Assist the patient into semi-Fowler's or high Fowler's position. Drape a linen-saver pad or towel across the patient's chest.

• Put on gloves.

• Clamp the tube and disconnect it from the suction. *This prevents the patient from aspirating any gastric contents that leak from the tube during withdrawal.*

• If your patient has a double-lumen Miller-Abbott tube or a triple-lumen Dennis tube, attach a 10-ml syringe to the balloon port and withdraw the mercury. Place the mercury in a specimen container and follow your hospital's protocol for safe disposal. (If you're working with a single-lumen Cantor or Harris tube, you'll withdraw the mercury after you remove the tube.)

• Slowly withdraw between 6″ and 8″ (15.2 and 20.3 cm) of the tube. Wait 10 minutes and withdraw another 6″ to 8″. Wait another 10 minutes. Continue this procedure until the tube reaches the patient's esophagus (with about 18″ [45.7 cm] of the tube remaining inside the patient). At this point, you can gently withdraw the tube completely with the mercury in the balloon.

Special considerations

For a double- or triple-lumen tube, note which lumen accommodates balloon inflation and which accommodates drainage.

An alternate method for removing a single-lumen tube is to withdraw it gently into the pharynx. Ask the patient to open his mouth. Then grasp the tube and mercury balloon and gently pull them outside of the patient's mouth. Remove mercury from the bag with a needle and syringe. Then pull the tube and empty balloon through the patient's nose. Never forcibly remove a tube if you meet resistance. Notify the doctor.

Apply a local anesthetic, if ordered, to the nostril or the back of the throat *to dull sensations and the gag reflex for intubation.* Letting the patient gargle with a liquid anesthetic or hold ice chips in his mouth for a few minutes serves the same purpose.

Mercury can be disposed of only by a licensed hazardous-waste disposal company. Put the container of mercury into a plastic bag, and send it to the appropriate department for disposal.

Complications

Nasoenteric-decompression tubes may cause reflux esophagitis, nasal or oral inflammation, and nasal, laryngeal, or esophageal ulceration.

Documentation

Record the date and time the nasoenteric-decompression tube was inserted and by whom. Note the patient's tolerance of the procedure; the type of tube used; the suction type and amount; and the color, amount, and consistency of drainage. Also note the date, time, and name of the person removing the tube and the patient's tolerance of the removal procedure.

Nasoenteric-decompression tube care

The patient with a nasoenteric-decompression tube needs special care and continuous monitoring to ensure tube patency, to maintain suction and bowel decompression, and to detect such complications as fluid-electrolyte imbalances related to aspiration of intestinal contents. Precise intake and output records form an integral part of the patient's care. Frequent mouth and nose care is also essential to provide comfort and to prevent skin breakdown. Finally, a patient with a nasoenteric-decompression tube will need encouragement and support during insertion and removal of the tube and while the tube is in place.

Equipment

Suction apparatus with intermittent suction capability (stationary or portable unit) ▪ container of water ▪ intake and output record sheets ▪ mouthwash and water mixture ▪ lemon-glycerin swabs ▪ petroleum jelly or water-soluble lubricant ▪ cotton-tipped applicators ▪ safety pin ▪ tape or rubber band ▪ disposable irrigation set ▪ irrigant ▪ labels for tube lumens ▪ optional: throat comfort measures such as gargle, viscous lidocaine, sour hard candy, throat lozenges, ice collar, or chewing gum.

Preparation of equipment

Assemble the suction apparatus and set up the suction unit. If indicated, test the unit by turning it on and placing the end of the suction tubing in a container of water. If the tubing draws in water, the unit works.

Implementation

● Explain to the patient and his family the purpose of the procedure. Answer questions clearly and thoroughly *to ease anxiety and enhance cooperation.*
● After inserting the tube, have the patient lie quietly on his right side for about 2 hours *to promote the tube's passage.* After the tube advances past the pylorus, the patient's activity level may increase, as ordered.
● After the tube advances to the desired position, coil the excess external tubing and secure it to the patient's gown or bed linens with a safety pin attached to tape or a rubber band looped around the tubing. *This may prevent kinks in the tubing, which would interrupt suction.* And once in the desired location, the tube may be taped to the patient's face.
● Maintain slack in the tubing *so the patient can move comfortably and safely in bed.* Show him how far he can move without dislodging the tube.
● After securing the tube, connect it to the tubing on the suction machine *to begin decompression.*
● Check the suction machine at least every 2 hours *to confirm proper functioning and to ensure continued tube patency and bowel decompression.* Excessive negative pressure may draw the mucosa into the tube openings, impair the suction's effectiveness, and injure the mucosa. By using intermittent suction, you may circumvent these problems. To check functioning in an intermittent suction unit, look for drainage in the connecting tube and for drainage dripping into the collecting container. Empty the container every 8 hours and measure the contents.
● After decompression and before extubation, as ordered, provide a clear-to-full liquid diet *to assess bowel function.*
● Record intake and output accurately *to monitor the patient's fluid balance.* If you irrigate the tube, its length may prohibit aspiration of the irrigant, so record the amount of instilled irrigant as "intake." Typically, normal saline solution supersedes water as the preferred irrigant *because water, which is hypotonic, may increase electrolyte loss through osmotic action, especially if you irrigate the tube often.*
● Observe the patient for signs and symptoms of disorders related to suctioning and intubation. These signs and symptoms may suggest dehydration, a fluid-volume deficit, or a fluid-electrolyte imbalance: dry skin and mucous membranes, decreased urine output, lethargy, exhaustion, and fever.
● Watch for signs and symptoms of pneumonia related to the patient's inability to clear his pharynx or cough effectively with a tube in place. Be alert for fever, chest pain, tachypnea or labored breathing, and diminished breath sounds over the affected area.
● Observe drainage characteristics, including amount, color, consistency, odor, and any unusual changes.

• Provide mouth care frequently (at least every 4 hours). *This increases patient comfort and promotes a healthy oral cavity. If the tube remains in place for several days, mouth-breathing will leave the patient's lips, tongue, and other tissues dry and cracked.*

• Encourage the patient to brush his teeth or rinse his mouth with the mouthwash and water mixture.

• Lubricate the patient's lips with either lemon-glycerin swabs or petroleum jelly applied with a cotton-tipped applicator.

• At least every 4 hours, gently clean and lubricate the patient's external nostrils with either petroleum jelly or water-soluble lubricant on a cotton-tipped applicator *to prevent skin breakdown.*

• Watch for peristalsis to resume, signaled by bowel sounds, passage of flatus, decreased abdominal distention, and possibly, a spontaneous bowel movement. *These signs may require tube removal.*

Special considerations

For a Miller-Abbott tube, clamp the lumen leading to the mercury balloon and label DO NOT TOUCH. Label the other lumen SUCTION. *Marking the tube in this way may prevent accidentally instilling irrigant into the wrong lumen and possibly rupturing the mercury balloon.*

If the suction machine works improperly, replace it immediately. If the machine works properly but no drainage accumulates in the collection container, suspect an obstruction in the tube.

As ordered, irrigate the tube with the irrigation set *to clear the obstruction.* (See *Clearing a nasoenteric-decompression tube obstruction.*)

If your patient is ambulatory and his tube connects to a portable suction unit, he may move short distances while connected to the unit. Or, if feasible and ordered, the tube can be disconnected and clamped for a brief time while he moves about.

If the tubing irritates the patient's throat or makes him hoarse, offer relief with mouthwash, gargles, viscous lidocaine, sour hard candy, throat lozenges, an ice collar, or chewing gum, as appropriate.

If the balloon at the end of the tube protrudes from the anus, notify the doctor. Most likely, the tube can be disconnected from suction, the proximal end severed, and the remaining tube removed gradually through the anus either manually or by peristalsis.

Complications

Besides fluid-volume deficit, electrolyte imbalance, and pneumonia, potential complications include mercury poisoning (from a ruptured mercury-filled balloon) and in-

Clearing a nasoenteric-decompression tube obstruction

If your patient's nasoenteric-decompression tube appears to be obstructed, notify the doctor right away. He may order measures, such as these, to restore patency quickly and efficiently.

First, disconnect the tube from the suction source and irrigate with normal saline solution. Use gravity flow to help clear the obstruction unless ordered otherwise.

If irrigation doesn't reestablish patency, the tube may be obstructed by its position against the gastric mucosa. To rectify this, tug slightly on the tube to move it away from the mucosa.

If gentle tugging doesn't restore patency, the tube may be kinked and may need additional manipulation. Before proceeding, though, take these precautions:

• Never reposition or irrigate a nasoenteric-decompression tube (without a doctor's order) in a patient who has had GI surgery.

• Avoid manipulating a tube in a patient who had the tube inserted during surgery. To do so may disturb new sutures.

• Don't try to reposition the tube in a patient who was difficult to intubate (because of an esophageal stricture, for example).

---

tussusception of the bowel (from the weight of the mercury in the balloon).

Documentation

Record the frequency and type of mouth and nose care given. Describe the therapeutic effect, if any. Document in your notes the amount, color, consistency, and odor of the drainage obtained each time you empty the collection container.

Record the amount of drainage on the intake and output sheet. Always write down the amount of any irrigant or other fluid introduced through the tube or taken orally by the patient.

If the suction machine malfunctions, note the length of time it didn't appear to be functioning and the nursing action taken. Document the amount and character of any vomitus. Also note the patient's tolerance of the tube's insertion and removal.

Esophageal tube insertion and removal

Used to control hemorrhage from esophageal or gastric varices, an esophageal tube is inserted nasally or orally and advanced into the esophagus or stomach. Ordinarily, a doctor inserts and removes the tube. In an emergency situation, a nurse may remove it.

Once the tube is in place, a gastric balloon secured at the end of the tube can be inflated and drawn tightly against the cardia of the stomach. The inflated balloon secures the tube and exerts pressure on the cardia. The pressure, in turn, controls the bleeding varices.

Most tubes also contain an esophageal balloon to control esophageal bleeding. (See *Types of esophageal tubes.*) Usually, gastric or esophageal balloons are deflated after 24 hours. If the balloon remains inflated longer than 24 hours, pressure necrosis may develop and cause further hemorrhage or perforation.

Other procedures to control bleeding include irrigation with tepid or iced saline solution and drug therapy with a vasopressor. Used with the esophageal tube, these procedures provide effective, temporary control of acute variceal hemorrhage.

Equipment

Esophageal tube ▪ nasogastric (NG) tube (if using a Sengstaken-Blakemore tube) ▪ two suction sources ▪ basin of ice ▪ irrigation set ▪ 2 liters of normal saline solution ▪ two 60-ml syringes ▪ water-soluble lubricant ▪ ½" or 1" adhesive tape ▪ stethoscope ▪ foam nose guard ▪ four rubber-shod clamps (two clamps and two plastic plugs for a Minnesota tube) ▪ anesthetic spray (as ordered) ▪ traction equipment (football helmet or a basic frame with traction rope, pulleys, and a 1-lb [0.5-kg] weight) ▪ mercury aneroid manometer ▪ Y connector tube (for a Sengstaken-Blakemore or a Linton tube) ▪ basin of water ▪ cup of water with straw ▪ scissors ▪ gloves ▪ gown ▪ waterproof marking pen ▪ goggles ▪ tape ▪ sphygmomanometer.

Preparation of equipment

Keep the traction helmet at the bedside or attach traction equipment to the bed, so that either is readily available after tube insertion. Place the suction machines nearby and plug them in. Open the irrigation set and fill the container with normal saline solution. Place all equipment within reach.

Test the balloons on the esophageal tube for air leaks by inflating them and submerging them in the basin of water. If no bubbles appear in the water, the balloons are

intact. Remove them from the water and deflate them. Clamp the tube lumens, so that the balloons stay deflated during insertion.

To prepare the Minnesota tube, connect the mercury manometer to the gastric pressure monitoring port. Note the pressure when the balloon fills with 100, 200, 300, 400, and 500 cc of air.

Check the aspiration lumens for patency, and make sure that they are labeled according to their purpose. If they aren't identified, label them carefully with the marking pen.

Chill the tube in a basin of ice. *This will stiffen it and facilitate insertion,* as ordered.

Implementation

• Explain the procedure and its purpose to the patient, and provide privacy.

• Wash your hands, and put on gloves, gown, and goggles *to protect yourself from splashing blood.*

• Assist the patient into semi-Fowler's position and turn him slightly toward his left side. *This position promotes stomach emptying and helps prevent aspiration.*

• Explain that the doctor will inspect the patient's nostrils (for patency).

• *To determine the length of tubing needed,* hold the balloon at the patient's xiphoid process, extend the tube to the patient's ear and forward to his nose. Using a waterproof pen, mark this point on the tubing.

• Inform the patient that the doctor will spray the patient's posterior pharynx (throat) and nostril with an anesthetic *to minimize discomfort and gagging during intubation.*

• After lubricating the tip of the tube with water-soluble lubricant *to reduce friction and facilitate insertion,* the doctor will pass the tube through the more patent nostril. As he does, he will direct the patient to tilt his chin toward his chest and to swallow when he senses the tip of the tube in the back of his throat. *Swallowing helps to advance the tube into the esophagus and prevents intubation of the trachea.* (If the doctor introduces the tube orally, he will direct the patient to swallow immediately.) As the patient swallows, the doctor quickly advances the tube at least ½" (1.3 cm) beyond the previously marked point on the tube.

• *To confirm tube placement,* the doctor will aspirate stomach contents through the gastric port. He will also auscultate the stomach with a stethoscope as he injects air. After partially inflating the gastric balloon with 50 to 100 cc of air, he will order an X-ray of the abdomen *to confirm correct placement of the balloon.* Before fully inflating the balloon, he will use the 60-ml syringe to irrigate the stomach with normal saline solution and empty the stomach as completely as possible. *This helps*

Types of esophageal tubes

When working with patients who have an esophageal tube, remember the advantages of the most common types.

Sengstaken-Blakemore tube
This triple-lumen, double-balloon tube has a gastric aspiration port, which allows you to obtain drainage from below the gastric balloon and also to instill medication.

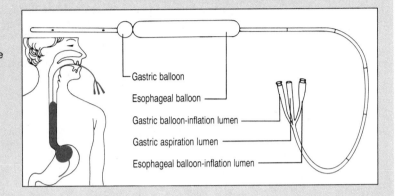

Gastric balloon

Esophageal balloon

Gastric balloon-inflation lumen

Gastric aspiration lumen

Esophageal balloon-inflation lumen

Linton tube
This triple-lumen, single-balloon tube has a port for gastric aspiration and one for esophageal aspiration, too. Additionally, the Linton tube reduces the risk of esophageal necrosis because it doesn't have an esophageal balloon.

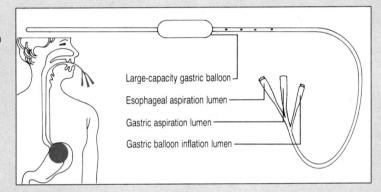

Large-capacity gastric balloon

Esophageal aspiration lumen

Gastric aspiration lumen

Gastric balloon inflation lumen

Minnesota esophagogastric tamponade tube
This esophageal tube has four lumens and two balloons. The device provides pressure-monitoring ports for both balloons without the need for Y connectors. One port is used for gastric suction, the other for esophageal suction.

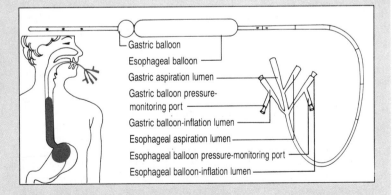

Gastric balloon

Esophageal balloon

Gastric aspiration lumen

Gastric balloon pressure-monitoring port

Gastric balloon-inflation lumen

Esophageal aspiration lumen

Esophageal balloon pressure-monitoring port

Esophageal balloon-inflation lumen

Securing an esophageal tube

To reduce the risk of the gastric balloon's slipping down or away from the cardia of the stomach, secure an esophageal tube to a football helmet. Tape the tube, as shown, to the face guard, and fasten the chin strap.

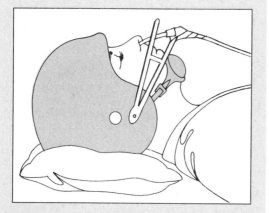

To remove the tube quickly, unfasten the chin strap and pull the helmet slightly forward. Cut the tape and the gastric balloon and esophageal balloon lumens. Be sure to hold onto the tube near the patient's nostril.

the patient avoid regurgitating gastric contents when the balloon inflates.

• After confirming tube placement, the doctor fully inflates the gastric balloon (250 to 500 cc of air for the Sengstaken-Blakemore tube; 700 to 800 cc of air for the Linton tube) and clamps the tube. If he's using the Minnesota tube, he connects the pressure-monitoring port for the gastric balloon lumen to the mercury manometer and then inflates the balloon in 100-cc increments until it fills with up to 500 cc of air. As he introduces the air, he monitors the intragastric balloon pressure *to make sure the balloon stays inflated.* Then, he clamps the ports. For the Sengstaken-Blakemore or Minnesota tube, the doctor gently pulls on the tube until he feels resistance, *which indicates that the gastric balloon is inflated and exerting pressure on the cardia of the stomach.* When he senses that the balloon is engaged, the doctor places the foam nose guard around the area where the tube emerges from the nostril.

• Be ready to tape the nose guard in place around the tube. *This helps to minimize pressure on the nostril from the traction and decreases the risk of necrosis.*

• With the nose guard secured, traction can be applied to the tube with a traction rope and a 1-lb weight, or the tube can be pulled gently and taped securely to the face guard of a football helmet. (See *Securing an esophageal tube.*)

• With pulley-and-weight traction, lower the head of the bed to about 25 degrees *to produce countertraction.*

• Lavage the stomach through the gastric aspiration lumen with normal saline solution (iced or tepid) until the return fluid is clear. *The vasoconstriction thus achieved stops the hemorrhage; the lavage empties the stomach. Any blood detected later in the gastric aspirate indicates that bleeding remains uncontrolled.*

• Attach one of the suction sources to the gastric aspiration lumen. *This empties the stomach, helps prevent nausea and possible vomiting, and allows continuous observation of the gastric contents for blood.*

• If the doctor inserted a Sengstaken-Blakemore or a Minnesota tube, he'll inflate the esophageal balloon as he inflates the gastric balloon *to compress the esophageal varices and control bleeding.*

To do this with a Sengstaken-Blakemore tube, attach the Y connector tube to the esophageal lumen. Then, attach a sphygmomanometer inflation bulb to one end of the Y connector and the manometer to the other end. Inflate the esophageal balloon until the pressure gauge ranges between 30 and 40 mm Hg and clamp the tube.

To do this with a Minnesota tube, attach the mercury manometer directly to the esophageal pressure-monitoring outlet. Then, using the 60-ml syringe and pushing the air slowly into the esophageal balloon port, inflate the balloon until the pressure gauge ranges between 35 and 45 mm Hg.

• Set up esophageal suction *to prevent accumulation of secretions that may cause vomiting and pulmonary aspiration.* This is important, because swallowed secretions can't pass into the stomach if the patient has an inflated esophageal balloon in place. If the patient has a Linton or a Minnesota tube, attach the suction source to the esophageal aspiration port. If the patient has a Sengstaken-Blakemore tube, advance an NG tube through the other nostril into the esophagus to the point where the esophageal balloon begins, and attach the suction source as ordered.

To remove the tube

• The doctor deflates the esophageal balloon by aspirating the air with a syringe. (He may order the esophageal balloon to be deflated at 5 mm Hg increments every 30 minutes for several hours.) Then if bleeding does not recur, he will remove the traction from the gastric tube and deflate the gastric balloon (also by aspiration). The gastric balloon is always deflated just before removing the tube *because the balloon may ride up into the esophagus or pharynx and obstruct the airway or, possibly, cause asphyxia or rupture.*

• After disconnecting all suction tubes, the doctor gently removes the esophageal tube. If he feels resistance, he aspirates the balloons again. (To remove a Minnesota tube, he grasps it near the patient's nostril and cuts across all four lumens approximately 3″ [7.6 cm] below that point. *This ensures deflation of all balloons.*)

• After the tube is removed, assist the patient with mouth care.

Special considerations
If the patient appears cyanotic or if other signs of airway obstruction develop during tube placement, remove the tube immediately *because it may have entered the trachea instead of the esophagus.* After intubation, keep scissors taped to the head of the bed. If respiratory distress occurs, cut across all lumens while holding the tube at the nares, and remove the tube quickly. Unless contraindicated, the patient can sip water through a straw during intubation *to facilitate tube advancement.*

Keep in mind that the intraesophageal balloon pressure varies with respirations and esophageal contractions. Baseline pressure is the important pressure.

The balloon on the Linton tube should stay inflated no longer than 24 hours *because necrosis of the cardia may result.* Usually, the doctor removes the tube only after a trial period (at least 12 hours) with the esophageal balloon deflated or with the gastric balloon tension released from the cardia, *to check for rebleeding.* In some centers, the doctor may deflate the esophageal balloon for 5 to 10 minutes every hour to temporarily relieve pressure on the esophageal mucosa.

Complications
Erosion and perforation of the esophagus and gastric mucosa may result from the tension placed on these areas by the balloons during traction. Esophageal rupture may result if the gastric balloon accidentally inflates in the esophagus. Acute airway occlusion may result if the balloon dislodges and moves upward into the trachea. Other erosions, nasal tissue necrosis, and aspiration of oral secretions may also complicate the patient's condition.

Documentation
Record the date and time of insertion and removal, the type of tube used, and the name of the doctor who performed the procedure. Also document the intraesophageal balloon pressure (for the Sengstaken-Blakemore or Minnesota tubes), the intragastric balloon pressure (for the Minnesota tube), or the amount of air injected (for the Sengstaken-Blakemore and the Linton tubes). Also record the amount of fluid used for gastric irrigation and the color, consistency, and amount of gastric returns, both before and after lavage.

Esophageal tube care

Although the doctor inserts an esophageal tube, the nurse cares for the patient during and after intubation. Typically, the patient is in the intensive care unit for close observation and constant care. The environment may help to increase the patient's tolerance for the procedure and may help to control bleeding. Sedatives may be contraindicated, especially for a patient with portal systemic encephalopathy.

Most importantly, the patient who has an esophageal tube in place to control variceal bleeding (typically from portal hypertension) must be observed closely for possible esophageal rupture because varices weaken the esophagus. Additionally, possible traumatic injury from intubation or esophageal balloon inflation increases the chance of rupture. Usually, emergency surgery is performed if a rupture occurs. The operation has a low success rate.

Equipment
Manometer ▪ two 2-liter bottles of normal saline solution ▪ irrigation set ▪ water-soluble lubricant ▪ several cotton-tipped applicators ▪ mouth-care equipment ▪ nasopharyngeal suction apparatus ▪ several #12 French suction catheters ▪ intake and output record sheets ▪ gloves ▪ sedatives ▪ traction weights ▪ foam nose guard.

Implementation
• *To help ease the patient's anxiety,* explain the care that you'll give.
• Provide privacy. Wash your hands and put on gloves.
• Monitor the patient's vital signs every 5 minutes to 1 hour, as ordered. *A change in vital signs may signal complications or recurrent bleeding.*
• If the patient has a Sengstaken-Blakemore or a Minnesota tube, check the pressure gauge on the manometer every 30 to 60 minutes *to detect any leaks in the esophageal balloon and to verify the set pressure.*
• Maintain drainage and suction on gastric and esophageal aspiration ports, as ordered. This is important because *fluid accumulating in the stomach may cause the*

patient to regurgitate the tube; fluid accumulating in the esophagus may lead to vomiting and aspiration.

• Irrigate the gastric aspiration port, as ordered, using the irrigation set and normal saline solution. *Frequent irrigation keeps the tube from clogging. Obstruction in the tube can lead to regurgitation of the tube and vomiting.*

• *To prevent pressure ulcers,* clean the patient's nostrils, and apply water-soluble lubricant frequently. Use warm water to loosen crusted nasal secretions before applying the lubricant with cotton-tipped applicators.

• Give mouth care often *to rid the patient's mouth of foul-tasting matter and to relieve dryness from mouth breathing.*

• Use #12 French catheters to provide gentle oral suctioning, if necessary, *to help remove secretions.*

• Offer emotional support. Keep the patient as quiet as possible, and administer sedatives, if ordered.

• Be sure that the traction weights hang from the foot of the bed at all times. Never rest them on the bed. Instruct housekeepers and other co-workers not to move the weights *because reduced traction may change the position of the tube.*

• Elevate the head of the bed about 25 degrees *to ensure countertraction for the weights.*

• Keep the patient on complete bed rest *because exertion, such as coughing or straining, increases intra-abdominal pressure, which may trigger further bleeding.*

• Keep the patient in semi-Fowler's position *to reduce blood flow into the portal system and to prevent reflux into the esophagus.*

• Monitor intake and output, as ordered.

Special considerations

Observe the patient carefully for esophageal rupture indicated by signs and symptoms of shock, increased respiratory difficulties, and increased bleeding. Tape scissors to the head of the bed *so you can cut the tube quickly to deflate the balloons if asphyxia develops.* When performing this emergency intervention, hold the tube firmly close to the nostril before cutting.

If using traction, be sure to release the tension before deflating any balloons. If weights and pulleys supply traction, remove the weights. If a football helmet supplies traction, untape the esophageal tube from the face guard before deflating the balloons. *Deflating the balloon under tension triggers a rapid release of the entire tube from the nose, which may injure mucous membranes, initiate recurrent bleeding, and obstruct the airway.*

If the doctor orders an X-ray study to check the tube's position or to view the chest, lift the patient in the direction of the pulley, and then place the X-ray film behind his back. Never roll him from side to side *because pressure exerted on the tube in this way may shift the tube's position.*

Similarly lift the patient to make the bed or to assist him with the bedpan.

Complications

Esophageal rupture, the most life-threatening complication associated with esophageal balloon tamponade, can occur at any time but is most likely to occur during intubation or inflation of the esophageal balloon. Asphyxia may result if the balloon moves up the esophagus and blocks the airway. Aspiration of pooled esophageal secretions may also complicate this procedure.

Documentation

Read the manometer hourly, and record the esophageal pressures. Note when the balloons are deflated and by whom. Document vital signs, the condition of the patient's nostrils, routine care, and any drugs administered. Also note the color, consistency, and amount of gastric returns. Record any signs and symptoms of complications and the nursing actions taken. Document gastric port and nasogastric tube irrigations. Maintain accurate intake and output records.

RECTAL ACCESS
Rectal tube insertion and removal

Whether GI hypomotility simply slows the normal release of gas and feces or results in paralytic ileus, inserting a rectal tube may relieve the discomfort of distention and flatus.

Decreased motility may result from various medical or surgical conditions, certain medications (such as atropine sulfate), or even swallowed air.

Conditions that contraindicate using a rectal tube include recent rectal or prostatic surgery, recent myocardial infarction, and diseases of the rectal mucosa.

Equipment

Stethoscope ■ linen-saver pads ■ drape ■ water-soluble lubricant ■ commercial kit or #22 to #32 French rectal tube of soft rubber or plastic ■ container (emesis basin, plastic bag, or water bottle with vent) ■ tape ■ gloves.

Implementation

• Bring all equipment to the patient's bedside, provide privacy, and wash your hands.

• Explain the procedure and encourage the patient to relax.

• Check for abdominal distention. Using the stethoscope, auscultate for bowel sounds.
• Place the linen-saver pads under the patient's buttocks *to absorb any drainage that may leak from the tube.*
• Position the patient in left-lateral Sims' position *to facilitate rectal tube insertion.*
• Put on gloves.
• Drape the patient's exposed buttocks.
• Lubricate the rectal tube tip with water-soluble lubricant *to ease insertion and prevent rectal irritation.*
• Lift the patient's right buttock *to expose the anus.*
• Insert the rectal tube tip into the anus, advancing the tube 2″ to 4″ (5 to 10 cm) into the rectum. Direct the tube toward the umbilicus *along the anatomic course of the large intestine.*
• As you insert the tube, tell the patient to breathe slowly and deeply, or suggest that he bear down as he would for a bowel movement *to relax the anal sphincter and ease insertion.*
• Using tape, secure the rectal tube to the buttocks. Then attach the tube to the container *to collect possible leakage.*
• Remove the tube after 15 to 20 minutes. If the patient reports continued discomfort or if gas wasn't expelled, you can repeat the procedure in 2 or 3 hours if ordered.
• Clean the patient, and replace soiled linens and the linen-saver pad. Be sure the patient feels as comfortable as possible. Again, check for abdominal distention and listen for bowel sounds.
• If you will reuse the equipment, clean it and store it in the bedside cabinet; otherwise discard the tube.

Special considerations
Inform the patient about each step and reassure him throughout the procedure *to encourage cooperation and promote relaxation.*

Fastening a plastic bag (like a balloon) to the external end of the tube lets you observe gas expulsion. Leaving a rectal tube in place indefinitely does little to promote peristalsis, can reduce sphincter responsiveness, and may lead to permanent sphincter damage or pressure necrosis of the mucosa.

Repeat insertion periodically *to stimulate GI activity.* If the tube fails to relieve distention, notify the doctor.

Documentation
Record the date and time that you insert the tube. Jot down the amount, color, and consistency of any evacuated matter. Describe the patient's abdomen—hard, distended, soft, or drumlike on percussion. Note bowel sounds before and after insertion.

Administration of an enema

This procedure involves instilling a solution into the rectum and the colon. In a retention enema, the patient holds the solution within the rectum or colon for 30 minutes to 1 hour. In an irrigating enema, the patient expels the solution almost completely within 15 minutes. Both types of enema stimulate peristalsis by mechanically distending the colon and stimulating rectal wall nerves.

Enemas are used to clean the lower bowel in preparation for diagnostic or surgical procedures; to relieve distention and promote expulsion of flatus; to lubricate the rectum and colon; and to soften hardened stool for removal. They're contraindicated, however, after recent colon or rectal surgery or myocardial infarction, and in the patient with an acute abdominal condition of unknown origin, such as suspected appendicitis. They should be administered cautiously to a patient with arrhythmia.

Equipment
Prescribed solution ∎ bath (utility) thermometer ∎ enema administration bag with attached rectal tube and clamp ∎ I.V. pole ∎ gloves ∎ linen-saver pads ∎ bath blanket ∎ two bedpans with covers, or bedside commode ∎ water-soluble lubricant ∎ toilet tissue ∎ bulb syringe or funnel ∎ plastic bag for equipment ∎ water ∎ gown ∎ washcloth ∎ soap and water ∎ if observing enteric precautions: plastic trash bags, labels ∎ optional (for patients who can't retain solution): plastic rectal tube guard, Foley indwelling catheter or Verden rectal catheter with 30-ml balloon and syringe.

Prepackaged disposable enema sets are available, as are small-volume enema solutions in both irrigating and retention types and in pediatric sizes.

Preparation of equipment
Prepare the prescribed type and amount of solution, as indicated. (See *Carminative, cleansing, and emollient enemas,* page 538.) Standard irrigating enema volumes are 750 to 1,000 ml for an adult; 500 to 1,000 ml for a school-aged child; 250 to 500 ml for a toddler or preschooler; and 50 to 250 ml or less for an infant or for a retention enema.

Because some ingredients may be mucosal irritants, be sure the proportions are correct and the agents are thoroughly mixed *to avoid localized irritation.*

Warm the solution *to reduce patient discomfort.* Note that some enemas, such as the milk and molasses, must be heated to high temperatures for proper mixing and

Carminative, cleansing, and emollient enemas

SOLUTION	PREPARATION	PURPOSE
Irrigating enemas		
Harris flush	Instill 1,000 ml of tap water.	Cleansing
Magnesium sulfate	Add 2 tbs of magnesium sulfate to 3 tbs of salt in 1,000 ml of tap water.	Carminative
Saline	If a commercially prepared solution isn't available, add 2 tsp of salt to 1,000 ml of tap water.	Cleansing
Soap and water	Add 1 packet of mild soap to 1,000 ml of tap water and remove all bubbles before administering solution.	Cleansing
Retention enemas		
Milk and molasses	Heat 175 to 200 ml of milk to 140° F (60° C). Slowly add the same amount of molasses. Stir well, to blend ingredients thoroughly. Cool to 100° F (37.8° C) before administering.	Carminative
Oil	Instill 150 ml of mineral, olive, or cottonseed oil.	Cleansing and emollient
1-2-3	Add 30 ml of 50% magnesium sulfate to 60 ml of glycerin. Add mixture to 90 ml of warm tap water.	Cleansing

then cooled to about 100° to 105° F (37.8° to 40.5° C). Test the solution's temperature with the bath thermometer. Administer an adult's enema at 100° to 105° F and a child's enema at 100° F *to avoid burning rectal tissues.*

Clamp the tubing and fill the solution bag with the prescribed solution. Unclamp the tubing, flush the solution through the tubing, then reclamp it. *Flushing detects leaks and removes air that could cause discomfort if introduced into the colon.*

Hang the solution container on the I.V. pole and take all supplies to the patient's room. If you're using a Foley or Verden catheter, fill the syringe with 30 ml of water.

Implementation
• Check the doctor's order and assess the patient's condition.
• Provide privacy and explain the procedure. If you're administering an enema to a child, familiarize him with the equipment and allow a parent or another relative to remain with him during the procedure *to provide reassurance.* Instruct the patient to breathe through the mouth

to relax the anal sphincter, which will facilitate catheter insertion.
• Ask the patient if he's had previous difficulty retaining an enema *to determine whether you need to use a rectal tube guard or a catheter.*
• Wash your hands and put on gloves.
• Assist the patient, as necessary, in putting on a hospital gown. *The gown makes enema administration easier, and the patient worries less about soiling it.*
• Assist the patient into the left-lateral Sims' position. *This will facilitate the solution's flow by gravity into the descending colon.* (See *Giving an enema.*) If contraindicated or if the patient reports discomfort, reposition him on his back or right side.
• Place linen-saver pads under the patient's buttocks *to prevent soiling the linens.* Replace the top bed linens with a bath blanket *to provide privacy and warmth.*
• Have a bedpan or commode nearby for the patient to use. If the patient may use the bathroom, be sure that it will be available when the patient needs it. Have toilet tissue within the patient's reach.

• Lubricate the distal tip of the rectal catheter with water-soluble lubricant *to facilitate rectal insertion and reduce irritation.*

• Separate the patient's buttocks and touch the anal sphincter with the rectal tube *to stimulate contraction.* Then, as the sphincter relaxes, tell the patient to breathe deeply through the mouth as you gently advance the tube.

• If the patient feels pain or the tube meets continued resistance, notify the doctor. *This may signal an unknown stricture or abscess.* If the patient has poor sphincter control, use a plastic rectal tube guard, or slip the tube through the cut end of a baby bottle nipple.

• You can also use a Foley or Verden catheter as a rectal tube *if your hospital's policy permits.* Insert the lubricated catheter as you would a rectal tube. Then, gently inflate the catheter's balloon with 20 to 30 ml of water. Gently pull the catheter back against the patient's internal anal sphincter *to seal off the rectum.* If leakage still occurs with the balloon in place, add more water to the balloon in small amounts. When using either catheter, avoid inflating the balloon above 45 ml *because overinflation can compromise blood flow to the rectal tissues and cause possible necrosis from pressure on the rectal mucosa.*

• If you're using a rectal tube, hold it in place throughout the procedure *because bowel contractions and the pressure of the tube against the anal sphincter can promote tube displacement.*

• Hold the solution container slightly above bed level and release the tubing clamp. Then raise the container gradually to start the flow—usually at a rate of 75 to 100 ml/minute for an irrigating enema, but at the slowest possible rate for a retention enema *to avoid stimulating peristalsis and to promote retention.* Adjust the flow rate of an irrigating enema by raising or lowering the solution container according to the patient's retention ability and comfort. However, be sure not to raise it higher than 18″ (46 cm) for an adult, 12″ (31 cm) for a child, and 6″ to 8″ (15 to 20 cm) for an infant, *because excessive pressure can force colon bacteria into the small intestine or rupture the colon.*

• Assess the patient's tolerance frequently during instillation. If he complains of discomfort, cramps, or the need to defecate, stop the flow by pinching or clamping the tubing. Then hold the patient's buttocks together or firmly press toilet tissue against the anus. Instruct him to gently massage his abdomen and breathe slowly and deeply through his mouth *to help relax abdominal muscles and promote retention.* Resume administration at a slower flow rate after a few minutes when discomfort passes, but interrupt the flow any time the patient feels uncomfortable.

• If the flow slows or stops, the catheter tip may be clogged with feces or pressed against the rectal wall.

Giving an enema

Unless contraindicated, help the patient into the left-lateral Sims' position. After lubricating the end of the tube, separate the patient's buttocks and push the tube gently into the anus, aiming it toward the umbilicus. For an adult, insert the tube 2″ to 4″ (5 to 10 cm); for a child, insert it only 2″ to 3″ (5 to 7.6 cm); for an infant, insert it only 1″ to 1½″ (2.5 to 3.8 cm). Avoid forcing the tube *to prevent rectal wall trauma.* If it doesn't advance easily, allow a little solution to flow in *to relax the inner sphincter enough to allow passage.*

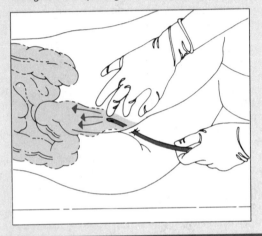

Gently turn the catheter slightly *to free it without stimulating defecation.* If the catheter tip remains clogged, withdraw the catheter, flush with solution, and reinsert.

• After administering most of the prescribed amount of solution, clamp the tubing. Stop the flow before the container empties completely *to avoid introducing air into the bowel.*

• To administer a commercially prepared, small-volume enema, first remove the cap from the rectal tube. Insert the rectal tube into the rectum and squeeze the bottle *to deposit the contents in the rectum.* Remove the rectal tube, replace the used enema unit in its original container, and discard.

• For a flush enema, stop the flow by lowering the solution container below bed level and allowing gravity to siphon the enema from the colon. Continue to raise and lower the container until gas bubbles cease or the patient feels more comfortable and abdominal distention subsides. Don't allow the solution container to empty completely before lowering it *because this may introduce air into the bowel.*

• For an irrigating enema, instruct the patient to retain the solution for 15 minutes, if possible.

• For a retention enema, instruct the patient to avoid defecation for the prescribed time or as follows: 30 minutes or longer for oil retention and milk and molasses; and 15 to 30 minutes for anthelmintic and emollient enemas. If you're using an indwelling catheter, leave the catheter in place *to promote retention.*

• If the patient's apprehensive, position him on the bedpan and allow him to hold toilet tissue or a rolled washcloth against his anus. Place the call signal within his reach. If he will be using the bathroom or the commode, instruct him to call for help before attempting to get out of bed *because the procedure may make the patient — particularly an elderly patient — feel weak or faint.* Also instruct him to call you if he feels weak at any time.

• When the solution has remained in the colon for the recommended time or for as long as the patient can tolerate it, assist the patient onto a bedpan or to the commode or bathroom, as required.

• If an indwelling catheter is in place, deflate the balloon and remove the catheter, if applicable.

• Provide privacy while the patient expels the solution. Instruct the patient not to flush the toilet.

• While the patient uses the bathroom, remove and discard any soiled linen and linen-saver pads.

• Assist the patient with cleaning, if necessary, and help him to bed. Make sure he feels clean and comfortable and can easily reach the call signal. Place a clean linen-saver pad under him *to absorb rectal drainage,* and tell him that he may need to expel additional stool or flatus later. Encourage him to rest for a while *because the procedure may be tiring.*

• Cover the bedpan or commode and take it to the utility room for observation, or observe the contents of the toilet, as applicable. Carefully note fecal color, consistency, amount (minimal, moderate, or generous), and foreign matter, such as blood, rectal tissue, worms, pus, mucus, or other unusual matter.

• Send specimens to the laboratory, if ordered.

• Rinse the bedpan or commode with cold water, then wash it in hot soapy water. Return it to the patient's bedside.

• Properly dispose of the enema equipment. If additional enemas are scheduled, store clean, reusable equipment in a closed plastic bag in the patient's bathroom. Discard your gloves and wash your hands.

• Ventilate the room or use an air freshener, if necessary.

Special considerations

Because patients with salt-retention disorders, such as congestive heart failure, may absorb sodium from the saline enema solution, administer the solution to such patients cautiously and monitor electrolyte status.

Schedule a retention enema before meals *because a full stomach may stimulate peristalsis and make retention difficult.* Follow an oil-retention enema with a soap and water enema 1 hour later *to help expel the softened feces completely.*

Administer less solution when giving a hypertonic enema *because osmotic pull moves fluid into the colon from body tissues, increasing the volume of colon contents.* Alternate means of instilling the solution include using a bulb syringe or a funnel with the rectal tube.

For the patient who cannot tolerate a flat position (for example, a patient with shortness of breath), administer the enema with the head of the bed in the lowest position he can safely and comfortably maintain. For a bedridden patient who needs to expel the enema into a bedpan, raise the head of the bed to approximate a sitting or squatting position. Don't give an enema to a patient who's in a sitting position, unless absolutely necessary, *because the solution won't flow high enough into the colon and will only distend the rectum and trigger rapid expulsion.* If the patient has hemorrhoids, instruct him to bear down gently during tube insertion. *This causes the anus to open and facilitates insertion.*

If the patient fails to expel the solution within 1 hour *because of diminished neuromuscular response,* you may need to remove the enema solution. First, review your hospital's policy *because you may need a doctor's order.* Inform the doctor when a patient can't expel an enema spontaneously *because of possible bowel perforation or electrolyte imbalance.* To siphon the enema solution from the patient's rectum, assist him to a side-lying position on the bed. Place a bedpan on a bedside chair so it rests below mattress level. Disconnect the tubing from the solution container, place the distal end in the bedpan, and reinsert the rectal end into the patient's anus. If gravity fails to drain the solution into the bedpan, instill 30 to 50 ml of warm water through the tube (105° F [40.6° C] for an adult patient; 100° F [37.8° C] for a child or infant). Then quickly direct the distal end of the tube into the bedpan. In both cases, measure the return *to be sure all solution has drained.*

In patients with fluid and electrolyte disturbances, measure the amount of expelled solution *to assess for retention of enema fluid.*

Double-bag all enema equipment and label it as isolation equipment if the patient is on enteric precautions.

If the doctor orders enemas until returns are clear, give no more than three *to avoid excessive irritation of the rectal mucosa.* Notify the doctor if the returned fluid isn't clear after three administrations.

Home care

Describe the procedure to the patient and his family. Emphasize that administering an enema to a person in a sitting position or on the toilet could injure the rectal wall. Tell the patient how to prepare and care for the equipment. Discuss relaxation techniques, and review measures for preventing constipation, including regular exercise, dietary modifications, and adequate fluid intake.

Complications

Enemas may produce dizziness or faintness; excessive irritation of the colonic mucosa resulting from repeated administration or from sensitivity to the enema ingredients; hyponatremia or hypokalemia from repeated administration of hypotonic solutions; and cardiac arrhythmias resulting from vasovagal reflex stimulation after insertion of the rectal catheter. Colonic water absorption may result from prolonged retention of hypotonic solutions, which may, in turn, cause hypervolemia or water intoxication.

Documentation

Record the date and time of enema administration; special equipment used; type and amount of solution; retention time; approximate amount returned; color, consistency, and amount of the return; abnormalities within the return; any complications that occurred; and the patient's tolerance of the treatment.

TRANSABDOMINAL ACCESS
Transabdominal tube feeding and care

To access the stomach, duodenum, or jejunum, the doctor may place a tube through the patient's abdominal wall. This may be done surgically or percutaneously.

Gastrostomy or jejunostomy tubes are usually placed during intra-abdominal surgery. The tube may be used for feeding during the immediate postoperative period or it may provide long-term enteral access, depending on what type of surgery the patient had. Typically, the doctor will suture the tube in place to prevent gastric contents from leaking.

In contrast, a percutaneous endoscopic gastrostomy (PEG) or jejunostomy (PEJ) tube can be inserted endoscopically without the need for laparotomy or general anesthesia. Typically, the insertion is done in the endoscopy suite or at the patient's bedside. A PEG or PEJ tube may be used for nutrition, drainage, and decompression. Contraindications to endoscopic placement include obstruction (such as an esophageal stricture or duodenal blockage), previous gastric surgery, morbid obesity, and ascites. These conditions would necessitate surgical placement.

With either type of tube placement, feedings may begin after about 24 hours (or when peristalsis resumes).

After a time, the tube may need replacement, and the doctor may recommend a similar tube, such as a Foley or a mushroom catheter, or a gastrostomy button — a skin-level feeding tube. (See "Gastrostomy feeding button care" in this chapter.)

Nursing care includes providing skin care at the tube site, maintaining the feeding tube, administering feeding, monitoring the patient's response to feeding, adjusting the feeding schedule, and preparing the patient for self-care after discharge.

Equipment

For feeding: feeding formula ▪ large-bulb or catheter-tip syringe ▪ 120 ml of water ▪ $4'' \times 4''$ gauze pads ▪ soap ▪ skin protectant ▪ antibacterial ointment ▪ nonallergenic tape ▪ gravity-drip administration bags ▪ mouthwash, toothpaste, or mild salt solution ▪ gloves ▪ optional: enteral infusion pump.

For decompression: suction apparatus with tubing and straight drainage collection set.

Preparation of equipment

Always check the expiration date on commercially prepared feeding formulas. If the formula has been prepared by the dietitian or pharmacist, check the preparation time and date. Discard any opened formula or solution that's more than 1 day old.

Commercially prepared administration sets and enteral pumps allow continuous formula administration. Place the desired amount of formula into the gavage container and purge air from the tubing. To avoid formula contamination, hang only a 4- to 6-hour supply of formula at a time.

Implementation

• Provide privacy and wash your hands.

• Explain the procedure to the patient. Tell him, for example, that feedings usually start at a slow rate and increase as tolerated. After he tolerates continuous feed-

ings, he may progress to intermittent feedings to prepare him for home management, as ordered.
- Assess for bowel sounds before feeding, and monitor for abdominal distention.
- Ask the patient to sit, or assist him into the semi-Fowler's position, for the entire feeding. *This helps to prevent esophageal reflux and pulmonary aspiration of the formula.* For an intermittent feeding, have the patient maintain this position throughout the feeding and for 1 hour after.
- Put on gloves. Before starting the feeding, measure residual gastric contents. Attach the syringe to the feeding tube and aspirate. If the contents measure more than twice the amount infused, hold the feeding and recheck in 1 hour. Then, if residual contents remain too high, notify the doctor. Chances are the formula isn't being absorbed properly.
- With PEJ or jejunostomy tube feedings, keep in mind that residual contents will be minimal.
- Allow 30 ml of water to flow into the feeding tube *to establish patency.*
- Be sure to administer formula at room temperature. *Cold formula may cause cramping.*

Intermittent feedings
- Allow gravity to help the formula flow over 30 to 45 minutes. *Faster infusions may cause bloating, cramps, or diarrhea.*
- Begin intermittent feeding with a low volume (200 ml) daily. According to the patient's tolerance, increase the volume per feeding, as needed, *to reach the desired calorie intake.*
- When the feeding finishes, flush the feeding tube with 30 to 60 ml of water. *This maintains patency and provides hydration.*
- Cap the tube *to prevent leakage.*
- Rinse the feeding administration set thoroughly with hot water *to avoid contaminating subsequent feedings.* Allow the tube to dry between feedings.

Continuous feedings
- Measure residual gastric contents every 4 hours.
- To administer the feeding with a pump, set up the equipment according to the manufacturer's guidelines, and fill the feeding bag. To administer the feeding by gravity, fill the container with formula and purge air from the tubing.
- Monitor the gravity drip rate or pump infusion rate frequently *to ensure accurate delivery of formula.*
- Flush the feeding tube with 30 to 60 ml of water every 4 hours *to maintain patency and to provide hydration.*
- Monitor intake and output *to anticipate and detect fluid or electrolyte imbalances.*

Decompression
- To decompress the stomach, connect the PEG port to the suction device with tubing or straight gravity drainage tubing. Jejunostomy feeding may be given simultaneously via the PEJ port of the dual-lumen tube.

Tube exit site care
- Provide daily skin care.
- Gently remove the dressing by hand. Never cut away the dressing over the catheter because *you may inadvertently cut the tube or the sutures holding the tube in place.*
- At least daily and as needed, clean the skin around the tube's exit site using a $4'' \times 4''$ gauze pad soaked in the prescribed cleaning solution. When healed, wash the skin around the exit site daily with soap. Rinse the area with water and pat dry. Apply skin protectant, if necessary, and antibacterial ointment to the catheter at the exit site *to prevent or treat skin maceration.*
- Anchor a gastrostomy or jejunostomy tube to the skin with nonallergenic tape *to prevent peristaltic migration of the tube.* This also prevents tension on the suture anchoring the tube in place.
- Coil the tube, if necessary, and tape it to the abdomen *to prevent pulling and contamination of the tube.* PEG and PEJ tubes have toggle-bolt-like internal and external bumpers that make tape anchors unnecessary. (See *Caring for the PEG or PEJ site.*)

Special considerations
If the patient vomits, stop the feeding immediately and assess his condition. Also stop the feeding if he complains of nausea, feeling too full, or regurgitation. Flush the feeding tube and attempt to restart the feeding again in 1 hour (measure residual gastric contents first). You may have to decrease the volume or rate of feedings. If dumping syndrome develops, which includes nausea, vomiting, cramps, pallor, and diarrhea, the feedings may have been given too quickly.

Provide oral hygiene frequently. Brush all surfaces of the teeth, gums, and tongue at least twice daily using mouthwash, toothpaste, or mild salt solution.

You can administer most tablets and pills through the tube by crushing them and diluting as necessary. (The exception: enteric-coated or sustained-released drugs, which lose their effectiveness when crushed.) Medications should be in liquid form for administration.

Control diarrhea resulting from dumping syndrome by using continuous pump or gravity-drip infusions, diluting the feeding formula, or adding antidiarrheal medications.

Home care
Instruct the patient and family members or other caregivers in all aspects of enteral feedings, including tube

Caring for the PEG or PEJ site

The exit site of a percutaneous endoscopic gastrostomy (PEG) or percutaneous endoscopic jejunostomy (PEJ) tube requires routine observation and care. Follow these care guidelines:
• Change the dressing daily while the tube is in place.
• After removing the dressing, carefully slide the tube's outer bumper away from the skin about ½" (1 cm).

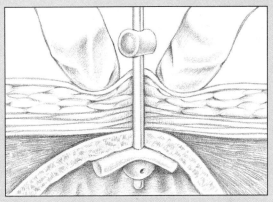

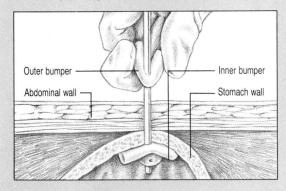

• Clean the site with the prescribed cleaning solution. Then apply povidone-iodine ointment over the exit site, according to your hospital's guidelines.
• Rotate the outer bumper 90 degrees *(to prevent repeating the same tension on the same skin area),* and slide the outer bumper back over the exit site.
• If leakage appears at the PEG site, or if the patient risks dislodging the tube, apply a sterile gauze dressing over the site. Do not put sterile gauze underneath the outer bumper. Loosening the anchor in this way allows the feeding tube free play, which could lead to wound abscess.
• Write the date and time of the dressing change on the tape.

• Examine the skin around the tube. Look for redness and other signs of infection or erosion.
• Gently depress the skin surrounding the tube and inspect for drainage (see illustration at right). Initially after implantation, expect minimal wound drainage. This should subside in about 1 week.
• Inspect the tube for wear and tear. (A tube that wears out will need replacement.)

maintenance and site care. Specify signs and symptoms to report to the doctor, define emergency situations, and review actions to take.

When the tube needs replacement, advise the patient that the doctor may insert a replacement gastrostomy button or a latex, indwelling, or mushroom catheter after removing the initial feeding tube. The procedure may be done in the doctor's office or the hospital endoscopy suite.

As the patient's tolerance to tube feeding improves, he may wish to try syringe feedings rather than intermittent feedings. If appropriate, teach him how to feed himself by this method. (See *Teaching the patient about syringe feeding,* page 544.)

Complications

Common complications related to transabdominal tubes include GI or other systemic problems, mechanical malfunction, and metabolic disturbances.

Cramping, nausea, vomiting, bloating, and diarrhea may be related to medication; rapid infusion rate; formula contamination, osmolarity, or temperature (too cold or too warm); fat malabsorption; or intestinal atrophy from malnutrition.

Constipation may result from inadequate hydration, or insufficient exercise.

Systemic problems may be caused by pulmonary aspiration, infection at the tube exit site, or contaminated formula. Proper positioning during feeding, verification of tube placement, meticulous skin care, and aseptic formula preparation are ways to prevent these complications.

Teaching the patient about syringe feeding

If the patient plans to feed himself by syringe when he returns home, you'll need to teach him how to do this before he's discharged. Here are some points to emphasize.

Initial instructions
First, show the patient how to clamp the feeding tube, remove the syringe's bulb or plunger, and place the tip of the syringe into the feeding tube. Then, instill between 30 and 60 ml of water into the feeding tube to be sure it stays open and patent.

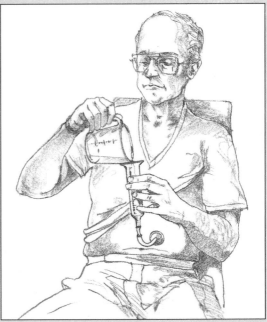

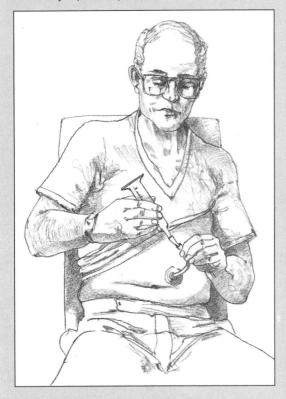

Next, tell him to pour the feeding solution into the syringe and begin the feeding (see illustration at top right). As the solution flows into the stomach, show him how to tilt the syringe to allow air bubbles to escape. Describe the discomfort that air bubbles may cause.

Tips for free flow
When about one-fourth of the feeding solution remains, direct the patient to refill the syringe. Caution him to avoid letting the syringe empty completely. Doing so may result in abdominal cramping and gas.

Demonstrate how to increase and decrease the solution's flow rate by raising or lowering the syringe. Explain also that he may need to dilute a thick solution to promote free flow.

Finishing up
Inform the patient that the feeding infusion process should take about 15 minutes or more. If the process takes less than 15 minutes, dumping syndrome may result.

Show the patient the steps needed to finish the feeding, including how to flush the tube with water, clamp the tube, and clean the equipment for later use. Naturally, if he's using disposable gear, urge him to discard it properly. Review how to store unused feeding solution if appropriate.

Typical mechanical problems include tube dislodgment, obstruction, or impairment. For example, a PEG or PEJ tube may migrate if the external bumper loosens. Occlusion may result from incompletely crushed and liquefied medication particles or inadequate tube flushing. Further, the tube may rupture or crack from age, drying, or frequent manipulation.

Monitor the patient for vitamin and mineral deficiencies, glucose tolerance, and fluid and electrolyte imbalances, which may follow bouts of diarrhea or constipation.

Documentation

On the intake and output record, note the date, time, and amount of each feeding and the water volume instilled. Maintain total volumes for nutrients and water separately to allow calculation of nutrient intake. In your notes, document the type of formula, the infusion method and rate, the patient's tolerance of the procedure and formula, and the amount of residual gastric contents. Also record complications and abdominal assessment findings. Note patient-teaching topics covered, and note the patient's progress in self-care.

Gastrostomy feeding button care

The gastrostomy feeding button serves as an alternative feeding device for an ambulatory patient receiving long-term enteral feedings. Approved by the Food and Drug Administration for 6-month implantation, the feeding button can be used to replace the gastrostomy tube if necessary.

The button has a mushroom dome at one end and two wing tabs and a flexible safety plug at the other. When inserted into an established stoma, the button lies almost flush with the skin, with only the top of the safety plug visible.

The button usually can be inserted into a stoma in less than 15 minutes. Besides its cosmetic appeal, the device is easily maintained, reduces skin irritation and breakdown, and has a smaller risk of dislodgment and migration than an ordinary feeding tube. A one-way, antireflux valve mounted just inside the mushroom dome prevents accidental leakage of gastric contents. The device usually requires replacement after 3 to 4 months, most often because the antireflux valve wears out.

Equipment

Gastrostomy feeding button of the correct size (all three sizes, if the correct one isn't known) ■ obturator ■ water-soluble lubricant ■ gloves ■ feeding accessories, including adapter, feeding catheter, food syringe or bag, and formula ■ catheter clamp ■ cleaning equipment, including water, a syringe, cotton-tipped applicator, pipe cleaner, and mild soap or povidone-iodine solution ■ optional: pump to provide continuous infusion over several hours.

Implementation

• Explain the insertion, reinsertion, and feeding procedure to the patient. Tell him the doctor will perform the initial insertion.

• Wash your hands and put on gloves. (See *How to reinsert a gastrostomy feeding button,* page 546.)

• Attach the adapter and feeding catheter to the syringe or feeding bag. Clamp the catheter and fill the syringe or bag and catheter with formula. Refill the syringe before it's empty. *These steps prevent air from entering the stomach and distending the abdomen.*

• Open the safety plug and attach the adapter and feeding catheter to the button. Elevate the syringe or feeding bag above stomach level, and gravity-feed the formula for 15 to 30 minutes, varying the height as needed *to alter the flow rate.* Use a pump for continuous infusion or for feedings lasting several hours.

• After feeding, flush the button with 10 ml of water and clean the inside of the feeding catheter with a cotton-tipped applicator and water *to preserve patency and to dislodge formula or food particles,* and lower the syringe or bag below stomach level *to allow burping.* Remove the adapter and feeding catheter. The antireflux valve should prevent gastric reflux. Then snap the safety plug in place *to keep the lumen clean and prevent leakage if the antireflux valve fails.* If the patient feels nauseated or vomits after feeding, vent the button with the adapter and feeding catheter *to control emesis.*

• Wash the catheter and syringe or feeding bag in warm soapy water and rinse thoroughly. Clean the catheter and adapter with a pipe cleaner. Rinse well before using for the next feeding. Soak the equipment once a week according to manufacturer's recommendations.

Special considerations

If the button pops out while feeding, reinsert it, estimate the formula already delivered, and resume feeding.

Once daily, clean the peristomal skin with mild soap and water or povidone-iodine, and let the skin air-dry for 20 minutes, *to avoid skin irritation.* Also clean the site whenever spillage from the feeding bag occurs.

Home care

Before discharge, be sure the patient can insert and care for the gastrostomy feeding button. If necessary, teach him or a family member how to reinsert the button by

How to reinsert a gastrostomy feeding button

If your patient's gastrostomy feeding button pops out (with coughing for instance), either you or he will need to reinsert the device. Here are some steps to follow.

Prepare the equipment
Collect the feeding button, an obturator, and water-soluble lubricant. If the button will be reinserted, wash it with soap and water and rinse it thoroughly.

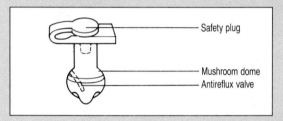

Safety plug

Mushroom dome
Antireflux valve

Insert the button
• Check the depth of the patient's stoma *to make sure you have a feeding button of the correct size.* Then, clean around the stoma.
• Lubricate the obturator with a water-soluble lubricant, and distend the button several times *to ensure patency of the antireflux valve within the button.*
• Lubricate the mushroom dome and the stoma. Gently push the button through the stoma into the stomach.

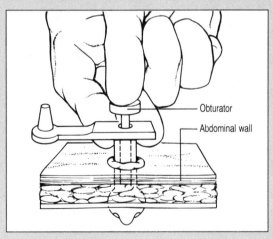

Obturator
Abdominal wall

• Remove the obturator by gently rotating it as you with-draw it, *to keep the antireflux valve from adhering to it.* If the valve sticks nonetheless, gently push the obturator back into the button until the valve closes.
• After removing the obturator, check the valve to make sure it's closed. Then close the flexible safety plug, which should be relatively flush with the skin surface.

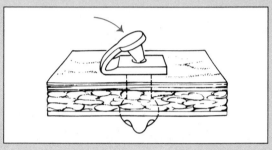

• If you need to administer a feeding right away, open the safety plug and attach the feeding adapter and feeding tube. Deliver the feeding as ordered.

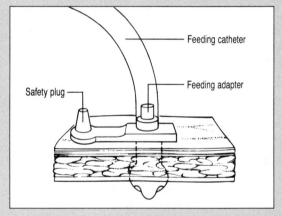

Feeding catheter

Feeding adapter

Safety plug

first practicing on a model. Offer written instructions and answer his questions on obtaining replacement supplies.

Documentation

Record feeding time and duration, amount and type of feeding formula used, and patient tolerance. Maintain intake and output records, as necessary. Note the appearance of the stoma and surrounding skin.

 # Colostomy and ileostomy care

A patient with an ascending or transverse colostomy or an ileostomy may wear an external pouch to collect emerging fecal matter, which will be watery or pasty. Besides collecting waste matter, the pouch helps to control odor and to protect the stoma and peristomal skin. Most disposable pouching systems can be used from 2 to 7 days. Some models last even longer—up to 14 days.

Any pouching system needs immediate changing if a leak develops. And every pouch needs emptying when it's one-third to one-half full. The patient with an ileostomy may need to empty his pouch four or five times daily.

Naturally, the best time to change the pouching system is when the bowel is least active, usually between 2 and 4 hours after meals. After a few months, most patients can predict the best changing time.

Pouching-system selection should consider which system provides the best adhesive seal and skin protection for the individual patient. The type of pouch selected depends on the stoma's location and structure, availability of supplies, wear time, consistency of effluent, personal preference, and finances.

Equipment

Pouching system ■ stoma measuring guide ■ stoma paste (if drainage is watery to pasty or stoma secretes excess mucus) ■ plastic bag ■ water ■ washcloth and towel ■ closure clamp ■ toilet or bedpan ■ water or pouch cleaning solution ■ gloves ■ facial tissues ■ optional: ostomy belt, paper tape, mild nonmoisturizing soap, skin shaving equipment, liquid skin sealant, pouch deodorant.

Pouching systems may be drainable or closed-bottomed, disposable or reusable, adhesive-backed, and one-piece or two-piece. (See *Comparing ostomy pouching systems*, page 548.)

Implementation

Begin the following procedures by providing privacy and emotional support.

To fit the pouch and skin barrier

• For a pouch with an attached skin barrier, measure the stoma with the stoma measuring guide. Select the opening size that matches the stoma.

• For an adhesive-backed pouch with a separate skin barrier, measure the stoma with the measuring guide and select the opening that matches the stoma. Trace the selected size opening onto the paper back of the skin barrier's adhesive side. Cut out the opening. (If the pouch has precut openings, which can be handy for a round stoma, select an opening that's ⅛″ larger than the stoma. If the pouch comes without an opening, cut the hole ⅛″ wider than the measured tracing.) The cut-to-fit system works best for an irregularly shaped stoma.

• For a two-piece pouching system with flanges, see *Applying a skin barrier and pouch*, page 549.

• Avoid fitting the pouch too tightly *because the stoma has no pain receptors. A constrictive opening could injure the stoma or skin tissue without the patient feeling warning discomfort. Also avoid cutting the opening too big because this may expose the skin to fecal matter and moisture.*

• The patient with a descending or sigmoid colostomy who has formed stool and whose ostomy doesn't secrete much mucus may choose to wear only a pouch. In this case, make sure that the pouch opening closely matches the stoma size.

• Between 6 weeks and 1 year after surgery, the stoma will shrink to its permanent size. Then pattern-making preparations will be unnecessary unless the patient gains weight, has additional surgery, or injures the stoma.

To apply or change the pouch

• Collect all equipment.

• Wash your hands and provide privacy.

• Explain the procedure to the patient. As you perform each step, explain what you are doing and why *because the patient will eventually perform the procedure himself.*

• Put on gloves.

• Remove and discard the old pouch. Wipe the stoma and peristomal skin gently with a facial tissue.

• Carefully wash and dry the peristomal skin. Inspect the peristomal skin and stoma. Shave surrounding hair, if necessary, *to promote a better seal and avoid skin irritation from hair pulling against the adhesive.*

• If applying a separate skin barrier, peel off the paper backing of the prepared skin barrier, center the barrier over the stoma, and press gently to ensure adhesion.

• You may want to outline the stoma or the back of the skin barrier (depending on the product) with a thin ring of stoma paste *to provide extra skin protection.* (Skip this step if the patient has a sigmoid or descending colostomy, formed stool, and little mucus.)

(Text continues on page 550.)

Comparing ostomy pouching systems

Manufactured in many shapes and sizes, ostomy pouches are fashioned for comfort, safety, and easy application. For example, a disposable closed-end pouch may meet the needs of a patient who irrigates, who wants added security, or who wants to discard the pouch after each bowel movement. Another patient may prefer a reusable, drainable pouch. Some commonly available pouches are described below.

Disposable pouches

The patient who must empty his pouch often (because of diarrhea or a new colostomy or ileostomy) may prefer a one-piece, drainable, disposable pouch with a closure clamp attached to a skin barrier (below, left). These transparent or opaque, odor-proof, plastic pouches come with attached adhesive or karaya seals. Some pouches have microporous adhesive or belt tabs. The bottom opening allows for easy draining. This pouch may be used permanently or temporarily, until stoma size stabilizes.

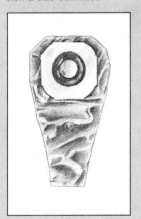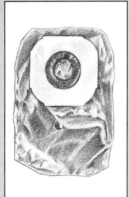

Also disposable and also made of transparent or opaque odor-proof plastic, a one-piece disposable closed-end pouch (above, right) may come in a kit with adhesive seal, belt tabs, skin barrier, or carbon filter for gas release. A patient with a regular bowel elimination pattern may choose this style for additional security and confidence.

A two-piece disposable drainable pouch with separate skin barrier, shown below, permits frequent changes and also minimizes skin breakdown. Also made of transparent or opaque odor-proof plastic, this style comes with belt tabs and usually snaps to the skin barrier with a flange mechanism.

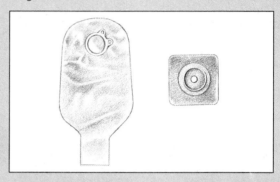

Reusable pouches

Typically manufactured from sturdy, opaque, nonallergenic plastic, the reusable pouch comes with a separate custom-made faceplate and O-ring, as shown below. Some pouches have a pressure valve for releasing gas. The device has a 1- to 2-month life span, depending on how frequently the patient empties the pouch.

Reusable equipment may benefit a patient who needs a firm faceplate or who wishes to minimize cost. However, many reusable ostomy pouches aren't odor-proof.

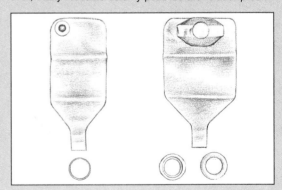

Applying a skin barrier and pouch

Fitting a skin barrier and ostomy pouch properly can be done in a few steps. Shown below is a two-piece pouching system with flanges, which is in common use.

Measure the stoma using a measuring guide.

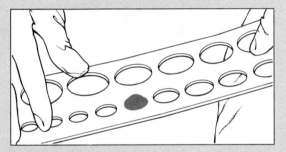

Trace the appropriate circle carefully on the back of the skin barrier.

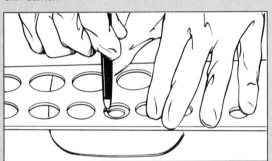

Cut the circular opening in the skin barrier. Bevel the edges to keep them from irritating the patient.

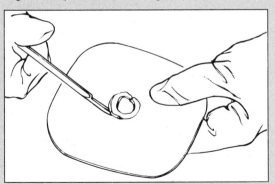

Remove the backing from the skin barrier and moisten it or apply barrier paste, as needed, along the edge of the circular opening.

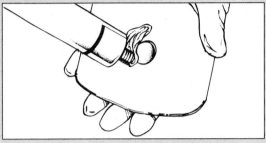

Center the skin barrier over the stoma, adhesive side down, and gently press it to the skin.

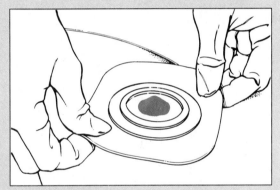

Gently press the pouch opening onto the ring until it snaps into place.

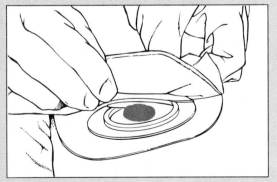

• Remove the paper backing from the adhesive side of the pouching system and center the pouch opening over the stoma. Press gently to secure.
• For a pouching system with flanges, align the lip of the pouch flange with the bottom edge of the skin barrier flange. Gently press around the circumference of the pouch flange, beginning at the bottom, until the pouch securely adheres to the barrier flange. (The pouch will click into its secured position.) Holding the barrier against the skin, gently pull on the pouch *to confirm the seal between flanges.*
• Encourage the patient to stay quietly in position for about 5 minutes *to improve adherence. The patient's body warmth also helps to improve adherence and soften a rigid skin barrier.*
• Attach an ostomy belt to further secure the pouch, if desired. (Some pouches have belt loops, and others have plastic adapters for belts.)
• Leave a bit of air in the pouch *to allow drainage to fall to the bottom.*
• Apply the closure clamp, if necessary.
• If desired, apply paper tape in a picture-frame fashion to the pouch edges *for additional security.*

To empty the pouch
• Tilt the bottom of the pouch upward and remove the closure clamp.
• Turn up a cuff on the lower end of the pouch and allow it to drain into the toilet or bedpan.
• Wipe the bottom of the pouch and reapply the closure clamp.
• If desired, the bottom portion of the pouch can be rinsed with cool tap water. Do not aim water up near the top of the pouch *because this may loosen the seal on the skin.*
• A two-piece flanged system can also be emptied by unsnapping the pouch. Let the drainage flow into the toilet.
• Release flatus through the gas release valve if the pouch has one. Otherwise, release flatus by tilting the pouch bottom upward, releasing the clamp, and expelling the flatus. To release flatus from a flanged system, loosen the seal between the flanges. (Some pouches have gas release valves.)
• Never make a pinhole in a pouch to release gas. *This destroys the odor-proof seal.*

Special considerations
After performing and explaining the procedure to the patient, encourage the patient's increasing involvement in self-care.

Use adhesive solvents and removers only after patch-testing the patient's skin because *some products may irritate the skin or produce hypersensitivity reactions.* Con-sider using a liquid skin sealant, if available, *to give skin tissue additional protection from drainage and adhesive irritants.*

Remove the pouching system if the patient reports burning or itching beneath it or purulent drainage around the stoma. Notify the doctor or therapist of any skin irritation, breakdown, rash, or unusual appearance of the stoma or peristomal area.

Use commercial pouch deodorants, if desired. However, most pouches are odor-free, and odor should only be evident when you empty the pouch or if it leaks. Before discharge, suggest that the patient avoid odor-causing foods such as fish, eggs, onions, and garlic.

If the patient wears a reusable pouching system, suggest that he obtain two or more systems *so he can wear one while the other dries after cleaning with soap and water or a commercially prepared cleaning solution.*

Complications
Failing to fit the pouch properly over the stoma or improper use of a belt can injure the stoma. Be alert for a possible allergic reaction to adhesives and other ostomy products.

Documentation
Record the date and time of the pouching system change; note the character of drainage, including color, amount, type, and consistency. Also describe the appearance of the stoma and the peristomal skin. Document patient teaching. Describe the teaching content. Record the patient's response to self-care, and evaluate his learning progress.

 # Colostomy irrigation

This procedure can serve two purposes: it allows a patient with a descending or sigmoid colostomy to regulate bowel function, and it's used to clean the large bowel before and after tests, surgery, or other procedures.

Colostomy irrigation may begin as soon as bowel function resumes after surgery. However, most clinicians recommend waiting until bowel movements are more predictable. Initially, the nurse or the patient irrigates the colostomy at the same time every day, recording the amount of output and any spillage between irrigations. Between 4 and 6 weeks may pass before colostomy irrigation establishes a predictable elimination pattern.

Equipment

Colostomy irrigation set (contains an irrigation drain or sleeve, an ostomy belt [if needed] to secure the drain or sleeve, water-soluble lubricant, drainage pouch clamp, and irrigation bag with clamp, tubing, and cone tip) ▪ 1,000 ml (about 30 oz or 1 quart) of tap water irrigant warmed to about 100° F (37.8° C) ▪ normal saline solution (for cleansing enemas) ▪ I.V. pole or wall hook ▪ washcloth and towel ▪ water ▪ ostomy pouching system ▪ linen-saver pad ▪ gloves ▪ optional: bedpan or chair, mild non-moisturizing soap, rubber band or clip, small dressing or bandage, stoma cap.

Preparation of equipment

Depending on the patient's condition, colostomy irrigation may be performed in bed using a bedpan or in the bathroom using the chair and the toilet.

Set up the irrigation bag with tubing and cone tip. If irrigation will take place with the patient in bed, place the bedpan beside the bed and elevate the head of the bed between 45 and 90 degrees, if allowed. If irrigation will take place in the bathroom, have the patient sit on the toilet or on a chair facing the toilet, whichever he finds more comfortable.

Fill the irrigation bag with warmed tap water (or normal saline solution, if the irrigation is for bowel cleansing). Hang the bag on the I.V. pole or wall hook. The bottom of the bag should be at the patient's shoulder level *to prevent the fluid from entering the bowel too quickly.* Most irrigation sets also have a clamp that regulates the flow rate.

Prime the tubing with irrigant *to prevent air from entering the colon and possibly causing cramps and gas pains.*

Implementation

• Explain every step of the procedure to the patient *for teaching purposes, especially since the patient will most likely be irrigating the colostomy himself.*
• Provide privacy and wash your hands.
• If the patient's in bed, place a linen-saver pad under him *to protect the sheets from soiling.*
• Put on gloves.
• Remove the ostomy pouch if the patient uses one.
• Place the irrigation sleeve over the stoma. If the sleeve doesn't have an adhesive backing, secure the sleeve with an ostomy belt. If the patient has a two-piece pouching system with flanges, snap off the pouch and save it. Snap on the irrigation sleeve.
• Place the open-ended bottom of the irrigation sleeve in the bedpan or toilet *to promote drainage by gravity.* If necessary, cut the sleeve so that it meets the water level inside the bedpan or toilet. *Effluent may splash from a short sleeve. From a long sleeve, it may not drain.*

• Lubricate your gloved small finger with water-soluble lubricant and insert the finger into the stoma. If you're teaching the patient, have him do this *to determine the bowel angle at which to insert the cone safely.* Expect the stoma to tighten when the finger enters the bowel and then to relax in a few seconds.
• Lubricate the cone with water-soluble lubricant *to prevent it from irritating the mucosa.*
• Insert the cone into the top opening of the irrigation sleeve and then into the stoma. Angle the cone to match the bowel angle. Insert it gently but snugly.
• Unclamp the irrigation tubing and allow the water to flow slowly. If you don't have a clamp to control the irrigant's flow rate, pinch the tubing *to control the flow.* The water should enter the colon over 10 to 15 minutes. (If the patient reports cramping, slow or stop the flow, keep the cone in place, and have the patient take a few deep breaths until the cramping stops.) Cramping during irrigation may result from a bowel that's ready to empty, water that's too cold, a rapid flow rate, or air in the tubing.
• Have the patient remain stationary for 15 or 20 minutes *so the initial effluent can drain.*
• If the patient's ambulatory, he can stay in the bathroom until all effluent empties, or he can clamp the bottom of the drainage sleeve with a rubber band or clip and return to bed. Explain that *ambulation and activity stimulate elimination.* Suggest that the nonambulatory patient lean forward or massage his abdomen *to stimulate elimination.*
• Wait about 45 minutes for the bowel to finish eliminating the irrigant and effluent. Then remove the irrigation sleeve.
• If the irrigation was intended to clean the bowel, repeat the procedure with warmed normal saline solution until the return solution appears clear.
• Using a washcloth, mild soap, and water, gently clean the area around the stoma. Rinse and dry the area thoroughly with a clean towel.
• Inspect the skin and stoma for changes in appearance. Usually dark pink to red, stoma color may change with the patient's status. Notify the doctor of marked stoma color changes because *a pale hue may result from anemia, and substantial darkening suggests a change in blood flow to the stoma.*
• Apply a clean pouch. Or if the patient has a regular bowel elimination pattern, he may prefer a small dressing, bandage, or commercial stoma cap.
• Discard a disposable irrigation sleeve. Rinse a reusable irrigation sleeve and hang it to dry along with the irrigation bag, tubing, and cone.

Special considerations

Irrigating a colostomy to establish a regular bowel elimination pattern doesn't work for all patients. If the bowel continues to move between irrigations, try decreasing the volume of irrigant. *Increasing the irrigant will not help because it serves only to stimulate peristalsis.* Keep a record of results. Also consider irrigating every other day.

Irrigation may help to regulate bowel function in patients with a descending or sigmoid colostomy *because this is the bowel's stool storage area.* However, a patient with an ascending or transverse colostomy won't benefit from irrigation. Also, a patient with descending or sigmoid colostomy who is missing part of the ascending or transverse colon may not be able to irrigate successfully because his ostomy may function like an ascending or transverse colostomy.

If diarrhea develops, discontinue irrigations until stools form again. Keep in mind that irrigation alone won't achieve regularity for the patient. He must also observe a complementary diet and exercise regimen.

If the patient has a strictured stoma that prohibits cone insertion, remove the cone from the irrigation tubing and replace it with a soft silicone catheter. Angle the catheter gently 2″ to 4″ (5 to 10 cm) into the bowel to instill the irrigant. Don't force the catheter into the stoma, and don't insert it further than the recommended length *because you may perforate the bowel.*

Complications

Bowel perforation may result if a catheter is incorrectly inserted into the stoma. Fluid and electrolyte imbalances may result from using too much irrigant.

Documentation

Record the date and time of irrigation and the type and amount of irrigant. Note the stoma's color and the character of drainage, including the drainage color, consistency, and amount. Record any patient teaching. Describe teaching content and patient response to self-care instruction. Evaluate the patient's learning progress.

Continent ileostomy care

An alternative to conventional ileostomy, a continent or pouch ileostomy (also called a Koch ileostomy or an ileal pouch) features an internal reservoir fashioned from the terminal ileum. This procedure may be used for a patient who requires proctocolectomy for chronic ulcerative colitis or multiple polyposis. Other patients may have a traditional ileostomy converted to a pouch ileostomy.

This procedure is contraindicated in Crohn's disease or gross obesity. Patients who need emergency surgery and those who cannot care for the pouch are also unlikely to have this procedure.

The length of preoperative hospitalization varies with the patient's condition. Nursing responsibilities include providing bowel preparation, antibiotic therapy, and emotional support. After surgery, nursing responsibilities include ensuring patency of the drainage catheter, assessing GI function, caring for the stoma and peristomal skin, managing pain resulting from surgery, and if necessary, perineal skin care.

Usually, daily patient teaching on pouch intubation and drainage begins soon after surgery. Continuous drainage is maintained for about 2 to 6 weeks to allow the suture lines to heal. During this period, a drainage catheter is attached to low intermittent suction. After the suture line heals, the patient learns how to drain the pouch himself.

Equipment

Leg drainage bag ▪ bedside drainage bag ▪ normal saline solution ▪ 50-ml catheter-tip syringe ▪ extra continent ileostomy catheter ▪ 20-ml syringe with adapter ▪ 4″ × 4″ × 1″ foam dressing and Montgomery straps ▪ precut drain dressing ▪ gloves ▪ water-soluble lubricant ▪ graduated container ▪ skin sealant ▪ optional: commercial catheter securing device.

Implementation

Nursing interventions for the patient having a continent ileostomy range from standard preoperative and postoperative care to pouch care and patient teaching.

Preoperative care

• Reinforce and, if necessary, supplement the doctor's explanation of a continent ileostomy and its implications for the patient. (See *Understanding pouch construction.*)
• Assess patient and family attitudes related to the operation and to the forthcoming change in the patient's body image.
• Provide encouragement and support.

Postoperative care

• When the patient returns to his room, attach the drainage catheter emerging from the ileostomy to continuous gravity drainage.
• A leg drainage bag may be attached to the patient's thigh during ambulation.
• Irrigate the catheter with 30 ml of normal saline solution, as ordered and as necessary, *to prevent catheter obstruction and to allow fluid return by gravity.* During the early postoperative period, keep the pouch empty *to allow*

the suture lines to heal and to prevent rapid pouch expansion. At first, drainage will be serosanguineous.

• Monitor fluid intake and output.

• Check the catheter frequently once the patient begins eating solid food *to ensure that mucus or undigested food particles don't block it.*

• If the patient complains of abdominal cramps, distention, and nausea — symptoms of bowel obstruction — the catheter may be clogged. Gently irrigate with 20 to 30 ml of water or normal saline solution until the catheter drains freely. Then move the catheter slightly or rotate it gently *to help clear the obstruction.* Finally, try milking the catheter. If these measures fail, notify the doctor.

• Check the stoma frequently for color, edema, and bleeding. Normally pink to red, a stoma that turns dark red or blue-red may have a compromised blood supply.

• To care for the stoma and peristomal skin, put on gloves. Remove the dressing, gently clean the peristomal area with water, and pat dry. Use a skin sealant around the stoma *to prevent skin irritation.*

• One way to apply a stoma dressing is to slip a precut drain dressing around the catheter to cover the stoma. Cut a hole slightly larger than the lumen of the catheter in the center of a $4'' \times 4'' \times 1''$ piece of foam. Disconnect the catheter from the drainage bag and insert the distal end of the catheter through the hole in the foam. Slide the foam pad onto the dressing. Secure the foam in place with Montgomery straps. Secure the catheter by wrapping the strap ties around it or by using a commercial catheter securing device. Then reconnect the catheter to the drainage bag. (The drainage catheter will be removed by the surgeon when he determines that the suture line has healed.)

• Assess the peristomal skin for irritation from moisture.

• *To reduce discomfort from gas pains,* encourage ambulation. Also recommend that the patient avoid swallowing air (*to minimize gas pains*) by chewing food well, limiting conversation while eating, and not drinking from a straw.

Draining the pouch

• Provide privacy, carefully explain the procedure to the patient, and wash your hands.

• Put on gloves.

• Have the patient with a pouch conversion sit on the toilet *to help him feel more at ease during the procedure.*

• Remove the stoma dressing.

• Encourage the patient to relax his abdominal muscles *to allow the catheter to slide easily into the pouch.*

• Lubricate the tip of the drainage catheter tip with the water-soluble lubricant and insert it in the stoma. Gently push the catheter downward. (The direction of insertion may vary depending on the patient.)

Understanding pouch construction

Depending on the patient and related factors during intestinal surgery, the doctor may construct a pouch to collect fecal matter internally. To make such a pouch, the doctor loops about 12" (30.5 cm) of ileum and sutures the inner sides together.

He opens the loop with a U-shaped cut and seams the inside to create a smooth lining. Then he fashions a nipple or valve between what is becoming the pouch and what will be the stoma.

He folds the open ileum over, sews the pouch closed, and fixes the pouch to the abdominal wall.

Because the pouch holds fecal matter in reserve, the patient benefits from not having to change and empty ostomy equipment. Instead, he empties and irrigates the pouch as needed by inserting a catheter though the stoma and into the pouch.

Initially after surgery, the nurse performs this procedure until the patient can do it himself.

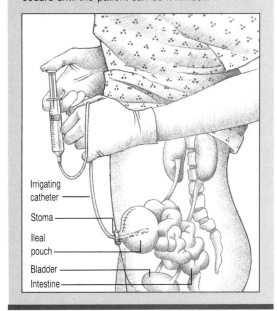

Irrigating catheter

Stoma

Ileal pouch

Bladder

Intestine

• When the catheter reaches the nipple valve of the internal pouch or reservoir (after about 2" or 2½" [5 or 6.4 cm]), you'll feel resistance. Instruct the patient to take a deep breath as you exert gentle pressure on the catheter to insert it through the valve. If this fails, have the patient lie supine and rest for a few minutes. Then, with the patient still supine, try to insert the catheter again.

• Gently advance the catheter to the suture marking made by the surgeon.

• Let the pouch drain completely. This usually takes 5 to 10 minutes. With thick drainage or a clogged catheter, the process may take 30 minutes.

• If the tube clogs, irrigate using the 50-ml catheter-tip syringe with 30 ml of water or normal saline solution. Also, rotate and milk the tube. If these measures fail, then remove, rinse, and reinsert the catheter.

• Remove the catheter after completing drainage.

• Measure output, subtracting the amount of irrigant used.

• Rinse the catheter thoroughly with warm water.

• Clean the peristomal area and apply a fresh stoma dressing.

Predischarge teaching

• Be sure the patient can properly intubate and drain the pouch himself.

• Provide the patient with the appropriate equipment. If the postoperative drainage catheter is still in place, teach the patient how to care for it properly.

• Be sure the patient has a pouch-draining schedule, and give him appropriate pamphlets or video instructions on pouch care.

• Make sure he feels comfortable calling the doctor, nurse, or appropriate other caregivers with questions or problems.

• Tell the patient where to obtain supplies.

• Refer the patient to a local ostomy group.

• Provide dietary counseling.

Special considerations

Never aspirate fluid from the catheter *because the resulting negative pressure may damage inflamed tissue.*

The first few times you intubate the pouch, the patient may be tense, making insertion difficult. Encourage relaxation. To shorten drainage time, have the patient cough, press gently on his abdomen over the pouch, or suddenly tighten his abdominal muscles and then relax them.

Keep an accurate record of intake and output *to ensure fluid and electrolyte balance.* The average daily output should be 1,000 ml. Report inadequate or excessive output (more than 1,400 ml daily).

Complications

Common postoperative complications include obstruction, fistula, pouch perforation, nipple valve dysfunction, abscesses, and bacterial overgrowth in the pouch.

Documentation

Record the date, time, and all aspects of preoperative and postoperative care including condition of the stoma and peristomal skin, diet, medications, intubations, patient teaching, and discharge planning.

 # T-tube care

The T tube may be placed in the common bile duct after cholecystectomy. This tube facilitates biliary drainage during healing. The surgeon inserts the short end (the crossbar) of the T tube in the common bile duct and draws the long end through the incision. The tube then connects to a closed gravity drainage system. (See *Understanding T-tube placement.*) Postoperatively, the tube remains in place between 7 and 14 days.

Equipment

Graduated collection container ■ small plastic bag ■ sterile gloves and clean gloves ■ clamp ■ sterile 4″ × 4″ gauze pads ■ transparent dressings ■ rubber band ■ normal saline solution ■ sterile cleaning solution ■ two sterile basins ■ povidone-iodine sponges ■ sterile precut drain dressings ■ nonallergenic paper tape ■ skin protectant, such as petroleum jelly, zinc oxide, or aluminum-based gel ■ optional: Montgomery straps.

Preparation of equipment

Assemble equipment at the bedside. Open all sterile equipment. Place one sterile 4″ × 4″ gauze pad in each sterile basin. Using sterile technique, pour 50 ml of cleaning solution into one basin and 50 ml of normal saline into the other basin. Tape a small plastic bag on the table to use for refuse.

Implementation

• Provide privacy and explain the procedure to the patient. Wash your hands thoroughly.

To empty drainage

• Put on clean gloves.

• Place the graduated collection container under the outlet valve of the drainage bag. Without contaminating the clamp, valve, or outlet valve, empty the bag's contents completely into the container and reseal the outlet valve. Carefully measure and record the character, color, and amount of drainage. Discard gloves.

Understanding T-tube placement

The T tube is placed in the common bile duct, anchored to the abdominal wall, and connected to a closed drainage system.

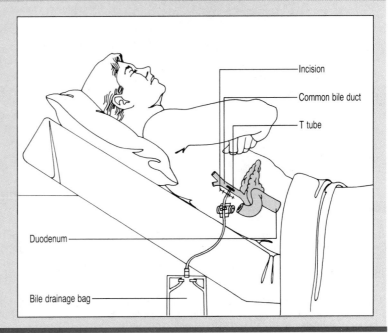

- Incision
- Common bile duct
- T tube
- Duodenum
- Bile drainage bag

To re-dress the T tube

- Wash your hands thoroughly *to prevent bacterial contamination of the incision.* Put on clean gloves.
- Without dislodging the T tube, remove old dressings, and dispose of them in the small plastic bag. Remove the clean gloves.
- Wash your hands again and put on sterile gloves. From this point on, follow strict aseptic technique *to prevent bacterial contamination of the incision.*
- Inspect the incision and tube site for signs of infection, including redness, edema, warmth, tenderness, induration, or skin excoriation. Assess for wound dehiscence or evisceration.
- Use sterile cleaning solution as prescribed to clean and remove dried matter or drainage from around the tube. Always start at the tube site and gently wipe outward in a continuous motion *to prevent recontamination of the incision.*
- Use normal saline solution to rinse off the prescribed cleaning solution. Dry the area with a sterile 4″ × 4″ gauze pad and discard all used materials.
- Using a circular motion, wipe the incision site with a povidone-iodine sponge. Allow the area to dry thoroughly.

- Lightly apply a skin protectant, such as petroleum jelly, zinc oxide, or aluminum-based gel *to protect the skin from injury caused by draining bile.*
- Apply a sterile precut drain dressing on each side of the T tube *to absorb drainage.*
- Apply a sterile 4″ × 4″ gauze pad or transparent dressing over the T tube and the drain dressings. Be careful not to kink the tubing, *which may block the drainage.* Also be careful not to put the dressing over the open end of the T tube *because it connects to the closed drainage system.*
- Secure the dressings with the nonallergenic paper tape or Montgomery straps if necessary.

To clamp the T tube

- As ordered, occlude the tube lightly with a clamp or wrap a rubber band around the end. *Clamping the tube 1 hour before and after meals diverts bile back to the duodenum to aid digestion.*
- *To ensure patient comfort and safety,* check bile drainage amounts regularly. Be alert for such signs of obstructed bile flow as chills, fever, tachycardia, nausea, right-upper-quadrant fullness and pain, jaundice, dark foamy

Managing T-tube obstruction

If your patient's T tube blocks after cholecystectomy, notify the doctor and take these steps while
you wait for him to arrive.
• Unclamp the T tube (if it was clamped before and
after a meal) and connect the tube to a closed
gravity-drainage system.
• Inspect the tube carefully to detect any kinks or
obstructions.
• Prepare the patient for possible T-tube irrigation
or direct X-ray of the common bile duct (cholangi-
ography). Briefly describe these measures to reduce the patient's apprehension and promote
cooperation.
• Provide encouragement and support.

urine, and clay-colored stools. Report them immediately.
(See *Managing T-tube obstruction*.)

Special considerations

Normal daily bile drainage ranges from 500 to 1,000 ml
of viscous, green-brown liquid. The T tube usually drains
300 to 500 ml of blood-tinged bile in the first 24 hours
after surgery. Report drainage that exceeds 500 ml in
the first 24 hours after surgery. This amount typically
declines to 200 ml or less after 4 days. Monitor fluid,
electrolyte, and acid-base status carefully.

To prevent excessive bile loss (over 500 ml in first
24 hours) or backflow contamination, secure the T-tube
drainage system at abdominal level. Bile will flow into
the bag only when biliary pressure increases. As ordered,
return excessive bile drainage (between 1,000 and 1,500
ml daily) to the patient mixed with chilled fruit juice or,
if possible, through a nasogastric tube.

Provide meticulous skin care and frequent dressing
changes. Observe for bile leakage, which may indicate
obstruction. Assess tube patency and site condition hourly
for the first 8 hours and then every 4 hours until the
doctor removes the tube. Protect the skin edges and avoid
excessive taping *to prevent shearing the skin.*

Monitor all urine and stools for color changes. Assess
for icteric skin and sclera, *which may signal jaundice.*

Loose bowels occur commonly in the first few weeks
after surgery. Teach the patient about signs and symptoms of T-tube and biliary obstruction, which he should
report to the doctor.

Complications

Obstructed bile flow, skin excoriation or breakdown, tube
dislodgment, drainage reflux, and infection are the most
common complications related to a biliary T tube.

Documentation

Record the date and time of each dressing change. Note
the appearance of the wound and surrounding skin. Write
down the color, character, and volume of bile collected.
Also record the color of skin and mucous membranes
around the T tube. Record any complaints of nausea or
pain. Keep a precise record of temperature trends, the
patient's coloring, and the amount and frequency of urination and bowel movements.

 Abdominal paracentesis

A bedside procedure, abdominal paracentesis involves the
aspiration of fluid from the peritoneal space through a
needle, trocar, or cannula inserted in the abdominal wall.
Used for diagnosis and therapy, the procedure helps the
health care team determine the cause of ascites and, at
the same time, relieves the pressure created by ascites.
With abdominal paracentesis, the health care team can
also detect intra-abdominal bleeding after traumatic injury and obtain a peritoneal fluid specimen for laboratory
analysis. The procedure must be performed cautiously in
pregnant patients and in patients with bleeding tenden-
cies or unstable vital signs.

Nursing responsibilities during abdominal paracentesis include preparing the patient, monitoring his condition and providing emotional support during the
procedure, assisting the doctor, and obtaining specimens
for laboratory analysis.

Equipment

Tape measure ■ sterile gloves ■ clean gloves ■ linen-saver
pads ■ four Vacutainer laboratory tubes ■ two large glass
Vacutainer bottles (1,000 ml or larger) ■ dry, sterile
pressure dressing ■ laboratory request forms ■ povidone-
iodine solution ■ local anesthetic (multidose vial of 1%
or 2% lidocaine with epinephrine) ■ 4″ × 4″ sterile gauze
pads ■ sterile paracentesis tray (containing needle, trocar, cannula, three-way stopcock) ■ sterile drapes ■ marking pen ■ 5-ml syringe with 22G or 25G needle ■ optional:
povidone-iodine ointment, alcohol sponge, 50-ml syringe,
suture materials, salt-poor albumin.

Implementation

- Explain the procedure to the patient *to ease his anxiety and promote cooperation.* Reassure him that he should feel no pain but that he may feel a stinging sensation from the local anesthetic injection and pressure from the needle or trocar and cannula insertion. He may also sense pressure when the doctor aspirates abdominal fluid.
- Be sure to obtain the patient's signed consent form.
- Instruct the patient to void before the procedure. Or insert an indwelling (Foley) catheter, if ordered, *to minimize the risk of accidental bladder injury from the needle or trocar and cannula insertion.*
- Identify and record baseline values, including the patient's vital signs, weight, and abdominal girth. (Use the tape measure to gauge the patient's abdominal girth at the umbilical level.) Indicate the abdominal area measured with a felt-tipped marking pen. *Baseline data will be used to monitor the patient's status during and after the procedure.*
- Help the patient sit up in bed *so that fluid accumulates in the lower abdomen.* Or help him sit on the side of the bed and use pillows to support his back. (See *Positioning the patient for abdominal paracentesis.*)
- Expose the patient's abdomen from diaphragm to pubis. Keep the rest of the patient covered *to avoid chilling him.*
- Make the patient as comfortable as possible, and place a linen-saver pad under him *for protection from drainage.*
- Remind the patient to stay as still as possible during the procedure *to prevent injury from the needle or trocar and cannula.*
- Wash your hands. Open the paracentesis tray using aseptic technique *to ensure a sterile field.* Next, put on gloves before assisting the doctor as he prepares the patient's abdomen with povidone-iodine solution, drapes the operative site with sterile drapes, and administers the local anesthetic.
- If the paracentesis tray doesn't contain a sterile ampule of anesthetic, wipe the top of a multidose vial of anesthetic solution with an alcohol sponge, and invert the vial at a 45-degree angle. *This allows the doctor to insert the sterile 5-ml syringe with the 22G or 25G needle and withdraw the anesthetic without touching the nonsterile vial.*
- Using the scalpel, the doctor may make a small incision before inserting the needle or trocar and cannula (usually 1″ to 2″ [2.5 to 5 cm] below the umbilicus). Listen for a popping sound. This signifies that the needle or trocar has pierced the peritoneum.
- Assist the doctor with specimen collection in the appropriate containers. Wear clean gloves *to protect you from possible body fluid contamination.* If the doctor orders substantial drainage, connect the three-way stopcock and tubing to the cannula. Run the other end of the tubing to a large sterile Vacutainer collection bottle. Or

Positioning the patient for abdominal paracentesis

Help the patient sit up in bed, or allow the patient to sit on the side of the bed with additional support for his back and arms.

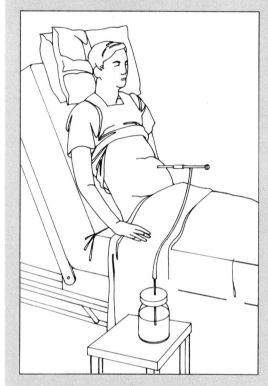

When the patient takes this position, gravity helps fluid to accumulate in the lower abdominal cavity. The internal abdominal structures provide counterresistance and additional pressure to facilitate fluid flow.

aspirate the fluid with a three-way stopcock and 50-ml syringe.
- Gently turn the patient from side to side *to enhance drainage* if necessary.
- As the fluid drains, monitor the patient's vital signs every 15 minutes. Observe him closely for vertigo, faintness, diaphoresis, pallor, heightened anxiety, tachycardia, dyspnea, and hypotension—especially if more than

1,500 ml of peritoneal fluid was aspirated at one time. *This loss may induce a fluid shift and hypovolemic shock.*
• Immediately report signs of shock to the doctor, who may order you to administer salt-poor albumin intravenously to replace aspirated fluid and to prevent hypovolemia.
• When the procedure ends and the doctor removes the needle or trocar and cannula, he may suture the incision. Wearing sterile gloves, apply the dry, sterile pressure dressing and povidone-iodine ointment to the site. Help the patient assume a comfortable position.
• Monitor the patient's vital signs and check the dressing for drainage every 15 minutes for 1 hour, every 30 minutes for 2 hours, every hour for 4 hours, and then every 4 hours for 24 hours *to detect delayed reactions to the procedure.* Note drainage color, amount, and character.
• Label the Vacutainer specimen tubes, and send them to the laboratory with the appropriate laboratory request forms. If the patient is receiving antibiotics, note this on the request form. *This information will be considered during fluid analysis.*
• Remove and dispose of all equipment properly.

Special considerations
Throughout this procedure, explain each step thoroughly to the patient and provide emotional support. Help the patient remain still *to prevent accidental perforation of abdominal organs.*

If the patient shows any signs of hypovolemic shock, reduce the vertical distance between the needle or the trocar and cannula and the drainage collection container *to slow the drainage rate.* If necessary, stop the drainage.

To prevent fluid shifts and hypovolemia, limit aspirated fluid to between 1,500 and 2,000 ml. If peritoneal fluid doesn't flow easily, try repositioning the patient *to facilitate drainage.* Also verify suction in the Vacutainer collection bottle when you connect it to the drainage tubing, and be sure to use macrodrip tubing without a backflow device.

After the procedure, observe for peritoneal fluid leakage. If this develops, notify the doctor. Always maintain daily patient weight and abdominal girth records. Compare these values with the baseline figures *to detect recurrent ascites.*

Complications
Hypovolemic shock may result from the sudden shift of fluid from the circulatory system to the peritoneum to replace aspirated fluid. Other possible complications include perforation of abdominal organs by the needle or the trocar and cannula, hepatic coma from decreased systemic circulation and reduced tissue perfusion, wound infection, and peritonitis.

Documentation
Record the date and time of the procedure, the puncture site location, and whether the wound was sutured. Document the amount, color, viscosity, and odor of aspirated fluid in your notes and in the fluid intake and output record. Record the patient's vital signs, weight, and abdominal girth measurements before and after the procedure. Also note his tolerance of the procedure, vital signs, and any signs and symptoms of complications during the procedure. Note the number of specimens sent to the laboratory.

 ## Peritoneal lavage

Used as a diagnostic procedure in a patient with blunt abdominal trauma, peritoneal lavage helps detect bleeding in the peritoneal cavity. The test may proceed through several steps. Initially, the doctor inserts a catheter through the abdominal wall into the peritoneal cavity and aspirates the peritoneal fluid with a syringe. If he cannot see blood in the aspirated fluid, he then infuses a balanced saline solution and siphons the fluid from the cavity. He inspects the siphoned fluid for blood and also sends fluid samples to the laboratory for microscopic examination.

The medical team maintains strict aseptic technique throughout this procedure to avoid introducing microorganisms into the peritoneum and causing peritonitis. (See *Tapping the peritoneal cavity.*)

Peritoneal lavage is contraindicated in a patient who has had multiple abdominal operations (adhesions), who is unstable and needs immediate surgery, or who cannot be catheterized before the procedure. The procedure requires great caution and a different technique if the patient is pregnant.

Equipment
Indwelling (Foley) catheter and drainage bag ▪ nasogastric (NG) tube ▪ gastric suction machine ▪ shaving kit ▪ I.V. pole ▪ macrodrip I.V. tubing ▪ I.V. solutions (1 liter of balanced saline solution, usually lactated Ringer's solution or normal saline solution) ▪ peritoneal dialysis tray ▪ sterile gloves ▪ antiseptic solution (such as povidone-iodine) ▪ 3-ml syringe with 25G 1″ needle ▪ bottle of 1% lidocaine with epinephrine ▪ 8″ (20.3 cm) #14 intracatheter extension tubing and a small sterile hemostat (to clamp tubing) ▪ 30-ml syringe ▪ one 20G 1½″ needle ▪ sterile towels ▪ three containers for specimen collection, including one sterile tube for a culture and sensitivity

specimen ■ labels ■ antiseptic ointment ■ 4″ × 4″ gauze pads ■ alcohol sponges ■ 1″ nonallergenic tape.

If using a commercially prepared peritoneal dialysis kit (containing a #15 peritoneal dialysis catheter, trocar, and extension tubing with roller clamp), be sure the macrodrip I.V. tubing doesn't have a reverse flow (or backcheck) valve that prevents infused fluid from draining out of the peritoneal cavity.

Implementation

• Provide privacy and wash your hands. Reinforce the doctor's explanation of the procedure.
• Before the procedure, advise the patient to expect a sensation of abdominal fullness. Also inform him that he may experience a chill if the lavage solution isn't warmed or doesn't reach his body temperature.
• Catheterize the patient with the indwelling bladder catheter, and connect this catheter to the drainage bag. *This decreases bladder fullness, thereby reducing the risk of accidental bladder puncture from the trocar or catheter used for the peritoneal lavage.*
• Insert the NG tube. Attach this tube to the gastric suction machine (set for low intermittent suction) to drain the patient's stomach contents. *Decompressing the stomach prevents vomiting and subsequent aspiration and minimizes the possibility of bowel perforation during trocar or catheter insertion.*
• Using the shaving kit, clip or shave the hair, as ordered, from the area between the patient's umbilicus and pubis.
• Set up the I.V. pole. Attach the macrodrip tubing to the lavage solution container, and clear air from the tubing *to avoid introducing air into the peritoneal cavity during lavage.*
• Using aseptic technique, open the peritoneal dialysis tray.
• The doctor will wipe the patient's abdomen from the costal margin to the pubic area and from flank to flank with the antiseptic solution. He will drape the area with sterile towels from the dialysis tray *to create a sterile field.*
• Using aseptic technique, hand the doctor the 3-ml syringe and the 25G 1″ needle. If the peritoneal dialysis tray doesn't contain a sterile ampule of anesthetic, wipe the top of a multidose vial of 1% lidocaine with epinephrine with an alcohol sponge, and invert the vial at a 45-degree angle. *This allows the doctor to insert the needle and withdraw the anesthetic without touching the nonsterile vial.*
• The doctor injects the anesthetic directly below the umbilicus (or at an adjacent site if the patient has a surgical scar). Once the area is numb, he makes an incision, inserts the catheter or trocar, withdraws fluid, and checks the findings. With positive findings, the pro-

Tapping the peritoneal cavity

After administering a local anesthetic to numb the area near the patient's navel, the surgeon will make a small incision (about ¾″ [2 cm]) through the skin and subcutaneous tissues of the abdominal wall. He will retract the tissue, ligate severed blood vessels, and use 4″ × 4″ gauze pads to absorb and keep incisional blood from entering the wound and producing a false-positive test result. Next, he will direct the trocar through the incision into the pelvic midline until the instrument enters the peritoneum. Then, he will advance the peritoneal catheter (via the trocar) 6″ to 8″ (15.2 to 20.3 cm) into the pelvis.

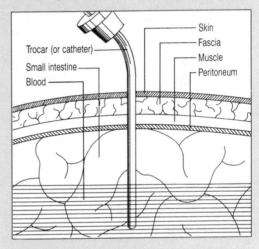

Using a syringe attached to the catheter, he will aspirate fluid from the peritoneal cavity and look for blood or other abnormal findings.

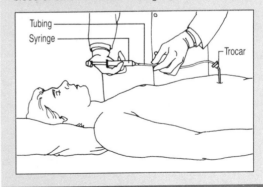

Interpreting peritoneal lavage results

With abnormal test findings in peritoneal lavage, your patient may need laparotomy and further treatment. The most common abnormal findings include the following:

• unclotted blood, bile, or intestinal contents in aspirated peritoneal fluid (20 ml in an adult or 10 ml in a child)

• bloody or pinkish-red fluid returned from lavage — dark enough to obscure reading newsprint through it (if you can read newsprint through the fluid, test results are considered negative, although the doctor may order more tests)

• green, cloudy, turbid, or milky peritoneal fluid return (normal peritoneal fluid appears clear to pale yellow)

• red blood cell count over 100,000/mm³

• white blood cell count exceeding 500/mm³

• bacteria in fluid (identified by culture and sensitivity testing or Gram stain).

If the patient's condition is stable, borderline positive results may suggest the need for additional tests, such as echography and arteriography.

If test results are questionable or inconclusive, the doctor may leave the catheter in place to repeat the procedure.

cedure ends, and you'll prepare the patient for laparotomy and further measures. Even if retrieved fluid looks normal, lavage will continue. (See *Interpreting peritoneal lavage results*.)

• Wearing gloves, connect the catheter extension tubing to the I.V. tubing, if ordered, and instill 500 to 1,000 ml (10 ml/kg body weight) of the warmed I.V. solution into the peritoneal cavity over 5 to 10 minutes. Then clamp the tubing with the hemostat.

• Unless contraindicated by the patient's injuries (such as a spinal cord injury, fractured ribs, or unstable pelvic fracture), gently tilt the patient from side to side *to distribute the fluid throughout the peritoneal cavity.* (If the patient's condition contraindicates tilting, the doctor may gently palpate the sides of the abdomen *to distribute the fluid.*)

• After 5 to 10 minutes, place the I.V. container below the level of the patient's body, and open the clamp on the I.V. tubing. *Lowering the container helps excess fluid to drain.* Gently drain as much of the fluid as possible from

the peritoneal cavity to the container. Be careful not to disconnect the tubing from the catheter. The peritoneal cavity may take 20 to 30 minutes to drain completely.

• Although you don't need to vent a plastic bag container, be sure to vent glass I.V. containers with a needle *to promote flow.*

• To obtain a fluid specimen, put on gloves and use a 30-ml syringe and 20G 1½" needle to withdraw between 25 and 30 ml of fluid from a port in the I.V. tubing. Clean the top of each specimen container with an alcohol sponge. Deposit fluid specimens in the containers, and send the specimens to the laboratory for culture and sensitivity analysis, Gram stain, red and white blood cell counts, amylase and bile level determinations, and spun-down sediment evaluation. *Note:* If you didn't obtain the culture and sensitivity specimen first, change the needle before drawing this fluid sample *to avoid contaminating the specimen.*

• Label the specimens, and send them to the laboratory immediately. With positive test results, the doctor will usually perform a laparotomy. If test results are normal, the doctor will close the incision.

• Wearing sterile gloves, apply antiseptic ointment to the site, and dress the incision with a 4″ × 4″ gauze pad secured with 1″ nonallergenic tape.

• Discard disposable equipment. Return reusable equipment to the appropriate department for cleaning and sterilization.

Special considerations

After the lavage, monitor the patient's vital signs frequently. Report symptoms of shock, such as tachycardia, decreased blood pressure, diaphoresis, dyspnea or shortness of breath, and vertigo immediately. Assess the incisional site frequently for bleeding.

If the doctor orders abdominal X-rays, they will probably precede peritoneal lavage. *X-ray films made after lavage may be unreliable because of air introduced into the peritoneal cavity.*

Complications

Bleeding from lacerated blood vessels may occur at the incisional site or intra-abdominally. A visceral perforation causes peritonitis and necessitates laparotomy for repair. If the patient has respiratory distress, infusion of a balanced saline solution may cause additional stress and trigger respiratory arrest.

The bladder may be lacerated or punctured if it isn't emptied completely before peritoneal lavage. Infection may develop at the incision site without strict aseptic technique.

Documentation

Record the type and size of the peritoneal dialysis catheter used, the type and amount of solution instilled and withdrawn from the peritoneal cavity, and the amount and color of fluid returned. Document whether the fluid flowed freely into and out of the abdomen. Note which specimens were obtained and sent to the laboratory. Also note any complications encountered and the nursing action taken to handle them.

Selected references

Advanced Trauma Life Support Manual for Students. Chicago: American College of Surgeons, 1989.

Andrus, C., and Ponsky, J. "The Effects of Irrigant Temperature in Upper Gastrointestinal Hemorrhage: A Requiem for Iced Saline Lavage," *American Journal of Gastroenterology* 82(10):1062-64, October 1987.

Brunner, L., and Suddarth, D. *Textbook of Medical-Surgical Nursing,* 6th ed. Philadelphia: J.B. Lippincott Co., 1988.

Camp, D., and Otten, N. "How to Insert and Remove Nasogastric Tubes," *Nursing90* 20(9):59-64, September 1990.

Cardona, V., et al. *Trauma Nursing: From Resuscitation to Rehabilitation.* Philadelphia: W.B. Saunders Co., 1988.

Carlson, C., et al. *Rehabilitation Nursing Procedures Manual.* Rockville, Md.: Aspen Pubs., Inc., 1990.

Dees, G. "Difficult Nasogastric Tube Insertions," *Emergency Medicine Clinics of North America* 7(1):177-82, February 1989.

Eaves, D. "Making Sense of Gastric Lavage," *Nursing Times* 84(16):52-53, April 20-26, 1988.

Hudak, C.M., et al. *Critical Care Nursing: A Holistic Approach,* 5th ed. Philadelphia: J.B. Lippincott Co., 1990.

Luckmann, J., and Sorenson, K. *Medical-Surgical Nursing: A Psychophysiologic Approach,* 3rd ed. Philadelphia: W.B. Saunders Co., 1987.

McCormick, P., and Burroughs, A.K. "How to Insert a Sengstaken-Blakemore Tube," *British Journal of Hospital Medicine* 43(4):274-77, April 1990.

Metheny, N. "Measures to Test Placement of Nasogastric and Nasointestinal Feeding Tubes," *Nursing Research* 37(6):324-29, November-December 1988.

Persons, C. *Critical Care Procedures and Protocols: A Nursing Process Approach.* Philadelphia: J.B. Lippincott Co., 1987.

Rolstad, B.S. "Innovative Surgical Procedures and Stoma Care in the Future," *Nursing Clinics of North America* 22(2):341-56, June 1987.

Rombeau, J., and Caldwell, M. *Clinical Nutrition: Enteral and Tube Feeding,* 2nd ed. Philadelphia: W.B. Saunders Co., 1990.

Rombeau, J., et al. *Atlas of Nutritional Support Techniques.* Boston: Little, Brown & Co., 1989.

Silberman, H. *Parenteral and Enteral Nutrition,* 2nd ed. Norwalk, Conn.: Appleton & Lange, 1989.

Sleisenger, M., and Fordtran, J. *Gastrointestinal Disease: Pathophysiology, Diagnoses, and Management,* 4th ed. Philadelphia: W.B. Saunders Co., 1989.

Starkey, J., et al. "Taking Care of Percutaneous Endoscopic Gastrostomy," *AJN* 88(1):42-45, January 1988.

Ulrich, S.P., et al. "Nursing Care of the Client with Disturbances of the Liver, Biliary Tract and Pancreas," in *Nursing Care Planning Guides: A Nursing Diagnosis Approach,* 2nd ed. Philadelphia: W.B. Saunders Co., 1990.

RENAL AND
UROLOGIC CARE

MARY BETH MODIC, RN, MSN

Based on the results of continued patient assessment, you can make valid clinical decisions and establish priorities that will contribute to a positive outcome. Your ability to assess a situation, analyze it critically, and establish priorities probably has the greatest impact on the success of the nursing process.

Introduction
Because the renal and urologic systems produce, transport, collect, and excrete urine, their dysfunction will impair fluid, electrolyte, and acid-base balance and the elimination of waste. To restore or facilitate effective function of these systems, treatment of renal and urologic disorders usually involves temporary or permanent insertion of a urinary, peritoneal, or vascular catheter or tube. Catheterization also allows monitoring of renal and urologic systems and aids diagnosis of dysfunction.

Helping the patient cope
One goal in caring for a patient with a renal or urologic disorder is helping him accept an invasive procedure or adjust to a new body image. Begin to meet this goal by assessing the amount and kind of information he needs and can absorb about the procedure. Then present or reinforce this information and tell him what to expect.

For example, before insertion of an indwelling catheter, tell the patient that he'll feel pressure during insertion, that the catheter will cause a sense of fullness or the urge to void, that he must avoid dislodging the catheter, and that the collection bag must be at lower-than-bladder level.

In a patient with a severe and chronic disorder, treatment usually requires permanent changes, such as urinary diversion, which may seriously affect his body image. To manage such a patient effectively, you must help him cope with any distressing changes by helping him recognize the health benefits of the treatment. For example, a stoma may be initially unappealing, but you can help the patient see that living with the stoma is easier than living with the disease or symptoms that caused him to seek treatment in the first place.

Managing the procedure
Performing procedures skillfully is only one aspect of successfully managing renal and urologic disorders. You must also understand the purpose of each step of the procedure, the physiologic and scientific principles that support the procedure, and the associated indications, contraindications, and clinical ramifications.

Additionally, you must accurately assess the patient's status, plan the appropriate approach to the procedure, implement the procedure, and evaluate its overall effect on the patient.

URINARY CATHETERS
Insertion of an indwelling catheter

Also known as a Foley or retention catheter, an indwelling catheter remains in the bladder to provide continuous urine drainage. A balloon inflated at the catheter's distal end prevents it from slipping out of the bladder after insertion. Indwelling catheters are used most often to relieve bladder distention caused by urine retention and to allow continuous urine drainage when the urinary meatus is swollen from childbirth, surgery, or local trauma. Other indications for an indwelling catheter include urinary tract obstruction (by a tumor or enlarged prostate), urine retention or infection from neurogenic bladder paralysis caused by spinal cord injury or disease, and any illness in which the patient's urine output must be monitored closely.

An indwelling catheter is inserted using sterile technique and only when absolutely necessary. Insertion should be performed with extreme care to prevent injury and infection.

Equipment
Sterile indwelling catheter (latex or silicone #10 to #22 French [average adult sizes are #16 to #18 French]) ▪ syringe filled with 5 to 8 ml of normal saline solution ▪ washcloth ▪ towel ▪ soap and water ▪ two linen-saver pads ▪ sterile gloves ▪ sterile drape ▪ sterile fenestrated drape ▪ sterile cotton-tipped applicators (or cotton balls and plastic forceps) ▪ povidone-iodine or other antiseptic cleaning agent ▪ urine receptacle ▪ sterile water-soluble lubricant ▪ sterile drainage collection bag ▪ intake and output sheet ▪ adhesive tape ▪ optional: urine-specimen container and laboratory request form, leg band with Velcro closure, gooseneck lamp.

Prepackaged sterile disposable kits are available and usually contain all the necessary equipment. The syringes in these kits are prefilled with normal saline solution.

Preparation of equipment
Check the order on the patient's chart *to determine if a catheter size or type has been specified*. Then wash your

hands, select the appropriate equipment, and assemble it at the patient's bedside.

Implementation

• Explain the procedure to the patient and provide privacy. Check his chart and ask when he voided last. Percuss and palpate the bladder *to establish baseline data.* Ask if he feels the urge to void.

• *So that you can see the urinary meatus clearly in poor lighting,* place a gooseneck lamp next to the patient's bed.

• Place the female patient in the supine position, with her knees flexed and separated and her feet flat on the bed, about 2′ (61 cm) apart. If she finds this position uncomfortable, have her flex one knee and keep the other leg flat on the bed. You may need an assistant to help the patient stay in position or to direct the light. Place the male patient in the supine position with his legs extended and flat on the bed. Ask the patient to hold the position *to give you a clear view of the urinary meatus and to prevent contamination of the sterile field.*

• Use the washcloth to clean the patient's genital area and perineum thoroughly with soap and water. Dry the area with the towel. Then, wash your hands.

• Place the linen-saver pads on the bed between the patient's legs and under the hips. *To create the sterile field,* open the prepackaged kit or equipment tray and place it between the female patient's legs or next to the male patient's hip. If the sterile gloves are the first item on the top of the tray, put them on. Place the sterile drape under the patient's hips. Then drape the patient's lower abdomen with the sterile fenestrated drape so that only the genital area remains exposed. Take care not to contaminate your gloves.

• Open the rest of the kit or tray. Put on the sterile gloves if you haven't already done so.

• Tear open the packet of povidone-iodine or other antiseptic cleaning agent, and use it to saturate the sterile cotton balls or applicators. Be careful not to spill the solution on the equipment.

• Open the packet of water-soluble lubricant and apply it to the catheter tip; attach the drainage bag to the other end of the catheter. (If you're using a commercial kit, the drainage bag may be attached.) Make sure all tubing ends remain sterile, and be sure the clamp at the emptying port of the drainage bag is closed *to prevent urine leakage from the bag.* Some drainage systems have an air-lock chamber *to prevent bacteria from traveling to the bladder from urine in the drainage bag.*

• Before inserting the catheter, inflate the balloon with normal saline solution *to inspect it for leaks.* To do this, attach the saline-filled syringe to the luer-lock, then push the plunger and check for seepage as the balloon expands. Aspirate the saline *to deflate the balloon.* Also inspect the

catheter for resiliency. *Rough, cracked catheters can injure the urethral mucosa during insertion, which can predispose the patient to infection.*

• For the female patient, separate the labia majora and labia minora as widely as possible with the thumb, middle, and index fingers of your nondominant hand *so you have a full view of the urinary meatus.* Keep the labia well separated throughout the procedure, *so they don't obscure the urinary meatus or contaminate the area once it's cleaned.*

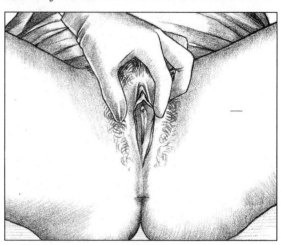

• With your dominant hand, use a sterile, cotton-tipped applicator (or pick up a sterile cotton ball with the plastic forceps) and wipe one side of the urinary meatus with a single downward motion. Wipe the other side with another sterile applicator or cotton ball in the same way. Then wipe directly over the meatus with still another sterile applicator or cotton ball. Take care not to contaminate your sterile glove.

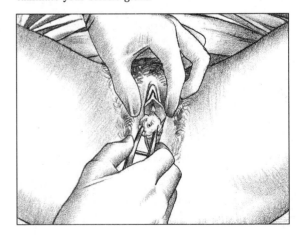

• For the male patient, hold the penis with your nondominant hand. If he's uncircumcised, retract the foreskin. Then gently lift and stretch the penis to a 60-degree to 90-degree angle. Hold the penis in this way throughout the procedure *to straighten the urethra and maintain a sterile field.*

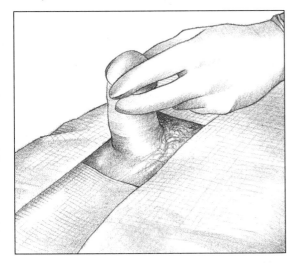

• Use your dominant hand to clean the glans with a sterile cotton-tipped applicator or a sterile cotton ball held in forceps. Clean in a circular motion, starting at the urinary meatus and working outward.
• Repeat the procedure using another sterile applicator or cotton ball and taking care not to contaminate your sterile glove.
• Pick up the catheter with your dominant hand and prepare to insert the lubricated tip into the urinary meatus. *To facilitate insertion by relaxing the sphincter,* ask the patient (male or female) to cough as you insert the catheter. Tell the patient to breathe deeply and slowly *to further relax the sphincter and prevent spasms.* Hold the catheter close to its tip *to ease insertion and control its direction.*
◆ *Nursing alert.* Never force a catheter during insertion. Maneuver it gently as the patient bears down or coughs. If you still meet resistance, stop the procedure and notify the doctor. Strictures, sphincter spasms, misplacement in the vagina (in females), or an enlarged prostate (in males) may cause resistance. ◆
• For the female patient, advance the catheter about 2" to 3" (5 to 7.6 cm) — while continuing to hold the labia apart — until urine begins to flow (top right).

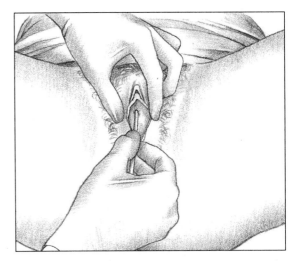

• For the male patient, advance the catheter about 6" to 8" (15.2 to 20.3 cm) until urine begins to flow. If the foreskin was retracted, be sure to replace it *to prevent compromised circulation and painful swelling.*

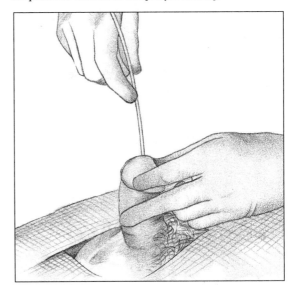

• When urine stops flowing, attach the saline-filled syringe to the luer-lock.
• Push the plunger and inflate the balloon *to keep the catheter in place in the bladder* (see top left illustration, page 566).

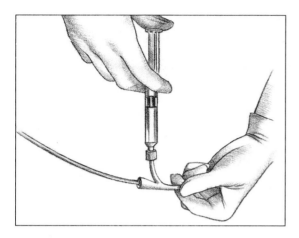

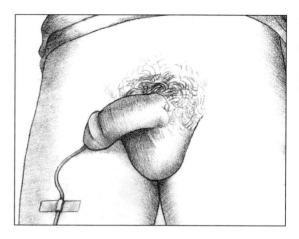

♦ ***Nursing alert.*** Never inflate a balloon without first establishing urine flow, *which assures you that the catheter is in the bladder, not in the urethral channel.* ♦

• Hang the collection bag below bladder level *to prevent urine reflux into the bladder, which can cause infection, and to facilitate gravity drainage of the bladder.* Make sure the tubing doesn't get tangled in the bed's side rails.

• Tape the catheter to the female patient's thigh *to prevent possible tension on the urogenital trigone.*

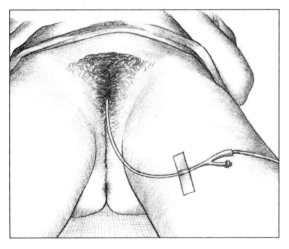

• Tape the catheter to the male patient's thigh or lower abdomen *to prevent pressure on the urethra at the penoscrotal junction, which can lead to formation of urethrocutaneous fistulas* (see illustration at top right).

• Also tape the catheter, as stated, to prevent traction on the bladder and alteration in the normal direction of urine flow in males.

• As an alternative, secure the catheter to the patient's thigh using a leg band with a Velcro closure. *This decreases skin irritation, especially in patients with long-term indwelling catheters.*

• Dispose of all used supplies properly.

Special considerations

Several types of catheters are available with balloons of various sizes. Each type has its own method of inflation and closure. For example, in one type of catheter, sterile solution or air is injected through the inflation lumen; then the end of the injection port is folded over itself and fastened with a clamp or rubber band.

Note: Injecting a catheter with air makes identifying leaks difficult and doesn't guarantee deflation of the balloon for removal.

A similar catheter is inflated by penetrating a seal in the end of the inflation lumen with a needle or the tip of the solution-filled syringe. Another type of balloon catheter self-inflates when a prepositioned clamp is loosened. The balloon size determines the amount of solution needed for inflation, and the exact amount is usually printed on the distal extension of the catheter used for inflating the balloon.

If necessary, ask the female patient to lie on her side with her knees drawn up to her chest during the catheterization procedure. *This position may be especially helpful for elderly or disabled patients, such as those with severe contractures* (see illustration on page 567).

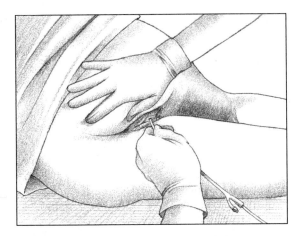

If the doctor orders a urine specimen for laboratory analysis, obtain it from the urine receptacle with a specimen collection container at the time of catheterization, and send it to the laboratory with the appropriate laboratory request form. Connect the drainage bag when urine stops flowing.

Inspect the catheter and tubing periodically while they're in place *to detect compression or kinking that could obstruct urine flow.* Explain the basic principles of gravity drainage *so that the patient realizes the importance of keeping the drainage tubing and collection bag lower than his bladder at all times.* If necessary, provide the patient with detailed instructions for performing clean intermittent self-catheterization. (See "Intermittent self-catheterization" in this chapter.)

For monitoring purposes, empty the collection bag at least every 8 hours. Excessive fluid volume may require more frequent emptying *to prevent traction on the catheter,* which would cause the patient discomfort, and *to prevent injury to the urethra and bladder wall.* Some hospitals encourage changing catheters at regular intervals, such as every 30 days, if the patient will have long-term continuous drainage.

♦ *Nursing alert.* Observe the patient carefully for adverse reactions, such as hypovolemic shock, caused by removing excessive volumes of residual urine. Check the hospital's policy beforehand to determine the maximum amount of urine that may be drained at one time (some hospitals limit the amount to 700 to 1,000 ml). Whether or not to limit the amount of urine drained is currently controversial. Clamp the catheter at the first sign of an adverse reaction, and notify the doctor. ♦

Home care
If the patient will be discharged with a long-term indwelling catheter, teach him and his family all aspects of daily catheter maintenance, including care of the skin and urinary meatus, signs and symptoms of urinary tract infection or obstruction, how to irrigate the catheter (if appropriate), and the importance of adequate fluid intake to maintain patency. Explain that a home care nurse should visit every 4 to 6 weeks, or more often if needed, to change the catheter.

Complications
Urinary tract infection can result from the introduction of bacteria into the bladder. Improper insertion can cause traumatic injury to the urethral and bladder mucosa. Bladder atony or spasms can result from rapid decompression of a severely distended bladder.

Documentation
Record the date, time, and size and type of indwelling catheter used. Also describe the amount, color, and other characteristics of urine emptied from the bladder. Your hospital may require only the intake and output sheet for fluid-balance data. If large volumes of urine have been emptied, describe the patient's tolerance for the procedure. Note whether a urine specimen was sent for laboratory analysis.

 Care of an indwelling catheter

Intended to prevent infection and other complications by keeping the catheter insertion site clean, routine catheter care typically is performed daily after the patient's morning bath and immediately after perineal care. (Bedtime catheter care may have to be performed before perineal care.)

Because some studies suggest that catheter care increases the risk of infection and other complications rather than lowers it, many hospitals don't recommend daily catheter care. Thus, individual hospital policy dictates whether or not a patient receives such care. Regardless of the catheter care policy, the equipment and the patient's genitalia require inspection twice daily.

Equipment
For catheter care: povidone-iodine (or other antiseptic cleaning agent) ■ sterile gloves ■ basin ■ eight sterile 4″ × 4″ gauze pads ■ sterile absorbent cotton balls or cotton-tipped applicators ■ leg bag ■ collection bag ■ adhesive tape ■ waste receptacle ■ optional: safety pin, rubber band, gooseneck lamp or flashlight, adhesive remover, antibiotic ointment, specimen container.

For perineal cleaning: washcloth ■ additional basin ■ soap and water.

Commercially prepared catheter care kits containing all necessary supplies are available.

Preparation of equipment
Wash your hands and bring all equipment to the patient's bedside. Open the gauze pads, place several in the first basin, and pour some povidone-iodine or other cleaning agent over them.

Some hospitals specify that, after wiping the urinary meatus with cleaning solution, you should wipe it off with wet, sterile gauze pads *to prevent possible irritation from the cleaning solution.* If this is your hospital's policy, pour water into the second basin, and moisten three more gauze pads.

Implementation
• Explain the procedure and its purpose to the patient.
• Provide privacy and make sure that the lighting is adequate *so you can see the perineum and catheter tubing clearly.* Place a gooseneck lamp at the bedside if needed.
• Inspect the catheter for any problems, and check the urine drainage for mucus, blood clots, sediment, and turbidity. Then pinch the catheter between two fingers *to determine if the lumen contains any material.* If you notice any of these conditions (or if hospital policy requires it), obtain a urine specimen (about 6 oz or 174 ml), and notify the doctor.
• Inspect the outside of the catheter where it enters the urinary meatus *for encrusted material and suppurative drainage.* Also inspect the tissue around the meatus for irritation or swelling.
• Remove any adhesive tape securing the catheter to the patient's thigh or abdomen. Inspect the area for signs of adhesive burns — redness, tenderness, or blisters.
• Put on the sterile gloves. Then use a saturated, sterile gauze pad or cotton-tipped applicator to clean the outside of the catheter and the tissue around the meatus. *To avoid contaminating the urinary tract,* always clean by wiping away from — never toward — the urinary meatus. Use a dry gauze pad to remove encrusted material.
♦ *Nursing alert.* Don't pull on the catheter while you're cleaning it. *This can injure the urethra and the bladder wall. It can also expose a section of the catheter that was inside the urethra, so that when you release the catheter, the newly contaminated section will reenter the urethra, introducing potentially infectious organisms.* ♦
• Remove your gloves and tear a piece of adhesive tape from the roll.
• *To prevent skin hypersensitivity or irritation,* retape the catheter to the other thigh or opposite side of the abdomen.

♦ *Nursing alert.* Provide enough slack before securing the catheter to prevent tension on the tubing *to avoid injuring the urethral lumen or bladder wall.* ♦
• Most drainage bags have a plastic clamp on the tubing to attach them to the sheet. If this isn't available, wrap a rubber band around the drainage tubing, insert the safety pin through a loop of the rubber band, and pin the tubing to the sheet below bladder level. Then attach the collection bag, below bladder level, to the bed frame.
• If necessary, clean residue from the previous tape site with adhesive remover. Then dispose of all used supplies in a waste receptacle.

Special considerations
Your hospital may require the use of specific cleaning agents for catheter care, so check the policy manual before beginning this procedure. A doctor's order will also be needed to apply antibiotic ointments to the urinary meatus after cleaning.

Avoid raising the drainage bag above bladder level. *This prevents reflux of urine, which may contain bacteria. To avoid damaging the urethral lumen or bladder wall,* always disconnect the drainage bag and tubing from the bed linen and bed frame before helping the patient out of bed.

When possible, attach a leg bag *to allow the patient greater mobility.* If the patient will be discharged with an indwelling catheter, teach him how to use a leg bag. (See *Teaching about leg bags.*)

Encourage patients with unrestricted fluid intake to increase intake to at least 3,000 ml per day. *This helps flush the urinary system and reduces sediment formation. To prevent urinary sediment and calculi from obstructing the drainage tube,* some patients are placed on an acid-ash diet to acidify the urine. Cranberry juice, for example, may help to promote urinary acidity.

Home care
Instruct patients discharged with indwelling catheters to wash the urinary meatus and perineal area with soap and water twice daily and the anal area after each bowel movement.

Complications
Sediment buildup, such as casts or mucus plugs, can occur anywhere in a catheterization system, especially in bedridden and dehydrated patients. *To prevent sediment buildup,* keep the patient well hydrated if he's not on fluid restriction. Change the indwelling catheter as ordered or when malfunction, obstruction, or contamination occurs.

Acute renal failure may result from a catheter obstructed by sediment. Be alert for sharply reduced urine

Teaching about leg bags

A urine drainage bag attached to the leg provides the catheterized patient with greater mobility. Because the bag is hidden under clothing, it may also help him feel more comfortable about catheterization. Leg bags are usually worn during the day and are replaced at night with a standard collection device.

If your patient will be discharged with an indwelling catheter, teach him how to attach and remove a leg bag. To demonstrate, you'll need a bag with a short drainage tube, two straps, an alcohol sponge, adhesive tape, and a screw clamp or hemostat.

Attaching the leg bag
• Provide privacy and explain the procedure. Describe the advantages of a leg bag, but caution the patient that a leg bag is smaller than a standard collection device and may have to be emptied more frequently.
• Remove the protective covering from the tip of the drainage tube. Then show the patient how to clean the tip with an alcohol sponge, wiping away from the opening to avoid contaminating the tube. Show him how to attach the tube to the catheter.
• Place the drainage bag on the patient's calf or thigh. Have him fasten the straps securely, and then show him how to tape the catheter to his leg. Emphasize that he must leave slack in the catheter to minimize pressure on the bladder, urethra, and related structures. Explain that excessive pressure or tension can lead to tissue breakdown.
• Also tell him not to fasten the straps too tightly to avoid interfering with his circulation.

Avoiding complications
• Although most leg bags have a valve in the drainage tube that prevents urine reflux into the bladder, urge the

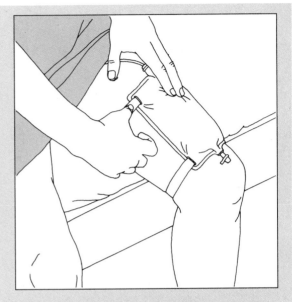

patient to keep the drainage bag lower than his bladder at all times because urine in the bag is a perfect growth medium for bacteria. Caution him also not to go to bed or take long naps while wearing the drainage bag.
• To prevent a full leg bag from damaging the bladder wall and urethra, encourage the patient to empty the bag when it's only half full. He should also inspect the catheter and drainage tube periodically for compression or kinking, which could obstruct urine flow and result in bladder distention.
• Tell the patient to wash the leg bag with soap and water or a bacteriostatic solution before each use to prevent infection.

flow from the catheter. Assess for bladder discomfort or distention.

Urinary tract infection is caused by endogenous or exogenous bacteria introduced into the urethra. This can occur during catheter insertion or from intraluminal or extraluminal migration of bacteria up the catheter. Signs and symptoms vary but may include cloudy urine, hematuria, fever, malaise, tenderness over the bladder, and flank pain.

Documentation
Record the care you performed, any necessary modifications in technique, any patient complaints or comments, and the condition of the perineum and urinary meatus. Note the character of the urine in the drainage bag, any sediment buildup, and whether a specimen was sent for laboratory analysis. Also record fluid intake and output. An hourly record is usually necessary for critically ill patients and those with renal insufficiency who are hemodynamically unstable.

Catheter irrigation

To avoid introducing microorganisms into the bladder, the nurse irrigates an indwelling catheter only to remove an obstruction, such as a blood clot that develops after bladder, kidney, or prostate surgery.

Equipment

Ordered irrigating solution (such as normal saline solution) ■ sterile graduated receptacle or emesis basin ■ sterile bulb syringe or 50-ml catheter-tip syringe ■ two alcohol sponges ■ sterile gloves ■ linen-saver pad ■ intake-output sheet ■ optional: basin of warm water.

Commercially packaged sterile irrigating kits are available and usually include irrigating solution, a graduated receptacle, and a bulb or 50-ml catheter-tip syringe. If the volume of irrigating solution instilled must be measured, use a graduated syringe instead of a noncalibrated bulb syringe.

Preparation of equipment

Check the expiration date on the irrigating solution. *To prevent vesical spasms during instillation of solution,* warm it to room temperature. If necessary, place the container in a basin of warm water. Never heat the solution on a burner or in a microwave oven. *Hot irrigating solution can injure the patient's bladder.*

Implementation

• Wash your hands, and assemble the equipment at the bedside. Explain the procedure to the patient, and provide privacy.
• Place the linen-saver pad under the patient's buttocks *to protect the bed linens.*
• Create a sterile field at the patient's bedside by opening the sterile equipment tray or commercial kit. Using aseptic technique, clean the lip of the solution bottle by pouring a small amount of solution into a sink or waste receptacle. Then pour the prescribed amount of solution into the graduated receptacle or emesis basin.
• Place the tip of the syringe into the solution. Squeeze the bulb or pull back the plunger (depending on the type of syringe), and fill the syringe with the appropriate amount of solution (usually 30 ml).
• Open the alcohol sponges; then put on the sterile gloves. Clean the juncture of the catheter and drainage tube with an alcohol sponge *to remove as many bacterial contaminants as possible.*
• Disconnect the catheter and drainage tube by twisting them in opposite directions and carefully pulling them apart without creating tension on the catheter. Do not

let go of the catheter — hold it in your nondominant hand. Then place the end of the drainage tube on the sterile field, making sure not to contaminate the tube.
• Twist the bulb syringe or catheter-tip syringe onto the catheter's distal end.
• Squeeze the bulb or slowly push the plunger of the syringe *to instill the irrigating solution through the catheter.* If necessary, refill the syringe and repeat this step until you've instilled the prescribed amount of irrigating solution.
• Remove the syringe and direct the return flow from the catheter into a graduated receptacle or emesis basin. Don't let the catheter end touch the drainage in the receptacle or become contaminated in any other way.
• Wipe the end of the drainage tube and catheter with the remaining alcohol sponge.
• Wait a few seconds until the alcohol evaporates; then reattach the drainage tubing to the catheter.
• Dispose of all used supplies properly.

Special considerations

Catheter irrigation requires strict aseptic technique to prevent bacteria from entering the bladder. The ends of the catheter and drainage tube and the tip of the syringe must be kept sterile throughout this procedure.

If you encounter any resistance during instillation of the irrigating solution, do not try to force the solution into the bladder. Instead, stop the procedure and notify the doctor. If an indwelling catheter becomes totally obstructed, obtain an order to remove it and replace it with a new one *to prevent bladder distention, acute renal failure, urinary stasis, and subsequent infection.*

The doctor may order a continuous irrigation system. *This decreases the risk of infection by eliminating the need to disconnect the catheter and drainage tube repeatedly.* (See "Continuous bladder irrigation.")

Encourage catheterized patients not on restricted fluid intake to increase intake to 3,000 ml per day *to help flush the urinary system and reduce sediment formation. To keep the patient's urine acidic and help prevent calculus formation,* tell the patient to eat foods containing ascorbic acid, including citrus fruits and juices, cranberry juice, and dark green and deep yellow vegetables.

Documentation

Note the amount, color, and consistency of return urine flow, and document the patient's tolerance for the procedure. Also note any resistance during instillation of the solution. If the return flow volume is less than the amount of solution instilled, note this on the intake and output balance sheets and in your notes.

EQUITMENT

Setup for continuous bladder irrigation

In continuous bladder irrigation, a triple-lumen catheter allows irrigating solution to flow into the bladder through one lumen and flow out through another, as shown in the inset. The third lumen is used to inflate the balloon that holds the catheter in place.

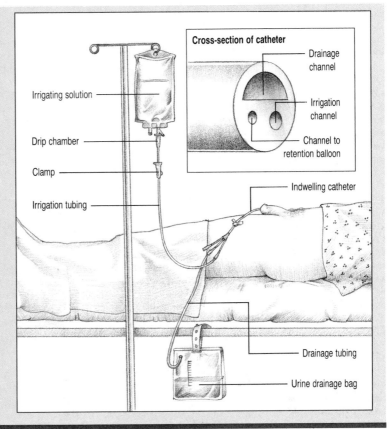

Irrigating solution

Drip chamber

Clamp

Irrigation tubing

Cross-section of catheter

Drainage channel

Irrigation channel

Channel to retention balloon

Indwelling catheter

Drainage tubing

Urine drainage bag

Continuous bladder irrigation

Continuous bladder irrigation can help prevent urinary tract obstruction by flushing out small blood clots that form after prostate or bladder surgery. It may also be used to treat an irritated, inflamed, or infected bladder lining.

This procedure requires placement of a triple-lumen catheter. One lumen controls balloon inflation, one allows irrigant inflow, and one allows irrigant outflow. The continuous flow of irrigating solution through the bladder also creates a mild tamponade that may help prevent venous hemorrhage. (See *Setup for continuous bladder irrigation.*) Although the patient typically receives the catheter while he's in the operating room after prostate or bladder surgery, he may have it inserted at bedside if he's not a surgical patient.

Equipment

One 4,000-ml container or two 2,000-ml containers of irrigating solution (usually normal saline solution) or the prescribed amount of medicated solution ▪ Y-type tubing made specifically for bladder irrigation ▪ alcohol or povidone-iodine sponge.

Normal saline solution is usually prescribed for bladder irrigation after prostate or bladder surgery. Large volumes of irrigating solution are usually required during the first 24 to 48 hours after surgery. *This explains the use of Y-type tubing, which allows immediate irrigation with reserve solution.*

Preparation of equipment

Before starting continuous bladder irrigation, double-check the irrigating solution against the doctor's order. If the solution contains an antibiotic, check the patient's chart *to make sure he's not allergic to the drug.*

Implementation

• Wash your hands. Assemble all equipment at the patient's bedside. Explain the procedure and provide privacy.

• Insert the spike of the Y-type tubing into the container of irrigating solution. (If you have a two-container system, insert one spike into each container.)

• Squeeze the drip chamber on the spike of the tubing.

• Open the flow clamp and flush the tubing *to remove air, which could cause bladder distention.* Then close the clamp.

• To begin, hang the irrigating solution on the I.V. pole.

• Clean the opening to the inflow lumen of the catheter with the alcohol or povidone-iodine sponge.

• Insert the distal end of the Y-type tubing securely into the inflow lumen (third port) of the catheter.

• Attach the outflow lumen to the tubing leading to the drainage bag.

• Open the flow clamp under the container of irrigating solution, and set the drip rate, as ordered.

• *To prevent air from entering the system,* don't allow the primary container to empty completely before replacing it.

• If you have a two-container system, simultaneously close the flow clamp under the nearly empty container and open the flow clamp under the reserve container. *This prevents reflux of irrigating solution from the reserve container into the nearly empty one.* Hang a new reserve container on the I.V. pole and insert the tubing, maintaining asepsis.

• Empty the drainage bag about every 4 hours, or as often as needed. Use sterile technique *to avoid the risk of contamination.*

Special considerations

Check the inflow and outflow lines periodically for kinks *to make sure the solution is running freely.* If the solution flows rapidly, check the lines frequently.

Measure the outflow volume accurately. It should equal or, allowing for urine production, slightly exceed inflow volume. If inflow volume exceeds outflow volume postoperatively, suspect bladder rupture at the suture lines, or renal damage, and notify the doctor immediately.

Also assess outflow for changes in appearance and for blood clots, especially if irrigation is being performed postoperatively to control bleeding. If drainage is bright red, irrigating solution should usually be infused rapidly *with the clamp wide open* until drainage clears. Notify the

doctor immediately if you suspect hemorrhage. If drainage is clear, the solution is usually given at a rate of 40 to 60 drops/minute. The doctor typically specifies the rate for antibiotic solutions.

Complications

Interruptions in a continuous irrigation system can predispose the patient to infection. Obstruction in the catheter's outflow lumen can cause bladder distention.

Documentation

Each time you finish a container of solution, record the date, time, and amount of fluid given on the intake and output record. Also record the time and the amount of fluid each time you empty the drainage bag. Note the appearance of the drainage and any complaints the patient has.

 ## Removal of an indwelling catheter

An indwelling catheter should be removed when bladder decompression is no longer necessary, when the patient can resume voiding, or when the catheter is obstructed. Depending on how long the patient was catheterized, the doctor may order bladder retraining before catheter removal.

Equipment

Absorbent cotton ■ gloves ■ alcohol sponge ■ 10-ml syringe with a luer-lock ■ bedpan ■ optional: clamp for bladder retraining.

Preparation of equipment

If the doctor orders bladder retraining, follow these steps: Clamp the catheter for 2 hours; then release it for 5 minutes *to empty the bladder.* Repeat the procedure. *This gradual filling and emptying helps restore the bladder's muscle tone.*

Implementation

• Wash your hands. Assemble the equipment at the patient's bedside. Explain the procedure to the patient, and tell him that he may feel slight discomfort. Tell him that you'll check him periodically during the first 8 to 24 hours after catheter removal *to make sure he resumes voiding.* Provide adequate privacy.

• Put on gloves. Attach the syringe to the luer-lock mechanism on the catheter.

• Pull back on the plunger of the syringe. *This deflates the balloon by aspirating the fluid injected at the time of catheter insertion.* The amount of fluid injected is usually indicated on the tip of the catheter's balloon lumen — it should also be noted on the Kardex and the patient's chart.

• Grasp the catheter with the absorbent cotton and gently pull it from the urethra. Before doing so, offer the patient a bedpan *because catheter removal typically creates a desire to void.*

• Measure and record the amount of urine in the collection bag before discarding it.

Special considerations

Encourage fluid intake *to stimulate urine production, dilute the urine, and help decrease the patient's discomfort when he begins voiding.*

Within 24 hours, the patient should be voiding normally (300 to 400 ml at a time), depending on fluid intake. If he's voiding small amounts (30 to 100 ml every 30 minutes to 1 hour), he's not emptying his bladder completely. Report this to the doctor. He may order a post-voiding catheterization *to remove residual urine.*

After catheter removal, assess the patient for incontinence (or dribbling), urgency, persistent dysuria or bladder spasms, fever, chills, or palpable bladder distention. Report any such findings to the doctor.

Complications

Major complications in removing an indwelling catheter are failure of the balloon to deflate and rupture of the balloon. If the balloon ruptures, cystoscopy is usually performed to ensure removal of any balloon fragments.

Documentation

For bladder retraining, record the date and time the catheter was clamped, the time it was released, and the volume and appearance of the urine. For catheter removal, record the date and time the catheter was removed and the patient's tolerance for the procedure. Record when and how much the patient voided after catheter removal and any problems associated with voiding.

 # Intermittent self-catheterization

A patient with impaired or absent bladder function may catheterize himself for routine bladder drainage. Called intermittent self-catheterization, this procedure requires thorough and careful teaching by the nurse. The patient will probably use clean technique for self-catheterization at home, but he must use sterile technique in the hospital because of the increased risk of infection.

Equipment

Rubber catheter ▪ washcloth ▪ soap and water ▪ small packet of water-soluble lubricant ▪ plastic storage bag ▪ optional: drainage container, paper towels, deodorant (such as Diaparene), rubber or plastic sheets, gooseneck lamp, catheterization record.

Preparation of equipment

Instruct the patient to keep a supply of catheters at home and to use each catheter only once before cleaning it. When all but the last one has been used, he should boil the catheters for 20 minutes in a pan of water, drain the water, and store the catheters in the pan or in a freshly laundered towel. *Catheters become brittle with repeated use,* so tell the patient to check them often and to order a new supply well in advance.

Implementation

• Tell the patient to begin by trying to urinate into the toilet or, if a toilet's not available or he needs to measure urine quantity, into a drainage container. Then he should wash his hands thoroughly with soap and water and dry them.

• Demonstrate how the patient should perform the catheterization, explaining each step clearly and carefully. Position a gooseneck lamp nearby if room lighting is inadequate *to make the urinary meatus clearly visible.* Arrange the patient's clothing so it's out of the way.

Teaching a woman

• Demonstrate and explain to the female patient that she should separate the vaginal folds as widely as possible with the fingers of her nondominant hand *to obtain a full view of the urinary meatus.* Ask if she's right- or left-handed and then tell her which is her nondominant hand. While holding her labia open with the nondominant hand, she should use the dominant hand to wash the perineal area thoroughly with a soapy washcloth, using downward strokes. Tell her to rinse the area with the washcloth, using downward strokes as well.

• Show her how to squeeze some lubricant onto the first 3″ (7.6 cm) of the catheter and then how to insert the catheter. (See *Teaching self-catheterization,* page 574.)

• When the urine stops draining, tell her to remove the catheter slowly, get dressed, and wash the catheter with warm, soapy water. Then she should rinse it inside and out and dry it with a paper towel.

Teaching a man

• Tell a male patient to wash and rinse the end of his penis thoroughly with soap and water, pulling back the foreskin if appropriate. He should keep the foreskin pulled back during the procedure.

Teaching self-catheterization

Teach a woman to hold the catheter in her dominant hand as if it were a pencil or a dart, about ½" (1.3 cm) from its tip. Keeping the vaginal folds separated, she should slowly insert the lubricated catheter about 3" (7.6 cm) into the urethra. Tell her to press down with her abdominal muscles to empty the bladder, allowing all urine to drain through the catheter and into the toilet or drainage container.

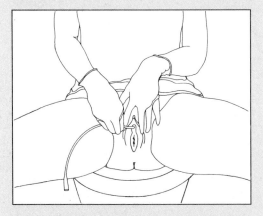

Teach a man to hold his penis in his nondominant hand, at a right angle to his body. He should hold the catheter in his dominant hand as if it were a pencil or a dart and slowly insert it 7" to 10" (17.8 to 25 cm) into the urethra until urine begins flowing. Then he should gently advance the catheter about 1" (2.5 cm) farther, allowing all urine to drain into the toilet or drainage container.

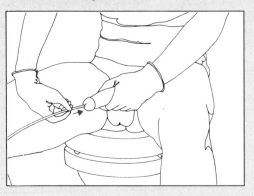

• Show him how to squeeze lubricant onto a paper towel and have him roll the first 7" to 10" (17.8 to 25 cm) of the catheter in the lubricant. Tell him that copious lubricant will make the procedure more comfortable for him. Then show him how to insert the catheter.
• When the urine stops draining, tell him to remove the catheter slowly and, if necessary, pull the foreskin forward again. Have him get dressed and wash and dry the catheter as described above.

Special considerations

Impress upon the patient that the timing of catheterization is critical *to prevent overdistention of the bladder, which can lead to infection.* Intermittent self-catheterization usually occurs every 4 to 6 hours around the clock (or more often at first).

Female patients should be able to identify the body parts involved in self-catheterizaton: labia majora, labia minora, vagina, and urinary meatus.

Keep in mind the difference between boiling and sterilization. Boiling kills bacteria, viruses and fungi, but does not kill spores, whereas sterilization does. However, because catheter cleaning will be done in the patient's home, boiling provides sufficient safeguard against spreading infections.

Advise the patient to store cleaned catheters only after they're completely dry *to prevent growth of gram-negative organisms.*

Stress the importance of regulating fluid intake, as ordered, *to prevent incontinence while maintaining adequate hydration.* However, explain that incontinent episodes may occur occasionally. For managing incontinence, the doctor or a home health care nurse can help develop a plan, such as more frequent catheterizations. After an incontinent episode, tell the patient to wash with soap and water, pat himself dry with a towel, and expose the skin to the air for as long as possible. He can reduce urine odor by putting methylbenzethonium chloride (Diaparene) or cornstarch on his skin. Bedding and furniture can be protected by covering them with rubber or plastic sheets and then covering the rubber or plastic with fabric.

Also stress the importance of taking medications as ordered *to increase urine retention and help prevent incontinence.* The patient should avoid calcium-rich and phosphorus-rich foods, as ordered, *to reduce the chance of renal calculus formation.*

Complications

Overdistention of the bladder can lead to urinary tract infection and urine leakage. Improper hand washing or equipment cleaning can also cause urinary tract infection. Incorrect catheter insertion can injure the urethral or bladder mucosa.

Urinary diversion techniques

Nephrostomy and cystostomy can be used to create permanent diversion, to relieve obstruction from an inoperable tumor, or to provide an outlet for urine after cystectomy. Temporary diversion can relieve obstruction from a calculus or ureteral edema. In *cystostomy*, a catheter is inserted percutaneously through the suprapubic area into the bladder. In *nephrostomy*, a catheter is inserted percutaneously through the flank into the renal pelvis.

Cystostomy

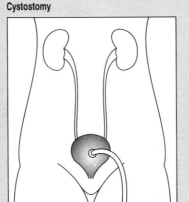

Nephrostomy

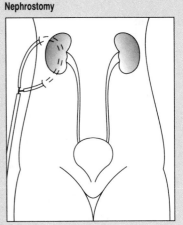

Documentation
Record the date and times of catheterization, character of the urine (color, odor, clarity, presence of particles or blood), the amount of urine (increase, decrease, no change), and any problems encountered during the procedure. Note whether the patient has difficulty performing a return demonstration.

SURGICAL URINARY DIVERSION

Care of nephrostomy and cystostomy tubes

Two urinary diversion techniques — nephrostomy and cystostomy — ensure adequate drainage from the kidneys or bladder and help prevent urinary tract infection or kidney failure. (See *Urinary diversion techniques.*)

A nephrostomy tube drains urine directly from a kidney when a disorder inhibits the normal flow of urine. The tube is usually placed percutaneously, though sometimes it is surgically inserted through the renal cortex and medulla into the renal pelvis from a lateral incision in the flank. The usual indication is obstructive disease, such as calculi in the ureter or ureteropelvic junction, or an obstructing tumor. Draining urine with a nephrostomy

tube also allows kidney tissue damaged by obstructive disease to heal.

A cystostomy tube drains urine from the bladder, diverting it from the urethra. This type of tube is used after certain gynecologic procedures, bladder surgery, prostatectomy, and for severe urethral strictures or traumatic injury. Inserted about 2″ (5 cm) above the symphysis pubis, a cystostomy tube may be used alone or with an indwelling urethral catheter.

Equipment
For dressing changes: 4″ × 4″ gauze pads ■ povidone-iodine solution or povidone-iodine sponges ■ sterile cup or emesis basin ■ paper bag ■ linen-saver pad ■ clean gloves (for dressing removal) ■ sterile gloves (for new dressing) ■ forceps ■ precut 4″ × 4″ drain dressings or transparent semipermeable dressings ■ adhesive tape (preferably hypoallergenic).

For nephrostomy-tube irrigation: 3-ml syringe ■ alcohol sponge or povidone-iodine sponge ■ normal saline solution ■ optional: hemostat.

Commercially prepared sterile dressing kits and povidone-iodine sponges may be available.

Preparation of equipment
Wash your hands and assemble all equipment at the patient's bedside. Open several packages of gauze pads, place them in the sterile cup or emesis basin, and pour the povidone-iodine solution over them. Or open several packages of povidone-iodine sponges. If you're using a

commercially packaged dressing kit, open it using aseptic technique. Fill the cup with antiseptic solution.

Open the paper bag and place it away from the other equipment *to avoid contaminating the sterile field.*

Implementation

• Wash your hands, provide privacy, and explain the procedure to the patient.

To change a dressing

• Help the patient to lie on his back (for a cystostomy tube) or the side opposite the tube (for a nephrostomy tube) *so you can see the tube clearly and change the dressing more easily.*
• Place the linen-saver pad under the patient *to absorb excess drainage and keep him dry.*
• Put on the clean gloves. Carefully remove the tape around the tube, and then remove the wet or soiled dressing. Discard the tape and dressing in the paper bag. Remove the gloves and discard them in the bag.
• Put on the sterile gloves. Pick up a saturated pad or dip a dry one into the cup of antiseptic solution.
• To clean the wound, wipe only once with each pad or sponge, moving from the insertion site outward. Discard the used pad or sponge in the paper bag. Don't touch the bag *to avoid contaminating your gloves.*
• Pick up a sterile 4″ × 4″ drain dressing and place it around the tube. If necessary, overlap two drain dressings *to provide maximum absorption.* Or, depending on your hospital's policy, apply a transparent semipermeable dressing over the site and tubing *to allow observation of the site without removing the dressing.*
• Use hypoallergenic tape *to secure the dressing.* Then tape the tube to the patient's lateral abdomen *to prevent tension on the tube.* (See *Taping a nephrostomy tube.*)
• Dispose of all equipment appropriately. Clean the patient as necessary.

To irrigate a nephrostomy tube

• Fill the 3-ml syringe with the normal saline solution.
• Clean the junction of the nephrostomy tube and drainage tube with the alcohol sponge or povidone-iodine sponge, and disconnect the tubes.
• Insert the syringe into the nephrostomy tube opening, and instill 2 to 3 ml of saline solution into the tube.
• Slowly aspirate the solution back into the syringe. *To avoid damaging the renal pelvis tissue,* never pull back forcefully on the plunger.
• If the solution doesn't return, remove the syringe from the tube and reattach it to the drainage tubing *to allow the solution to drain by gravity.*
• Dispose of all equipment appropriately.

Special considerations

Change dressings once a day or more often if needed.
♦ *Nursing alert.* Never irrigate a nephrostomy tube with more than 5 ml of solution *because the capacity of the renal pelvis is usually between 4 and 8 ml.* (Remember: The purpose of irrigation is to keep the tube patent, not to lavage the renal pelvis.) ♦

When necessary, irrigate a cystostomy tube as you would an indwelling catheter. Be sure to perform the irrigation gently *to avoid damaging any suture lines.*

Check a nephrostomy tube frequently for kinks or obstructions. Kinks are likely to occur if the patient lies on the insertion site. Suspect an obstruction when the amount of urine in the drainage bag decreases or the amount of urine around the insertion site increases. Pressure created by urine backing up in the tube can damage nephrons. Gently curve a cystostomy tube *to prevent kinks.*

If a blood clot or mucus plug obstructs a nephrostomy or cystostomy tube, try milking the tube *to restore its patency.* With your nondominant hand, hold the tube securely above the obstruction *to avoid pulling the tube out of the incision.* Then place the flat side of a closed hemostat under the tube, just above the obstruction, pinch the tube against the hemostat, and slide both your finger and the hemostat toward you, away from the patient.

Typically, cystostomy tubes for postoperative urologic patients should be checked hourly for 24 hours *to ensure adequate drainage and tube patency.* To check tube patency, note the amount of urine in the drainage bag and check the patient's bladder for distention.

Home care

Tell the home care patient that he must clean the insertion site with soap and water, check for skin breakdown, and change the dressing daily; then show him how to take these steps. Also teach him how to change the leg bag or drainage bag. He can use a leg bag during the day and a larger drainage bag at night.

Stress the importance of reporting to the doctor signs of infection (red skin or white, yellow, or green drainage at the insertion site) or tube displacement (drainage that smells like urine).

Whether he uses a drainage bag or larger container, explain that he must wash the device daily with a 1:3 vinegar and water solution, rinse it with plain water, and dry it on a clothes hanger or over the towel rack. *This prevents crystalline buildup.*

Complications

The patient has an increased risk of infection because nephrostomy and cystostomy tubes provide a direct opening to the kidneys and bladder.

Taping a nephrostomy tube

To tape a nephrostomy tube directly to the skin, cut a wide piece of hypoallergenic adhesive tape twice lengthwise to its midpoint.

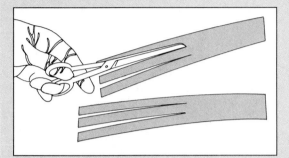

Apply the uncut end of the tape to the skin so that the midpoint meets the tube. Wrap the middle strip around the tube in spiral fashion. Tape the other two strips to the patient's skin on both sides of the tube.

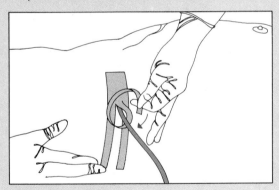

For greater security, repeat this step with a second piece of tape, applying it in the reverse direction. You may also apply two more strips of tape perpendicular to and over the first two pieces.

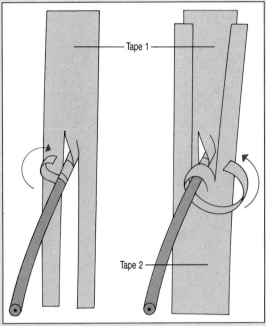

Tape 1

Tape 2

In any case, always apply another strip of tape lower down on the tube in the direction of the drainage tube to further anchor the tube. Don't put tension on any sutures that prevent tube dislocation.

Documentation

Describe the color and amount of drainage from the nephrostomy or cystostomy tube, and record any color changes as they occur.

Similarly, if the patient has more than one tube, describe the drainage (color, amount, and character) from each tube separately. If irrigation is necessary, record the amount and type of irrigant used and whether or not you obtained a complete return.

Care of a urinary diversion stoma

Urinary diversions provide an alternative route for urine flow when a disorder, such as an invasive bladder tumor, impedes normal drainage. A permanent urinary diversion is indicated in any condition that requires a total cystectomy. In conditions requiring temporary urinary drainage or diversion, a suprapubic or urethral catheter is usually inserted to divert the flow of urine temporarily. The catheter remains in place until the incision heals.

Urinary diversions may also be indicated for patients with neurogenic bladder, congenital anomaly, traumatic injury to the lower urinary tract, or severe chronic urinary tract infection.

Three types of permanent urinary diversions can be created: ureterostomy, ileal conduit, and continent urinary diversion. (See *Types of permanent urinary diversion.*) Most require the patient to wear a urine-collection appliance and to care for the stoma created during surgery.

Equipment

Soap and warm water ■ waste receptacle (such as an impervious or wax-coated bag) ■ linen-saver pad ■ nonallergenic paper tape ■ povidone-iodine sponges ■ urine collection container ■ rubber catheter (usually #14 or #16 French) ■ ruler ■ scissors ■ urine-collection appliance (with or without antireflux valve) ■ graduated cylinder ■ cottonless gauze pads (some rolled, some flat) ■ washcloth ■ skin barrier in liquid, paste, wafer, or sheet form ■ appliance belt ■ stoma covering (nonadherent gauze pad or panty liner) ■ two pairs of gloves ■ optional: adhesive solvent, irrigating syringe, tampon, hair dryer, electric razor, regular gauze pads, vinegar, deodorant tablets.

Commercially packaged stoma care kits are available.

In place of soap and water, you can use adhesive remover pads, if available, or cotton gauze saturated with adhesive solvent.

Some appliances come with a semipermeable skin barrier (impermeable to liquid but permeable to vapor and oxygen, which is essential for maintaining skin integrity). Wafer-type barriers may offer more protection against irritation than adhesive appliances. For example, a carbon-zinc barrier is economical and easy to apply. Its puttylike consistency allows it to be rolled between the palms to form a "washer" that can encircle the base of the stoma. This barrier can withstand enzymes, acids, and other damaging discharge material. All semipermeable barriers are easily removed along with the adhesive, causing less damage to the skin.

Preparation of equipment

Assemble all the equipment on the patient's overbed table. Tape the waste receptacle to the table for ready access. Provide privacy for the patient, and wash your hands. Measure the diameter of the stoma with a ruler. Cut the opening of the appliance with the scissors — it shouldn't be more than ¹⁄₁₆″ to ⅛″ larger than the diameter of the stoma. Moisten the faceplate of the appliance with a small amount of solvent or water *to prepare it for adhesion.* Performing these preliminary steps at the bedside *allows you to demonstrate the procedure and show the patient that it's not difficult, which will help him relax.*

Implementation

• Wash your hands again. Explain the procedure to the patient as you go along, and offer constant reinforcement and reassurance *to counteract negative reactions that may be elicited by stoma care.*

• Place the bed in a low Fowler's position so the patient's abdomen is flat. *This position eliminates skin folds that could cause the appliance to slip or irritate the skin and allows the patient to observe or participate.*

• Put on the gloves and place the linen-saver pad under the patient's side, near the stoma. Open the drain valve of the appliance being replaced *to empty the urine into the graduated cylinder.* Then, *to remove the appliance,* apply soap and water or adhesive solvent as you gently push the skin back from the pouch. If the appliance is disposable, discard it into the waste receptacle. If it's reusable, clean it with soap and lukewarm water and let it air-dry.

♦ *Nursing alert. To avoid irritating the patient's stoma, avoid touching it with adhesive solvent. If adhesive remains on the skin, gently rub it off with a dry gauze pad. Discard used gauze pads in the waste receptacle.* ♦

• *To prevent a constant flow of urine onto the skin while you're changing the appliance,* wick the urine with an absorbent, lint-free material. (See *Wicking urine from a stoma,* page 580.)

• Use water to carefully wash off any crystal deposits that may have formed around the stoma. If urine has stagnated and has a strong odor, use soap to wash it off. Be sure to rinse thoroughly *to remove any oily residue that could cause the appliance to slip.*

• Follow hospital skin care protocol to treat any minor skin problems.

• Dry the peristomal area thoroughly with a gauze pad *because moisture will keep the appliance from sticking.* Use a hair dryer if you wish. Remove any hair from the area with scissors or an electric razor *to prevent hair follicles from becoming irritated when the pouch is removed, which can cause folliculitis.*

• Inspect the stoma *to see if it's healing properly and to detect complications.* Check the color and the appearance of the suture line, and examine any moisture or effluent. Inspect the peristomal skin for redness, irritation, and intactness.

• Apply the skin barrier. If you apply a wafer or sheet, cut it to fit over the stoma. Remove any protective backing and set the barrier aside with the adhesive side up. If you apply a liquid barrier (such as Skin-Prep), saturate a gauze pad with it and coat the peristomal skin. Move in concentric circles outward from the stoma until you've covered an area 2″ (5 cm) larger than the wafer. Let the skin dry for several minutes — it should feel tacky. Gently

Types of permanent urinary diversion

The types of permanent urinary diversion with stomas include ureterostomy, ileal conduit, and continent urinary diversion.

Ureterostomy
A stoma or stomas are formed when ureters are diverted to the abdominal wall or flank. There are five different types of ureterostomy:
• *Flank loop ureterostomy:* Ureters loop as they are brought to the skin surface, forming a stoma.
• *Double-barrel ureterostomy:* Both ureters are brought to the skin surface to form side-by-side stomas.
• *Transureteroureterostomy:* One ureter is anastomosed to the other, which is then brought to the skin surface to form a stoma.
• *Bilateral ureterostomy:* Both ureters are brought to the skin surface to form stomas.
• *Unilateral ureterostomy:* One ureter is brought to the skin surface to form a stoma.

Ileal conduit
A segment of the ileum is excised, and the two ends of the ileum that result from excision of the segment are sutured closed. Then the ureters are dissected from the bladder and anastomosed to the ileal segment. One end of the ileal segment is closed with sutures; the opposite end is brought through the abdominal wall, thereby forming a stoma.

Continent urinary diversion
A tube is formed from part of the bladder wall. One end of the tube is brought to the skin to form the stoma. At the internal end of this tube, a nipple valve is created from the bladder wall so urine won't drain out unless a catheter is inserted through the stoma into the bladder pouch. The urethral neck is sutured closed.

Flank loop ureterostomy

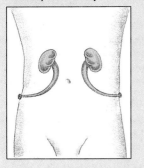

Double-barrel ureterostomy

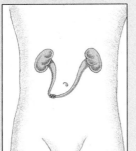

Transureteroureterostomy

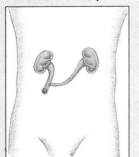

Bilateral ureterostomy

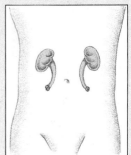

Unilateral ureterostomy

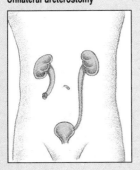

Ileal conduit

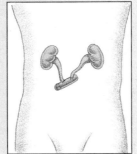

Continent urinary diversion

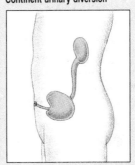

Wicking urine from a stoma

Use a piece of rolled, cottonless gauze or a tampon to wick urine from a stoma. Working by capillary action, wicking absorbs urine while you prepare the patient's skin to hold a urine-collection appliance.

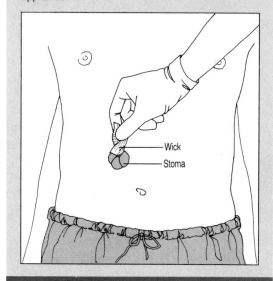

press the wafer around the stoma, sticky side down, smoothing from the stoma outward.
• If you're using a barrier paste, open the tube, squeeze out a small amount, and then discard it. Then squeeze a ribbon of paste directly onto the peristomal skin about ½″ (1.3 cm) from the stoma, making a complete circle. Make several more concentric circles outward. Dip your fingers into lukewarm water, and smooth the paste until the skin is completely covered from the edge of the stoma to 3″ to 4″ (7.6 to 10.2 cm) outward. The paste should be ¼″ to ½″ (0.6 to 1.3 cm) thick. Then discard the gloves, wash your hands, and put on new gloves.
• Remove the material used for wicking urine, and place it in the waste receptacle.
• Now place the appliance over the stoma, leaving only a small amount (⅜″ to ¾″ [1 to 2 cm]) of skin exposed.
• Secure the faceplate of the appliance to the skin with paper tape, if recommended. To do this, place a piece of tape lengthwise on each edge of the faceplate so that the tape overlaps onto the skin.
• Apply the appliance belt. Be sure that it's on a level with the stoma. *Applied above or below the stoma, the belt*

can break the bag's seal, or it can rub or injure the stoma. The belt should be loose enough for you to insert two fingers between the skin and the belt. *If the belt is too tight, it can irritate the skin or cause internal damage.*
• Dispose of the used materials appropriately.

Special considerations

The patient's attitude toward his urinary diversion stoma plays a big part in determining how well he'll adjust to it. *To encourage a positive attitude,* help him get used to the idea of caring for his stoma and the appliance as though they are natural extensions of himself. When teaching him to perform the procedure, give him written instructions and provide positive reinforcement after he completes each step. Suggest that he perform the procedure in the morning when urine flows most slowly.

Help the patient choose between disposable and reusable appliances by telling him the advantages and disadvantages of each. Emphasize the importance of correct placement and of a well-fitted appliance *to prevent seepage of urine onto the skin.* When positioned correctly, most appliances remain in place for at least 3 days and for as long as 5 days if no leakage occurs. After 5 days, the appliance should be changed. With the improved adhesives and pouches available, belts aren't always necessary.

Because urine flows constantly, it accumulates quickly, becoming even heavier than stools. *To prevent the weight of the urine from loosening the seal around the stoma and separating the appliance from the skin,* tell the patient to empty the appliance through the drain valve when it is one-third to one-half full.

Instruct the patient to connect his appliance to a urine-collection container before he goes to sleep. *The continuous flow of urine into the container during the night prevents the urine from accumulating and stagnating in the appliance.*

Teach the patient sanitary and dietary measures that can protect the peristomal skin and control the odor that commonly results from alkaline urine, infection, or poor hygiene. Reusable appliances should be washed with soap and lukewarm water, then air-dried thoroughly *to prevent brittleness.* Soaking the appliance in vinegar and water or placing deodorant tablets in it can further dissipate stubborn odors. An acid-ash diet that includes ascorbic acid and cranberry juice may raise urinary acidity, thereby reducing bacterial action and fermentation (the underlying causes of odor). Generous fluid intake also helps to reduce odors by diluting the urine.

If the patient has a continent urinary diversion, be sure you know how to meet his special needs. (See *Caring for the patient with a continent urinary diversion.*)

Caring for the patient with a continent urinary diversion

In this procedure, an alternative to the traditional ileal conduit, a pouch created from the ascending colon and the terminal ileum serves as a new bladder, which empties through a stoma. To drain urine continuously, several drains are inserted into this reconstructed bladder and left in place for 3 to 6 weeks until the new stoma heals. The patient will be discharged from the hospital with the drains in place. He will return to have them removed and to learn how to catheterize his stoma.

During first hospitalization
• Immediately after surgery, monitor intake and output from each drain. Be alert for decreased output, which may indicate that urine flow is obstructed.
• Watch for common postoperative complications, such as infection or bleeding. Also watch for signs of urinary leakage, which include increased abdominal pain, decreased urine output from the drains, increased abdominal distention, and urine appearing around the drains or midline incision.
• Irrigate the drains as ordered.
• Clean the area around the drains daily—first with povidone-iodine solution and then with sterile water. Apply a dry sterile dressing to the area. Use precut 4″ × 4″ drain dressings around the drain *to absorb leakage.*
• *To increase the patient's mobility and comfort,* connect the drains to a leg bag.

During second hospitalization
• After the patient's drains are removed, teach the patient how to catheterize the stoma. Begin by gathering the following equipment on a clean towel: rubber catheter (usually #14 or #16 French), water-soluble lubricant, washcloth, stoma covering (nonadherent gauze pad or panty liner), nonallergenic adhesive tape, and an irrigating syringe (optional).
• Apply water-soluble lubricant to the catheter tip *to facilitate insertion.*

• Remove and discard the stoma cover. Using the washcloth, clean the stoma and the area around it, starting at the stoma and working outward in a circular motion.
• Hold the urine-collection container under the catheter; then slowly insert the catheter into the stoma. Urine should begin to flow into the container. If it doesn't, gently rotate the catheter or redirect its angle. If the catheter drains slowly, it may be plugged with mucus. Irrigate with sterile saline solution or sterile water *to clear it.* When the flow stops, pinch the catheter closed and remove it.
• Dry the skin if necessary. Apply a sterile gauze pad over the stoma *to keep it clean,* and secure the pad with tape. Alternatively, secure a panty liner to the patient's underwear.

Home care
• Teach the patient how to care for the drains and their insertion sites during the 3 to 6 weeks he'll be at home before their removal, and teach him how to attach them to a leg bag. Also teach him to recognize the signs of infection and obstruction.
• After the drains are removed, teach the patient how to empty the pouch, and direct him to do so on a schedule. Initially, he should catheterize the stoma and empty the pouch every 2 to 3 hours. Later, he should catheterize every 4 hours while awake and also irrigate the pouch each morning and evening. Instruct him to empty the pouch whenever he feels a sensation of fullness.
• Tell the patient that catheters are reusable, but only after they are cleaned. He should clean the catheter thoroughly with warm, soapy water, rinse it thoroughly, and hang it to dry over a clean towel. He should store cleaned and dried catheters in plastic bags. Tell him he can reuse catheters for up to 1 month before discarding them. However, he should immediately discard any catheter that becomes discolored or cracked.

Tell the patient about ostomy clubs and the American Cancer Society. Members of these organizations routinely visit hospitals to explain ostomy care and the types of appliances available and to help patients learn to function normally with a stoma.

Home care
The patient or a family member can learn to care for a urinary diversion stoma at home. However, the patient's

emotional adjustment to the stoma must be given special consideration before he can be expected to maintain it properly. Arrange for a visiting nurse or an enterostomal therapist to assist the patient at home.

Complications
Because intestinal mucosa is delicate, an ill-fitting appliance can cause bleeding. This is especially likely with

Principles of peritoneal dialysis

Peritoneal dialysis works by a combination of diffusion and osmosis.

Diffusion

In this process, particles move through a semipermeable membrane from an area of high concentration to an area of low concentration.

In peritoneal dialysis, the water-based dialysate being infused contains glucose, sodium chloride, calcium, magnesium, acetate or lactate, and no waste products. Therefore, the waste products and excess electrolytes in the blood cross through the semipermeable peritoneal membrane into the dialysate. Removing the waste-filled dialysate and replacing it with fresh solution keeps the waste concentration low and encourages further diffusion. Potassium may be added occasionally to maintain serum levels of this element. However, because failing kidneys can't excrete potassium, levels must be monitored closely and adjusted as needed.

Osmosis

In this process, fluids move through a semipermeable membrane from an area of low-solute concentration to an area of high-solute concentration. In peritoneal dialysis, osmosis removes excess water from the patient's blood. Dextrose in the dialysate encourages fluid movement by giving the dialysate a higher solute-particle concentration than the blood.

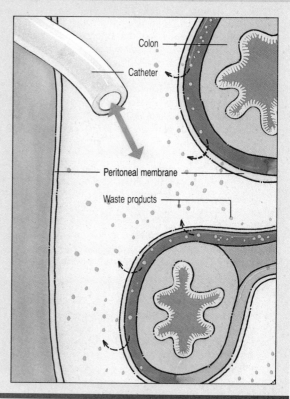

Colon

Catheter

Peritoneal membrane

Waste products

---

an ileal conduit, the most common urinary diversion stoma, *because a segment of the intestine forms the conduit.*

Peristomal skin may become reddened or excoriated from too-frequent changing or improper placement of the appliance, poor skin care, or allergic reaction to the appliance or adhesive. Constant leakage around the appliance can result from improper placement of the appliance or from poor skin turgor.

Documentation

Record the appearance and color of the stoma and whether it's inverted, flush with the skin, or protruding. If it protrudes, note by how much it protrudes above the skin. (The normal range is ½″ to ¾″ [1.3 to 2 cm].) Record the appearance and condition of the peristomal skin, noting any redness or irritation or complaints by the patient of itching or burning.

Document the patient's adjustment to the stoma, and note his participation in stoma care and application of the appliance.

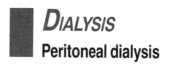

DIALYSIS
Peritoneal dialysis

In patients with acute or chronic renal failure, peritoneal dialysis performs the kidneys' function of removing impurities from the blood. Dialysate—the solution instilled into the peritoneal cavity by a catheter—draws waste products, excess fluid, and electrolytes from the blood across the semipermeable peritoneal membrane. (See *Principles of peritoneal dialysis.*) After a prescribed period, the dialysate is drained from the peritoneal cavity, removing impurities with it. The dialysis procedure is then repeated, using a new dialysate each time, until waste removal is complete and fluid, electrolyte, and acid-base balance have been restored.

The catheter is inserted in the operating room or at the patient's bedside with a nurse assisting. With special preparation, the nurse may perform dialysis, either manually or using an automatic or semiautomatic cycle machine. (Or, in some cases, she may assist the patient with continuous ambulatory peritoneal dialysis. See "Continuous ambulatory peritoneal dialysis" later in this chapter.)

Equipment

For catheter placement and dialysis: prescribed dialysate (in 1- or 2-liter bottles or bags, as ordered) ▪ warmer, heating pad, or water bath ▪ at least three face masks ▪ medication, such as heparin, if ordered ▪ dialysis administration set with drainage bag ▪ two pairs of sterile gloves ▪ I.V. pole ▪ fenestrated sterile drape ▪ vial of 1% or 2% lidocaine ▪ povidone-iodine pads ▪ 3-ml syringe with 25G 1″ needle ▪ scalpel (with #11 blade) ▪ ordered type of multi-eyed, nylon, peritoneal catheter (see *Comparing peritoneal dialysis catheters,* page 584) ▪ peritoneal stylet ▪ sutures or nonallergenic tape ▪ povidone-iodine solution (for doctor to prepare abdomen) ▪ precut drain dressings ▪ protective cap for catheter ▪ small, sterile plastic clamp ▪ 4″ × 4″ gauze pads ▪ optional: 10-ml syringe with 22G 1½″ needle, protein or potassium supplement, specimen container, label, laboratory request form.

For dressing changes: one pair of sterile gloves ▪ ten sterile cotton-tipped applicators or sterile 2″ × 2″ gauze pads ▪ povidone-iodine ointment ▪ two precut drain dressings ▪ adhesive tape ▪ povidone-iodine solution or normal saline solution ▪ two sterile 4″ × 4″ gauze pads.

All equipment must be sterile. Commercially packaged dialysis kits or trays are available and contain all the equipment needed for catheter placement and dressing changes.

Preparation of equipment

Bring all equipment to the patient's bedside. Make sure the dialysate is at body temperature. *This decreases patient discomfort during the procedure and reduces vasoconstriction of the peritoneal capillaries. Dilated capillaries enhance blood flow to the peritoneal membrane surface, increasing waste clearance into the peritoneal cavity.* To warm the solution, place the container in a warmer or wrap it in a heating pad set at 105° F (40.6° C) for 30 to 60 minutes. You can also place the container in a water bath at 98.6° to 100.4° F (37° to 38° C) for 30 to 60 minutes.

Implementation

● Explain the procedure to the patient. Weigh him and record his vital signs *to establish baseline levels.*

For catheter placement and dialysis

● Have the patient try to urinate. *This reduces the risk of bladder perforation during insertion of the peritoneal catheter and also reduces patient discomfort.* If he can't urinate, and if you suspect that his bladder isn't empty, obtain an order for straight catheterization *to empty his bladder.*
● Place the patient in the supine position, and have him put on one of the sterile face masks.
● Wash your hands.
● Inspect the warmed dialysate, which should appear clear and colorless.
● Put on a sterile face mask. Prepare to add any prescribed medication to the dialysate, using strict aseptic technique *to avoid contaminating the solution.* Commonly, heparin is added *to prevent accumulation of fibrin in the catheter.*
● Prepare the dialysis administration set. (See *Setup for peritoneal dialysis,* page 585.)
● Close the clamps on all lines. Place the drainage bag below the patient *to facilitate gravity drainage,* and connect the drainage line to it. Connect the dialysate infusion lines to the bottles or bags of dialysate. Hang the bottles or bags on the I.V. pole at the patient's bedside. *To prime the tubing,* open the infusion lines and allow the solution to flow until all lines are primed. Then close all clamps.
● At this point, the doctor puts on a mask and a pair of sterile gloves. He cleans the patient's abdomen with povidone-iodine solution and drapes it with a sterile drape.
● Wipe the stopper of the lidocaine vial with povidone-iodine and allow it to dry. Invert the vial and hand it to the doctor so he can withdraw the lidocaine, using the 3-ml syringe with the 25G 1″ needle.
● The doctor anesthetizes a small area of the patient's abdomen below the umbilicus. He then makes a small incision with the scalpel, inserts the catheter into the peritoneal cavity—using the stylet to guide the catheter—and sutures or tapes the catheter in place.
● Connect the catheter to the administration set, using strict aseptic technique *to prevent contamination of the catheter and the solution, which could cause peritonitis.*
● Open the drain dressing and the 4″ × 4″ gauze pad packages. Put on the other pair of sterile gloves. Apply the precut drain dressings around the catheter. Cover them with the gauze pads and tape them securely.
● Unclamp the lines to the patient. Rapidly instill 500 ml of dialysate into the peritoneal cavity *to test the catheter's patency.*

Comparing peritoneal dialysis catheters

The first step in any type of peritoneal dialysis is insertion of a catheter to allow instillation of dialyzing solution. The surgeon may insert one of three different catheters described below.

Tenckhoff catheter
To implant a Tenckhoff catheter, the surgeon inserts the first 6¾″ (17 cm) of the catheter into the patient's abdomen. The next 2¾″ (7-cm) segment, which may have a Dacron cuff at one or both ends, is imbedded subcutaneously. Within a few days after insertion, the patient's tissues grow around the cuffs, forming a tight barrier against bacterial infiltration. The remaining 3⅞″ (10 cm) of the catheter extends outside of the abdomen and is equipped with a metal adapter at the tip that connects to dialyzer tubing.

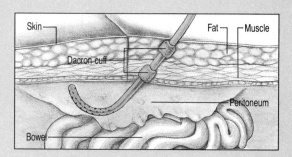

Flanged-collar catheter
To insert this kind of catheter, the surgeon positions its flanged collar just below the dermis so that the device extends through the abdominal wall. He keeps the distal end of the cuff from extending into the peritoneum, where it could cause adhesions.

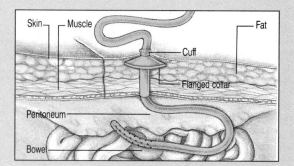

Column-disk peritoneal catheter
To insert a column-disk peritoneal catheter (CDPC), the surgeon rolls up the flexible disk section of the implant, inserts it into the peritoneal cavity, and retracts it against the abdominal wall. The implant's first cuff rests just outside the peritoneal membrane, while its second cuff rests just beneath the skin. Because the CDPC doesn't float freely in the peritoneal cavity, it keeps inflowing dialyzing solution from being directed at the sensitive organs—which increases patient comfort during dialysis.

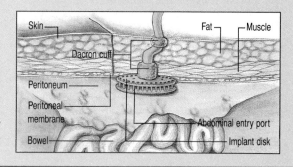

• Clamp the lines to the patient. Immediately unclamp the lines to the drainage bag *to allow fluid to drain into the bag.* Outflow should be brisk.
• Having established the catheter's patency, clamp the lines to the drainage bag and unclamp the lines to the patient *to infuse the prescribed volume of solution over a period of 5 to 10 minutes.* As soon as the dialysate container empties, clamp the lines to the patient immediately *to prevent air from entering the tubing.*
• Allow the solution to dwell in the peritoneal cavity for the prescribed time (10 minutes to 4 hours). *This lets excess fluid, electrolytes, and accumulated wastes move from the blood through the peritoneal membrane and into the dialysate.*

- Warm the solution for the next infusion.
- At the end of the prescribed dwell time, unclamp the line to the drainage bag and allow the solution to drain from the peritoneal cavity into the drainage bag.
- Repeat the infusion-dwell-drain cycle immediately after outflow until the prescribed number of fluid exchanges have been completed.
- If the doctor or hospital policy requires a dialysate specimen, you'll usually collect one after every 10 infusion-dwell-drain cycles (*always* during the drain phase), after every 24-hour period, or as ordered. To do this, attach the 10-ml syringe to the 22G 1½″ needle and insert it into the injection port on the drainage line, using strict aseptic technique, and aspirate the drainage sample. Transfer the sample to the specimen container, label it appropriately, and send it to the laboratory with a laboratory request form.
- After completing the prescribed number of exchanges, clamp the catheter, and put on sterile gloves. Disconnect the administration set from the peritoneal catheter. Place the sterile protective cap over the catheter's distal end. (Or the doctor may remove the catheter and place a Deane's prosthesis in its place *to maintain the patency of the tract and to simplify reinsertion of the catheter for the next dialysis treatment.*)
- Dispose of all used equipment appropriately.

Dressing changes

- Explain the procedure to the patient and wash your hands.
- If necessary, carefully remove the old dressings *to avoid putting tension on the catheter and accidentally dislodging it and to avoid introducing bacteria into the tract through movement of the catheter.*
- Put on the sterile gloves.
- Saturate the sterile applicators or the 2″ × 2″ gauze pads with povidone-iodine, and clean the skin around the catheter, moving in concentric circles from the catheter site outward. Remove any crusted material carefully.
- Inspect the catheter site for drainage and the tissue around the site for redness and swelling.
- Apply povidone-iodine ointment to the catheter site with a sterile gauze pad.
- Place two precut drain dressings around the catheter site. Tape the 4″ × 4″ gauze pads over them to secure the dressing.

Special considerations

During and after dialysis, monitor the patient and his response to treatment. Peritoneal dialysis is usually contraindicated in patients who have had extensive abdominal or bowel surgery or extensive abdominal trauma.

Setup for peritoneal dialysis

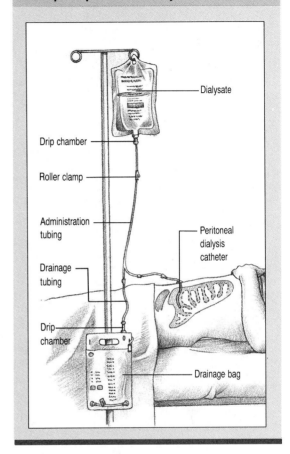

- Dialysate
- Drip chamber
- Roller clamp
- Administration tubing
- Drainage tubing
- Drip chamber
- Peritoneal dialysis catheter
- Drainage bag

Monitor the patient's vital signs every 10 to 15 minutes for the first 1 to 2 hours of exchanges, then every 2 to 4 hours, or more frequently if necessary. Notify the doctor of any abrupt changes in the patient's condition.

To reduce the risk of peritonitis, use strict aseptic technique during catheter insertion, dialysis, and dressing changes. Masks should be worn by all personnel in the room whenever the dialysis system is opened or entered. Change the dressing at least every 24 hours or whenever it becomes wet or soiled. Frequent dressing changes will also help prevent skin excoriation from any leakage.

To prevent respiratory distress, position the patient for maximal lung expansion. Promote lung expansion through turning and deep-breathing exercises.

♦ *Nursing alert.* If the patient suffers severe respiratory distress during the dwell phase of dialysis, drain the peritoneal cavity and notify the doctor. Monitor any patient on peritoneal dialysis who's being weaned from a ventilator. ◆

To prevent protein depletion, the doctor may order a high-protein diet or a protein supplement. He will also monitor serum albumin levels.

Dialysate is available in three concentrations—4.25% dextrose, 2.5% dextrose, and 1.5% dextrose. The 4.25% solution usually removes the largest amount of fluid from the blood because its glucose concentration is highest. If your patient receives this concentrated solution, monitor him carefully *to prevent excess fluid loss.* Also, some of the glucose in the 4.25% solution may enter the patient's bloodstream, causing hyperglycemia severe enough to require an insulin injection or an insulin addition to the dialysate.

Patients with low serum potassium levels may require the addition of potassium to the dialysate solution *to prevent further losses.*

Monitor fluid volume balance, blood pressure, and pulse *to help prevent fluid imbalance.* Assess fluid balance at the end of each infusion-dwell-drain cycle. Fluid balance is positive if less than the amount infused was recovered; it's negative if more than the amount infused was recovered. Notify the doctor if the patient retains 500 ml or more of fluid for three consecutive cycles or if he loses at least 1 liter of fluid for three consecutive cycles.

Weigh the patient daily *to help you determine how much fluid is being removed during dialysis treatment.* Note the time and any variations in the weighing technique next to his weight on his chart.

If inflow and outflow are slow or absent, check the tubing for kinks. You can also try raising the I.V. pole or repositioning the patient *to increase the inflow rate.* Repositioning the patient or applying manual pressure to the lateral aspects of the patient's abdomen may also help increase drainage. If these maneuvers fail, notify the doctor. Improper positioning of the catheter or an accumulation of fibrin may obstruct the catheter.

Always examine outflow fluid (effluent) for color and clarity. Normally it's clear or pale yellow, but pink-tinged effluent may appear during the first three or four cycles. If the effluent remains pink-tinged, or if it's grossly bloody, suspect bleeding into the peritoneal cavity and notify the doctor. Also notify the doctor if the outflow contains feces, which suggests bowel perforation, or if it's cloudy, which suggests peritonitis. Obtain a sample for culture and Gram stain. Send the sample in a labeled specimen container to the laboratory with a laboratory request form.

Patient discomfort at the start of the procedure is normal. If the patient experiences pain during the procedure, determine when it occurs, its quality and duration, and whether it radiates to other body parts. Then notify the doctor. Pain during infusion usually results from a dialysate that's too cool or acidic. Pain may also result from rapid inflow; slowing the inflow rate may reduce the pain. Severe, diffuse pain with rebound tenderness and cloudy effluent may indicate peritoneal infection. Pain that radiates to the shoulder often results from air accumulation under the diaphragm. Severe, persistent perineal or rectal pain can result from improper catheter placement.

The patient undergoing peritoneal dialysis will require a great deal of assistance in his daily care. *To minimize his discomfort,* perform daily care during a drain phase in the cycle, when the patient's abdomen is less distended.

Complications

Peritonitis, the most common complication, usually follows contamination of the dialysate, but it may develop if solution leaks from the catheter exit site and flows back into the catheter tract.

Protein depletion may result from the diffusion of protein in the blood into the dialysate solution through the peritoneal membrane. As much as ½ oz (15 g) of protein may be lost daily—more in patients with peritonitis.

Respiratory distress may result when dialysate in the peritoneal cavity increases pressure on the diaphragm, which decreases lung expansion.

Constipation is a major cause of inflow-outflow problems; therefore, *to ensure regular bowel movements,* give a laxative or stool softener, as needed.

Excessive fluid loss from the use of 4.25% solution may cause hypovolemia, hypotension, and shock. Excessive fluid retention may lead to blood volume expansion, hypertension, peripheral edema, and even pulmonary edema and congestive heart failure.

Other possible complications include electrolyte imbalance and hyperglycemia, which can be identified by frequent blood tests.

Documentation

Record the amount of dialysate infused and drained, any medications added to the solution, and the color and character of effluent. Also record the patient's daily weight and fluid balance.

Use a peritoneal dialysis flowchart to compute total fluid balance after each exchange. Note the patient's vital signs and tolerance of the treatment and other pertinent observations.

Three major steps of continuous ambulatory peritoneal dialysis

A bag of dialysate is attached to the tube entering the patient's abdominal area so the fluid flows into the peritoneal cavity.

While the dialysate remains in the peritoneal cavity, the patient can roll up the bag, place it under his shirt, and go about his normal activities.

Unrolling the bag and suspending it below the pelvis allows the dialysate to drain from the peritoneal cavity back into the bag.

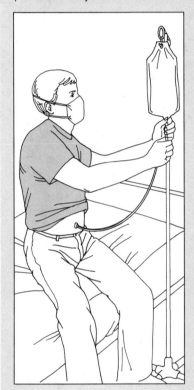 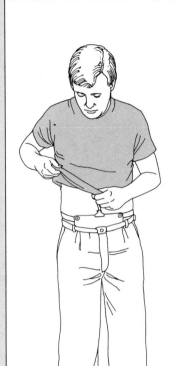 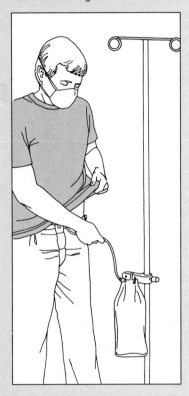

Continuous ambulatory peritoneal dialysis

This procedure requires insertion of a permanent peritoneal catheter (such as a Tenckhoff catheter) to circulate dialysate in the peritoneal cavity constantly. Inserted under local anesthetic, the catheter is sutured in place and its distal portion tunneled subcutaneously to the skin surface. There it serves as a port for the dialysate, which flows in and out of the peritoneal cavity by gravity.

(See *Three major steps of continuous ambulatory peritoneal dialysis.*)

Continuous ambulatory peritoneal dialysis (CAPD) is used most commonly for patients with end-stage renal disease. CAPD can be a welcome alternative to hemodialysis, because it gives the patient more independence and requires less travel for treatments. It also provides more stable fluid and electrolyte levels than conventional hemodialysis.

Patients or family members can usually learn to perform CAPD after only 2 weeks of training. And because the patient can resume normal daily activities between solution changes, CAPD helps promote independence and a return to a near-normal life-style. CAPD has the added advantage of costing less than hemodialysis.

Conditions that may prohibit CAPD include recent abdominal surgery, abdominal adhesions, an infected abdominal wall, diaphragmatic tears, ileus, and respiratory insufficiency.

Equipment
To infuse dialysate: prescribed amount of dialysate (usually in 2-liter bags) ■ basin of hot water or commercial warmer ■ three face masks ■ 42″ (106.7-cm) connective tubing with drain clamp ■ six to eight packages of sterile 4″ × 4″ gauze pads ■ medication, if ordered ■ povidone-iodine sponges ■ nonallergenic tape ■ plastic snap-top container ■ povidone-iodine solution ■ sterile basin ■ container of alcohol ■ sterile gloves ■ belt or fabric pouch ■ two sterile waterproof paper drapes (one fenestrated) ■ optional: syringes, labeled specimen container.

To discontinue dialysis temporarily: three sterile waterproof paper barriers (two fenestrated) ■ 4″ × 4″ gauze pads (for cleaning and dressing the catheter) ■ two face masks ■ sterile basin ■ nonallergenic tape ■ povidone-iodine solution ■ sterile gloves ■ sterile rubber catheter cap ■ alcohol sponges.

All equipment for infusing the dialysate and discontinuing the procedure must be sterile. Commercially prepared sterile CAPD kits are available.

Preparation of equipment
Check the concentration of the dialysate against the doctor's order. Also check the expiration date and appearance of the solution — it should be clear, not cloudy. Warm the solution to body temperature by placing it in a sink or basin of hot water, or use a commercial warmer if one is available. Don't warm the solution in a microwave oven, *because the temperature is unpredictable.*

To minimize the risk of contaminating the bag's port, leave the dialysate container's wrapper in place. *This also keeps the bag dry, which makes examining it for leakage easier after you remove the wrapper.*

Wash your hands and put on a surgical mask. Remove the dialysate container from the warming setup, and remove its protective wrapper. Squeeze the bag firmly *to check for leaks.*

If ordered, use a syringe to add any prescribed medication to the dialysate, using sterile technique *to avoid contamination.* (The ideal approach is to add medication under a laminar flow hood.)

Insert the connective tubing into the dialysate container. Open the drain clamp *to prime the tube.* Then close the clamp.

Place a povidone-iodine sponge on the dialysate container's port. Cover the port with a dry gauze pad, and

secure the pad with tape. Remove and discard the surgical mask. Tear the tape *so it will be ready to secure the new dressing.* Commercial devices with povidone-iodine sponges are available for covering the dialysate container and tubing connection.

Implementation
● Weigh the patient *to establish a baseline level.* Weigh him at the same time every day *to help monitor fluid balance.*

To infuse dialysate
● Assemble all equipment at the patient's bedside, and explain the procedure to him. Prepare the sterile field by placing a waterproof, sterile paper drape on a dry surface near the patient. Take care to maintain the drape's sterility.

● Fill the snap-top container with povidone-iodine solution, and place it on the sterile field. Place the basin on the sterile field. Then place four pairs of sterile gauze pads in the sterile basin, and saturate them with the povidone-iodine solution. Drop the remaining gauze pads on the sterile field. Loosen the cap on the alcohol container, and place it next to the sterile field.

● Put on a clean surgical mask and provide one for the patient.

● Carefully remove the dressing covering the peritoneal catheter and discard it. Be careful not to touch the catheter or skin. Check skin integrity at the catheter site, and look for signs of infection, such as purulent drainage. If drainage is present, obtain a swab specimen, put it in a labeled specimen container, and notify the doctor.

● Put on the sterile gloves and palpate the insertion site and subcutaneous tunnel route for tenderness or pain. If these symptoms occur, notify the doctor.

◆ *Nursing alert.* If the patient has drainage, tenderness, or pain, don't proceed with the infusion without specific orders. ◆

● Wrap one gauze pad saturated with povidone-iodine solution around the distal end of the catheter, and leave it in place for 5 minutes. Clean the catheter and insertion site with the rest of the gauze pads, moving in concentric circles away from the insertion site. Use straight strokes to clean the catheter, beginning at the insertion site and moving outward. Use a clean area of the pad for each stroke. Loosen the catheter cap one notch and clean the exposed area. Place each used pad at the base of the catheter *to help support it.* After using the third pair of pads, place the fenestrated paper drape around the base of the catheter. Continue cleaning the catheter for another minute with one of the remaining pads soaked with povidone-iodine.

● Remove the povidone-iodine sponge on the catheter cap, remove the cap, and use the remaining povidone-iodine sponge to clean the end of the catheter hub. Attach the connective tubing from the dialysate container to the catheter. Be sure to secure the luer-lock connector tightly.

• Open the drain clamp on the dialysate container *to allow solution to enter the peritoneal cavity by gravity* over a period of 5 to 10 minutes. Leave a small amount of fluid in the bag *to make folding it easier.* Close the drain clamp.

• Fold the bag and secure it with a belt, or tuck it in the patient's clothing or a small fabric pouch.

• After the prescribed dwell time (usually 4 to 6 hours), unfold the bag, open the clamp, and allow peritoneal fluid to drain back into the bag by gravity.

• When drainage is complete, attach a new bag of dialysate and repeat the infusion.

• Discard used supplies appropriately.

To discontinue dialysis temporarily

• Wash your hands, put on a surgical mask, and provide one for the patient. Explain the procedure to him.

• Using sterile gloves, remove and discard the dressing over the peritoneal catheter.

• Set up a sterile field next to the patient by covering a clean, dry surface with a waterproof drape. Be sure to maintain the drape's sterility. Place all equipment on the sterile field, and place the $4'' \times 4''$ gauze pads in the basin. Saturate them with the povidone-iodine solution. Open the $4'' \times 4''$ gauze pads to be used as the dressing, and drop them onto the sterile field. Tear pieces of tape as needed.

• Tape the dialysate tubing to the side rail of the bed *to keep the catheter and tubing off the patient's abdomen.*

• Change to another pair of sterile gloves. Then place one of the fenestrated drapes around the base of the catheter.

• Use a pair of povidone-iodine sponges to clean about 6″ (15.2 cm) of the dialysis tubing. Clean for 1 minute, moving in one direction only, away from the catheter. Then clean the catheter, moving from the insertion site to the junction of the catheter and dialysis tubing. Place used sponges at the base of the catheter *to prop it up.* Use two more pairs of sponges to clean the junction for a total of 3 minutes.

• Place the second fenestrated paper drape over the first at the base of the catheter. With the fourth pair of sponges, clean the junction of the catheter and 6″ of the dialysate tubing for another minute.

• Disconnect the dialysate tubing from the catheter. Pick up the catheter cap and fasten it to the catheter, making sure it fits securely over both notches of the hard plastic catheter tip.

• Clean the insertion site and a 2″ (5-cm) radius around it with povidone-iodine sponges, working from the insertion site outward. Let the skin air-dry before applying the dressing.

• Discard used supplies appropriately.

Special considerations

Carefully monitor the patient and his response to treatment.

If the patient suffers severe respiratory distress during the dwell phase of CAPD, drain the peritoneal cavity and notify the doctor.

If inflow and outflow are slow or absent, check the tubing for kinks. You can also try raising the solution or repositioning the patient *to increase the inflow rate.* Repositioning the patient or applying manual pressure to the lateral aspects of the patient's abdomen may also help increase drainage. If these maneuvers fail, notify the doctor. Improper positioning of the catheter or an accumulation of fibrin may obstruct the catheter.

Home care

The patient or family will be entirely responsible for performing CAPD at home, so make sure they understand all steps of the procedure thoroughly and can perform them confidently before discharge. (The patient may also be taught at home or in an outpatient setting.) Teach how to use sterile technique throughout the procedure, especially for cleaning and dressing changes, *to prevent such complications as peritonitis.* Teach them the signs and symptoms of peritonitis — cloudy fluid, fever, abdominal pain, and tenderness — and stress the importance of notifying the doctor immediately if such symptoms arise. Also tell them to call the doctor if redness and drainage occur; these are also signs of infection. Assess the patient's and family's personal hygiene. Reemphasize sterile technique as appropriate.

Instruct the patient to follow a regular schedule of fluid exchanges each day *to maintain optimal fluid balance.* Tell him to record his weight and blood pressure daily and to check regularly for swelling of the extremities. Teach him to keep an accurate record of intake and output. Exchanges are usually done at 4- to 6-hour intervals, except at night; encourage the patient to resume his normal activities between them.

Complications

Peritonitis is the most frequent complication of CAPD. Although treatable, it can permanently scar the peritoneal membrane, decreasing its permeability and reducing dialysis efficiency. Untreated peritonitis can cause septicemia and death.

Protein depletion may result from the diffusion of protein from the blood, through the peritoneal membrane, and into the dialysate solution.

Excessive fluid loss may result from a concentrated (4.25%) dialysate solution, improper or inaccurate monitoring of inflow and outflow, or inadequate oral fluid intake. Excessive fluid retention may result from improper or inaccurate monitoring of inflow and outflow, or excessive salt or oral fluid intake.

Documentation

Record the type and amount of fluid instilled and returned for each exchange, the time and duration of the exchange, and any medications added to the dialysate. Note the color and clarity of the returned exchange fluid and check it for mucus, pus, and blood. Also note any discrepancy in the balance of fluid intake and output, as well as any signs or symptoms of fluid imbalance, such as weight changes, decreased breath sounds, peripheral edema, ascites, and changes in skin turgor. Record the patient's weight, blood pressure, and pulse rate after his last fluid exchange for the day.

Hemodialysis

Hemodialysis is performed to remove toxic wastes from the blood of patients in renal failure. This potentially life-saving procedure removes blood from the body, circulates it through a purifying dialyzer, and then returns the blood to the body. Various access sites can be used for this procedure. (See *Hemodialysis access sites.*) The most common access device for long-term treatment is an arteriovenous (AV) fistula.

The underlying mechanism in hemodialysis is differential diffusion across a semipermeable membrane, which extracts by-products of protein metabolism, such as urea and uric acid, as well as creatinine and excess body water. This process restores or maintains the balance of the body's buffer system and electrolyte level. Hemodialysis thus promotes a rapid return to normal serum values and helps prevent complications associated with uremia. (See *How hemodialysis works,* page 592.)

Hemodialysis provides temporary support for patients with acute reversible renal failure. It's also used for regular long-term treatment of patients with chronic end-stage renal disease. A less common indication for hemodialysis is acute poisoning, such as barbiturate or analgesic overdose. The patient's condition and the equipment available determine the number and duration of hemodialysis treatments.

Specially prepared personnel usually perform this procedure in a hemodialysis unit. However, if the patient is acutely ill, hemodialysis can be done at bedside. Special hemodialysis units are available for home use.

Equipment

For preparing the hemodialysis machine: hemodialysis machine with appropriate dialyzer ■ I.V. solutions, administration sets and filters, and related equipment ■ dialysate ■ optional: heparin, 3-ml syringe with needle, medication label, clamp.

For hemodialysis with a double-lumen catheter: povidone-iodine sponges ■ sterile drape ■ two sterile 4″ × 4″ gauze pads ■ two 5-ml syringes ■ tape ■ heparin bolus syringe ■ sterile gloves.

For hemodialysis with an AV fistula: two winged fistula needles (each attached to a 10-ml syringe filled with heparinized normal saline solution) ■ linen-saver pad ■ povidone-iodine sponges ■ sterile 4″ × 4″ gauze pads ■ tourniquet ■ sterile gloves ■ two sterile hemostats ■ povidone-iodine ointment ■ adhesive tape.

For hemodialysis with an AV shunt: sterile drape or barrier shield ■ alcohol sponges ■ sterile gloves ■ two sterile shunt adapters ■ sterile Teflon connector ■ two bulldog clamps ■ two 10-ml syringes ■ normal saline solution ■ four short strips of adhesive tape ■ optional: sterile shunt spreader.

For discontinuing hemodialysis with a double-lumen catheter: sterile drape ■ two sterile 4″ × 4″ gauze pads ■ alcohol sponge ■ povidone-iodine sponge ■ precut gauze dressing ■ sterile gloves ■ normal saline solution ■ sterile gauze sponges ■ heparin flush solution ■ luer-lock injection caps ■ optional: transparent occlusive dressing, skin barrier preparation, tape, materials for culturing drainage.

For discontinuing hemodialysis with an AV fistula: clean gloves ■ four hemostats ■ sterile absorbable gelatin sponges (Gelfoam) ■ sterile 4″ × 4″ gauze pads ■ topical thrombin solution ■ two adhesive bandages.

For discontinuing hemodialysis with an AV shunt: sterile gloves ■ two bulldog clamps ■ two hemostats ■ povidone-iodine solution ■ sterile 4″ × 4″ gauze pads ■ alcohol sponges ■ elastic gauze bandages.

Preparation of equipment

Prepare the hemodialysis equipment following the manufacturer's instructions and your hospital's protocol. Maintain strict aseptic technique *to prevent introducing pathogens into the patient's bloodstream during dialysis.* Be sure to test the dialyzer and dialysis machine for residual disinfectant after rinsing. Also test all the alarms.

Implementation

• Weigh the patient. *To determine ultrafiltration requirements,* compare his present weight to his weight after

Hemodialysis access sites

Hemodialysis requires vascular access. The site and type of access may vary, depending on the expected duration of dialysis, the surgeon's preference, and the patient's condition.

Subclavian vein catheterization

Using the Seldinger technique, the doctor or surgeon inserts an introducer needle into the subclavian vein. He then inserts a guidewire through the introducer needle and removes the needle. Using the guidewire, he then threads a 5″ to 12″ (12.7- to 30.4-cm) plastic or Teflon catheter (with a Y hub) into the patient's vein.

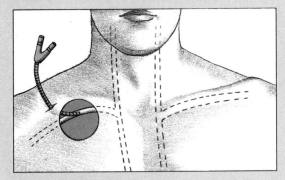

Femoral vein catheterization

Using the Seldinger technique, the doctor or surgeon inserts an introducer needle into the left or right femoral vein. He then inserts a guidewire through the introducer needle and removes the needle. Using the guidewire, he then threads a 5″ to 12″ plastic or Teflon catheter with a Y hub or two catheters, one for inflow and another placed about ½″ (1.3 cm) distal to the first for outflow.

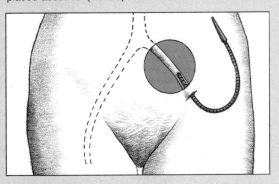

Arteriovenous fistula

To create a fistula, the surgeon makes an incision into the patient's wrist or lower forearm, then a small incision in the side of an artery and another in the side of a vein. He sutures the edges of these incisions together to make a common opening 3 to 7 mm long.

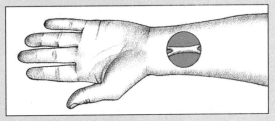

Arteriovenous shunt

To create a shunt, the surgeon makes an incision in the patient's wrist, lower forearm, or (rarely) an ankle. He then inserts a 6″ to 10″ (15.2- to 25.4-cm) transparent Silastic cannula into an artery and another into a vein. Finally, he tunnels the cannulas out through stab wounds and joins them with a piece of Teflon tubing.

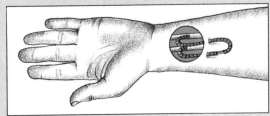

Arteriovenous graft

To create a graft, the surgeon makes an incision in the patient's forearm, upper arm, or thigh. He then tunnels a natural or synthetic graft under the skin and sutures the distal end to an artery and the proximal end to a vein.

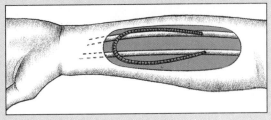

How hemodialysis works

In hemodialysis, blood flows from the patient to an external dialyzer (or artificial kidney) through an arterial access site. Inside the dialyzer, blood and dialysate flow countercurrently, divided by a semipermeable membrane. The composition of the dialysate resembles normal extracellular fluid. The blood contains an excess of specific solutes (metabolic waste products and some electrolytes), and the dialysate contains electrolytes that may be at abnormal levels in the patient's bloodstream. The dialysate's electrolyte composition can be modified to raise or lower electrolyte levels, depending on need.

Excretory function and electrolyte homeostasis are achieved by *diffusion,* the movement of a molecule across the dialyzer's semipermeable membrane, from an area of higher solute concentration to an area of lower solute concentration. Water (solvent) crosses the membrane from the blood into the dialysate by *ultrafiltration.* This process removes excess water, waste products, and other metabolites through *osmotic pressure* and *hydrostatic pressure.* Osmotic pressure is the movement of water across the semipermeable membrane from an area of lesser solute concentration to one of greater solute concentration. Hydrostatic pressure forces water from the blood compartment into the dialysate compartment. Cleaned of impurities and excess water, the blood returns to the body through a venous site.

Types of dialyzers

There are three types of dialyzers: the *hollow-fiber,* the *flat-plate* or *parallel flow-plate,* and the *coil.*

The *hollow-fiber* dialyzer, the most common type, contains fine capillaries, with a semipermeable membrane enclosed in a plastic cylinder. Blood flows through these capillaries as the system pumps dialysate in the opposite direction on the outside of the capillaries.

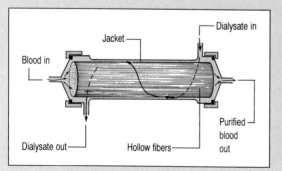

The *flat-plate* or *parallel flow-plate* dialyzer has two or more layers of semipermeable membrane, bound by a semirigid or rigid structure. Blood ports are located at both ends, between the membranes. Blood flows between the membranes, and dialysate flows in the opposite direction along the outside of the membranes.

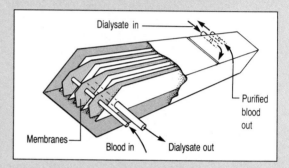

The *coil* dialyzer (no longer widely used) consists of one or more semipermeable membrane tubes supported by mesh and wrapped concentrically around a central core. Blood passes through the coils as dialysate circulates at high speed around the coils and meshwork.

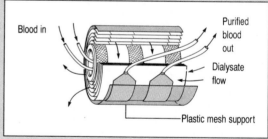

The flat-plate and hollow-fiber dialyzers may be used several times on each patient. Heparin is used to prevent clot formation during hemodialysis.

Three system types can be used to deliver dialysate. The *batch* system uses a reservoir for recirculating dialysate. The *regenerative* system uses sorbents to purify and regenerate recirculating dialysate. The *proportioning* system (the most common) mixes concentrate with water to form dialysate, which then circulates through the dialyzer and goes down a drain after a single pass, followed by fresh dialysate.

the last dialysis and his target weight. Record his baseline vital signs, taking his blood pressure while he's supine and standing. Auscultate his heart for rate, rhythm, and abnormalities. Observe respiratory rate, rhythm, and quality. Assess for edema. Check his mental status and the condition and patency of the access site. Also check for problems since the last dialysis, and evaluate previous laboratory data.

• Help the patient into a comfortable position (supine or sitting in recliner chair with feet elevated). Be sure the access site is well supported and resting on a sterile drape or sterile barrier shield.

• If the patient is undergoing hemodialysis for the first time, explain the procedure in detail.

• Use universal precautions in all cases *to prevent transmission of infection*. Wash your hands before beginning.

To begin hemodialysis with a double-lumen catheter

• Prepare venous access. If extension tubing is not already clamped, clamp it *to prevent air from entering the catheter*. Then clean each catheter extension tube, clamp, and luer-lock injection cap with povidone-iodine sponges *to remove contaminants*. Next, place a sterile drape under the extension tubing, and place two 5-ml syringes and two sterile gauze pads on the drape.

• Prepare anticoagulant regimen as ordered.

• Identify arterial and venous blood lines and place them near the drape. Put on sterile gloves.

• *To remove clots and ensure catheter patency*, remove catheter caps, attach syringes to each catheter port, open one clamp, and aspirate 3 to 5 ml of blood. Close the clamp and repeat the procedure with the other port.

• Attach blood lines to patient access. First, remove the syringe from the arterial port, grasp the blood line with sterile gauze pads, and attach the line to the arterial port. Next, attach the heparin bolus syringe to the venous port, remove the clamp, administer the heparin, and reclamp. *This prevents clotting in the extracorporeal circuit.*

• Remove the bolus syringe, grasp the venous blood line with a sterile gauze pad, and attach the line to the venous port. Open the clamps on the extension tubing, and secure the tubing to the patient's extremity with tape *to reduce tension on the tube and minimize trauma to the insertion site*.

• Begin hemodialysis according to your unit's protocol.

To begin hemodialysis with an AV fistula

• Flush the fistula needles, using attached syringes containing heparinized saline solution, and set them aside.

• Place a linen-saver pad under the patient's arm.

• Using aseptic technique, clean a 3″ × 10″ (7.6 × 25.4 cm) area of skin over the fistula with povidone-iodine sponges. Discard each pad after one wipe. (If the patient is sensitive to iodine, use chlorhexidine gluconate [Hibiclens] instead.)

• Apply a tourniquet above the fistula *to distend the veins and facilitate venipuncture.*

• Put on sterile gloves. Perform the venipuncture with a venous fistula needle. Remove the needle guard and squeeze the wing tips firmly together. Insert the venous needle at least 1″ (2.5 cm) above the fistula, being careful not to puncture the fistula.

• Release the tourniquet and flush the needle with heparinized normal saline solution *to prevent clotting*. Clamp the venous needle tubing with a hemostat, apply povidone-iodine ointment to the insertion site, and secure the wing tips of the needle to the skin with adhesive tape *to prevent it from dislodging within the vein.*

• Perform another venipuncture with the arterial needle a few inches below the venous needle. Flush the needle with heparinized saline solution. Clamp the arterial needle tubing, apply ointment, and secure the wing tips of the arterial needle as you did the venous needle.

• Remove the syringe from the end of the arterial tubing, uncap the arterial line from the hemodialysis machine, and connect the two lines. Tape the connection securely *to prevent it from separating during the procedure*. Repeat these two steps for the venous line.

• Release the hemostats and start hemodialysis.

To begin hemodialysis with an AV shunt

• Remove the bulldog clamps and place them within easy reach of the sterile field. Remove the shunt dressing, and clean the shunt, using aseptic technique, as you would for daily care. (See "Care of an arteriovenous shunt" later in this chapter.) Clean the bulldog clamps with an alcohol sponge.

• Assemble the shunt adapters according to the manufacturer's directions.

• Clean the arterial and venous shunt connection with povidone-iodine sponges *to remove contaminants*. Use a separate sponge for each tube, and wipe in one direction only, from the insertion site to the connection sites. Allow the tubing to air-dry.

• Put on sterile gloves.

• Clamp the arterial side of the shunt with a bulldog clamp *to prevent blood from flowing through it*. Clamp the venous side *to prevent leakage when the shunt is opened.*

• Open the shunt by separating its sides with your fingers or with a sterile shunt spreader, if available. Both sides of the shunt should be exposed. Always inspect the Teflon connector on one side of the shunt *to see if it's damaged or bent*. If necessary, replace it before proceeding. Note which side contains the connector *so you can use the new one to close the shunt after treatment.*

• *To adapt the shunt to the lines of the machine,* attach a shunt adapter and 10-ml syringe filled with about 8 ml of normal saline solution to the side of the shunt containing the Teflon connector. Attach the new Teflon connector to the other side of the shunt with the second adapter. Attach the second 10-ml syringe filled with about 8 ml of saline solution to the same side.

• Flush the shunt's arterial tubing by releasing its clamp and gently aspirating it with the saline solution-filled syringe. Then flush the tubing slowly, observing it for signs of fibrin buildup. Repeat the procedure on the venous side of the shunt.

• Secure the shunt to the adapter connection with adhesive tape *to prevent separation during treatment.*

• Connect the arterial and venous lines to the adapters and secure the connections with tape. Tape each line to the patient's arm *to prevent unnecessary strain on the shunt during treatment.*

• Begin hemodialysis according to your unit's protocol.

To discontinue hemodialysis with a double-lumen catheter

• Wash your hands.

• Clamp the extension tubing *to prevent air from entering the catheter.* Clean all connection points on the catheter and blood lines, as well as the clamps, *to reduce the risk of systemic or local infections.*

• Place a sterile drape under the catheter, and place two sterile 4″ × 4″ gauze pads on the drape. Then prepare the catheter flush solution with normal saline or with heparin-saline solution, as ordered.

• Put on sterile gloves.

• Grasp each blood line with a sterile gauze pad and disconnect each line from the catheter.

• Flush each port with saline solution *to clean the extension tubing and catheter of blood.* Administer additional heparin flush solution as ordered *to ensure catheter patency.* Then attach luer-lock injection caps *to prevent entry of air or loss of blood.*

• Clamp the extension tubing.

• When hemodialysis is complete, re-dress the catheter insertion site; also re-dress it if it is occluded, soiled, or wet. Position the patient supine with his face turned away from the insertion site *so he doesn't contaminate the site by breathing on it.*

• Wash your hands and remove the outer occlusive dressing. Then put on sterile gloves, remove the old inner dressing, and discard the gloves and the inner dressing.

• Set up a sterile field, and observe the site for drainage. Obtain a drainage sample for culture if necessary. Notify the doctor if the suture appears to be missing.

• Put on sterile gloves and clean the insertion site with an alcohol sponge *to remove skin oils.* Then clean the site with a povidone-iodine sponge and allow it to air-dry.

Then apply povidone-iodine ointment to the insertion site and the suture site.

• Put a precut gauze dressing over the ointment and under the catheter, and place another gauze dressing over the catheter.

• Apply a skin barrier preparation to the skin surrounding the gauze dressing. Then cover the gauze and catheter with a transparent occlusive dressing.

• Apply a 4- to 5-inch piece of 2-inch tape over the cut edge of the dressing *to reinforce the lower edge.*

To discontinue hemodialysis with an AV fistula

• Wash your hands. Turn the blood pump on the hemodialysis machine to 50 to 100 ml/minute.

• Put on sterile gloves and remove the tape from the connection site of the arterial lines. Clamp the needle tubing with the hemostat and disconnect the lines. The blood in the machine's arterial line will continue to flow toward the dialyzer, followed by a column of air. Just before the blood reaches the point where the saline solution enters the line, clamp the blood line with another hemostat.

• Unclamp the saline solution *to allow a small amount to flow through the line.* Reclamp the saline line and unclamp the hemostat on the machine line. *This allows all blood to flow into the dialyzer where it's circulated through the filter and back to the patient through the venous line.*

• Just before the last volume of blood enters the patient, clamp the venous needle tubing and the machine's venous line with hemostats.

• Remove the tape from the connection site of the venous lines. Turn off the blood pump and disconnect the lines.

• Remove the venipuncture needle and apply pressure to the site with a folded 4″ × 4″ gauze pad until all bleeding stops, usually 10 minutes. Apply an adhesive bandage. Repeat the procedure on the arterial line.

• When hemodialysis is complete, assess the patient's weight, vital signs (including standing blood pressure) and mental status. Then compare your findings with your predialysis assessment data. Document your findings.

• Disinfect and rinse the delivery system according to the manufacturer's instructions.

To discontinue hemodialysis with an AV shunt

• Wash your hands. Turn the blood pump on the hemodialysis machine to 50 to 100 ml/minute.

• Put on the sterile gloves and remove the tape from the connection site of the arterial lines. Clamp the arterial cannula with a bulldog clamp, and then disconnect the lines. The blood in the machine's arterial line will continue to flow toward the dialyzer, followed by a column of air. Just before the blood reaches the point where the normal saline solution enters the line, clamp the blood line with a hemostat.

• Unclamp the saline solution *to allow a small amount to flow through the line.* Reclamp the saline solution line and unclamp the hemostat on the machine line. *This allows all blood to flow into the dialyzer where it's circulated through the filter and back to the patient through the venous line.*

• Just before the last volume of blood enters the patient, clamp the venous cannula with a bulldog clamp and the machine's venous line with a hemostat.

• Remove the tape from the connection site of the venous lines. Turn off the blood pump and disconnect the lines.

• Reconnect the shunt cannula. Remove the older of the two Teflon connectors and discard it. Connect the shunt, taking care to position the Teflon connector equally between the two cannulas. Remove the bulldog clamps.

• Secure the shunt connection with plasticized or non-allergenic tape *to prevent accidental disconnection.*

• Clean the shunt and its site with the gauze pads soaked with povidone-iodine solution. When the cleaning procedure is finished, remove the povidone-iodine with alcohol sponges.

• Make sure blood flows through the shunt adequately.

• Apply a dressing to the shunt site and wrap it securely (but not too tightly) with elastic gauze bandages. Attach the bulldog clamps to the outside dressing.

• When hemodialysis is complete, assess the patient's weight, vital signs, and mental status. Then compare your findings with your predialysis assessment data. Document your findings.

• Disinfect and rinse the delivery system according to the manufacturer's instructions.

Special considerations

Obtain blood samples from the patient, as ordered. Samples are usually drawn before beginning hemodialysis.

♦ *Nursing alert. To avoid pyrogenic reactions and bacteremia with septicemia resulting from contamination,* use strict aseptic technique during preparation of the machine. Discard equipment that has fallen on the floor or that has been disconnected and exposed to the air. ♦

Immediately report any machine malfunction or equipment defect.

Avoid unnecessary handling of shunt tubing. However, be sure to inspect the shunt carefully for patency by observing its color. Also look for clots and serum and cell separation, and check the temperature of the Silastic tubing. Assess the shunt insertion site for signs of infection, such as purulent drainage, inflammation, and tenderness, which may indicate the body's rejection of the shunt. Also check to see if the shunt insertion tips are exposed.

Make sure you complete each step in this procedure correctly. *Overlooking a single step or performing it incorrectly can cause unnecessary blood loss or inefficient treatment from poor clearances or inadequate fluid removal.* For example, never allow a saline solution bag to run dry while priming and soaking the dialyzer. *This can cause air to enter the patient portion of the dialysate system.* Ultimately, failure to perform accurate hemodialysis therapy can lead to patient injury and even death.

If bleeding continues after you remove an AV fistula needle, apply pressure with a sterile, absorbable gelatin sponge. If bleeding persists, apply a similar sponge soaked in topical thrombin solution.

Throughout hemodialysis, carefully monitor the patient's vital signs. Read blood pressure at least hourly or as often as every 15 minutes, if necessary. Monitor the patient's weight before and after the procedure *to ensure adequate ultrafiltration during treatment.* (Many dialysis units are equipped with bed scales.)

Perform periodic tests for clotting time on the patient's blood samples and samples from the dialyzer. If the patient receives meals during treatment, make sure they're light.

Continue necessary drug administration during dialysis unless the drug would be removed in the dialysate; if so, administer the drug after dialysis.

Home care

Before the patient leaves the hospital, teach him how to care for his vascular access site. Instruct him to keep the incision clean and dry *to prevent infection,* and to clean it daily until it heals completely and the sutures are removed (usually 10 to 14 days after surgery). He should notify the doctor of pain, swelling, redness, or drainage in the accessed arm. Teach him how to use a stethoscope to auscultate for bruits and how to palpate a thrill.

Explain that once the access site heals, he may use the arm freely. In fact, exercise is beneficial because it helps stimulate vein enlargement. Remind him not to allow any treatments or procedures on the accessed arm, including blood pressure monitoring or needle punctures. Also tell him to avoid putting excessive pressure on the arm. He shouldn't sleep on it, wear constricting clothing on it, or lift heavy objects or strain with it. He also should avoid getting wet for several hours after dialysis.

Teach the patient exercises for the affected arm *to promote vascular dilation and enhance blood flow.* He may start by squeezing a small rubber ball or other soft object for 15 minutes, when advised by the doctor.

If the patient will be performing hemodialysis at home, thoroughly review all aspects of the procedure with the patient and family. Give them the phone number of the dialysis center. Emphasize that training for home hemodialysis is a complex process requiring 2 to 3 months to ensure that the patient or family member performs it safely and competently. Keep in mind that this procedure is stressful.

Complications

Bacterial endotoxins in the dialysate may cause fever. Rapid fluid removal and electrolyte changes during hemodialysis can cause early dialysis disequilibrium syndrome. Signs and symptoms include headache, nausea, vomiting, restlessness, hypertension, muscle cramps, backache, and seizures.

Excessive removal of fluid during ultrafiltration can cause hypovolemia and hypotension. Diffusion of the sugar and sodium content of the dialysate solution into the blood can cause hyperglycemia and hypernatremia. These conditions, in turn, can cause hyperosmolarity.

Cardiac arrhythmias can occur during hemodialysis as a result of electrolyte and pH changes in the blood. They can also develop in patients taking antiarrhythmic drugs because the dialysate removes these drugs during treatment. Angina may develop in patients with anemia or preexisting arteriosclerotic cardiovascular disease because of the physiologic stress on the blood during purification and ultrafiltration.

Reduced oxygen levels resulting from extracorporeal blood flow or membrane sensitivity may require increasing oxygen administration during hemodialysis.

Some complications of hemodialysis can be fatal. For example, an air embolism can result if the dialyzer retains air, if tubing connections become loose, or if the saline solution container empties. Symptoms include chest pain, dyspnea, coughing, and cyanosis.

Hemolysis can result from obstructed flow of the dialysate concentrate or from incorrect setting of the conductivity alarm limits. Symptoms include chest pain, dyspnea, cherry red blood, arrhythmias, acute decrease in hematocrit, and hyperkalemia.

Hyperthermia, another potentially fatal complication, can result if the dialysate becomes overheated. Exsanguination can result from separations of the blood lines or from rupture of the blood lines or dialyzer membrane.

Documentation

Record the time treatment began and any problems with it. Note the patient's vital signs and weight before and during treatment. Note the time blood specimens were taken for testing, the test results, and treatment for complications. Record the time the treatment was completed and the patient's response to it.

Care of an arteriovenous shunt

An arteriovenous (AV) shunt consists of two segments of tubing joined (in a U-shape) to divert blood from an artery to a vein. Inserted surgically, usually in a forearm or (rarely) an ankle, the AV shunt provides access to the circulatory system for hemodialysis. After insertion, an AV shunt requires regular assessment for patency and examination of the surrounding skin for signs of infection.

AV shunt care also includes aseptically cleaning the arterial and venous exit sites, applying antiseptic ointment, and dressing the sites with sterile bandages. When done just before hemodialysis, this procedure prolongs the life of the shunt, helps prevent infection, and allows early detection of clotting. Shunt site care is done more often if the dressing becomes wet or nonocclusive.

Equipment

Drape ■ stethoscope ■ sterile gloves ■ sterile 4″ × 4″ gauze pads ■ sterile cotton-tipped applicators ■ antiseptic (usually povidone-iodine solution) ■ bulldog clamps ■ plasticized or nonallergenic tape ■ optional: swab specimen kit, prescribed antimicrobial ointment (usually povidone-iodine), sterile elastic gauze bandage, 2″ × 2″ gauze pads, hydrogen peroxide.

Kits containing all the necessary equipment can be prepackaged and stored for use.

Implementation

• Explain the procedure to the patient, provide privacy, and wash your hands.

• Place the drape on a stable surface, such as a bedside table, *to reduce the risk of traumatic injury to the shunt site.* Then place the shunted extremity on the draped surface.

• Remove the two bulldog clamps from the elastic gauze bandage, and unwrap the bandage from the shunt area.

• Carefully remove the gauze dressing covering the shunt. Remove the 4″ × 4″ gauze pad under the shunt.

• Assess the arterial and venous exit sites for signs of infection, such as erythema, swelling, excessive tenderness, or drainage. Obtain a swab specimen of any purulent drainage, and notify the doctor immediately of any signs of infection.

• Check blood flow through the shunt by inspecting the color of the blood and comparing the warmth of the shunt with that of the surrounding skin. The blood should be bright red; the shunt should feel as warm as the skin.

◆ *Nursing alert.* If the blood is dark purple or black and the temperature of the shunt is lower than the surrounding skin, clotting has occurred. Notify the doctor immediately. ◆

• Use the stethoscope to auscultate the shunt between the arterial and venous exit sites. A bruit confirms normal blood flow. Palpate the shunt for a thrill, which also indicates normal blood flow. Don't use a Doppler device to auscultate *because it will detect peripheral blood flow as well as shunt-related sounds.*

• Open a few packages of $4'' \times 4''$ gauze pads and cotton-tipped applicators and soak them with the antiseptic. Put on the sterile gloves.

• Using a soaked $4'' \times 4''$ gauze pad, start cleaning the skin at one of the exit sites. Wipe away from the site *to remove bacteria and reduce the chance of contaminating the shunt.*

• Use the soaked cotton-tipped applicators to remove any crusted material from the exit site *because the encrustations provide a medium for bacterial growth.*

• Clean the other exit site, using fresh, soaked $4'' \times 4''$ gauze pads and cotton-tipped applicators.

• Clean the rest of the skin that was covered by the gauze dressing with fresh, soaked $4'' \times 4''$ gauze pads.

• If ordered, apply antimicrobial ointment to the exit sites *to help prevent infection.*

• Place a dry, sterile $4'' \times 4''$ gauze pad under the shunt. *This prevents the shunt from contacting the skin, which could cause skin irritation and breakdown.*

• Cover the exit sites with a dry, sterile $4'' \times 4''$ gauze pad, and tape it securely *to keep the exit sites clean and protected.*

• For routine daily care, wrap the shunt with an elastic gauze bandage. Leave a small portion of the shunt cannula exposed *so the patient can check for patency without removing the dressing.*

• Place the bulldog clamps on the edge of the elastic gauze bandage *so the patient can use them quickly to stop hemorrhage in case the shunt separates.*

• For care before hemodialysis, don't re-dress the shunt, but keep the bulldog clamps readily accessible.

Special considerations

◆ **Nursing alert.** Make sure the AV junction of the shunt is secured with plasticized or nonallergenic tape. *This prevents separation of the two halves of the shunt, minimizing the risk of hemorrhage.* ◆

Always handle the shunt and dressings carefully. Don't use scissors or other sharp instruments to remove the dressing *because you may accidentally cut the shunt.* Never remove the tape securing the AV junction during dressing changes.

When cleaning the shunt exit sites, use each $4'' \times 4''$ gauze pad only once and avoid wiping any area more than once *to minimize the risk of contamination.* When re-dressing the site, make sure the tape doesn't kink or occlude the shunt. If the exit sites are heavily encrusted, place a $2'' \times 2''$ hydrogen peroxide-soaked gauze pad on the area for about 1 hour *to loosen the crust.* Make sure the patient isn't allergic to iodine before using povidone-iodine solution or ointment.

Home care

Ask the patient how he cares for the shunt at home. Then teach proper home care, if necessary.

Documentation

Record that shunt care was administered, the condition of the shunt and surrounding skin, any ointment used, and any instructions given to the patient.

Continuous arteriovenous hemofiltration

A relatively new procedure, continuous arteriovenous hemofiltration (CAVH) is used to treat patients who have fluid overload but who don't require dialysis. CAVH filters fluid, solutes, and electrolytes from the patient's blood and infuses a replacement solution.

The hemofilter, composed of about 5,000 hollow fiber capillaries, filters blood at a rate of about 250 ml/minute and is driven by the patient's arterial blood pressure (a systolic blood pressure of 60 mm Hg is adequate for the procedure). Some of the ultrafiltrate collected during CAVH is replaced with a filter replacement fluid (FRF). This fluid can be lactated Ringer's solution or any solution that resembles plasma. Because the amount of fluid removed is greater than the amount replaced, the patient gradually loses fluid (12 to 15 liters daily).

CAVH carries a much lower risk of hypotension from fluid withdrawal than conventional hemodialysis because it withdraws fluid more slowly — at only 5 to 10 ml/minute (compared with 200 ml/minute for hemodialysis). CAVH can be performed in hypotensive patients who require fluid removal, who cannot have peritoneal dialysis, or whose requirements for parenteral nutrition would make fluid volume control problematic. Additionally, CAVH reduces the risk of other complications — cramps, nausea, vomiting, and headache, for example. And because it withdraws fluid slowly, CAVH makes maintaining a stable fluid volume and regulating fluid and electrolyte balance easier. The procedure costs less than hemodialysis, and the equipment is easier to operate.

A similar procedure, continuous arteriovenous filtration and hemodialysis (CAVH-D), combines hemodialysis

Continuous arteriovenous hemofiltration setup

During continuous arteriovenous hemofiltration (CAVH), the patient's arterial blood pressure serves as a natural pump, driving blood through the arterial line. A hemofilter removes water and toxic solutes (ultrafiltrate) from the blood. Filter replacement fluid is infused into a port on the arterial side; this same port can be used to infuse heparin. The venous line carries the replacement fluid, along with purified blood, to the patient. The illustration shows one of several CAVH setups.

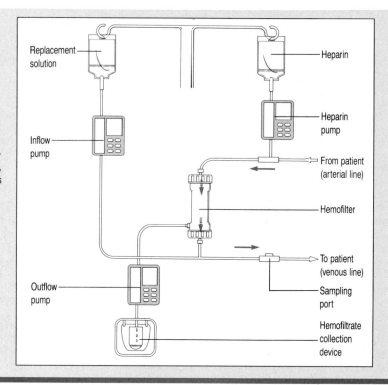

with hemofiltration. Like CAVH, it can also be performed in patients with hypotension and fluid overload.

Commonly used to treat patients in acute renal failure, CAVH is also used for treating fluid overload that doesn't respond to diuretics and for some electrolyte and acid-base disturbances.

Equipment

CAVH equipment (see *Continuous arteriovenous hemofiltration setup*) ▪ heparin flush solution ▪ occlusive dressings for catheter insertion sites ▪ sterile gloves ▪ sterile mask ▪ povidone-iodine solution ▪ sterile 4″ × 4″ gauze pads ▪ tape ▪ FRF, as ordered ▪ infusion pump.

Preparation of equipment

Prime the hemofilter and tubing according to the manufacturer's instructions.

Implementation

• Wash your hands. Assemble your equipment at the patient's bedside, and explain the procedure.
• If necessary, assist with inserting the catheters into the femoral artery and vein, using strict aseptic technique. (In some cases, an internal arteriovenous fistula or external arteriovenous shunt may be used instead of the femoral route.)
• If ordered, flush both catheters with the heparin flush solution *to prevent clotting.*
• Apply occlusive dressings to the insertion sites, and mark the dressings with the date and time. Secure the tubing and connections with tape.
• Assess all pulses in the affected leg every hour for the first 4 hours, then every 2 hours afterwards.
• Weigh the patient, take baseline vital signs, and make sure that all necessary laboratory studies have been done (usually, electrolyte levels, coagulation factors, complete blood count, blood urea nitrogen, and creatinine studies). Monitor the patient's weight and vital signs hourly.

• Put on the sterile gloves and mask. Prepare the connection sites by cleaning them with gauze pads soaked in povidone-iodine solution, then connect them to the exit port of each catheter.
• Connect the arterial and venous lines to the hemofilter. Use aseptic technique.
• Turn on the hemofilter and monitor the blood flow rate through the circuit. The flow rate is usually kept between 500 and 900 ml/hour.
• Inspect the ultrafiltrate during the procedure. It should remain clear yellow, with no gross blood. Pink-tinged or bloody ultrafiltrate may signal a membrane leak in the hemofilter, which would leave the blood compartment open to contamination from bacteria. If a leak occurs, notify the doctor so he can have the hemofilter replaced.
• Assess the affected leg for signs of obstructed blood flow, such as coolness, pallor, and weak pulse. Check the groin area on the affected side *for signs of hematoma.* Also ask the patient if he has pain at the insertion sites.
• Calculate the amount of FRF every hour, or as ordered, according to your hospital's policy. Then infuse the prescribed amount and type of FRF through the infusion pump into the arterial side of the circuit.

Special considerations
Because blood flows through an extracorporeal circuit during CAVH, the blood in the hemofilter may need to be anticoagulated. To do this, infuse heparin in low doses (usually starting at 500 units/hour) into an infusion port on the arterial side of the setup. Then measure thrombin clotting time or the activated clotting time (ACT). *This ensures that the circuit, not the patient, is anticoagulated.* A normal ACT is 100 seconds; during CAVH, keep it between 100 and 300 seconds, depending on the patient's clotting times. If the ACT is too high or too low, the doctor will adjust the heparin dose accordingly.

Another way to prevent clotting in the hemofilter is not to infuse medications or blood through the venous line. This line may be used in emergencies to infuse I.V. fluids, but will slow the return of dialyzed blood to the patient, increasing the risk of clotting. Run infusions through another line if possible.

A third way to help prevent clots in the hemofilter, and also to prevent kinks in the catheter, is to make sure the patient doesn't bend the affected leg more than 30 degrees at the hip.

To prevent infection, perform skin care at the catheter insertion sites every 48 hours, using aseptic technique. Cover the sites with an occlusive dressing.

Check the connection sites *to be sure they're taped securely.* Blood loss from a sudden disconnection in the circuit could cause serious complications.

If the ultrafiltrate flow rate decreases, raise the bed *to increase the distance between the collection device and the hemofilter.* Lower the bed *to decrease the flow rate.* (Clamping the ultrafiltrate line is contraindicated with some types of hemofilters *because pressure may build up in the filter, clotting it and collapsing the blood compartment.*)

Complications
Possible complications include bleeding, hemorrhage, hemofilter occlusion, infection, and thrombosis.

Documentation
Record the time the treatment began and ended, fluid balance information, times of dressing changes, complications, medications given, and the patient's tolerance.

Selected references

Daugirdas, J.T., and Ing, T.S. *Handbook of Dialysis.* Boston: Little, Brown & Co., 1988.

Dirkes, S.M. "Making a Critical Difference with CAVH," *Nursing89* 19(11):57-60, November 1989.

Guyton, A. *Textbook of Medical Physiology,* 7th ed. Philadelphia: W.B. Saunders Co., 1986.

Heneghan, G., et al. "The Indiana Pouch: A Continent Urinary Diversion," *Journal of Enterostomal Therapy* 17(6):231-36, November-December 1990.

Illustrated Manual of Nursing Practice. Springhouse, Pa.: Springhouse Corp., 1991.

Norris, M. "Action Stat! Dialysis Disequilibrium Syndrome," *Nursing89* 19(4):33, April 1989.

Phillips, R.H. *Coping with Kidney Failure: A Guide to Living with Kidney Failure for You and Your Family.* Wayne, N.J.: Avery Pub. Group, 1987.

Rake, R.F., ed. *Conn's Current Therapy.* Philadelphia: W.B. Saunders Co., 1988.

Rowland, R.G. "Continent Urinary Reservoirs," *Surgical Clinics of North America* 68(5):891-907, October 1988.

Snyder, T.E. "An Exercise Program for Dialysis Patients," *AJN* 89(3):362-64, March 1989.

Ulrich, B.T., ed. *Nephrology Nursing: Concepts and Strategies.* Norwalk, Conn.: Appleton & Lange, 1988.

ORTHOPEDIC CARE

DORI TAYLOR, RN, PhD, CNA

Introduction

Orthopedics began as a specialty for the prevention and treatment of children's musculoskeletal deformities. However, this branch of medicine has expanded dramatically to include the prevention, treatment, and care of musculoskeletal conditions affecting patients of all ages.

The American Nurses' Association defines orthopedic nursing as the diagnosis and treatment of human responses to actual and potential health problems related to musculoskeletal function. More specifically, orthopedic nursing focuses on promoting wellness and self-care and on preventing further injury and illness in patients with degenerative, traumatic, inflammatory, neuromuscular, congenital, metabolic, and oncologic disorders.

Traditionally, orthopedic nurses have needed to operate special mechanical and traction equipment. Today, such nurses need to understand principles of internal and external fixation, prosthetics, orthotics, immobilization, and implantation.

Despite the evolution of complex surgical procedures and mechanical devices that characterize modern orthopedic care, some things remain the same. A patient hospitalized for any orthopedic procedure—whether it's cast application, traction, or arthroplasty—is vulnerable to similar complications, such as:
• joint stiffness and skin breakdown from impaired physical mobility
• fractures from mishandling of osteoporotic extremities
• neurovascular compromise from pressure on major blood vessels and nerves caused by immobilization devices or compartmental edema
• infection of surgical wounds or skeletal pin tracts
• prolonged healing time from failure to observe sound principles of immobilization.

In addition, the patient's level of understanding and effectiveness of coping skills must be assessed.

Consistent care

Without exception, orthopedic complications can be prevented or minimized by appropriate and consistent assessment, monitoring, and therapy. For example, it's essential to assess the orthopedic patient's neurovascular status at regular intervals; otherwise, the signs and symptoms of neurovascular compromise may go undetected until irreversible damage occurs. Consistent orthopedic care remains the surest way to promote rapid healing and successful rehabilitation.

Ready for an emergency

Orthopedic nursing care is characterized by the high incidence of emergency procedures that you're likely to perform. The first step—always—in administering emergency care at the scene of an accident is immediate assessment for a life-threatening condition. Do not move the patient unless danger is imminent, because this might worsen the injury and increase pain. If the patient must be moved, assess him for possible spinal injury so that appropriate transfer techniques can be used. After determining that no life-threatening injury exists, conduct an initial head-to-toe assessment, comparing bilaterally where applicable.

Always evaluate neurovascular status. (Check the five P's: pain, pallor, pulse, paresthesia, and paralysis.) Assess the injury thoroughly, and use strict aseptic technique when caring for all open wounds to prevent infection. If you suspect bone injury, apply a splint to reduce injury and immobilize the bone.

In nonemergencies, performing orthopedic procedures correctly can ease pain, prevent further injury, and encourage proper healing.

SUPPORT PROCEDURES
Triangular sling

Made from a triangular piece of muslin, canvas, or cotton, a sling supports and immobilizes an injured arm, wrist, or hand, and thereby facilitates healing. It may be applied to restrict movement of a fracture or dislocation or to support a muscle sprain. A sling can also support the weight of a splint or help secure dressings.

Equipment

Triangular bandage or commercial sling ▪ gauze (for padding) ▪ safety pins (tape for children under age 7).

Implementation

• Explain the procedure to the patient and wash your hands.
• If the patient is a child, fold the bandage in half *to make a smaller triangle.* Then follow the steps shown in *Making a sling,* page 602.
• If you anticipate prolonged use of a sling, pad the area under the knot with gauze *to prevent skin irritation.* Place

Making a sling

Place the apex of a triangular bandage behind the patient's elbow on the injured side. Hold one end of the bandage so it extends up toward the patient's neck on the uninjured side and let the other end hang straight down. The bandage's long side should parallel the midline of the patient's body (upper left).

Loop the top corner of the bandage over the shoulder on the uninjured side and around the back of the patient's neck. Then bring the lower end of the bandage over the flexed forearm and up to the shoulder on the injured side (upper right).

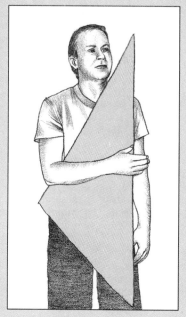 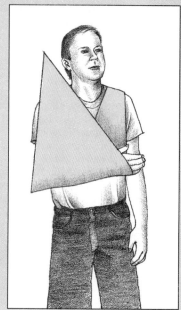

Adjust the bandage so that the forearm and upper arm form an angle of slightly less than 90 degrees *to increase venous return from the hand and forearm* and *to facilitate drainage from swelling.* Then tie the two bandage ends at the side of the patient's neck, rather than at the back, *to prevent neck flexion and avoid irritation and pressure over a cervical vertebra* (lower left).

Carefully secure the sling with a safety pin above and behind the elbow. See the illustration (lower right). (For a child under age 7, use tape instead of a pin *to avoid the chance of an injury.*)

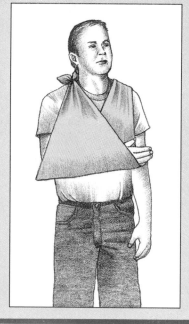 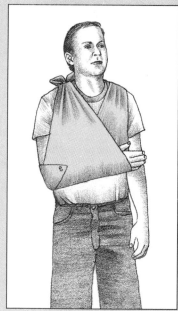

the sling outside the shirt collar *to reduce direct pressure on the neck and shoulder.*

If the arm requires complete immobilization, apply a swathe after placing the arm in a sling. (See *Applying a swathe.*) At regular intervals, check to be sure that the sling stays in proper position. Also assess patient comfort and circulation to the fingers.

Special considerations
Before the patient leaves the hospital, provide an extra triangular bandage. Teach him and a family member or friend how to change the sling. If appropriate, instruct him to change the sling regularly *because a soiled sling can cause irritation and infection.* Also, teach him how to check periodically for axillary skin breakdown.

Documentation
In the patient's chart, record the date, time, and location of sling application, and describe the patient's tolerance of the procedure. Also document circulation to the fingers, noting color and temperature.

 ## Clavicle strap

Also called a figure-eight strap, a clavicle strap reduces and immobilizes fractures of the clavicle. It does this by elevating, extending, and supporting the shoulders in position for healing, known as the *position of attention.* A commercially available figure-eight strap or a 4" elastic bandage may serve as a clavicle strap. This strap is contraindicated for an uncooperative patient.

Equipment
Powder or cornstarch ■ figure-eight clavicle strap or 4" elastic bandage ■ safety pins, if necessary ■ tape ■ cotton batting or padding ■ marking pen ■ analgesics, as ordered.

Implementation
• Explain the procedure to the patient and provide privacy.
• Help the patient take off his shirt.
• Assess neurovascular integrity by palpating skin temperature; noting the color of the hand and fingers; palpating the radial, ulnar, and brachial pulses bilaterally; and then comparing the affected with the unaffected side. Also, ask the patient about any numbness or tingling distal to the injury, and assess his motor function. Determine the patient's degree of comfort and administer analgesics, as ordered.

Applying a swathe

To further immobilize an arm after applying a sling, wrap a folded triangular bandage or wide elastic bandage around the patient's upper torso and the upper arm on the injured side. Don't cover the patient's uninjured arm. Make the swathe just tight enough to secure the injured arm to the body. Tie or pin the ends of the bandage just in front of the axilla on the uninjured side.

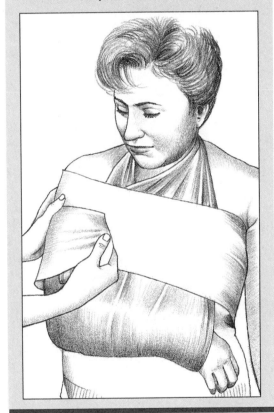

• Demonstrate how to assume the position of attention. Instruct the patient to sit upright and assume the position of attention gradually *to minimize pain.*
• Gently apply powder or cornstarch, as appropriate, to the axillae and shoulder area *to reduce friction from the clavicle strap.* You can use cornstarch if the patient is allergic to powder.

Types of clavicle straps

Clavicle straps provide support to the shoulder to help heal a fractured clavicle. These straps are available ready-made. They can also be made from a bandage.

Commercially made clavicle straps have a short back panel and long straps that extend around the patient's shoulders and axillae. They have Velcro pads or buckles on the ends for easy fastening.

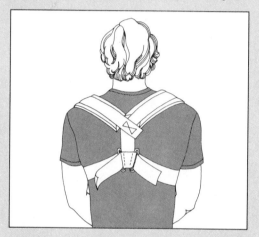

When making a clavicle strap with a wide elastic bandage, start in the middle of the patient's back. After wrapping the bandage around the shoulders, fasten the ends with safety pins.

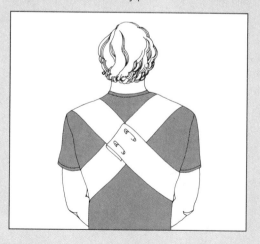

To apply a figure-eight strap
• Place the apex of the triangle between the scapulae and drape the straps over the shoulders. Bring the strap with the Velcro or buckle end under one axilla and through the loop; then pull the other strap under the other axilla and through the loop. (See *Types of clavicle straps*.)
• Gently adjust the straps so they support the shoulders in the position of attention.
• Bring the straps back under the axillae toward the anterior chest, making sure they maintain the position of attention.

To apply a 4″ elastic bandage
• Roll both ends of the elastic bandage toward the middle, leaving between 12″ and 18″ (30.5 to 45.7 cm) unrolled.
• Place the unrolled portion diagonally across the patient's back, from right shoulder to left axilla.
• Bring the lower end of the bandage under the left axilla and back over the left shoulder; loop the upper end over the right shoulder and under the axilla.
• Pull the two ends together at the center of the back *so the bandage supports the position of attention.*

To complete a figure-eight strap or elastic bandage
• Secure the ends using safety pins, Velcro pads, or a buckle, depending on the equipment. Make sure a buckle or any sharp edges face away from the skin. Tape the secured ends to the underlying strap or bandage.
• Place cotton batting or padding under the straps, as well as under the buckle or pins, *to avoid skin irritation.*
• Use a pen to mark the strap at the site of the loop of the figure-eight strap, or the site where the elastic bandage crosses on the patient's back. *If the strap loosens, this mark helps you tighten it to the original position.*
• Assess neurovascular integrity, *which may be impaired by a strap that's too tight.* If neurovascular integrity is compromised when the strap is correctly applied, notify the doctor. *He may want to change the treatment.*

Special considerations
If possible, perform the procedure with the patient standing. However, this may not be feasible, because the pain from the fracture can cause syncope.

An adult with a clavicle strap made from an elastic bandage may require a triangular sling *to help support the weight of the arm, enhance immobilization, and reduce pain.* (See "Triangular sling.") For a small child or a confused adult, a well-molded plaster jacket is needed to ensure immobilization. *Inadequate immobilization can cause improper healing.*

Instruct the patient not to remove the clavicle strap. Explain that, with help, he can maintain proper hygiene by lifting segments of the strap to remove the cotton and by washing and powdering the skin daily. Explain that fresh cotton should be applied after cleaning.

For a hospitalized patient, monitor the position of the strap by checking the pen markings every 8 hours. Also assess neurovascular integrity. Teach the outpatient how to assess his own neurovascular integrity and to recognize symptoms to report promptly to the doctor.

Documentation
In the appropriate section of the emergency department sheet or in your notes, record the date and time of strap application, type of clavicle strap, use of powder and padding, bilateral neurovascular integrity before and after the procedure, and instructions to the patient.

Cervical collar

A cervical collar may be used for an acute injury (such as strained cervical muscles) or a chronic condition (such as arthritis or cervical metastasis). Or it may augment such splinting devices as a spine board to prevent potential cervical spine fracture or spinal cord damage.

Designed to hold the neck straight with the chin slightly elevated and tucked in, the collar immobilizes the cervical spine, decreases muscle spasms, and relieves some pain; it also prevents further injury and promotes healing. As symptoms of an acute injury subside, the patient may gradually discontinue wearing the collar, alternating periods of wear with increasing periods of removal, until he no longer needs the collar.

Equipment
Cervical collar, in the appropriate size. (See *Types of cervical collars.*)

Implementation
• Check the patient's neurovascular status before application.
• Instruct the patient to position his head slowly to face directly forward.
• Place the cervical collar in front of the patient's neck *to ensure that the size is correct.*
• Fit the collar snugly around the neck and attach the Velcro fasteners or buckles at the back of the neck.
• Check the patient's airway and his neurovascular status *to ensure that the collar isn't too tight.*

Types of cervical collars

Cervical collars are used to support an injured or weakened cervical spine and to maintain alignment during healing.

Made of rigid plastic, the molded cervical collar holds the patient's neck firmly, keeping it straight, with the chin slightly elevated and tucked in.

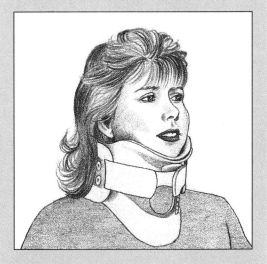

The soft cervical collar, made of spongy foam, provides gentler support and reminds the patient to avoid cervical spine motion.

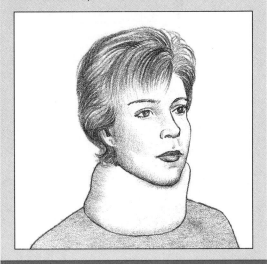

Special considerations

For a sprain or a potential cervical spine fracture, make sure the collar isn't too high in front *because this may hyperextend the neck.* In a neck sprain, such hyperextension may cause ligaments to heal in a shortened position. In a potential cervical spine fracture, hyperextension may cause serious neurologic damage.

Home care

Teach the patient how to apply the collar and how to do a neurovascular check. Name symptoms to report to the doctor. If indicated, advise sleeping without a pillow.

Documentation

Note the type and size of the cervical collar and the time and date of application in your notes. Record the results of neurovascular checks. Document patient comfort, the collar's snugness, and all patient instruction.

Splints

By immobilizing the site of an injury, a splint alleviates pain and allows the injury to heal in proper alignment. It also minimizes possible complications, such as excessive bleeding into tissues, restricted blood flow caused by bone pressing against vessels, and possible paralysis from an unstable spinal cord injury. In cases of multiple serious injuries, a splint or spine board allows caretakers to move the patient without risking further damage to bones, muscles, nerves, blood vessels, and skin.

A splint can be applied to immobilize a simple or compound fracture, a dislocation, or a subluxation. (See *Types of splints.*) During an emergency, any injury even suspected of being a fracture, dislocation, or subluxation should be splinted. No contraindications exist for rigid splints; traction splints are contraindicated for upper extremity injuries and open fractures.

Equipment

Rigid splint, Velcro support splint, spine board, or traction splint ■ bindings ■ padding ■ sandbags or rolled towels or clothing ■ optional: roller gauze, cloth strips, sterile or clean compress, ice bag.

Several commercial splints are available. In an emergency, any long, sturdy object, such as a tree limb, mop handle, or broom—even a magazine or newspaper—can be used to make a rigid splint for an extremity; a door can be used as a spine board.

Velcro straps, 2″ roller gauze, or 2″ cloth strips can be used as bindings. When improvising, avoid using twine or rope, if possible, *because they can restrict circulation.*

An inflatable semirigid splint, called an air splint, sometimes can be used to secure an injured extremity. (See *Using an air splint,* page 608.)

Implementation

● Obtain a complete history of the injury, if possible, and begin a thorough head-to-toe assessment, inspecting for obvious deformities, swelling or bleeding.
● Ask the patient if he can move the injured area (typically an extremity). Compare it bilaterally with the uninjured extremity, where applicable. Gently palpate the injured area; inspect for swelling, obvious deformities, bleeding, discoloration, and evidence of fracture or dislocation.
● Remove or cut away clothing from the injury site, if necessary. Check neurovascular integrity distal to the site. Explain the procedure to the patient to allay his fears.
● If an obvious bone misalignment causes the patient acute distress or severe neurovascular problems, align the extremity in its normal anatomic position, if possible. Stop doing this, however, if the action causes further neurovascular deterioration. Don't attempt to straighten a dislocation *because movement may damage displaced vessels and nerves.* Also, don't attempt reduction of a contaminated bone end *because this may cause additional laceration of soft tissues, vessels, and nerves, and also may cause gross contamination of deep tissues.*
● Choose a splint that will immobilize the joints above and below the fracture; pad the splint as necessary *to prevent excessive pressure over bony prominences.*

To apply a rigid splint

● Support the injured extremity and apply firm, gentle traction.
● Have an assistant place the splint under, beside, or on top of the extremity, as ordered.
● Tell the assistant to apply the bindings *to secure the splint.* Make sure they don't obstruct circulation.

To apply a spine board

● Pad the spine board (or door) carefully, especially the areas that will support the lumbar region and knees, *to prevent uneven pressure and discomfort.*
● If the patient is lying on his back, place one hand on each side of his head and apply gentle traction to the head and neck, keeping the head aligned with the body. Have one assistant logroll the patient onto his side while another slides the spine board under the patient. Then instruct the assistants to roll the patient onto the board while you maintain traction and alignment.

Types of splints

Three kinds of splints are commonly used to help provide support for injured or weakened limbs, or to help correct deformities.

A *rigid splint* can be used to immobilize a fracture or dislocation in an extremity, as shown. Ideally, two people should apply a rigid splint to an extremity.

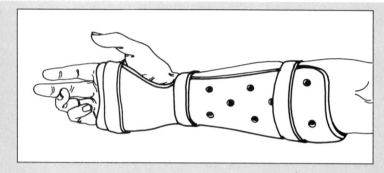

A *traction splint* immobilizes a fracture and exerts a longitudinal pull that reduces muscle spasms, pain, and arterial and neural damage. Used primarily for femoral fractures, a traction splint may also be applied for a fractured hip or tibia. Two trained people should apply a traction splint.

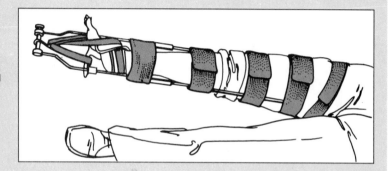

A *spine board,* applied for a suspected spinal fracture, is a rigid splint that supports the injured person's entire body. Three people should apply a spine board.

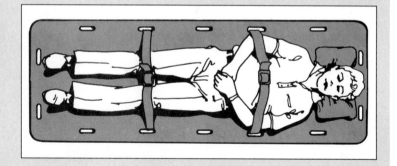

• If the patient is prone, logroll him onto the board so he ends up in a supine position.
• *To maintain body alignment,* use strips of cloth to secure the patient on the spine board; *to keep head and neck aligned,* place sandbags or rolled towels or clothing on both sides of his head.

To apply a traction splint
• Place the splint beside the injured leg. (Never use a traction splint on an arm *because the major axillary plexus of nerves and blood vessels can't tolerate countertraction.*) Adjust the splint to the correct length, and then open and adjust the Velcro straps.

Using an air splint

In an emergency, an air splint can be applied to immobilize a fracture or control bleeding, especially from a forearm or lower leg. This compact, comfortable splint is made of double-walled plastic and provides gentle, diffuse pressure over an injured area. The appropriate splint is wrapped around the affected extremity, secured with Velcro or other strips, then inflated. The fit should be snug enough to immobilize the extremity without impairing circulation.

An air splint may actually control bleeding better than a local pressure bandage. The device's clear plastic construction simplifies inspection of the affected site for bleeding, pallor, or cyanosis. An air splint also allows the patient to be moved without further damage to the injured limb.

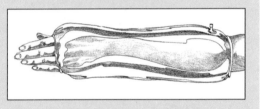

• Have an assistant keep the leg motionless while you pad the ankle and foot and fasten the ankle hitch around them. (You may leave the shoe on.)
• Tell the assistant to lift and support the leg at the injury site, as you apply firm, gentle traction.
• While you maintain traction, instruct the assistant to slide the splint under the leg, pad the groin *to avoid excessive pressure on external genitalia,* and gently apply the ischial strap.
• Have the assistant connect the loops of the ankle hitch to the end of the splint.
• Adjust the splint to apply enough traction *to secure the leg comfortably in the corrected position.*
• After applying traction, fasten the Velcro support splints *to secure the leg closely to the splint.*
• ◆ *Nursing alert.* Don't use a traction splint for a severely angulated femur or knee fracture. ◆

Special considerations
At the scene of an accident, always examine the patient completely for other injuries. Avoid unnecessary movement or manipulation *that may cause additional pain or injury.*

Always consider the possibility of cervical injury in an unconscious patient. If possible, apply the splint before repositioning the patient.

If the patient requires a rigid splint but one isn't available, use another body part as a splint. To splint a leg in this manner, pad its inner aspect and secure it to the other leg with roller gauze or cloth strips.

After applying any type of splint, monitor vital signs frequently *because bleeding in fractured bones and surrounding tissues may cause shock.* Also monitor the neurovascular status of the fractured limb by assessing skin color and checking for numbness in the fingers or toes. *Numbness or paralysis distal to the injury indicates pressure on nerves.* (See *Assessing neurovascular status.*)

Transport the patient as soon as possible to a medical facility. Apply ice to the injury. Regardless of the apparent extent of the patient's injury, don't allow him to eat or drink anything until the doctor evaluates him.

Indications for removal of a splint include evidence of improper application or vascular impairment. Apply gentle traction, and remove the splint carefully under a doctor's direct supervision.

Complications
Multiple transfers and repeated manipulation of a fracture may result in fat embolism, indicated by shortness of breath, agitation, and irrational behavior. This complication usually occurs within 24 to 72 hours of injury or manipulation.

Documentation
Record the circumstances and cause of the injury. Document the patient's complaints, noting whether symptoms are localized. Also record neurovascular status before and after applying the splint. Note the type of wound and the amount and type of drainage, if any. Document the time of splint application. If the bone end should slip into surrounding tissue or if transportation causes any change in the degree of dislocation, be sure to note it.

 Casts

A cast is a hard mold that encases a body part, usually an extremity, to provide immobilization without discomfort. It can be used to treat injuries (including fractures), correct orthopedic conditions (such as deformities), or promote healing after general or plastic surgery, amputation, or nerve and vascular repair. (See *Types of cylindrical casts,* page 610.)

Casts may be constructed of plaster, fiberglass, or synthetic materials. Plaster—a commonly used material—is inexpensive, nontoxic, nonflammable, easy to mold, and rarely causes allergic reactions or skin irritation. However, fiberglass is lighter, stronger, and more resilient than plaster. Because fiberglass dries rapidly, it is more difficult to mold, but it can bear body weight immediately, if necessary.

Typically, a doctor applies a cast and a nurse prepares the patient and the equipment and assists during the procedure. With special preparation, a nurse may apply or change a standard cast, but an orthopedist must reduce and set the fracture.

Contraindications for casting may include skin diseases, peripheral vascular disease, diabetes mellitus, open or draining wounds, and susceptibility to skin irritations. However, these aren't strict contraindications; the doctor must weigh the potential risks and benefits for each patient.

Equipment
Tubular stockinette ■ casting material ■ plaster rolls ■ plaster splints (if necessary) ■ bucket of water ■ sink equipped with plaster trap ■ linen-saver pad ■ sheet wadding ■ sponge or felt padding (if necessary) ■ cast scissors, cast saw, and cast spreader (if necessary) ■ pillows or bath blankets ■ optional: rubber gloves, cast stand, moleskin or adhesive tape.

Gather the tubular stockinette, cast material, and plaster splints in the appropriate sizes. Tubular stockinettes range from 2″ to 12″ (5 to 30.5 cm) wide; plaster rolls, from 2″ to 6″ (5 to 15.2 cm) wide; and plaster splints, from 3″ to 6″ (7.6 to 15.2 cm) wide. Wear rubber gloves, especially if applying a fiberglass cast.

Preparation of equipment
Gently squeeze the packaged casting material *to make sure the envelopes don't have any air leaks*. Humid air penetrating such leaks can cause plaster to become stale, which could make it set too quickly, form lumps, fail to bond with lower layers, or set as a soft, friable mass. (Baking a stale plaster roll at a medium temperature for 1 hour can make it usable again.)

Follow the manufacturer's directions for water temperature when preparing plaster. Usually, room temperature or slightly warmer water is best *because it allows the cast to set in about 7 minutes without excessive exothermia.* (Cold water retards the rate of setting and may be used to facilitate difficult molding; warm water speeds the rate of setting and raises skin temperature under the cast.) Place all equipment within the doctor's reach.

Assessing neurovascular status

When assessing an injured extremity, always include the following steps and compare your findings bilaterally:
• Inspect the color of fingers or toes.
• To detect edema, note the size of the digits.
• Simultaneously touch the digits of the affected and unaffected extremities and compare temperature.
• Check capillary refill by pressing on the distal tip of one digit until it's white. Then release the pressure and note how soon the normal color returns. It should return quickly in both the affected and the unaffected extremities.
• Check sensation by touching the fingers or toes and asking the patient how they feel. Note reports of any numbness or tingling.
• To check proprioception, tell the patient to close his eyes; then move one digit and ask him which position it's in.
• To test movement, tell the patient to wiggle his toes or move his fingers.
• Palpate the distal pulses to assess vascular patency.

Record your findings for the affected and the unaffected extremities, using standard terminology to avoid ambiguity. Warmth, free movement, rapid capillary refill, and normal color, sensation, and proprioception indicate sound neurovascular status.

Implementation
• *To allay the patient's fears,* explain the procedure. If plaster is being used, make sure he understands that heat will build under the cast because of a chemical reaction between the water and plaster. Also begin explaining some aspects of proper cast care *to prepare him for patient teaching and to assess his knowledge level.*
• Cover the appropriate parts of the patient's bedding and gown with a linen-saver pad.
• If the cast is applied to the wrist or arm, remove rings that may interfere with circulation in the fingers.
• Assess the condition of the skin in the affected area, noting any redness, contusions, or open wounds. *This will make it easier to evaluate any complaints the patient may have after the cast is applied.*
• If the patient has severe contusions or open wounds, prepare him for a local anesthetic if the doctor will administer one.

Types of cylindrical casts

Made of plaster, fiberglass, or synthetic material, casts may be applied almost anywhere on the body to support a single finger or the entire body. Common casts are shown here.

Hanging arm cast

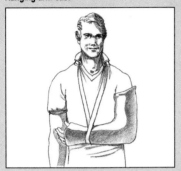

Shoulder spica

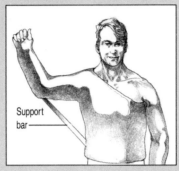

Support bar

Short arm cast

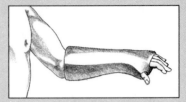

One-and-one-half hip spica

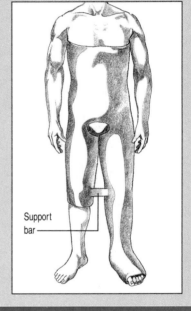

Support bar

Long leg cast

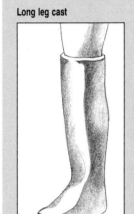

Short leg cast

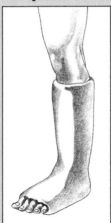

Single hip spica

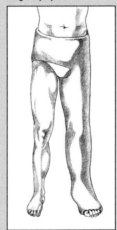

• *To establish baseline measurements,* assess neurovascular status. Palpate the distal pulses; assess the color, temperature, and capillary refill of the appropriate fingers or toes; and check neurologic function, including sensation and motion in the affected and unaffected extremities.
• Help the doctor position the limb, as ordered. (Commonly, the limb is immobilized in the neutral position.)
• Support the limb in the prescribed position while the doctor applies the tubular stockinette and sheet wadding. The stockinette, if used, should extend beyond the ends of the cast *to pad the edges.* (If the patient has an open wound or a severe contusion, the doctor may not use the stockinette.) He then wraps the limb in sheet wadding, starting at the distal end, and applies extra wadding to the distal and proximal ends of the cast area, as well as any points of prominence. As he applies the sheet wadding, check for wrinkles.
• If needed, assist the doctor to place an extra layer of sponge or felt padding over the area where the cast scissors will be used.
• Prepare the various cast materials as ordered.

To prepare plaster casting

• Place a roll of plaster casting on its end in the bucket of water. Make sure to immerse it completely. When air bubbles stop rising from the roll, remove it, gently squeeze out the excess water, and hand the casting material to the doctor, who will begin applying it to the extremity. As he applies the first roll, prepare a second roll in the same manner. (Stay at least one roll ahead of the doctor during the procedure.)

• After the doctor applies each roll, he'll smooth it to remove wrinkles, spread the plaster into the cloth webbing, and empty air pockets. If he's using plaster splints, he'll apply them in the middle layers of the cast. Before wrapping the last roll, he'll pull the ends of the tubular stockinette over the cast edges *to create padded ends, prevent cast crumbling, and reduce skin irritation.* He will then use the final roll to keep the ends of the stockinette in place.

To prepare cotton and polyester casting

• Open these casting materials one roll at a time *because cotton and polyester casting must be applied within 3 minutes—before humidity in the air hardens the tape.*

• Immerse the roll in cold water, and squeeze it four times *to ensure uniform wetness.*

• Remove the dripping wet material from the bucket. Tell the patient that it will be applied immediately. Forewarn him that the material will feel warm, giving off heat as it sets.

To prepare fiberglass casting

• If you're using water-activated fiberglass, immerse the tape rolls in tepid water for 10 to 15 minutes *to initiate the chemical reaction that causes the cast to harden.* Open one roll at a time. Avoid squeezing out excess water before application.

• If you're using light-cured fiberglass, you can unroll the material more slowly. This casting remains soft and malleable until it's exposed to ultraviolet light, which sets it.

To complete casting

• As necessary, "petal" the cast's edges *to reduce roughness and to cushion pressure points.* (See *How to petal a cast.*)

• Use a cast stand or the palm of your hand to support the cast in the therapeutic position until it becomes firm to the touch (usually 6 to 8 minutes).

• *To check circulation in the casted limb,* palpate the distal pulse and assess the color, temperature, and capillary refill of the fingers or toes. Determine neurologic status by asking the patient if he's experiencing paresthesia in the extremity or decreased motion of the extremity's

How to petal a cast

Rough cast edges can be cushioned by petaling them with adhesive tape or moleskin. To do this, first cut several 4" × 2" (10.2 × 5 cm) strips. Round off one end of each strip to keep it from curling. Then, making sure the rounded end of the strip is on the outside of the cast, tuck the straight end just inside the cast edge.

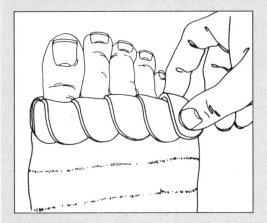

Smooth the moleskin with your finger until you're sure it's secured inside and out. Repeat the procedure, overlapping the moleskin pieces until you've gone all the way around the cast edge.

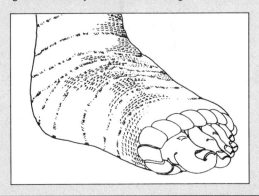

uncovered joints. Assess the unaffected extremity in the same manner and compare findings.

• Elevate the limb above heart level with pillows or bath blankets, as ordered, *to facilitate venous return and reduce*

edema. To prevent molding, make sure pressure is evenly distributed under the cast.
• The doctor will then send the patient for X-rays *to ensure proper positioning.*
• Instruct the patient to notify the doctor of any pain, foul odor, drainage, or burning sensation under the cast. (After the cast hardens, the doctor may cut a window in it to inspect the painful or burning area.)
• Pour water from the plaster bucket into a sink containing a plaster trap. Don't use a regular sink *because plaster will block the plumbing.*

Special considerations
A fiberglass cast dries immediately after application. A plaster extremity cast dries in approximately 24 to 48 hours; a plaster spica or body cast, in 48 to 72 hours. During this drying period, the cast must be properly positioned to prevent a surface depression that could cause pressure areas or dependent edema. Neurovascular status must be assessed, drainage monitored, and the condition of the cast checked periodically.

After the cast dries completely, it looks white and shiny and no longer feels damp or soft. Care consists of monitoring for changes in the drainage pattern, preventing skin breakdown near the cast, and averting the complications of immobility.

Patient teaching must begin immediately after the cast is applied and should continue until the patient or a family member can care for the cast.

Never use the bed or a table to support the cast as it sets *because molding can result, causing pressure necrosis of underlying tissue.* Also, don't use rubber- or plastic-covered pillows before the cast hardens *because they can trap heat under the cast.*

If a cast is applied after surgery or traumatic injury, remember that the most accurate way to assess for bleeding is to monitor vital signs. A visible blood spot on the cast can be misleading: One drop of blood can produce a circle 3″ (7.6 cm) in diameter.

The doctor usually removes the cast at the appropriate time, with a nurse assisting. (See *Removing a plaster cast.*) Tell the patient that when the cast is removed, his casted limb will appear thinner and flabbier than the uncasted limb. What's more, his skin will appear yellowish or gray from the accumulated dead skin and oils from the glands near the skin surface. Reassure the patient that with exercise and good skin care, his limb will return to normal.

Home care
Before the patient goes home, teach him how to care for his cast. Tell him to keep the casted limb elevated above heart level to minimize swelling. Raise a casted leg by having the patient lie supine with his leg on top of pillows. Prop a casted arm so that the hand and elbow are higher than the shoulder.

Instruct the patient to call the doctor if he can't move his fingers or toes, if he has numbness or tingling in the affected limb, or if he has symptoms of infection such as a fever, unusual pain, or a foul odor from the cast.

Instruct the patient to maintain muscle strength by continuing any recommended exercises.

If the cast needs repair (if it loosens and slips) or if the patient has any questions about cast care, advise him to notify his doctor.

Warn the patient not to get the cast wet. Moisture will weaken or destroy it.

Urge the patient not to insert anything (such as a back scratcher or powder) into the cast to relieve itching. Foreign matter can damage the skin and cause an infection. Tell him, though, that he can use alcohol on the skin at the cast edges.

Warn the patient not to chip, crush, cut, or otherwise break any area of the cast and not to bear weight on the cast unless instructed to do so by the doctor.

If the patient must use crutches, instruct him to remove throw rugs from the floor and to rearrange furniture to reduce the risk of tripping and falling.

If the patient has a cast on his dominant arm, he may need help with bathing, toileting, eating, and dressing.

Complications
Complications of improper cast application include compartment syndrome, palsy, paresthesia, ischemia, ischemic myositis, pressure necrosis and, eventually, misalignment or nonunion of fractured bones.

Documentation
Record the date and time of cast application and skin condition of the extremity before the cast was applied. Note any contusions, redness, or open wounds; results of neurovascular checks, before and after application, for the affected and unaffected extremities; location of any special devices, such as felt pads or plaster splints; and any patient teaching.

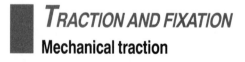

TRACTION AND FIXATION
Mechanical traction

Mechanical traction exerts a pulling force on a part of the body — usually the spine, pelvis, or long bones of the arms and legs. It can be used to reduce fractures, treat

Removing a plaster cast

Typically, a cast is removed when a fracture heals or requires further manipulation. Less common indications include cast damage, a pressure ulcer under the cast, excessive drainage or bleeding, and a constrictive cast.

Explain the procedure to the patient. Tell him he'll feel some heat and vibration as the cast is split with the cast saw. If the patient is a child, tell him the saw is very noisy but will not cut the skin beneath. Warn the patient that when the padding is cut, he'll see discolored skin and signs of poor muscle tone. Reassure him that you'll stay with him. The pictures show how a plaster cast is removed.

First, the doctor cuts one side of the cast, then the other. As he does so, closely monitor the patient's anxiety level.

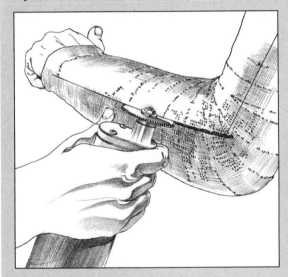

Next, the doctor opens the cast pieces with a spreader.

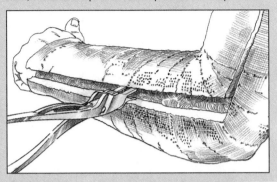

Finally, using cast scissors, the doctor cuts through the cast padding.

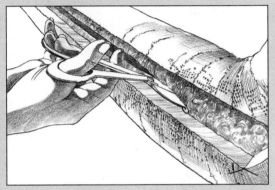

When the cast is removed, give skin care to remove accumulated dead skin and to begin restoring the extremity's normal appearance.

dislocations, correct or prevent deformities, improve or correct contractures, or decrease muscle spasms. Depending on the injury or condition, an orthopedist may order either skin or skeletal traction.

Applied directly to the skin and thus indirectly to the bone, skin traction is ordered when a light, temporary, or noncontinuous pulling force is required. Contraindications for skin traction include a severe injury with open wounds, an allergy to tape or other skin traction equipment, circulatory disturbances, dermatitis, and varicose veins.

In skeletal traction, an orthopedist inserts a pin or wire through the bone and attaches the traction equipment to the pin or wire to exert a direct, constant, longitudinal pulling force. Indications for skeletal traction include fractures of the tibia, femur, and humerus. Infections such as osteomyelitis contraindicate skeletal traction.

Nursing responsibilities for this procedure include setting up the traction frame. (See *Traction frames,* page 614.) The design of the patient's bed usually dictates whether to use a claw clamp or I.V.-post-type frame.

Traction frames

You may encounter three types of traction frames, as described below.

Claw-type basic frame
With this frame, claw attachments secure the uprights to the footboard and headboard.

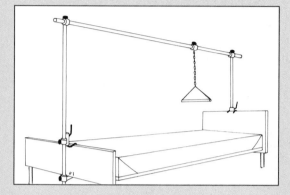

I.V.-type basic frame
With this frame, I.V. posts, placed in I.V. holders, support the horizontal bars across the foot and head of the bed. These horizontal bars then support the two uprights.

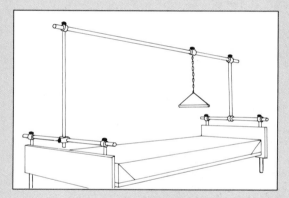

I.V.-type Balkan frame
This frame features I.V. posts and horizontal bars (secured in the same manner as those for the I.V.-type basic frame) that support four uprights.

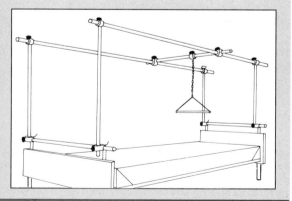

(However, the claw-type Balkan frame is rarely used.) Setup of the specific traction can be done by a nurse with special skills, an orthopedic technician, or by the doctor. Instructions for setting up these traction units usually accompany the equipment. (See *Comparing traction types*.) After the patient is placed in the specific type of traction ordered by the orthopedist, the nurse is responsible for preventing complications from immobility; for routinely inspecting the equipment; for adding traction weights, as ordered; and, in patients with skeletal traction, for monitoring the pin insertion sites for signs of infection.

Equipment
For a claw-type basic frame: 102″ (259-cm) plain bar ▪ two 66″ (168-cm) swivel-clamp bars ▪ two upper-panel clamps ▪ two lower-panel clamps.

   For an I.V.-type basic frame: 102″ plain bar ▪ 27″ (68.6-cm) double-clamp bar ▪ 48″ (122-cm) swivel-clamp bar ▪ two 36″ (91.4-cm) plain bars ▪ four 4″ (10-cm) I.V. posts with clamps ▪ cross clamp.

   For an I.V.-type Balkan frame: two 102″ plain bars ▪ two 48″ swivel-clamp bars ▪ five 36″ plain bars ▪ two 27″ double-clamp bars ▪ four 4″ I.V. posts with clamps ▪ eight cross clamps.

   For all frame types: trapeze with clamp ▪ wall bumper or roller.

   For skeletal traction care: sterile cotton-tipped applicators ▪ prescribed antiseptic solution ▪ sterile gauze pads ▪ povidone-iodine solution ▪ optional: antimicrobial ointment.

Preparation of equipment
Arrange with central supply or the appropriate department to have the traction equipment transported to the patient's room on a traction cart. If appropriate, gather the equipment for pin-site care at the patient's bedside. Pin-site care protocols may vary with each hospital or doctor.

Implementation
• Explain the purpose of traction to the patient. Emphasize the importance of maintaining proper body alignment after the traction equipment is set up.

To set up a claw-type basic frame
• Attach one lower-panel and one upper-panel clamp to each 66″ swivel-clamp bar.
• Fasten one bar to the footboard and one to the headboard by turning the clamp knobs clockwise until they are tight and then pulling back on the upper clamp's rubberized bar until it is tight.

Comparing traction types

Traction therapy restricts movement of a patient's affected limb or body part and may confine the patient to bed rest for an extended period. The limb is immobilized by pulling with equal force on each end of the injured area—an equal mix of traction and countertraction. Weights provide the pulling force. Countertraction is produced by using other weights or by positioning the patient's body weight against the traction pull.

Skin traction
This procedure immobilizes a body part intermittently over an extended period through direct application of a pulling force on the patient's skin. The force may be applied using adhesive or nonadhesive traction tape or other skin traction devices, such as a boot, belt, or halter.

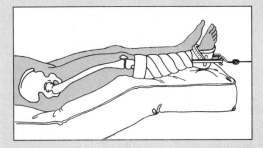

Adhesive attachment allows more continuous traction, whereas nonadhesive attachment allows easier removal for daily skin care.

Skeletal traction
This procedure immobilizes a body part for prolonged periods by attaching weighted equipment directly to the patient's bones. This may be accomplished with pins, screws, wires, or tongs.

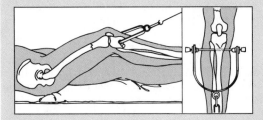

● Secure the 102″ horizontal plain bar atop the two vertical bars, making sure the clamp knobs point up.
● Using the appropriate clamp, attach the trapeze to the horizontal bar about 2′ (0.6 m) from the head of the bed.

To set up an I.V.-type basic frame

● Attach one 4″ I.V. post with clamp to each end of both 36″ horizontal plain bars.
● Secure an I.V. post in each I.V. holder at the bed corners. Using a cross clamp, fasten the 48″ vertical swivel-clamp bar to the middle of the horizontal plain bar at the foot of the bed.
● Fasten the 27″ vertical double-clamp bar to the middle of the horizontal plain bar at the head of the bed.
● Attach the 102″ horizontal plain bar to the tops of the two vertical bars, making sure the clamp knobs point up.
● Using the appropriate clamp, attach the trapeze to the horizontal bar about 2′ from the head of the bed.

To set up an I.V.-type Balkan frame

● Attach one 4″ I.V. post with clamp to each end of two 36″ horizontal plain bars.
● Secure an I.V. post in each I.V. holder at the bed corners.
● Attach a 48″ vertical swivel-clamp bar, using a cross clamp, to each I.V. post clamp on the horizontal plain bar at the foot of the bed.
● Fasten one 36″ horizontal plain bar across the midpoints of the two 48″ swivel-clamp bars, using two cross clamps.
● Attach a 27″ vertical double-clamp bar to each I.V. post clamp on the horizontal bar at the head of the bed.
● Using two cross clamps, fasten a 36″ horizontal plain bar across the midpoints of two 27″ double-clamp bars.
● Clamp a 102″ horizontal plain bar onto the vertical bars on each side of the bed, making sure the clamp knobs point up.
● Use two cross clamps to attach a 36″ horizontal plain bar across the two overhead bars, about 2′ from the head of the bed.
● Attach the trapeze to this 36″ horizontal bar.

After setting up any frame

● Attach a wall bumper or roller to the vertical bar or bars at the head of the bed. *This protects the walls from damage caused by the bed or equipment.*

Caring for the traction patient

● Show the patient how much movement he's allowed and instruct him not to readjust the equipment. Also tell him to report any pain or pressure from the traction equipment.

● At least once a shift, make sure that the traction equipment connections are tight and that no parts touch the bedding, the patient, or other inappropriate portions of the apparatus. Check for impingements, such as ropes rubbing on the footboard or getting caught between pulleys. *Friction and impingement reduce the effectiveness of traction.*
● Inspect the traction equipment *to ensure the correct alignment.*
● Inspect the ropes for fraying, *which can eventually cause a rope to break.*
● Make sure the ropes are positioned properly in the pulley track. *An improperly positioned rope changes the degree of traction.*
● *To prevent tampering and aid stability and security,* make sure that all rope ends are taped above the knot.
● Inspect the equipment regularly to make sure that the traction weights hang freely. *Weights that touch the floor, bed, or each other reduce the amount of traction.*
● About every 2 hours, check the patient for proper body alignment and reposition the patient as necessary. *Misalignment causes ineffective traction and may keep the fracture from healing properly.*
● *To prevent complications from immobility,* assess neurovascular integrity routinely. The patient's condition, the hospital routine, and the doctor's orders determine the frequency of neurovascular assessments.
● Provide skin care, encourage coughing and deep breathing exercises, and assist with ordered range-of-motion exercises for unaffected extremities. Typically, an order for elastic support stockings is written. Check elimination patterns and provide laxatives, as ordered.
● For the patient with skeletal traction, make sure that the protruding pin or wire ends are covered with cork *to prevent them from tearing the bedding or injuring the patient and staff.*
● Check the pin site and surrounding skin regularly for signs of infection.
● If ordered, clean the pin site and surrounding skin. Pin-site care varies, but you'll usually follow guidelines like these: Use sterile technique; avoid digging at pin sites with the cotton-tipped applicator; if ordered, clean the pin site and surrounding skin with a cotton-tipped applicator dipped in ordered antiseptic; if ordered, apply antimicrobial ointment to the pin sites; apply a loose sterile dressing, or dress with sterile gauze pads soaked in povidone-iodine solution. Perform pin-site care as often as necessary, depending on the amount of drainage.

Special considerations

When using skin traction, apply ordered weights slowly and carefully *to avoid jerking the affected extremity. To avoid injury in case the ropes break,* arrange the weights so they don't hang over the patient.

Complications

Immobility during traction may result in pressure ulcers, muscle atrophy, weakness, or contractures; and osteoporosis. Immobility can also cause GI disturbances, such as constipation; urinary problems, including stasis and calculi; respiratory problems, such as stasis of secretions and hypostatic pneumonia; and circulatory disturbances, including stasis and thrombophlebitis. Prolonged immobility, especially after traumatic injury, may promote depression or other emotional disturbances. Skeletal traction may cause osteomyelitis originating at the pin or wire sites.

Documentation

In the patient record, document the amount of traction weight used daily, noting the application of additional weights and the patient's tolerance. Document equipment inspections and patient care, including routine checks of neurovascular integrity, skin condition, respiratory status, and elimination patterns. If applicable, note the condition of the pin site and any care given.

 External fixation

In external fixation, a doctor inserts metal pins through skin and muscle layers into the broken bones and fixes them to an adjustable external frame that maintains their proper alignment. (See *Types of external fixation devices.*) This procedure is used most commonly to treat open, unstable fractures with extensive soft tissue damage, comminuted closed fractures, and septic, nonunion fractures and to facilitate surgical immobilization of a joint. Specialized types of external fixators may be used to lengthen leg bones or immobilize the cervical spine.

An advantage of external fixation over other immobilization techniques is that it stabilizes the fracture while allowing full visualization and access to open wounds. It also facilitates early ambulation, thus reducing the risk of complications from immobilization.

Equipment

Sterile cotton-tipped applicators ▪ prescribed antiseptic cleaning solution ▪ sterile gauze pads ▪ povidone-iodine solution ▪ optional: antimicrobial ointment.

Equipment varies with the type of fixator used, and the type and location of the fracture. Typically, sets of

 ## Types of external fixation devices

The illustrations below show how some common external fixation devices work. The doctor's selection of a device will depend on the severity of the patient's fracture and on the type of bone alignment needed.

Universal day frame

This device is used to manage tibial fractures. The frame allows the doctor to readjust the position of bony fragments by angulation and rotation. The compression-distraction device allows compression and distraction of bony fragments.

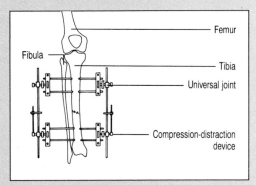

Portsmouth external fixation bar

This device is used to manage complicated tibial fractures. The locking nut adjustment on the mobile carriage only allows bone compression, so the doctor must accurately reduce bony fragments before applying the device.

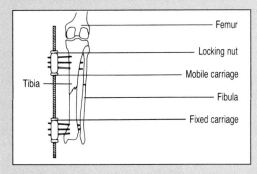

pins, stabilizing rods, and clips are available from manufacturers. Do not reuse pins.

Preparation of equipment
Make sure that the external fixation set includes all the equipment it's supposed to include. Also make sure that the equipment has been sterilized according to hospital procedure.

Implementation
• Explain the procedure to the patient *to reduce his anxiety.* Emphasize that he'll feel little pain once the fixation device is in place. Assure the patient that his feelings of anxiety are normal and that he will be able to adjust to the apparatus.

• Tell the patient that he will be able to move about with the apparatus in place, which may help him resume normal activities more quickly.

• After the fixation device is in place, perform neurovascular checks every 2 to 4 hours for 24 hours, then every 4 to 8 hours, as appropriate, *to assess for possible neurologic damage.* Assess color, motion, sensation, digital movement, edema, capillary refill, and pulses of the affected extremity. Compare with the unaffected side.

• Apply an ice bag to the surgical site, as ordered, *to reduce swelling, relieve pain, and lessen bleeding.*

• Administer analgesics or narcotics, as ordered, before exercising or mobilizing the affected extremity *to promote comfort.*

• Monitor the patient for pain not relieved by analgesics or narcotics, or for burning, tingling, or numbness, *which may indicate nerve damage or circulatory impairment.*

• Elevate the affected extremity, if appropriate, *to minimize edema.*

• Perform pin-site care, as ordered, *to prevent infection.* Pin-site care varies, but you'll usually follow guidelines like these: Use sterile technique; avoid digging at pin sites with the cotton-tipped applicator; if ordered, clean the pin site and surrounding skin with a cotton-tipped applicator dipped in ordered antiseptic solution; if ordered, apply antimicrobial ointment to pin sites; apply a loose sterile dressing, or dress with sterile gauze pads soaked in povidone-iodine solution. Perform pin-site care as often as necessary, depending on the amount of drainage.

• Also check for redness, tenting of the skin, prolonged or purulent drainage from the pin site, swelling, elevated body or pin-site temperature, and any bowing or bending of pins, which may stress the skin.

Special considerations
Before discharge, teach the patient and family members how to give pin-site care. Although this is a sterile procedure in the hospital, the patient can use clean technique at home. Teach the patient to recognize warning signs of pin-site infection. Tell him to keep the affected limb elevated when sitting or lying down.

Complications
Complications of external fixation include loosening of pins and loss of fracture stabilization, infection of the pin tract or wound, skin breakdown, nerve damage, and muscle impingement.

Documentation
Record the patient's reaction to the apparatus. Assess and document the condition of the pin sites and skin. Also document the patient's reaction to ambulation and understanding of teaching instructions.

Internal fixation

In this procedure, also known as surgical reduction or open reduction-internal fixation, the doctor implants fixation devices—using no external framework—to stabilize the fracture. Internal fixation devices include nails, screws, pins, wires, and rods, all of which may be used in combination with metal plates. These devices remain in the body indefinitely unless the patient experiences adverse reactions after the healing process is complete. (See *Reviewing internal fixation devices.*)

Typically, internal fixation is used to treat fractures of the face and jaw, spine, bones of the arms and legs, and fractures involving a joint (most commonly, the hip). Internal fixation permits earlier mobilization and can shorten hospitalization, particularly in elderly patients with hip fractures.

Equipment
Ice bag ▪ pain medication (analgesic or narcotic) ▪ incentive spirometer or intermittent positive-pressure breathing (IPPB) device ▪ elastic stockings.

Patients with leg fractures may also need the following: overhead frame with trapeze ▪ pressure-relief mattress ▪ crutches or walker ▪ pillow (hip fractures may require abductor pillows).

Preparation of equipment
Equipment is collected and prepared in the operating room.

Reviewing internal fixation devices

Choice of a specific internal fixation device depends on the location, type, and configuration of the fracture. In trochanteric or subtrochanteric fractures, for instance, the surgeon may use a hip pin or nail, with or without a screw plate. A pin or plate with extra nails stabilizes the fracture by impacting the bone ends at the fracture site.

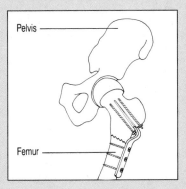

In an uncomplicated fracture of the femoral shaft, the surgeon may use an intramedullary rod, as shown at the top of the next column. This device permits early ambulation with partial weight bearing.

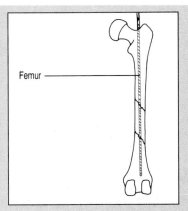

Another choice for fixation of a long-bone fracture is a screw plate, shown here on the tibia.

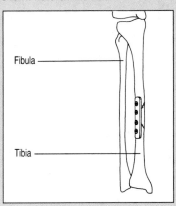

In an arm fracture, the surgeon may fix the involved bones with a plate, rod, or nail. Most radial and ulnar fractures may be fixed with plates, whereas humeral fractures are commonly fixed with rods.

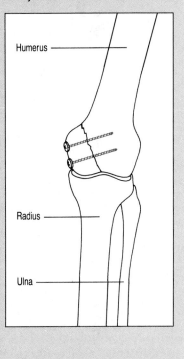

Implementation
• Explain the procedure to the patient *to allay his fears.* Tell him what to expect during postoperative assessment and monitoring; teach him how to use an IPPB device or incentive spirometer; and prepare him for proposed exercise and progressive ambulation regimens, if necessary. Instruct him to tell the doctor if he feels pain.
• After the procedure, monitor the patient's vital signs every 2 to 4 hours for 24 hours, then every 4 to 8 hours, according to hospital protocols. *Changes in vital signs may indicate hemorrhage or infection.*

• Monitor fluid intake and output every 4 to 8 hours.
• Perform neurovascular checks every 2 to 4 hours for 24 hours, then every 4 to 8 hours as appropriate. Assess color, motion, sensation, digital movement, edema, capillary refill, and pulses of the affected area. Compare findings with the unaffected side.
• Apply an ice bag to the operative site, as ordered, *to reduce swelling, relieve pain, and lessen bleeding.*
• Administer analgesics or narcotics, as ordered, before exercising or mobilizing the affected area *to promote comfort.*

• Monitor the patient for pain unrelieved by analgesics or narcotics, or for burning, tingling, or numbness, *which may indicate infection or impaired circulation.*
• Elevate the affected limb on a pillow, if appropriate, *to minimize edema.*
• Check surgical dressings for excessive drainage or bleeding. Also check the incision site for signs of infection, such as erythema, drainage, edema, and unusual pain.
• Assist and encourage the patient to perform range-of-motion and other muscle strengthening exercises, as ordered, *to promote circulation, improve muscle tone, and maintain joint function.*
• Teach the patient to perform progressive ambulation and mobilization using an overhead frame with trapeze, or crutches or a walker, as appropriate.

Special considerations
To avoid the complications of immobility after surgery, have the patient use an incentive spirometer or IPPB device. Apply elastic stockings, as appropriate. The patient may also require a pressure-relief mattress.

Home care
Before discharge, instruct the patient and family members about caring for the incisional site, recognizing signs and symptoms of wound infection, administering pain medication, practicing an exercise regimen (if any), and using assistive ambulation devices (such as crutches or a walker), if appropriate.

Complications
Wound infection and, more critically, infection involving metal fixation devices may require reopening the incision, draining the suture line and, possibly, removing the fixation device. Any such infection would require wound dressings and antibiotic therapy. Other complications may include malunion, nonunion, fat or pulmonary embolism, and neurovascular impairment.

Documentation
In the patient record, document perioperative findings on cardiovascular, respiratory, and neurovascular status. Name pain management techniques used. Describe wound appearance and alignment of the affected bone. Document the patient's response to teaching about appropriate exercise, care of the infection site, use of assistive devices (if appropriate), and symptoms that should be reported to the doctor.

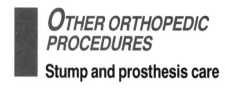

OTHER ORTHOPEDIC PROCEDURES
Stump and prosthesis care

Patient care immediately after limb amputation includes monitoring drainage from the stump, positioning the affected limb, assisting with exercises prescribed by a physical therapist, and wrapping and conditioning the stump. Postoperative care of the stump will vary slightly, depending on the amputation site (arm or leg) and the type of dressing applied to the stump (elastic bandage or plaster cast).

After the stump heals, it requires only routine daily care, such as proper hygiene and continued muscle-strengthening exercises. The prosthesis — once the patient begins to use it — also requires daily care. Typically, a plastic prosthesis, the most common type, must be cleaned and lubricated and checked for proper fit. As the patient recovers from the physical and psychological trauma of amputation, he will need to learn correct procedures for routine daily care of the stump and the prosthesis.

Equipment
For postoperative stump care: pressure dressing ■ tourniquet ■ ABD pad ■ suction equipment, if ordered ■ overhead trapeze ■ 1″ adhesive tape, bandage clips or safety pins ■ sandbags or trochanter roll (for a leg) ■ elastic stump shrinker or 4″ elastic bandage ■ optional: tourniquet (as last resort to control bleeding).

For stump and prosthesis care: mild soap or alcohol sponges ■ stump socks or athletic tube socks ■ two washcloths ■ two towels ■ appropriate lubricating oil.

Implementation
• Perform routine postoperative care — frequently assessing respiratory status and level of consciousness, monitoring vital signs and I.V. infusions, checking tube patency, and providing for the patient's comfort and safety.

Monitor stump drainage
• *Because gravity causes fluid to accumulate at the stump,* frequently check the amount of blood and drainage on the dressing. Notify the doctor if accumulations of drainage or blood increase rapidly. If excessive bleeding occurs, notify the doctor immediately and apply a pressure dressing or compress the appropriate pressure points. If this doesn't control bleeding, use a tourniquet only as a last resort. Keep a tourniquet available, if needed.

• Tape the ABD pad over the moist part of the dressing, as necessary. *This provides a dry area to help prevent bacterial infection.*
• Monitor the suction drainage equipment and note the amount and type of drainage.

Position the extremity
• *To prevent contractures,* position an arm with the elbow extended and the shoulder abducted.
• *To correctly position a leg,* elevate the foot of the bed slightly and place sandbags or a trochanter roll against the hip *to prevent external rotation.*
♦ *Nursing alert.* Don't place a pillow under the thigh to flex the hip *because this can cause hip flexion contracture.* For the same reason, tell the patient to avoid prolonged sitting. ♦
• After a below-the-knee amputation, maintain knee extension *to prevent hamstring muscle contractures.*
• After any leg amputation, place the patient on a firm surface in the prone position for at least 4 hours a day, with his legs close together and without pillows under his stomach, hips, knees, or stump, unless this position is contraindicated. *This position helps prevent hip flexion, contractures, and abduction; it also stretches the flexor muscles.*

Assist with prescribed exercises
• After arm amputation, encourage the patient to exercise the remaining arm *to prevent muscle contractures.* Help the patient perform isometric and range-of-motion (ROM) exercises for both shoulders, as prescribed by the physical therapist, *because use of the prosthesis requires both shoulders.*
• After leg amputation, stand behind the patient and, if necessary, support him with your hands at his waist during balancing exercises.
• Instruct the patient to exercise the affected and unaffected limbs *to maintain muscle tone and increase muscle strength.* The patient with a leg amputation may perform push-ups, as ordered (in the sitting position, arms at his sides), or pull-ups on the overhead trapeze *to strengthen his arms, shoulders, and back in preparation for using crutches.*

Wrap and condition the stump
• If the patient doesn't have a rigid cast, apply an elastic stump shrinker *to prevent edema and shape the limb in preparation for the prosthesis.* Wrap the stump so that it narrows toward the distal end. *This helps to ensure comfort when the patient wears the prosthesis.*
• Instead of using an elastic stump shrinker, you can wrap the stump in a 4″ elastic bandage. To do this, stretch the bandage to about two-thirds its maximum length as you wrap it diagonally around the stump, with the greatest pressure distally. (Depending on the size of the leg, you may need to use two 4″ bandages.) Secure the bandage with clips, safety pins, or adhesive tape. Make sure the bandage covers all portions of the stump smoothly *because wrinkles or exposed areas encourage skin breakdown.* (See *Wrapping a stump,* page 622.)
• If the patient experiences throbbing after the stump is wrapped, remove the bandage immediately and reapply it less tightly. *Throbbing indicates impaired circulation.*
• Check the bandage regularly. Rewrap it when it begins to bunch up at the end (usually about every 12 hours for a moderately active patient) or every 24 hours.
• After removing the bandage to rewrap it, massage the stump gently, always pushing toward the suture line rather than away from it. *This stimulates circulation and prevents scar tissue from adhering to the bone.*
• When healing begins, instruct the patient to push the stump against a pillow. Then have him progress gradually to pushing against harder surfaces, such as a padded chair, then a hard chair. *These conditioning exercises will help the patient adjust to experiencing pressure and sensation in the stump.*

Care for the healed stump
• Bathe the stump, but never shave it *because a rash or irritation may result.* If possible, bathe the stump at the end of the day *because the warm water may cause swelling, making reapplication of the prosthesis difficult.*
• Rub the stump with alcohol daily *to toughen the skin, reducing the risk of skin breakdown.* (Avoid using powders or lotions *because they can soften or irritate the skin.) Because alcohol may cause severe irritation in some patients,* instruct the patient to watch for and report this sign.
• Inspect the stump for redness, swelling, irritation, and calluses. Report any of these to the doctor. Tell the patient to avoid putting weight on the stump. (The skin should be firm but not taut over the bony end of the limb.)
• Continue muscle-strengthening exercises *so the patient can build the strength he'll need to control the prosthesis.*
• Change the patient's stump socks as necessary *to avoid exposing the skin to excessive perspiration, which can be irritating.* Wash the socks in warm water and gentle nondetergent soap; lay them flat on a towel to dry. *Machine washing or drying may shrink the socks.*

Care for the plastic prosthesis
• Wipe the plastic socket of the prosthesis with a damp cloth and mild soap or alcohol *to prevent bacterial accumulation.*
• Wipe the insert (if the prosthesis has one) with a dry cloth.

Wrapping a stump

Proper stump care helps protect the limb, reduces swelling, and prepares the limb for a prosthesis. As you perform the procedure, teach it to the patient. Start by obtaining two 4″ elastic bandages. Center the end of the first 4″ bandage at the top of the patient's thigh. Unroll the bandage downward over the stump and to the back of the leg, as shown here.

Make three figure-eight turns to adequately cover the ends of the stump. As you wrap, be sure to include the roll of flesh in the groin area. Use enough pressure to ensure that the stump narrows toward the end so that it fits comfortably into the prosthesis.

Use the second 4″ bandage to anchor the first bandage around the waist. For a below-the-knee amputation, use the knee to anchor the bandage in place. Secure the bandage with clips, safety pins, or adhesive tape. Check the stump bandage regularly, and rewrap it if it bunches at the end.

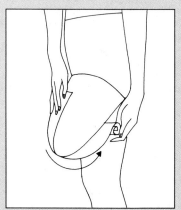
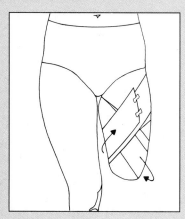
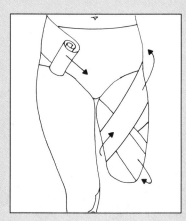

- Dry the prosthesis thoroughly; if possible, allow it to dry overnight.
- Maintain and lubricate the prosthesis, as instructed by the manufacturer.
- Check for malfunctions and adjust or repair the prosthesis as necessary *to prevent further damage.*
- Check the condition of the shoe on a foot prosthesis frequently and change it as necessary.

Apply the prosthesis
- Apply a stump sock. Keep the seams away from bony prominences.
- If the prosthesis has an insert, remove it from the socket, place it over the stump, and insert the stump into the prosthesis.
- If it has no insert, merely slide the prosthesis over the stump. Secure the prosthesis onto the stump according to the manufacturer's directions.

Special considerations
If a patient arrives at the hospital with a traumatic amputation, the amputated part may be saved for possible reimplantation. (See *Caring for an amputated body part.*)

Teach the patient how to care for his stump and prosthesis properly. Make sure he knows the signs and symptoms that indicate problems in the stump. Explain that a 10-lb (4.5-kg) change in body weight will alter his stump size and require a new prosthesis socket *to ensure a correct fit.*

Exercise of the remaining muscles in an amputated limb must begin the day after surgery. A physical therapist will direct these exercises. For example, arm exercises progress from isometrics to assisted ROM to active ROM. Leg exercises include rising from a chair, balancing on one leg, and ROM exercises of the knees and hips.

For a below-the-knee amputation, you may substitute an athletic tube sock for a stump sock by cutting off the elastic band. If the patient has a rigid plaster of paris dressing, perform normal cast care. Check the cast frequently to make sure it doesn't slip off. If it does, apply

Caring for an amputated body part

After traumatic amputation, a surgeon may be able to reimplant the severed body part through microsurgery. The chance of successful reimplantation is much greater if the amputated part has received proper care.

If a patient arrives at the hospital with a severed body part, first make sure that bleeding at the amputation site has been controlled. Then follow these guidelines for preserving the body part.
• Put on sterile gloves. Place several sterile gauze pads and an appropriate amount of sterile roller gauze in a sterile basin, and pour sterile normal saline or sterile lactated Ringer's solution over them. *Never* use any other solution, and don't try to scrub or debride the part.
• Holding the body part in one gloved hand, carefully pat it dry with sterile gauze. Place saline-soaked gauze pads over the stump; then wrap the whole body part with saline-soaked roller gauze. Wrap the gauze with a sterile towel, if available. Then put this package in a watertight container or bag and seal it.
• Fill another plastic bag with ice and place the part, still in its watertight container, inside. Seal the outer bag. (Always protect the part from direct contact with ice—and *never* use dry ice—*to prevent irreversible tissue damage, which would make the part unsuitable for reimplantation.*) Keep this bag ice-cold until the doctor's ready to do the reimplantation surgery.

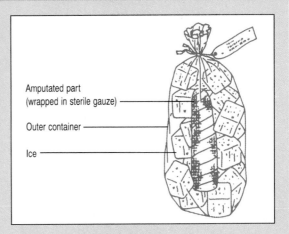

Amputated part (wrapped in sterile gauze)

Outer container

Ice

• Label the bag with the patient's name, identification number, identification of the amputated part, the hospital identification number, and the date and time when cooling began.

Note: The body part must be wrapped and cooled quickly. Irreversible tissue damage occurs after only 6 hours at ambient temperature. However, hypothermic management seldom preserves tissues for more than 24 hours.

---

an elastic bandage immediately and notify the doctor *because edema will develop rapidly.*

Home care
Emphasize to the patient that proper care of his stump can speed healing. Tell the patient to inspect his stump carefully every day, using a mirror. Instruct him to call the doctor if the incision appears to be opening, looks red or swollen, feels warm, is painful to touch, or is seeping drainage. Instruct him to continue proper daily stump care.

Tell the patient to massage the stump *toward the suture line* to mobilize the scar and prevent its adherence to bone. Advise him to avoid exposing the skin around the stump to excessive perspiration, which can be irritating. Tell him to change his elastic bandages or stump socks during the day to avoid this.

Tell the patient that he may experience twitching, spasms, or phantom limb pain as his stump muscles adjust to amputation. Advise him that he can decrease these symptoms with heat, massage, or gentle pressure.

If his stump is sensitive to touch, tell him to rub it with a dry washcloth for 4 minutes three times a day.

Stress the importance of performing prescribed exercises to help minimize complications, maintain muscle strength and tone, prevent contractures, and promote independence. Also stress the importance of positioning to prevent contractures and edema.

Complications
The most common postoperative complications include hemorrhage, stump infection, contractures, and a swollen or flabby stump. Complications that may develop at any time after an amputation include skin breakdown or irritation from lack of ventilation; friction from an irritant in the prosthesis; a sebaceous cyst or boil from tight socks; psychological problems, such as denial, depression, or withdrawal; and phantom limb pain caused by stimulation of nerves that once carried sensations from the distal part of the extremity.

Looking at total hip replacement

To form a totally artificial hip (here, the McKee-Far-rar total hip replacement), the surgeon cements a femoral head prosthesis in place to articulate with a studded cup, which he then cements into the deepened acetabulum. He may avoid using cement by implanting a prosthesis with a porous coating that promotes bony ingrowth.

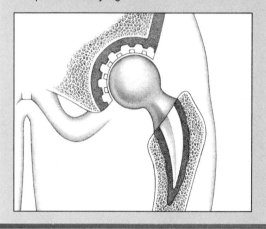

Documentation

Record the date, time, and specific procedures of all postoperative care, including amount and type of drainage, condition of the dressing, need for dressing reinforcement, and appearance of the suture line and surrounding tissue. Also note any signs of skin irritation or infection, any complications and the nursing action taken, the patient's tolerance for exercises, and his psychological reaction to the amputation.

During routine daily care, document the date, time, type of care given, and condition of the skin and suture line, noting any signs of irritation, such as redness or tenderness. Also note the patient's progress in caring for the stump or prosthesis.

Arthroplasty care

Care of the patient after arthroplasty — surgical replacement of all or part of a joint — helps restore mobility and normal use of the affected extremity; it also helps prevent such complications as infection, phlebitis, and respiratory problems. Arthroplasty care includes maintaining alignment of the affected joint, assisting with exercises, and providing routine postoperative care. An equally important nursing responsibility is teaching home care and exercises that may continue for several years, depending on the type of arthroplasty performed and the patient's condition.

The two most common arthroplastic procedures are cup arthroplasty and total joint replacement. In *cup arthroplasty,* the surgeon inserts a movable cup between the hip joint surfaces. The prosthesis has a porous coating that promotes bone regrowth. This procedure is usually indicated for a young patient who has rheumatoid arthritis, degenerative joint disease from traumatic injury, or an acetabulum fracture.

Total joint replacement (usually of the hip or knee) is commonly performed on patients over age 50. Total hip replacement may be used to treat osteoarthritis and severe crippling rheumatoid arthritis; total knee replacement is commonly used to treat severe pain, joint contractures, and deterioration of joint surfaces, conditions that prohibit full extension or flexion. (See *Looking at total hip replacement.*)

Nursing care after these operations — as well as care after less common surgical procedures (such as shoulder, elbow, wrist, ankle, or finger joint replacement) — requires similar skills.

Equipment

Balkan frame with trapeze ▪ comfort device (such as foam mattress, static air mattress overlay, low-air-loss bed, or sheepskin) ▪ bed sheets ▪ ordered traction apparatus (for example, for Buck's extension) ▪ incentive spirometer or intermittent positive-pressure breathing (IPPB) machine ▪ continuous passive motion (CPM) machine ▪ elastic stocking ▪ sterile dressings ▪ hypoallergenic tape ▪ ice bag ▪ skin lotion ▪ warm water ▪ crutches or walker ▪ pain medications ▪ closed-wound drainage system ▪ I.V. antibiotics ▪ pillow ▪ optional: abduction splint.

Traction is not usually applied after cup arthroplasty or total hip replacement. Instead, the patient may be given CPM treatments, which permit passive joint flexion.

After total knee replacement, a knee immobilizer may be applied in the operating room, or the leg may be placed in CPM.

Preparation of equipment

After the patient goes to the operating room, construct a Balkan frame with a trapeze on his bed frame. *This will allow him some mobility after the operation.* Then make the bed, using a comfort device and clean sheets. If the doctor orders postoperative traction, have the bed taken to the operating room. *This enables immediate placement of the patient on his hospital bed after surgery and eliminates the need for an additional move from his recovery room bed.*

Implementation

• Check vital signs every 30 minutes until they stabilize, then every 2 to 4 hours and routinely thereafter, according to hospital protocol. Report any changes in vital signs *because they may indicate infection and hemorrhage.*
• Encourage the patient to perform deep-breathing and coughing exercises. Assist with incentive spirometry or IPPB treatments, as ordered, *to prevent respiratory complications.*
• Assess neurovascular status every 2 hours for the first 48 hours and then every 4 hours *for signs of complications.* Specifically, check the affected leg for color, temperature, toe movement, sensation, edema, capillary filling, and pedal pulse. Also investigate any complaints of pain, burning, numbness, or tingling.
• Apply the elastic stocking to the unaffected leg, as ordered, *to promote venous return and prevent phlebitis and pulmonary emboli.* Once every 8 hours, remove the stocking, inspect the leg for pressure ulcers, and reapply it.
• Administer pain medications, as ordered.
• For at least 48 hours after surgery, administer I.V. antibiotics, as ordered, *to minimize the risk of wound infection.* Also observe the site for symptoms of phlebitis, such as warmth, swelling, tenderness, redness, and positive Homans' sign.
• Administer anticoagulant therapy, as ordered, *to minimize the risk of thrombophlebitis and embolus formation.* Observe for bleeding.
• Check dressings for excessive bleeding. Circle any drainage on the dressing and mark it with your initials, the date, and the time. As appropriate, apply more sterile dressings, using hypoallergenic tape. Report any excessive bleeding to the doctor.
• Observe the closed-wound drainage system for discharge color. *Proper drainage prevents hematoma. Purulent discharge and fever may indicate infection.* Empty and measure drainage, as ordered, using aseptic technique *to prevent infection.* (For more information, see "Closed-wound drain management," Chapter 4.)
• Monitor fluid intake and output daily, making sure to include wound drainage in the output measurement.
• Apply an ice bag, as ordered, to the affected site for the first 48 hours *to reduce swelling, relieve pain, and control bleeding.*
• Every 2 hours, turn the patient no more than 45 degrees toward each side and keep him in this position as long as he's comfortable. *These position changes enhance comfort, prevent pressure ulcers, and help prevent respiratory complications.*

• Help the patient use the trapeze to lift himself every 2 hours. Then provide skin care for his back and buttocks, using warm water and lotion, as indicated.
• Instruct the patient to perform muscle-strengthening exercises for affected and unaffected extremities, as ordered, *to help maintain muscle strength and range of motion and to help prevent phlebitis.*
• Before ambulation exercises, administer a mild analgesic, as ordered, *because movement is very painful.* Encourage the patient during the exercises.
• Assist the patient with progressive ambulation, using adjustable crutches or a walker when needed for support.

After cup arthroplasty

• Maintain balanced suspension and, if appropriate, Buck's extension traction *to support the leg, reduce muscle spasms, maintain abduction, and increase patient comfort.*
• Keep the affected leg in abduction and in the neutral position *to stabilize the hip and keep the cup and femur head in the acetabulum.* Place a pillow between the patient's legs *to maintain hip abduction.*
• On the day after surgery, teach the patient about CPM exercises, as ordered, *to maintain muscle strength and prepare him for eventual ambulation.* Exercises include quadriceps setting, ankle rotation, and plantar flexion and dorsiflexion of the feet.

After total hip replacement

• If ordered, maintain balanced suspension *to increase patient comfort, reduce muscle spasms, and maintain hip abduction.* Place a pillow or abduction splint between the patient's legs *to help maintain hip abduction.*
• If the patient desires, elevate the head of the bed 45 degrees for comfort. (Some doctors permit 60-degree elevation.) Keep the bed elevated no more than 30 minutes at a time *to prevent excessive hip flexion.*
♦ *Nursing alert.* Don't let the hip flex more than 90 degrees *because the prosthesis may dislocate.* ♦
• Keep the patient in the supine position, with the affected hip in full extension, for 1 hour three times a day and at night. *This will help prevent hip flexion contracture.*
• On the day after surgery, have the patient begin plantar flexion and dorsiflexion exercises of the foot on the affected leg. When ordered, instruct him to begin quadriceps exercises. Progressive ambulation protocols vary. Most patients are permitted to dangle their feet on the first day after surgery and to begin transfer and progressive ambulation with assistive devices on the second day.

After total knee replacement

• Keep the knee immobilized in full extension immediately after surgery. Many hospitals start CPM in the recovery room.

• Elevate the affected leg, as ordered, *to reduce swelling.*

• Instruct the patient to begin quadriceps exercises and straight leg-raising, when ordered (usually on the second postoperative day). Encourage flexion-extension exercises, when ordered (usually after the first dressing change).

• If the doctor orders use of the CPM machine, he will adjust the machine daily *to gradually increase the degree of flexion of the affected leg.* Typically, patients can dangle their feet on the first day after surgery and begin ambulation with partial weight-bearing as tolerated (cemented knee) or toe-touch ambulation only (uncemented knee) by the second day. The patient may need to wear a knee immobilizer for support when walking; otherwise, he should be in CPM for most of the day and night or during waking hours only. Check your hospital's protocol.

Special considerations

Before surgery, explain the procedure to the patient. Emphasize that frequent assessment — including the monitoring of vital signs, neurovascular integrity, and wound drainage — is normal after the operation.

Inform the patient that he'll receive I.V. antibiotics for about 2 days. Also be sure he understands that he'll receive medication around the clock for pain control. Explain the need for immobilizing the affected leg and exercising the unaffected one.

Before discharge, instruct the patient regarding home care and exercises.

Complications

Immobility after arthroplasty may result in such complications as shock, pulmonary embolism, pneumonia, phlebitis, paralytic ileus, urine retention, and bowel impaction. A deep wound or infection at the prosthesis site is a serious complication that may force removal of the prosthesis. Dislocation of a total hip prosthesis may occur after violent hip flexion or adduction or during internal rotation. Signs of dislocation include inability to rotate the hip or bear weight, shortening of the leg, and increased pain.

Fat embolism, a potentially fatal complication resulting from release of fat molecules in response to increased intermedullary canal pressure from the prosthesis, may develop within 72 hours after surgery. Watch for such signs and symptoms as apprehension, diaphoresis, fever, dyspnea, pulmonary effusion, tachycardia, cyanosis, seizures, decreased level of consciousness, and a petechial rash on the chest and shoulders.

Documentation

Record the patient's neurovascular status, maintenance of traction (for cup arthroplasty and hip replacement), or knee immobilization (for knee replacement). Note also the condition of the dressings and the drainage system and the application of ice bags. Describe the patient's position (especially the position of the affected leg), skin care and condition, respiratory care and condition, and the use of elastic stockings. Document all exercises performed and their effect; also record ambulatory efforts, the type of support used, and the amount of traction weight.

On the appropriate flowchart, record vital signs and fluid intake and output. Note the turning and skin care schedule and the current exercise and ambulation program. Also include the doctor's orders for the amount of traction weight and the degree of flexion permitted; update these orders as necessary. Record discharge instructions and how well the patient seems to understand them.

Electrical bone growth stimulation

By imitating the body's natural electrical forces, this procedure initiates or accelerates the healing process in a fractured bone that fails to heal. About 1 in 20 fractures may fail to heal properly, possibly as a result of infection, insufficient reduction or fixation, pseudarthrosis, or severe tissue trauma around the fracture.

Recent discoveries about the stimulating effects of electrical currents on osteogenesis have led to using electrical bone stimulation to promote healing. The technique is also being investigated for treating spinal fusions.

Three basic electrical bone stimulation techniques are available: fully implantable direct current stimulation; semi-invasive percutaneous stimulation; and noninvasive electromagnetic coil stimulation. (See *Methods of electrical bone growth stimulation.*) Choice of technique depends on the fracture type and location, the doctor's preference, and the patient's ability and willingness to comply. The invasive device requires little or no patient involvement. With the other two methods, however, the patient must manage his own treatment schedule and maintain the equipment. Treatment time averages 3 to 6 months.

Equipment

For direct current stimulation: The equipment set consists of a small generator and lead wires that connect to a titanium cathode wire that is surgically implanted into the nonunited bone site.

For percutaneous stimulation: The set consists of an external anode skin pad with a lead wire, lithium battery pack, and one to four Teflon-coated stainless steel cathode wires that are surgically implanted.

For electromagnetic stimulation: The set consists of a generator that plugs into a standard 110-volt outlet and 2 strong electromagnetic coils placed on either side of the injured area. The coils can be incorporated into a cast, cuff, or orthotic device.

Preparation of equipment

All equipment comes in sets with instructions provided by the manufacturer. Follow the instructions carefully. Make sure that all parts are included and are sterilized according to hospital policy and procedure.

Implementation

• Tell the patient whether he will have an anesthetic and, if possible, which kind.

Direct current stimulation

• Implantation is performed with the patient under general anesthesia. Afterward, the doctor may apply a cast or external fixator to immobilize the limb. The patient is usually hospitalized for 2 to 3 days after implantation. Weight bearing may be ordered as tolerated.

• Once the bone fragments join, the generator and lead wire can be removed under local anesthesia. The titanium cathode remains implanted.

Percutaneous stimulation

• Remove excessive body hair from the injured site before applying the anode pad. Avoid stressing or pulling on the anode wire. Instruct the patient to change the anode pad every 48 hours. Tell him to report any local pain to his doctor. The patient must not bear weight for the duration of treatment.

Electromagnetic stimulation

• Show the patient where to place the coils, and tell him to apply them for 3 to 10 hours each day, as ordered by his doctor. Many patients find it most convenient to perform the procedure at night.

• Urge the patient not to interrupt the treatments for more than 10 minutes at a time.

• Teach the patient how to use and care for the generator.

• Relay the doctor's instructions for weight bearing. Usually, the doctor will advise against bearing weight until evidence of healing appears on X-rays.

Methods of electrical bone growth stimulation

Electrical bone growth stimulation may be invasive or noninvasive.

Invasive system

An invasive system (shown below) involves placing a spiral cathode inside the bone at the fracture site. A wire leads from the cathode to a battery-powered generator, also implanted in local tissues. The patient's body completes the circuit.

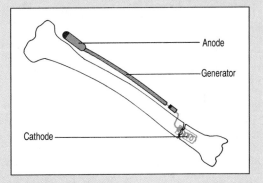

Noninvasive system

A noninvasive system may include a cufflike transducer or fitted ring that wraps around the patient's limb at the level of the injury. Electric current penetrates the limb.

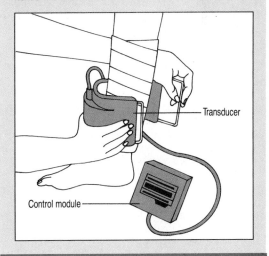

Special considerations

A patient with a direct current electrical bone stimulation should not undergo electrocauterization, diathermy, or magnetic resonance imaging (MRI). *Electrocautery may "short" the system; diathermy may potentiate the electrical current, possibly causing tissue damage; and MRI will interfere with or stop the current.*

Percutaneous electrical bone stimulation is contraindicated if the patient has any kind of inflammatory process. Ask the patient if he is sensitive to nickel or chromium *because both are present in the electrical bone stimulation system.*

Electromagnetic coils are contraindicated for a pregnant patient, a patient with a tumor, or a patient with an arm fracture and a pacemaker.

Home care

Teach the patient how to care for his cast or external fixation devices. Also tell him how to care for the electrical generator. Urge him to follow treatment instructions faithfully.

Complications

Complications associated with any surgical procedure, including increased risk of infection, may occur with direct current electrical bone stimulation equipment. Local irritation or skin ulceration may occur around cathode pin sites with percutaneous devices. No complications are associated with use of electromagnetic coils.

Documentation

Record the type of electrical bone stimulation equipment provided, including date, time, and location, as appropriate. Note the patient's skin condition and tolerance of the procedure. Also record instructions given to the patient and family members, as well as their ability to understand and act on those instructions.

Selected references

Adams, J.C., and Hamblen, D.L. *Outline of Orthopaedics,* 11th ed. New York: Churchill Livingstone, 1990.

American Nurses' Association Staff and National Association of Orthopaedic Nurses. *Orthopaedic Nursing Practice: Process and Outcome Criteria for Selected Diagnoses.* Kansas City, Mo.: American Nurses' Association, 1986.

Arandottir, G. *Neurobehavioral Assessment in Adult CNS Dysfunction.* St. Louis: C.V. Mosby Co., 1989.

Barangan, J.D. "Factors That Influence Recovery from Hip Fracture During Hospitalization," *Orthopaedic Nursing* 9(5):19-30, September-October 1990.

Barden, R.M., and Sinkora, G.L. "Bone Stimulators for Fusions and Fractures," *Nursing Clinics of North America* 26(1):89-103, March 1991.

Barr, N., and Swan, D. *The Hand: Principles and Techniques of Splintmaking,* 2nd ed. Stoneham, Mass.: Butterworth Pubs., 1988.

Barris, R., et al. *Occupational Therapy in Psychosocial Practice.* Thorofare, N.J.: Charles B. Slack, Inc., 1988.

Basmajian, J. *Therapeutic Exercise,* 5th ed. Baltimore: Williams & Wilkins Co., 1989.

Baum, C., et al. *Human Performance Deficits: Occupational Therapy Assessment and Intervention.* Thorofare, N.J.: Charles B. Slack, Inc., 1989.

Cailliet, R. *Low Back Pain Syndrome,* 4th ed. Philadelphia: F.A. Davis Co., 1988.

Cailliet, R. *Soft Tissue Pain and Disability,* 2nd ed. Philadelphia: F.A. Davis Co., 1988.

Ceccio, C.M., and Horosz, J.E. "Teaching the Elderly Amputee to Meet the World," *RN* 51(9):70-72, 74, 76-77, September 1988.

Crenshaw, A.H., ed. *Campbell's Operative Orthopaedics,* 8th ed. St. Louis: Mosby-Year Book, Inc., 1991.

Davis, C.M. *Patient/Practitioner Interaction: An Experiential Manual for Developing the Art of Health Care.* Thorofare, N.J.: Charles B. Slack, Inc., 1989.

Dubrovskis, V., and Wells, D. "Hip Fracture in the Elderly: Program Planning Puts These Patients on Their Feet Again," *Canadian Nurse* 84(5):20-22, May 1988.

Errico, T.J., et al., eds. *Spinal Trauma.* Philadelphia: J.B. Lippincott Co., 1991.

Hansell, M.J. "Fractures and the Healing Process," *Orthopaedic Nursing* 7(1):43-50, January-February 1988.

Illustrated Manual of Nursing Practice. Springhouse, Pa.: Springhouse Corp., 1991.

"Internal Fixation for Open Fractures," *Patient Care* 21(14):25, September 15, 1988.

Mansfield, F. "Neck Pain: Whiplash, Infection, or Worse," *Emergency Medicine* 19(21):20-24, 36, December 15, 1987.

Medhat, A., et al. "Factors That Influence the Level of Activities in Persons with Lower Extremity Amputation," *Rehabilitation Nursing* 15(1):13-18, January-February 1990.

Moncor, C., and Williams, H.J. "Cervical Spine Management in Patients with Rheumatoid Arthritis," *Physical Therapy* 68(4):509-15, April 1988.

Morton, P.G. *Health Assessment in Nursing.* Springhouse, Pa.: Springhouse Corp., 1989.

Mourad, L. *Nursing Care of Adults with Orthopedic Conditions,* 2nd ed. New York: John Wiley & Sons, 1988.

Mourad, L., and Droste, M. *The Nursing Process in the Care of Adults with Orthopaedic Conditions*, 2nd ed. New York: John Wiley & Sons, 1988.

Osborne, L.J., and DiGiacomo, I. "Traction: A Review with Nursing Diagnoses and Interventions," *Orthopaedic Nursing* 6(4):13-19, July-August 1987.

Pastorino, C., et al. "Scope of Orthopaedic Nursing Practice," *Orthopaedic Nursing* 9(6):11-13, November-December 1990.

Patient Teaching Loose-leaf Library. Springhouse, Pa.: Springhouse Corp., 1990.

Reiner, A., and Brown, B. *Manual of Patient Care Standards.* Rockville, Md.: Aspen Pubs., Inc., 1988.

Rockwood, C.A., and Green, D.P., eds. *Fractures in Adults,* 3rd ed. Philadelphia: J.B. Lippincott Co., 1990.

Rockwood, C.A., and Matsen, F.A., eds. *The Shoulder.* Philadelphia: W.B. Saunders Co., 1990.

Sherk, H.H., ed. *Lasers in Orthopaedics.* Philadelphia: J.B. Lippincott Co., 1990.

Treatments. Nurse's Reference Library. Springhouse, Pa.: Springhouse Corp., 1988.

Weinstein, J.N., and Wiesel, S.W., eds. *The Lumbar Spine.* Philadelphia: W.B. Saunders Co., 1990.

Zaslav, K., et al. "General Principles of Management of Fractures and Dislocations," in *Principles of Orthopaedic Practice,* vol. 1. Edited by Dee, R., et al. New York: McGraw-Hill Book Co., 1988.

SKIN CARE

FLORENCE JONES, RN, MSN

Introduction

Besides helping to shape a patient's self-image, the skin performs many physiologic functions. For instance, it protects internal body structures from the environment and from potential pathogens. It also regulates body temperature and homeostasis and serves as an organ of sensation and excretion. As a result, meticulous skin care is essential to overall health. When skin integrity is compromised by pressure ulcers, burns, or other lesions, you'll need to take steps to prevent or control infection, promote new skin growth, control pain, and provide emotional support.

Controlling infection

Because the skin is the body's first line of defense against infection, any damage to its integrity increases the risk of infection, which could delay healing, worsen pain, and even threaten the patient's life. Most burn deaths, for example, result from complications of infection rather than from the burns themselves.

Infection control requires sterile techniques to avoid introducing new pathogens into an already contaminated wound. It's achieved by thorough hand washing with an antiseptic agent and by using sterile equipment during wound care.

Promoting new skin growth

To enhance natural healing, skin wounds need regular dressing changes (extra changes for soiled dressings), thorough cleaning and, if necessary, debridement to remove debris, reduce bacterial growth, and encourage tissue repair. Using warm solutions for wound cleaning increases circulation to the site, which promotes delivery of oxygen and nutrients required to support tissue repair.

Controlling pain

To control pain effectively, you need to evaluate each patient's response to pain and adapt your techniques accordingly. If the patient has minor skin discomfort, such as pruritus, an analgesic or topical medication, reassurance, or distraction techniques may offer him adequate relief. If he has moderate pain, he may benefit from comfortable positioning and ample rest. However, if he has severe pain, only strong narcotic analgesics may provide relief.

Providing emotional support

A patient with a painful and disfiguring skin disorder may have to deal with depression, frustration, and anger. Along with physical support, such a patient needs continuing emotional support as he develops coping mechanisms to accommodate an altered self-image. Severe disfigurement — common in a burn patient — may require emotional support and psychological counsel throughout a slow and painful recovery period. The expectation and reality of scars (or other evidence of skin injury or disease) influence the patient's self-acceptance as well as his acceptance by others. Sensitivity to the patient's needs and respect for his manner of coping are among your most important challenges.

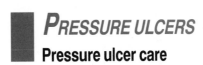

PRESSURE ULCERS
Pressure ulcer care

As their name implies, pressure ulcers result when pressure — applied with great force for a short period or with less force over a longer period — impairs circulation, depriving tissues of oxygen and other life-sustaining nutrients. This process damages skin and underlying structures. Untreated, these ischemic lesions can lead to serious infection.

Most pressure ulcers develop over bony prominences, where friction and shearing force combine with pressure to break down skin and underlying tissues. Common sites include the sacrum, coccyx, ischial tuberosities, and greater trochanters. Other common sites include the skin over the vertebrae, scapulae, elbows, knees, and heels in bedridden and relatively immobile patients. (See *Pressure ulcers: Who's at risk?* page 632.)

Successful pressure ulcer treatment involves relieving pressure, restoring circulation, and — if possible — resolving or managing related disorders. Typically, treatment effectiveness and duration depend on wound severity. (See *Grading pressure ulcers*, page 633.)

Ideally, prevention is the key to avoiding extensive therapy. Preventive measures include ensuring adequate nourishment and mobility to relieve pressure and promote circulation.

When a pressure ulcer develops despite preventive efforts, treatment includes pressure relief with mechanical devices, such as air therapy beds and pressure-relieving cushions, and frequent patient repositioning and exercise. (See Chapter 1, Fundamental procedures.) Other therapeutic measures include meticulous wound cleaning

Pressure ulcers: Who's at risk?

Assess every patient for signs of developing pressure ulcers. At greatest risk for these ulcers are elderly patients and those with the following conditions:
• poor circulation
• diabetes mellitus
• malnutrition
• immunosuppression
• dehydration
• incontinence
• significant obesity or thinness
• paralysis
• diminished pain awareness
• history of corticosteroid therapy
• previous pressure ulcers
• chronic illness that requires bed rest
• mental impairment, possibly related to coma, altered level of consciousness, sedation, confusion, or use of restraints.

and dressings with appropriate medications. Dressings come in various forms for various uses.

A recent treatment — platelet-derived growth factor — may hasten recovery as well. Applied to the pressure ulcer, this agent stimulates wound healing at the cellular level. (See *Understanding platelet-derived growth factor therapy,* page 634.)

Additionally, debridement, hydrotherapy, and skin grafting supplement measures to promote healing. The enterostomal nurse usually performs or coordinates these treatments according to hospital policy. The procedures detailed below address cleaning and dressing the pressure ulcer.

Equipment

Nonallergenic tape or elastic netting ▪ overbed table ▪ sterile irrigation set with bulb syringe ▪ two pairs of gloves ▪ normal saline or other cleaning solution, as ordered ▪ sterile 4″ × 4″ gauze pads ▪ selected topical dressing (see *Choosing an ulcer dressing,* page 635) ▪ linen-saver pads ▪ impervious plastic trash bag ▪ disposable wound-measuring device ▪ sterile cotton-tipped applicators ▪ optional: skin sealant, convoluted foam mattress, or Clinitron therapy bed.

Preparation of equipment

Assemble equipment at the patient's bedside. Cut tape into strips for securing dressings. Loosen lids on cleaning

solutions and medications for easy removal. Loosen existing dressing edges and tapes before putting on gloves. Attach an impervious plastic trash bag to the overbed table to hold used dressings and refuse.

Implementation

• Before any dressing change, wash your hands and review the principles of universal precautions. (See Chapter 2, Infection control.)

To clean the pressure ulcer

• Provide privacy, and explain the procedure to the patient *to allay his fears and promote cooperation.*

• Position the patient *to increase his comfort* but be sure that his position allows you easy access to the pressure ulcer site.

• Cover the bed linens with a linen-saver pad *to prevent soiling.*

• Open the sterile irrigation set. Carefully pour normal saline solution into the irrigation container *to avoid splashing.* Put the bulb syringe into the opening provided in the irrigation container.

• Open packages of sterile supplies and arrange them on the sterile field in order of use.

• Put on gloves to remove the old dressing and expose the pressure ulcer. Discard the soiled dressing in the impervious plastic trash bag *to avoid contaminating the sterile field and spreading infection.*

• Inspect the wound. Note color, amount, and odor of any drainage and necrotic debris. Measure the wound perimeter with the disposable wound-measuring device (a square, transparent card with concentric circles arranged in bull's-eye fashion and bordered with a straight-edge ruler).

• Using the bulb syringe, gently irrigate the pressure ulcer. If the wound contains necrotic debris, select a 30-ml syringe fitted with a 19G needle or a catheter instead of a bulb syringe.

• Remove and discard your soiled gloves and put on a fresh pair.

• Insert a sterile cotton-tipped applicator into the wound *to assess wound tunneling.* Gauge tunnel depth by determining how far the applicator can be inserted. (Use the measuring guide. *To avoid contamination,* don't let the applicator touch the guide.) *Tunneling usually signals wound extension and possible infection of underlying tissues.*

• Using the gauze pads, blot the skin dry around the ulcer. Begin blotting at the center of the ulcer. Work with a spiral motion toward the edges *to avoid contaminating the wound with microorganisms from the skin.*

Grading pressure ulcers

To select the most effective treatment for a pressure ulcer, you first need to assess its severity. The following pressure ulcer grades describe wound depth and character. Keep in mind that, if the wound contains necrotic tissue, you won't be able to determine a grade until you can see the wound base.

Grade 1

Intact skin appears red and fails to return to normal color even after 30 minutes without pressure. When the skin is pressed and released, capillaries refill more slowly than normal—or the skin may not blanch at all. The condition can be reversed by removing pressure.

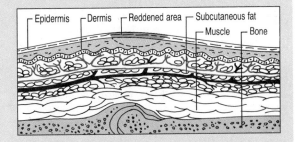

Grade 2

Blistering with erythema or induration may appear. The epidermis may or may not be intact. The ulcer develops into a partial-thickness wound with skin erosion involving the epidermis and part of the dermis. The ulcer base appears pink and moist but not necrotic. The patient usually reports pain. After pressure is relieved, healing may be complete within 2 weeks.

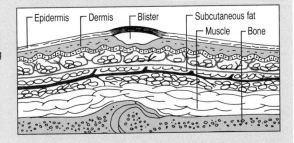

Grade 3

The ulcer constitutes a full-thickness wound, penetrating the subcutaneous layer down to muscle. Resembling a shallow crater, the ulcer may have tunnels extending from it. Infection or exudate may appear, although the base of the wound may not be painful. Healing may take up to 3 months.

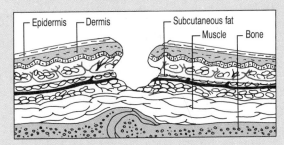

Grade 4

The ulcer extends through skin, fat, and muscle and may reach the bone. Like a grade 3 lesion, the ulcer base usually doesn't cause pain, although tunneling, infection, or exudate may appear. At best, expect healing to take months or even a year.

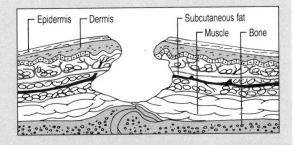

Understanding platelet-derived growth factor therapy

Current pressure ulcer treatments rely on protecting the wound from injury and maintaining an infection-free environment to promote healing. But in some patients, underlying infection, poor circulation, or other problems may delay or prohibit healing. In these patients, a promising experimental therapy uses growth factors derived from the patient's own platelets (platelet-derived wound healing formula, or Procuren Solution) to stimulate granulation tissue, capillaries, and skin growth. The procedure complements rather than replaces standard wound-management procedures.

Preparing for the procedure

Treatment begins with measures to control underlying infections, correct poor circulation, and relieve contributing conditions.

Then, platelets extracted from a small sample of the patient's blood are processed and resuspended in solution. These platelets are returned to the patient in a series of single-tube doses. One 60-ml blood sample produces enough growth factor solution for a 10-week treatment course.

Applying growth factor

• Wash your hands and put on gloves.
• Saturate a piece of sterile gauze with a single dose of growth factor solution.
• Pack the wet gauze into the wound. Be sure to cover all wound surfaces.
• Cover the packing with a petroleum-gauze dressing to keep the wound moist.
• Keep the solution-soaked gauze on the wound for 12 hours (usually overnight).
• Replace the packing with a normal saline solution or antibiotic dressing, as ordered, during the day.

• Next, reassess the condition of the skin and the ulcer. Note the character of the cleaned wound bed and the surrounding skin.
• Prepare to apply the appropriate topical dressing. Directions for typical hydrocolloid, transparent, and calcium alginate dressings follow. For other dressings or topical agents, follow your hospital's protocol or the supplier's instructions. (See *Guide to topical agents for pressure ulcers,* page 636.)

To apply a hydrocolloid dressing

• Choose a pre-sized dressing or cut one to overlap the pressure ulcer by about 1″ (2.5 cm). Remove the dressing from its package, pull the release paper from the adherent side of the dressing, and apply the dressing to the wound. *To minimize irritation,* carefully smooth out wrinkles as you apply the dressing.
• If the dressing's edges need to be secured with tape, apply a skin sealant to the intact skin around the ulcer. After the area dries, tape the dressing to the skin. *The sealant protects the skin and promotes tape adherence.* Never use tension or pressure when applying the tape.
• Remove your gloves and discard them in the impervious trash bag. Dispose of refuse according to your hospital's policy, and wash your hands.
• Change a hydrocolloid dressing every 1 to 7 days as needed; for example, if the dressing tears, the patient complains of pain, or leakage or foul odor occurs.

To apply a transparent dressing

• Clean and dry the wound as described above.
• Select a dressing to overlap the ulcer by 2″ (5 cm).
• Gently lay the dressing over the ulcer. *To prevent shearing force,* do not stretch the dressing. Press firmly on the edges of the dressing to promote adherence. Though these dressings are self-adhesive, you may have to tape the edges *to prevent them from curling.*
• If necessary, aspirate accumulated fluid with an 18G to 20G needle and syringe using aseptic technique *to preserve dressing integrity.* After aspirating the pocket of fluid, clean the aspiration site with an alcohol sponge and cover it with another strip of transparent dressing.
• Change the dressing every 3 to 7 days depending on whether the ulcer is infected and whether drainage is minimal or profuse.

To apply a calcium alginate dressing

• Irrigate the pressure ulcer with normal saline solution. Blot the surrounding skin dry.
• Apply the calcium alginate to the ulcer surface. Cover the area with a second dressing, such as gauze pads, as ordered. Secure the dressing with tape or elastic netting.
• If the wound is draining heavily, change the dressing once or twice daily for the first 3 to 5 days. As drainage decreases, change the dressing less frequently — every 2 to 4 days, or as ordered.

To prevent pressure ulcers

• Turn and reposition the patient every 1 to 2 hours unless contraindicated. For patients who can't turn themselves or who are turned on a schedule, use pressure-relieving and pressure-reducing devices, such as a 4″ (10-cm) convoluted foam mattress or a low-air-loss or Clinitron therapy bed. As appropriate, implement active or passive range-of-motion exercises *to relieve pressure and promote circulation. To save time,* combine these exercises with bathing if applicable.

• When turning the patient, lift him rather than slide him *because sliding increases friction and shear.* Use a turning sheet and get help from co-workers if necessary.

• Use pillows *to position your patient and increase his comfort.* Be sure to eliminate sheet wrinkles that could increase pressure and cause discomfort.

• Post a turning schedule at the patient's bedside. Adapt position changes to the patient's situation. Emphasize the importance of regular position changes to the patient and his family. Encourage their participation in treatment and pressure ulcer prevention by having them perform a position change correctly after you demonstrate how.

• Except for brief periods, avoid raising the head of the bed more than 30 degrees *to prevent shearing pressure.*

• Direct the patient confined to a chair or wheelchair to shift his weight every 30 minutes *to promote blood flow to compressed tissues.* Show a paraplegic patient how to shift his weight by doing push-ups in the wheelchair. If the patient needs your help, sit next to him and help him shift his weight to one buttock for 60 seconds, then repeat the procedure on the other side. Provide him with pressure-relieving cushions as appropriate. However, avoid seating the patient on a rubber or plastic doughnut, *which can increase localized pressure at vulnerable points.*

• Adjust or pad appliances, casts, or splints as needed *to ensure proper fit and avoid increased pressure and impaired circulation.*

• Tell the patient to avoid heat lamps and harsh soaps *because they dry the skin.* Lotion applied after bathing will help keep his skin moist. Also tell him to avoid vigorous massage *because it can damage capillaries.*

• If the patient's condition permits, recommend a diet that includes adequate calories, protein, and vitamins. Dietary therapy may involve nutritional consultation, food supplements, enteral feeding, or total parenteral nutrition.

• If diarrhea develops or if the patient is incontinent, clean and dry soiled skin. Then, apply a protective moisture barrier *to prevent skin maceration.*

Special considerations
Avoid using elbow and heel protectors that fasten with a single narrow strap. *The strap may impair neurovascular function in the involved hand or foot.*

As a rule, avoid using tincture of benzoin compound as a skin sealant. *This agent triggers an allergic reaction in some patients.*

Choosing an ulcer dressing

Should a patient with a grade 2 pressure ulcer receive the same kind of dressing as a patient with a grade 4 ulcer? This review of common protective dressings will help you decide.

Hydrocolloid dressings
Known by such trade names as DuoDERM, Restore, and Tegasorb, these occlusive coverings are water-resistant and block exogenous microorganisms and contaminants. Hydrocolloid dressings absorb exudates and form a hydrated gel that protects developing tissue, but they can't break down dry, leathery eschar.

Transparent film dressings
Made of a clear plastic-like material, popular transparent dressings include Bioclusive, Op-Site, and Tega-derm. These dressings allow some exchange of air and moist vapor but keep water out. Their transparency permits visual inspection.

However, because these dressings can't absorb drainage, they're used on partial- or full-thickness wounds with minimal exudate. (The DuoDERM extra-thin dressing is transparent but retains hydrocolloid properties on superficial wounds with minimal exudate.)

Absorptive dressings
Gauze, karaya powder, and dextranomer beads may benefit patients who have pressure ulcers with copious exudate and deep tissue loss. Powder and bead dressings absorb drainage and maintain a moist surface by interacting with the exudate to form a gelatinous mass. This matter then conforms to the wound surface and eliminates dead space.

Calcium alginate dressings
Available as soft, white sterile pads or ropes, calcium alginate dressings can absorb up to 20 times their weight in exudate. And they can be used when the ulcer contains infection. As the dressing absorbs exudate, it turns into a gel that maintains moisture in the wound bed and promotes healing.

Hydrogel dressings
These highly flexible, absorptive sheets liquefy necrotic tissue and cover partial-thickness wounds. They have a cooling effect that eases pain.

Guide to topical agents for pressure ulcers

TOPICAL AGENTS	NURSING CONSIDERATIONS
Antibiotics bacitracin, Neosporin Ointment, Polysporin Ointment	• Use only for early ulcers because these agents may not penetrate sufficiently to kill deeper bacterial colonies.
Antiseptics hydrogen peroxide, povidone-iodine (Betadine), sodium hypochlorite (Dakin's solution)	• Dilute the standard 3% hydrogen peroxide solution to half or quarter strength. • Avoid using hydrogen peroxide after granulation tissue develops because its foaming action may cause blistering. Also avoid cleaning deep or tunneled wounds with this agent because the wound may retain and absorb oxygen bubbles, creating air emboli. • Avoid using povidone-iodine on open wounds because it may damage granulation tissue, retard collagen synthesis, and irritate surrounding skin. • Apply diluted sodium hypochlorite, as directed, only to debride the wound initially. • Avoid multiple applications of sodium hypochlorite because it inhibits granulation tissue growth, delays epithelialization, and irritates surrounding skin.
Circulatory stimulants (Granulex, Proderm)	• Use these agents to promote blood flow. Both contain balsam of Peru and castor oil, but Granulex also contains trypsin, an enzyme that facilitates debridement.
Enzymes collagenase (Santyl), fibrinolysin and desoxyribonuclease (Elase), sutilains (Travase)	• Apply collagenase in thin layers after cleaning the wound with normal saline solution. • Promote effectiveness by avoiding conjoint use of collagenase with agents that decrease enzymatic activity, including detergents, hexachlorophene, antiseptics with heavy-metal ions, iodine, or such acid solutions as Burow's solution. • Use collagenase cautiously near the patient's eyes. If contact occurs, flush the eyes repeatedly with normal saline solution or sterile water. • Use fibrinolysin only after surgical removal of dry eschar. • If using sutilains and topical antibacterials, apply sutilains ointment first. • Avoid applying sutilains to ulcers in major body cavities, to areas with exposed nerve tissue, or to fungating neoplastic lesions. Do not use sutilains in women of childbearing age or in patients with limited cardiopulmonary reserve. • Store sutilains at cool temperature range: 35.6° to 50° F (2° to 10° C). • Use sutilains cautiously near the patient's eyes. If contact occurs, flush the eyes repeatedly with normal saline solution or sterile water.
Exudate absorbers dextranomer beads (Debrisan)	• Use dextranomer on secreting ulcers. Discontinue use when secretions stop. • Clean but don't dry the ulcer before applying dextranomer beads. Don't use in tunneling ulcers. • Remove gray-yellow beads (which indicate saturation) by irrigating with sterile water or saline. • Use cautiously near the eyes. If contact occurs, flush the eyes repeatedly with normal saline solution or sterile water.
Isotonic solutions normal saline solution	• This agent moisturizes tissue without injuring cells.

Complications

Infection, the most common complication, causes foul-smelling drainage, persistent pain, severe erythema, induration, and elevated skin and body temperatures. Ongoing infection can lead to septicemia and osteomyelitis.

Documentation

Record the date and time of initial and subsequent treatments. Note the specific treatment given. Detail preventive strategies performed. Document the pressure ulcer's location; size (length, width, and depth); color and appearance of the wound bed; amount, odor, color, and consistency of drainage; and condition of the surrounding skin.

Update the care plan as required. Note any change in the condition or size of the pressure ulcer and any elevation of skin temperature on the progress record. Document when the doctor was notified of any pertinent abnormal observations. Record the patient's temperature daily on the graphic sheet to allow easy assessment of body temperature patterns.

Unna's boot

Named for dermatologist Paul Gerson Unna, this boot can be used to treat uninfected, nonnecrotic leg and foot ulcers that result from conditions such as venous insufficiency and stasis dermatitis. A commercially prepared, medicated gauze compression dressing, the boot wraps around the affected foot and leg. Alternatively, a preparation known as Unna's paste (gelatin, zinc oxide, and glycerin) may be applied to the ulcer and covered with lightweight gauze. The boot's effectiveness results from compression applied by the bandage combined with moisture supplied by the paste.

Unna's boot is contraindicated in patients allergic to any ingredient used in the paste and in patients with arterial ulcers, weeping eczema, or cellulitis.

Equipment

Scrub sponge with ordered cleaning agent ▪ normal saline solution ▪ commercially prepared gauze bandage saturated with Unna's paste (or Unna's paste and lightweight gauze) ▪ bandage scissors ▪ gloves ▪ optional: elastic bandage to cover Unna's boot.

Implementation

• Explain the procedure to the patient and provide privacy.
• Wash your hands and put on gloves.

• Assess the ulcer and the surrounding skin. Evaluate ulcer size, drainage, and appearance. Perform a neurovascular assessment of the affected foot *to ensure adequate circulation.*
• Clean the affected area gently with the sponge and cleaning agent *to retard bacterial growth and to remove dirt, which may create pressure points after you apply the bandage.* Rinse with normal saline solution.
• Position the patient's leg in a slightly flexed position *to ease application.* Put on clean gloves.
• If a commercially prepared gauze bandage isn't ordered, spread Unna's paste evenly on the leg and foot. Then cover the leg and foot with the lightweight gauze. Apply three to four layers of paste interspersed with layers of gauze. In a prepared bandage, the paste is impregnated into the bandage.
• Apply gauze or the prepared bandage in a circular motion from the foot to the knee. The wrap should be snug but not tight. *To cover the area completely,* be sure each turn overlaps the previous one by half the bandage's width. (See *How to wrap Unna's boot,* page 638.)
• Continue wrapping the patient's leg up to the knee, using firm, even pressure. Mold the boot with your free hand as you apply the bandage *to make it smooth and even.*
• If using a commercially prepared bandage, you may cover the boot with an elastic bandage *to protect the patient's clothing and bed linens from the paste.*
• Instruct the patient to remain in bed with his leg outstretched and elevated on a pillow until the paste dries (approximately 30 minutes). Observe the patient's foot for signs of impairment, such as cyanosis, loss of feeling, or swelling. *This indicates that the bandage is too tight and should be rewrapped.*
• Leave the boot on for 5 to 7 days, or as ordered. Instruct the patient to walk on and handle the wrap carefully *to avoid damaging it.* Tell him the boot will stiffen, but won't be as hard as a cast.
• Change the boot weekly or as ordered *to assess the underlying skin and ulcer healing.* Remove the boot by unwrapping the bandage from the knee back to the foot.

Special considerations

Never apply the boot to a swollen leg *because the boot will loosen as the edema subsides. This, in turn, reduces the therapeutic effect of pressure on the veins.*

Don't make reverse turns while wrapping the bandage. *This could create excessive pressure areas that may cause discomfort as the bandage hardens.*

For bathing, instruct the patient to cover the boot with a plastic kitchen trash bag sealed at the knee with an elastic bandage *to avoid wetting the boot. A wet boot softens and loses its effectiveness.*

How to wrap Unna's boot

After cleaning the patient's skin thoroughly, flex his knee. Then, starting with the foot positioned at a right angle to the leg, wrap the medicated gauze bandage firmly — not tightly — around the patient's foot in overlapping turns. Continue overlapping the wrap up the leg. Smooth the boot with your free hand as you go, as shown below.

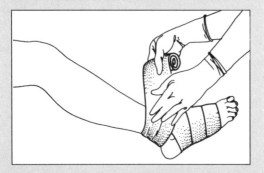

Stop wrapping about 1″ (2.5 cm) or 2″ (5 cm) below the knee. If necessary, you may make a 2″ slit in the boot just below the knee *to relieve constriction that may develop as the dressing hardens.*

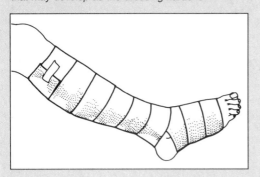

Repeat this procedure until the patient's leg has a three-layer boot.

Complications
Contact dermatitis may result from hypersensitivity to Unna's paste.

Documentation
Record the date and time of application. Specify which leg you bandaged. Describe the appearance of the pa-

tient's skin before and after boot application. Name the equipment used (commercially prepared bandage or Unna's paste and lightweight gauze). Describe any allergic reaction.

BURNS
Burn care

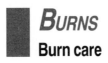

The goals of burn care are to encourage regrowth of burned tissue, prevent infection, and maintain the patient's physiologic stability. Infection can increase wound depth, cause rejection of skin grafts, delay healing, worsen pain, prolong hospitalization, and even lead to death. In fact, whenever possible, the health care team avoids invasive procedures in burn patients because these procedures heighten the patient's risk for infection. Procedures to prevent infection include using strict aseptic technique during care, dressing the burn site, monitoring and rotating I.V. lines regularly, and carefully assessing body system function, emotional status, and burn extent (see *Estimating burn surfaces in adults and children* and *Evaluating burn severity,* page 640).

To promote patient stability, you'll aim to control body temperature because skin loss interferes with temperature regulation. Additionally, you'll frequently review laboratory values, such as serum electrolyte levels, to detect early changes in the patient's condition.

Other interventions, such as careful positioning and regular exercise for burned extremities, help maintain joint function, prevent contractures, and minimize deformity (see *Positioning the burn patient to prevent deformity,* page 641).

Although some burns respond to topical medications and exposure to air (to limit bacterial growth), most need greater protection from the environment. Burn dressings encourage healing by barring germ entry and by removing exudate, eschar, and other debris that host infection. Dressing materials — natural or synthetic — are applied in layers. Typically, the first layer consists of nonadherent fine-mesh gauze moistened with water, normal saline solution, or a topical antibacterial agent. Subsequent layers consist of absorptive coarse mesh. An outer, elastic gauze layer typically secures the dressing in place.

Equipment
Ordered topical medication ▪ ordered pain medication ▪ 4″ × 4″ gauze pads ▪ two basins ▪ two pairs of gloves ▪ rolls or sheets of fine-mesh gauze ▪ roller gauze ▪ elastic

Estimating burn surfaces in adults and children

You need to use different formulas to compute burned body surface areas in adults and children because the proportion of body surface areas varies with growth.

Rule of nines

You can quickly estimate the extent of an adult patient's burn by using the "rule of nines." This method quantifies body surface area in percentages either in fractions of nine or in multiples of nine. To use this method, mentally assess your patient's burns by the body chart shown below. Add the corresponding percentages for each body section burned. Use the total—a rough estimate of burn extent—to calculate initial fluid replacement needs.

Lund and Browder

The rule of nines isn't accurate for infants and children because their body shapes differ from those of adults. An infant's head, for example, accounts for about 17% of his total body surface area, compared with 7% for an adult. Instead, use the Lund and Browder chart shown here.

Percentage of burned body surface by age

	AT BIRTH	0 TO 1 YR	1 TO 4 YR	5 TO 9 YR	10 TO 15 YR	ADULT
A: Half of head						
	9½%	8½%	6½%	5½%	4½%	3½%
B: Half of thigh						
	2¾%	3¼%	4%	4¼%	4½%	4¾%
C: Half of leg						
	2½%	2½%	2¾%	3%	3¼%	3½%

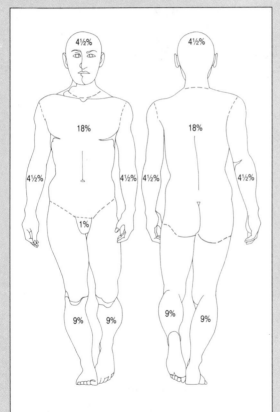

Evaluating burn severity

To judge a burn's severity, assess its size, depth, and character.

Superficial (first-degree) burn
Does the burned area appear pink or red with minimal edema? Is the area sensitive to touch and temperature changes? If so, your patient most likely has a first-degree, or partial-thickness, burn affecting just one or two layers of his skin.

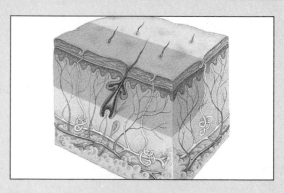

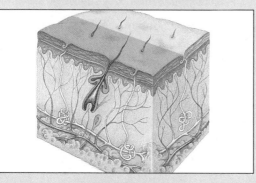

Deep (third-degree) burn
Does the burned area appear waxy white, red, brown, or black? Does red skin remain red with no blanching when you touch it? Is the skin leathery with extensive subcutaneous edema? Is the skin insensitive to touch? If so, your patient has a third-degree, or full-thickness, burn that affects all skin layers.

Moderate (second-degree) burn
Does the burned area appear pink or red? Do red areas blanch when you touch them? Does the skin have large thick-walled blisters with subcutaneous edema? Is the burned area itself firm or leathery? Does touching the burn cause severe pain? If so, your patient has a second-degree, or partial-thickness, burn (shown above, at right) affecting at least two skin layers.

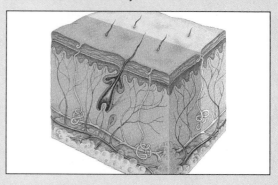

gauze dressing ▪ cotton-tipped applicators ▪ antiseptic cleaning agent ▪ normal saline solution ▪ towels ▪ scissors ▪ tissue forceps ▪ bath blanket ▪ gown ▪ mask ▪ surgical cap ▪ heat lamps ▪ impervious plastic trash bag.

All equipment except cap and mask should be sterile.

Preparation of equipment
Assemble equipment on the dressing table. Make sure the treatment area has adequate light *to allow accurate wound assessment.* Open equipment packages using aseptic technique. Arrange supplies on a sterile field in order of use. Warm the normal saline solution by immersing unopened bottles in warm water.

Implementation
• Administer ordered pain medication about 20 minutes before beginning wound care *to maximize patient comfort and cooperation.*
• Explain the procedure to the patient and provide privacy.
• Turn on overhead heat lamps *to keep the patient warm.* Be sure that they don't overheat the patient.
• Wash your hands.

To remove a dressing without hydrotherapy
• Put on a gown (a clean gown if you're in a burn unit, a sterile gown if you're not), mask, and sterile gloves.

Positioning the burn patient to prevent deformity

BURNED AREA	POTENTIAL DEFORMITY	PREVENTIVE POSITIONING	NURSING INTERVENTIONS
Neck	• Flexion contracture of neck • Extensor contracture of neck	• Extension • Prone with head slightly raised	• Remove pillow from bed. • Place pillow or rolled towel under upper chest to flex cervical spine. Or apply cervical collar.
Axilla	• Adduction and internal rotation • Adduction and external rotation	• Shoulder joint in external rotation and 100- to 130-degree abduction • Shoulder in forward flexion and 100- to 130-degree abduction	• Use an I.V. pole, bedside table, or sling to suspend arm. • Use an I.V. pole, bedside table, or sling to suspend arm.
Pectoral region	• Shoulder protraction	• Shoulders abducted and externally rotated	• Remove pillow from bed.
Chest or abdomen	• Kyphosis	• As for pectoral region, with hips neutral (not flexed)	• Use no pillow under head or legs.
Lateral trunk	• Scoliosis	• Supine; affected arm abducted	• Put pillows or blanket rolls at sides.
Elbow	• Flexion and pronation	• Arm extended and supinated	• Use an elbow splint, armboard, or bedside table.
Wrist	• Flexion • Extension	• Splint in 15-degree extension • Splint in 15-degree flexion	• Apply a hand splint. • Apply a hand splint.
Fingers	• Adhesions of the extensor tendons, loss of palmar grasp	• Metacarpophalangeal joints in maximum flexion; interphalangeal joints in slight flexion; thumb in maximum abduction	• Apply a hand splint; wrap fingers separately.
Hip	• Internal rotation, flexion, and adduction; possibly joint subluxation if contracture is severe	• Neutral rotation and abduction; maintain extension by prone position	• Put a pillow under buttocks (if supine) or use trochanter rolls or knee or long leg splints.
Knee	• Flexion	• Maintain extension	• Use a knee splint with no pillows under legs.
Ankle	• Plantar flexion if foot muscles are weak or their tendons are divided	• 90-degree dorsiflexion	• Use a footboard or ankle splint.

• Remove dressing layers down to the innermost, fine-mesh layer by cutting the outer dressings with sterile blunt scissors. Lay open these dressings.
• Soak the fine-mesh inner layer with warm normal saline solution or other ordered solution *to ease removal*.
• Remove the inner dressing with sterile tissue forceps or your sterile gloved hand.
• *Because soiled dressings harbor infectious microorganisms*, dispose of the dressings carefully in an impervious bag according to your hospital's policy.
• Gently remove any exudate and old topical medication with 4″ × 4″ gauze pads moistened with an ordered antiseptic cleaning agent or saline solution.
• Carefully remove all loose eschar with sterile forceps and scissors, if ordered. (See "Mechanical debridement" in this chapter.)
• Assess wound condition. The wound should appear clean, with no debris, loose tissue, purulence, inflammation, or darkened margins.
• Before applying a new dressing, remove your gown, gloves, and mask. Discard them properly, and put on a fresh, clean mask, surgical cap, gown (clean if you're in a burn unit, sterile if you're not), and sterile gloves.

To apply a wet dressing
• Soak fine-mesh gauze and the elastic gauze dressing in a large sterile basin containing the ordered solution (for example, silver nitrate).
• Wring out the fine-mesh gauze until it's moist — not dripping — and apply it to the wound. Warn the patient that he may feel transient pain when you apply the dressing.
• Wring out the elastic gauze dressing, and position it *to hold the fine-mesh gauze in place*.
• Roll an elastic gauze dressing over the dressing *to keep dressings intact*.
• Cover the patient with a cotton bath blanket *to prevent chills*. Change the blanket if it becomes damp. Use an overhead heat lamp if necessary.
• Change the dressings frequently, as ordered, *to keep the wound moist* — especially if you're using silver nitrate. *Silver nitrate becomes ineffective and the silver ions may damage tissue if the dressings become dry. (To maintain moisture,* some protocols call for irrigating the dressing with solution at least every 4 hours through small slits cut into the outer dressing.)

To apply a dry dressing with a topical medication
• Remove old dressings, and clean the wound (as described previously).
• If the fine-mesh gauze doesn't already hold topical medication, apply the ordered medication to the wound in a thin layer — about 2 to 4 mm thick — with your sterile gloved hand. Then apply fine-mesh gauze over the wound *to contain the medication but allow exudate to escape*. (If you apply an occlusive dressing, wrap it with elastic gauze dressing *to hold the fine-mesh gauze in place and absorb any drainage*.)
• Remember to cut the dressing to fit only the wound areas; do not cover unburned areas.
• Apply several layers of coarse absorptive gauze. Then cover the entire dressing with elastic or stockinette gauze *to secure the dressing and prevent evaporation of body fluid*.

To provide arm and leg care
• Apply the dressings from the distal to the proximal area *to stimulate circulation and prevent constriction*. Wind the dressings once around the arm or leg, so the edges overlap slightly. Continue wrapping in this way until the dressing covers the wound. Then cut the bandage.
• Apply a dry roller gauze or elastic gauze bandage to hold the bottom layers in place.

To provide hand and foot care
• Wrap each finger separately with a single layer of fine-mesh gauze *to allow the patient to use his hands and to prevent webbing contractures*.
• Place the hand in a functional position and secure this position using a dressing.
• Put gauze between each toe, as appropriate, *also to prevent webbing contractures*.

To provide chest, abdomen, and back care
• Cover the wound with a large gauze sheet and a layer of coarse gauze saturated with the ordered medication.
• Place sterile towels on top of the gauze and pin other sterile towels to the dressing so that the bandage wraps around the chest, abdomen, or back. Or wrap the wound area with an elastic gauze dressing *to avoid restricting respiratory motion, especially in very young or elderly patients or those with circumferential injuries*.

To provide facial care
• If the patient has scalp burns, clip or shave the hair around the burn, as ordered. Clip other hair until it's about 2″ (5 cm) long *to prevent contamination of burned scalp areas*.
• Be sure not to cover the eyes, nostrils, or mouth with the final elastic gauze dressing.

To provide ear care
• Clip or shave the hair around the affected ear.
• Remove exudate and crusts with cotton-tipped applicators dipped in a saline solution.
• Place a layer of fine-mesh gauze behind the auricle *to prevent webbing*.

Burn care at the scene

By acting promptly when a burn injury occurs, you can improve a patient's chance of uncomplicated recovery. Emergency care at the scene should include steps to stop the burn from worsening; assessment of the patient's airway, breathing, and circulation (ABCs); a call for help from an emergency medical team; and emotional and physiologic support for the patient.

Stop the process
• If the victim is on fire, tell him to fall to the ground and roll to put out the flames. (If he panics and runs, air will fuel the flames, worsening the burn and increasing the risk of inhalation injury.) Or, if you can, wrap the person in a blanket or other large covering to smother the flames and protect the burned area from dirt. Keep the patient's head outside the blanket so he doesn't breathe toxic fumes.
• If you have water handy, pour it directly on the burned area to cool the involved tissue, stop the burn from growing deeper or larger, and decrease pain.
• If possible, remove any potential sources of continued heat, such as jewelry, belt buckles, and some types of clothing. Besides adding to the burn process, these items may cause constriction as edema develops. If the patient's clothing adheres to his skin, don't try to remove it. Rather, cut around it.
• Cover the wound with a tablecloth, sheet, or other smooth, nonfuzzy material. If the burn covers less than 9% of the body surface and is superficial, cover it with a moist towel. (For a more serious or extensive burn, this tactic could induce hypothermia.)

Assess the damage
• Assess the patient's ABCs and perform cardiopulmonary resuscitation if necessary. Then check for other serious injuries, such as fractures, a spinal cord injury, lacerations, blunt trauma, or head contusions.
• Estimate the extent and depth of burns. If flames caused the burn, assess the patient for signs of inhalation injury, such as singed nasal hairs, burns on the face or mouth, soot-stained sputum, coughing or hoarseness, crackles, rhonchi or wheezes, or respiratory distress.
• Call for help as quickly as possible. Send someone to contact the emergency medical service.
• If the patient is conscious and alert, try to get a brief medical history as soon as possible.
• Offer no fluids to drink because someone with major burns may vomit, which can lead to aspiration pneumonia, or an ileus may develop.
• Reassure the patient and tell him that help is on the way. By explaining everything, you may be able to keep him calm.
• When help arrives, give the emergency service a report on the patient's status.

• Apply fine-mesh gauze and $4'' \times 4''$ gauze pads to the burned area. Dampen the pads with the ordered topical medication. (*To prevent pooling in the middle ear*, don't soak the pads.) Before securing the dressing with a bandage, position the patient's ears normally *to avoid damaging auricular cartilage.*
• Assess the patient's hearing ability.

To provide eye care
• Clean the area around the eyes and the eyelids with a cotton-tipped applicator and normal saline solution every 4 to 6 hours or as needed *to remove crusts and drainage.*
• Administer ordered eye ointments or drops.
• If the patient can't close his eyes, apply lubricating ointments or drops as ordered.
• Be sure to close the patient's eyes before applying eye pads, *to prevent corneal abrasion.* Don't apply any topical ointments near the eyes without a doctor's order.

To provide nasal care
• Check the nostrils for inhalation injury, inflamed mucosa, and singed vibrissae.
• Clean the nostrils with cotton-tipped applicators dipped in normal saline solution.
• Remove crusts.
• Apply the ordered ointments.
• Small plexiglass inserts may be placed in the nostrils *to prevent contractures.*
• If the patient has a nasogastric tube, use tracheostomy ties to secure the tube.
• Clean the area around the tube every 4 to 6 hours.

Special considerations
Competent care delivered immediately after a burn occurs can make a dramatic difference to the success of overall treatment. (See *Burn care at the scene.*)

All second- and third-degree burns are serious, especially when the patient is older than age 60 or younger

Successful burn care after discharge

You can help the patient make a successful transition from hospital to home by encouraging him to follow certain wound and skin care guidelines.

Wound care
• Tell the patient or a family member to clean the bathtub, shower, or wash basin thoroughly before using them for wound care.
• Advise the patient to wash the wound using mild soap and warm water unless ordered otherwise. To remove topical creams, scales, or loose skin, he can apply gentle friction with a clean washcloth and pat the skin dry with a clean towel.
• Instruct him to check the burn for signs of infection and call the doctor if he thinks infection is setting in. Show him how to apply a new dressing.
• If the patient uses a splint, tell him to wash it with soap and cold water to avoid harming the splint.
• To enhance healing, encourage the patient to consume adequate carbohydrates and proteins. Advise him to have three well-balanced meals and three between-meal snacks daily. Emphasize that he should include one protein source with each meal and snack.

Skin care
• Remind the patient that regenerated skin tissue is delicate and needs protection. He should avoid bumping or scratching it.
• Tell the patient that he can wash the new skin with mild soap and water, but that he should apply lotions sparingly and only if they contain no alcohol or perfume.
• Recommend nonrestrictive, unabrasive clothing. The patient should launder it in a mild detergent.
• Warn the patient not to expose new skin to strong sunlight or such irritants as paint, solvent, strong detergent, and antiperspirants.
• Recommend cool baths or ice packs to relieve itching.
• Advise the patient to eliminate from his diet substances that constrict peripheral blood flow, such as tobacco, alcohol, and caffeine.
• To minimize scar formation, the patient may need to wear a pressure garment as instructed — usually for 23 hours a day for 6 months to 1 year. Suspect that the garment is too tight if it causes cold, numbness, or discoloration (cyanosis) in the fingers or toes or if the garment's seams and zippers leave deep, red impressions more than 10 minutes after removing the garment.

than age 2. Of increased concern are burns of the patient's hands, feet, or genitalia, and burns that cover 10% or more of an adult's body, 5% or more of a child's.

Systemic problems can complicate burns. These include renal, respiratory, GI, and other disorders that compromise the patient's ability to compensate for fluid shifts and to resist infection (such as diabetes mellitus, congestive heart failure, and cirrhosis).

An overly dry wound suggests dehydration, and a purulent wound or a green-grey exudate indicates infection. Suspect septicemia with a blue-black wound edge, cellulitis with a swollen red edge, and fungal infection with a white, powdery wound. Healthy granulation tissue appears clean, pinkish, faintly shiny, and free of exudate.

Blisters protect underlying tissue, so leave them intact and protected as long as they don't impede joint motion, become infected, or cause the patient discomfort. Keep in mind that the patient with healing burns has greater nutritional needs. He'll require extra proteins and carbohydrates *to accommodate an almost doubled basal metabolism.*

If you must manage a burn with topical medication, exposure to air, and no dressing, watch for such problems

as wound adherence to bed linens, poor drainage control, and partial loss of topical medications.

Home care
Begin discharge planning as soon as the patient enters the hospital *to help the patient make a smooth transition from the burn unit to home. To encourage therapeutic compliance,* prepare the patient for scarring, teach about wound management and pain control, and urge him to follow the prescribed exercise regimen. Provide encouragement and emotional support. Teach the patient's family or caregivers how to encourage, support, and care for him. (See *Successful burn care after discharge.*)

Complications
Infection is the most common burn complication.

Documentation
Record the date and time of all care provided. Describe wound condition, special dressing-change techniques, topical medications administered, positioning of the burned area, and the patient's tolerance of the procedure.

Biological dressings

TYPE	DESCRIPTION AND USES	NURSING CONSIDERATIONS
Cadaver (homograft)	• Obtained at autopsy up to 24 hours after death • Available as fresh cryopreserved homografts in tissue banks nationwide • Applied by the doctor to debrided untidy wounds • Provides protection, especially to granulation tissue after escharotomy • May be used in some patients as a test graft for autografting • Covers excised wounds immediately	• Observe for exudate. • Watch for signs of rejection. • Keep in mind that the gauze dressing may be removed every 8 hours to observe the graft.
Pigskin (heterograft or xenograft)	• Applied by the nurse • Comes fresh or frozen in rolls or sheets • Can cover and protect debrided untidy wounds, mesh autografts, clean (eschar-free) partial-thickness burns, and exposed tendons	• Reconstitute frozen form with normal saline solution 30 minutes before use. • Watch for signs of rejection. • Cover with gauze dressing or leave exposed to air, as ordered. • Note that pigskin dressings are typically changed every 2 to 5 days.
Amniotic membrane (homograft)	• Available from the obstetric department • Must be sterile and come from an uncomplicated birth • Bacteriostatic condition doesn't require antimicrobials • May be used to protect partial-thickness burns or (temporarily) granulation tissue before autografting • Applied by the doctor to clean wounds only	• The membrane will be changed every 48 hours. • Cover the membrane with a gauze dressing or leave exposed as ordered. • If you apply a gauze dressing, change it every 48 hours.
Biobrane (biosynthetic membrane)	• Comes in sterile, prepackaged sheets in various sizes and in glove form for hand burns • Applied by the nurse • Used to cover donor graft sites, superficial partial-thickness burns, debrided wounds awaiting autograft, or meshed autograft • Provides significant pain relief	• Leave the membrane in place for 3 to 14 days, possibly longer. • Do not use this dressing for preparing a granulation bed for subsequent autografting.

Biological burn dressings

Biological dressings provide a temporary protective covering for burn wounds and for clean granulation tissue. They also temporarily secure fresh skin grafts and protect graft donor sites. In common use are three organic materials and one synthetic material: pigskin, cadaver skin, amniotic membrane, and Biobrane. (See *Biological dressings*.) Besides stimulating new skin growth, these dressings act like normal skin: they minimize fluid, electrolyte, and protein losses; reduce heat loss; and block infection.

A doctor will apply amniotic membrane or fresh cadaver skin to the patient in the operating room. The nurse may apply pigskin or Biobrane to small wounds. Before applying a biological dressing, the caregiver must clean and debride the wound. The frequency of dressing changes will depend on the type of wound and the dressing's specific function.

Equipment

Ordered analgesic ▪ cap ▪ mask ▪ two pairs of sterile gloves ▪ sterile or clean gown ▪ shoe covers ▪ biological dressing ▪ normal saline solution ▪ sterile basin ▪ 18″ × 18″ fine-mesh gauze (impregnated with a topical medication, if ordered) ▪ elastic gauze dressing ▪ stockinette or elastic bandage ▪ sterile forceps ▪ sterile scissors ▪ sterile hemostats.

Preparation of equipment

Place the biological dressing in the sterile basin (or open the Biobrane package). Using aseptic technique, open the sterile dressing packages. Arrange the equipment on the dressing cart and keep the cart readily accessible. Be sure the treatment area has adequate light *to allow accurate wound assessment and dressing placement.*

Implementation

• If this is the patient's first treatment, explain the procedure *to allay fears and promote cooperation.* Provide privacy.

• If ordered, administer an analgesic to the patient 20 minutes before beginning the procedure, or give an analgesic I.V. immediately before the procedure *to increase the patient's comfort and tolerance levels.*

• Wash your hands and put on cap, mask, gown (clean if in a burn unit, sterile if not), shoe covers, and sterile gloves.

• Clean and debride the wound *to reduce bacteria.* Change to a fresh pair of sterile gloves.

• Place the dressing directly on the wound surface. Apply pigskin dermal (shiny) side down; apply Biobrane nylon-backed (dull) side down.

• Roll the dressing directly onto the skin, if applicable.

• Place the dressing strips so that the edges touch but don't overlap. Use sterile forceps if necessary.

• Smooth the dressing. Eliminate folds and wrinkles by rolling out the dressing with the hemostat handle, the forceps handle, or your sterile-gloved hand *to cover the wound completely and ensure adherence.*

• Use the scissors to trim the dressing around the wound *so that the dressing fits the wound without overlapping adjacent areas.*

• Place 18″ × 18″ fine-mesh gauze (impregnated with a topical medication, if ordered) over the biological dressing *to avoid disturbing the biological dressing during the first dressing change.*

• Cover the 18″ × 18″ fine-mesh gauze with an elastic gauze dressing *to hold the biological dressing in place.*

• Put a stockinette bandage over the entire area or wrap the area with an elastic bandage *to protect the dressing layers and to secure them.*

• Position the patient comfortably.

• Remove the dressing cart. Take off gloves, gown, mask, cap, and shoe covers. Discard disposable items according to hospital policy.

Special considerations

Handle the biological dressing as little as possible. The procedure for applying cadaver skin or amniotic membrane is similar. However these dressings are applied in the operating room by the doctor.

Home care

If a discharged patient goes home with a biological dressing, advise him to avoid disturbing it. Inform him that the dressing will slough off in 7 to 10 days or when the wound heals.

If the dressing isn't covered, tell the patient to observe the area daily for redness, swelling, blisters, drainage, and separation. Inform him that he must notify the doctor if signs of infection develop.

Complications

Infection may develop under the dressing. Observe the wound carefully during dressing changes for infection signs. If wound drainage appears purulent, remove the dressing, clean the area with normal saline solution or another prescribed cleaning solution as ordered, and apply a fresh biological dressing.

Suspect an allergic reaction to the dressing if the patient develops a fever within the first 48 hours.

Documentation

Record the time and date of dressing changes. Note areas of application, quality of adherence, and purulent drainage or other infection signs. Also describe the patient's tolerance of the procedure.

Hydrotherapy

Treating diseases or injuries by immersing part or all of the patient's body in water is known as hydrotherapy. Commonly used to debride serious burns and to hasten healing, hydrotherapy also promotes circulation and comfort in patients with peripheral vascular disease and musculoskeletal disorders, such as arthritis. Historically, this therapy has been used to relieve the pain of sprains, strains, and various other complaints. Although hydrotherapy usually involves immersing the patient in a tub of water ("tubbing"), showers or other water-spray techniques may replace tubbing in some hospitals and burn centers. (See *Positioning the patient for hydrotherapy.*)

Positioning the patient for hydrotherapy

To perform hydrotherapy, you'll immerse the patient in a tub or Hubbard tank as shown. Alternatively, you may spray the patient's wounds with water as he lies on a special shower table. Either way, hydrotherapy is traumatic and painful for the burn patient. Provide continual support and encouragement as you proceed.

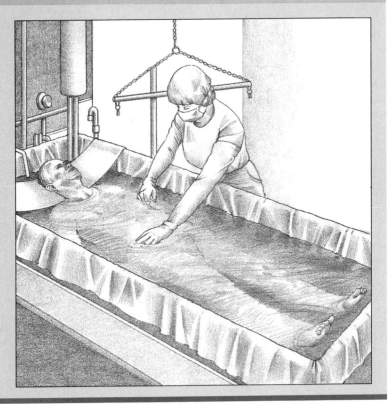

The nurse or physical therapist usually assists the patient into the tub or shower area if he's ambulatory. If he's not ambulatory, he can enter the water by a stretcher or hoist device.

Hydrotherapy is contraindicated if the patient's condition reflects sudden changes, such as fever, electrolyte or fluid imbalance, or unstable vital signs. Immersion isn't recommended for patients with mending fractures, endotracheal tubes, tracheostomy tubes (or other respiratory aids), or for patients with skin grafts less than 5 days old.

Equipment

Water tank or tub or shower table (may be sized for extremities or total body immersion — a Hubbard tank, for example) ▪ plastic tub liner ▪ chemical additives, as ordered ▪ plinth (padded table for patient to sit or lie on while performing exercises) ▪ stretcher ▪ headrest ▪ hydraulic hoist ▪ gown ▪ cap ▪ mask ▪ gloves (for removing dressings) ▪ shoulder-length gloves (for tubbing) ▪ apron ▪ debridement instruments (see "Mechanical debridement" in this chapter) ▪ razor, shaving cream, mild soap, shampoo, washcloth (for general cleaning) ▪ gauze or foam-rubber surgical pads ▪ cotton-tipped applicators ▪ sterile sheets ▪ warm, sterile bath blankets.

Barriers, sheets, and bath blankets may be sterile or clean depending on the patient's condition and your hospital's infection-control policies.

Preparation of equipment

The tub or shower, its equipment, and the tub or shower room must be thoroughly cleaned and disinfected before each treatment *to prevent cross-contamination.* After cleaning, place the tub liner in the tub and fill the tub with warm water between 98° and 104° F (36.6° to 40° C).

Attach the headrest to the sides of the tub. Add prescribed chemicals, such as sodium chloride, *to maintain normal isotonic level (usually 0.9%) and prevent dialysis and tissue irritation.* Also add potassium chloride *to prevent potassium loss,* calcium hypochlorite detergent *to help prevent infection,* and an antifoaming agent *to reduce sudsing during water agitation,* as ordered.

Warm the sterile bath blankets and be sure that the room is warm enough to avoid chilling the patient.

Implementation

• If this is the patient's first treatment, explain the procedure to him *to allay his fears and promote cooperation.* As necessary (before debridement, for example) administer an analgesic about 20 minutes before the procedure.
• Check the patient's vital signs.
• If the patient is receiving an I.V. infusion, be sure that he has enough I.V. solution to last through the procedure.
• If the patient has an indwelling urinary catheter, drain and clamp the tubing *to maintain a closed system and prevent contamination.*
• Transfer the patient to a stretcher, and transport him to the therapy room. Ambulatory patients may walk unassisted to the therapy room if the room is nearby.
• Wash your hands and put on your gown, gloves, mask, and surgical cap.
• Remove the outer dressings and dispose of them properly before immersing the patient. Leave the inner, fine-mesh gauze layer on the wound.
• If the patient's ambulatory, direct him to sit on the plinth for transfer to the tub, or assist him into the tub and situate him on the already lowered plinth.
• If the patient's not ambulatory, attach the stretcher to the overhead hydraulic hoist. Ensure that the hoist hooks are fastened securely. Use the hoist to transfer the patient to and from the tub.
• Lower the patient into the tub. Position him so that the headrest supports his head. Allow him to soak for 3 to 5 minutes.
• Remove your gloves and put on the shoulder-length tubbing gloves and apron.
• Remove remaining gauze dressings, if any, from the patient's wounds.
• If ordered, place the tub's agitator into the water and turn it on. (The motor may burn out if turned on out of water.) Some tubs have aerators to agitate the water.
• Clean all unburned areas first (encourage the patient to do this himself if he can). Wash unburned skin, and clip or shave hair near the wound. Shave facial hair, shampoo the scalp, and give mouth care as appropriate. Provide perineal care, and clean inside the patient's nose and the folds of the ears and eyes with cotton-tipped applicators.
• Gently scrub burned areas with gauze or foam-rubber pads *to remove topical agents, exudates, necrotic tissue, and*

other debris. Debride the wound after turning off the agitator.
• Exercise the patient's extremities with active or passive range of motion, depending on his condition and exercise tolerance. Or have the physical therapist exercise the patient.
• Once you complete the treatment, use the hoist to raise the patient above the water.
• With the patient still suspended over the water, spray-rinse his body *to remove debris from shaving, cleaning, and debridement.*
• Transfer the patient to a stretcher covered with a sterile sheet and bath blanket, and cover him with a warm, sterile sheet (a blanket may be added for warmth). Pat dry unburned areas and warm him *to prevent chilling.*
• Remove the wet or damp linens, and cover the patient with dry linens. Remove your gown, gloves, and mask before transporting the patient to the dressing area for further debridement, if needed, and new sterile dressings.
• Have the tub drained, cleaned, and disinfected according to hospital policy.

Special considerations

Remain with the patient at all times, *to prevent accidents in the tub.* Limit hydrotherapy to 20 or 30 minutes. Watch the patient closely for adverse reactions. Take care to position body parts carefully *because edema may develop if a body part dangles for too long in warm water.*

Patients with endotracheal tubes may receive hydrotherapy but cannot be immersed in the tub. Instead, spray their wounds while they remain on a plinth suspended over the tub. Immerse patients with long-standing tracheostomies only if you have a doctor's order.

If necessary, weigh the patient during hydrotherapy *to assess nutritional status, possible electrolyte imbalance, and fluid shift.* Use a hoist that has a table scale.

Complications

Incomplete disinfection of tub, drains, and faucets, or cross-contamination from members of the tubbing team may cause infection. The patient may chill easily from decreased resistance to temperature changes. And a fluid or electrolyte imbalance (or both) may result from a chemical imbalance between the patient and the tub solution. For example, if the bath solution contains insufficient sodium chloride, osmotic action may cause dialysis.

Documentation

Record the date, time, and patient's reaction to hydrotherapy. Note the patient's condition (vital signs and wound appearance). Document any wound infection or bleeding. Note treatments given, such as debridement and dressing changes. Record any special treatments in the nursing care plan.

Mechanical debridement

Debridement involves removing necrotic tissue by mechanical, chemical, or surgical means to allow underlying healthy tissue to regenerate. Mechanical debridement procedures include irrigation, hydrotherapy, and excising dead tissue with forceps and scissors. The procedure may be done at bedside or in a specially prepared room.

Depending on the type of burn, a combination of debridement techniques may be used. Besides mechanical methods, they may include chemical debridement (with wound-cleaning beads or topical agents that absorb exudate and debris) or surgical excision and skin grafting (usually reserved for deep burns or ulcers). Typically, the patient receives a local or general anesthetic.

Burn wound debridement removes eschar (hardened, dead tissue). This prevents or controls infection, promotes healing, and prepares the wound surface to receive a graft. Ideally, the wound should be debrided daily during the dressing change. Frequent, regular debridement guards against possible hemorrhage resulting from more extensive and forceful debridement. What's more, it reduces the need to conduct extensive debridement under anesthesia.

Closed blisters over partial-thickness burns should not be debrided. (For additional information, see "Hydrotherapy" in this chapter.)

Equipment

Ordered pain medication ▪ two pairs of sterile gloves ▪ two gowns or aprons (clean if the procedure takes place in a burn unit, sterile if elsewhere) ▪ mask ▪ cap ▪ sterile scissors ▪ sterile forceps ▪ 4″ × 4″ sterile gauze pads ▪ sterile solutions and medications as ordered ▪ hemostatic agent, as ordered.

Be sure to have the following equipment immediately available to control hemorrhage: ▪ needle holder ▪ gut suture with needle.

Preparation of equipment

Assemble all supplies. Check expiration dates on sterile solutions and medications.

Implementation

• Explain the procedure to the patient *to allay his fears and promote cooperation.* Teach distraction and relaxation techniques, as possible, *to minimize his discomfort.*

• Provide privacy. Administer an analgesic 20 minutes before debridement begins, or give an I.V. analgesic immediately before the procedure.

• Keep the patient warm. Expose only the area to be debrided *to prevent chilling and fluid and electrolyte loss.*

• Wash your hands and put on cap, mask, gown, or apron (clean if the procedure occurs in a burn unit, sterile if not), and sterile gloves.

• Remove the burn dressings and clean the wound (for detailed directions, see "Burn care" in this chapter).

• Remove your gown or apron and dirty gloves, and change to another gown or apron (again, clean if in a burn unit, sterile if not) and sterile gloves.

• Lift loosened edges of eschar with forceps. Use the blunt edge of scissors or forceps to probe the eschar. Cut the dead tissue from the wound with the scissors. Leave a ¼″ (0.6-cm) edge on remaining eschar *to avoid cutting into viable tissue.*

• Because debridement removes only dead tissue, bleeding should be minimal. If bleeding occurs, apply gentle pressure on the wound with sterile, 4″ × 4″ gauze pads. Then apply the hemostatic agent. If bleeding persists, notify the doctor, and maintain pressure on the wound until he arrives. Excessive bleeding or spurting vessels may require ligation.

• Perform additional procedures, such as application of topical medications and dressing replacements, as ordered.

Special considerations

Work quickly with an assistant, if possible, to complete this painful procedure as soon as possible. Acknowledge the patient's discomfort and provide emotional support. Debride no more than a 4″ (10-cm) square area at one time. Keep the procedure time to 20 minutes or less, if possible.

Complications

Because burns damage or destroy the protective skin barrier, infection may develop despite aseptic techniques and equipment. And some blood loss may occur if debridement exposes an eroded blood vessel or if you inadvertently cut a vessel. Fluid and electrolyte imbalances may result from exudate lost during the procedure.

Documentation

Record the date and time of wound debridement, the area debrided, and solutions and medications used. Describe wound condition, noting signs of infection or skin breakdown. Record the patient's tolerance of and reaction to the procedure. Note indications for additional therapy.

Skin graft care

A skin graft consists of healthy skin taken either from the patient (autograft) or a donor (allograft) and applied to a part of the patient's body. There the graft resurfaces an area damaged by burns, traumatic injury, or surgery. Care procedures for an autograft or an allograft are essentially the same. However, an autograft requires care for two sites: the graft site and the donor site.

The graft itself may be one of several types: split-thickness, full-thickness, or pedicle-flap. (See *Understanding graft types*.) Successful grafting depends on various factors, including clean wound granulation with adequate vascularization; complete contact of the graft with the wound bed; aseptic technique to prevent infection; adequate graft immobilization; and skilled care.

Understanding graft types

A burn patient may receive one or more of the graft types described below.

Split-thickness
The type used most commonly for covering open burns, a split-thickness graft includes the epidermis and part of the dermis. It may be applied as a sheet (usually on the face or neck to preserve the cosmetic result) or as a mesh. A mesh graft has tiny slits cut in that allow the graft to expand up to nine times its original size. Mesh grafts prevent fluids from collecting under the graft and typically are used over extensive full-thickness burns.

Full-thickness
This graft type includes the epidermis and the entire dermis. Consequently, the graft contains hair follicles, sweat glands, and sebaceous glands, which typically aren't included in split-thickness grafts. Full-thickness grafts usually are used for small burns that cause deep wounds.

Pedicle-flap
This full-thickness graft includes not only skin and subcutaneous tissue, but also subcutaneous blood vessels to ensure a continued blood supply to the graft. Pedicle-flap grafts may be used during reconstructive surgery to cover previous defects.

The size and depth of the patient's burns determine whether they will require grafting. Grafting usually occurs at the completion of wound debridement — about 14 to 21 days after the injury. With enzymatic debridement, grafting may be performed 5 to 7 days after debridement is complete; with surgical debridement, grafting can occur the same day as the surgery.

Depending on hospital policy, a doctor or a nurse with special preparation may change graft dressings. Usually they stay in place for 3 to 5 days after surgery to avoid disturbing them. Meanwhile, the donor graft site needs diligent care. (See *How to care for a donor graft site*.)

Equipment
Ordered analgesic ▪ clean and sterile gloves ▪ sterile gown ▪ cap ▪ mask ▪ sterile forceps ▪ sterile scissors ▪ sterile scalpel ▪ sterile 4" × 4" gauze pads ▪ elastic gauze dressing ▪ sterile fine-mesh gauze ▪ warm, normal saline solution ▪ moisturizing cream ▪ topical medication (such as micronized silver sulfadiazine cream) ▪ optional: sterile cotton-tipped applicators.

Preparation of equipment
Assemble the equipment on the dressing cart.

Implementation
• Explain the procedure to the patient and provide privacy. Administer an analgesic, as ordered, 20 to 30 minutes before beginning the procedure. Alternatively, give an I.V. analgesic immediately before the procedure.
• Wash your hands.
• Put on the sterile gown and the clean mask, cap, and gloves.
• Gently lift off all outer dressings. Soak the middle dressings with warm saline solution. Remove these carefully and slowly *to avoid disturbing the graft site*. Leave the first-layer dressing of fine-mesh gauze intact *to avoid dislodging the graft*.
• Remove and discard the clean gloves and put on the sterile gloves.
• Assess the condition of the graft. If you see purulent drainage, notify the doctor.
• Remove the first layer of fine-mesh gauze with sterile forceps and clean the area gently. If necessary, soak the gauze with the warm saline solution *to facilitate removal.*
• Inspect an allograft for signs of rejection, such as infection and delayed healing.
• Inspect a sheet graft frequently for blebs. If ordered, evacuate them carefully with a sterile scalpel. (See *Evacuating fluid from a sheet graft*, page 652.)
• Place fresh mesh gauze saturated with the ordered topical agent over the site *to promote wound healing and*

prevent infection. Cover this with an elastic gauze dressing.

• Clean any completely healed areas and apply a moisturizing cream to them *to keep the skin pliable and to retard scarring.*

Special considerations

To avoid dislodging the graft, hydrotherapy should be discontinued, as ordered, usually for 3 to 4 days after grafting. Avoid using a blood pressure cuff over the graft. Don't tug or pull dressings during dressing changes. Keep the patient from lying on the graft.

If the graft dislodges, apply sterile skin compresses *to keep the area moist until the surgeon reapplies the graft.* If the graft affects an arm or a leg, elevate the affected extremity *to reduce postoperative edema.* Check for bleeding and signs of neurovascular impairment — increasing pain, numbness or tingling, coolness, and pallor.

Teach the patient how to apply moisturizing cream. Emphasize the importance of using a sunscreen on all grafted areas *to avoid sunburn and discoloration.*

Complications

Graft failure may result from traumatic injury, hematoma or seroma formation, infection, an inadequate graft bed, or rejection.

Documentation

Record the time and date of all dressing changes. Document all medications used, and note the patient's response to the medications. Describe the condition of the graft and note any signs of infection or rejection. Record any additional treatment, and note the patient's reaction to the graft.

OTHER LESIONS
Ultraviolet light therapy

Ultraviolet (UV) light reduces basal cell proliferation by suppressing mitosis. As a result, such skin conditions as psoriasis, mycosis fungoides, atopic dermatitis, and uremic pruritus may respond to therapy that uses timed exposure to UV light rays.

UV light comprises various wavelengths, none of which are visible to the human eye and each of which affects skin somewhat differently. UVA, the shortest UV wavelength, has no known effect on skin. UVB, which includes the middle UV wavelengths, causes sunburn. And UVC, which includes the longest UV wavelengths, is lethal to

---

How to care for a donor graft site

Autografts are usually taken from another area of the patient's body with a dermatome. This instrument cuts uniform, split-thickness skin portions — typically, about 0.005″ to 0.02″ (0.013 to 0.05 cm) thick. Essentially, autografting makes the donor site a partial-thickness wound, which may bleed, drain, and cause pain.

This site needs scrupulous care *to prevent infection that could convert the site to a full-thickness wound.* Depending on the graft's thickness, tissue may be obtained from the donor site again in as few as 10 days.

Usually, you can apply a transparent dressing (such as Op-Site or Tegaderm) to a small donor site. For larger sites, a biological dressing may give effective protection.

Care for the donor site as you care for the autograft, using dressing changes at the initial stages *to prevent infection and promote healing.* Follow the guidelines below.

Dressing the wound

• Choose a dressing 1½″ to 2″ (3.8 to 5 cm) larger than the donor site *to cover the wound adequately.*
• Wash your hands and put on sterile gloves.
• Clean the wound periphery with an antibacterial solution, if ordered.
• Apply the transparent film dressing snugly, and smooth away wrinkles.
• Apply a pressure dressing (or elastic wrap) for 24 hours *to reduce fluid accumulation and wound exudate.*
• Leave small amounts of fluid accumulation alone. Using aseptic technique, aspirate larger amounts through the dressing with a small-gauge needle and syringe. After aspiration, patch the needle hole with a small transparent dressing.
• Apply a lanolin-based cream daily to completely healed donor sites *to keep skin tissue pliable and to remove crusts.*

---

plants and animals. Fortunately, the atmospheric ozone layer filters this light, preventing it from reaching the earth's surface.

The drug methoxsalen, a psoralens agent, creates artificial sensitivity to UVA. It does this by binding with the deoxyribonucleic acid in epidermal basal cells. Treating skin with a photosensitizing agent, such as meth-

Evacuating fluid from a sheet graft

When small pockets of fluid (called blebs) accumulate beneath a sheet graft, you'll need to evacuate the fluid using a sterile scalpel and cotton-tipped applicators. First, carefully perforate the center of the bleb with the scalpel.

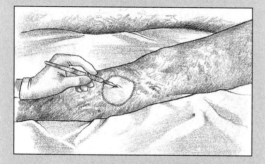

Gently express the fluid with cotton-tipped applicators.

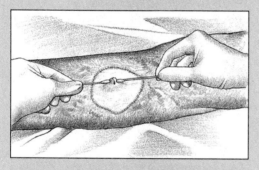

Never express fluid by rolling the bleb to the edge of the graft. This would disturb healing in other areas.

oxsalen, and UVA is called PUVA therapy (or photochemotherapy). Administered before a UV light treatment, methoxsalen photosensitizes the skin to enhance therapeutic effect.

Other drugs used in photochemotherapy include etretinate (Tegison) — an oral vitamin A derivative — and topical preparations, such as crude coal tar ointment (Goeckerman therapy) or carbonis detergens, a coal tar derivative.

Contraindications to PUVA and UVB therapy include photosensitivity diseases, use of photosensitivity-induc-

ing drugs, history of skin cancer, previous skin irradiation (which can induce skin cancer), and cataracts or cataract surgery.

Equipment
For UVA radiation: fluorescent black-light lamp ■ high-intensity UVA fluorescent bulbs.

For UVB radiation: fluorescent sunlamp or hot quartz lamp ■ sunlamp bulbs.

For all UV treatments: oral or topical phototherapeutic medications if necessary ■ body-sized light chamber or smaller light box ■ dark, polarized goggles ■ sunscreen if necessary ■ hospital gown ■ towels.

Preparation of equipment
The patient can have UV light therapy in the hospital, a doctor's office, or at home. Typically set into a reflective cabinet, the light source comprises a bank of high-intensity fluorescent bulbs. (At home, the patient may use a small fluorescent sunlamp.)

Check the doctor's orders to confirm the light treatment type and dose. For PUVA, the initial dose is usually 0.5 joules/cm^2, which requires between 1 and 8 minutes of exposure depending on the patient's skin type and pigmentation. The doctor calculates the UVB dose based on exposure duration and distance from the light source to ensure maximal dermatologic benefit with minimal adverse effect.

Implementation
• Inform the patient that UV light treatments produce a mild sunburn that will help reduce or resolve skin lesions.
• Review the patient's health history *for contraindications to UV light therapy.* Also ask if he's currently taking photosensitizing drugs, such as anticonvulsants, certain antihypertensives, phenothiazines, salicylates, sulfonamides, tetracyclines, tretinoin, and various cancer drugs.
• If the patient will have PUVA therapy, be sure he took methoxsalen (with food) 2 hours before treatment.
• To begin therapy, instruct the patient to disrobe and put on a hospital gown. Have him remove the gown or expose just the treatment area once he's in the phototherapy unit. Be sure that he wears goggles *to protect his eyes* and a sunscreen, towels, or the hospital gown *to protect vulnerable skin areas.*
• If the patient's having local UVB treatment, position him at the correct distance from the light source. For instance, for facial treatment with a sunlamp, position the patient's face 12" (30.5 cm) from the lamp. For body treatment, position the patient's body about 30" (76 cm) from either the sunlamp or the hot quartz lamp.
• During therapy, be sure the patient wears goggles at all times. And if you're observing him through light-

chamber windows, you should wear goggles, too. If the patient must stand for the treatment, ask him to report any dizziness *to ensure his safety.*

• After delivering the prescribed UVB dose, help the patient out of the unit.

Special considerations
Overexposure to UV light (sunburn) can result from prolonged treatment and an inadequate distance between the patient and light source. It can also result from use of photosensitizing drugs or overly sensitive skin.

Prevent eye damage by using gray or green polarized lenses during UVB therapy or UV-opaque sunglasses during PUVA therapy. The patient undergoing PUVA therapy should wear these glasses after treatment because methoxsalen can cause photosensitivity.

Tell the patient to look for marked erythema, blistering, peeling, or other signs of overexposure 4 to 6 hours after UVB and 24 to 48 hours after UVA therapy. In either case, the erythema should disappear within another 24 hours. Inform him that mild dryness and desquamation will occur in 1 or 2 days. Advise him to notify the doctor if overexposure occurs. Typically, the doctor recommends stopping treatment for a few days and then starting over at a lower exposure level.

Before administering methoxsalen or etretinate, check to ensure that baseline liver function studies have been done. Keep in mind that *both drugs are hepatotoxic agents and are never given together.*

If the doctor prescribes tar preparations with UVB treatment, watch for signs of sensitivity, such as erythema, pruritus, or eczematous reactions. If you apply carbonis detergens to the patient's skin before UV light therapy, be sure to remove it completely with mineral oil just before treatment begins *to allow the light to penetrate the skin properly.*

Home care
Encourage the patient to use emollients and drink plenty of fluids *to combat dry skin and maintain adequate hydration.* Warn him to avoid hot baths or showers and to use soap sparingly. *Heat and soap promote dry skin.*

Review your PUVA patient's methoxsalen dosage schedule. Explain that deviating from it could result in burns or ineffective treatment. Urge him to wear appropriate sunglasses outdoors for at least 12 hours after taking methoxsalen. Similarly, recommend yearly eye examinations *to detect possible cataract formation.*

Instruct the patient to notify his doctor before taking any medication, including aspirin, *to prevent heightened photosensitivity.*

If the patient uses a sunlamp at home, advise him to let the lamp warm for 5 minutes before treatment. Then stress that he expose his skin to the light for the exact time prescribed by the doctor. Instruct the patient to protect his eyes with goggles and to use a dependable timer or have someone else time his therapy. Above all, urge him never to use the sunlamp when he's tired *to avoid falling asleep under the lamp and sustaining a burn.*

Discuss first aid for localized burning: Apply cool water soaks for 20 minutes or until skin temperature cools. For more extensive burns, recommend tepid tap water baths after notifying the doctor about the burn. After the patient bathes, suggest using an oil-in-water moisturizing lotion (not a petroleum-jelly-based product that can trap radiant heat).

Tell the patient to limit natural-light exposure, to use a sunscreen when he's outdoors, and to notify his doctor immediately if he discovers any unusual skin lesions. Instruct the patient having PUVA therapy to report the absence of erythema, which suggests that the doctor needs to increase the methoxsalen dosage.

Advise the patient to avoid contact with harsh soaps and chemicals, such as paints and solvents, and to discuss ways to manage physical and psychological stress, which may exacerbate skin disorders.

Complications
Septicemia may result from impaired skin integrity. Be alert for changes in vital signs and severe skin irritation. Long-term treatment effects are similar to those from excessive sun exposure: skin atrophy and aging and an increased risk for skin cancer. The patient can minimize adverse effects by using emollients, sunscreens, and cover-ups.

Documentation
Record the date and time of initial and subsequent treatments, the UV wavelength used, and the name and dose of any oral or topical medications given. Record the exact duration of therapy, the distance between the light source and the skin, and the patient's tolerance of the treatment. Note safety measures used, such as eye protection. Also describe the patient's skin condition before and after treatment. Note improvements and adverse reactions, such as increased pruritus, oozing, or scaling.

 # Laser therapy

Using the highly focused and intense energy of a laser beam, the surgeon can treat various skin lesions. Laser surgery has several advantages. As a surgical instrument, the laser offers precise control. It spares normal tissue, speeds healing, and deters infection by sterilizing the operative site. What's more, by sealing tiny blood vessels as it vaporizes tissue, the laser beam leaves a nearly bloodless operative field. And the procedure can be performed on an outpatient basis.

The two lasers used most commonly to treat skin lesions are the argon and carbon dioxide (CO_2) lasers. The argon laser emits a blue or green light that's readily absorbed by the red pigment of hemoglobin. Therefore, blood vessels absorb much more energy from the argon laser than do surrounding tissues. As the vascular tissue absorbs the laser energy, the small blood vessels coagulate, ablating superficial vascular lesions but leaving surrounding tissues nearly unaffected.

An important argon laser application includes removing port wine stains, which are otherwise untreatable. In addition, the argon laser's relatively superficial action makes it useful for removing birthmarks, tattoos, hemangiomas, and keloids.

Less selective than the argon laser, the CO_2 laser is absorbed by water in the cells and tissues. Besides treating port wine stains, facial telangiectases, spider angiomas, and tattoos (like the argon laser), the CO_2 laser also destroys warts and tumors.

In general, laser surgery is safe, although bleeding and scarring can result. One pronounced hazard—to the patient and treatment staff alike—is eye damage or other injury caused by unintended laser beam reflection. For this reason, anyone in the surgical suite, including the patient, must wear special goggles to filter laser light. And the surgeon must use special nonreflective instruments. Access to the room must be strictly controlled, and all windows must be covered.

Equipment
Argon or CO_2 laser ▪ filtration face masks ▪ protective eyewear ▪ smoke evacuator (vacuum) ▪ extra vacuum filters ▪ antibiotic ointment ▪ surgical drape ▪ sterile gauze ▪ nonadherent dressings ▪ surgical tape ▪ cotton-tipped applicators ▪ hydrogen peroxide solution ▪ nonreflective surgical instruments ▪ gowns, masks, and gloves.

Preparation of equipment
Before the procedure begins, prepare the tray. It should include a local anesthetic, as ordered, and dry and wet gauze. The gauze will be used to control bleeding, protect healthy tissue, and abrade and remove any eschar, which would otherwise inhibit laser absorption. Prepare surgical instruments as needed.

Implementation
• Tell the patient how the laser works and name its benefits. Point out the equipment and outline the procedure *to help allay the patient's concerns.*
• Just before the surgeon begins, position the patient comfortably, drape him, and place protective gauze around the operative site. Confirm that everyone in the room—including the patient—has safety goggles on *to filter the laser light.*
• Lock the door to the surgical suite *to keep unprotected persons from inadvertently entering the room.*
• After the surgeon administers the anesthetic and it takes effect, activate the laser vacuum. The CO_2 laser has a vacuum hose attached to a separate apparatus. Use this apparatus *to clear the surgical site.* The vacuum has a filter that traps and collects most of the vaporized tissue. Change the filter whenever suction decreases, and follow your hospital's guidelines for filter disposal.
• When the surgeon finishes the procedure, apply direct pressure with a sterile gauze pad to any bleeding wound for 20 minutes. (Wear sterile gloves.) If the wound continues to bleed, notify the doctor.
• Once the bleeding is controlled, use sterile technique to clean the area with a cotton-tipped applicator dipped in the prescribed cleaning solution. Then size and cut a nonadherent dressing. Spread a thin layer of antibiotic ointment on one side of the dressing. Place the ointment side over the wound and secure the dressing with surgical tape.

Special considerations
The surgeon uses the laser beam much as he would a scalpel to excise the lesion. Explain that the laser causes a burnlike wound that can be deep. Tell the patient the wound will appear charred. Also, inform the patient that some of the eschar will be removed during the initial postoperative cleaning, and that more will gradually dislodge at home.

Warn the patient to expect a burning odor and smoke during the procedure. A machine called a smoke evacuator, which sounds like a vacuum cleaner, will clear it away. Advise the patient that he may sense heat from the laser. Urge him to tell the doctor at once if pain develops.

Home care
Teach the patient how to dress his wound daily as ordered by the surgeon. Tell him that he can take showers but that he must not immerse the wound site in water *to promote wound healing and prevent infection.*

If the wound bleeds at home, demonstrate how to apply direct pressure on the site with clean gauze or a washcloth for 20 minutes. If pressure doesn't control the bleeding, tell the patient to call his doctor.

If the patient's foot or leg was operated on, urge him to keep the extremity elevated and to use it as little as possible *because pressure can inhibit healing.*

Warn the patient to protect the wound from exposure to the sun *to avoid changes in pigmentation.* Tell him to call the doctor if a fever of 100° F (37.8° C) or higher persists longer than 1 day.

Complications

Rarely, bleeding, scarring, and infection may follow laser surgery.

Documentation

Most patients who have laser surgery for skin lesions are treated as outpatients. Note the patient's skin condition before and after the procedure. Also document any bleeding, record the type of dressing applied, and list the patient's complaints of pain. Note whether the patient comprehends home care instructions.

Selected references

Alvarez, O., et al. "Moist Environment for Healing: Matching the Dressing to the Wound," *Wounds: A Compendium of Clinical Research and Practice* 1:35, 1989.

Atwater, E. "Care of the Surgically Created Granulating Wound," *Dermatology Nursing* 1:43, 1989.

Bayley, E. "Wound Healing in the Patient with Burns," *Nursing Clinics of North America* 25(1):205-22, March 1990.

Boswick, J., ed. *The Art and Science of Burn Care.* Rockville, Md.: Aspen Pubs., Inc., 1987.

Fowler, E. "Equipment and Products Used in Management and Treatment of Pressure Ulcers," *Nursing Clinics of North America* 22(2):449-61, June 1987.

Gosnell, D. "Assessment and Evaluation of Pressure Sores," *Nursing Clinics of North America* 22(2):399-415, June 1987.

Hess, C., and Miller, P. "The Management of Open Wounds: Acute and Chronic," *Ostomy/Wound Management* 31:58-69, November-December 1990.

Illustrated Manual of Nursing Practice. Springhouse, Pa.: Springhouse Corp., 1991

International Association for Enterostomal Therapy. *Standards of Care, Dermal Wounds: Pressure Sores.* Irvine, Calif.: IAET, 1990.

Lehr, P. "Surgical Lasers," *AORN Journal* 50(5):972-77, November 1989.

Martin, L. "Nursing Implications of Today's Burn Care Techniques," *RN* 52(5):26-33, May 1989.

Motta, G. "Calcium Alginate Topical Wound Dressings: A New Dimension in the Cost-effective Treatment for Exudating Dermal Wounds and Pressure Sores," *Ostomy/Wound Management* 25:52-56, Winter 1989.

Nursing92 Drug Handbook. Springhouse, Pa.: Springhouse Corp., 1992.

Porth, C., ed. *Pathophysiology: Concepts of Altered Health States,* 3rd ed. Philadelphia: J.B. Lippincott Co., 1990.

Preston, K. "Dermal Ulcers: Simplifying a Complex Problem," *Rehabilitation Nursing* 12(1):17-21, January 1987.

Tan, O., et al. "Treatment of Children with Port-Wine Stains Using the Flashlight-pulsed Tunable Dye Laser," *New England Journal of Medicine,* 320(7):416-21, February 16, 1989.

Thomas, C. "Nursing Alert: Wound Healing Halted with the Use of Povidone-Iodine," *Ostomy/Wound Management* 18:30-33, Spring 1988.

Thomason, S. "Pressure Ulcers: Considerations of Intervention Strategies," *Ostomy/Wound Management* 19:48-54, Summer 1988.

Trelease, C. "Developing Standards for Wound Care," *Ostomy/Wound Management* 20:46-56, Fall 1988.

Van Dover, D. "Topical Wound Management: To Betadine or Not to Betadine?" *Ostomy/Wound Management* 32:40-41, January-February 1991.

Wilkerson, N. "Treating Hyperbilirubinemia," *MCN* 14(1):32-36, January-February 1989.

EYE, EAR, AND NOSE CARE

REBECCA McCASKEY, RN, BA, MEd

Always provide thorough explanations. A simple fact or tip that seems, to you, almost too obvious to mention may actually offer valuable insight to the patient. When the patient leaves you, he should be better able to prevent, cope with, and manage not only the sensory disorder he has, but also any that could arise in the future.

Introduction

Because the eyes transmit about 70% of the sensory information reaching the brain, visual impairment can severely limit a patient's ability to function independently and to perceive and react to his surroundings. Similarly, untreated hearing loss can drastically impair communication and social interaction. Inner-ear disorders may disrupt equilibrium and the ability to move freely. And nasal disorders can interfere with respiration, reduce vitality, and cause marked discomfort.

When caring for a patient with a sensory loss, remember that he's actually experiencing multiple impairments. That's because sensory impairment brings about perceptual impairment. The combined loss significantly alters a person's daily activities and threatens his security and self-image.

Because eye, ear, and nose disorders are as common as they are troublesome, you're likely to perform the procedures presented in this chapter whether you practice in a hospital, clinic, extended-care facility, or other setting. You may be called on to assist with or perform eye, ear, or nose procedures in situations ranging from emergencies to routine checkups. These procedures call for the utmost care and precision to prevent infection and injury and to preserve function.

Overcome perceptual barriers

Performing procedures that diagnose, treat, or even briefly cause sensory impairment requires you to give clear, simple instructions and explanations. You'll also need to give ample reassurance to a patient who's certain to feel apprehensive about his ability to care for himself and function independently. In an emergency, effective communication becomes even more important because you'll be dealing with a patient suddenly disoriented by sensory and perceptual impairments.

Provide clear patient teaching

You can make an important contribution to the patient's understanding of eye, ear, and nasal disorders. As you implement various procedures, inform your patient about preventive care measures. Help him to recognize signs and symptoms of sensory disorders. Urge him to schedule regular examinations to detect problems early. And remind him to use safety equipment at work and, as appropriate, at home.

EYE CARE
Hot and cold eye compresses

Whether applied hot or cold, eye compresses are soothing and therapeutic. Hot compresses may be used to relieve discomfort. Because heat increases circulation (which enhances absorption and decreases inflammation), hot compresses may promote drainage of superficial infections. On the other hand, cold compresses can reduce swelling or bleeding and relieve itching. Because cold numbs sensory fibers, cold compresses may be ordered to ease periorbital discomfort between prescribed doses of pain medication. Typically, a hot or cold compress should be applied for 20-minute periods, four to six times a day. Ocular infection calls for the use of aseptic technique.

Equipment

For hot compresses: gloves ■ prescribed solution, usually sterile water or normal saline solution ■ sterile bowl ■ sterile 4″ × 4″ gauze pads ■ towel.

For cold compresses: small plastic bag (such as a sandwich bag) or glove ■ ice chips ■ ½″ (1.3 cm) nonallergenic tape ■ towel ■ sterile 4″ × 4″ gauze pads ■ sterile water, normal saline solution, or prescribed ophthalmic irrigant ■ gloves.

Preparation of equipment

For hot compresses: Place a capped bottle of sterile water or normal saline solution in a bowl of hot water or under a stream of hot, tap water. Allow the solution to become warm, not hot (no higher than 120° F [49° C]). Pour the warm water or saline solution into a sterile bowl, filling the bowl about halfway. Place some sterile gauze pads in the bowl.

For cold compresses: Place ice chips in a plastic bag (or a glove if necessary) to make an ice pack. Keep the ice pack small *to avoid excessive pressure on the eye.* Remove excess air from the bag or glove and knot the open end. Cut a piece of nonallergenic tape *to secure the ice pack.* Place all equipment on the bedside stand near the patient.

Implementation
• Explain the procedure to the patient, make him comfortable, and provide privacy.
• When applying hot compresses, have the patient sit, if possible. When applying cold compresses, have the patient lie supine. Support his head with a pillow, and turn his head slightly to the unaffected side. *This position will help to hold the compress in place.*
• If the patient has an eye patch, remove it.
• Drape a towel around the patient's shoulders *to catch any spills*. Wash your hands and put on gloves.

To apply hot compresses
• Take two 4″ × 4″ gauze pads from the basin. Squeeze out the excess solution.
• Instruct the patient to close his eyes. Gently apply the pads—one on top of the other—to the affected eye. (If the patient complains that the compress feels too hot, remove it immediately.)
• Change the compress every few minutes, as necessary, for the prescribed length of time. After removing each compress, check the skin for signs that the compress solution is too hot.

To apply cold compresses
• Moisten the middle of one of the sterile 4″ × 4″ gauze pads with the sterile water, normal saline solution, or ophthalmic irrigating solution. *This helps to conduct the cold from the ice pack.* Keep the edges dry *so that they can absorb excess moisture.*
• Tell the patient to close his eyes; then place the moist gauze pad over the affected eye.
• Place the ice pack on top of the gauze pad and tape it in place. If he complains of pain, remove the ice pack. Some patients may have an adverse reaction to cold.
• After 15 to 20 minutes, remove the tape, ice pack, and gauze pad and discard them.

To conclude the procedure
• Use the remaining sterile 4″ × 4″ gauze pads to clean and dry the patient's face.
• If ordered, apply ophthalmic ointment.
• If ordered, apply an eye patch. (See *Applying an eye patch.*)

Special considerations
When applying hot compresses, change the prescribed solution as frequently as necessary *to maintain a constant temperature.*

If ordered to apply moist, cold compresses directly to the patient's eyelid, fill a bowl with ice and water and soak 4″ × 4″ gauze pads in it. Place a compress directly on the lid; change compresses every 2 to 3 minutes.

Home care
When teaching a patient to apply warm compresses at home, explain that he can substitute a clean bowl and washcloth for the sterile equipment.

If both eyes are infected, emphasize using separate equipment for each eye (two bowls of prescribed solution and individual compresses). Inform the patient that this will keep him from passing infection back and forth between eyes. Also direct him to wash his hands thoroughly after treating each eye.

Documentation
Record the time and duration of the procedure. Describe the eye's appearance before and after treatment. Name any ointments (and amounts) or dressings applied to the eye. Also note the patient's tolerance of the procedure.

 # Eye irrigation

Used mainly to flush secretions, chemicals, and foreign bodies from the eye, eye irrigation also provides a way to administer medications for corneal and conjunctival disorders. In an emergency, tap water may serve as an irrigant.

The amount of solution needed to irrigate an eye depends on the contaminant. Secretions require a moderate volume; major chemical burns require a copious amount. Usually, an I.V. bottle or bag of normal saline solution (with I.V. tubing attached) supplies enough solution for continuous irrigation of a chemical burn. (See *Three devices for eye irrigation*, page 660.)

Equipment
Gloves ■ towels ■ eyelid retractor ■ cotton balls or facial tissues ■ optional: litmus paper, proparacaine hydrochloride topical anesthetic.

For moderate-volume irrigation: prescribed sterile ophthalmic irrigant ■ cotton-tipped applicators.

For copious irrigation: one or more 1,000-ml bottles or bags of normal saline solution ■ standard I.V. infusion set without needle.

Commercially prepared bottles of sterile ophthalmic irrigant are available. All solutions should be at body temperature: 98.6° F (37° C).

Preparation of equipment
Read the label on the sterile ophthalmic irrigant. Double-check its sterility, strength, and expiration date.

For moderate-volume irrigation: Remove the cap from the irrigant container and place the container within

Applying an eye patch

With a doctor's order, you may apply an eye patch for various reasons: to protect the eye after injury or surgery, to prevent accidental damage to an anesthetized eye, to promote healing, to absorb secretions, or to prevent the patient from touching or rubbing his eye.

A thicker patch, called a pressure patch, may be used to help corneal abrasions heal, compress postoperative edema, or control hemorrhage from traumatic injury. Application requires an ophthalmologist's prescription and supervision.

To apply a patch, choose a gauze pad of appropriate size for the patient's face, place it gently over the closed eye, and secure it with two or three strips of tape. Extend the tape from midforehead across the eye to below the earlobe.

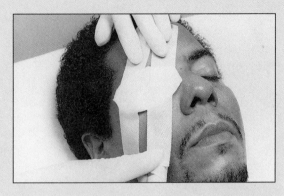

For increased protection of an injured eye, you should place a plastic or metal shield (as shown below) on top of the gauze pads and apply tape over the shield.

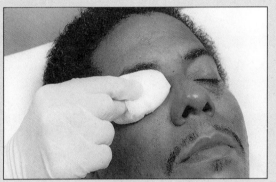

A pressure patch, which is markedly thicker than a single-thickness gauze patch, exerts extra tension against the closed eye. After placing the initial gauze pad, you'll need to build it up with additional gauze pieces (as shown above, at right). Tape it firmly so that the patch exerts even pressure against the closed eye.

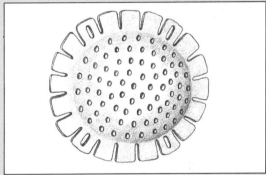

Occasionally, you may use a head dressing to secure a pressure patch. The dressing applies additional pressure or, in burn patients, holds the patch in place without tape.

---

easy reach. (Be sure to keep the tip of the container sterile.)

For copious irrigation: Use sterile technique to set up the I.V. tubing and the bag or bottle of normal saline solution. Hang the container on an I.V. pole, fill the I.V. tubing with the solution, and adjust the drip regulator valve *to ensure an adequate but not forceful flow.* Place all other equipment within easy reach.

Implementation
● Wash your hands, put on gloves, and explain the procedure to the patient. If the patient has a chemical burn, ease his anxiety by explaining that irrigation prevents further damage.
● Assist the patient in lying supine. Turn his head slightly toward the affected side *to prevent solution flowing over his nose and into the other eye.*
● Place a towel under the patient's head, and let him hold another towel against his affected side *to catch excess solution.*

Three devices for eye irrigation

Depending on the type and extent of injury, the patient's eye may need to be irrigated using different devices.

Squeeze bottle

For moderate-volume irrigation—to remove eye secretions, for example—apply sterile ophthalmic irrigant to the eye directly from the squeeze bottle container. Direct the stream at the inner canthus and position the patient so the stream washes across the cornea and exits at the outer canthus.

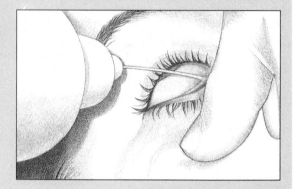

I.V. tube

For copious irrigation—to treat chemical burns, for example—set up an I.V. bag and tubing without a needle. Use the procedure described for moderate irrigation to flush the eye for at least 15 minutes.

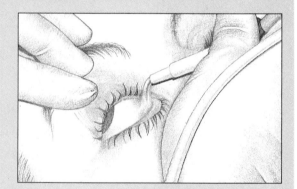

Morgan lens

Connected to irrigation tubing, a Morgan lens permits continuous lavage and also delivers medication to the eye. Use an adapter to connect the lens to the I.V. tubing and the solution container. Begin the irrigation at the prescribed flow rate. To insert the device, ask the patient to look down as you insert the lens under the upper eyelid. Then have her look up as you retract and release the lower eyelid over the lens.

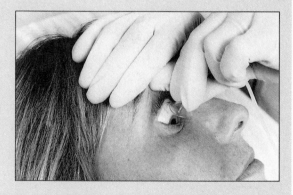

• Using the thumb and index finger of your nondominant hand, separate the patient's eyelids.
• If ordered, instill proparacaine hydrochloride eyedrops *as a comfort measure.* Use them only once *because repeated use retards healing.*
• *To irrigate the conjunctival cul-de-sac,* continue holding the eyelids apart with your thumb and index finger.
• *To irrigate the upper eyelid (the superior fornix)* use an eyelid retractor. Steady the hand holding the retractor by resting it on the patient's forehead. *The retractor prevents the eyelid from closing involuntarily when solution touches the cornea and conjunctiva.*

Moderate irrigation
• Holding the bottle of sterile ophthalmic irrigant about 1″ (2.5 cm) from the eye, direct a constant, gentle stream at the inner canthus *so that the solution flows across the cornea to the outer canthus.*
• Evert the lower eyelid and then the upper eyelid *to inspect for retained foreign particles.*
• Remove any foreign particles by gently touching the the conjunctiva with sterile, wet, cotton-tipped applicators. Do not touch the cornea.
• Resume irrigating the eye until it's clean of all visible foreign particles.

Copious irrigation
• Hold the control valve on the I.V. tubing about 1″ above the eye, and direct a constant, gentle stream of normal saline solution at the inner canthus *so that the solution flows across the cornea to the outer canthus.*
• Ask the patient to rotate his eye periodically while you continue the irrigation. This action may dislodge foreign particles.
• Evert the lower and then the upper eyelid to inspect for retained foreign particles. (This inspection is especially important when the patient has caustic lime in his eye.)

Aftercare
• After eye irrigation, gently dry the eyelids with cotton balls or facial tissues, wiping from the inner to the outer canthus. Use a new cotton ball or tissue for each wipe. *This reduces the patient's need to rub his eye.*
• Remove and discard your gloves.
• When indicated, arrange for follow-up care.
• Wash your hands *to avoid burning from residual chemical contaminants.*

Special considerations
When irrigating both eyes, have the patient tilt his head toward the side being irrigated to avoid cross-contamination.

For chemical burns, irrigate each eye for at least 15 minutes with normal saline solution *to dilute and wash out the harsh chemical.* If the patient can't identify the specific chemical, use litmus paper *to determine if the chemical is acidic or alkaline, or to be sure that the eye has been irrigated adequately.* (After irrigating any chemical, note the time, date, and chemical for your own reference *in case you develop contact dermatitis.*)

Documentation
Note the duration of irrigation, the type and amount of solution, and characteristics of the drainage. Record your assessment of the patient's eye before and after irrigation. Also note his response to the procedure.

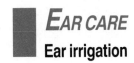

EAR CARE
Ear irrigation

Irrigating the ear involves washing the external auditory canal with a stream of solution to clean the canal of discharges, to soften and remove impacted cerumen, or to dislodge a foreign body. Sometimes, irrigation aims to relieve localized inflammation and discomfort. The procedure must be performed carefully to avoid causing the patient discomfort or vertigo, to prevent maceration of tissue that lines the canal, and to avoid increasing the risk of otitis externa. Because irrigation may contaminate the middle ear if the tympanic membrane is ruptured, an otoscopic examination always precedes ear irrigation.

This procedure is contraindicated when a vegetable foreign body (such as a pea, a bean, or a corn kernel) obstructs the auditory canal. These foreign bodies are *hygroscopic* — that is, they attract and absorb moisture. In contact with an irrigant or other solution, they swell, causing intense pain and complicating removal of the object by irrigation. The procedure is contraindicated also if the patient has a cold, fever, ear infection, or an injured or ruptured tympanic membrane.

Equipment
Ear irrigation syringe (rubber bulb) ▪ otoscope ▪ prescribed irrigant ▪ large basin ▪ linen-saver pad and bath towel ▪ emesis basin ▪ cotton balls or cotton-tipped applicators ▪ 4″ × 4″ gauze pad ▪ optional: adjustable light (such as a gooseneck lamp), container for irrigant, tubing, clamp, and catheter with ear tip.

Wear gloves if you expect contact with infected matter.

How to irrigate the ear canal

Follow these guidelines for irrigating the ear canal.
• Gently pull the auricle up and back *to straighten the ear canal.* (For a child, pull the ear down and back.)
• Have the patient hold an emesis basin beneath the ear to catch returning irrigant. Position the tip of the irrigating syringe at the meatus of the auditory canal. Be sure not to occlude the meatus *because you'll impede backflow and increase pressure in the canal.*

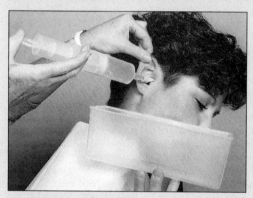

• Point the tip of the syringe upward and toward the posterior ear canal. *This angle prevents damage to the tympanic membrane and also guards against pushing debris farther into the canal.*

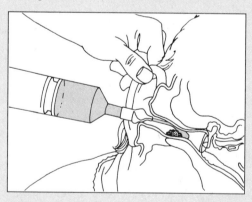

• Direct a steady stream of irrigant against the side of the ear canal and inspect the return fluid for cloudiness, cerumen, blood, or foreign matter.

Preparation of equipment
Select the appropriate syringe, and obtain the prescribed irrigant. Put the container of irrigant into the large basin filled with hot water *to warm the solution to body temperature:* 98.6° F (37° C). Avoid extreme temperature changes *because they can affect inner ear fluids, causing nausea and dizziness.*

Test the temperature of the solution by sprinkling a few drops on your inner wrist. Inspect equipment (syringe or catheter tips) for breaks or cracks; inspect all metal tips for roughness.

Implementation
• Explain the procedure to the patient, provide privacy, wash your hands, and put on gloves (if necessary).
• If you haven't already done so, use the otoscope to inspect the auditory canal to be irrigated.
• Help the patient to a sitting position. *To prevent the solution from running down his neck,* tilt his head slightly forward and toward the affected side. If he can't sit, have him lie on his back and tilt his head slightly forward and toward the affected ear.
• Make sure that you have adequate lighting.
• If the patient is sitting, place the linen-saver pad — covered with the bath towel — on his shoulder and upper arm, under the affected ear. If he's lying down, cover his pillow and the area under the affected ear.
• Have the patient hold the emesis basin close to his head under the affected ear.
• *To avoid getting foreign matter into the ear canal,* clean the auricle and the meatus of the auditory canal with a cotton ball or cotton-tipped applicator moistened with normal saline or the prescribed irrigating solution.
• Draw the irrigant into the syringe and expel any air.
• Straighten the auditory canal; then insert the syringe tip and start the flow. (See *How to irrigate the ear canal.*)
• During the irrigation, observe the patient for signs of pain or dizziness. If he reports either, stop the procedure immediately.
• When the syringe is empty, remove it and inspect the return flow. Then, refill the syringe, and continue the irrigation until the return flow is clear. Never use more than 500 ml of irrigant during this procedure.
• Remove the syringe, and inspect the ear canal for cleanliness with the otoscope.
• Dry the patient's auricle and neck.
• Remove the bath towel and linen-saver pad. Help the seated patient lie on his affected side with the 4″ × 4″ gauze pad under his ear *to promote drainage of residual debris and solution.*

Special considerations

Avoid dropping or squirting irrigant on the tympanic membrane. *This may startle the patient and cause discomfort.* If you're using an irrigating catheter instead of a syringe, adjust the flow of solution to a steady, comfortable rate with a flow clamp. Don't raise the container more than 6″ (15.2 cm) above the ear. *If the container is higher, the resulting pressure may damage the tympanic membrane.*

If the doctor directs you to place a cotton pledget in the ear canal *to retain some of the solution,* pack the cotton loosely. Instruct the patient not to remove it.

If irrigation doesn't dislodge impacted cerumen, the doctor may order you to instill several drops of glycerin, carbamide peroxide (Debrox), or a similar preparation two to three times daily for 2 to 3 days, and then to irrigate the ear again.

Complications

Possible complications include vertigo, nausea, skin maceration, otitis externa, and otitis media (if the patient has a perforated or ruptured tympanic membrane). Forceful instillation of irrigant can rupture the tympanic membrane.

Documentation

Record the date and time of irrigation. Note which ear you irrigated. Also note the volume and the solution used, the appearance of the canal before and after irrigation, the appearance of the return flow, the patient's tolerance of the procedure, and any comments he made about his condition, especially related to his hearing acuity.

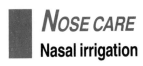

NOSE CARE
Nasal irrigation

Irrigation of the nasal passages with warm normal saline solution soothes irritated mucous membranes and washes away crusted mucus, secretions, and foreign matter. Left unattended, these deposits may impede sinus drainage and airflow and cause headaches, infections, and unpleasant odors. Routine irrigation reduces the infection risk and increases comfort and ease of breathing. Irrigation may be done with a bulb syringe or an electronic oral irrigating device.

Nasal irrigation benefits patients with chronic nasal conditions—such as sinusitis, rhinitis, Wegener's granulomatosis, and Sjögren's syndrome. In addition, it may help long-term users of some inhalant drugs (such as cocaine or nose drops containing phenylephrine chloride) and those who regularly inhale toxins or allergens—paint fumes, sawdust, pesticides, or coal dust, for example.

Contraindications to nasal irrigation may include recent sinus surgery, advanced destruction of the sinuses, frequent nosebleeds, and foreign bodies in the nasal passages (which could be driven farther into the passages by the irrigant). However, some patients with these conditions may benefit from irrigation.

Equipment

Bulb syringe or an oral irrigating device (such as a Water Pik) ▪ rigid or flexible disposable irrigation tips (for one-patient use) ▪ normal saline solution ▪ plastic sheet ▪ apron or towels ▪ facial tissues ▪ bath basin ▪ gloves.

Preparation of equipment

Warm the normal saline solution to about 105° F (40.5° C). If you're irrigating with a bulb syringe, draw some irrigant into the bulb and then expel it. *This will rinse any residual solution from the previous irrigation and warm the bulb.*

If you're using an oral irrigating device, plug the instrument into an electrical outlet in an area near the patient. Then, run about 1 cup of normal saline solution through the tubing *to rinse residual solution from the lines and warm the tubing.* Next, fill the reservoir of the device with warm normal saline solution.

Implementation

• Wash your hands and put on gloves.
• Explain the procedure to the patient.
• Have the patient sit comfortably near the equipment in a position that allows the bulb or catheter tip to enter his nose and the returning irrigant to flow into the bath basin or sink. (See *Positioning the patient for nasal irrigation,* page 664.)
• Remind him to keep his mouth open and to breathe rhythmically during irrigation. *This causes the soft palate to seal the throat, allowing the irrigant to stream out the opposite nostril and carry discharge with it.*
• *Instruct the patient not to speak or swallow during the irrigation to avoid forcing infectious material into the sinuses or eustachian tubes.*
• *To avoid injuring the nasal mucosa,* remove the irrigating tip from the patient's nostril if he has to sneeze or cough.

To use a bulb syringe

• Fill the bulb syringe with normal saline solution and insert the tip about ½″ (1.3 cm) into the patient's nostril.
• Squeeze the bulb until a gentle stream of warm irrigant washes through the nose. Avoid forceful squeezing, *which*

Positioning the patient for nasal irrigation

Whether you're teaching a patient to perform nasal irrigation with a bulb syringe or an oral irrigating device, the irrigation will progress more easily once the patient learns how to hold her head for safety, comfort, and effectiveness.

Help the patient to sit upright with her head bent forward over the basin or sink and well-flexed on her chest. Her nose and ear should be on the same vertical plane.

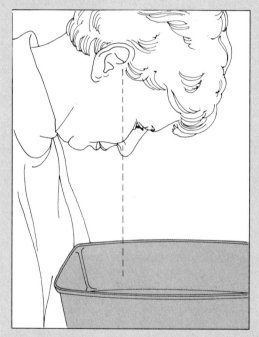

Explain that she's less likely to breathe in the irrigant when holding her head in this position. Additionally, this position should keep the irrigant from entering the eustachian tubes, which will now lie above the level of the irrigation stream.

may drive debris from the nasal passages into the sinuses or eustachian tubes and introduce infection. Alternate nostrils until the return irrigant runs clear.
• Inspect returning irrigant. Changes in color, viscosity, or volume may signal an infection and should be reported to the doctor. Also report blood or necrotic material.

To use an oral irrigation device
• Insert the irrigation tip into the nostril about ½" to 1" (1.3 to 2.5 cm) and turn on the irrigating device. Begin with a low pressure setting (increasing the pressure as needed) *to obtain a gentle stream of irrigant.* Again, be careful not to drive material from the nose into the sinuses or eustachian tubes. Irrigate both nostrils.
• Inspect returning irrigant. Changes in color, viscosity, or volume may signal an infection and should be reported to the doctor. Also report blood or necrotic material.

To conclude the procedure
• After irrigation, have the patient wait for a few minutes before blowing excess fluid from both nostrils at once. *Gentle blowing through both nostrils prevents fluid or pressure buildup in the sinuses. This action also helps to loosen and expel crusted secretions and mucus.*
• Clean the bulb syringe and irrigating device with disinfectant as recommended. Rinse and dry.

Special considerations
Expect fluid to drain from the patient's nose for a brief time after the irrigation and before he blows his nose.

Be sure to insert the irrigation tip far enough to ensure that the irrigant cleans the nasal membranes before draining out. The amount of normal saline solution used for an irrigation varies depending on the amount of crusted mucus. A typical amount ranges from 500 to 1,000 ml.

Home care
To continue nasal irrigations at home, teach the patient how to prepare normal saline solution. Tell him to fill a clean 1-liter plastic bottle with tap water or distilled water (4 cups + 1 oz = 1 liter), add 1½ tsp of table salt, and shake the solution until the salt dissolves. Teach him how to disinfect used irrigation devices.

Documentation
Write down the time and duration of the procedure and the amount of irrigant used. Describe the appearance of the returned solution. Record your assessment of the patient's comfort level and breathing ease before and after the procedure. Document patient-teaching content.

Nasal packing

In the highly vascular nasal mucosa, even seemingly minor injuries can cause major bleeding and blood loss. When routine therapeutic measures — such as direct pressure, cautery, or vasoconstrictive medications — fail to control epistaxis (nosebleed), the patient's nose may have to be packed to stop anterior bleeding (which runs out of the nose) or posterior bleeding (which runs down the throat). If blood drains into the nasopharyngeal area or the lacrimal ducts, the patient may appear to bleed from the mouth and eyes as well.

Most nasal bleeding originates at a plexus of arterioles and venules in the anteroinferior septum. Only about 1 in 10 nosebleeds occurs in the more vascular posterior nose, which usually bleeds more heavily than the anterior location.

A nurse typically assists a doctor with anterior or posterior nasal packing, depending on the bleeding site. (See *Types of nasal packing,* page 666.) Or she may assist with nasal balloon catheterization, a procedure that applies pressure to a posterior bleeding site. (See *Nasal balloon catheters,* page 667.)

Whichever procedure the patient undergoes, the nurse should provide ongoing encouragement and support to reduce his discomfort and anxiety. In addition, the nurse should perform ongoing assessment to determine the procedure's success and detect possible complications.

Equipment

For anterior and posterior packing: gowns ▪ goggles ▪ masks ▪ sterile gloves ▪ prepackaged nasal packing kit, head and neck examination kit, or sterile tray ▪ nasal speculum ▪ headlamp ▪ sterile bayonet forceps ▪ suction apparatus (with sterile suction-connecting tubing and sterile nasal aspirator tip) ▪ two sterile towels ▪ normal saline solution ▪ sterile bowl ▪ local anesthetic spray or vial of local anesthetic solution (such as lidocaine with epinephrine or a decongestant with a vasoconstrictor, such as phenylephrine) ▪ cotton pledgets ▪ electrocautery device or silver nitrate pledgets ▪ antibiotic ointment ▪ 10-ml syringe with a 22G 1½" needle ▪ sedative or tranquilizer ▪ water-soluble lubricant ▪ sterile cotton-tipped applicators ▪ nonallergenic tape ▪ emesis basin ▪ facial tissues ▪ mouth care supplies.

For anterior packing: ½" (1.3 cm) petroleum gauze (3′ to 4′ [0.9- to 1.2-m] strip), nasal tampons, or absorbable nasal pack (Surgicel, Gelfoam, or thrombin) ▪ small flexible catheter ▪ normal saline solution or antibiotic solution.

For posterior packing: sterile 4″ × 4″ gauze pads or dental roll ▪ sterile 2″ × 2″ gauze pads ▪ long heavy silk sutures ▪ two small flexible catheters ▪ two single- or double-chamber nasal balloon catheters ▪ normal saline solution ▪ two hemostats ▪ 30-ml syringe.

For emergency bedside use: flashlight ▪ scissors ▪ hemostat.

Preparation of equipment

Wash your hands. Assemble all equipment at the patient's bedside. Be sure the headlamp works. Plug in the suction apparatus and connect the tubing from the collection bottle to the suction source. Test the suction equipment to be sure it works properly. At the bedside, create a sterile field. (Use the sterile towels or the sterile tray.) Using sterile technique, place all sterile equipment on the sterile field.

If the doctor will inject a local anesthetic rather than spray it, place the 22G 1½" needle attached to the 10-ml syringe on the sterile field. When the doctor readies the syringe, clean the stopper on the anesthetic vial and hold the vial so he can withdraw the anesthetic. *This practice allows the doctor to avoid touching his sterile gloves to the nonsterile vial.*

Open the packages containing sterile suction-connecting tubing and aspirating tip and place them on the sterile field. Fill the sterile bowl with the normal saline solution *so the suction tubing can be flushed as necessary.*

If the patient needs posterior packing and you don't have premade packing, wash your hands, put on sterile gloves, and make a posterior pack by rolling a sterile 2″ × 2″ gauze pad. The pack should be 1½" (3.75 cm) long and 1″ (2.5 cm) in diameter. Trim excess gauze with sterile scissors. Secure the roll with the three 18″ (46-cm) lengths of silk suture. Tie a suture at each end and one in the middle of the roll; don't trim the suture ends. Thoroughly lubricate the anterior or posterior packing with antibiotic ointment.

If the patient needs a nasal balloon catheter, test the balloon for leaks by inflating the catheter with normal saline solution. Remove the solution before insertion.

Implementation

● Ensure that all persons caring for the patient wear gowns, gloves, and eye protection during insertion of packing *to prevent possible contamination from splattered blood.*
● Check the patient's vital signs and observe for hypotension with postural changes. *Hypotension suggests significant blood loss.* Also monitor airway patency *because the patient will be at risk for aspirating or vomiting swallowed blood.*
● Explain the procedure to the patient and offer reassurance *to reduce his anxiety and promote cooperation.*
● If ordered, administer a sedative or tranquilizer *to reduce the patient's anxiety and decrease sympathetic stimulation, which can exacerbate a nosebleed.*

(Text continues on page 668.)

Types of nasal packing

Depending on its source, your patient's nosebleed may be controlled with anterior or posterior nasal packing.

Anterior nasal packing
The doctor may treat an anterior nosebleed by packing the anterior nasal cavity with a 3′ to 4′ (0.9- to 1.2-m) strip of antibiotic-impregnated petroleum gauze or with a nasal tampon.

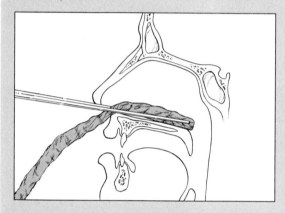

A nasal tampon is made of tightly compressed absorbent material with a central breathing tube. The doctor inserts a lubricated tampon along the floor of the nose and, with the patient's head tilted backward, instills 5 to 10 ml of antibiotic or normal saline solution. The tampon expands as a result, stopping the bleeding. It should be moistened periodically, and the central breathing tube should be suctioned regularly.

In a child or a patient with blood dyscrasias, the doctor may fashion an absorbable pack by moistening a gauzelike, regenerated cellulose material with a vasoconstrictor. Applied to a visible bleeding point, this substance will swell to form a clot. Because it's absorbable, the packing doesn't need removal.

Posterior nasal packing
Posterior packing consists of a gauze roll shaped and secured by three sutures (one suture at each end and one in the middle) or a balloon-type catheter. To insert the packing, the doctor advances one or two soft catheters into the patient's nostrils. When the catheter tips appear in the nasopharynx, the doctor grasps them with a Kelly clamp or bayonet forceps and pulls them forward

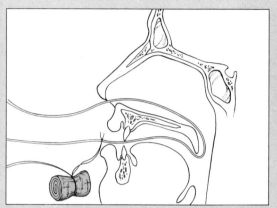

through the patient's mouth. He secures the two end sutures to the catheter tip and draws the catheter back through the patient's nostrils.

This step brings the packing into place with the end sutures hanging from the patient's nostril. (The middle suture emerges from the patient's mouth to free the packing, when needed.)

The doctor may weight the nose sutures with a clamp. Then he will pull the packing securely into place behind the soft palate and against the posterior end of the septum (nasal choana).

Finally, after he examines the patient's throat (to ensure that the uvula hasn't been forced under the packing), he will insert anterior packing and secure the whole apparatus by tying the posterior pack strings around rolled gauze or a dental roll at the nostrils.

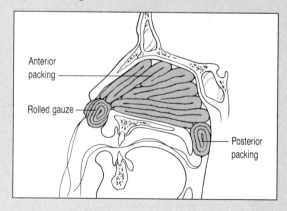

Anterior packing

Rolled gauze

Posterior packing

Nasal balloon catheters

To control posterior epistaxis, the doctor may use a balloon catheter instead of nasal packing. Self-retaining and disposable, the catheter may have a single or a double balloon to apply pressure to bleeding nasal tissues. Less commonly, the doctor may insert a balloon-tipped urinary drainage catheter (a #14 to #16 French with a 30-ml balloon for an adult). If bleeding remains uncontrolled, arterial ligation, cryotherapy, or arterial embolization may be needed.

Once inserted and inflated, the single-balloon catheter shown below compresses the blood vessels while a soft, collapsible external bulb prevents the catheter from dislodging posteriorly.

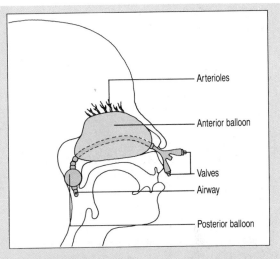

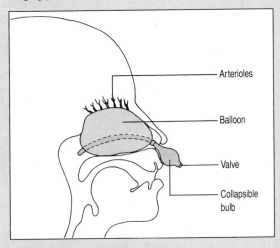

After placement and inflation with saline solution (not air because it will leak slowly), the posterior portion of the double-balloon device (shown at the top of the next column) secures the catheter in the nasopharynx while the anterior balloon compresses bleeding vessels. This catheter has a central airway for breathing comfort.

Assisting with insertion

To assist with inserting a single- or double-balloon catheter, prepare the patient as you would for nasal packing. Take care to discuss the procedure thoroughly to alleviate the patient's anxiety and promote his cooperation.

Explain that the catheter tip will be lubricated with an antibiotic or water-soluble lubricant to ease passage and to prevent infection.

Providing routine care

The tip of the single-balloon catheter will be inserted in the nostrils until it reaches the posterior pharynx. Then, the balloon will be inflated with normal saline solution, pulled gently into the posterior nasopharynx and secured at the nostrils with the collapsible bulb (or with a hemostat). With a double-balloon catheter, the posterior balloon is inflated with normal saline solution; then the anterior balloon is inflated.

Check catheter placement routinely. Assess the nostrils for irritation or erosion. Remove secretions by gently suctioning the airway of a double-balloon catheter or by dabbing away crusted external secretions if the patient has a catheter without an airway.

To prevent damage to nasal tissue, the doctor may order the balloon deflated for 10 minutes every 24 hours. If bleeding recurs or remains uncontrolled, reinflate the balloon and contact the doctor. He may add packing in front of or around the balloon.

Recognizing complications

Complications associated with nasal balloon catheters are similar to those associated with nasal packing. The patient may report difficulty breathing, swallowing, or eating, and the nasal mucosa may sustain damage from pressure. Balloon deflation may dislodge clots and nasal debris into the oropharynx, which could prompt coughing, gagging, or vomiting.

Preventing recurrent nosebleeds

Before your patient's discharge, review the following self-care guidelines to minimize his chances for recurrent nosebleeds at home, on the job, or in school.

• Because nosebleeds can result from dry mucous membranes, suggest that the patient use a cool-mist room vaporizer or humidifier as needed, especially in dry environments.

• Teach the patient how to minimize pressure on nasal passages. Advise him, for instance, to avoid constipation and consequent straining at stool. Recommend maintaining a fiber-rich diet and adequate fluid intake. Also warn him to forgo extreme physical exertion for 24 hours after the nosebleed stops.

• Other precautionary measures include avoiding aspirin (which has anticoagulant properties) for about 5 days and alcoholic beverages and tobacco as well for at least 5 days.

• If the patient develops a nosebleed despite these precautions, tell him to keep his head higher than his heart. He should use a thumb and forefinger to press the soft portion of the nostrils together and against the facial bones. (Recommend against direct pressure if he has a facial injury or nasal fracture.) He should maintain pressure for up to 10 minutes and then apply ice wrapped in a plastic bag or washcloth to his nose (because cold facilitates coagulation).

• Assist the patient to sit with his head tilted forward *to minimize blood drainage into the throat and prevent aspiration.*

• Turn on the suction apparatus and attach the connecting tubing *so the doctor can aspirate the nasal cavity to remove clots before locating the bleeding source.*

• To inspect the nasal cavity, the doctor will insert a nasal speculum. He will open the speculum *to dilate the cavity.* If he can see the bleeding site, the doctor calls the episode an "anterior bleed."

For anterior nasal packing
• Help the doctor try to control bleeding by chemical cautery with silver nitrate pledgets, electrocautery, or a vasoconstricting agent such as phenylephrine (topical), lidocaine with epinephrine (injected), or cocaine (topical).

• To enhance the vasoconstrictor's action, apply manual pressure to the nose for about 10 minutes. (See *Preventing recurrent nosebleeds.*)

• If bleeding persists, you may assist with insertion of an absorbable nasal pack directly on the bleeding site. The material will swell, forming an artificial clot.

• If these methods prove unsuccessful, prepare to assist the doctor with insertion of anterior nasal packing. (Even if only one side is bleeding, both sides may require packing to apply sufficient pressure to the bleeding site.)

• While the patient has the anterior pack in place, use the cotton-tipped applicators to apply petroleum jelly to his lips and nostrils *to prevent drying and cracking.*

For posterior nasal packing
• Wash your hands and put on sterile gloves.

• If the doctor identifies the bleeding source in the posterior nasal cavity, lubricate the soft catheters *to ease insertion.*

• Instruct the patient to open his mouth and pant during catheter insertion *to minimize gagging as the doctor advances the catheters into the patient's nostrils.*

• Assist the doctor, as directed, to insert the packing.

• Tape the sutures that protrude from the patient's mouth to his cheek. Leave enough slack to permit comfortable talking, chewing, and swallowing. *The slack also prevents stress on the sutures, which could cut the patient's lips or soft palate or cause the posterior pack to slip into the airway.*

• Help the patient assume a comfortable position. Assess him for airway obstruction or any respiratory changes.

• Monitor his vital signs *to detect hemodynamic changes that may indicate hypovolemia or hypoxemia.*

Special considerations
Test the patient's call bell to be sure he can summon help if needed. Also keep emergency equipment (a flashlight, scissors, and hemostats) at the patient's bedside *to speed packing removal in case the posterior pack slides and obstructs the airway.* To remove a posterior pack quickly, cut the sutures and pull the pack out through the patient's mouth.

Once the packing is in place, compile your assessment data carefully to help detect the underlying cause of nosebleeds. Mechanical factors include a deviated septum, traumatic injury, or a foreign body that produces pressure necrosis. Environmental factors include drying and erosion of the nasal mucosa. Other possible causes are upper respiratory tract infection, anticoagulant therapy, blood dyscrasias, cardiovascular disorders, tumors of the nasal cavity or paranasal sinuses, hepatic disease, chronic nephritis, and familial hemorrhagic telangiectasis.

If significant blood loss occurs or if the underlying cause remains unknown, expect the doctor to order a complete blood count and coagulation profile as soon as possible. Blood transfusion may be necessary. After the procedure, the doctor may order arterial blood gas analysis to detect any pulmonary complications and arterial oxygen saturation monitoring to assess for hypoxemia. If necessary, prepare to administer supplemental oxygen with a face mask, and give antibiotics and decongestants as ordered.

Because a patient with nasal packing must breathe through his mouth, provide thorough mouth care frequently.

The doctor usually removes anterior nasal packs after 2 days. However, absorbable packs may remain in place for 3 to 5 days. Posterior packing typically remains in place for 4 days. Until the pack is removed, the patient should be on modified bed rest. As ordered, administer moderate doses of nonaspirin analgesics and sedatives along with prophylactic antibiotics *to prevent sinusitis or related infections.*

After an anterior pack is removed, instruct the patient to avoid rubbing or picking his nose, inserting any object (such as a handkerchief or tissue) into his nose, and blowing his nose forcefully for 48 hours or as ordered.

Home care

To boost the patient's confidence in his self-care ability, offer applicable home care guidelines. Try to emphasize nosebleed prevention, if possible.

Complications

The pressure of a posterior pack on the soft palate may lead to hypoxemia. Patients with posterior nosebleeds are at special risk for hypoxemia because they commonly aspirate blood and because posterior packing partially obstructs the upper airway. Hypoxemia can be detected with pulse oximetry. Signs and symptoms include tachycardia, confusion, cyanosis, and restlessness.

Airway obstruction may occur if a posterior or anterior nasal pack slips backward. The patient may complain of difficulty swallowing and pain or discomfort. In patients with posterior packs, otitis media may develop because the pack blocks the eustachian tube openings. Other possible complications include hematotympanum and pressure necrosis of nasal structures, especially the septum.

Sedation may cause hypotension or hypertension in a patient with significant blood loss and may also increase the patient's risk of aspiration.

Documentation

Record the type of pack used to ensure its removal at the appropriate time. On the intake and output record, document the estimated blood loss and all fluid administered. Also note the patient's vital signs, his response to sedation or position changes, results of any laboratory tests, and any drugs administered, including topical agents. Record any unusual findings or complications. Document discharge instructions and clinical follow-up plans.

Selected references

Adams, G., et al. *Fundamentals of Otolaryngology,* 6th ed. Philadelphia: W.B. Saunders Co., 1989.

Blakely, B., and Swanson, R. *Otolaryngology for the House Officer.* Baltimore: Williams & Wilkins Co., 1989.

Brunner, L., and Suddarth, D. *Textbook of Medical-Surgical Nursing,* 6th ed. Philadelphia: J.B. Lippincott Co., 1988.

Flynn, J., and Hackel, R. *Technological Foundations in Nursing.* Norwalk, Conn.: Appleton & Lange, 1990.

Herrin, M. *Ophthalmic Examination and Basic Skills.* Thorofare, N.J.: Charles B. Slack, Inc., 1990.

Illustrated Manual of Nursing Practice. Springhouse, Pa.: Springhouse Corp., 1991.

Malseed, R.T., and Harrigan, G.S. *Textbook of Pharmacology and Nursing Care.* Philadelphia: J.B. Lippincott Co., 1989.

McConnell, E. "How to Irrigate the Eye," *Nursing91* 21(3):28, March 1991.

Newell, F.W. *Ophthalmology: Principles and Concepts,* 7th ed. St. Louis: Mosby-Year Book, Inc., 1991.

Nursing92 Drug Handbook. Springhouse, Pa.: Springhouse Corp., 1992.

Paparella, M.M., et al. *Otolaryngology: Head & Neck,* vol. 3, 3rd ed. Philadelphia: W.B. Saunders Co., 1991.

Perry, A., and Potter, P. *Clinical Nursing Skills and Techniques,* 2nd ed. St. Louis: C.V. Mosby Co., 1990.

Phipps, W., et al. *Medical-Surgical Nursing: Concepts and Clinical Practice,* 4th ed. St. Louis: Mosby-Year Book, Inc., 1991.

Riley, M. *Nursing Care of the Client with Ear, Nose, and Throat Disorders.* New York: Springer Publishing Co., 1987.

Sands, J. *Clinical Manual of Medical-Surgical Nursing,* 2nd ed. St. Louis: Mosby-Year Book, Inc., 1991.

Timby, B. *Clinical Nursing Procedures.* Philadelphia: J.B. Lippincott Co., 1989.

U.S. Public Health Service. Office of Clinical Center Communications. *Facts About the Nose and Nasal Irrigation.* Washington, D.C.: U.S. Department of Health and Human Services, 1990.

MATERNAL-NEONATAL CARE

SARAH WHITAKER, RN, MSN

Introduction

Because of its profound emotional implications for mother and child, maternal-neonatal care requires expertise that goes beyond clinical skills. Such care must combine clinical competence, sensitivity, and good judgment. It must consider the patient's sexuality and self-image and recognize changing social attitudes and values — especially those concerning conventional conception and childbirth and modern alternatives.

Changing maternity care

More than 4 million infants were born in the United States in 1991. Many of them were born with considerably less medical intervention than was customary in the previous decades and many of them were conceived with considerably more intervention. As a result, nurses today must be prepared to implement or assist with a wide range of procedures.

If you're working with a pregnant patient, you'll need to use your teaching skills. For instance, you may be called on to organize and direct natural childbirth classes or to teach the mother-to-be how to breathe and control pain during childbirth. Or you may teach fathers and other support persons to participate in childbirth by providing comfort and direction.

What's more, you may be asked to give information about childbirth options. Although most births still occur in a hospital, many parents inquire about delivery in a birth center. Usually located in the maternity unit of a hospital or sponsored by a childbirth association, a birth center combines the advantages of a homelike setting with the emergency medical and nursing interventions available in a hospital. Today's nurse may staff or direct the birth center.

Historically, the midwife has been a fixture in remote or poor communities. Today's professional nurse-midwife, however, brings advanced technical skills and certification to diverse communities — urban center to country town alike. She may work in collaboration with — or be supervised by — a doctor or a group. In some areas, she may even practice independently. In fact, several states permit insurers to make direct payment to the nurse-midwife for her services.

Changing neonatal care

Accompanying the changes in maternity care are changes in neonatal care — thanks to advanced knowledge and techniques for improving fetal monitoring and promoting neonatal survival. Until recently, for example, admission to a neonatal care unit depended solely on birth weight. A neonate weighing less than 5.5 lb (2.5 kg) was considered premature. A neonate exceeding this weight was considered full-term. Today, it's possible to identify the 8-lb (3.62 kg), 35-week neonate of a diabetic mother as premature and large for gestational age.

New clinical evaluation methods, combined with new electronic and biochemical monitoring techniques, allow improved neonatal care. To apply these advances, you must be familiar with neonatal physiology, procedures, and equipment.

 ## *FETAL ASSESSMENT*
Fetal heart rate

A major clue to fetal well-being during gestation and labor, fetal heart rate (FHR) may be assessed by auscultating with a fetoscope or a Doppler ultrasound stethoscope placed on the maternal abdomen. This ultrasound device emits low-energy, high-frequency sound waves that rebound from the fetal heart to a transducer, which transmits the impulses to a monitor strip for recording.

Because FHR normally ranges from 120 to 160 beats/minute, auscultation yields only an average rate at best. However, because auscultation can detect gross (but often late) fetal distress signs (tachycardia or bradycardia), the technique remains useful in an uncomplicated, low-risk pregnancy. In a high-risk pregnancy, indirect external or direct internal electronic fetal monitoring gives more accurate information on fetal status.

Equipment

Fetoscope or Doppler stethoscope (see *Instruments for hearing fetal heart tones,* page 672) ▪ water-soluble lubricant (for ultrasound instrument) ▪ watch with second hand.

Implementation

• Explain the procedure to the patient, wash your hands, and provide privacy. Reassure the patient that you may reposition the listening instrument frequently *to hear the loudest fetal heart tones.*
• Assist the patient to a supine position, and drape her appropriately *to minimize exposure.* If you're using the

Instruments for hearing fetal heart tones

The fetoscope and the Doppler stethoscope are basic instruments for auscultating fetal heart tones and assessing fetal heart rates.

Fetoscope

This instrument can detect fetal heartbeats as early as the 18th gestational week. As an assessment tool during labor, it's helpful for hearing fetal heart tones when contractions are mild and infrequent.

Doppler stethoscope

This instrument can detect fetal heartbeats as early as the 10th gestational week. Useful throughout labor, the Doppler stethoscope has greater sensitivity than the fetoscope.

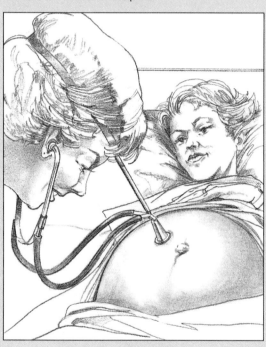

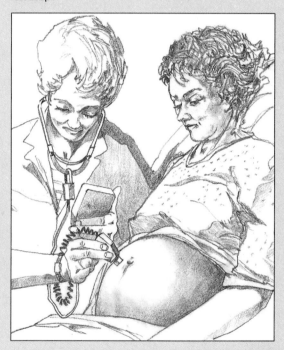

Doppler stethoscope, apply the water-soluble lubricant to the patient's abdomen. *This gel or paste creates an airtight seal between the skin and the instrument and promotes optimal ultrasound wave conduction and reception.*

To calculate FHR during gestation

• To assess FHR in a fetus age 20 weeks or less, place the earpieces in your ears and position the bell of the fetoscope or Doppler stethoscope on the abdominal midline above the pubic hairline. After 20 weeks, when you can palpate fetal position, use Leopold's maneuvers *to locate the back of the fetal thorax.* Then position the listening instrument over the fetal back. (For more infor-

mation, see *Performing Leopold's maneuvers,* pages 674 and 675.)

• Using a Doppler stethoscope, place the earpieces in your ears, and press the bell gently on the patient's abdomen. Start listening at the midline, midway between the umbilicus and the symphysis pubis. Or, using a fetoscope, place the earpieces in your ears with the fetoscope positioned centrally on your forehead. Gently press the bell about ½″ (1.3 cm) into the patient's abdomen. Remove your hands from the fetoscope *to avoid extraneous noise.*

• Move the bell of either instrument slightly from side to side, as necessary, *to locate the loudest heart tones.* After locating these tones, palpate the maternal pulse.
• While monitoring the maternal pulse rate (*to avoid confusing maternal heart tones with fetal heart tones*), count the fetal heartbeats for at least 15 seconds. If the maternal radial pulse and the FHR are the same, try to locate the fetal thorax by using Leopold's maneuvers; then reassess FHR. Usually, the fetal heart beats faster than the maternal heart. Record the FHR.

To count FHR during labor
• Allow the mother and her support person to listen to the fetal heart if they wish. *This helps to make the fetus a greater reality for them.* Record their participation.
• Position the fetoscope or Doppler stethoscope on the abdomen — midway between the umbilicus and symphysis pubis *for cephalic presentation,* or at the umbilicus or above *for breech presentation.* Locate the loudest heartbeats, and simultaneously palpate the maternal pulse *to ensure that you're monitoring fetal rather than maternal pulse.*
• Monitor maternal pulse rate and count fetal heartbeats for 60 seconds during the relaxation period between contractions *to determine baseline FHR.* In a low-risk labor, assess FHR every 60 minutes during the latent phase, every 30 minutes during the active phase, and every 15 minutes during the second stage of labor. In a high-risk labor, assess FHR every 30 minutes during the latent phase, every 15 minutes during the active phase, and every 5 minutes during the second stage of labor.
• Notify the doctor or nurse-midwife immediately if you observe marked changes in FHR from baseline values, (especially during or immediately after a contraction when signs of fetal distress typically occur). If fetal distress develops, begin indirect or direct electronic fetal monitoring.
• Repeat the procedure, as ordered.

Special considerations
If you're auscultating FHR with a Doppler stethoscope, be aware that obesity and hydramnios can interfere with sound-wave transmission, making accurate results more difficult to obtain. If the doctor orders continuous FHR monitoring, strap the ultrasound transducer to the patient's abdomen. The monitor will provide a printed record of the FHR.

Documentation
Record both the FHR and the maternal pulse rate on the flowchart.

 # Amniocentesis

A needle aspiration of amniotic fluid for laboratory analysis, amniocentesis is usually performed between the 16th and 20th gestational weeks. This procedure can detect neural tube or chromosomal defects and certain metabolic and other disorders. What's more, the procedure can identify the sex of the fetus and assist in assessing fetal health. When performed in the final trimester, amniocentesis helps to evaluate fetal lung maturity and detect Rh hemolytic disease.

Indications for amniocentesis include maternal age over 35 (associated with Down's syndrome), a family history of neural tube or chromosomal defects, or inborn errors of metabolism. Another test, chorionic villi sampling, may also detect fetal disorders (see *Understanding chorionic villi sampling,* page 676). Either procedure may be performed in a labor and delivery suite, in the ultrasound department, or in a doctor's office.

Contraindications for amniocentesis include an anterior uterine wall completely covered by the placenta and insufficient amniotic fluid. Risks of this procedure must be weighed against expected benefits if the mother tests positive for acquired immunodeficiency syndrome.

Equipment
Preassembled amniocentesis tray or ▪ hospital gown ▪ two sets of sterile gloves, sterile gowns, and masks ▪ stethoscope ▪ Doppler stethoscope and other appropriate ultrasound equipment ▪ fetoscope or electronic fetal monitor ▪ antiseptic solution with sterile container ▪ local anesthetic ▪ alcohol ▪ 10-ml syringe ▪ sterile 20G or 22G 4″ spinal needle with stylet ▪ 22G or 25G needle ▪ sterile 20-ml glass syringe ▪ clean amber glass specimen container for Rh sensitization and lecithin/sphingomyelin (L/S) ratio tests ▪ three sterile, glass specimen tubes (for genetic tests) ▪ laboratory request forms ▪ adhesive bandage.

Preparation of equipment
If you don't have an amber specimen container, cover the outside of a clean test tube or glass container with adhesive tape or aluminum foil. *Protecting aspirated amniotic fluid from light prevents the breakdown of such pigments as bilirubin.* Properly label all specimen containers or tubes.

Implementation
• Explain the procedure to the patient. Confirm that she understands the risk of complications. Emphasize that the doctor may need to repeat the procedure and that amniotic fluid analysis can't rule out all birth defects.

Performing Leopold's maneuvers

You can determine fetal position by performing Leopold's maneuvers. Ask the patient to empty her bladder, assist her to a supine position, and expose her abdomen. Then perform the four maneuvers in order.

First maneuver
Face the patient and warm your hands. Place them on her abdomen to determine fetal position in the uterine fundus. Curl your fingers around the fundus. With the fetus in vertex position, you'll feel the buttocks — irregularly shaped and firm. With the fetus in breech position, you'll feel the head — hard, round, and movable.

Second maneuver
Move your hands down the sides of the abdomen and apply gentle pressure. If the fetus lies in vertex position, you'll feel a smooth, hard surface on one side — the fetal back. On the other side, you'll feel lumps and knobs — the knees, hands, feet, and elbows. If the fetus lies in breech position, you may not feel the back at all.

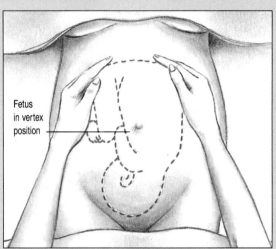

Fetus
in vertex
position

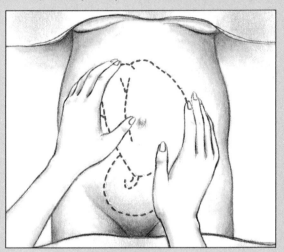

- Reaffirm that you have the patient's signed informed consent form.
- *To reduce the risk of bladder puncture,* ensure that the patient voids before the procedure if the pregnancy exceeds 20 weeks (before 20 weeks, a full bladder may help to hold the uterus steady).
- Provide privacy and instruct the patient to put on a hospital gown. Assist her to a supine position and obtain baseline maternal vital signs. Next, determine the baseline fetal heart rate (FHR) with the Doppler stethoscope or the fetoscope.
- Instruct the patient to fold her hands on her chest, or have her rest her hands behind her head. Remind her to stay still.
- The doctor will use ultrasonography to locate the fetus and placenta. Once he identifies an amniotic fluid pocket, he can determine the appropriate needle-insertion depth.

Next, he will put on the sterile gown, sterile gloves, and mask and clean the skin with an antiseptic solution.
- If the patient's receiving a local anesthetic, clean the diaphragm of the multidose vial of anesthetic solution with alcohol. Provide a 10-ml syringe and 22G or 25G needle. Then invert the bottle *to allow the doctor to withdraw the anesthetic.*
- Scrub your hands, and put on a sterile gown, sterile gloves, and mask to assist the doctor with amniocentesis, an aseptic procedure.
- After the anesthetic takes effect, the doctor, guided by ultrasonographic imaging, will advance the 20G needle with a stylet through the abdomen and uterine wall into the amniotic sac. Then he will remove the stylet. When a drop of amniotic fluid appears, he'll attach the 20-ml glass syringe to the needle and aspirate the fluid.
- If the patient's having genetic studies, open the sterile glass specimen tubes. After the doctor transfers amniotic

Third maneuver

Spread apart the thumb and fingers of one hand. Place them just above the patient's symphysis pubis. Bring your fingers together. If the fetus lies in vertex position (and hasn't descended), you'll feel the head. If the fetus lies in vertex position (and has descended), you'll feel a less distinct mass.

Fourth maneuver

Use this maneuver in late pregnancy. Place your hands on both sides of the lower abdomen. Apply gentle pressure with your fingers as you slide your hands downward, toward the symphysis pubis. If the head presents, one hand's descent will be stopped by the cephalic prominence. The other hand will be unobstructed.

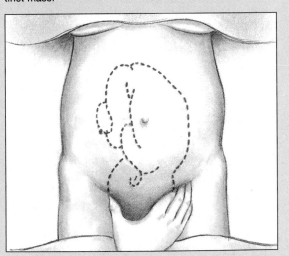

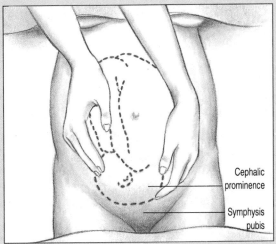

Cephalic prominence

Symphysis pubis

fluid to the tubes, use aseptic technique when closing the tubes *to avoid contamination, which can yield aberrant test results.*

• If the patient's having the Rh sensitization or L/S ratio tests, open the amber or covered specimen container *so the doctor can transfer the amniotic fluid.* Close the container at once *to protect the fluid from light, which may cause pigments in the fluid, such as bilirubin, to break down and skew test results.*

• When the doctor withdraws the needle, place an adhesive bandage over the insertion site.

• Complete the laboratory request forms, and send the specimens to the laboratory immediately. Speedy transport is important *because if the amniotic fluid contains blood or meconium, immediate centrifugation can preserve the specimen for analysis.*

• If the patient is in the final trimester of pregnancy, direct her to lie on her side *to avoid hypotension from pressure of the gravid uterus on the vena cava.*

• Assess maternal vital signs and FHR every 15 minutes for 30 minutes *to detect changes from the baseline values.* FHR changes, such as tachycardia or bradycardia, signal distress. If these signs appear, notify the doctor, and continue to monitor FHR.

• Electronically monitor the patient for uterine irritability and the fetus for changes in heart rate pattern. Monitoring should continue for a few hours after the procedure *to allow early intervention if complications occur.* Normally, maternal vital signs should remain stable.

• Instruct the patient to report signs and symptoms of complications: a vaginal discharge (fluid or blood), decreased fetal movement, contractions, or fever and chills.

• Help the patient dress *in preparation for discharge.*

Understanding chorionic villi sampling

Laboratory analysis of chorionic villi samples can detect genetic, metabolic, and blood disorders — such as Down's syndrome, Duchenne's muscular dystrophy, sickle cell anemia, alpha (and some beta) thalassemias, and phenylketonuria. Performed at 9 to 12 weeks' gestation, the procedure can yield results in just a few days.

To obtain the tissue samples, the doctor typically uses ultrasound or endoscopic imaging to guide a plastic catheter through the cervical canal into the uterus, as shown. He aspirates a small portion of chorionic tissue from the fetus, taking care not to contaminate the sample with maternal tissue.

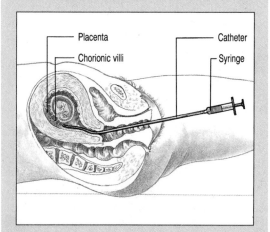

Placenta   Catheter
Chorionic villi   Syringe

Before the test, verify the patient's written consent, provide emotional support, and answer any questions. Arrange for ordered blood studies. Instruct the patient to drink 1 quart (about 1 liter) of water 30 minutes before the test *because a full bladder allows a better view of the uterus.*

Assess vital signs before, during, and after the procedure.

Special considerations

Provide emotional support for the patient during the procedure, and explain the key steps as the doctor performs them. Monitor her for signs and symptoms of supine hypotension, such as light-headedness, nausea, and diaphoresis.

If the patient will receive a dose of RhoGAM, explain that this passive immunizing agent may help prevent an Rh incompatibility between the patient and the fetus that would cause antibody formation in the mother's blood. This condition is known as erythroblastosis fetalis (hydrops fetalis or hemolytic disease of the newborn).

Inform the patient, her family, and her support person, as appropriate, that test results should be available in 2 to 4 weeks. Provide emotional support as needed.

Complications

Although amniocentesis is an invasive procedure, it rarely produces maternal or fetal complications. Maternal complications, which affect fewer than 1% of patients, include amniotic fluid embolism, hemorrhage, infection, premature labor, abruptio placentae, placenta or umbilical cord trauma, bladder or intestinal puncture, or Rh isoimmunization. Rare fetal complications include intrauterine fetal death, amnionitis, injury from needle puncture, amniotic fluid leakage, bleeding, spontaneous abortion, or premature birth.

Documentation

Record the doctor's name and the procedure's date and time. Record baseline maternal vital sign values and the FHR. Note any changes in these baseline data. Name the ordered laboratory tests. Describe the amount and appearance of the specimen fluid and time of transport to the laboratory. Document discharge instructions to the patient. Also document how the patient tolerated the procedure.

 # External fetal monitoring

An indirect, noninvasive procedure, external fetal monitoring uses two devices strapped to the mother's abdomen to evaluate fetal well-being during labor.

One device, an ultrasound transducer, transmits high-frequency sound waves through soft body tissues to the fetal heart. The waves rebound from the heart through the abdominal wall, where the transducer relays them to a monitor. The other, a pressure-sensitive tocotransducer, responds to the pressure exerted by uterine contractions and simultaneously records their duration and frequency (see *Applying external fetal monitoring devices*). The monitoring apparatus traces fetal heart rate (FHR) and uterine contraction data onto the same printout paper.

Indications for external fetal monitoring include high-risk pregnancy, oxytocin-induced labor, and antepartal

Applying external fetal monitoring devices

To ensure clear tracings that define fetal status and labor progress, be sure to precisely position external monitoring devices, such as an ultrasound transducer and a tocotransducer.

Fetal heart monitor

Palpate the uterus to locate the fetus's back. If possible, place the ultrasound transducer over this site where the fetal heartbeat sounds the loudest. Then tighten the belt. Use the fetal heart tracing on the monitor strip to validate the transducer's position.

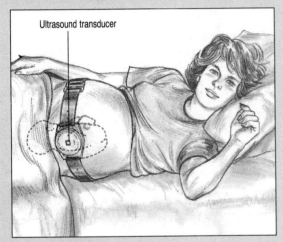

Ultrasound transducer

Labor monitor

A tocotransducer records uterine motion during contractions. Place the tocotransducer over the uterine fundus where it contracts, either midline or slightly to one side. Place your hand on the fundus and palpate a contraction to verify proper placement. Secure the tocotransducer's belt; then adjust the pen set so that the baseline values read between 5 and 15 mm Hg on the monitor strip.

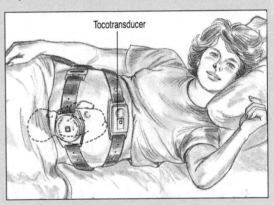

Tocotransducer

---

nonstress and contraction stress tests. Many labor and delivery units use external fetal monitoring for all patients. The procedure has no contraindications, but may be difficult to perform on patients with hydramnios, on obese patients, or on hyperactive or premature fetuses.

Equipment

Electronic fetal monitor ■ ultrasound transducer ■ tocotransducer ■ conduction gel ■ transducer straps ■ damp cloth ■ printout paper.

Monitoring devices, such as phonotransducers and abdominal electrocardiogram transducers, are commercially available. However, hospitals use these devices less frequently than the ultrasound transducer.

Preparation of equipment

Because fetal monitor features and complexity vary, review the operator's manual before proceeding. If the monitor has two paper speeds, select the slower speed

(typically 3 cm/minute) *to ensure an easy-to-read tracing.* At higher speeds (for example, 1 cm/minute), the printed tracings are condensed, making results difficult to decipher and interpret accurately.

Next, plug the tocotransducer cable into the uterine activity jack and the ultrasound transducer cable into the phono-ultrasound jack. Attach the straps to the tocotransducer and the ultrasound transducer.

Label the printout paper with the patient's hospital number or birthdate and name, the date, maternal vital signs and position, the paper speed, and the number of the strip paper *to maintain accurate, consecutive monitoring records.*

Implementation

● Explain the procedure to the patient, and provide emotional support. Inform her that the monitor may make noise if the pen set tracer moves above or below the grids on the printout paper. Reassure her that this doesn't

indicate fetal distress. As appropriate, explain other aspects of the monitor *to help reduce maternal anxiety about fetal well-being.*
• Make sure the patient has signed a consent form, if required.
• Wash your hands and provide privacy.

To begin the procedure
• Assist the patient to a semi-Fowler's or a left-lateral position with her abdomen exposed. Don't let her lie supine *because pressure from the gravid uterus on the maternal inferior vena cava may cause maternal hypotension, decrease uterine perfusion, and induce fetal hypoxia.*
• Palpate the patient's abdomen to locate the fundus — the area of greatest muscle density in the uterus. Then, using transducer straps, secure the tocotransducer over the fundus.
• Adjust the pen set tracer controls so that the baseline values read between 5 and 15 mm Hg on the monitor strip. *This prevents triggering the alarm that indicates the tracer has dropped below the paper's margins.* The proper setting varies among tocotransducers.
• Apply conduction gel to the ultrasound transducer crystals *to promote an airtight seal and optimal sound-wave transmission.*
• Use Leopold's maneuvers to palpate the fetal back, through which fetal heart tones resound most audibly.
• Start the monitor. Then apply the ultrasound transducer directly over the site having the strongest heart tones.
• Activate the control that begins the printout. On the printout paper, note any coughing, position changes, drug administration, vaginal examinations, and blood pressure readings that may affect interpretation of the tracings.
• Explain to the patient and her support person how to time and control contractions with the monitor. To time contractions, inform them that the distance from one dark vertical line to the next on the printout grid represents 1 minute. The support person can use this information to prepare the patient for the onset of a contraction and to guide and slow her breathing as the contraction subsides.

To monitor the patient
• Observe the tracings *to identify frequency and duration of uterine contractions,* but palpate the uterus *to determine intensity of contractions.*
• Mentally note the baseline FHR — the rate between contractions — *to compare with suspicious-looking deviations.* FHR normally ranges from 120 to 160 beats/minute.
• Assess periodic accelerations or decelerations from the baseline FHR. Compare the FHR patterns with those of the uterine contractions. Note the time relationship between the onset of an FHR deceleration and the onset of

a uterine contraction, the time relationship of the lowest level of an FHR deceleration to the peak of a uterine contraction, and the range of FHR deceleration. *These data help distinguish fetal distress from benign head compression.*
• Move the tocotransducer and the ultrasound transducer *to accommodate changes in maternal or fetal position.* Readjust both transducers every hour and assess the patient's skin for reddened areas caused by the strap pressure. Document skin condition.
• Clean the ultrasound transducer periodically with a damp cloth *to remove dried conduction gel that can interfere with ultrasound transmission.* Apply fresh gel, as necessary. After use, place the cover over the ultrasound transducer.

Special considerations
If the monitor fails to record uterine activity, palpate for contractions. Check for equipment problems as the manufacturer directs and readjust the tocotransducer.

If the patient reports discomfort in the position that provides the clearest signal, try to obtain a satisfactory 5- or 10-minute tracing with the patient in this position before assisting her to a more comfortable position. As the patient progresses through labor and abdominal pressure increases, the pen set tracer may exceed the alarm boundaries.

Documentation
Check to be sure you numbered each monitor strip in sequence and labeled each printout sheet with the patient's hospital number or birthdate and name, the date, the time, and the paper speed. Record the time of any vaginal examinations, membrane rupture, drug administration, and maternal or fetal movements. Record maternal vital signs and the intensity of uterine contractions. Document each time that you moved or readjusted the tocotransducer and ultrasound transducer, and summarize this information in your notes.

 Internal electronic fetal monitoring

Also known as direct fetal monitoring, internal electronic fetal monitoring utilizes a spiral electrode and an intrauterine catheter to evaluate fetal status during labor. A doctor or a nurse with special skills performs this invasive procedure only after the amniotic sac ruptures and the cervix dilates at least 2 cm. Typically used when external (indirect) fetal monitoring provides insufficient or unusual information about fetal well-being, internal monitoring furnishes information on beat-to-beat varia-bility and precisely measures intrauterine pressure and labor progress. This helps the health care team determine the need for intervention. For more information, see *Understanding internal electronic fetal monitoring devices*, page 680.

Contraindications to direct fetal monitoring include maternal blood dyscrasias, suspected fetal immune deficiency, placenta previa, face presentation or uncertainty regarding the presenting part, and cervical or vaginal herpetic lesions.

Equipment

Electronic fetal monitor ■ printout paper ■ strain gauge and mounting bracket ■ 20-ml syringe ■ intrauterine catheter and guide ■ three-way stopcock ■ sterile water for injection ■ conduction gel ■ spiral electrode with drive tube and guide tube ■ leg plate ■ Velcro straps or 2-inch tape ■ nonallergenic tape ■ two pairs of sterile gloves ■ sterile drape ■ optional: antiseptic solution.

Commercially available kits for direct fetal monitoring contain the intrauterine catheter and guide, syringe, and three-way stopcock.

Preparation of equipment

Because fetal monitor models vary in features and complexity, review the operator's manual before proceeding.

If the monitor has two paper speeds, set the monitor to 3 cm/minute *to ensure a readable tracing.* You may interpret a 1 cm/minute tracing less accurately because it's more condensed.

On the printout paper, record the number of the strip, the date, the patient's name and hospital number or birthdate, the printing speed, the type of procedure, and the reason for the procedure.

Place the strain gauge on the appropriate mounting bracket. Then attach this bracket to the side of the monitor. Connect the strain-gauge cable to the uterine activity outlet on the monitor.

Wash your hands and open the sterile equipment, maintaining aseptic technique. Fill the 20-ml syringe with sterile water.

Implementation

• Explain the procedure to the patient and provide emotional support.
• Confirm that the patient has signed a consent form, if required.

To monitor uterine contractions

• Assist the patient to the lithotomy position as the doctor or specially skilled nurse puts on sterile gloves. Inform the patient that she'll have a vaginal examination *to identify the position of the fetus.* During the examination, the intrauterine catheter will be inserted.
• Cover the perineum with a sterile drape. Then clean the perineum with antiseptic solution according to hospital policy. Using aseptic technique, the doctor or nurse will insert the uterine end of the catheter into a catheter guide *to advance the catheter.*
• Attach the syringe holding 20 ml of sterile water to the three-way stopcock at the monitor end of the catheter. Avoid touching the inside of the catheter *to prevent contamination.*
• Flush the catheter with about 5 ml of water and leave the syringe in place.
• Secure the three-way stopcock to the angle fitting of the strain gauge. Avoid touching the stopcock ports *to prevent contamination.*
• Position the strain gauge level with the patient's xiphoid process *to ensure accurate measurements.*
• Prepare the patient for catheter insertion. Explain that the guide will be placed about ¾″ (2 cm) into the cervical opening. The catheter will be advanced into the uterus alongside the fetus for about 18″ (45.7 cm) until a premarked level (on the tubing) reaches the introitus. Then the catheter guide will be removed and the catheter attached to the side fitting on the three-way stopcock.
• Refill the syringe with 20 ml of sterile water and secure the syringe to the upright fitting of the stopcock.
• Tape the catheter to the patient's inner thigh with the nonallergenic tape.
• Turn the stopcock lever to the right *to open the connection between the syringe and the catheter.* Inject 5 ml of sterile water *to clear air bubbles or vernix that could invalidate pressure measurements.*
• Turn the stopcock lever to the left *to close off the catheter.* Then lift the pressure-release cap, and inject water *to flush air bubbles from the strain gauge's dome.*
• Test the monitoring system. First, disconnect the syringe from the stopcock fitting *to open the strain gauge to atmospheric pressure.* Next, turn on the monitor. Observe the lower grid on the printout paper. (This shows uterine activity and contraction pressures.) Look for a zero level reading, which indicates a properly operating system. Reconnect the syringe to the stopcock fitting.
• Turn the stopcock lever to the upright position *to open the connection between the strain gauge and the catheter.* Begin monitoring.
• Inform the patient that the monitor may make noise if the tracer arm swings off the printout paper. Reassure her that this doesn't indicate fetal distress.
• Adjust the strain gauge level with the patient's xiphoid process *to ensure accurate pressure readings.*

Understanding internal electronic fetal monitoring devices

In direct contact with the fetus, an internal electronic fetal monitoring device provides the most accurate and sensitive information about fetal status. This invasive device has an electrode and a catheter.

Spiral electrode

A spiral electrode attaches directly to the presenting fetal part (usually the scalp) for recording the fetal heart rate (FHR). During a vaginal examination, the doctor or a nurse with advanced skills inserts the electrode about 1.5 mm into the presenting fetal part, usually the scalp or buttocks, and then connects the cable end of the electrode wire to the monitor. The spiral electrode may be used alone or with the intrauterine catheter.

Intrauterine catheter

A sterile, water-filled intrauterine catheter connects to a strain gauge that measures uterine activity including frequency, duration, and pressure of uterine contractions. The catheter also facilitates amniotic fluid withdrawal for laboratory analysis, if needed. During a vaginal examination, the doctor or nurse inserts the catheter. The catheter's monitoring end is then attached to the strain gauge, which connects to the monitor.

Data delivery

Both sensing devices connect to the same monitor. The monitor can produce FHR or uterine pressure readings individually or simultaneously, as needed.

Printed data appear on the same paper but on different grids.

Monitoring FHR with a spiral electrode

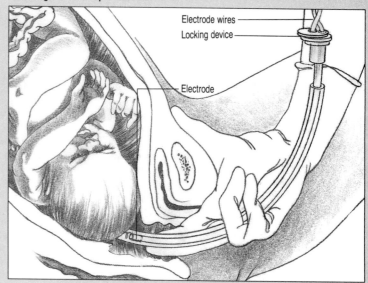

Electrode wires

Locking device

Electrode

Monitoring uterine contractions with an intrauterine catheter

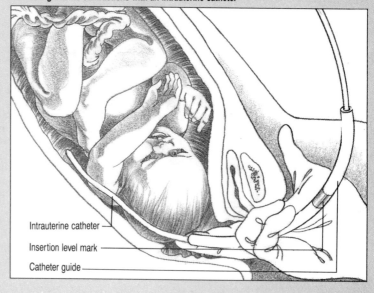

Intrauterine catheter

Insertion level mark

Catheter guide

Reading a fetal monitor strip

Presented in two parallel recordings, the fetal monitor strip records the fetal heart rate (FHR) in beats per minute in the top recording and uterine activity (UA) in mm Hg in the bottom recording. You can obtain information on fetal status and labor progress by reading the strips horizontally and vertically.

Reading horizontally on the FHR or the UA strip, each small block represents 10 seconds. Six consecutive small blocks, separated by a dark vertical line, represent 1 minute. Reading vertically on the FHR strip, each block represents an amplitude of 10 beats/minute. Reading vertically on the UA strip, each block represents 5 mm Hg of pressure.

Assess the baseline FHR—the "resting" heart rate—between uterine contractions when fetal movement diminishes. This baseline FHR (normal range: 120 to 160 beats/minute) pattern serves as a reference for subsequent FHR tracings produced during contractions.

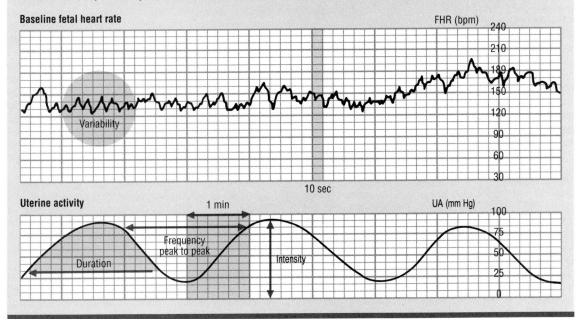

To monitor fetal heart rate
• Apply conduction gel to the leg plate. Then secure the leg plate to the patient's inner thigh with Velcro straps or 2-inch tape. Next, connect the leg plate to the electrocardiogram outlet on the monitor.
• Tell the patient that she will have a vaginal examination *to identify the fetal presenting part and determine its level of descent and to apply the electrode. Explain that this examination ensures against attaching the electrode to fetal suture lines or fontanels, the face, or the genitalia. The spiral electrode will be engaged in a drive tube and advanced through the vagina to the fetal presenting part. To secure the electrode, mild pressure will be applied and the drive tube turned clockwise 360 degrees.*

• After the electrode's in place and the drive tube removed, connect the color-coded electrode wires to the corresponding color-coded leg plate posts.
• Turn on the recorder. Note the time on the printout paper.
• Assist the patient to a comfortable position, and read the strip.

To monitor the patient
• Note the frequency, duration, and intensity of uterine contractions. (See *Reading a fetal monitor strip.*) Normal intrauterine pressure ranges between 8 and 12 mm Hg.
• Check the baseline fetal heart rate (FHR)—the rate between contractions. FHR normally ranges between 120 and 160 beats/minute.

• Assess periodic accelerations or decelerations from the baseline FHR. Compare the FHR pattern with the uterine contraction pattern. Note the time between the onset of an FHR deceleration and the onset of a uterine contraction; the time between the lowest level of an FHR deceleration and the peak of a uterine contraction; and the range of FHR deceleration.

• Check for FHR variability, a measure of fetal reserve and neurologic integrity and stability.

Special considerations

Take care to ensure a level strain-gauge position when monitoring contractions. Positioning the strain gauge too low will yield false-high values; positioning the strain gauge too high will yield false-low values.

During labor, clean the leg plate and reapply conduction gel, as necessary. Periodically flush the intrauterine catheter *to remove air and vernix that prevent accurate pressure measurement.* Also flush the catheter if the monitor stops recording contractions. If the FHR tracing diminishes, tug gently on the electrode wire *to ensure electrode attachment.* Internal electronic fetal monitoring is often used without internal uterine monitoring. However, internal electronic uterine monitoring is seldom used without internal fetal monitoring.

Complications

Possible maternal complications include uterine perforation and intrauterine infection. Possible fetal complications include abscess, hematoma, or infection.

Documentation

Be sure you've numbered each printout sheet and labeled it with the patient's hospital number or birthdate and name, the date, the time, the printing speed, the type of procedure, and the reason for the procedure.

Record any information related to the insertion of the catheter or electrode or both, drug administration, vaginal examinations, or position changes on the printout.

Periodically summarize this information in your notes. Follow hospital policy for required documentation.

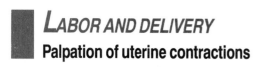

LABOR AND DELIVERY
Palpation of uterine contractions

Periodic, involuntary uterine contractions characterize normal labor and cause progressive cervical effacement and dilation, impelling the fetus to descend. Uterine pal-

pation can tell you the frequency, duration, and intensity of contractions and the relaxation time between them. The character of contractions varies with the stage of labor and the body's response to labor-inducing drugs, if administered.

As labor advances, contractions become more intense, occur more often, and last longer (see *Quick guide to the stages of labor*).

Equipment

Watch with a second hand ■ sheet (for draping).

Implementation

• Review the patient's admission history *to determine the onset, frequency, duration, and intensity of contractions.* Also note where contractions feel strongest or exert the most pressure.

• Wash your hands and provide privacy.

• Describe the palpation procedure to the patient. *Because she may be ticklish or sensitive to touch,* forewarn her that you'll palpate her abdominal area over the uterus.

• Assist the patient to a comfortable side-lying position *to relieve pressure on the inferior vena cava and promote uteroplacental circulation. This position also relieves direct pressure on the sacral area from the fetal head and eases backache.*

• Drape the patient with a sheet.

• Plant the palmar surface of your fingers on the uterine fundus and palpate lightly *to assess contractions.* Note the uterine tightening and abdominal lifting that occur with contractions. Each contraction has three phases: increment (rising), acme (peak), and decrement (letting down or ebbing).

• Palpate several contractions. Simultaneously use the second hand on your watch *to assess and measure such contraction qualities as frequency, duration, and intensity.*

To assess frequency, time the interval between the beginning of one contraction and the beginning of the next. In normal labor, contractions begin slowly and gradually occur more frequently with briefer relaxation intervals.

To assess duration, time the period from when the uterus begins tightening until it begins relaxing. Commonly, as labor progresses so does the duration of each contraction.

To assess intensity, press your fingertips into the uterine fundus when the uterus tightens. During mild contractions, the fundus indents easily and feels like a chin; during moderate contractions, the fundus indents less easily and feels like a nose; during strong contractions, the fundus resists indenting and feels like a forehead.

Quick guide to the stages of labor

Normal labor advances through the four stages summarized below. Offer your patient encouragement and progress reports through the stages.

First stage

Regular contractions, which repeat at 15- to 20-minute intervals and last between 10 and 30 seconds, signal the onset of labor's first stage. This stage has three phases: latent, active, and transitional. In primiparous patients, this stage of labor may average 3.3 to 19.7 hours; in multiparous patients, it may average 0.1 to 14.3 hours.

In the latent phase (characterized by irregular, brief, and mild contractions), the cervix dilates to 3 or 4 cm. Other signs and symptoms include abdominal cramping and backache. The patient may expel the mucus plug during this phase. This phase averages 8.6 hours in primiparous patients and 5.3 hours in multiparous patients.

During the active phase, cervical dilation increases to between 5 and 7 cm. Contractions occur every 3 to 5 minutes, last 30 to 45 seconds, and become moderately intense. In primiparous patients, this phase averages 5.8 hours; in multiparous patients, 2.5 hours.

In the transitional phase, the cervix dilates completely (8 to 10 cm). Uterine contractions grow intense, last between 45 and 60 seconds, and repeat at least every 2 minutes. The patient may thrash about, lose control of breathing techniques, and experience nausea and vomiting. This phase typically lasts less than 3 hours in primiparous patients and less than 1 hour in multiparous patients.

Second stage

In the second stage of labor, contractions occur often (every 1½ to 2 minutes) and last longer—up to 90 seconds. This stage commonly ends within 1 hour for a primiparous patient and possibly 15 minutes for a multiparous patient.

Signs and symptoms signaling onset of the second stage include increased bloody show, rupture of membranes (if they're still intact), severe rectal pressure and flaring, and reflexive bearing down with each contraction. The fetal head approaches the perineal floor and emerges at the vaginal opening.

The second labor stage concludes with birth.

Third stage

Strong but less painful contractions expel the placenta, which normally emerges within 30 minutes after the neonate emerges.

Signs indicating normal separation of the placenta from the uterine wall include lengthening of the umbilical cord, a sudden gush of dark blood from the vagina, and a palpable change in uterine shape from disclike to globular.

Fourth stage

This stage begins with placental expulsion and extends through the next 4 hours, while the patient's body rests and begins adjusting to the postpartum state.

• Determine how the patient copes with discomfort by assessing her breathing and relaxation techniques, if any. *This may help guide your intervention choices.* Naturally, you'll provide ongoing emotional support in any event.
• Observe the patient's response to contractions *to evaluate whether she needs an analgesic, anesthetic, or other appropriate measure, such as repositioning or back massage.*
• Assess contractions at least hourly during the latent phase of first-stage labor and every 30 minutes throughout the active phase. During second-stage labor, assess contractions every 15 minutes.

Special considerations

Because the patient may become irritable or anxious during the transitional phase of first-stage labor—when the cervix dilates fully—and because abdominal palpation may aggravate her distress, assess contractions only as necessary. If appropriate, teach her support person to palpate and record contractions.

If any contraction lasts longer than 90 seconds and isn't followed by uterine muscle relaxation, notify the doctor immediately *so he may evaluate maternal and fetal well-being. Keep in mind that hypertonic contractions can cause uterine rupture and fetal hypoxia.*

Also report a brief relaxation period between contractions. *This period allows the intervillous uterine spaces to fill with oxygen and nutrients. Inadequate relaxation intervals increase the risk of fetal hypoxia and exhaust the mother.*

Documentation
Record the frequency, duration, and intensity of contractions. Keep track of the relaxation time between contractions. In your notes, describe the patient's response to contractions.

 Vaginal examination

During first-stage labor, a doctor or a nurse with special skills performs a vaginal examination to assess cervical dilation, effacement, membrane status, and fetal presentation, position, and engagement.

Important considerations during the examination include respecting the patient's privacy, providing simple explanations for her and her support person, maintaining eye contact when possible, and using aseptic technique. With experience, the typical examiner develops a well-honed routine for collecting necessary information. This enables the examination to proceed precisely and efficiently.

Contraindications to a vaginal examination include excessive vaginal bleeding, which may signal placenta previa.

Equipment
Sterile gloves ▪ sterile, water-soluble lubricant or sterile water ▪ mild soap and water or cleaning solution ▪ linen-saver pads ▪ antiseptic solution ▪ sterile gauze.

Implementation
• Explain the procedure to the patient, and give her an opportunity to empty her bladder. *A distended bladder may interfere with accurate examination findings.*
• Use Leopold's maneuvers to identify the fetal presenting part and position. Then help the patient into a lithotomy position for the vaginal examination.
• Place a linen-saver pad under the patient's buttocks, and put on sterile gloves.
• Inform the patient when you are about to touch her *to avoid startling her.*
• Clean the perineum with mild soap and water or cleaning solution, spreading the labia with your independent hand *to avoid contaminating your examining hand.*
• Lubricate the index and middle fingers of your examining hand with sterile water or sterile water-soluble lubricant *to facilitate insertion.* If the membranes are ruptured, use an antiseptic solution.
• Ask the patient to relax by taking several deep breaths and slowly releasing the air. Then insert your lubricated fingers (palmar surface down) into the vagina. Keep your

uninserted fingers flexed *to avoid the rectum* (see *Step-by-step vaginal examination*).
• Palpate the cervix, keeping in mind that the cervix may assume a posterior position in early labor and be difficult to locate. Once you find the cervix, however, note its consistency. Throughout pregnancy, the cervix gradually softens, reaching a buttery consistency before labor begins (for more information, see *Cervical effacement and dilation,* page 686).
• After identifying the presenting fetal part and position, evaluating dilation and effacement, assessing fetal engagement and station, and verifying membrane status, gently withdraw your fingers. Let the patient clean her perineum herself with sterile gauze if she can walk to the bathroom. If she's confined to bed, you can clean her perineum and change the linen-saver pad.
• Describe how labor progresses, and define the patient's stage and phase, if appropriate, *to encourage her and help reduce her anxiety.*

Special considerations
In early labor, perform the vaginal examination between contractions, focusing primarily on the extent of cervical dilation and effacement. At the end of first-stage labor, perform the examination during a contraction, when the uterine muscle pushes the fetus downward. This examination will focus on assessing fetal descent.

If the amniotic membrane ruptures during the examination, record the fetal heart rate (FHR). Then note the time and describe the color, odor, and approximate amount of fluid. If FHR becomes unstable, notify the doctor, determine fetal station, and check for umbilical cord prolapse. After the membranes rupture, perform the vaginal examination only when labor changes significantly *to minimize the risk of introducing intrauterine infection.*

Documentation
After each examination, record the percentage of effacement, dilation, the station of the presenting fetal part, amniotic membrane status, and the patient's tolerance of the procedure.

 Oxytocin administration

The hormone oxytocin stimulates the uterine smooth-muscle fibers to contract, thereby facilitating cervical dilation. The doctor may order synthetic oxytocin (Pitocin, Syntocinon) to induce or augment labor or to control bleeding and enhance uterine contraction after the pla-

Step-by-step vaginal examination

Begin the vaginal examination — usually in early labor — by inserting your gloved index and middle fingers palm side down into the vagina. Use your nondominant hand to gently but firmly press on the uterus *to steady the fetal presenting part against the cervix for examination.*

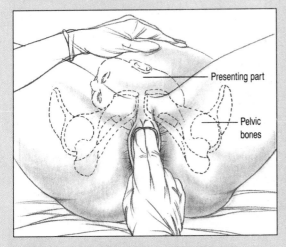

Presenting part

Pelvic bones

Confirm the presenting part and position

Rotate your fingers to palpate and confirm the fetal presenting part (a fetal head feels firm, the buttocks soft) and position (left, right, anterior, posterior, or transverse) identified by using Leopold's maneuvers.

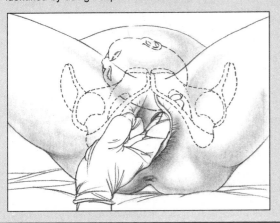

Assess cervical effacement and dilation

Estimate cervical dilation by palpating the internal os. Each fingerbreadth of dilation averages 1.5 to 2 cm, depending on the width of the examiner's finger.

Next, determine the percentage of effacement by palpating the ridge of tissue around the cervix. Assign a low percentage of effacement to defined and thick cervical tissue. Indistinct, wafer-thin cervical tissue scores 100%.

Assess fetal engagement and station

Estimate the extent of fetal engagement (descent of the fetal presenting part into the pelvis).

Then palpate the presenting part and grade the fetal station (where the presenting part lies in relation to the ischial spines of the maternal pelvis). A zero grade indicates that the presenting part lies level with the ischial spine.

Station grades range from −3 (3 cm above the maternal ischial spines) to +4 (4 cm below the maternal ischial spines, causing the perineum to bulge).

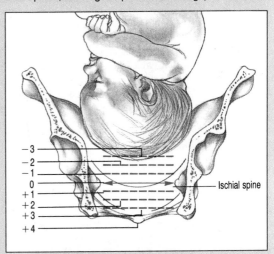

−3
−2
−1
0
+1
+2
+3
+4

Ischial spine

Evaluate membrane status

If appropriate, also check amniotic membrane status. If you feel a bulging, slick surface over the presenting fetal part, you know the membranes remain intact.

Cervical effacement and dilation

As labor advances, so do cervical effacement and dilation, thereby facilitating birth. During effacement, the cervix shortens and its walls become thin, progressing from 0% effacement (palpable and thick) to 100% effacement (fully indistinct—or effaced—and paper thin). Full effacement obliterates the constrictive uterine neck to create a smooth, unobstructed passage for the fetus.

At the same time, dilation occurs. This progressive widening of the cervical canal—from the upper internal cervical os to the lower external cervical os—advances from 0 to 10 cm. As the cervical canal opens, resistance decreases. This further eases fetal descent.

No effacement or dilation

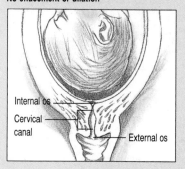

Internal os
Cervical canal
External os

Early effacement and dilation

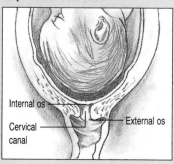

Internal os
Cervical canal
External os

Full effacement and dilation

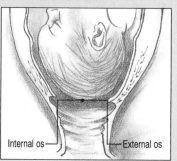

Internal os
External os

centa is delivered. Usually, the nurse administers oxytocin intravenously. To regulate dosage (which will vary depending on uterine sensitivity) and to help prevent uterine hyperstimulation (which may retard fetal blood flow), she typically uses an infusion pump. Additional nursing responsibilities include managing the infusion and monitoring maternal and fetal responses and possible complications.

Indications for oxytocin include pregnancy-induced hypertension, prolonged gestation, maternal diabetes, Rh sensitization, premature or prolonged rupture of membranes, incomplete or inevitable abortion, and evaluation of fetal distress after 31 weeks.

Oxytocin is contraindicated in such conditions as placenta previa and diagnosed cephalopelvic disproportion. Oxytocin should be administered cautiously to a patient who has an overdistended uterus or a history of cervical surgery, uterine surgery, or grand multiparity.

Equipment

Administration set for primary I.V. line ■ infusion pump and tubing ■ I.V. solution, as ordered ■ external or internal fetal monitoring equipment (see "External fetal monitoring" and "Internal electronic fetal monitoring" in this chapter) ■ oxytocin ■ 20G 1″ needle ■ label ■ venipuncture equipment with an 18G over-the-needle catheter ■ optional: autosyringe.

Preparation of equipment

Prepare the oxytocin solution, as ordered. Rotate the I.V. bag *to disperse the drug throughout the solution.* Label the I.V. container with the name of the medication. Then attach the infusion pump tubing to the I.V. container, and connect the tubing to the pump. *Because infusion pump features vary,* review the operator's manual before proceeding. Next, attach the 20G 1″ needle to the tubing *to piggyback it to the primary I.V. line,* or use an autosyringe connected to the primary I.V. line. Then set up the equipment for internal or external fetal monitoring.

Implementation

● Explain the procedure to the patient and provide privacy. Wash your hands. Describe the equipment, and forewarn the patient that she may feel a pinch from the venipuncture.

To administer oxytocin in labor and delivery
● Assist the patient to a lateral-tilt position and support her hip with a pillow. Don't let her lie supine. *In this position the gravid uterus presses on the maternal great vessels, producing maternal hypotension and reducing uterine perfusion.*
● Identify and record the fetal heart rate (FHR) and assess uterine contractions occurring in a 20-minute span.

to establish baseline fetal status and evaluate spontaneous maternal uterine activity.

• Start the primary I.V. line using an 18G over-the-needle catheter throughout labor and delivery. *Use this line to deliver not only oxytocin but also fluids, blood, or other medications as needed.*

• Piggyback the oxytocin solution (metered by the infusion pump) to the primary I.V. line at the Y injection site closest to the patient. *Piggybacking maintains I.V. line patency (which you'll need to preserve should you discontinue the oxytocin infusion). Besides, using the Y injection site nearest the venipuncture ensures that the primary line holds the lowest concentration of oxytocin if you must stop the infusion.*

• Begin the oxytocin infusion, as ordered. The typical recommended labor-starting dose ranges between 0.5 and 1.0 milliunit (mU)/minute. (The maximum dose is 20 mU/minute.)

• *Because oxytocin begins acting immediately,* be prepared to start monitoring uterine contractions.

• Increase the oxytocin as ordered. As a rule, each increase should range no more than 1 to 2 mU/minute infused once every 15 to 30 minutes. When induced labor simulates normal labor (contractions occur every 2 to 3 minutes and last 40 to 60 seconds) and cervical dilation progresses at least 1 cm/hour in first-stage, active-phase labor, you can stop increases. However, continue the infusion at the dosage and rate that maintain the activity closest to normal labor.

• Before each increase, be sure to time the frequency and duration of contractions, palpate the uterus to identify contraction intensity, and assess maternal vital signs and fetal heart rhythm and rate *to ensure safety and to anticipate possible complications.* If you're using an external fetal monitor, the uterine activity strip or grid should show contractions occurring every 2 to 3 minutes. The contractions should last for about 60 seconds and be followed by uterine relaxation. If you're using an internal fetal monitor, look for an optimal baseline value ranging from 5 to 15 mm Hg. Your aim is to verify uterine relaxation between contractions.

• Intervene with comfort measures as needed. For example, reposition the patient on her other side.

• Continue assessing maternal and fetal responses to the oxytocin. For example, every 10 to 15 minutes, evaluate FHR; maternal response to increased contraction activity and subsequent discomfort; and maternal pulse rate and pattern, blood pressure, respiration rate and quality, and uterine contractions; and review the infusion rate *to prevent uterine hyperstimulation.* Signs of hyperstimulation include contractions less than 2 minutes apart and lasting 90 seconds or longer; uterine pressure values that

don't return to baseline between contractions; and intrauterine pressure that rises over 75 mm Hg.

• *To reduce uterine irritability,* try to increase uterine blood flow. Do this by changing the patient's position and increasing the infusion rate of the primary I.V. line. Avoid exceeding the maximum total infusion of 20 mU/minute.

• *To manage hyperstimulation,* discontinue the infusion, administer oxygen, and notify the doctor.

• After hyperstimulation resolves, resume the oxytocin infusion. Depending on maternal and fetal conditions, select one of the following methods: resume the infusion beginning with oxytocin 0.5 mU/minute, increase the dosage to 1 mU/minute every 15 minutes, and increase the rate, as before; or resume the infusion at one-half of the last dosage given and increase the rate as before; or resume the infusion at the dosage given before hyperstimulation signs occurred. Check your hospital's policy for the appropriate method.

• Monitor and record intake and output. At rates of 16 mU/minute and more, oxytocin has an antidiuretic effect, so you may need to administer an electrolyte-containing I.V. solution *to maintain electrolyte balance.*

To administer oxytocin after delivery

• As ordered after delivery, administer 10 to 40 units of oxytocin added to 1,000 ml of physiologic electrolyte solution. Infuse at a rate titrated to decrease postpartum bleeding or uterine atony after placental delivery. As an alternative, administer 10 units of oxytocin intramuscularly until you can establish the I.V. line.

Special considerations

You can administer oxytocin without an electronic fetal monitor or an infusion pump. However, most hospitals require use of a pump to ensure accurate dosage and titration. (See *Conversion formulas for oxytocin administration,* page 688.) Without an infusion pump, administer oxytocin through a minidrop system (60 drops/ml) or an autosyringe, and observe the patient closely. Without an electronic fetal monitor, frequently palpate and assess contractions. Auscultate FHR every 5 to 15 minutes (see "Fetal heart rate" in this chapter).

Complications

Oxytocin can cause uterine hyperstimulation that may progress to tetanic contractions, which last longer than 2 minutes. Other complications include fetal distress, abruptio placentae, and uterine rupture.

Watch for signs of oxytocin hypersensitivity, such as elevated blood pressure. Rarely, oxytocin leads to maternal seizures or coma from water intoxication.

Conversion formulas for oxytocin administration

To ensure that all members of the health care team talk the same language when administering oxytocin, use the following formulas, as needed, to convert milliliters (ml) per minute or drops (gtt) per minute to milliunits (mU) per minute. Conversion to mU per minute gives the actual drug dosage instead of the fluid dosage.

Which conversion formula you use may be dictated by the infusion pump you use.

Synthetic oxytocin for I.V. administration comes in a concentration of 10 units/ml in 10-ml vials, in 0.5- and 1-ml ampules, and in 1-ml disposable syringes.

To calculate oxytocin dilution (in mU/ml):

$$\frac{\# \text{ of units oxytocin}}{\text{ml of fluid}} \times 1{,}000 = \text{mU/ml}$$

To convert ml/minute to mU/minute:

$$\frac{\text{mU}}{\text{ml}} \times \frac{\text{ml}}{\text{minute}} = \frac{\text{mU}}{\text{minute}}$$

To convert gtt/minute to mU/minute:

$$\frac{\text{gtt}}{\text{minute}} \times \frac{\text{mU}}{\text{ml}} \times \frac{\text{ml}}{\text{gtt}} = \frac{\text{mU}}{\text{minute}}$$

Documentation
Record maternal response to contractions, blood pressure, pulse rate and pattern, and respiratory rate and quality on the patient's labor progression chart. Also record FHR, oxytocin infusion rate, and intake and output amounts. Describe uterine activity as well.

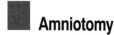

Amniotomy

When the doctor or a nurse with special skills (a nurse-midwife, for example) uses a sterile amniohook to rupture the amniotic membranes, she's performing an amniotomy. This controversial but common procedure prompts amniotic fluid drainage, which enhances the intensity, frequency, and duration of uterine contractions by reducing uterine volume.

Amniotomy induces or augments labor if the membranes fail to rupture spontaneously. It helps to expedite labor after the dilation begins, and it facilitates insertion of an intrauterine catheter and a spiral electrode for direct fetal monitoring.

Oxytocin infusion may precede amniotomy or follow it by 6 to 8 hours if labor fails to progress. If birth doesn't occur within 12 to 24 hours after amniotomy, the doctor may perform a cesarean section to reduce the risk of infection.

When deciding whether to perform amniotomy, the doctor or nurse-midwife considers such factors as fetal presentation, position, and station; the degree of cervical dilation and effacement; contraction frequency and intensity; the fetus's gestational age; existing complications; and maternal and fetal vital signs.

Amniotomy is contraindicated in high-risk pregnancies, unless more accurate fetal assessment using internal fetal monitoring is necessary. It's also contraindicated when the presenting fetal part is unengaged because of the risk of transverse lie and umbilical cord prolapse. For more information, see *Managing umbilical cord prolapse.*

Equipment
Povidone-iodine solution ▪ linen-saver pads ▪ bedpan ▪ soap and water ▪ 4″ × 4″ gauze pads ▪ external electronic fetal monitoring equipment or a fetoscope or Doppler stethoscope ▪ sterile gloves ▪ sterile amniohook.

Preparation of equipment
Assemble the equipment at the patient's bedside.

Implementation
● Reinforce the doctor or nurse-midwife's explanation of the procedure, and answer the patient's questions. Wash your hands and put on sterile gloves.
● Clean the perineum with soap and water or 4″ × 4″ gauze pads moistened with povidone-iodine solution.
● Position the patient and the bedpan *so that the bedpan receives the amniotic fluid.* Then elevate the head of the bed about 25 degrees *to tilt the pelvis for easier vaginal access.*
● Note the baseline fetal heart rate (FHR) *to evaluate fetal status before and after amniotomy.* Use external fetal monitoring throughout the procedure. Otherwise, use the fetoscope or Doppler stethoscope.

Managing umbilical cord prolapse

If not identified and corrected with 5 minutes, umbilical cord prolapse may cause fetal hypoxia, central nervous system damage, and possibly death. Fortunately, rapid detection and intervention by the health care team can help the mother and fetus survive. Be alert for the following signs and symptoms of cord prolapse, especially after amniotomy. Then intervene as appropriate until the patient undergoes an emergency cesarean or forceps delivery.

Signs and symptoms
• The patient reports feeling the cord "slither" down after membrane rupture.
• A visible or palpable umbilical cord enters the birth canal.
• Violent fetal activity occurs.
• Fetal monitoring detects bradycardia with variable deceleration during contractions.

Nursing interventions
• Immediately summon another health care team member who can notify the doctor and prepare for immediate delivery or emergency surgery.
• Move the patient into the Trendelenburg's or knee-chest position with hips elevated. *Either position will shift fetal weight from the cord.* While waiting to enter the operating room, push the fetal presenting part away from the cord with two gloved fingers.
• Do not attempt to return the cord to the uterus. *This may injure the cord, stop blood flow to the fetus, or introduce intrauterine infection.* Instead, lift it with gloved hands and gently wrap it in loose, sterile towels saturated with sterile saline solution.
• Be prepared to administer supplemental oxygen by face mask (10 to 12 liters/minute) and initiate or increase I.V. fluids with 5% dextrose in lactated Ringer's solution *to enhance fluid volume and circulation.*
• Anticipate drawing and sending blood for type and crossmatch if the information isn't already available.
• Prepare to assist in monitoring fetal heart tones by connecting an internal spiral electrode to the presenting fetal part.
• Reassure and inform the patient throughout this emergency. Calmly convey the seriousness of the situation and the importance of cooperation.
• Accompany the patient to the operating room. Continue interventions to relieve the cord of pressure. Continue monitoring for maternal and fetal distress.

• Using sterile technique, open the amniohook package. Then, wearing sterile gloves, the doctor or nurse-midwife removes the amniohook from the package.
• If ordered, apply pressure to the uterine fundus as the doctor or nurse-midwife inserts the amniohook vaginally to the cervical os. *This helps to keep the fetal presenting part engaged and reduces the risk of cord prolapse.* Then, carefully avoiding contact with the fetal presenting part, the doctor or nurse-midwife ruptures the amniotic membrane at the internal os.
• Without external electronic fetal monitoring equipment, use a fetoscope or Doppler stethoscope to evaluate FHR for at least 60 seconds after the membrane ruptures *to detect bradycardia.* Otherwise, check the monitor tracing for large, variable decelerations in FHR that suggest cord compression. If these FHR changes occur, the doctor or nurse-midwife will perform a vaginal examination *to check for cord prolapse.*
• Clean and dry the perineal area and remove the bedpan. When necessary, replace the linen-saver pad under the patient's buttocks *to promote comfort and hygiene.*

• Inspect the amniotic fluid for meconium, blood, or foul odor. Note the color and measure the amount of fluid.
• Take the patient's temperature every 2 hours *to detect possible infection.* If her temperature rises to 100° F (38° C), begin hourly checks. Continue to monitor uterine contractions and labor progress.

Special considerations
During a vaginal examination after amniotomy, maintain strict aseptic technique *to prevent uterine infection.* For the same reason, minimize the number of examinations.

Complications
Umbilical cord prolapse—a life-threatening potential complication of amniotomy—is an emergency requiring immediate cesarean delivery to prevent fetal death. It occurs when amniotic fluid, gushing from the ruptured sac, sweeps the cord down through the cervix. The risk of prolapse is higher if the fetal head is not engaged in the pelvis before the rupture occurs.

Intrauterine infection can result from failure to use aseptic technique for amniotomy. Infection may also result from prolonged labor after amniotomy.

Documentation

Record FHR before and at frequent intervals immediately after amniotomy (every 5 minutes for 20 minutes and then every 30 minutes). Note any meconium or blood in the amniotic fluid. Measure the amount of fluid, and note whether the fluid has an odor. Record maternal temperature every 2 hours and labor progress as appropriate.

⚑⚑ Emergency delivery

Emergency delivery—the unplanned birth of a neonate outside of a hospital—may occur when labor progresses very quickly or when circumstances prevent the mother from entering a medical facility. Whether assisting at an emergency delivery or instructing the person who is, your objectives include establishing a clean, safe, and private birth area; promoting a controlled delivery; and preventing injury, infection, and hemorrhage.

Equipment

Unopened newspaper or large, clean cloth (such as a tablecloth, towel, or curtain) ▪ bath towel, blanket, or coat (to cushion and support the patient's buttocks) ▪ gloves ▪ at least two small, clean cloths ▪ clean, sharp object (such as a crochet hook, scissors, new razor blade, knife, or nail file) ▪ ligating material (such as string, yarn, ribbon, or new shoelaces) ▪ clean blanket or towel (to cover the newborn) ▪ boiling water.

Preparation of equipment

Boil the ligating and cutting materials for at least 5 minutes, if possible.

Implementation

• Offer support and reassurance *to help relieve the patient's anxiety*. Encourage the patient to pant during contractions *to promote a controlled delivery*. As possible, provide privacy, wash your hands, and put on gloves.

• Position the patient comfortably on a bed, a couch, or the ground. Open the newspaper or the large, clean cloth and place it under the patient's buttocks *to provide a clean delivery area*. Elevate the buttocks slightly with the bath towel, blanket, or coat *to provide additional room for delivery.*

• Check for signs of imminent delivery—bulging perineum, an increase in bloody show, urgency to push, and crowning of the presenting part.

• As the fetal head reaches and begins to pass the perineum, instruct the patient to pant or blow through the contractions *because forceful bearing down could cause extensive maternal lacerations*. Place one hand gently on the perineum *to cover the fetal head, control birth speed, and prevent sudden expulsion.*

• Avoid forcibly restraining fetal descent because *undue pressure can cause cephalohematoma or scalp lacerations, head trauma, and vagal stimulation. Undue pressure may also occlude the umbilical cord, which may cause fetal bradycardia, circulatory depression, and hypoxia.*

• As the fetal head emerges, immediately break the amniotic sac if it's intact. Support the head as it emerges. Instruct the patient to continue blowing and panting.

• Locate the umbilical cord. Insert one or two fingers along the back of the emergent head *to be sure the cord isn't wrapped around the neck*. If the cord's wrapped loosely around the neck, slip it over the head *to prevent strangulation during delivery*. If it's wrapped tightly around the neck, ligate the cord in two places. Then carefully cut between the ligatures, using a clean, sharp object, or, if possible, a sterile one.

• Carefully support the head with both hands as it rotates to one side (external rotation). Gently wipe mucus and amniotic fluid from the nose and mouth with a clean, small cloth *to prevent aspiration.*

• Instruct the patient to bear down with the next contraction *to aid delivery of the shoulders*. Position your hands on either side of the neonate's head and support the neck. Exert gentle downward pressure *to deliver the anterior shoulder*. Then exert gentle upward pressure *to deliver the posterior shoulder.*

• Remember that amniotic fluid and vernix are slippery, so take care to support the neonate's body securely after freeing the shoulders.

• Keep the neonate in a slightly head-down position *to encourage mucus to drain from the respiratory tract*. Wipe excess mucus from the face. If the neonate doesn't breathe spontaneously, gently pat the soles of his feet or stroke his back. *Never suspend a neonate by his feet.*

• Dry and cover him quickly with the blanket or towel. Ensure that the head is well covered *to minimize exposure and prevent heat loss.*

• Cradle the neonate at the level of the maternal uterus until the umbilical cord stops pulsating. *This prevents the neonatal blood from flowing to or from the placenta and leading to hypovolemia or hypervolemia, respectively. Hypovolemia can lead to circulatory collapse and neonatal death; hypervolemia can cause hyperbilirubinemia.*

• Place the neonate on the mother's abdomen in a slightly head-down position.

• If this hasn't been done, ligate the umbilical cord at two points, 1″ to 2″ (2.5 to 5 cm) apart. Place the first ligature 4″ to 6″ (10 to 15 cm) from the neonate. *Ligation prevents autotransfusion, which may cause hemolysis and hyperbilirubinemia.*

• Cut the umbilical cord between the two ligatures, using sterile equipment if available. *Using unsterile instruments may cause infection.*

• Watch for signs of placental separation, such as a slight gush of dark blood from the vagina, cord lengthening, and a firm uterine fundus rising within the abdominal area. Usually, the placenta separates from the uterus within 5 minutes after delivery (though it may take as long as 30 minutes). When you see these signs, encourage the patient to bear down *to expel the placenta.* As she does, apply gentle downward pressure on her abdomen *to aid placental delivery.* Never tug on the umbilical cord to initiate or aid placental delivery *because this may invert the uterus or sever the cord from the placenta.*

• Examine the expelled placenta for intactness. *Retained placental fragments may cause hemorrhage or lead to intrauterine infection.*

• Place the cord and the placenta inside the towel or blanket covering the neonate *to provide extra warmth and also to ensure that the cord and placenta will be transported to the hospital for closer examination.*

• Palpate the maternal uterus *to make sure it's firm.* Gently massage the atonic uterus *to encourage contraction and prevent hemorrhage.* Encourage breast-feeding, if appropriate, *to stimulate uterine contraction.*

• Check the patient for excessive bleeding from perineal lacerations. Apply a perineal pad, if available, and instruct the patient to press her thighs together. Provide comfort and reassurance, and offer fluids, if available. Have someone summon an emergency medical service or arrange transportation to the hospital for the mother and neonate. Make sure that the mother and neonate are warm and dry while they await transport.

Special considerations

Never introduce any object into the vagina to facilitate delivery. *This increases the risk of intrauterine infection as well as injury to the cervix, uterus, fetus, cord, or placenta.*

In a *breech presentation,* make every effort to transport the patient to a nearby medical facility. If the patient begins to deliver, carefully support the fetal buttocks with both hands. Gently lift the body to deliver the posterior shoulder. Then lower the neonate slightly to deliver the anterior shoulder. Flexion of the head usually follows. Never apply traction to the body *to avoid lodging the head*

in the cervix. Allow the neonate to rotate and emerge spontaneously.

If the umbilical cord emerges first, elevate the presenting part throughout delivery *to prevent occluding the cord and causing fetal hypoxia.* Because this obstetric emergency usually necessitates a cesarean section, arrange for immediate transport to a nearby medical facility.

If the neonate fails to breathe spontaneously after birth, begin to breathe for him. Place your open mouth over his nose and mouth. Using air collected in your cheeks, deliver four short puffs. Next, check the umbilical cord for pulsation. If you find no pulse, begin cardiopulmonary resuscitation (CPR). Place your index and middle fingers over the lower third of the neonate's sternum. Administer a breath of air; then use your fingers gently but firmly to pump the heart. Pump five times for each breath of air delivered. Continue performing CPR until the neonate breathes and his heart beats.

Documentation

Give the medical care team the following information, if possible: the time of delivery and the presentation and position of the fetus. Describe any delivery complications, such as the cord wrapped around the neonate's neck. Describe the color, character, and amount of amniotic fluid. Note the time of placental expulsion, the placental appearance and intactness, the amount of postpartum bleeding, the status of uterine firmness (tone) and contractions, and the mother's response. If known, name the mother's blood type and Rh factor. Document the sex of the neonate, estimate the Apgar score, and define any resuscitative measures used. Record whether the mother began breast-feeding the neonate. Also identify and quantify any fluids given to the mother.

Postpartum fundal assessments

After delivery, the uterus gradually shrinks and descends into its prepregnancy position in the pelvis — a process known as involution. The nurse evaluates normal involutional progress by palpating and massaging the uterus to identify uterine size, firmness, and descent. (See *Hand placement for fundal palpation and massage*, page 692.)

Involution normally begins immediately after delivery, when the firmly contracted uterus lies midway between the umbilicus and the symphysis pubis. Soon the uterus rises to the umbilicus and, after the first postpartum day, begins returning to the pelvis. The average descent

Hand placement for fundal palpation and massage

A full-term pregnancy stretches the ligaments supporting the uterus, placing the uterus at risk for inversion during palpation and massage. To guard against this, use your hands to support and fix the uterus in a safe position. Here's how.

Place one hand against the patient's abdomen at the symphysis pubis level. This steadies the fundus and prevents downward displacement.

Place the other hand at the top of the fundus, cupping it.

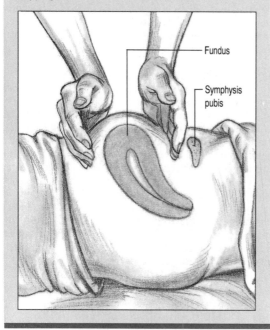

rate is 1 fingerbreadth or centimeter daily — slightly slower if the patient had a cesarean section. By the 10th postpartum day the now unpalpable uterus lies deep in the pelvis, either at or below the symphysis pubis.

When the uterus fails to contract or remain firm during involution, uterine bleeding or hemorrhage can result. That's because placental separation after delivery exposes large uterine blood vessels, which uterine contractions close off (like a tourniquet). Fundal massage, synthetic oxytocic therapy, or natural oxytocic substances released during breast-feeding help to maintain or stimulate contraction.

Typical nursing procedures that coincide with fundal palpation and massage include caring for the perineum and evaluating healing (see *Postpartum perineal care*).

Equipment
Gloves ■ analgesics ■ perineal pad ■ optional: urinary catheter.

Implementation
● Explain the procedure to the patient, and provide privacy. Wash your hands and put on gloves.
● Schedule fundal assessments (unless the doctor orders otherwise) every 15 minutes for the first hour after delivery, every 30 minutes for the next 2 to 3 hours, every hour for the next 4 hours, every 4 hours for the rest of the first postpartum day, and every 8 hours until the patient's discharge. Give prescribed analgesics before fundal checks, if indicated. Teach her relaxation techniques (deep breathing) to help her cope with discomfort.
● Encourage the patient's efforts to urinate *because bladder distention impairs uterine contraction by pushing the uterus up and aside.* You may need to catheterize the patient if she can't urinate or if the uterus becomes displaced with increased bleeding.
● Lower the head of the bed until the patient lies supine. If she reports discomfort in this position — especially if she's had cesarean surgery — keep the head of the bed slightly elevated.
● Expose the abdomen for palpation and the perineum for observation. You'll watch for bleeding, clots, and tissue expulsion as you massage the fundus.
● Gently compress the uterus between both hands *to evaluate uterine firmness.* Note the level of the fundus above or below the umbilicus in fingerbreadths or centimeters.
● If the uterus seems soft and boggy, gently massage the fundus with a circular motion until it becomes firm. Simply cupping the uterus between your hands may also stimulate contraction.
    Alternatively, massage the fundus with the side of the hand above the fundus. Without digging into the abdomen, gently compress and release, always supporting the lower uterine segment with the other hand. Observe for lochia flow during massage.
● Massage long enough to produce firmness. The sensitive and tender fundus needs only gentle pressure. *This should produce desired results without causing excessive discomfort.*
● Notify the doctor or nurse-midwife immediately should the uterus fail to contract and should heavy bleeding occur. If the fundus becomes firm after massage, keep one hand on the lower uterus and press gently toward the pubis *to help expel any clots.*
● Clean the perineum and apply a clean perineal pad. Help the patient into a comfortable position.

Special considerations

Because incisional pain makes fundal palpation uncomfortable for the patient who has had a cesarean section, provide pain medication beforehand, as ordered. If the lochia flow diminishes after 4 hours, the doctor may permit fewer fundal checks than usual, especially if the patient's receiving oxytocin.

Beware if no lochia appears. *This may signal a clot blocking the cervical os. Subsequent heavy bleeding may result if a position change dislodges the clot.* Take vital signs *to assess for signs of hypovolemic shock.*

Complications

Because the uterus and its supporting ligaments are usually tender after delivery, pain is the most common complication of fundal palpation and massage. Excessive massage can stimulate premature uterine contractions, causing undue muscle fatigue and leading to uterine atony or inversion.

Documentation

Record vital signs, fundal height in fingerbreadths or centimeters, and also record position (midline or off-center) and tone (firm or soft and boggy). Document massage and note passage of any clots. Record excessive bleeding and your notification of the doctor or nurse-midwife.

NEONATAL MONITORING

Apgar scoring

Named after its developer, Virginia Apgar, the Apgar score quantifies the neonatal heart rate, respiratory effort, muscle tone, reflexes, and color. Each category is assessed 1 minute after birth and again 5 minutes later. Scores in each category range from 0 to 2. The highest Apgar score is 10 — the greatest possible sum of the five categories.

The evaluation at 1 minute indicates the neonate's initial adaptation to extrauterine life. The evaluation at 5 minutes gives a clearer picture of overall status. If the neonate doesn't breathe or his heart beats fewer than 100 times a minute, call for help and begin resuscitation at once. Don't wait for a 1-minute Apgar test score.

Equipment

Apgar score sheet or neonatal assessment sheet (see *Recording the Apgar score*, page 694) ▪ stethoscope ▪ clock with second hand or Apgar timer ▪ gloves.

Postpartum perineal care

Vaginal birth (which stretches and sometimes tears the perineal tissues) and episiotomy (which may minimize tissue injury) usually leave the patient with perineal edema and tenderness. Postpartum perineal care aims to relieve this discomfort, promote healing, and prevent infection.

Performed after the patient eliminates, perineal hygiene involves cleaning and drying the perineum and assessing the wound area and the lochia (blood and debris sloughed from the placental site and the decidua). Red immediately after delivery, this discharge turns pinkish-brown in 4 to 7 days. Postpartum the lochia appears white. Lochia decreases gradually but may continue for as long as 6 weeks.

Put on gloves. To assess healing progress, inspect the perineum regularly. Ensure adequate lighting, and position the patient *to best expose the perineum and anal area.*

Inspect the wound area and be alert for such signs of infection as unusual swelling, redness and, possibly, drainage with a foul odor.

Typically, you'll use a water-jet irrigation system or a peribottle to clean the perineum. Assist the patient to the bathroom, wash your hands, and put on gloves.

If you're using a water-jet irrigation system, insert the prefilled cartridge containing antiseptic or medicated solution into the handle, and push the disposable nozzle into the handle until you hear it click into place.

Instruct the patient to sit on the commode. Next, place the nozzle parallel to the perineum and turn on the unit. Rinse the perineum for at least 2 minutes from front to back. Then turn off the unit, remove the nozzle, and discard the cartridge. Dry the nozzle, and store it appropriately for subsequent use.

If you're using a peribottle, fill it with cleaning solution and instruct the patient to pour it over the perineal area.

Help the patient to stand up before you flush the commode *to avoid spraying the perineum with contaminated water.* Also assist her in applying a new perineal pad before returning to bed. Instruct her to apply the pad front to back to avoid infection. Provide her with a belt to keep the pad in place. If she had a cesarean section, offer safety pins to secure the pad to her underwear *because a belt may irritate the incisional site.* Before she's discharged, teach the patient how to perform perineal care.

Recording the Apgar score

Use this chart to record the neonatal Apgar score at 1 minute and at 5 minutes after birth. A score of 7 to 10 indicates good condition; 4 to 6, fair condition—the infant may have moderate central nervous system depression, muscle flaccidity, cyanosis, and poor respirations; 0 to 3, danger—the infant needs immediate resuscitation, as ordered.

| | APGAR SCORE | | |
SIGN	0	1	2
Heart rate	Absent	Less than 100 beats/minute (slow)	More than 100 beats/minute
Respiratory effort	Absent	Slow, irregular	Good crying
Muscle tone	Flaccid	Some flexion and resistance to extension of extremities	Active motion
Reflex irritability	No response	Grimace or weak cry	Vigorous cry
Color	Pallor, cyanosis	Pink body, blue extremities	Completely pink

Preparation of equipment
If you use Apgar timers, make sure both timers are on at the instant of birth.

Implementation
• Note the exact time of delivery. Wear gloves *for protection from blood and body fluids*. Dry the neonate *to prevent heat loss*.
• Place the neonate in a 15-degree Trendelenburg's position to promote mucus drainage. Then position his head with the nose slightly tilted upward *to straighten the airway*.
• Assess the neonate's respiratory efforts. If necessary, supply stimulation by rubbing his back or gently flicking his foot.
• With abnormal respiratory responses, begin neonatal resuscitation according to the guidelines of the American Heart Association and the American Academy of Pediatrics. Then, use the Apgar score to judge the progress and success of resuscitation efforts. Should resuscitation efforts prove futile, you'll need to implement measures for dealing with stillbirth (see *Dealing with a stillbirth*).
• If the neonate exhibits normal responses, proceed to assign the Apgar score at 1 minute after birth.

• Repeat the evaluation and record the score at 5 minutes after birth.

To assess neonatal heart rate
• Using a stethoscope, listen to the heartbeat for 30 seconds, and record the rate. To obtain beats/minute, double the rate. Or palpate the umbilical cord where it joins the abdomen. Monitor pulsations for 6 seconds and multiply by 10 to obtain beats/minute. Assign a 0 for no heart rate, a 1 for a rate under 100 beats/minute, and a 2 for a rate over 100 beats/minute.

To assess respiratory effort
• Count unassisted respirations for 60 seconds, noting quality and regularity (a normal rate is 30 to 50 respirations/minute). Assign a 0 for no respirations; a 1 for slow, irregular, shallow, or gasping respirations; and a 2 for regular respirations and vigorous crying.

To assess muscle tone
• Observe the extremities for flexion and resistance to extension. This can be done by extending the limbs and observing their rapid return to flexion—the neonate's normal state. Assign a 0 for flaccid muscle tone; a 1 for some flexion and resistance to extension; and a 2 for

normal flexion of elbows, knees, and hips, with good resistance to extension.

To assess reflex irritability
• Observe the neonate's response to nasal suctioning or to flicking the sole of his foot. Assign a 0 for no response, a 1 for a grimace or weak cry, and a 2 for a vigorous cry.

To assess color
• Observe skin color, especially at the extremities. Assign a 0 for complete pallor and cyanosis, a 1 for a pink body with blue extremities (acrocyanosis), and a 2 for a completely pink body. To assess color in a dark-skinned neonate, inspect the oral mucous membranes and conjunctiva, the lips, the palms, and the soles.

Special considerations
If the patient and her support person don't know about the Apgar score, discuss it with them during early labor, when they will be more receptive to new knowledge. *To prevent confusion or misunderstanding at delivery,* explain to them what will occur and why. Add that this is a routine procedure.

If the neonate requires emergency care, make sure that a member of the delivery team offers appropriate support.

Closely observe the neonate whose mother receives heavy sedation just before delivery. Despite a high Apgar score at birth, he may show secondary effects of sedation in the nursery. Be alert for depression or unresponsiveness.

Documentation
Record the Apgar score on the Apgar score sheet or the neonatal assessment sheet required by your hospital. Be sure to indicate the total score and the signs for which points were deducted *to guide postnatal care.*

Neonatal vital signs

Measuring vital signs establishes the baseline of any neonatal assessment. Typically, the nurse visually assesses the respiratory rate by watching and counting the neonate's breaths, although she may auscultate the lungs with a pediatric stethoscope and watch for labored or abnormal breathing. She measures the heart rate apically — also with a pediatric stethoscope — and takes the first neonatal temperature rectally to verify rectal patency. Subsequent temperature readings are axillary to

---

Dealing with a stillbirth

If a fetus that's mature enough to survive extrauterine life dies before or during delivery, the event is called a stillbirth and the fetus a stillborn. Features of maturity include gestational age of 16 weeks or more and length of 6¼" (15.8 cm) or more.

Delivery of a less-mature fetus is called a spontaneous abortion.

Nursing interventions
Besides measuring, weighing, identifying, and preparing the stillborn for the morgue, provide emotional support to the parents. Whether or not the parents expect the stillbirth, they will need comfort and care.

When the parents expect the stillbirth, focus on assisting them to continue working through their grief — especially if they've delayed grieving while waiting for delivery.

When the parents don't expect the stillbirth, supportive care involves helping them to express their anger and relieve grief in positive ways. Refer them to appropriate support groups.

Offer bereaved parents the opportunity to hold the stillborn. If possible, provide a photograph, identification bracelet, or other memento. If they refuse these mementos now, file them with the chart so that they may obtain them later if desired.

---

avoid injuring the rectal mucosa. Blood pressure may be assessed by sphygmomanometer or by palpation or auscultation. An electronic vital signs monitor may also be used. (See "Temperature," "Pulse," "Respiration," and "Blood pressure" in Chapter 1.)

When the neonate arrives in the nursery, additional procedures may be required. Depending on hospital protocol, some procedures to ensure the neonate's safety and progress in the nursery include an identification and weight check; placement in radiant warming equipment; rectal temperature measurement; a vitamin K_1 injection to stimulate neonatal clotting mechanisms; and eye treatments with an antibiotic or silver nitrate to guard against infections.

Equipment
Pediatric stethoscope ■ watch with second hand ■ thermometer (mercury or electronic with rectal probe and cover) ■ water-soluble lubricant ■ gloves ■ sphygmomanometer with 1" (2.5 cm) cuff ■ optional: Doppler ultra-

Normal vital signs in full-term neonates

Use these ranges (or those established by your hospital) to guide assessment of neonatal status.

Respiratory rate
30 to 50 breaths/minute

Heart rate (apical)
110 to 160 beats/minute

Temperature
Axillary: 97.5° to 99° F (36.4° to 37.2° C)
Rectal: one degree higher

Blood pressure
Systolic: 60 to 80 mm Hg
Diastolic: 40 to 50 mm Hg

sound device with conduction gel or an electronic vital signs monitor.

Preparation of equipment
Assemble the equipment beside the patient. If you're using a mercury thermometer, shake it until the mercury drops under 96° F (35.5° C). If you have an electronic thermometer, apply the cover to the rectal probe. Using water-soluble lubricant, coat the thermometer or probe cover before taking a rectal temperature.

Implementation
• Wash your hands.

To determine respiratory rate
• Observe respirations first, before the neonate becomes too active or agitated. Watch and count respiratory movements for 1 minute. Then record the result.
• Expect to see mostly diaphragmatic respirations. Also expect an irregular respiratory rate and pattern, varying from slow and shallow to rapid and deep (see *Normal vital signs in full-term neonates*). Abnormally fast breathing (tachypnea) may signal a perinatal problem. A lapse of 15 seconds or more after a complete respiratory cycle (one expiration and one inspiration) indicates apnea.
• Check for labored breathing (sometimes resulting from blocked nasal passages). Observe for uneven chest expansion, nasal flaring, visible chest retractions, expiratory grunts, and inspiratory stridor (a high-pitched sound audible without a stethoscope).

• *To evaluate breath sounds,* auscultate the anterior and posterior lung fields, placing the stethoscope over each lung lobe for at least 5 seconds for a total time of 1 minute. Normal breath sounds are clear and the same bilaterally. However, immediately after birth, you may hear a few crackles *resulting from retained fetal lung fluid.*
• Observe the chest as it rises and falls; normal movement should be symmetrical. Also, determine any difference between the anterior and posterior diameters of the chest, which normally should be equal. *Unequal diameters suggest hyperinflated lungs or respiratory distress.*

To assess heart rate
• Place the stethoscope over the apical impulse on the fourth or fifth intercostal space at the left midclavicular line over the cardiac apex. Listen to and count the heartbeats for 1 minute *to learn the heart rate and to detect any abnormalities in quality or rhythm.*
• If you hear an unorthodox rhythm, assess whether the irregularity follows a definite or random pattern. *This evaluation helps to identify the type of abnormality.* For example, atrial fibrillation is an irregular rhythm with an irregular pattern.
• Auscultate for variations from the normal "lub-dub" systole-diastole sounds. Determine whether the first and second heart sounds are separate and distinct or split into two sounds. Assess for extra heartbeats and sounds that stretch into the next sound. *Such abnormal sounds may indicate a heart murmur—from patent ductus arteriosus, for example, as blood rushes through the abnormal opening.*

To take temperature rectally
• Wash your hands and put on gloves.
• With the neonate lying supine, firmly grasp his ankles with your index finger between them *to prevent skin trauma.* Place a diaper over the penis of a male neonate *to absorb urine if he urinates.*
• Still holding the neonate's ankles, insert the lubricated thermometer no more than ½" (1.3 cm) — *any farther could cause rectal injury.* Place the palm of your hand on his buttocks and hold the thermometer between your index and middle fingers. *This stabilizes the thermometer and prevents breakage if the neonate moves suddenly. To inhibit the defecation response induced by inserting a rectal thermometer,* press the buttocks together. If you meet resistance during insertion, withdraw the thermometer, and notify the doctor.
• Hold a mercury thermometer in place for 3 minutes and an electronic thermometer until the temperature registers (see "Temperature," Chapter 1). Remove the thermometer and read the number on the scale where the

mercury stops or on the digital display panel. Record the result.

To take an axillary temperature
• Dry the axillary skin. Then place the thermometer in the axilla and hold it along the outer aspect of the neonate's chest between the axillary line and the arm for at least 3 minutes *because axillary temperature takes this long to register.* Hold an electronic thermometer in place until the temperature registers.
• Reassess axillary temperature in 15 to 30 minutes if it registers outside the normal range. If the temperature remains abnormal, notify the doctor. *A subnormal temperature may result from infection, and an elevated temperature may result from dehydration or reflect the environment, such as a malfunctioning overhead warmer.*
• Document the temperature.

To determine blood pressure
• Measure blood pressure in a quiet neonate.
• Be sure that the blood pressure cuff is small enough for the patient (cuff width: about half the circumference of the neonate's arm) because *the cuff size affects accurate readings.*
• Wrap the cuff one or two fingerbreadths above the antecubital or popliteal area. With the stethoscope held directly over the chosen artery, hold the cuffed extremity firmly *to keep it extended* and inflate the cuff no faster than 5 mm Hg/second. (For additional ways to assess neonatal blood pressure, see *Alternative methods for assessing neonatal blood pressure.*)
• *To determine whether subsequent blood pressures measure within the neonate's normal range,* compare the readings to baseline values. Report any significant deviation.

Special considerations
If desired, count respirations while auscultating the heart rate.

When listening to neonatal heart tones immediately after birth, you may hear murmurs. These may result from a delayed closing of fetal blood shunts.

Excessive neonatal activity — restlessness and crying during a vital signs assessment, for example — may elevate the heart rate above normal. For this reason, describe the neonate's activity along with measured findings.

Documentation
Record vital signs and related measurements in your notes, a special neonatal appraisal form, or a flowchart. Include any observations about the neonate's condition, such as abnormal breath sounds.

Alternative methods for assessing neonatal blood pressure

Besides using a standard sphygmomanometer for assessing neonatal blood pressure, you may use palpation or auscultation.

Palpation
Feel for the neonate's radial or brachial pulse, which is the systolic blood pressure.

Auscultation
If you're using a pediatric stethoscope with amplification, listen for diastolic and systolic sounds at the brachial artery.

If you're using a Doppler blood pressure monitor, place the cuff directly over the brachial or popliteal artery *to ensure an accurate reading.* The device automatically inflates the cuff. *For greatest accuracy,* keep the cuffed arm or leg extended during cuff inflation. (Also observe the extremity's color. *Duskiness signifies reduced blood flow.*)

Neonatal size and weight

A beginning point for many neonatal assessments, measuring anthropometric dimensions and weight establishes the baseline for accurately monitoring normal growth. Size and weight measurements help detect such disorders as failure to thrive, small for gestational age, hydrocephalus, and intracranial bleeding. The nurse takes the measurements in the nursery during routine checkups and sometimes at the neonate's home. She then compares the results with previous measurements and with normal values.

Normally the neonate's head circumference measures the same as or more than his chest circumference. The exception: the first 24 hours after birth when head molding leaves the head circumference slightly smaller than chest circumference. The head's contour usually returns to normal in 2 to 3 days.

The neonate's weight varies with sex, gestational age, heredity, and other factors. A firstborn usually weighs less at birth than his siblings. The neonate with a diabetic mother tends to be large. Because of an erratic feeding pattern and passage of urine and meconium, the normal neonate loses between 5% and 10% of his birth weight during the first few days. However, he usually regains this weight in 10 days. Normal weight gain for the neonate is 5 to 7 oz (142 to 198 g) weekly.

Equipment

Crib or examination table with a firm surface ▪ scale with tray ▪ scale paper, if necessary ▪ tape measure ▪ length board ▪ gloves, if the neonate hasn't been bathed yet.

Disposable paper tape measures are available. Cloth tapes aren't recommended because they can stretch, leading to inaccurate measurements.

Preparation of equipment

Put clean paper on the scale to promote warmth and prevent cold stress. Balance the scale at zero as directed by the manufacturer.

Implementation

• Explain the procedure to the parents, if present. Wash your hands, and put on gloves if you haven't bathed the neonate yet.
• To begin, position the neonate supine in the crib or on the examination table. Remove all clothing but his diaper (if he has one). Be sure to record all measurements. (See *Average neonatal size and weight.*)

To measure head circumference

• Slide the tape measure under the neonate's head at the occiput. *To arrive at the greatest circumference,* draw the tape snugly around, just above the eyebrows.

To measure chest circumference

• Place the tape under the back and wrap it snugly around the chest at the nipple line. *To ensure accuracy,* keep the back and front of the tape level.
• Take the measurement after the neonate inspires and before he begins to exhale.

To measure head-to-heel length

• Fully extend the neonate's legs with the toes pointing up. Measure the distance from the heel to the top of the head. If possible, have someone extend the legs by pressing down gently on the knees. Or use a length board, if available.

To measure crown-to-rump length

• Place the neonate on his side and measure from the crown of his head to his buttocks. This measurement should approximate the head circumference.

To weigh the neonate

• Take this measurement before, not after, a feeding. Remove the neonate's diaper before placing him in the middle of the scale tray.
• Note the neonate's weight. Keep one hand poised over him at all times *to prevent accidents.* Work quickly *to avoid having the scale become soiled or wet and to prevent neonatal heat loss.*
• Return the neonate to the crib or examination table.
• If the neonate has clothing or equipment on him (such as an I.V. armband), be sure to record this information.
• Clean the scale tray *to prevent cross-contamination between neonates.*

To measure abdominal girth

• Place the neonate supine, and measure his girth just above the umbilicus. Though not an anthropometric measurement, *the size of this expanse may suggest abnormalities — an obstruction, for example.*
• When you finish, dress and diaper the neonate. Return him to his crib, if necessary, or give him to a parent who can hold and comfort him.

Special considerations

Keep in mind that head swelling or molding after delivery may skew initial head circumference measurements.

Another way to measure length is to place the neonate on paper, such as that used on examination tables. Mark the paper at the heel, with the toes pointing straight up, and at the head; measure the distance between the marks.

Various scale models are available. Be sure to learn how to read and operate the one available to you. If you use a model that measures metrically, supply the parents with a table of metric equivalents for use at home.

Documentation

Record each weight and dimension measurement in your notes or neonatal assessment sheet.

During routine checkups, remember to share information with the parents, who may carry a booklet in which they also document weight and dimensions.

 # Apnea monitoring

If detected and treated at onset, apneic episodes may be reversed. Using an apnea monitor that signals when breathing rate falls dangerously low may save the neonate who's vulnerable to apnea.

Apnea monitors may be used for vulnerable neonates, such as those born prematurely or those with neurologic

Average neonatal size and weight

Besides weight, anthropometric measurements include head and chest circumferences, crown-to-rump length, and head-to-heel length (as shown below). These measurements serve as a baseline and show whether neonatal size is within normal ranges or whether there may be a significant problem or anomaly—especially if values stray far from the mean. Initial average anthropometric ranges for a neonate follow:

- Head circumference: 13″ to 14″ (33 to 35 cm)
- Chest circumference: 12″ to 13″ (30 to 33 cm)
- Crown to rump: about the same as head circumference
- Head to heel: 18″ to 21″ (45 to 53 cm)
- Weight: 5 lb 8 oz to 8 lb 13 oz (2,500 to 4,000 g)

Head circumference

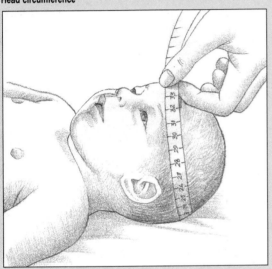

Chest circumference

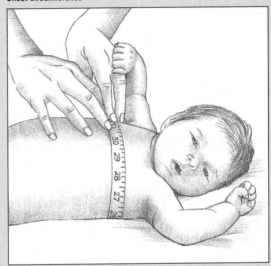

Crown to rump

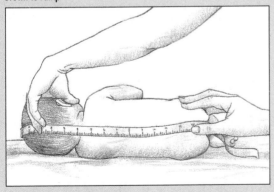

Head to heel

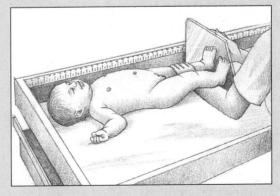

Using a home apnea monitor

When a neonate in your care will use home apnea monitoring equipment, you'll need to prepare his parents to operate it safely, correctly and confidently.

First, review the neonate's breathing problem with his parents. Explain that the monitor will warn them of breathing or heart rate changes. Then, offer the following guidelines.

• Advise parents to prepare their home and family for the equipment, for instance by providing a sturdy, flat surface for the monitor and by posting emergency telephone numbers (doctor, nurse, equipment supplier, ambulance) accessibly.

• Teach other responsible family members how to use the monitor safely. Also suggest that older siblings, grandparents, babysitters, and other caregivers learn cardiopulmonary resuscitation (CPR).

• Instruct parents to notify local service authorities — police, ambulance, telephone, and electric company — if their neonate uses an apnea monitor so that alternative power can be supplied if a failure occurs.

• Explain how a monitor with electrodes works. Teach parents to make sure the respirator indicator goes on each time the neonate breathes. If it doesn't, describe troubleshooting techniques, such as moving the electrodes slightly. Tell them to try this technique several times.

• Show parents how to respond to either the apnea or bradycardia alarm. Direct them to check the color of the neonate's oral tissues. If they appear bluish and the neonate isn't breathing, tell them to call loudly and touch him — gently at first, then more urgently as needed. Tell them to stop short of shaking him. If he doesn't respond, urge them to begin CPR.

• Also advise the parents to keep the operator's manual attached to or beside the monitor and to consult it as needed. Explain that an activated loose-lead alarm, for example, may indicate a dirty electrode, a loose electrode patch, a loose belt, or a disconnected or malfunctioning wire or monitor.

In most common use are two types of monitors. The *thoracic impedance monitor* uses chest electrodes to detect conduction changes caused by respirations. Some monitors of this type also detect bradycardia. The *apnea mattress,* or *underpad monitor,* relies on a transducer connected to a pressure-sensitive pad, which detects pressure changes resulting from altered chest movements.

To guard against potentially life-threatening apneic episodes in vulnerable neonates, monitoring begins in the hospital and continues at home. Parents need to learn how to operate the monitor, what actions to take when the alarm sounds, and how to revive a neonate or an infant with cardiopulmonary resuscitation (CPR). Crucial steps for correctly using a monitor include testing the alarm system, positioning the sensor properly, and setting the controls correctly. (See *Using a home apnea monitor.*)

Equipment

Monitor unit ■ electrodes ■ lead wires ■ electrode belt ■ electrode gel, if needed ■ pressure transducer pad, if using apnea mattress ■ stable surface for monitor placement.

Prepackaged and pretreated disposable electrodes are available.

Implementation

• Explain the procedure to the parents, as appropriate, and wash your hands.

• Plug the monitor's power cord into a grounded wall outlet. Attach the lead wires to the electrodes, and attach the electrodes to the belt. If appropriate, apply conduction gel to the electrodes. (Or apply gel to the neonate's chest, place the electrodes atop the gel, and attach the electrodes to the lead wires. Then secure the belt.)

• To hold the electrodes securely in position, wrap the belt snugly but not restrictively around the neonate's chest at the point of greatest movement — optimally at the right and left midaxillary line about ⅘" (2 cm) below the axilla. Be sure to position the lead wires according to the manufacturer's instructions.

• Follow the color code to connect the lead wires to the patient cable. Then connect the cable to the proper jack at the rear of the monitoring unit.

• Turn the sensitivity controls to maximum *to facilitate tuning when adjusting the system.*

• Set the alarms according to recommendations so that an apneic period lasting for a specified time activates the signal.

• Turn on the monitor. If the monitor has two alarms — one to signal apnea, one to signal bradycardia — both will sound until you adjust the monitor and reset the alarms according to the manufacturer's instructions.

disorders, neonatal respiratory distress syndrome, seizure disorders, congenital heart disease with congestive heart failure, a tracheostomy, a personal history of sleep-induced apnea, a family history of sudden infant death syndrome, or acute drug withdrawal.

• Adjust the sensitivity controls until the indicator lights blink with each breath and heartbeat.

• If you use an apnea mattress, assemble the monitor and pressure transducer pad according to the manufacturer's directions.

• Plug the monitor into a grounded wall outlet. Then plug the cable of the transducer pad into the monitor.

• Touch the pad to make sure it works. Watch for the monitor's respiration light to blink.

• Follow the manufacturer's instructions for pad placement.

• If you have difficulty obtaining a signal, place a foam rubber pad under the mattress, and sandwich the transducer pad between the foam pad and the mattress.

• If you hear the apnea or bradycardia alarm during monitoring, immediately check the neonate's respirations and color, but don't touch or disturb him *until you confirm apnea.*

• If he's still breathing and his color is good, readjust the sensitivity controls or reposition the electrodes, if necessary.

• If he isn't breathing, but his color looks normal, wait 10 seconds to see if he starts breathing spontaneously. If he isn't breathing and he appears pale, dusky, or blue, immediately try to stimulate breathing in these ways: Sequentially, place your hand on the neonate's back, rub him gently, or flick his soles gently. If he doesn't begin to breathe at once, start CPR (for detailed instructions see "Cardiopulmonary resuscitation" in Chapter 16).

Special considerations

To ensure accurate operation, don't put the monitor on top of any other electrical device. Make sure it's on a level surface and can't be bumped easily.

Avoid applying lotions, oils, or powders to the neonate's chest, *where they could cause the electrode belt to slip.* Periodically check the alarm by disconnecting the sensor plug. Then listen for the alarm to sound after the preset time delay.

Complications

An apneic episode resulting from upper airway obstruction may not trigger the alarm if the neonate continues to make respiratory efforts without gas exchange. However, the monitor's bradycardia alarm may be triggered by the decreased heart rate resulting from vagal stimulation (which accompanies obstruction).

If you're using a thoracic impedance monitor without a bradycardia alarm, you may interpret bradycardia during apnea as shallow breathing. That's because this type of monitor fails to distinguish between respiratory movement and the large cardiac stroke volume associated with

bradycardia. In this case, the alarm won't sound until the heart rate drops below the apnea limit.

Documentation

Record all alarm incidents. Document the time and duration of apnea. Describe the neonate's color, the stimulation measures implemented, and any other pertinent information.

Transcutaneous Po₂ monitoring

A transcutaneous partial oxygen pressure (TCPo₂) monitor measures the amount of oxygen diffusing through skin from capillaries directly beneath the surface. This measurement, which correlates closely with the neonate's partial pressure of oxygen in arterial blood (Pao₂), supplements traditional methods (observing skin color and taking periodic arterial blood gas measurements) for detecting hypoxemia and hyperoxemia.

The monitor relies on a tiny electrode sensor applied to the skin. This sensor—a metallic, oxygen-sensitive device—warms to between 107.6° and 115° F (42° and 46° C). As the electrode's temperature increases (typically, to slightly higher than skin temperature), so does capillary blood flow. The increased vasodilation in cutaneous vessels enhances oxygen diffusion, which the electrode measures. This procedure is widely used in neonatal intensive care units by staff nurses trained to use the monitor.

Because neonatal skin is thin with little subcutaneous fat, TCPo₂ monitoring produces accurate findings. However, in neonates with shock or hypoperfusion, the results seldom accurately reflect arterial oxygen levels. In these neonates, peripheral blood flow decreases as blood is shunted to the heart, brain, and lungs.

Another device for monitoring arterial oxygen levels is the pulse oximeter (see *Neonatal pulse oximetry,* page 702).

Equipment

TCPo₂ monitor and electrode ■ cotton balls ■ soap and water ■ alcohol sponge ■ adhesive ring for electrode.

Preparation of equipment

Set up the monitor, and calibrate it, if necessary, following manufacturer's instructions. Ensure that the strip chart recorder works properly.

Neonatal pulse oximetry

Another noninvasive technique for monitoring oxygenation is pulse oximetry. The sensor of the pulse oximeter, which is attached to the neonate's foot, measures beat-to-beat arterial oxygen saturation. Normally, oxygenation values should drop no lower than 90%.

Don't be guided only by oximetric findings, though. Every 3 to 4 hours, you'll need to correlate laboratory values (from arterial blood gas analyses) with oximetric values for a reliable overview of neonatal status.

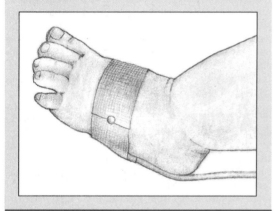

Implementation
• Wash your hands and decide where to place the electrode. Choose a flat site, with good capillary blood flow, few fatty deposits, and no bony prominences. Common sites include the neonate's upper chest, abdomen, and inner thigh.
• Clean the site first with a cotton ball and soap and water. Then wipe the site with an alcohol sponge *to remove dirt and oils and to ensure good electrode contact.*
• Dry the skin, attach the adhesive ring to the electrode, and moisten the skin site with a drop of water, according to the manufacturer's instructions, *to seal out all air.*
• Place the electrode on the site, and make sure that the adhesive ring is tight.
• Set the alarm switches and the electrode temperature according to the manufacturer's instructions or hospital policy.
• Expect the monitor reading to stabilize in 10 to 20 minutes. Normal oxygen pressures range from 50 to 80 mm Hg, but normal values also vary with the neonate

and the equipment. TCPO$_2$ monitors usually have digital readouts and strip chart recorders to show trends.
• Rotate the electrode site every 4 hours *to prevent skin irritation, breakdown, or burns.*

Special considerations
Expect TCPO$_2$ values to vary with neonatal movement and treatment. Also expect them to drop markedly whenever the neonate cries vigorously. But be prepared to start resuscitation if a sudden, significant drop in TCPO$_2$ pressure occurs.

Remember that TCPO$_2$ monitoring doesn't replace arterial blood gas measurements, because it doesn't give information about PaCO$_2$ and pH.

Complications
Be alert for burns and blisters from the electrode and skin reactions to the adhesive ring.

Documentation
Place graphic or printout results on the neonate's chart. Record the range of values observed during monitoring in your notes. Also record any skin disorders related to the electrode.

NEONATAL TREATMENTS
Neonatal eye prophylaxis (Credé's treatment)

Named for its developer, Credé's treatment prevents damage and blindness from conjunctivitis caused by *Neisseria gonorrhoeae* and transmitted during birth if the mother has gonorrhea.

Required by law in all states in the United States, the treatment consists of instilling a 1% silver nitrate solution into the neonate's eyes. Some states permit alternative treatment with 1% tetracycline ointment or 0.5% erythromycin ointment. By this method, the neonate may avoid chemical irritation from silver nitrate, yet benefit from the antimicrobial effects of broad-spectrum antibiotics.

The nurse instills the solution or ointment in the conjunctival sac (from the eye's inner canthus to its outer canthus). The treatment, which may cause conjunctival swelling, may also disturb the typically quiet but alert neonate at birth. So, although silver nitrate treatment is usually given at delivery, it can be delayed for up to 1 hour to allow initial parent-child bonding.

Silver nitrate prophylaxis may be ineffective if the neonate acquires the infection *in utero* after premature rupture of the membranes.

Equipment
Silver nitrate ampule or ophthalmic antibiotic ointment, as ordered ∎ sterile needle or pin supplied by silver nitrate manufacturer ∎ gloves ∎ gauze pads.

Preparation of equipment
Puncture one end of the wax silver nitrate ampule with the needle or pin. If you're administering ophthalmic antibiotic ointment, remove the cap from the ointment container. A single-dose ointment tube should be used *to prevent contamination and spread of infection.*

Implementation
• If the parents are present for the procedure, explain that state law mandates Credé's treatment. Forewarn them that the neonate may cry and that the treatment may irritate his eyes. Reassure them that these are temporary effects.
• Put on gloves. *For comfort and effectiveness,* shield the neonate's eyes from direct light, tilt his head slightly to the side of the intended treatment, and instill the medication (see *How to instill medication for Credé's treatment*).
• Close and manipulate the eyelids *to spread the medication over the eye.*
• Wait 15 seconds after instilling the medication. Then, *to prevent staining the skin,* remove excess silver nitrate with a gauze pad.

Special considerations
Instill another drop if the silver nitrate solution touches only the eyelid or eyelid margins *to ensure complete prophylaxis.*

If chemical conjunctivitis occurs or if the skin around the neonate's eyes discolors, reassure the parents that these temporary effects will subside within a few days.

Complications
Especially after silver nitrate instillation, chemical conjunctivitis may cause redness, swelling, and drainage.

Documentation
If you perform Credé's treatment in the delivery room, record the treatment on the delivery room form. If you do Credé's treatment in the nursery, document it in your notes.

How to instill medication for Credé's treatment

Using your nondominant hand, gently raise the neonate's upper eyelid with your index finger and pull down the lower eyelid with your thumb (as shown).

Using your dominant hand, instill 2 drops of silver nitrate solution into the lower conjunctival sac or apply the ordered ophthalmic antibiotic ointment in a line along the lower conjunctival sac.

Repeat the procedure for the other eye.

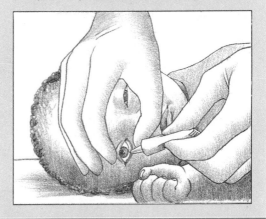

 ## Thermoregulation

A large body surface-to-mass ratio, reduced metabolism per unit area, limited amounts of insulating subcutaneous fat, vasomotor instability, and limited metabolic capacity make all neonates susceptible to hypothermia. To stay warm when he is cold-stressed, the neonate metabolizes brown fat. Unique to neonates, brown fat has energy-producing mitochondria in its cells, which enhances its capacity for heat production.

Brown fat metabolism effectively warms the body — but only within a narrow temperature range. Without careful external thermoregulation, the neonate may become chilled. Hypoxia, acidosis, hypoglycemia, pulmonary vasoconstriction, and even death may result.

Thermoregulation provides a neutral thermal environment that helps the neonate maintain a normal core temperature with minimal oxygen consumption and caloric expenditure. Although it varies with the neonate, the average core temperature is 97.7° F (36.5° C).

Understanding thermoregulators

Thermoregulators preserve neonatal body warmth in various ways. A radiant warmer maintains the neonate's temperature by *radiation*.

An incubator maintains the neonate's temperature by *conduction* and *convection*.

Temperature settings

Radiant warmers and incubators have two operating modes: *nonservo* and *servo*. Whereas the nurse manually sets temperature controls on nonservo equipment, a probe on the neonate's skin controls temperature settings on servo models.

Other features

Most thermoregulators come with alarms. Incubators have the added advantage of providing a stable, enclosed environment that protects the neonate from evaporative heat loss.

Radiant warmer

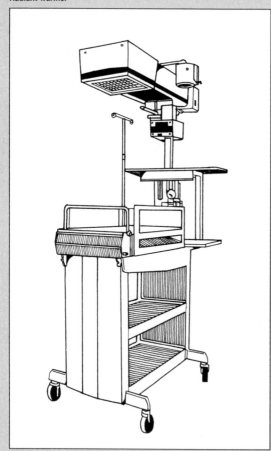

Incubator

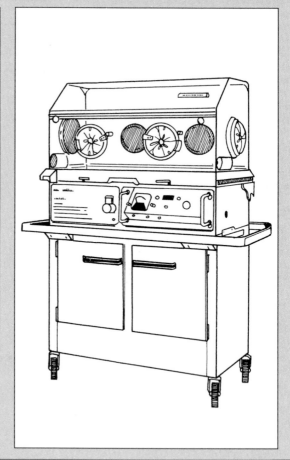

Two kinds of thermoregulators are common in the hospital nursery: radiant warmers and incubators. The radiant warmer controls environmental temperature while the nurse gives initial care in the delivery room. Then, when the neonate arrives in the nursery, another radiant warmer may be used until his temperature stabilizes and he can occupy a bassinet. If the temperature doesn't stabilize or if the neonate has a condition that affects thermoregulation, a temperature-controlled incubator will house him (see *Understanding thermoregulators*).

Equipment
Radiant warmer or incubator (if necessary) ■ blankets ■ washcloths or towels ■ skin probe ■ adhesive pad ■ water-soluble lubricant ■ thermometer ■ clothing (including a cap) ■ optional: stockinette gauze.

Preparation of equipment
Turn on the radiant warmer in the delivery room, and set the desired temperature. Warm the blankets, washcloths, or towels under a heat source.

Implementation
• Continue nursing measures to conserve neonatal body warmth until the patient's discharge.

In the delivery room
• Place the neonate under the radiant warmer and dry him with the warm washcloths or towels *to prevent heat loss by evaporation.*
• Pay special attention to drying his scalp and hair. Then cover his head with stockinette gauze or a ready-made cap *to prevent heat loss.* Because the head comprises about 25% of neonatal body surface, keep the cap on the neonate's head until his temperature stabilizes.
• Perform required procedures quickly *to reduce the neonate's exposure to cool delivery room air.*
• Wrap him in the warmed blankets. If his condition permits, give him to his parents *to promote bonding.*
• Transport the neonate to the nursery in the warmed blankets. Use a transport incubator when the nursery is far from the delivery room.

In the nursery
• Remove the blankets and place the neonate under the radiant warmer.
• Use the adhesive pad to attach the temperature control probe to his skin in the upper-right abdominal quadrant. *This lets the servo control maintain neonatal skin temperature between 96.8° and 97.7° F (36.0° and 36.5° C).* If the neonate will lie prone, put the skin probe on his back *to ensure accurate temperature control and avoid false-high*

readings from the neonate lying on the probe. Don't cover the device with anything *because this could interfere with the servo control.* Be sure to raise the warmer's side panels *to prevent accidents.*
• Lubricate the thermometer and take the neonate's rectal temperature on admission *to identify core temperature.* Take axillary temperatures thereafter *to avoid injuring delicate rectal mucosa.* Usually, axillary temperature readings are lower than the core temperature (see "Neonatal vital signs" in this chapter). Take axillary temperatures every 15 to 30 minutes until the temperature stabilizes, then every 4 hours *to ensure stability.*
• Sponge bathe the neonate under the warmer only after his temperature stabilizes, and leave him under the warmer until his temperature remains stable.
• Take appropriate action if the temperature doesn't stabilize. For example, place the neonate under a plastic heat shield or in a warmed incubator — depending on hospital policy. Look for objects, such as a phototherapy unit, that may be blocking the heat source. Also check for signs of infection, which can cause hypothermia.
• Apply a skin probe to the neonate in an incubator as you would for a neonate in a radiant warmer. Move the incubator away from cold walls or objects.
• Perform all required procedures quickly *to maintain a neutral thermal environment and to minimize heat loss.* Close portholes in the hood immediately after completing any procedure, *also to reduce heat loss.* If procedures must be performed outside the incubator, do them under a radiant warmer.
• To leave the hospital or to move to a bassinet, a neonate must be weaned from the incubator. Slowly reduce the incubator's temperature to that of the nursery. Check periodically for hypothermia. *To ensure temperature stability,* never discharge the neonate to home directly from an incubator.
• When the normal neonate's temperature stabilizes, dress him, put him in a bassinet, and cover him with a blanket.

Special considerations
Always warm oxygen before administering it to a neonate *to avoid initiating heat loss from his head and face.*

To prevent conductive heat loss, preheat the radiant warmer bed and linen; warm stethoscopes and other instruments before use; and pad the scale with paper or a preweighed, warmed sheet before weighing the neonate.

To avoid convective heat loss, place the neonate's bed out of direct line with an open window, a fan, or an air-conditioning vent.

To control evaporative heat loss, dry the neonate immediately after delivery. When bathing the neonate, ex-

Extracorporeal membrane oxygenation

Available in designated centers throughout the United States, extracorporeal membrane oxygenation (ECMO) derives from cardiopulmonary bypass methods used during heart surgery. In this procedure, a machine circulates the patient's venous blood outside his body, passes the blood through a membrane oxygenator, and returns the newly oxygenated blood to the circulation.

If the neonate meets stringent criteria, indications for ECMO include hyaline membrane disease, meconium aspiration, and congenital heart defects. Typically, the procedure is used as a last resort after maximum ventilatory support measures fail and when survival chances drop below 10%.

ECMO circuitry works by veno-arterial bypass or veno-venous bypass methods.

pose only one body part at a time; wash each part thoroughly, then dry it immediately.

Review the reasons for regulating body temperature with the neonate's family. Instruct them to keep him wrapped in a blanket and out of drafts when he's not in the bassinet—both in the hospital and at home. In a warm place, guard against overheating the neonate.

Complications

Hypothermia from ineffective natural or external thermoregulation can inhibit weight gain, because the neonate must use caloric energy to maintain his temperature. Hyperthermia can cause increased oxygen consumption and apnea. Both conditions can result from equipment failures or insufficient monitoring.

Documentation

Name the heat source, and record its temperature and the neonate's temperature, whenever taken. Document any complications that result from using thermoregulatory equipment.

Oxygen administration

The neonate with signs and symptoms of respiratory distress, such as cyanosis, pallor, tachypnea, nasal flaring, bradycardia, hypothermia, retractions, hypotonia, hyporeflexia, expiratory grunting, and blood gas levels indicating hypoxia, will most likely need oxygen. And because of his small size and special respiratory requirements, he'll need special equipment and administration techniques.

In an emergency, for instance, a hand-held resuscitation bag and a small oxygen mask may be sufficient until more permanent measures can be initiated. When the neonate requires additional oxygen above the ambient concentration, it can be delivered by means of an oxygen hood or nasal prongs. If he needs continuous positive airway pressure (CPAP) to prevent alveolar collapse at the end of a breath (as in respiratory distress syndrome), he may receive oxygen through a nasopharyngeal or an endotracheal tube. (Oxygenation typically improves with CPAP and any pulmonary shunting tends to decrease.) If the neonate can't breathe on his own or needs to conserve his energy, he may receive oxygen through a ventilator.

No matter which system delivers the oxygen, the therapy is potentially hazardous to the neonate. The gas must be warmed and humidified to prevent hypothermia and dehydration. In high concentrations over prolonged periods, oxygen can cause retrolental fibroplasia (which results in blindness). If the concentration's too low, hypoxia and central nervous system damage may occur. And depending on how it's delivered, oxygen can contribute to bronchopulmonary dysplasia.

In some cases, extracorporeal membrane oxygenation, an alternative to oxygen administration, may help neonates who have severe hypoxia. This technique also relies on a supplemental oxygen source (for more information, see *Extracorporeal membrane oxygenation*).

Equipment

Oxygen source (wall, cylinder, or liquid unit) ▪ compressed air source ▪ flowmeters ▪ nasal prongs ▪ blender or Y connector ▪ large- and small-bore oxygen tubing (sterile) ▪ warming-humidifying device ▪ blood gas analyzer ▪ thermometer ▪ stethoscope ▪ nasogastric (NG) tube.

For hand-held resuscitation bag and mask delivery: specially sized mask with manual resuscitation bag ▪ manometer with connectors. (The resuscitation bag must have a pressure-release valve.)

For oxygen hood delivery: appropriate-sized oxygen hood.

For nasal prong delivery: nasal prongs.

For CPAP delivery: manometer with connectors ▪ nasopharyngeal or endotracheal tube ▪ water-soluble lubricant ▪ hypoallergenic tape.

For delivery with a ventilator: ventilator unit with manometer and in-line thermometer ▪ specimen tubes for arterial blood gas (ABG) analyses ▪ endotracheal tube ▪

optional: pulse oximeter or transcutaneous oxygen monitor.

Preparation of equipment
Wash your hands, gather the necessary equipment, and assemble it conveniently.

To calibrate the oxygen analyzer: Turn the analyzer on and read the results. Room air should be about 21% oxygen. Check the analyzer power or battery level. Expose the analyzer probe to 100% oxygen and adjust sensitivity as necessary. Then recheck the amount of oxygen in room air.

To set up a manual resuscitation bag and mask: Place the resuscitation bag and mask in the crib. Connect the large-bore oxygen tubing to the mask outlet. Then use connectors and small-bore tubing to connect a manometer to the bag. Next, connect the free end of the oxygen tubing to the warming-humidifying device, and fill the device with sterile water. Turn on the device when ready to use it, or prepare the device according to the manufacturer's instructions.

Connect another piece of small-bore tubing to the inlet of the warming-humidifying device. Attach a Y connector to the opposite end of this tubing. Place a piece of small-bore tubing on each end of the Y connector, and connect the pieces of tubing to the flowmeters. Place an in-line thermometer as close as possible to the delivery end of the apparatus.

To set up an oxygen hood: Bring a clean oxygen hood and tubing if needed to the neonate's bedside. If the neonate was receiving oxygen via bag and mask, remove them from the connecting tubing. Attach the oxygen hood to this tubing. Place an in-line thermometer as close to the neonate as possible whenever using warmed oxygen.

Implementation
• Always wash your hands before working with a neonate *to prevent cross-contamination after handling other neonates.*

To administer emergency oxygen through a hand-held resuscitation bag and mask
• Turn on the oxygen and compressed air flowmeters to the prescribed flow rates.
• Place the mask on the neonate's face. Do not cover the neonate's eyes. Check pressure settings and mask size *to ensure that air doesn't leak from the mask's edges.*
• As you work to stabilize the neonate, have another staff member notify the doctor immediately.
• Provide 40 breaths/minute. Use enough pressure to cause a visible rise and fall of the neonate's chest. Provide enough oxygen to maintain pink nail beds and mucous membranes. If you can't reach the doctor during the emergency, deliver the oxygen percentage defined by hospital emergency policy.
• Continuously watch the neonate's chest movements and listen to breath sounds. Avoid overventilation, *which will blow off too much carbon dioxide and cause apnea.* If the neonate's heart rate falls below 110 beats/minute and doesn't rise, continue to use the hand-held resuscitation bag until the heartbeat rises to 110 beats/minute or higher.
• Insert an NG tube *to vent air from the neonate's stomach.*

To administer oxygen through an oxygen hood
• Remove the connecting tubing from the face mask and connect it to the oxygen hood. Activate oxygen and a compressed air source, if needed, at ordered flow rates.
• Place the oxygen hood over the neonate's head.
• Measure the amount of oxygen the neonate is receiving with the oxygen analyzer. Be sure to place the analyzer probe close to the neonate's nose. Adjust the oxygen to the prescribed amount.

To administer oxygen with nasal prongs
• Match the prong size to the neonate's nose. Apply a small amount of water-soluble lubricant to the outside of the prongs. Turn on the oxygen and compressed air, if necessary. Connect the prongs to the oxygen tubing. Insert the prongs into the nose and steady them. Be sure to clean the prongs each shift *to ensure patency.*

To administer oxygen with CPAP
• Position the neonate on his back with a rolled towel under his neck *to keep the airway open without hyperextending the neck.*
• If you're administering oxygen through a nasopharyngeal or an endotracheal tube, obtain the correct size tube. Turn on the oxygen and compressed air source. Then assist the doctor in inserting the endotracheal tube, attaching the oxygen delivery system (as set up for mask and bag delivery), and taping the tube in place. Next, insert an NG or orogastric tube, and leave it in place *to keep the stomach decompressed,* if ordered. Leave it open unless the neonate is receiving gavage feedings. Suction the nasal passages and oropharynx every 2 hours or as needed *to maintain an open airway.* Apply suction only while removing the suction catheter.

To administer oxygen through a ventilator
• Turn on the ventilator and set the controls, as ordered.
• Assist the doctor with inserting the endotracheal tube, if appropriate.
• Connect the endotracheal tube to the ventilator and tape the tube securely.

• As with any delivery system, carefully watch the manometer *to maintain pressure at the prescribed level.* Also monitor the in-line thermometer *for correct temperature.*

• Monitor ABG levels every 15 to 20 minutes — or other reasonable interval — after any changes in oxygen concentration or pressure. Draw blood samples for ABG analysis from an umbilical artery catheter, radial artery catheter, or radial artery puncture. If desired, obtain capillary blood by warmed heel stick — this gives accurate levels of pH and carbon dioxide, but not oxygen. If ordered, monitor oxygen perfusion with transcutaneous oxygen monitoring, pulse oximetry, or $S\bar{v}O_2$ monitoring.

• Keep the doctor aware of ABG levels so he can order appropriate changes in oxygen concentration. Usually, oxygen partial pressure is maintained between 60 and 90 mm Hg for an arterial sample and 40 and 60 mm Hg for a capillary sample.

• Auscultate the lungs for crackles, rhonchi, and bilateral breath sounds.

Special considerations

When administering oxygen, always take safety precautions *to avoid fire or explosion.* As soon as possible, explain the situation and the procedures to the parents. Take measures to keep the neonate warm *because hypothermia impedes respiration.*

Check ABG levels at least every hour whenever the unstable neonate receives high oxygen concentrations and whenever there's a clinical change. If he doesn't respond to oxygen administration, check for congenital anomalies.

Perform neonatal chest auscultation carefully *to hear subtle respiratory changes.* Also be alert for respiratory distress signs, and be prepared to perform emergency procedures. If required, perform chest physiotherapy and percussion, as ordered. Follow with suctioning *to remove secretions.* As ordered, discontinue oxygen when the neonate's fraction of inspired oxygen (FIO_2) reaches room air level and his arterial oxygen stabilizes between 60 and 90 mm Hg. Repeat ABG analysis 20 to 30 minutes after discontinuing oxygen and thereafter as ordered by the doctor or by hospital policy.

If the neonate will receive oxygen over a lengthy time span, prepare his parents or other caregivers to administer oxygen at home (see *Comparing oxygen delivery systems*).

Complications

Infection or "drowning" can result from overhumidification, which allows water to collect in tubing and then suffocate the neonate or provide a growth medium for bacteria. Hypothermia and increased oxygen consumption can result from administering cool oxygen. Metabolic and respiratory acidosis may follow inadequate ventilation. Pressure ulcers may develop on the neonate's head, face, and around the nose during prolonged oxygen therapy. Pulmonary air leak (pneumothorax, pneumomediastinum, pneumopericardium, interstitial emphysema) may develop spontaneously with respiratory distress or result from forced ventilation. Decreased cardiac output may come from excessive CPAP.

Documentation

Note any respiratory distress that requires oxygen administration, the oxygen concentration given, and the delivery method. Record each change in oxygen concentration and the neonate's FIO_2 as measured by the oxygen analyzer. Note all routine checks of oxygen concentration. Document all ABG values, the times that samples were obtained, the neonate's condition during therapy, times suctioned, the amount and consistency of mucus, the type of continuous oxygen monitoring (if any), and any complications. Note respiratory rate and describe breath sounds and any signs of additional respiratory distress.

Phototherapy

Phototherapy involves exposing the neonate to high-intensity fluorescent light that breaks down bilirubin (a pigment of red blood cells) for transport to the GI system and excretion in urine and feces. The treatment is commonly given to neonates with hyperbilirubinemia — a symptom of physiologic jaundice, breast-milk jaundice, or hemolytic disease. Phototherapy continues until bilirubin drops to normal levels because unchecked hyperbilirubinemia can lead to kernicterus (deposits of unconjugated bilirubin in the brain cells), permanent brain damage, and even death.

Physiologic jaundice — resulting from the neonate's high red blood cell (RBC) count and short RBC life span — may develop in 2 to 3 days after delivery in about 50% of full-term neonates and in 3 to 5 days in about 80% of premature neonates.

Breast-milk jaundice may develop 3 to 4 days after delivery in about 25% of breast-feeding neonates and 4 to 5 days after delivery in less than 5%. Experts think that this hyperbilirubinemia results from reduced calorie and fluid intake (before the mother develops an adequate milk supply) or from constituents in breast milk that reduce bilirubin decomposition. They encourage frequent breast-feeding to increase fluid and calorie intake until bilirubin levels reach about 15 mg/dl. Then breast-feeding discontinues for 48 hours while bilirubin levels decrease.

Comparing oxygen delivery systems

If a neonate in your care is discharged on oxygen, the delivery system prescribed may depend on such factors as equipment availability and parental skill levels. Other factors to consider include the liter flow (or oxygen concentration) required and appropriate administration equipment, for example, nasal cannula or catheter, oxyhood, tent, high-flow mask, or nebulizer.

The nasal cannula, which provides a direct flow of oxygen to the nostrils, is the most common oxygen delivery device for home use. It imposes the fewest restrictions on a child attempting to interact with the environment. For instance, attaching extension tubing (up to 50′ [15.2 m]) to the cannula allows the child to move freely from room to room. However, the cannula can become dislodged from the nostrils with extensive manipulation. Velcro straps or adhesive dressings can reduce this risk by securing the cannula in the proper position.

Common oxygen sources include the oxygen concentrator, cylinder oxygen, and liquid oxygen. When selecting the appropriate system for home care, the health care team looks at advantages and disadvantages, such as those that follow.

Oxygen concentrator
This system separates oxygen from ambient air and provides low-flow oxygen.

Advantages
• Cost-effective for the neonate who needs continuous, low-flow oxygen

Disadvantages
• Cannot be used with a high-flow mask or nebulizer
• Requires electricity
• Requires an oxygen cylinder as a backup in case of malfunction or power failure
• Bulky and noisy
• Emits heat

Cylinder oxygen
This system uses oxygen stored as a gas in a cylinder with a valve.

Advantages
• Cost-effective for the neonate who requires high-flow oxygen or intermittent oxygen for up to 12 hours daily
• Can be used with a high-flow oxygen mask, a nasal cannula, a nasal catheter, or a nebulizer
• Portable when a small cylinder is used

Disadvantages
• Requires a humidification source if the flow must exceed ¾ liter
• Must be used with caution and kept in a stand or cart; safety cap must be fastened securely in case the neonate falls

Liquid oxygen
This system uses oxygen stored in a liquid state under high pressure in a cylinder with a valve.

Advantages
• Cost-effective for the neonate who needs continuous low- to moderate-flow oxygen
• Usually can be used with any oxygen delivery method
• Smaller and more lightweight than other oxygen systems
• Refillable, portable units available for when the neonate travels

Disadvantages
• Humidification source required if flow must exceed ¾ liter
• May cause burns if oxygen comes into contact with skin during transfer from a stationary to a portable unit
• Cylinder must be used in an upright position

Treatment for hemolytic disease, a much more serious condition, includes phototherapy and exchange transfusions. In pathologic jaundice, which occurs within 24 hours of birth and raises serum bilirubin levels above 13 mg/dl, phototherapy may be used with appropriate treatment for the underlying cause.

Equipment
Phototherapy unit ■ photometer ■ opaque eye mask ■ thermometer ■ urimeter ■ surgical face mask or small diaper ■ optional: thermistor (if the phototherapy unit is combined with a temperature-controlled radiant heat warmer) or incubator (if the neonate is small for gestational age), bilimeter.

Prepackaged eye coverings are available.

Understanding the phototherapy unit

Whether you use fluorescent or daylight bulbs, blue lights, or high-intensity quartz lamps in your neonatal phototherapy unit, you'll prepare the neonate in much the same way. You'll position the unit at a correct distance according to whether the neonate is in a crib, radiant warmer, or incubator (as shown). You'll also take care to expose as much skin surface as possible to as much light as possible. That's because the light decomposes harmful, excess bilirubin in the skin and subcutaneous tissues to a more water-soluble form that's easily excreted from the body.

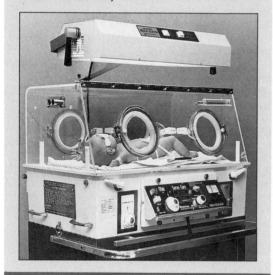

Preparation of equipment

Set up the phototherapy unit about 18 inches above the neonate's crib. Verify placement of the light-bulb shield *because this device filters ultraviolet rays and protects the neonate from broken bulbs.* If the neonate's in an incubator, place the phototherapy unit at least 3″ (7.6 cm) above the incubator *to promote sufficient air flow and prevent overheating.* (See *Understanding the phototherapy unit.*)

Turn on the lights. Place a photometer probe in the middle of the crib *to measure the energy emitted by the lights.* The energy should range between 6 and 8 microwatts per square centimeter per nanometer.

Implementation

• Explain the procedure to the parents *to reduce their anxiety and guilt and to ensure cooperation.*
• Record the neonate's initial bilirubin level and his axillary temperature *to establish baseline measurements.*
• Cover the neonate's closed eyes with the opaque eye mask. Fasten the mask securely enough to stay in place and to prevent the neonate from opening his eyes, but loosely enough to ensure circulation and avoid pressure on the eyeballs. *This protects the eyes from light-related retinal damage and prevents reflex bradycardia, head molding, and corneal abrasions.*
• Clean the eyes periodically *to remove drainage and check circulation.*
• Undress the neonate *to expose the most skin to the most light.* Remember to place a diaper under him and to cover male genitalia with a surgical mask or a small diaper *to catch urine and to prevent possible testicular damage from the heat and light waves.*
• Take the neonate's axillary temperature every 2 hours *to make sure the neonate maintains a normal and stable body temperature.*
• If the neonate uses a servo-controlled incubator or a radiant warmer, place the thermistor on the neonate's side and cover it with opaque or reflective tape. *This prevents frequent sensor changes and protects the sensor from direct energy.*
• Provide additional warmth, if necessary, by adjusting the warming unit's thermostat.
• Monitor elimination. Note urine and stool amounts and frequency. Weigh the neonate twice daily, and watch for dehydration signs (dry skin, poor turgor, depressed fontanels) *because phototherapy increases fluid loss through stools and evaporation.*
• Clean the neonate carefully after each bowel movement *because the loose green stools that result from phototherapy can excoriate the skin.* Don't apply ointment *because this can cause burns under phototherapy lights.*
• Check urine specific gravity with a urimeter *to gauge the neonate's hydration status.*
• Feed the neonate every 3 to 4 hours and offer water between feedings *to ensure adequate hydration and to boost gastric motility.* Make sure water intake doesn't replace breast milk or formula. Take the neonate out of the crib, turn off the phototherapy lights, and unmask his eyes at least every 8 hours, if possible, *to provide visual stimulation and human contact.* Also assess his eyes *for inflammation or injury.*
• Reposition the neonate every 2 hours *to expose all body surfaces to the light and to prevent head molding and skin breakdown from pressure.*
• Check the bilirubin level at least every 24 hours — more often if levels rise significantly. If you don't use a bili-

meter, turn off the phototherapy unit before drawing venous blood for testing *because the lights may degrade bilirubin in the blood sample and thereby produce inaccurate test results.*
• Notify the doctor if the bilirubin level nears 20 mg/dl in full-term neonates, or 15 mg/dl in premature neonates *because these levels may lead to kernicterus.*
• Review the neonatal and maternal histories for clues to possible hyperbilirubinemia causes. Also watch for signs of infection and metabolic disorders, and check the neonate's hematocrit for polycythemia. Inspect the neonate for hematoma, bruising, petechiae, and cyanosis. If the phototherapy unit has blue lights, turn them off for the examination *because these lights can mask cyanosis.*

Special considerations
If the neonate cries excessively during phototherapy, place a blanket roll at each side *to give him a feeling of security.*

If the doctor diagnoses breast-feeding jaundice (suspending breast-feeding temporarily), teach the mother to express milk manually or with a pump. Encourage continued breast-feeding when indicated. Reassure the parents by explaining the transitory nature of jaundice. If possible, give phototherapy treatment in the mother's room *to facilitate bonding and decrease parental anxiety and guilt feelings.*

Home care
Home phototherapy programs are safe and effective alternatives for treating uncomplicated neonatal jaundice. Teach families how to perform the procedure and encourage their compliance. Explain that testing will continue until results show serum bilirubin at acceptable levels. Provide written instructions at discharge.

Complications
Bronze baby syndrome (an idiopathic darkening of the skin, serum, and urine) may occur. Changes in feeding and activity patterns and hormonal secretions may follow prolonged therapy.

Documentation
At least once every 2 hours, note the progress of phototherapy and that the neonate's eyes remain protected. Record the time of all bilirubin testing, and plot results. Document eye covering changes and eye care given. Keep records of measured radiant energy — initially and then every 8 hours. Document neonatal time away from lights, for example, for feeding or other procedures. Note fluid intake and the amount of urine and feces eliminated. Describe any changes in skin appearance and character, in feeding patterns, and in activity level.

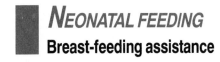

NEONATAL FEEDING
Breast-feeding assistance

Breast-feeding is the safest, simplest, and least expensive way to provide complete infant nourishment. Components of successful and satisfying breast-feeding include proper breast care, normal milk flow, and a comfortably positioned mother and infant.

Breast-feeding is contraindicated for a mother with a severe chronic condition, such as active tuberculosis, human immunodeficiency virus (HIV) infection, or hepatitis.

Equipment
Nursing or support bra ▪ pillow ▪ protective cover, such as cloth diaper or small towel ▪ optional: commercially available breast pads without plastic liners, or pads made from sanitary napkins, gauze, cloth diapers, or cotton handkerchiefs; instructional materials.

Implementation
• Explain the procedure to the mother and provide privacy.
• Encourage the mother to drink a beverage before and during or after breast-feeding. *This ensures adequate fluid intake, which helps to maintain milk production.*
• Encourage the mother to attend to personal needs and to change the infant's wet or soiled diaper before breast-feeding begins *to avoid interruptions during feeding time.*
• Wash your hands. Also instruct the mother to wash her hands.
• Help the mother find a comfortable position, for example, the cradle or side-lying position, *to promote the letdown reflex* (see *Breast-feeding positions,* page 712). Have her expose one breast and rest the nape of the infant's neck at the antecubital space of her arm, supporting his back with her forearm.
• Urge the mother to relax during breast-feeding *because relaxation also promotes the letdown reflex.* Inform her that she may feel a tingling sensation when it occurs and that milk may drip or spray from her breasts. Tell her the reflex may also be initiated by hearing the infant's cry.
• Guiding the mother's free hand, have her place her thumb on top of the exposed breast's areola and her first two fingers beneath it, forming a "C" with her hand. Turn the infant so that he faces the breast.
• Tell the mother to stroke the infant's cheek located nearest her exposed breast or the infant's mouth with the nipple. *This stimulates the rooting instinct.* Emphasize that she shouldn't touch the infant's other cheek *because*

Breast-feeding positions

Ordinarily, a maternity patient chooses a breast-feeding position that's comfortable and efficient. If the patient experiences discomfort in one position, she can choose another position. In fact, by changing positions periodically, she can alter the infant's grasp on the nipple and thereby avoid constant friction on the same area. As appropriate, suggest these typical breast-feeding positions.

Cradle position

This is the most common position for breast-feeding. The mother sits in a comfortable chair and cradles the infant's head in the crook of her arm. If desired, she can support her elbow with pillows *to minimize tension and fatigue.* She can also tuck the infant's lower arm alongside her body *so it stays out of the way.* The infant's mouth should remain even with the nipple and his stomach should face and touch the mother's stomach.

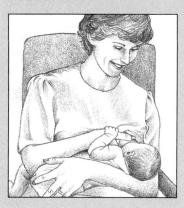

Side-lying position

The mother may choose this position for breast-feeding at night or during recovery from a cesarean section. She lies on her side with her stomach facing the infant's and the infant's head near her breast. She then lifts her breast, and as the infant's mouth opens, she pulls him toward her nipple.

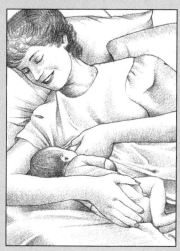

Football position

Often selected by mothers with large breasts or by those who have had a cesarean section, this position is also useful for feeding twins or infants who are small or premature. The mother sits in a comfortable chair with a pillow under her arm on the nursing side. She places her hand under the infant's head and brings it close to the breast, while placing the fingers of her other hand above and below the nipple. As the infant's mouth opens, she pulls his head close to her breast.

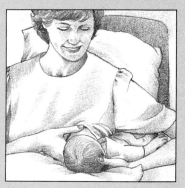

he may turn his head toward the touch and away from the breast.
- When the infant opens his mouth and roots for the nipple, instruct the mother to insert the nipple and as much of the areola as possible into the infant's mouth. *This helps him to exert sufficient pressure with his lips, gums, and cheek muscles on the milk sinuses below the areola.*
- Check for occlusion of the infant's nostrils by the mother's breast. If this happens advise the mother to press her finger on her breast below the infant's nose to give him room to breathe.
- Suggest that the mother begin nursing the infant for 15 minutes on each breast.

- To alternate breasts, instruct the mother to slip a finger into the side of the infant's mouth *to break the seal and move him to the other breast.*
- *To burp the infant,* show the mother how to hold him in an upright forward-tilting position with one hand supporting his chest and chin.
- Tell the mother to gently pat or rub the infant's back *to expel any ingested air.* Help her place a protective cover, such as a cloth diaper, under the infant's chin.
- Instruct the mother to feed the infant at the other breast. If she wishes, and if the infant remains awake, she may nurse him longer. *A demand-feeding routine, in which the infant feeds according to his hunger and desire,*

establishes an abundant, steady milk supply appropriate for the infant's requirements (the more the infant feeds, the more milk the mother produces). What's more, frequent nursing satisfies the infant's need to suck. It also promotes bonding.
• When the mother finishes breast-feeding, have her place the infant prone or on his side with a blanket roll at his back *to provide stability.* Instruct her not to place him supine *because if he throws up, he may aspirate vomitus.* However, if the mother wishes to hold the infant longer, encourage her to do so. *Touching enhances bonding.*
• Instruct the mother to air-dry her nipples for 15 minutes after feeding finishes, and give additional breast-care instructions (see *Breast care for new mothers*).
• Encourage the mother's breast-feeding efforts. *To boost these efforts,* urge her to eat balanced meals, to drink at least eight, 8-oz glasses of fluid daily, and to nap daily for at least the first 2 weeks after giving birth. Answer her questions about breast-feeding, and provide instructional materials, if available. Before she goes home, inform her about local breast-feeding and parenting support groups—La Leche League, for example.
• Observe the mother for breast engorgement. If traditional relief measures fail to trigger the letdown reflex, administer an analgesic to relieve discomfort. Also notify the doctor.
• Discuss signs of mastitis to report—red, tender, or warm breast, and fever—should they occur after discharge.

Special considerations

Instruct the mother to use the side-lying position for breast-feeding on the delivery table. *This reduces discomfort from pressure on the episiotomy (if she had one).* Or you can adjust the table so that she can sit up. Because the mother will probably be exhausted from delivery or drowsy from medication, stay with her during this time.

Inform the mother that infants routinely lose weight (several ounces) during the first days of extrauterine life. Advise her that colostrum, her first milk, is yellow, rich in protein and antibodies, and secreted in small amounts. Her true milk, which is thin and bluish, won't appear until several days after delivery.

Advise a mother who's breast-feeding twins that using the football position allows her to feed both infants at once. Instruct her to alternate breasts and infants at each feeding. If the mother prefers to nurse one infant at a time, make sure the nursery and the mother both keep track of which infant came first during each feeding.

Reassure her that there is no standard schedule for breast-feeding and that developing a comfortable routine takes time.

Tell her to expect uterine cramping (contractions) during breast-feeding until her uterus returns to its original

Breast care for new mothers

If a mother plans to breast-feed her infant, she can prepare her breasts as directed by her doctor. After the infant's birth, she'll need to maintain breast tissue integrity, the keratin layer that builds protectively on the areola, and the natural lubricant that the breast produces as well.

Although postpartum care varies for the breast-feeding and non-breast-feeding mother, both may need a few guidelines.

For the breast-feeding mother

• Instruct the mother to wash the areolae and nipples with water, without soap or a washcloth, to avoid washing away the natural oils and keratin.
• Advise the mother with sore or irritated nipples to apply ice compresses just before breast-feeding. This numbs and firms the nipples, making them less sensitive and easier for the infant to grasp.
• Suggest that lubricating the nipple with a few drops of expressed breast milk before feeding may help prevent tenderness.
• Recommend placing breast pads over the nipples to collect colostrum or milk, which commonly leaks during the first few breast-feeding weeks. Advise replacing pads often to guard against infection.
• Inform the mother that breast milk comes in 2 to 5 days after delivery and is accompanied by a slight temperature elevation and breast changes—increased size, warmth, and firmness.
• Tell the mother that a well-fitting support bra may help control engorgement.
• Advise the mother with engorged breasts to apply warm compresses, massage the breasts, take a warm shower, or express some milk before feeding. This dilates the milk ducts, promotes letdown, and makes the nipples more pliable.

For the non-breast-feeding mother

• Instruct the mother to clean her breasts using the same technique as the breast-feeding mother. Add that she may use soap.
• Advise her to wear a support bra to help minimize engorgement and to decrease nipple stimulation.
• Advise her to avoid stimulating the nipples or manually expressing her milk to minimize further milk production. Instead, provide pain medication, as ordered, ice packs, or a breast binder.

size. These contractions result from released oxytocin, a natural hormone that prompts the uterus to return to its prepregnancy state. Oxytocin also initiates the letdown reflex, thereby allowing milk to flow from the alveoli into the ducts.

During breast-feeding, milk leakage in the nonnursing breast may be controlled by applying light pressure to the nipple with the fingers or the palm of the hand.

If the infant shows little interest in breast-feeding, reassure the mother that he may need several days to learn and to adjust. If the infant is sleepy, encourage the mother to offer the breast frequently but to refrain from forcing the infant to nurse. Instead, advise her to try rubbing the infant's feet, unwrapping his blanket, changing his diaper, changing her position or the infant's, or manually expressing milk and then allowing the infant to suckle. A balky infant may suck eagerly if milk is already flowing.

If the infant fails to nurse sufficiently and dehydration seems likely, have the mother give him expressed milk through a medicine dropper or small syringe. Instruct her to avoid frequent feeding with a bottle *because the infant may become used to the artificial nipple and subsequently reject the mother's.* Only rarely does a breast-fed infant need supplemental glucose and water.

Advise the mother to start breast-feeding with the breast she used last at the previous feeding *to help avoid engorgement of the breast.* Suggest attaching a safety pin to the bra strap supporting the breast she last used *to serve as a reminder.*

Complications

Breast engorgement may result from venous and lymphatic stasis and alveolar milk accumulation. Mastitis occurs postpartum in about 1% of mothers. It usually results from a pathogen that passes from the infant's nose or pharynx into breast tissue through a cracked or fissured nipple.

Documentation

After assisting the mother to breast-feed, note the areas in which she needs further instruction and help. Document patient teaching.

 Breast pumps

By creating suction, manual and electric breast pumps stimulate lactation. Indicated for a mother who wants to maintain milk production while she and her infant are separated or while illness temporarily incapacitates one

or the other, or both, a breast pump also can relieve engorgement or collect milk for a premature infant with a weak sucking reflex.

Having many uses, the electric pump is more effective and efficient than the manual pump (see *Comparing breast pumps*). The mother can use it to reduce pressure on sore or cracked nipples or to reestablish maternal milk supply when a weaned infant becomes allergic to formula. Or she can use it to collect milk from inverted nipples or to express milk mechanically when she can't express milk by hand or with a manual pump.

Equipment

Manual cylinder or electric breast pump ■ sterile collection bag or bottle (to store milk if desired) ■ optional: warm compresses.

An electric breast pump should come with a sterile, single-use accessory kit, which many pump manufacturers supply. The kit contains shields, milk cups, an overflow bottle, and tubing. These parts can be washed with soap and water and then sterilized for repeated use.

Preparation of equipment

Assemble the breast pump according to the manufacturer's instructions. If milk will be stored or frozen, thoroughly clean any removable parts the milk will touch.

Implementation

• Explain the procedure to the patient.

• Give her time to attend to personal needs first *so she won't have to interrupt the procedure for this purpose.* Also advise her to wash her hands.

• Instruct the patient to drink a beverage before and after breast pumping. *This ensures sufficient fluid intake to maintain adequate milk production.*

• Assist the patient to assume a comfortable position and to relax. Offer pillows for support. Provide privacy, and instruct her to uncover her breast completely *to prevent lint and dirt from entering the milk-collection container.*

• If the patient's breasts are engorged, have her apply warm compresses for 5 minutes or take a warm shower *to dilate the milk ducts and stimulate the letdown reflex.*

• *To help trigger the release of milk-producing hormones,* instruct the patient to use her thumb and forefinger to stimulate the nipple and areola for 1 to 2 minutes.

To use a manual cylinder pump

• Instruct the patient to place the flange or shield against her breast with the nipple in the center of the device. Then tell her to move the outer cylinder of the pump toward and then away from the breast, using a pistonlike motion, *to draw the milk from the breast.* Have her pump each breast in this manner until it's empty.

Comparing breast pumps

Breast pumps are available as battery-operated, electric, and hand-operated models. The pump that's best for your patient depends on such factors as the pump's purpose and the patient's situation. A description of common pumps and their features follows.

Battery-powered pump
Having a battery-powered motor, this pump can be operated with one hand. Easy to clean, it's a good choice for mothers who work outside the home or who need a breast pump only for short-term use.

Electric pump
Usually used in hospitals, this efficient, gentle pump plugs into an electrical outlet and can be operated with one hand. It's available as a small, 2-lb model or as a larger model about the size of a small sewing machine. Inform your patient that the larger model can be rented from a pharmacy or medical supply company.

Cylinder pump
This pump operates with two plastic cylinders, one inside the other, that create gentle suction as the outer cylinder is moved back and forth. Because two hands are needed to operate it, it may be tiring to use. Easily cleaned and portable, however, this pump proves relatively efficient for short-term or intermittent use.

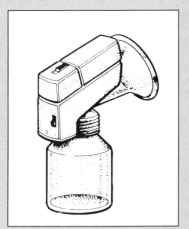
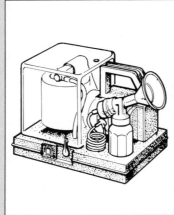
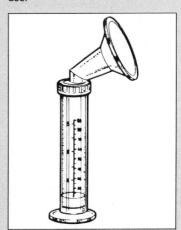

• If the milk will be stored or frozen, direct the patient to fill a sterile bottle with the milk from the cylinder. If the infant will drink the milk directly, instruct the patient to attach a rubber nipple to the cylinder.

To use a battery-powered or electric breast pump
• Unless the pump is battery-powered, be sure the pump has a three-pronged plug to ground it *to prevent electric shock.*
• Instruct the patient to set the suction regulator on low. Tell her to hold the collection unit upright *to prevent milk from being sucked into the machine.* Have her center her nipple in the shield, which she will place against the breast.

• Direct her to activate the machine and adjust the suction regulator to achieve a comfortable pressure. Have her check the operator's manual to determine the pressure setting at which the pump functions most efficiently.
• Instruct her to pump each breast for 5 to 8 minutes or until the spray grows scant. Then pump each breast again for 3 to 5 minutes and then again for 2 to 3 minutes. (Usually, 8 oz, or 237 ml, can be pumped within 15 to 30 minutes.)
• Tell the patient to remove the shield from the breast by inserting a finger between the breast and the shield *to break the vacuum seal.* Then she should return the suction regulator to the low setting and turn off the machine.

• If the milk will be stored or frozen, pour it from the collection unit into a sterile container. (If it's to be frozen, place it in the freezer immediately.)
• If the infant will drink the milk directly, pour it into a sterile bottle.
• Label the collected milk with the date, the time of collection, and the amount. Also be sure the label contains the infant's name, if applicable.

To conclude the procedure
• Instruct the patient to air-dry her nipples for about 15 minutes.
• Instruct her to disassemble the removable parts of the pump and wash them according to the manufacturer's directions.

Special considerations
Provide emotional support *to alleviate the mother's distress related to the infant's absence at feeding time.*

If the patient will use a breast pump for some time, have her pump her breasts every 2 to 3 hours *because neonates nurse 8 to 12 times every 24 hours.* Remind her to pump her breasts at night *because the breasts need round-the-clock stimulation to produce milk and maintain an adequate supply.*

Once the milk supply is established, some mothers may need to pump once nightly; others find that they can sleep for 6 hours and still maintain the milk supply.

Breast milk can be stored in the refrigerator for 48 hours and in the freezer at 0° F (−17.8° C) for up to 6 months.

Complications
Common complications include nipple injury from suction and contaminated milk from improperly cleaned equipment or incorrect storage.

Documentation
Record the duration that the patient pumped each breast, the amount of milk collected, and the patient's tolerance of the procedure.

Bottle-feeding

When a neonate requires a special diet or when a mother cannot or chooses not to breast-feed, formula is the next-best food source. Formula preparations supply all needed vitamins and nutrients and can be administered by anyone. Most formulas used in hospitals come ready-to-feed in disposable containers. Some formulas and equipment, however, may require advance preparation, such as mixing and sterilizaton. The American Academy of Pediatrics recommends commercially prepared formula over animal milks or homemade preparations for the infant's first year.

Because formulas for the neonate must be sterile, they are prepared either by the aseptic method (in which all articles used in formula preparation are sterilized before mixing) or by the terminal heat method (in which the formula is prepared with clean technique and then sterilized using a home sterilizer). In the United States, some pediatricians recommend clean technique and tap water for formulas because water supplies are clean and safe in most areas.

A normal neonate takes 15 to 20 minutes to consume a 1- to 1½-oz portion of formula. He usually feeds every 3 to 4 hours.

Equipment
Commercially prepared formula or ingredients ■ bottle, nipple, and cap ■ tissue or cloth ■ gown.

Hospitals commonly use disposable bottle and nipple units for neonatal feeding.

Preparation of equipment
If you're using commercially prepared formula, uncap the formula bottle and make sure the seal wasn't previously broken *to ensure sterility and freshness.* Then screw on the nipple and cap. Keep the protective sterile cap over the nipple until the neonate is ready to feed. If you're preparing formula, follow the manufacturer's instructions or the doctor's prescription. Administer the formula at room temperature or slightly warmer.

Implementation
• Wash your hands.
• Invert the bottle and shake some formula on your wrist *to test the patency of the nipple hole and the formula's temperature.* The nipple hole should allow formula to drip freely but not to stream out. *If the hole is too large, the neonate may aspirate formula; if it's too small, the extra sucking effort he expends may tire him before he can empty the bottle.*
• Sit comfortably in a semireclining position, and cradle the neonate in one arm to support his head and back. *This position allows swallowed air to rise to the top of the stomach where it's more easily expelled.* If he can't be held, sit by him and elevate his head and shoulders slightly.
• Place the nipple in the neonate's mouth while making sure the tongue is down, but don't insert it so far as to stimulate the gag reflex. He should begin to suck, pulling in as much nipple as is comfortable. If he doesn't start to suck, stroke him under the chin or on his cheek, or

touch his lips with the nipple *to stimulate his sucking reflex.*

• As the neonate feeds, tilt the bottle upward *to keep the nipple filled with formula and to prevent him from swallowing air.* Watch for a steady stream of bubbles in the bottle. This indicates proper venting and flow of formula. If the neonate pushes out the nipple with his tongue, reinsert the nipple. *Expelling the nipple is a normal reflex. It doesn't necessarily mean that the neonate is full.*

• Always hold the bottle for a neonate. If left to feed himself, he may aspirate formula or swallow air if the bottle tilts or empties. *Experts link bottle propping with an increased incidence of otitis media and dental caries in older infants.*

• Burp the neonate after each ½ oz of formula, because he will typically swallow some air even when fed correctly. Hold the neonate upright in a slightly forward position, supporting his head and chest with one hand. Or, position a clean cloth *to protect your clothing,* and hold the neonate upright over your shoulder, or place him face down across your lap. *The change in position helps the gas to rise or "bring up the bubble."* In either case, rub or gently pat his back until he expels the air.

• After you finish feeding and burping the neonate, place him on his stomach or right side *to prevent aspiration if he regurgitates.* Neonates are prone to regurgitation because of an immature cardiac sphincter.

• Discard any remaining formula, and properly dispose of all equipment.

Special considerations

Change feeding duration by changing the size of the nipple or the nipple hole *because the neonate tires if he feeds too long, and his sucking needs aren't met if he doesn't feed long enough.*

Be sure to note how much formula is in the bottle before and after the feeding. Use the calibrations along the side of the container to calculate the amount of formula consumed.

Be alert for aspiration in the neonate who has a diminished sucking or swallowing reflex and who may have difficulty feeding. Also take appropriate measures according to hospital policy to feed the neonate with cleft lip and palate.

Teach parents how to properly prepare and sterilize (if required) formula, bottles, and nipples, and how to feed and burp the neonate. Although most hospitals have a feeding schedule, advise the mother that she may switch to a more flexible demand-feeding schedule when at home. Forewarn her that the neonate may not feed well on his first day home because of the new activity and environment. Inform parents about the forms of formula available

(ready-to-feed, concentrate, powders) *so that they can choose the most convenient form.*

Prepare parents to expect the neonate to regurgitate formula. Explain that regurgitation (merely an overflow that typically follows feeding) shouldn't be confused with vomiting (a more complete emptying of the stomach accompanied by symptoms not associated with feeding).

Complications

Bottle-propping may allow the nipple to block the airway, causing suffocation; it may also lead to otitis media or dental caries. Lung infection or death may follow aspiration of regurgitated formula.

Documentation

Record the time of the feeding, the amount of formula consumed, how well the neonate fed, and whether he appeared satisfied. Note any regurgitation or vomiting. If the mother feeds him, observe and describe their interactions. Document any patient teaching.

Gavage feeding

Gavage feeding involves passing nutrients directly to the neonate's stomach by a tube advanced nasally or orally. If a neonate can't suck (because of prematurity, illness, or congenital deformity) or if a neonate risks aspiration (because of gastroesophageal reflux, ineffective gag reflex, or easy tiring), gavage feeding may supply nutrients until he can take food by mouth.

Unless the neonate has problems with the feeding tube, the nurse usually inserts it orally before each feeding and withdraws it after the feeding. This intermittent method stimulates the sucking reflex. If the neonate can't tolerate this, the nurse advances the tube nasally and leaves it in place for 24 to 72 hours.

Tube feeding is contraindicated for neonates without bowel sounds or with suspected intestinal obstruction, severe respiratory distress, or massive gastroesophageal reflux.

Equipment

Feeding tube (#3½ up to #6 French for nasogastric feeding of premature neonate; #8 French for others) ■ feeding reservoir or large (20- to 50-ml) syringe ■ prescribed formula or breast milk ■ sterile water ■ tape measure ■ tape ■ stethoscope ■ gloves ■ optional: bowl and pacifier.

A commercial feeding reservoir is available.

Preparation of equipment

Allow the formula or breast milk to warm to room temperature, if necessary. Wash your hands and open the sterile water, if it comes in a small-sized disposable container. Remove the syringe or reservoir and the feeding tube from the packaging.

Implementation

• Identify the neonate and verify the doctor's orders.
• Using a tape measure, determine the length of tubing needed to ensure placement in the stomach. Commonly, you'll measure from the tip of the nose to the tip of the earlobe to the xiphoid process. Mark the tube at the appropriate distance with a piece of tape. Measure from the bottom.
• Position the neonate supine. Elevate the head of his mattress one notch. Otherwise, place him supine or tilted slightly to his right with head and chest slightly elevated.
• Put on gloves. Stabilize the neonate's head with one hand and lubricate the feeding tube with sterile water with the other hand.
• Insert the tube smoothly and quickly up to the pre-measured tape mark. For oral insertion, pass the tube toward the back of the throat. For nasal insertion, pass the tube toward the occiput in a horizontal plane.
• Synchronize tube insertion with throat movement if the neonate swallows *to facilitate tube passage into the stomach.* During insertion, watch for choking and cyanosis, signs that a tube has entered the trachea. If these occur, remove the tube and reinsert it. Also watch for brady-cardia and apnea resulting from vagal stimulation.
• If the tube will remain in place, tape it flat to the neonate's cheek. *To prevent possible nasal skin breakdown,* don't tape the tube to the bridge of his nose.
• Make sure the tube is in the stomach (and not the lungs) by aspirating residual stomach contents with the syringe. Check the content's pH because gastric contents are highly acidic. *This helps confirm tube placement. Note the volume obtained, and then reinject it to avoid altering the neonate's buffer system and electrolyte balance.* Or, as ordered, reduce the feeding volume by the residual amount, or prolong the interval between feedings.
• Alternatively, or additionally, check placement of the feeding tube in the stomach by injecting 0.5 to 1 cc of air into the tube while listening with the stethoscope for air sounds in the stomach and on each side of the anterior chest.
• If you suspect that the tube's displaced, advance it several centimeters farther and test again. *Don't* begin feeding until you're certain the tube is in the stomach.
• When the tube is in place, fill the feeding reservoir or syringe with formula or breast milk. Connect the feeding reservoir or syringe to the top of the tube, and start the feeding.

reservoir or syringe to the top of the tube, and start the feeding.
• If the neonate's on your lap, hold the container about 4″ (10 cm) above his abdomen. If he's lying down, hold it between 6″ and 8″ (15 to 20 cm) above his head. When using a commercial feeding reservoir, look for air bubbles in the container, an indicator of formula passage.
• Regulate flow by raising and lowering the container, so that the feeding takes 15 to 20 minutes, the average time for a bottle-feeding. *To prevent stomach distention, reflux, and vomiting,* don't let the feeding proceed too rapidly.
• When the feeding is finished, pinch off the tubing before air enters the neonate's stomach. *This helps prevent distention, fluid leakage into the pharynx during tube removal, and consequent aspiration.*
• Withdraw the tube smoothly and quickly. If the tube will remain in place, flush it with several milliliters of sterile water, if ordered.
• Burp the neonate *to decrease abdominal distention.* Hold him upright or in a sitting position. Let your one hand support his head and chest and your other hand gently rub or pat his back until he expels the air.
• Place him on his stomach or right side for 1 hour after feeding *to facilitate gastric emptying and to prevent aspiration if he regurgitates.*
• Don't perform postural drainage and percussion until 1 hour or more after feeding.

Special considerations

Use the nasogastric approach for the neonate who must keep the feeding tube in place, *because the nasogastric approach holds the tube more securely than the orogastric approach.* Alternate the nostril used at each insertion *to prevent skin and mucosal irritation.*

Observe the premature neonate for indications that he's ready to begin bottle- or breast-feeding: strong sucking reflex, coordinated sucking and swallowing, alertness before feeding, and sleep after it.

Provide the neonate with a pacifier during feeding *to soothe him, to help prevent gagging, and to promote an association between sucking and the full feeling that follows feeding.*

Complications

Gagging with regurgitation causes loss of nutrients. An indwelling nasogastric tube can irritate mucous membranes and cause nasal airway obstruction, epistaxis, and stomach perforation. A feeding tube may kink, coil, or knot and become obstructed, preventing feeding.

Documentation

Record the amount of residual fluid and the amount currently taken. Note the type and amount of any vomitus, and any adverse reactions to tube insertion or feeding.

SPECIAL PROCEDURES
Circumcision

Steeped in controversy and history, circumcision (the removal of the penile foreskin) is thought to promote a clean glans and to minimize the risk of phimosis (tightening of the foreskin) in later life. It's also thought to reduce the risk of penile cancer or cervical cancer in sexual partners, although the American Academy of Pediatrics (AAP) has contended since 1971 that no valid medical reason exists for routine circumcision. Currently, the AAP is continuing its studies on the effects of circumcision.

In Judaism, circumcision (*bris*) is a religious rite performed by a *mohel* on the eighth day after birth, when the neonate officially receives his name. Because most neonates are discharged before this time, the bris rarely occurs in the hospital.

One method of circumcision involves removing the foreskin by using a Yellen clamp to stabilize the penis. With this device, a cone that fits over the glans provides a cutting surface and protects the glans penis. Another technique uses a plastic circumcision bell (Plastibell) over the glans and a suture tied tightly around the base of the foreskin. This method prevents bleeding. The resultant ischemia causes the foreskin to slough off within 5 to 8 days. This method is thought to be painless because it stretches the foreskin, which inhibits sensory conduction.

Circumcision is contraindicated in neonates who are ill or who have bleeding disorders, ambiguous genitalia, or congenital anomalies of the penis, such as hypospadias or epispadias, because the foreskin may be needed for later reconstructive surgery.

Equipment

Circumcision tray (contents vary but usually include circumcision clamps, various-sized cones, scalpel, probe, scissors, forceps, sterile basin, sterile towel, and sterile drapes) ■ povidone-iodine solution ■ restraining board with arm and leg restraints ■ sterile gloves ■ petroleum gauze ■ sterile 4″ × 4″ gauze pads ■ optional: sutures, plastic circumcision bell, antimicrobial ointment, topical anesthetic, and overhead warmer.

Preparation of equipment

For a circumcision using a Yellen clamp: Assemble the sterile tray and other equipment in the procedure area. Open the sterile tray and pour povidone-iodine solution into the sterile basin. Using sterile technique, place sterile 4″ × 4″ gauze pads and petroleum gauze on the sterile tray. Arrange the restraining board and direct adequate light on the area.

For circumcision with a plastic circumcision bell: You won't need to assemble a circumcision tray. Do assemble sterile gloves, sutures, restraining board, petroleum gauze and, if ordered, antibiotic ointment.

A mohel usually brings his own equipment.

Implementation

● Beforehand, make sure the parents understand the procedure and have signed the proper consent form.
● Withhold feeding for at least 1 hour before the procedure *to reduce the possibility of emesis or aspiration or both.*
● Place the neonate on the restraining board, and restrain his arms and legs. Don't leave him unattended.
● Assist the doctor as necessary throughout the procedure and comfort the neonate as needed.

For Yellen circumcision

● After putting on sterile gloves, the doctor will clean the penis and scrotum with povidone-iodine and drape the neonate.
● He will apply a Yellen clamp to the penis, loosen the foreskin, insert the cone under it *to provide a cutting surface and to protect the penis,* and remove the foreskin.
● He will cover the wound with sterile petroleum gauze *to prevent infection and control bleeding.*

For circumcision with a plastic bell

● The doctor will slide the plastic bell device between the foreskin and the glans penis.
● Then he will tie a suture tightly around the foreskin at the coronal edge of the glans. The foreskin distal to the suture will become ischemic, then atrophic. After 5 to 8 days, the foreskin will drop off with the plastic bell attached, leaving a clean, well-healed excision. No special care is required, but watch for swelling that may indicate infection or interfere with urination.

For care after circumcision

● Remove the neonate from the restraining board, and check for bleeding.
● Place him in a side-lying position, rather than prone, *to minimize pressure on the excisional area.* Leave him diaperless for 1 to 2 hours *to observe for bleeding and to reduce possible chafing and irritation.*

• Show the neonate to his parents *to reassure them that he is all right.*

• Once you rediaper the neonate, change his diaper as soon as he voids. If the dressing falls off, clean the wound with warm water *to minimize pain from urine on the circumcised area.* Don't remove the original dressing until it falls off (usually after the first or second voiding).

• Check for bleeding every 15 minutes for the first hour and then every hour for the next 24 hours. If bleeding occurs, apply pressure with sterile gauze pads. Notify the doctor if bleeding continues.

• Loosely diaper the neonate *to prevent irritation.* At each diaper change, apply ordered antimicrobial ointment, petroleum jelly, or petroleum gauze until the wound appears healed. Avoid leaving the neonate under the radiant warmer after placing petroleum gauze on the penis *because the area might burn.*

• Watch for drainage, redness, or swelling. Don't remove the thin, yellow-white exudate that forms over the healing area within 1 to 2 days—this normal incrustation protects the wound until it heals in 3 to 4 days.

• Don't discharge the neonate until he has voided.

Special considerations

Always be sure to show parents the circumcision before discharge *so they can ask any questions and so you can teach them how to care for the area.*

If the neonate's mother has human immunodeficiency virus (HIV) infection, circumcision will be delayed until the doctor knows the neonate's HIV status. The neonate whose mother has HIV infection has a higher-than-normal risk of infection.

Home care

Inform the mother that the circumcision site may appear yellow in light-skinned neonates and lighter than the surrounding skin in dark-skinned neonates. Tell her that this signifies healing and is not a cause for concern.

Instruct the mother to observe the circumcision site regularly for pus or bloody discharge, which may indicate delayed healing or infection. If these signs occur, she should notify the doctor.

Tell the mother that the rim of the device used for circumcision may remain in place after discharge from the hospital. Reassure her that the rim will fall off harmlessly in 3 or 4 days. However, if the rim doesn't fall off after 1 week, notify the doctor. *A retained rim may lead to infection.*

Complications

After a Yellen clamp procedure, infection and bleeding may occur. The skin of the penile shaft can adhere to the glans, resulting in scarring or fibrous bands. The most severe complications are urethral fistulae and edema. Incomplete amputation of the foreskin can follow application of the plastic circumcision bell.

Documentation

Note the time and date of the circumcision, any parent teaching, and any excessive bleeding.

 # RhoGAM administration

RhoGAM is a concentrated solution of immune globulin containing $Rh_o(D)$ antibodies. Intramuscular injection of RhoGAM keeps the Rh-negative mother from producing active antibody responses and forming anti-$Rh_o(D)$ to Rh-positive fetal blood cells and endangering future Rh-positive infants. Maternal immunization to the Rh antigen commonly results from transplacental hemorrhage during gestation or delivery. If unchecked during gestation, incompatible fetal and maternal blood can lead to hemolytic disease in the neonate.

RhoGAM is indicated for the Rh-negative mother after abortion, ectopic pregnancy, or delivery of a neonate having $Rh_o(D)$-positive or D^u-positive blood and Coombs'-negative cord blood, accidental transfusion of Rh-positive blood, amniocentesis, abruptio placentae, or abdominal trauma. A RhoGAM injection should be given within 72 hours to prevent future maternal sensitization.

Subsequent pregnancies of the Rh-negative mother require screening to detect previous inadequate RhoGAM administration or low Rh-positive antibody titers.

Administration of RhoGAM at approximately 28 weeks' gestation can also protect the fetus of the Rh-negative mother. Common in western Europe, Canada, and Australia, this practice is growing in the United States. The dose is determined according to the fetal packed red blood cell (RBC) volume that enters the mother's blood. A volume under 15 ml usually calls for 1 vial of RhoGAM; a significant feto-maternal hemorrhage calls for more than 1 vial if the fetal packed RBC volume is greater than 15 ml.

Equipment

3-ml syringe ▪ 22G 1½″ needle ▪ RhoGAM vial ▪ alcohol sponges ▪ gloves ▪ triplicate form and patient identification (from the blood bank or hospital laboratory).

Implementation

• Identify the patient. Explain RhoGAM administration to the patient, and answer her questions. If the patient refuses the injection, notify the doctor or nurse-midwife.

• Two nurses must check the vial's identification numbers and sign the triplicate form that comes with the RhoGAM. Complete the form as indicated. Attach the top copy to the patient's chart. Send the remaining two copies, along with the empty RhoGAM vial, to the laboratory or blood bank.
• Provide privacy, wash your hands, and put on gloves.
• Withdraw the RhoGAM from the vial with the needle and syringe. Clean the gluteal injection site, and administer the RhoGAM intramuscularly.
• Give the patient a card that identifies her Rh-negative status, and instruct her to carry it with her or keep it in a convenient location.

Special considerations
After the procedure, watch for redness and soreness at the injection site. Provide an opportunity for the patient to voice any guilt or anxiety she may feel if she perceives her body as acting against the fetus.

Complications
Complications of a single RhoGAM injection are rare, mild, and confined to the injection site. After multiple injections (given after Rh mismatch), complications may include fever, myalgia, lethargy, discomfort, splenomegaly, or hyperbilirubinemia.

Documentation
Record the date, the time, and the site of the RhoGAM injection. If applicable, note the patient's refusal to accept a RhoGAM injection. Document patient teaching about RhoGAM. Note whether the patient received a card identifying her Rh-negative status.

Selected references

Baer, C., and Williams, B. *Clinical Pharmacology and Nursing,* 2nd ed. Springhouse, Pa.: Springhouse Corp., 1992.

Bliss-Holtz, J. "Comparison of Rectal, Axillary, and Inguinal Temperatures in Full-term Newborn Infants," *Nursing Research* 38(2):85-87, March-April 1989.

Carlo, W., and Lough, M. *Neonatal Respiratory Care,* 2nd ed. Chicago: Year-book Medical Pubs., 1988.

Cohen, S.M., et al. *Maternal, Neonatal, and Women's Health Nursing.* Springhouse, Pa.: Springhouse Corp., 1991.

Cohen, W., et al. *Management of Labor,* 2nd ed. Rockville, Md.: Aspen Pubs., Inc., 1989.

Hodson, W., and Truog, W. *Critical Care of the Newborn,* 2nd ed. Philadelphia: W.B. Saunders Co., 1989.

Illustrated Manual of Nursing Practice. Springhouse, Pa.: Springhouse Corp., 1991.

Nursing92 Drug Handbook. Springhouse, Pa.: Springhouse Corp., 1992.

Schroeder, C. "Pulse Oximetry: A Nursing Care Plan," *Critical Care Nurse* 8(8):50-68, November-December 1988.

PEDIATRIC CARE

MYRTLE TAYLOR WILLIAMS, RN, MSN

Introduction

Caring for pediatric patients demands specialized knowledge and skills. A child's physiologic immaturity heightens his response both to illness and to treatment regimens. And his small size narrows the margin for error in treatment. What's more, although children tend to recover more rapidly from an illness than adults do, they have a higher risk for serious complications.

When you care for a child, you need to consider the child's level of growth and development. For example, young children have only rudimentary motor skills and limited comprehension. This makes them especially prone to injury. For this reason, you need to remain alert to possibly dangerous situations, and take steps to ensure the child's safety.

Keep in mind, too, that even though a child is ill, he still needs sensory and social stimulation. For this reason, you need to include play in your pediatric care plans. Besides promoting development and fostering a sense of security and well-being, play allows children to release the stress and tension that result from the unfamiliar surroundings and activities they encounter in the hospital.

Remember to include the parents in all aspects of the child's care. Encourage them to maintain their roles as caregivers and to continue including the child as a member of the family — especially during long-term hospitalization. Doing so will help to achieve the overall goal of pediatric care: to create a positive environment that promotes the physical and emotional health of the child and his family.

SPECIMEN COLLECTION
Urine collection

Collection of a urine specimen for laboratory analysis allows screening for urinary tract infection and renal disorders, evaluation of treatment, and detection of systemic and metabolic disorders.

Although a child without bladder control can't provide a clean-catch midstream urine specimen, the pediatric urine collection bag provides a simple, effective alter-native. It offers minimal risk of specimen contamination without resorting to invasive procedures that can introduce bacteria into the bladder — catheterization or suprapubic aspiration, for example. Because the collection bag is secured with adhesive flaps, its use is contraindicated in a patient who has extremely sensitive or excoriated perineal skin. Alternative methods of collecting urine from small children include using an inside-out disposable diaper or a test tube.

Equipment

For a random specimen: pediatric urine collection bag (individually packaged) ■ urine specimen container ■ label ■ laboratory request form ■ two disposable diapers of appropriate size ■ scissors ■ gloves ■ washcloth ■ soap ■ water ■ towel ■ bowl ■ linen-saver pad.

For a culture and sensitivity specimen: sterile pediatric urine collection bag ■ sterile urine specimen container ■ label ■ laboratory request form ■ two disposable diapers of appropriate size ■ scissors ■ gloves ■ sterile bowl ■ sterile or distilled water ■ antiseptic skin cleaner ■ sterile 4″ × 4″ gauze pads ■ alcohol sponge ■ 3-ml syringe with needle ■ linen-saver pad.

For a timed specimen: 24-hour pediatric urine collection bag (individually packaged) with evacuation tubing ■ 24-hour urine specimen container ■ label ■ laboratory request form ■ scissors ■ two disposable diapers of appropriate size ■ gloves ■ washcloth ■ soap ■ water ■ bowl ■ towel ■ sterile 4″ × 4″ gauze pads ■ compound benzoin tincture ■ small medicine cup ■ 35-ml luer-lock syringe or urimeter ■ tubing stopper ■ specimen preservative, such as formaldehyde solution ■ linen-saver pad.

Kits containing sterile supplies for clean-catch collections are commercially available and may be used to obtain a culture and sensitivity specimen.

Preparation of equipment

Check the doctor's order for the type of specimen needed and assemble the appropriate equipment. Check the patient's chart for allergies (for example, to iodine). Complete the laboratory request form *to avoid delay in sending the specimen to the laboratory.* Wash your hands. With scissors, make a 2″ (5-cm) slit in one diaper, cutting from the center point toward one of the shorter edges. Later, you'll pull the urine collection bag through this slit when you position the bag and diaper on the patient. Next, pour water into the bowl; use sterile water and a sterile bowl if you need to collect a specimen for culture and sensitivity.

If you do need a culture and sensitivity specimen, check the expiration date on each sterile package and inspect for tears. Put on new gloves and open several packages of sterile 4″ × 4″ gauze pads.

If you need a timed specimen and will use benzoin in liquid form, pour it into the medicine cup. Cut the tubing on the urine collection bag so only 6″ (15 cm) remain attached. Discard the excess. Place the stopper in the severed end of the tubing. If you're going to use a urimeter for the patient who voids large amounts, don't cut the tubing; simply attach the device.

Implementation

• Explain the procedure to the patient—if he's old enough to understand—and to his parents. Provide privacy, especially if the patient is beyond infancy.

To collect a random specimen

• Wash your hands.
• Place the patient on a linen-saver pad.
• Clean the perineal area with soap, water, and a washcloth, working from the urinary meatus outward *to prevent contamination of the urine specimen with flora from the surrounding skin.* Wipe gently *to prevent tissue trauma and stimulation of urination.* Be sure to separate the labia of the female patient and retract the foreskin of the uncircumcised male patient *to expose the urinary meatus for thorough cleaning.* Thoroughly rinse the area with clear water and dry with a towel. Don't use powder, lotion, or cream *because these counteract the adhesive.*
• Place the patient in the frog position, with his legs separated and knees flexed. If necessary, have the patient's parent hold him while you apply the collection bag.
• Remove the protective coverings from the collection bag's adhesive flaps. For the female patient, first separate the labia and gently press the bag's lower rim to the perineum. Then, working upward toward the pubis, attach the rest of the adhesive rim inside the labia majora. For the male patient, place the bag's opening over the penis and scrotum and press the adhesive rim to the skin.
• Once the bag is securely attached, gently pull it through the slit in the diaper *to prevent compression of the bag by the diaper and to allow observation of the specimen immediately after the patient voids.* Then fasten the diaper on the patient.
• When urine appears in the bag, put on gloves and gently remove the diaper and the bag. Hold the bag's bottom port over the collection container, remove the tab from the port, and let the urine flow into the container.
• Measure the output if necessary.
• Label the specimen and attach the laboratory request form to the container. Send the specimen directly to the laboratory. Remove and discard gloves.
• Put the second diaper on the patient and make sure he's comfortable.

To collect a culture and sensitivity specimen

Follow the procedure for collecting a random specimen, with these modifications.
• Use sterile or distilled water, an antiseptic skin cleaner, and sterile 4″ × 4″ gauze pads to clean the perineal area.
• After donning gloves, clean the urinary meatus; then work outward. Wipe only once with each gauze pad; then discard it.
• After the patient urinates, remove the bag and use an alcohol sponge to clean a small area of the bag's surface. Puncture the clean area with the needle and aspirate urine into the syringe.
• Inject the urine into the sterile specimen container. Be careful to keep the needle from touching the container's sides *to maintain sterility.* Remember, a large volume of urine is unnecessary *because only about 1 ml of urine is needed to perform the culture and sensitivity test.* Then remove and discard your gloves.

To collect a timed specimen

• Check the doctor's order for the duration of the collection and the indication for the procedure. Following the steps for random specimen collection, prepare the patient, put on gloves, and clean the perineum.
• If bag adhesion is difficult, apply compound benzoin tincture to the perineal area, if ordered, *so that the collection bag will adhere better and you won't have to reapply it during the collection period.* If you're using liquid benzoin, dip a gauze pad into the medicine cup containing the liquid. If you're using benzoin spray, cover the genitalia with a gauze pad before spraying *to prevent tissue trauma.*
• Allow the benzoin to dry. Then apply the collection bag, pull the bottom of the bag and the tubing through the slit in the diaper, and fasten the diaper. Remove and discard your gloves.
• Check the collection bag and tubing every 30 minutes *to ensure a proper seal, because any leak prevents collection of a complete specimen.*
• When urine appears in the bag, put on gloves and remove the stopper in the bag's tubing, then attach the syringe to the end of the tubing, and aspirate the urine. Remove the syringe and insert the stopper into the tubing.
• Discard the specimen and begin timing the collection.
• When the next urine specimen is obtained, add the preservative to the 24-hour specimen container along with the specimen and refrigerate, if ordered, *to keep the sample stable.*
• Periodically empty the collection bag *to prevent skin breakdown and infection and dislodgment of the collection bag from the weight of the urine.* Each time you remove urine, add it to the specimen container; then use the

syringe to inject a small amount of air into the collection bag *to prevent a vacuum that can block urine drainage.*

• When the prescribed collection period has elapsed (or as nearly as possible), stop the collection and send the total accumulated specimen to the laboratory.

• Put on gloves and wash the perineal area thoroughly with soap and water *to remove the benzoin;* then put the second diaper on the patient.

Special considerations

Whatever the collection method used, avoid forcing fluids *to prevent dilution of the specimen, which can alter test results.* For a random collection or a culture and sensitivity collection, obtain a first-voided morning specimen if possible.

If the collection bag becomes dislodged during timed collection, immediately reapply benzoin and attach another collection bag *to prevent loss of the specimen and the need to restart the collection.*

To collect a urine specimen from an infant or a young child with extremely sensitive or excoriated perineal skin, use the inside-out disposable diaper method. Place cotton balls in the perineal area of the diaper *to absorb urine as the patient voids.* After he has voided, remove the diaper and squeeze urine from the cotton balls into a specimen cup. Alternately, tape a test tube to a male patient's penis to collect urine.

Complications

Adhesive from the collection bag can cause skin excoriation.

Documentation

Record the date, time, and method of collection. Also record the name of the test, the amount of urine collected (if necessary), and the time of specimen transport to the laboratory. Document any use of restraints, any complications, and the patient's tolerance of the procedure. Note the patient's and family's responses to any patient teaching.

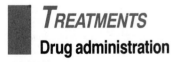

TREATMENTS
Drug administration

Because a child responds more rapidly — and unpredictably — to drugs than does an adult, pediatric drug administration requires special care. Such factors as age, weight, body surface area, and drug form and route may dramatically affect a child's response to a drug. For ex-

ample, because of his thin epithelium, a neonate or an infant absorbs topical medications much faster than an older child does.

Certain disorders also affect a child's response to medication. For example, gastroenteritis increases gastric motility, which in turn impairs absorption of certain oral medications. And liver or kidney disorders may hinder the metabolism of some medications.

Usual drug administration techniques may need adjustment to account for the child's age, size, and developmental level. A tablet for a young child, for example, may be crushed and mixed with a liquid for oral administration. And an injection site and needle size will vary depending on the child's age and physical development.

Equipment

For oral medications: prescribed medication ■ plastic disposable syringe, plastic medicine dropper, or spoon ■ medication cup ■ water, syrup, or jelly (for tablets) ■ optional: fruit juice.

For injectable medications: prescribed medication ■ appropriately sized syringe and needle ■ alcohol sponges or povidone-iodine solution ■ gloves ■ gauze pads ■ cold compresses ■ adhesive bandage.

Preparation of equipment

Check the doctor's order for the prescribed drug, dosage, and route. Compare the order with the drug label; check the drug expiration date; and review the patient's chart for drug allergies. Carefully calculate the dosage, if necessary, and have another nurse verify it. Typically, you'll double-check dosages for potentially hazardous or lethal drugs, such as insulin, heparin, digoxin, epinephrine, or narcotics. Check your hospital's policy *to learn which drugs must be calculated and checked by two nurses.*

For giving an injection, select the appropriate needle. Typically, for intramuscular (I.M.) injections in infants, you'll use a 25G ¾" needle, and in older children, a 23G 1" needle. For subcutaneous injections, select a ¾" or ½" needle and, for intradermal medications, a 27G ½" needle. To administer viscous medications, select a larger-gauge needle.

Implementation

• Assess the child's condition *to determine the need for the medication and therapy's effectiveness.*

• Carefully observe the child for a rash, pruritus, cough, or other signs of an adverse reaction to a previously administered drug.

• Identify the child by comparing the name on his wristband with the name on the medication card. If the child can talk and respond, ask him his name.

Giving oral medications to an infant

Use a dropper or syringe without a needle to administer an oral medication to an infant. Place the dropper or syringe at the corner of the infant's mouth so the medication will run into the pocket between the infant's cheek and gum. *This keeps him from spitting it out and reduces the risk of aspiration.*

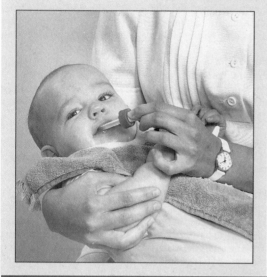

• Explain the procedure to the child and his parents. Use terms the child can understand.
• Provide privacy — especially for an older child.

To give oral medication to an infant
• Use a plastic syringe without a needle, or use a drug-specific medicine dropper to measure the dose. If the medication comes in tablet form, first crush the tablet (if appropriate) and mix it with water, syrup, or jelly. Then draw the mixture into the syringe or dropper.
• Pick up the infant, raising his head and shoulders or turning his head to one side *to prevent aspiration.* Hold the infant close to your body *to help restrain him.*
• Using your thumb, press down on the infant's chin *to open his mouth.*
• Slide the syringe or medicine dropper into the infant's mouth alongside his tongue (see *Giving oral medications to an infant*). Release the medication slowly *to allow the infant time to swallow and to prevent choking.* If appro-

priate, allow him to suck on the syringe as you expel the medication.
• If not contraindicated, give fruit juice after giving medication.
• Then, place a particularly small or inactive infant on his side or abdomen *to prevent aspiration.* Allow an active infant to assume the position comfortable for him; avoid forcing him into a side-lying position *to prevent agitation.*

To give oral medication to a toddler
• Use a plastic, disposable syringe or dropper to measure liquid medication. Then transfer the fluid to a medication cup.
• Elevate the toddler's head and shoulders *to prevent aspiration.*
• If possible, ask him to help hold the cup *to enlist his cooperation.* Otherwise, hold the cup to the toddler's lips, or use a syringe or a spoon to administer the liquid. Make sure that the toddler ingests all of the medication.

To give oral medication to an older child
• If possible, let the child choose both the liquid medication mixer and a beverage to drink after taking the medication.
• If appropriate, allow him to choose where he'll take the medication, for example, sitting in bed or sitting on a parent's lap.
• If the medication comes in tablet or capsule form, and if the child is old enough (between ages 4 and 6), teach him how to swallow solid medication. (If he already knows how to do this, review the procedure with him *for safety's sake.*) Tell him to place the pill on the back of his tongue and to swallow it immediately by drinking water or juice. Focus most of your explanation on the water or juice *to draw the child's attention away from the pill.* Make sure the child drinks enough water or juice *to keep the pill from lodging in his esophagus.* Afterward, look inside the child's mouth *to confirm that he swallowed the pill.*
• If the child can't swallow the pill whole, crush it and mix it with water, syrup, or jelly. Or, after checking with the child's doctor, order the medication in liquid form.

To give an I.M. injection
• Choose the injection site according to the child's age and muscle mass (see *I.M. injection sites in children*).
• Position the patient appropriately for the site chosen, and locate key landmarks, for example, the posterior superior iliac spine and the greater trochanter. Have someone help you restrain an infant; gain an older child's cooperation before enlisting assistance.
• Put on gloves. Clean the injection site with an alcohol or povidone-iodine sponge. Wipe outward from the center with a spiral motion *to avoid contaminating the clean area.*

I.M. injection sites in children

When selecting the best site for a child's intramuscular (I.M.) injection, consider the child's age, weight, and muscular development; the amount of subcutaneous fat over the injection site; the type of drug you're administering; and the drug's absorption rate.

Vastus lateralis and rectus femoris

For a child under age 3, you'll typically use the vastus lateralis or rectus femoris muscle for an I.M. injection. Constituting the largest muscle mass in this age-group, the vastus lateralis and rectus femoris have few major blood vessels and nerves.

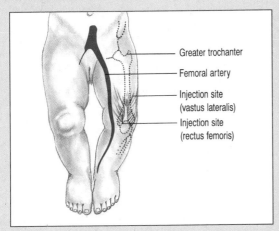

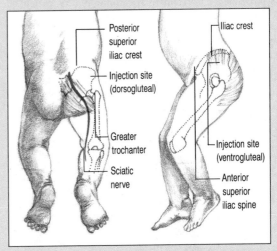

Ventrogluteal and dorsogluteal

For a child who can walk and who is over age 3, use the ventrogluteal and dorsogluteal muscles (top right). Like the vastus lateralis, the ventrogluteal site is relatively free of major blood vessels and nerves. Before you select either site, though, be sure that the child has been walking for at least 1 year to ensure sufficient muscle development.

Deltoid

For a child older than 18 months who needs rapid medication results, consider using the deltoid muscle for the injection. Because blood flows faster in the deltoid muscle than in other muscles, drug absorption should be faster. Be careful if you use this site, though. The deltoid doesn't develop fully until adolescence. In a younger child, it's small and close to the radial nerve, which may be injured during needle insertion.

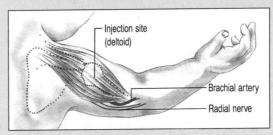

• Grasp the tissue surrounding the site between your index finger and thumb *to immobilize the site and to create a muscle mass for the injection.*
• Insert the needle quickly. Use a darting motion. If you're using the ventrogluteal site, insert the needle at a 45-degree angle toward the knee.
• Aspirate the plunger *to ensure that the needle isn't in a blood vessel.* If no blood appears, inject the medication slowly so the muscle can distend to accommodate the volume.
• Withdraw the needle and gently massage the area with a gauze pad *to stimulate circulation and enhance absorption.*
• Provide comfort and praise.

To give a subcutaneous injection
• Select from these possible sites: the middle third of the upper, outer arm; the middle third of the upper, outer

thigh; or the abdomen. You may apply a cold compress to the injection site *to minimize pain.*

• Put on gloves and prepare the injection site with alcohol or povidone-iodine solution according to the patient's needs and hospital policy.

• Pinch the tissue surrounding the site between your index finger and thumb *to ensure injection into the subcutaneous tissue.* Holding the needle at a 45- to 90-degree angle, quickly insert it into the tissue. Release your grasp on the tissue and slowly inject the medication. Remove the needle quickly *to decrease discomfort.* Unless contraindicated, gently massage the area *to facilitate absorption.*

To give an intradermal injection

• Put on gloves and pull the skin taut (the site of choice is the inner aspect of the forearm).

• Insert the needle, bevel up, at a 10- to 15-degree angle just beneath the outer skin layer.

• Slowly inject the medication, and watch for a bleb to appear. Quickly remove the needle, being careful to maintain the injection angle. If appropriate — for example, if the injection's related to allergy testing — draw a circle around the bleb, and avoid massaging the area *to avoid interfering with test results.*

Special considerations

Don't hesitate to consult the parents for tips on successfully administering medication to their child. If possible, have a parent administer prescribed oral medications while you supervise. However, avoid asking a parent to help with injections because the child may perceive the parent as a cause of pain.

Aim for a trusting relationship with the child and his parents *so that you can offer support and promote cooperation even when a medication causes discomfort.* If the child will receive one injection, allow him to choose from the appropriate sites. However, if the child will receive numerous injections, remember that site rotation must follow a set pattern. Allow the child to play with a medication cup or syringe and to pretend to give medication to a doll.

When giving medication to an older child, be honest. Reassure him that distaste or discomfort will be brief. Emphasize that he must remain still *to promote safety and minimize discomfort.* Explain to the child and his parent that an assistant will help the child remain still, if necessary. Keep your explanations brief and simple.

To divert the child's attention, have him start counting just before the injection, and challenge him to try to reach 10 before you finish the injection. If the child cries, don't scold him or allow the parents to scold him. Hold a younger child and praise him for allowing you to give

him the injection. Apply an adhesive bandage to the injection site *as a form of reward or badge.*

If the prescribed medication comes only in tablet form, consult the pharmacist (or an appropriate drug reference book) *to make sure that crushing the tablet won't invalidate its effectiveness.* Avoid adding medication to a large amount of liquid, such as the child's milk or formula, because the child may not drink the entire amount, resulting in an inaccurate dose of medication.

Because infants and toddlers can't tell you what effects they're experiencing from a medication, you must be alert for signs of an adverse reaction. Compile a list of appropriate emergency drugs, calculating the dosages to the patient's weight. Post the list near the patient's bed *for reference in an emergency.*

If you have any doubt about proper medication dosage, always consult the doctor who ordered the drug. Double-check information in a reliable drug reference.

Home care

Teach the parents about the proper dosage and administration of all prescribed medications. If the parents will administer a liquid medication, advise them to use a commercially available, disposable oral syringe to measure the dose. *To ensure an accurate dose,* advise them to avoid using a teaspoon. Teach them how to use the oral syringe. Use written materials — a medication instruction sheet, for example — to reinforce your teaching. If appropriate, teach the child and his parents about subcutaneous injectors (see *Using subcutaneous injectors*).

Documentation

Record the medication, form, dose, date, time, route, and site of administration. Also record the effect of the medication, the patient's tolerance to the procedure, complications, and nursing interventions. Note instructional activities related to medications.

I.V. therapy

In children, I.V. therapy may be prescribed to administer medications or to correct a fluid deficit, improve serum electrolyte balance, or provide nourishment. Primary nursing concerns related to pediatric I.V. therapy include correlating the I.V. site and equipment with the reason for therapy and the patient's age, size, and activity level. For example, a scalp vein is a typical I.V. site for an infant, whereas a peripheral hand, wrist, or foot vein may suit older children.

Using subcutaneous injectors

Currently available for use by patients at home, subcutaneous injectors feature disposable needles or pressure jets to deliver doses of prescribed medications, such as short-acting insulin. Appropriate for use in children, these devices deliver medication safely and accurately. The NovoPen, for instance, has disposable needles and replaceable cartridges. Preci-Jet, Vitajet, and Medi-Jector draw their medications from standard bottles. A pressure jet deposits the drug in subcutaneous tissue.

Although still relatively expensive, these devices are easy to use. For example, studies indicate that jet-injected insulin disperses faster and is absorbed more rapidly because it avoids the puddling effect common with needle delivery.

Needle injection

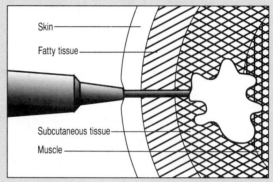

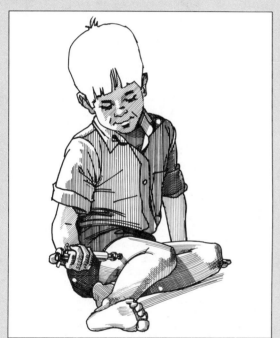

Pressure-jet injection

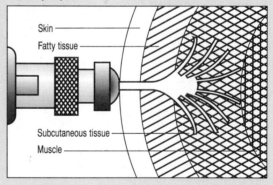

During I.V. therapy, the nurse must continually assess the patient and the infusion to prevent fluid overload and other complications.

Equipment

Prescribed I.V. fluid ▪ volume-control set with microdrip tubing ▪ infusion pump ▪ I.V. pole ▪ normal saline solution or sterile dextrose 5% in water for injection ▪ povidone-iodine solution ▪ alcohol sponges ▪ 3-ml syringe ▪ child-sized butterfly needle or I.V. catheter ▪ tourniquet ▪ ½" or 1" tape ▪ gloves ▪ optional: armboard, insulated foam or medicine cup, luer-lock cap, air eliminator I.V. filter.

Whenever possible, use a catheter instead of a needle. A flexible catheter is less likely to perforate the vein wall.

Preparation of equipment

Gather the I.V equipment, and take it to the patient's bedside. Check the expiration date on the I.V. fluid and inspect the I.V. container (an I.V. bag for leakage, a bottle for cracks). Examine the I.V. tubing for defects or cracks.

Common pediatric I.V. sites

Below are the most common sites for I.V. therapy in infants and children. Peripheral hand, wrist, or foot veins are typically used with older children, whereas scalp veins are used with an infant.

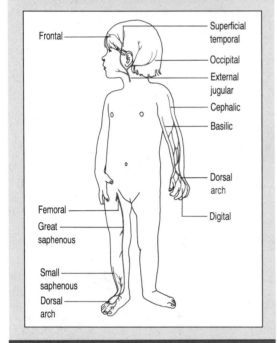

Make sure that the packaging surrounding the I.V. catheter or needle remains intact.

Open the wrappings on the I.V. solution and the volume-control tubing set. Close all clamps on the tubing set; then insert the tip of the tubing set into the entry port of the I.V. bag or bottle. (If you're using an I.V. bag, be sure to hold the bag upright when attaching the tubing. *This will keep the sterile air inside the bag from escaping and making the fluid level difficult to read.*)

Hang the bottle or bag from the I.V. pole. Open the clamp between the bag and the volume-control set and allow 30 to 50 ml of solution to flow into the calibrated chamber. Close the clamp.

Squeeze the drip chamber located below the calibrated chamber or volume-control set *to create a vacuum.* Release the drip chamber and allow it to fill halfway with solution.

Release the clamp below the drip chamber *so that fluid flows into the remaining tubing, removing any air.* After the tubing fills, close the clamp.

If you're using an infusion pump, attach the I.V. tubing to the infusion cassette, and insert the cassette into the infusion pump. Prime the cassette tubing according to the manufacturer's instructions. If you're using an air eliminator I.V. filter, attach the filter to the end of the cassette tubing. *To prevent any air bubbles from entering the patient's circulatory system,* place the filter as close to the patient as possible.

To minimize the risk of infection, maintain sterility at the tip of the I.V. tubing until you connect it to the I.V. needle.

Cut as many strips of ½" or 1" tape as you'll need to secure the I.V. line. Then prepare a syringe with 3 ml of flush solution—either the normal saline solution or dextrose 5% in water.

Implementation

• Match the name on the patient's wristband with the name on the doctor's order (or on the medication card). Ask the patient (or his parents) if he is allergic to povidone-iodine solution or to any type of tape.

• Explain the reason for the I.V. therapy. Reassure the parents, and enlist their assistance in explaining the procedure to the patient in terms he can understand.

• Be sure to have a staff member available to assist you. Inform the parents that the staff member will help the patient remain still, if necessary, during the procedure.

• Wash your hands and put on gloves.

• Select the insertion site for the butterfly needle or catheter (see *Common pediatric I.V. sites*). Aim for the most distal site possible, and avoid placing the I.V. line in the patient's dominant arm or in areas of flexion if possible. Avoid previously used or sclerotic veins.

• To locate an appropriate scalp vein, carefully palpate the site for arterial pulsations. If you feel these pulsations, select another site. Then, before inserting the I.V. line, prepare the selected site as ordered.

• To find an appropriate peripheral site, apply a tourniquet to the patient's arm or leg and palpate a suitable vein.

• If you're inserting a butterfly needle, flush the tubing connected to the butterfly with dextrose 5% in water or normal saline solution.

• Clean the insertion site. Unless contraindicated, use a pad containing povidone-iodine solution. Wipe with a circular motion from the insertion site's center to the outer rim. Let the solution dry.

• Insert the I.V. needle into the vein. Watch for blood to flow backward through the catheter or butterfly tubing, *which confirms that the needle is in the vein.*

• Loosen the tourniquet, and attach the I.V. tubing to the hub of the needle or catheter. Begin the infusion.
• Secure the device by applying a piece of ½" tape over the hub. Next, place a piece of tape, adhesive side up, underneath and perpendicular to the device. Lift the ends of the tape and crisscross them over the device. (For more information, see *Methods of taping a venipuncture site* in Chapter 6.) Further secure and protect the I.V. line as needed (see *Protecting an I.V. site,* page 732).
• Adjust the infusional flow, as ordered, by using the clamp on the I.V. volume-control tubing or by setting the infusion rate on the infusion pump.
• Add solution hourly (or as needed) from the I.V. bag to the volume-control set.
• Assess the I.V. site frequently for signs of infiltration, and check the I.V. bottle or bag for the amount of solution infused.
• Change the I.V. dressing every 24 hours, or as needed, *to prevent infection.* Also change the I.V. tubing every 48 to 72 hours and the I.V. solution bottle or bag every 24 hours. Label the I.V. bottle or bag, tubing, and volume control set with the time and date of change.
• Change the I.V. insertion site every 72 hours, if possible, *to minimize the risk of infection.* If you inserted the I.V. line without proper skin preparation (during an emergency, for example), change the site sooner.

Special considerations
When selecting an I.V. site, try not to use a site that impairs the patient's ability to seek comfort. For example, if an infant typically sucks the thumb or fingers on his right hand, avoid placing the I.V. needle or catheter in his right arm.

Forewarn parents if you will start the I.V. infusion in a scalp vein. Also tell them that you may have to shave hair from a small section of the infant's head.

Ask an older child to participate in selecting the I.V. site, if possible, *to give the patient a sense of control.* For a mobile patient, aim for an I.V. site on the upper extremity *so that he can still get out of bed.* Avoid starting the I.V. in the same arm as the patient's identification band, unless you first remove the band and replace it on the other arm, *to prevent potential circulatory impairment.*

Evaluate the need for restraints after inserting the I.V. line. Apply them only if I.V. needle displacement seems imminent. If you must use restraints, assess the patient's skin integrity and provide hourly skin care *to prevent skin breakdown.* Remove the restraints at frequent intervals *to let the patient move freely.* Encourage the parents to hold and comfort the patient when he's unrestrained.

For precise regulation of the I.V. infusion, use a volumetric infusion pump. These pumps infuse fluids at a predetermined rate regardless of temperature fluctuations, vessel variations, or fluid volume changes. Before using an infusion pump, review the operator's manual.

After inserting the I.V. needle or catheter, reward preschool and school-age patients. Popular rewards include colorful stickers to wear on clothes or on the I.V. dressing.

You may apply an antimicrobial ointment over the I.V. site *to prevent infection.*

Home care
Pediatric patients requiring long-term I.V. medications or nourishment may continue receiving I.V. therapy at home. Help the patient and parents assess conditions that promote successful home I.V. therapy. They include—first and foremost—a patient and parent (or other caregiver) who can and want to participate in home I.V. therapy. Other factors include the availability of relief caregivers to provide occasional assistance (especially in an emergency); and a conducive home environment with electricity, running water, a telephone, refrigeration, storage space for supplies, and an area set up for solution and tubing changes and I.V. site care. Additionally, a medical facility should be accessible should the patient need emergency assistance or routine reinsertion of an I.V. line.

Teach the parents (and the patient, if appropriate) how to identify and manage complications, such as site infiltration or clotting in the I.V. needle. Show them how to operate equipment, such as the infusion pump. Supplement verbal instructions with written patient-teaching materials for later reference. Before discharge, watch the parents operate the infusion pump for 24 hours *so that you can evaluate areas for further instruction and identify skills needing refinement.*

At discharge, arrange for a home health nurse to visit the patient daily for 2 or 3 days to support and guide initial home therapy. Inform the parents that after her daily visits, the home health nurse will probably visit every 2 to 3 days to assess the I.V. site, provide care, and answer questions.

Complications
Infection, fluid overload, electrolyte imbalance, infiltration, and circulatory impairment are complications of I.V. therapy.

Documentation
Record the date and time of the I.V. infusion. Document the insertion site and the type and size of I.V. needle or catheter. Note the patient's tolerance of the procedure. Describe patient- and parent-teaching activities. Document the condition of the I.V. site according to hospital policy. If infiltration affects the I.V. site, document the

Protecting an I.V. site

To prevent a child from dislodging an I.V. line or injuring himself, you'll need to secure the needle or catheter carefully. If the child is old enough to understand, you can warn him not to play with or jostle the equipment. And you can teach him how to walk with an I.V. pole to minimize tension on the line. If necessary, you can restrain the extremity.

Also create a protective barrier between the I.V. site and the environment using one of these methods.

Medicine cup

Cut a clean, empty medicine cup made of clear plastic in half lengthwise. Using nonallergenic tape, affix the half-cup over the I.V. site. The tape securing the I.V. line protects the skin from the cup's edges. Or, if you're using a butterfly needle, make a protective cover from the needle's plastic container.

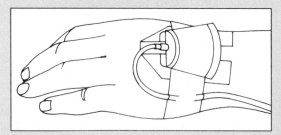

Paper cup

Consider using a small paper cup to protect a scalp site. First, cut off the cup's bottom. Next, cut a small slot through the top rim to accommodate the I.V. tubing. Place the cup upside down over the insertion site, so the I.V. tubing extends through the slot. Then, secure the cup with strips of tape (as shown). The opening you cut in the cup allows you to examine the site.

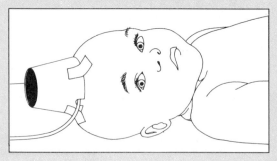

Stockinette

Cut a piece of 4″ stockinette the same length as the patient's arm. Slip the stockinette over the patient's arm, and lay the arm on an armboard. Then, grasp the stockinette at both sides of the arm, and stretch it under the armboard. Securely tape the stockinette beneath the armboard, as shown.

Note: You may also protect a scalp site by placing a stockinette on the patient's head, leaving a hole to allow access to the site.

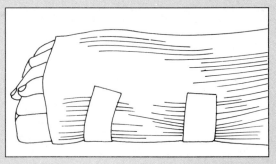

I.V. shield

Peel off the strips covering the adhesive backing on the bottom of the shield. Position the shield over the site, so that the I.V. tubing runs through one of the shield's two slots. Then, firmly press the shield's adhesive backing against the patient's skin. The shield's clear plastic composition allows you to see the I.V. site clearly.

If the shield's too large to fit securely over the site, just cut off the shield's narrow end below the two air holes. Now, you can easily shape the device to the patient's arm.

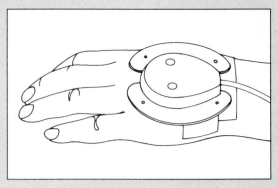

condition of the site at every shift change until the condition resolves.

Mist tent therapy

Also known as a croupette for infants or a cool-humidity tent for children, a mist tent houses a nebulizer that transforms distilled water into mist. Mist tent therapy benefits the patient by providing a cool, moist environment. This atmosphere eases breathing and helps to decrease respiratory tract edema, liquefy secretions, and reduce fever. Oxygen may also be administered along with the mist. Mist tents are commonly used to treat croup and such infections or inflammations as bronchiolitis and pneumonia.

Equipment
Mist tent frame and plastic tenting ■ bed sheets ■ plastic sheet or linen-saver pad ■ two bath blankets ■ nebulizer with water reservoir and filter ■ oxygen flowmeter and oxygen analyzer, if ordered ■ sterile distilled water ■ optional: stockinette cap or booties, infant seat.

Preparation of equipment
Review your hospital's policy to determine who sets up a mist tent. In some hospitals the nurse sets up the tent; in others a respiratory therapist may do so. Whoever sets up the tent will first place the tent frame and the plastic tenting at the head of the crib or bed. Then she'll cover the mattress with a bed sheet, cover the bed sheet with a plastic sheet or linen-saver pad (tucked under the mattress), and cover these layers with a bath blanket.

Next, she'll fill the reservoir of the nebulizer with sterile distilled water, and make sure that the inlet for air contains a clean filter. If the patient will have oxygen in the tent, be sure that the oxygen flowmeter connects to the tent. Then turn the flowmeter to the desired setting. Be sure to analyze the percentage of oxygen being delivered. Wait 2 minutes after mist begins filling the tent before placing the patient in it.

Implementation
• Carefully explain the mist tent's purpose to the patient and his parents *to alleviate anxiety and promote cooperation*. Use terms that both generations can understand. When talking with the parents, you might compare the mist tent with a vaporizer. When talking with the patient, however, you might compare the tent with a teepee or a spaceship cabin.

• Elevate the head of the bed to a position *that enhances patient comfort.* If the patient is an infant, consider placing him in an infant seat. *The more upright position will help him to mobilize secretions.* If the patient will be in the room alone, position him on his side or prone *to prevent him from aspirating mucus from liquefied secretions and productive coughing.*

• Use a stockinette cap, booties, and the other bath blanket, as needed, *to keep the patient from becoming chilled as the mist condenses inside the tent.*

• Change the patient's bed sheets and clothing as they dampen, and check his temperature frequently *to detect impending hypothermia.*

• Monitor the patient frequently for a change in condition, keeping in mind that the mist may make observation difficult.

• Encourage parents to stay with the patient. If he grows irritable and uncooperative while in the tent, take him out and let his parents comfort him because *excessive irritability causes labored breathing and increases oxygen consumption.* Return him to the tent when he calms down.

• If secretions coat the inside of the tent, wipe it down with a hospital-approved cleaner, such as soap and water. Also clean the reservoir with sterile water *to prevent bacterial growth.*

Special considerations
Allow the patient to have toys in the mist tent *to provide distraction.* To amuse infants, string plastic toys across the top bar of the tent. However, discourage playing with cloth or stuffed toys in the tent *because these objects absorb moisture and supply a medium for bacterial growth.*

To prevent a possible fire, forbid toys or games that may spark or trigger an electric shock, such as battery-operated toys. Also remove the electric call light, and give older children a hand bell instead. *To further minimize the risk of a fire or an explosion* — especially if the patient's receiving oxygen — prohibit smoking by anyone near the mist tent. Also if the patient's receiving oxygen, analyze the percentage at least every 4 hours.

For bathing, remove the patient from the tent *to prevent hypothermia.*

Home care
If the mist tent will be used at home, show the parents how to set up, use, and clean the tent properly.

Documentation
Record the date and time the patient was placed in the tent. Describe the patient's respiratory status, including breath sounds, sputum production, and perfusion. Record the patient's vital signs. Also note the date and time that the patient was removed from the tent. Record the per-

centage of oxygen being delivered, the date and time of all analyses, and the oxygen saturation.

◤◤ Cardiopulmonary resuscitation

When an adult needs cardiopulmonary resuscitation (CPR), she typically suffers from a primary cardiac disorder or arrhythmia that has stopped her heart. When an infant or child needs CPR, she typically suffers from hypoxia caused by respiratory difficulty or respiratory arrest.

Most pediatric crises requiring CPR are preventable. They include motor vehicle accidents, drowning, burns, smoke inhalation, falls, poisoning, suffocation, and choking (usually from inhaling a plastic bag or small foreign bodies, such as toys or food). Other causes of cardiopulmonary arrest in children include laryngospasm and edema from upper respiratory infections and sudden infant death syndrome.

Based on the same principle, CPR in adults, children, and infants aims to restore cardiopulmonary function by pumping the victim's heart and ventilating the lungs until natural function resumes. However, CPR techniques differ depending on whether the patient is an adult, a child, or an infant (see *Performing infant CPR,* pages 736 and 737). For CPR purposes, the American Heart Association defines a patient by age. An infant is under age 1; a child is ages 1 to 8; an adult is over age 8.

Survival chances improve the sooner CPR begins and the faster advanced life support systems are implemented. However speedily you undertake CPR for a child, though, first determine whether the patient's respiratory distress results from a mechanical obstruction or an infection, such as epiglottitis or croup. Epiglottitis or croup requires immediate medical attention, not CPR. CPR is appropriate only when the child isn't breathing.

Equipment
CPR requires no special equipment except a hard surface on which to place the patient.

Implementation
• Gently shake the apparently unconscious child's shoulder and shout at her *to elicit a response.* If the child is conscious but has difficulty breathing, help her into a position that best eases her breathing—if she hasn't naturally assumed this position already.
• Call for help *to alert others and to enlist emergency assistance.* If you're alone and the child isn't breathing, perform CPR for 1 minute before calling for help.

• Position the child supine on a firm, flat surface (usually the ground). *The surface should provide the resistance needed for adequate heart compression.* If you must turn the child from a prone position, support her head and neck and turn her as a unit *to avoid injuring her spine.*

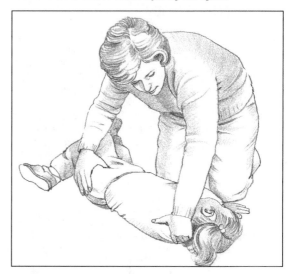

To establish a patent airway
• Kneel beside the child's shoulder. Place one hand on the child's forehead and gently lift her chin with your other hand *to open her airway.* (In infants, this is called the sniffing position.) Avoid fingering the soft neck tissue *to avoid obstructing the airway.* Never let the child's mouth close completely.

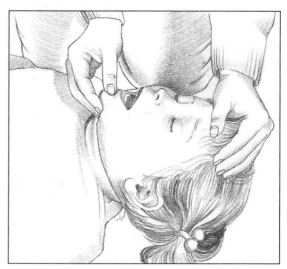

• If you suspect a neck injury, use the jaw-thrust maneuver to open the child's airway *to keep from moving the child's neck.* To do this, kneel beside the child's head. With your elbows on the ground, rest your thumbs at the corners of the child's mouth, and place two or three fingers of each hand under the lower jaw. Lift the jaw upward.

• While maintaining an open airway, place your ear near the child's mouth and nose *to evaluate her breathing status.* Look for chest movement, listen for exhaled air, and feel for exhaled air on your cheek.

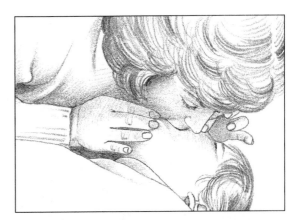

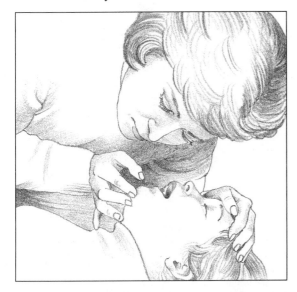

• If the child is breathing, maintain an open airway and monitor respirations.

• If you suspect that a mechanical airway obstruction blocks respiration (whether the child's conscious or not), attempt to clear the airway as you would in an adult — with two exceptions: Don't use the blind finger-sweep maneuver (*which could compound or relodge the obstruction*), and do adjust your technique to the child's size. (For directions, see "Obstructed airway management" in Chapter 8.)

To restore ventilation

• If the child isn't breathing, maintain the open airway position, and take a breath. Then pinch the child's nostrils shut, and cover the child's mouth with your mouth (top right). Give two slow breaths (1 to 1½ seconds/ breath), and pause between each.

• If your first attempt at ventilation fails to restore the child's breathing, reposition the child's head to open the airway and try again. If you're still unsuccessful, the airway may be obstructed by a foreign body.

• Repeat the steps for airway clearance.

• Once you free the obstruction, check for breathing and pulse. If absent, proceed with chest compressions.

To restore heartbeat and circulation

• Assess circulation by palpating the carotid artery for a pulse.

• Locate the carotid artery with two or three fingers of one hand. (You'll need the other hand to maintain the head-tilt position that keeps the airway open.) Place your fingers in the center of the child's neck on the side closest to you and slide your fingers into the groove formed by the trachea and the sternocleidomastoid muscles. Palpate the artery for 5 to 10 seconds *to confirm the child's pulse status.*

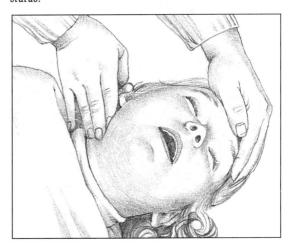

Performing infant CPR

Although the objective of cardiopulmonary resuscitation (CPR) in an infant is the same as in a child and an adult, the techniques for an infant vary.

Clear the airway
• To remove an airway obstruction, place the infant face-down on your forearm with his head lower than his trunk. Support your forearm on your thigh.
• Use the heel of your free hand to deliver four blows between the infant's shoulder blades. *Back blows are safer than abdominal thrusts in infants because of the size of the infant's liver, the close proximity of vital organs, and the poor abdominal muscle tone.*

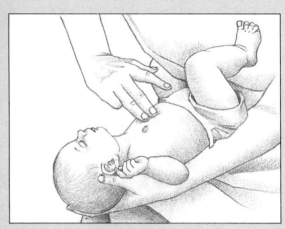

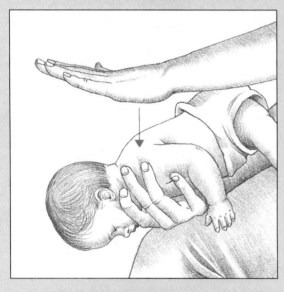

• If the airway remains obstructed, sandwich the infant between your hands and forearms and flip him over onto his back as shown (top right).
• Keeping the infant's head lower than his trunk, give four midsternal chest thrusts, using your middle and ring fingers only, *to raise intrathoracic pressure enough to force a cough that will expel the obstruction.* Remember to hold the head firmly *to avoid injury.*

• Repeat this sequence until the obstruction is dislodged or the infant loses consciousness.
  Caution: Do not do a blind finger-sweep to discover or remove an obstruction. In an infant, the maneuver may push the object back in the airway and cause further obstruction.

Restore consciousness
• If the infant loses consciousness, position him to open the airway. Deliver two breaths (as described below).
• If he doesn't regain consciousness, reposition his head and try breathing for him again.
• If this attempt fails, repeat the procedure for removing a foreign object.
• When the foreign object's removed, assess respirations and pulse. Continue revival efforts if needed.

Provide ventilation
• Take a breath, and tightly seal your mouth over the infant's nose and mouth.

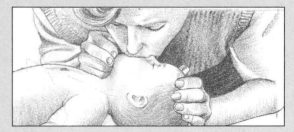

• Deliver a *gentle* puff of air *because an infant's lungs hold less air than an adult's.* If the infant's chest rises and falls, then the amount of air is probably adequate.
• Continue rescue breathing with one breath every 3 seconds (20 breaths/minute) if you can detect a pulse.

Restore heartbeat and circulation

• Assess the infant's pulse by palpating the brachial artery located inside the infant's upper arm between the elbow and the shoulder. If you find a pulse, continue rescue breathing but don't initiate heart compressions.

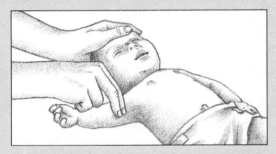

• Begin heart compressions if you find no pulse. To locate the infant's heart, draw an imaginary horizontal line between the infant's nipples. Place three fingers directly below — and perpendicular to — the nipple line. Then lift up your index finger so that the middle and ring fingers lie one finger's width below the nipple line. Use these two fingers to depress the sternum here ½" to 1" (1.3 to 2.5 cm) at least 100 compressions/minute.

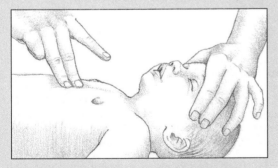

• Supply one breath after every five compressions. Maintain this ratio whether you're the helper or the lone rescuer. This ratio allows for about 100 compressions and 20 breaths/minute for an infant.

• If you feel the child's pulse, continue rescue breathing, giving one breath every 4 seconds (15 breaths/minute).
• If you can't feel a pulse, begin cardiac compressions.
• Kneel next to the child's chest. Using the hand closest to her feet, locate the lower border of the rib cage on the side nearest you.

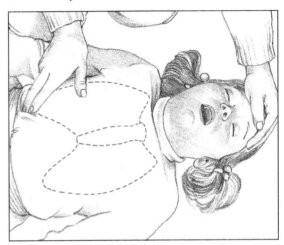

• Hold your middle and index fingers together and move them up the rib cage to the notch where the ribs and sternum join. Put your middle finger on the notch and your index finger next to it.

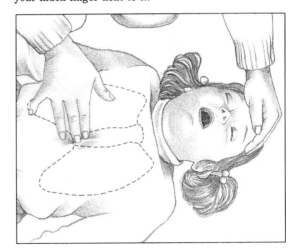

• Lift your hand and place the heel just above the spot where the index finger was. The heel of your hand should be aligned with the long axis of the sternum.

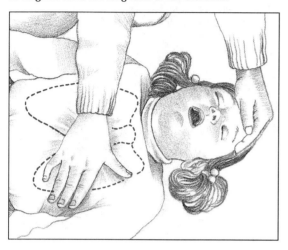

• Using the heel of one hand only, apply enough pressure to compress the child's chest downward 1″ to 1½″ (2.5 to 3.8 cm). Deliver five serial compressions at a rate of 80 to 100 compressions/minute.

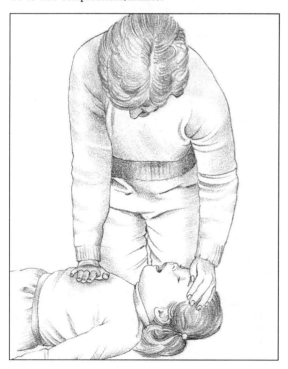

• After every five compressions, breathe one breath into the child. Deliver one breath for every five compressions whether you're working alone or with a partner.
• After 10 cycles (1 minute) of CPR, feel the pulse for 5 seconds *to detect a heartbeat.* If you can't detect a pulse, give one breath and continue CPR.
• If you can detect a pulse, check for spontaneous respirations. Without respirations, give one breath every 4 seconds (15 breaths/minute) and continue to monitor the pulse. If the child begins breathing spontaneously, keep the airway open and monitor both the respirations and pulse.

Special considerations
A child's small airway can be easily blocked by her tongue. If this occurs, simply opening the airway may eliminate the obstruction.

When performing cardiac compressions, take care to ensure smooth motions. Keep your fingers off and the heel of your hand on the child's chest at all times. Also time your motions so that the compression and relaxation phases are equal *to promote effective compressions.*

If the child has breathing difficulty and a parent is present, find out whether the child recently had a fever or an upper respiratory tract infection. If so, suspect epiglottitis. In this instance, do not attempt to manipulate the airway *because laryngospasm may occur and completely obstruct the airway.* Allow the child to assume a comfortable position and monitor her breathing until additional assistance arrives.

Persist in attempts to remove an obstruction. As hypoxia develops, the child's muscles will relax, allowing you to remove the foreign object.

During resuscitation efforts, make sure that someone communicates support and information to the parents.

Documentation
Document all the events of resuscitation, and name the persons present. Record whether the child had cardiac or respiratory arrest. Note where the arrest occurred, the time when CPR began, and how long the procedure continued. Note the outcome. Also note any complications—a fractured rib, bruised mouth, or gastric distention, for example. Describe actions taken to correct complications.

If the child received advanced cardiac life support, document which interventions were performed, who performed them, when they were performed, and what equipment was used.

Bryant's traction

Also called vertical suspension, Bryant's traction is used mostly to reduce congenital hip dislocations in children. With the patient lying supine in a bed or crib, the traction extends the legs vertically at a 90-degree angle to the body. Even if the disorder affects only one leg, the patient will have traction applied to both legs to prevent hip rotation and to ensure equal stress on the legs and even, bilateral bone growth.

Bryant's traction continues for about 2 to 4 weeks. Afterward, the patient may be immobilized in a hip spica cast (see "Hip spica cast care" in this chapter). Usually chosen for children under age 2 who weigh between 25 and 30 lb (11.3 and 16.3 kg), Bryant's traction is contraindicated for heavier children because the risk of positional hypertension rises with increased weight.

Equipment
Traction setup (supplied by the orthopedic department) ▪ moleskin traction straps ▪ elastic bandages ▪ foam rubber padding ▪ cotton balls ▪ compound benzoin tincture ▪ adhesive tape ▪ jacket restraint ▪ optional: safety razor, cotton batting, convoluted foam mattress, sheepskin pad.

Preparation of equipment
Assist the doctor and orthopedic technician with measuring and cutting the moleskin straps and with assembling the traction equipment.

Implementation
• Thoroughly explain the purpose and function of the traction *to enhance learning and alleviate patient and family anxiety.* If possible, use visual aids to illustrate your teaching. Keep a diagram handy for parents and a doll in traction for the patient.
• Ask the parents if the patient is sensitive or allergic to rubber or to adhesive tape.
• If the patient has hairy legs, shave or clip the hair with a safety razor *to ensure good contact between the moleskin traction straps and the skin.* Use soap, warm water, and long, downward strokes *to minimize nicking.*
• Apply the compound benzoin tincture, if ordered, to the patient's legs *to protect the skin.*
• Assist the doctor or orthopedic technician with placing foam rubber padding and moleskin traction straps against the patient's legs and securing the straps with elastic bandages from foot to thigh. If the patient's allergic to rubber or to adhesive tape, wrap the legs in cotton batting before applying the straps.

• If necessary to keep the patient positioned properly, apply a jacket restraint *to keep the weights from pulling the patient forward and altering the tractional force.*
• Carefully monitor the circulatory status of the patient's legs at 15 minutes and at 30 minutes after applying initial traction. Then check circulatory status every 4 hours *to detect any impairment caused by traction.* Assess capillary refill, skin color, sensation, movement, temperature, peripheral pulses, and bandage tightness. If you detect circulatory compromise, loosen the elastic bandages and notify the patient's doctor.
• Take care to position the elastic bandages precisely. Unless contraindicated, periodically remove the bandages from the unaffected leg to assess circulation and provide skin care. When doing so, have another person hold the traction straps in place *to prevent slipping.* Don't unwrap the affected leg unless ordered to do so by the patient's doctor.
• Check the patient's position regularly *to ensure optimum traction.* Be sure to raise the patient's buttocks high enough off the mattress to allow one hand to slide between the skin and the mattress. Avoid raising the buttocks too high, though, because *this may reduce the effectiveness of traction.*
• Try marking the bed sheet with an "X" at the correct shoulder position *as a guide to correct body alignment.* Near the patient's bed, post an illustration of the correct alignment to guide other nurses and caregivers (see *Maintaining body alignment and traction,* page 740).
• Give skin care every 4 hours, focusing especially on the back, buttocks, and elbows. *These areas are most prone to breakdown.* Place a convoluted foam mattress or a sheepskin pad — or both — beneath the patient *to help prevent or alleviate skin problems.*
• Inspect the traction apparatus at least every 2 hours to ensure the correct weight. Be sure that the weights hang freely, the pulleys glide easily, the ropes aren't frayed, and the knots remain snugly tied and taped.
• Encourage the patient to take deep breaths at least every 2 hours *to minimize his risk for hypostatic pneumonia.*
• Review the patient's diet to ensure that he consumes enough fiber and fluid *to prevent constipation and urinary stasis.* (Infants should consume about 130 ml of fluid for each kilogram of body weight every 24 hours; toddlers should consume about 115 ml per kilogram.)
• *Promote safety* by keeping the side rails raised on the patient's bed whenever you're not at the bedside.

Special considerations
To encourage regular deep breathing and guard against pneumonia, allow the patient to blow a horn, whistle, pinwheel, or bubbles heartily. Or urge him to sing. *This promotes lung expansion and enjoyment at the same time.*

Maintaining body alignment and traction

Keeping the patient's body in correct position with Bryant's traction requires precision and continual supervision and adjustment.

At the same time that the traction apparatus holds the patient's legs perpendicular to the mattress, you'll need to ensure that the patient's buttocks stay slightly elevated *to provide countertraction* and that his shoulders stay flat and in the same position on the mattress *to maintain body alignment.*

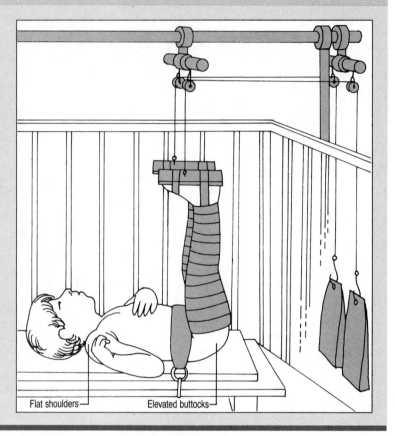

Flat shoulders ——   Elevated buttocks ——

Because a child can't always tell you that he's in pain, carefully observe his behavior, facial expression, and cry to judge discomfort levels. Besides needing an analgesic or sedative, the patient may need an antispasmodic medication to relieve irritable muscles and muscle spasms.

To foster development, diversion, and mobility, provide age-appropriate games and activities as permitted within the confines of traction. For infants, this can include mobiles, music boxes, and rattles. Toddlers may enjoy puppets, large-pieced puzzles, and dolls. Involve the family in the patient's care and recreational activities *to increase the patient's sense of security and minimize the family's sense of anxiety.* If hospital policy permits, consider moving the patient's crib to the playroom *so that he can be around other children.*

Eating and drinking is difficult and inconvenient for the patient in Bryant's traction because of the head-down

position. *To facilitate digestion and encourage eating* — especially if the patient refuses food — place a small pillow under his head at mealtime. If possible, allow him to choose his own foods, and encourage his family to bring food from home.

To minimize patient movement, change bed linens every other day unless the linens get wet or soiled. Keep sheets taut and wrinkle-free *to help prevent skin breakdown.*

Complications

Although generally safe, Bryant's traction may lead to pneumonia from restricted lung expansion resulting from the head-down position. Skin necrosis may result from bandages wrapped too tightly. Other complications include urinary stasis and constipation.

Documentation

Record the date and time that traction was applied; the amount of weight applied; and the patient's circulatory status, skin condition, and position. Note whether weights hang freely. Document changes in the patient's status, and describe the patient's and family's response to the traction. Also note the patient's and family's response to any patient teaching.

Hip spica cast care

After orthopedic surgery to correct a fracture or deformity, a patient may need a hip spica cast to immobilize both legs. Occasionally, the doctor may apply a hip spica cast to treat an orthopedic deformity that doesn't require surgery.

Caring for a patient in a hip spica cast poses several challenges, including protecting the cast from urine and feces, keeping the cast dry, ensuring proper blood supply to the legs, and teaching the patient and his parents to care for the cast at home.

Infants usually adapt more easily to the cast than do older children, but both need encouragement, support, and diversionary activity during their prolonged immobilization.

Equipment

Waterproof adhesive tape ■ moleskin or plastic petals ■ cast cutter or saw ■ scissors ■ nonabrasive cleaner ■ hair dryer ■ optional: disposable diaper or perineal pad.

Implementation

• Before the doctor applies the cast, describe the procedure to the patient and his parents. For patients ages 3 to 12, illustrate your explanation. Draw a picture, present a diagram, or use a doll with a cast or an elastic gauze dressing wrapped around its trunk and limbs (see *Understanding the hip spica cast*).

• Once the doctor constructs the cast, keep all but the perineal area uncovered. Provide privacy by draping a small cover over this opening. Turn the patient every 1 to 2 hours *to speed drying time.* Be sure to turn the patient to his unaffected side *to prevent adding pressure to the affected side.* If the patient's an infant, you can turn him by yourself. If the patient's an older child or an adolescent, seek assistance before attempting to turn him. When turning the patient, don't use the stabilizer bar between his legs for leverage. *Excessive pressure on this bar may disrupt the cast.* Handle a damp cast only with your palms *to avoid misshaping the cast material.*

Understanding the hip spica cast

As you talk with parents about their child's hip spica cast, describe how it will extend from the patient's lower rib margin (or sometimes from the nipple line) down to the tips of the toes on the affected side and to the knee on the opposite unaffected side. Also mention that it expands at the waist to allow the child to eat comfortably. A stabilizer bar positioned between the legs keeps the hips in slight abduction and separates the legs.

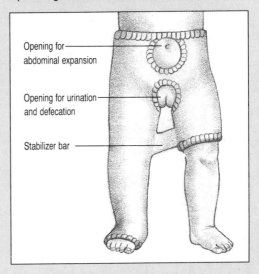

• After the cast dries, inspect the inside edges of the cast for stray pieces of casting material *that can irritate the skin.* (A traditional hip spica cast requires 24 to 48 hours to dry. However, a hip spica cast made from newer, quick-drying substances takes only 8 to 10 hours to dry. If made of fiberglass, it will dry in less than 1 hour.)

• Cut several petal-shaped pieces of moleskin and place them, overlapping, around the open edges of the cast *to protect the patient's skin.* Use waterproof adhesive tape around the perineal area.

• Give the patient a sponge bath *to remove any cast fragments from his skin.*

• Assess the patient's legs for coldness, swelling, cyanosis, or mottling. Also assess pulse strength, toe movement, sensation (numbness, tingling, or burning), and capillary refill. Perform these circulatory assessments every 1 to 2 hours while the cast is wet and every 2 to 4 hours after the cast dries.

• If the patient had surgery, check the cast for signs of bleeding or drainage (look for a stain or discoloration). If you notice a stain, outline it with a ballpoint pen. Note the date and time, and add your initials. Then observe whether the stain extends beyond the outline, *which could indicate continued bleeding.*

• Check the patient's exposed skin for redness or irritation, and observe the patient for pain or discomfort caused by hot spots (pressure-sensitive areas under the cast). Also be alert for a foul odor. *These signs and symptoms suggest a pressure ulcer or infection.*

• *To relieve itching,* set a hand-held hair dryer on "cool." Then blow air under the cast. Warn the patient and his parents not to insert any object (ruler, coat hanger, or knitting needle) into the cast to relieve itching by scratching *because these objects could disrupt the suture line, break adjacent skin, and introduce infection.* Also be vigilant *to ensure that small objects or food particles don't lodge under the cast and cause skin breakdown and infection.*

• Encourage the patient's family to visit and participate in his care and recreation. *This increases the patient's sense of security and the parents' sense of participation and control.*

Special considerations

If the patient is incontinent (or not toilet-trained), *protect the cast from soiling.* Tuck a folded disposable diaper or perineal pad around the perineal edges of the cast. Then apply a second diaper to the patient, over the top of the cast, to hold the first diaper in place. Also, tuck plastic petals into the cast *to channel urine and feces into a bedpan.* If the cast still becomes soiled, wipe it with a nonabrasive cleaner and a damp sponge or cloth. Then air-dry it with a hair dryer set on "cool."

Keep a cast cutter or saw available at all times *to remove the cast quickly in case of an emergency.*

During mealtimes, position older children on their abdomens *to promote safer eating and swallowing.*

Before removing the cast, reassure the parents and the patient that the noisy sawing process is painless. If necessary, explain how the saw works.

Home care

Before discharge, teach parents how to care for the cast, and give them an opportunity to demonstrate their understanding.

Include instructions for checking circulatory status, recognizing signs of circulatory impairment, and notifying the doctor. Also demonstrate how to turn the patient, apply moleskin, clean the cast, and ensure adequate nourishment.

Teach caregivers to treat dry, scaly skin around the cast by washing the patient's skin frequently. After the cast is removed, they may apply baby oil or other lotion to soothe the skin. Urge them to schedule and keep all follow-up medical appointments.

Complications

Complications associated with a hip spica cast come from immobility. They include constipation, urinary stasis, kidney stones, skin breakdown, respiratory compromise, and contractures. Frequent turnings, range-of-motion exercises, and adequate hydration and nutrition can minimize complications.

Documentation

Record the date and time of cast care. Describe circulatory status in the patient's legs, and record measurements of any bleeding or drainage. Note the condition of the cast and the patient's skin. Describe all skin care given.

Record findings of bowel and bladder assessments. Note patient and family tolerance of the cast. Document patient- and family-teaching topics discussed as well.

Selected references

Betz, C., and Poster, E. *Mosby's Pediatric Nursing Reference.* St. Louis: C.V. Mosby Co., 1989.

Blatz, S., and Paes, B. "Intravenous Infusion by Superficial Vein in the Neonate," *Journal of Intravenous Nursing* 13(2):122-28, March-April 1990.

Clarke, P.H., and Deeds, N.C. "The Child in a Mist Tent," *Pediatric Nursing* 14(6):446-50, November-December 1988.

Crockett, S.J. "The Family Team Approach to Fitness: A Proposal," *Public Health Reports* 102(5):546-51, September-October 1987.

Dickey, S. *A Guide to the Nursing of Children.* Baltimore: Williams & Wilkins Co., 1987.

Engel, J. *Pocket Guide to Pediatric Assessment.* St. Louis: C.V. Mosby Co., 1989.

Gomberg, S.M. "Mistaken Identity—Is It Epiglottitis or Croup?" *Pediatric Nursing* 16(6):567-70, November-December 1990.

Guyon, G. "Pharmacokinetic Considerations in Neonatal Drug Therapy," *Neonatal Network* 7(5):9-12, April 1989.

Humphrey, C., and Nuzzo, P., eds. *Home Care Nursing: An Orientation to Practice.* Norwalk, Conn.: Appleton & Lange, 1991.

James, S., and Mott, S. *Child Health Nursing: Essential Care of Children and Families.* Edited by Hunter, D. Reading, Mass.: Addison-Wesley Publishing Co., 1988.

Jowett, N.J., and Thompson, D.R. "Basic Life Support—The Forgotten Skills?" *Intensive Care Nurse* 4(1):9-17, March 1988.

Lenox, A.C. "I.V. Therapy: Reducing the Risk of Infection," *Nursing90* 20(3):60-61, March 1990.

Mott, S. *Nursing Care of Children and Families,* 2nd ed. Edited by Hunter, D. Reading, Mass.: Addison-Wesley Publishing Co., 1992.

Nelms, B.C. "Promoting Emotional Health: Role of the Nurse Practitioner," *Journal of Pediatric Health Care* 2(1):1-2, January-February 1988.

Nelson, N., and Beckel, J., eds. *Nursing Care Plans for the Pediatric Patient.* St. Louis: C.V. Mosby Co., 1987.

Nugent, K.E., et al. "A Model for Providing Health Maintenance and Promotion to Children from Low-income, Ethnically Diverse Backgrounds," *Journal of Pediatric Health Care* 2(4):175-80, July-August 1988.

Nursing92 Drug Handbook. Springhouse, Pa.: Springhouse Corp., 1992.

Pillitteri, A. *Child Health Nursing: Care of the Growing Family,* 3rd ed. Glenview, Ill.: Scott, Foresman & Co., 1987.

Professional Guide to Diseases, 4th ed. Springhouse, Pa.: Springhouse Corp., 1992.

Richardson, S.F. "Child Health Promotion Practices," *Journal of Pediatric Health Care* 2(2):73-78, March-April 1988.

Rose, M.H., and Thomas, R.B., eds. *Children with Chronic Conditions: Nursing in a Family and Community Context.* New York: Grune & Stratton, 1987.

Smith, M.J., et al. *Child and Family: Concepts of Nursing Practice.* St. Louis: Mosby-Year Book, Inc., 1991.

Textbook of Pediatric Life Support. Dallas: American Heart Association, 1988.

Treatments. Nurse's Reference Library. Springhouse, Pa.: Springhouse Corp., 1988.

Whaley, L.F, and Wong, D.L. *Essentials of Pediatric Nursing,* 3rd ed. St. Louis: C.V. Mosby Co., 1988.

GERIATRIC CARE

M. CATHERINE WOLLMAN, RN, MSN, CRNP

Introduction

Today, more people live to old age than ever before. Although 40% of people over age 65 may occasionally require a stay in an extended care facility, only 5% of elderly people require long-term supervised care; the rest can maintain their independence. However, about 80% of elderly people have at least one chronic health problem — usually arthritis, heart or respiratory disease, hypertension, or impaired vision or hearing. These problems often occur simultaneously, straining the patient's and his family's ability to cope.

When caring for an elderly patient, you'll usually implement procedures similar to those you'd use for any other adult. But you'll need to take into account the psychosocial, physiologic, and biological changes that normally occur during aging. Because age-related changes in body function may affect drug action, you'll need to recognize how certain drugs affect elderly patients. Your aim is to improve compliance and avoid adverse reactions and interactions.

You'll also help an elderly patient learn to deal with other age-related concerns, such as urinary or fecal incontinence and falls. This chapter will help you identify and treat these common gerontologic problems and avoid prolonging the patient's care unnecessarily. At the same time that you provide physical care, you may also alert your patient and his family to community health and social service agencies that can help improve the patient's quality of life and enable him to remain independent for as long as possible.

TREATMENTS
Management of incontinence

In elderly patients, incontinence commonly follows any loss or impairment of urinary or anal sphincter control. The incontinence may be transient or permanent. In all, about 10 million adults experience some form of urinary incontinence; this includes about 50% of the 1.5 million people in extended care facilities. And fecal incontinence affects up to 10% of the patients in such facilities.

Contrary to popular opinion, urinary incontinence is not a disease and not part of normal aging. It may be caused by confusion, dehydration, fecal impaction, or restricted mobility. It's also a sign of various disorders, such as prostatic hyperplasia, bladder calculus, bladder cancer, urinary tract infection (UTI), cerebrovascular accident, diabetic neuropathy, Guillain-Barré syndrome, multiple sclerosis, prostatic cancer, prostatitis, spinal cord injury, and urethral stricture. It may also result from urethral sphincter damage after prostatectomy. What's more, certain drugs, including diuretics, hypnotics, sedatives, anticholinergics, antihypertensives, and alpha antagonists, may trigger urinary incontinence.

Urinary incontinence is classified as acute or chronic. Acute urinary incontinence results from disorders that are potentially reversible, such as delirium, dehydration, urine retention, restricted mobility, fecal impaction, infection or inflammation, drug reactions, and polyuria. Chronic urinary incontinence occurs as four distinct types: stress, overflow, urge, or functional incontinence. With *stress incontinence*, leakage results from sudden physical strain, such as a sneeze, cough, or quick movement. In *overflow incontinence*, urine retention causes dribbling because the distended bladder cannot contract strongly enough to force a urine stream. In *urge incontinence*, the patient cannot control the impulse to urinate. Finally, *functional (total) incontinence* results when urine leakage occurs even though the bladder and urethra function normally. This condition is usually related to cognitive or environmental factors, such as mental impairment or lack of appropriate or timely care.

Fecal incontinence, the involuntary passage of feces, may occur gradually (as it does in dementia) or suddenly (as it does in spinal cord injury). It most commonly results from fecal stasis and impaction secondary to reduced activity, inappropriate diet, or untreated painful anal conditions. It can also result from chronic laxative use, reduced fluid intake, and neurologic deficit. Pelvic, prostatic, or rectal surgery can also cause fecal incontinence as can medications, including antihistamines, psychotropics, and iron preparations. Not usually a sign of serious illness, fecal incontinence can seriously impair an elderly patient's physical and psychological well-being.

Patients with urinary or fecal incontinence should be carefully assessed for underlying disorders. Most can be treated — some can be cured. Treatment aims to control the condition through bladder or bowel retraining or other behavior management techniques, diet modification, drug therapy, and possibly surgery. Corrective surgery for urinary incontinence includes transurethral resection of the prostate in men, repair of the anterior vaginal wall or retropelvic suspension of the bladder in women, urethral

Artificial urinary sphincter implant

An artificial urinary sphincter implant can help restore continence to a patient with a neurogenic bladder. Criteria for inserting an implant include:
• incontinence associated with a weak urinary sphincter
• incoordination between the detrusor muscle and the urinary sphincter (if drug therapy fails)
• inadequate bladder storage (if intermittent catheterization and drug therapy are unsuccessful).

Configuration and placement
An implant consists of a control pump, an occlusive cuff, and a pressure-regulating balloon. The cuff is placed around the bladder neck, and the balloon is placed under the rectus muscle in the abdomen. The balloon holds fluid that inflates the cuff. In men, the surgeon places the control pump in the scrotum; in women, the surgeon places the pump in the labium.

Using the implant
To void, the patient squeezes the bulb to deflate the cuff, which opens the urethra by returning fluid to the balloon. After voiding, the cuff reinflates automatically, sealing the urethra until the patient needs to void again.

Complications and care
If complications develop, the implant may need to be repaired or removed. Possible complications include cuff leakage (uncommon); trapped blood or other fluid contaminants (which can cause control pump problems); skin erosion around the bulb or erosion in the bladder neck or the urethra; infection; inadequate occlusion pressures; and kinked tubing. If the bladder holds residual urine, intermittent self-catheterization may be needed.

Care includes avoiding strenuous activity for about 6 months after surgery and having regular checkups.

Implant position in a man

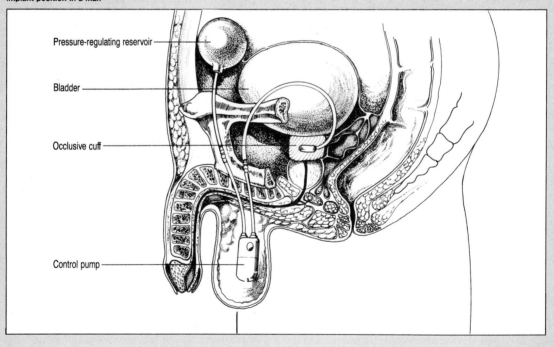

Correcting urinary incontinence with bladder retraining

The incontinent patient typically feels frustrated, embarrassed, and sometimes hopeless. Fortunately, though, his problem can usually be corrected by bladder retraining—a program that aims to establish a regular voiding pattern. To implement such a program, follow these guidelines.

Assess elimination patterns
First assess the patient's intake pattern, voiding pattern, and reason for each accidental voiding (for example, a coughing spell).

Establish a voiding schedule
Encourage the patient to void regularly—every 2 hours, for example. Once he can stay dry for 2 hours, increase the time between voidings by 30 minutes each day until he achieves a 3- to 4-hour voiding schedule.

Teach the patient to practice relaxation techniques, such as deep breathing, *which helps decrease the sense of urgency.*

Record results and remain positive
Keep a record of continence and incontinence for about 5 days—*this may reinforce your patient's efforts to remain continent.*

Remember, both your positive attitude and your patient's are crucial to his successful bladder retraining.

Take steps for success
Here are some additional tips to help boost the patient's success:
- Be sure to locate the patient's bed near a bathroom or portable toilet. Leave a light on at night. If the patient needs assistance getting out of a bed or a chair, promptly answer the call for help.
- Encourage the patient to wear his usual clothing. *This confirms your confidence in his ability to stay dry.* If necessary, use high quality incontinence products *to decrease the risk of skin breakdown.*
- Encourage the patient to drink 1,500 to 2,000 ml of fluid each day. Lowering fluid intake will not reduce or prevent incontinence; it will promote infection. Limiting fluid intake after 6 p.m., however, will help the patient remain continent during the night.
- Reassure your patient that periodic incontinent episodes don't signal failure of the program. Encourage persistence, tolerance, and a positive attitude.

---

sling, and bladder augmentation. (For more information, see *Artificial urinary sphincter implant.*)

Equipment
Bladder retraining record sheet ■ gloves ■ stethoscope (to assess bowel sounds) ■ lubricant ■ moisture barrier cream ■ antidiarrheal or laxative suppository ■ incontinence pads ■ bedpan ■ specimen container ■ label ■ laboratory request form ■ optional: stool collection kit, urinary catheter.

Implementation
- Whether the patient reports urinary or fecal incontinence, or both, you'll need to perform initial and continuing assessments to plan effective interventions. (See *Correcting urinary incontinence with bladder retraining.*)

For urinary incontinence
- Ask the patient when he first noticed urine leakage and whether it began suddenly or gradually. Have him describe his typical urinary pattern: Does incontinence usually occur during the day or at night? Ask him to

rate his urinary control: Does he have moderate control, or is he completely incontinent? If he sometimes urinates with control, ask him to identify when and how much he usually urinates.
- Evaluate related problems, such as urinary hesitancy, frequency, urgency, nocturia, and decreased force or interrupted urine stream. Ask the patient to describe any previous treatment he had for incontinence or measures he performed by himself. Also ask about medications, including nonprescription drugs.
- Assess the patient's environment. Is a toilet or commode readily available, and how long does the patient take to reach it? Once the patient is in the bathroom, assess manual dexterity — for example, how easily does he manipulate his clothes?
- Evaluate the patient's mental status and cognitive function.
- Quantify the patient's normal daily fluid intake.
- Review the patient's medication and diet history for drugs and foods that affect digestion and elimination.
- Review or obtain the patient's medical history, noting especially number and route of births and any incidence

Strengthening pelvic floor muscles

Stress incontinence is the most common kind of urinary incontinence in women and usually results from weakening of the urethral sphincter. In men, it may sometimes occur after a radical prostatectomy.

You can help a patient prevent or minimize stress incontinence by teaching about pelvic floor (Kegel) exercises to strengthen the pubococcygeal muscles. Here's how.

Learning the exercises

First, teach the patient how to locate the muscles of the pelvic floor. Instruct the patient to tense the muscles around the anus, as if to retain stool or intestinal gas.

Next, teach the patient to tighten the muscles of the pelvic floor to stop the flow of urine while urinating and then to release the muscles to restart the flow.

Once learned, these exercises can be done anywhere at any time.

Establishing a regimen

Suggest starting out by contracting the muscles and holding the contraction for 10 seconds. Then direct the patient to relax for 10 seconds before slowly tightening the muscles and then releasing them. Stress that contraction and relaxation exercises are essential to muscle retraining.

Typically, the patient starts with 15 contractions in the morning and afternoon and 20 at night. Or the patient may exercise for 10 minutes, three times a day, working up to 25 contractions at a time as strength improves.

Advise the patient not to use stomach, leg, or buttock muscles. Also discourage leg crossing or breath holding during these exercises.

• Obtain specimens for appropriate laboratory tests, as ordered. Label each specimen container and send it to the laboratory with a request form.

• Begin incontinence management by implementing an appropriate bladder retraining program.

• *To manage stress incontinence,* implement an exercise program to help strengthen the pelvic floor muscles. (See *Strengthening pelvic floor muscles.*)

• *To manage functional incontinence,* frequently assess the patient's mental and functional status. Regularly remind the patient to void. Respond to his calls promptly, and help him get to the bathroom as quickly as possible. Provide positive reinforcements.

• *To ensure healthful hydration and to prevent UTI,* be sure the patient maintains adequate daily fluid intake (six to eight 8-oz glasses of fluid). Restrict fluid intake after 6 p.m.

For fecal incontinence

• Ask the patient with fecal incontinence to identify its onset, duration, and severity. Also have him identify any discernible incontinence patterns — for instance, determine whether it occurs at night or with diarrhea. Focus the history on GI, neurologic, and psychological disorders.

• Note the frequency, consistency, and volume of stool passed within the last 24 hours and obtain a stool specimen, if ordered. Protect the patient's bed with an incontinence pad.

• Assess the patient for chronic constipation and GI and neurologic disorders, as well as laxative abuse. Also inspect the abdomen for distention, and auscultate for bowel sounds. If not contraindicated, check for fecal impaction (which may be a factor in overflow incontinence).

• Assess the patient's medication regimen. Check for medications that affect bowel activity, such as aspirin, some anticholinergic antiparkinson agents, aluminum hydroxide, calcium carbonate antacids, diuretics, iron preparations, opiates, tranquilizers, tricyclic antidepressants, and phenothiazines.

• For the neurologically capable patient with chronic incontinence, provide bowel retraining.

• Advise the patient to consume a fiber-rich diet, with raw, leafy vegetables (such as carrots and lettuce), unpeeled fruits (such as apples), and whole grains (such as wheat or rye breads and cereals). If the patient has a lactase deficiency, suggest calcium supplements to replace calcium lost by eliminating dairy products from the diet.

• Encourage adequate fluid intake.

• Teach the elderly patient to gradually eliminate laxative use, if necessary. Point out, as needed, that using laxative agents to promote regular bowel movement may have the

---

of UTI, prostate disorders, spinal injury or tumor, cerebrovascular accident, or bladder, prostate, or pelvic surgery. Also assess for disorders, such as delirium, dehydration, urine retention, restricted mobility, fecal impaction, infection, inflammation, or polyuria.

• Inspect the urethral meatus for obvious inflammation or anatomic defects. Have the female patient bear down while you note any urine leakage. Gently palpate the abdomen for bladder distention, signaling urine retention. If possible, have the patient examined by a urologist.

opposite effect—producing either constipation or incontinence over time. Suggest using natural laxatives, such as prunes or prune juice, instead.
• Promote regular exercise by explaining how it helps to regulate bowel motility. Even a nonambulatory patient can perform some exercises while sitting or lying in bed.

Special considerations
To rid the bladder of residual urine, teach the patient to perform Valsalva's or Credé's maneuver. Or institute clean intermittent catheterization. Use an indwelling urinary catheter only as a last resort *because of the risk of UTI.*

For fecal incontinence, maintain effective hygienic care *to increase the patient's comfort and prevent skin breakdown and infection.* Clean the perineal area frequently, and apply a moisture barrier cream. Control foul odors as well.

Schedule extra time to provide encouragement and support for the patient After all, he may feel shame, embarrassment, and powerlessness from loss of control.

Complications
Skin breakdown and infection may result from incontinence. Psychological problems resulting from incontinence include social isolation, loss of independence, lowered self-esteem, and depression.

Documentation
Record all bladder and bowel retraining efforts, noting scheduled bathroom times, food and fluid intake, and elimination amounts, as appropriate. Record duration of of continent periods. Note any complications, including emotional problems, and signs of skin breakdown and infection. Document treatment given for complications.

Drug therapy

Four of five persons over age 65 have one or more chronic disorders. This helps explain why elderly patients consume more drugs than any other age-group. Although elderly adults represent only 12% of the population, they take 30% to 40% of the prescription drugs issued. That's about 400 million prescriptions a year, or twice the number of prescriptions filled for persons under age 65.

Drug therapy for elderly patients presents a special set of problems rooted in age-related changes. These changes affect drug metabolism, absorption, distribution, and excretion. The changes also potentiate adverse reactions to drugs and may interfere with therapeutic compliance.

Physiologically, aging alters body composition and triggers changes in the digestive system, liver, and kidneys (see *How age affects drug action,* page 750). In turn, these changes may affect drug dosage and administration techniques (see *Modifying I.M. injections,* page 751).

Even though the elderly patient receives the optimum drug dosage, he's still at risk for an adverse drug reaction. Ongoing physiologic changes, poor compliance with the drug regimen, and greater drug consumption contribute to elderly patients experiencing twice as many adverse reactions as younger patients. In fact, about 40% of the people who experience adverse drug reactions are over age 60.

Signs and symptoms of adverse drug reactions (such as confusion, weakness, and lethargy) are typically blamed on disease. If the adverse reaction is unidentified or misidentified, the patient will probably continue taking the drug. To compound the problem, if the patient has multiple physical dysfunctions or adverse drug reactions, or both, he may consult several doctors or specialists who—unknown to one another—may prescribe more drugs. If the patient's drug history remains uninvestigated and if the patient takes additional nonprescription drugs to relieve common complaints (such as indigestion, dizziness, and constipation), he may innocently fall into a pattern of inappropriate and excessive drug use. Known as "polypharmacy," this pattern imperils the patient's safety and the drug regimen's effectiveness as well.

Although many drugs can cause adverse reactions, most serious reactions in elderly patients result from relatively few drugs. Commonly, these reactions result from diuretics, antihypertensives, digitalis glycosides, corticosteroids, sleeping aids, and nonprescription drugs.

Finally, the elderly patient may have difficulty complying with his drug regimen. Hearing and vision deficits, forgetfulness, the need for multiple drug therapy, poor understanding of dosage and directions, and various socioeconomic factors (such as poverty or social isolation) combine to make compliance a special problem. Ensuring successful compliance requires involving family members, the pharmacist, and other caregivers in supervision and teaching tailored to the patient's needs.

Equipment
Patient's medication record ■ appropriate drugs ■ written dosage instructions ■ optional: compliance aids (pill containers, calendar or other large-print teaching aids, premeasured injections).

Implementation
• Noncompliance in elderly patients is so prevalent that it's no wonder that most nurses rank handling it as a top priority when planning nursing care. Follow these

How age affects drug action

As the body ages, body structures and systems change. This affects how the body responds to medications. Some changes that commonly and significantly affect medication administration follow.

Body composition
As a person grows older, his total body mass and lean body mass tend to decrease while body fat tends to increase. These factors affect the relationship between a drug's concentration and solubility in the body.

Digestive system
Decreases in gastric acid secretion and GI motility lead to the body's decreased ability to absorb many drugs well. This can cause problems with certain drugs—for example, digoxin, whose narrow therapeutic range is tied closely to absorption.

Hepatic system
Advancing age reduces blood supply, and certain liver enzymes become less active. As a result, the liver loses some of its ability to metabolize drugs. With reduced liver function comes more intense drug effects as higher levels of a drug remain in circulation. This increases the incidence of drug toxicity.

Renal system
Kidney function diminishes with age. This alone may impair drug elimination by 50% or more. In many cases, decreased kidney function leads to increased blood levels of certain drugs.

procedures to assess the patient's ability or motivation to follow a drug regimen.

To assess compliance ability
• Review the patient's complaint and obtain a comprehensive health and drug history.
• Keeping in mind that discharge planning begins at admission, evaluate the patient's physical ability to take drugs. Can he read drug labels and directions? Does he identify drugs by sight or by touch? Can he open drug bottles easily? If he's disabled by Parkinson's disease or arthritis, for example, or if he lacks manual dexterity for any reason, advise him to ask his pharmacist for snap

or screw caps—rather than childproof closures—for his drug containers.
• Evaluate the patient's cognitive skills. Can he remember to take prescribed drugs on time and regularly? Can he remember where he stored his drugs? If not, refer him to appropriate community resources for supervision.
• Assess the patient's life-style. Does he live with family or friends? If so, include them in your patient-teaching sessions, if possible. Does he live alone or with a debilitated spouse? If so, he'll need continuing support from a visiting nurse or other caregiver. Keep in mind that inadequate supervision may result in drug misuse. Make appropriate referrals and contact appropriate social agencies *to ensure compliance and safety and to provide financial assistance if necessary.* Assess the patient's beliefs concerning drug use.

To prevent reactions that impede compliance
• Discuss the patient's drug therapy with him. As he receives drugs, name them, explain their intended effect, and describe possible adverse reactions to watch for and report (see *Recognizing common adverse reactions in elderly patients,* page 752).
• Tell the patient that you'll ask questions *to help identify (or reduce the risk of) possibly harmful food or drug interactions (such as those caused by alcohol or caffeine) that may interrupt or interfere with compliance.*
• Ask the patient about all drugs—prescription and nonprescription—he takes currently and those he's taken in the past. If possible, ask to see samples. Have the patient name each drug and tell you why, when, and how often he takes it. Remember, the patient may have drugs prescribed by more than one doctor. Also remember to ask if he's taking any drugs originally prescribed for another person or family member (this is not uncommon).
• If your hospital has a specially designed computer program, use it *to help prevent possible drug interactions.* Enter all the data you've collected on drug, dose, frequency, and administration route into a master file of drugs commonly used by elderly patients, for example, anticoagulants (warfarin), benzodiazepines (diazepam), beta blockers (propranolol), calcium channel blockers (verapamil), cardiac glycosides (digoxin), and diuretics (furosemide). From this information the computer compiles a list of the patient's drugs, possible adverse effects, potential interactions, and suggested interventions. Then review the findings with the patient. *If he knows what to expect, he's more likely to comply with treatment.* (If you don't have access to such technology, you can compile a similar list using a reputable drug reference.)
• Alternatively, encourage the patient to purchase drugs from only one pharmacy, preferably one that maintains a drug profile for each customer. Advise the patient to

Modifying I.M. injections

Before you give an intramuscular (I.M.) injection to an elderly patient, remember the physical changes that accompany aging and choose your equipment, site, and technique accordingly.

Choosing a needle
Remember that an elderly patient usually has less subcutaneous tissue and less muscle mass than a younger patient—especially in the buttocks and deltoids. So you may need to use a shorter needle than you would for a younger adult.

Selecting a site
Also remember that an elderly patient typically has more fat around the hips, abdomen, and thigh areas. This makes the vastus lateralis muscle and ventrogluteal area (gluteus medius and minimus, but not gluteus maximus muscles) primary injection sites.

You should be able to palpate the muscle in these areas easily. However, if the patient's extremely thin, gently pinch the muscle *to elevate it and to avoid putting the needle completely through it (which will alter the absorption and distribution of the drug).*

Caution: Never give an I.M. injection in an immobile limb *because of poor drug absorption and the risk that a sterile abscess will form at the injection site.*

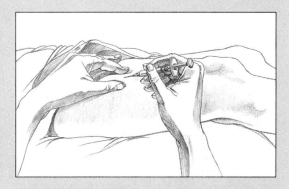

Checking technique
To avoid inserting the needle in a blood vessel, pull back on the plunger and look for blood before injecting the drug. Because of age-related vascular changes, elderly patients are also at greater risk for hematomas. *To check bleeding after an I.M. injection,* you may need to apply direct pressure over the puncture site for a longer time than usual. Gently massage the injection site *to aid drug absorption and distribution.* However, avoid site massage with certain drugs given by the Z-track injection technique, such as iron dextran or hydroxyzine hydrochloride.

---

consult the pharmacist, who can anticipate drug interactions before they occur.
• Advise the patient about specific food-drug interactions. Based on the information in your drug history, provide a list of food items to avoid.

To boost therapeutic compliance
• *To circumvent noncompliance caused by visual impairment,* provide dosage instructions in large print, if necessary.
• *To alter eating habits that lead to noncompliance,* emphasize which drugs the patient must take with food and which he must take on an empty stomach. Explain that taking some drugs on an empty stomach may cause nausea, whereas taking some drugs on a full stomach may interfere with absorption. Also find out whether the patient eats regularly or skips meals. If he skips meals, he may be skipping doses, too. As needed, help him coordinate his drug administration schedule with his eating habits.

• *To correct problems related to drug form and administration,* help the patient find easier ways to take medicine. For example, if he can't swallow pills or capsules, switch to a liquid or powdered form of the drug—if possible. Or suggest that he slide the tablet down with food, such as applesauce. Keep in mind which tablets you can crush and which you can't. For example, enteric-coated tablets, timed-release capsules, or sublingual or buccal tablets should not be crushed. *Doing so may affect absorption and effectiveness.* Some crushed drugs may taste bitter and may stain or irritate oral mucosa.
• If mobility or transportation deters compliance, help the patient locate a pharmacy that refills and delivers prescriptions. If appropriate, consider using a mail order pharmacy.
• If forgetfulness interferes with compliance, devise a system for helping the patient remember to take his drugs properly. Suggest that the patient or a family member purchase or make a scheduling aid, such as a calendar,

Recognizing common adverse reactions in elderly patients

Common signs and symptoms of adverse reactions to medications include hives, impotence, incontinence, stomach upset, and rashes. Elderly patients are especially susceptible and may experience serious adverse reactions such as orthostatic hypotension, altered mental status, anorexia, dehydration, blood disorders, and tardive dyskinesia.

Additional adverse reactions, such as anxiety, confusion, and forgetfulness may be dismissed as typical elderly behaviors rather than recognized as drug effects.

Orthostatic hypotension
Marked by light-headedness or faintness and unsteady footing, orthostatic hypotension occurs as a common adverse response to antidepressant, antihypertensive, antipsychotic, and sedative medications.

To prevent accidents, such as falls, warn the patient not to sit up or get out of bed too rapidly. Instruct him to call for assistance in walking if he feels dizzy or faint.

Altered mental status
Agitation or confusion may follow ingestion of alcohol or anticholinergic, antidiuretic, antihypertensive, and antidepressant medications. Paradoxically, depression is a common effect of antidepressant medications.

Anorexia
This is a warning sign of toxicity—especially from digitalis glycosides such as digoxin. That's why the doctor usually prescribes a very low initial dose.

Dehydration
If the patient's taking diuretics, such as hydrochlorothiazide, be alert for dehydration and electrolyte imbalance. Monitor blood levels and provide potassium supplements as ordered.

Oral dryness results from many medications. If anticholinergic medications cause dryness, suggest sucking on sugarless candy for relief.

Blood disorders
If the patient takes an anticoagulant, such as warfarin, watch for signs of easy bruising or bleeding (such as excessive bleeding after toothbrushing). Easy bruising or bleeding may be signs of other problems such as blood dyscrasias or thrombocytopenia. Drugs that may cause these reactions include several antineoplastic agents such as methotrexate, antibiotics like nitrofurantoin, and anticonvulsants such as valproic acid and phenytoin. A patient who bruises easily should report this sign to his doctor immediately.

Tardive dyskinesia
Characterized by abnormal tongue movements, lip pursing, grimacing, blinking, and gyrating motions of the face and extremities, this disorder may be triggered by psychotropic drugs such as haloperidol or chlorpromazine.

checklist, alarm wristwatch, or compartmented drug container. (See *Using compliance aids.*)
• If financial considerations prevent compliance, help the patient explore new ways to manage. In some cases, the patient may try to save money by not having prescriptions filled or refilled. Or he may try to save by taking fewer doses than ordered to make the drug last longer. Suggest using less expensive generic equivalents of name-brand drugs whenever possible. Also explore ways that family members can help, or refer the patient to the social service department and appropriate community agencies. For example, many states have programs to help low-income, elderly patients buy needed drugs.

Special considerations
Advise the patient to contact you or his doctor before taking any over-the-counter drugs *to avoid the risk of possible adverse drug interactions. If necessary, regularly monitor serum levels of drugs, such as digoxin or potassium, to avoid toxicity.*

When the doctor advises discontinuing a drug, instruct the patient to discard it—in the toilet, if possible. *This prevents others from using the drug and ensures that the patient won't continue taking it by mistake.*

To avoid improper storage and possible drug deterioration, advise the patient to keep all prescribed drugs in their original containers. Keep in mind that some drugs deteriorate when exposed to light; others decompose if they come in contact with other drugs—in a pillbox, for example. Before the patient stores drugs together, advise him to consult his pharmacist or doctor.

Suggest a storage area that's well-lighted (but protected from direct sunlight), not too warm or humid (not the bathroom medicine chest), and some distance from

Using compliance aids

To help your patient comply with oral or injectable drug therapy safely, you or a family member may premeasure doses for him, using compliance aids like those shown below or ones you create yourself. Most pharmacies or community service agencies can supply similar aids.

One-day pill pack
A plastic box with four lidded medication compartments marked "breakfast," "lunch," "dinner," and "bedtime" helps the patient see whether he's taken all medications prescribed for one day. The lids may also be embossed with braille characters if needed.

The patient, caregiver, or visiting nurse must remember to fill the device each day. Being small, the device doesn't hold many tablets or capsules.

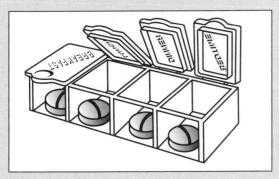

Seven-day pill reminder
The boxes shown here will help the patient remember if he has taken all the tablets and capsules prescribed for each day of the week. Each box has seven medication compartments marked with the initials for each day of the week (in both braille characters and printed letters).

Like the one-day pill container, this device is inappropriate for large numbers of tablets or capsules, or for tablets and capsules that must be taken at different times each day.

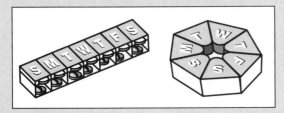

Homemade dosing aids
Show the patient and his caregivers how to make their own compliance aids by labeling clean, empty jars; extra prescription bottles (obtainable from the pharmacist); or envelopes with the drug name, the time of day, and the day of the week to take the medication. Recommend using a separate container for each time, and fill this container every morning with the correct dose of each medication.

Syringe-filling device
This device precisely measures insulin doses for a visually impaired diabetic. Designed for use with a disposable U-100 syringe and an insulin bottle, the device is set by the caregiver to accommodate the syringe's width. She then positions the plunger at the point determined by the dose and tightens the stop. When the device is set, the patient can draw up the precise dose ordered for each injection.

As with any device, several drawbacks must be considered. This device can't be used if insulin needs to be mixed or if doses vary. The settings must be checked and adjusted whenever the syringe size or type changes. The screws must be checked regularly because they loosen with repeated use.

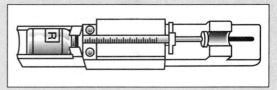

Syringe scale magnifier
This device helps a visually impaired diabetic read syringe markings, thereby enabling him to fill his own syringe. The plastic magnifier snaps onto the syringe barrel. This device may be impractical for a patient with arthritis who can't easily attach the magnifier to the syringe.

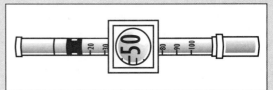

the patient's bedside (not on a bedside table). If he keeps drugs at his bedside, *he may give himself an accidental overdose by taking them before he's fully awake and alert.*

Home care
If the patient is discharged from the hospital with a new drug regimen, schedule him for follow-up care by a visiting nurse *to assess his ability to follow the regimen and to monitor his response to therapy.*

Documentation
Document all assessment findings and laboratory test results in the patient's chart. Record all instructions and teaching materials given to the patient, family members, or other caregivers. Keep a record of all drugs, dosages, and adverse reactions and interventions. Describe the patient's understanding of his drug regimen. Note all health and social service agency referrals.

Prevention and management of falls

Falls are a major cause of injury and death among elderly people. In fact, the older the person, the more likely he'll die of a fall or its complications. In people age 75 or older, falls account for three times as many accidental deaths as motor vehicle accidents.

Factors that contribute to falls include lengthy convalescent periods in elderly patients, higher risks of incomplete recovery, and increasing physical disability. Once impaired, equilibrium takes longer to restore in elderly people than in younger adults. And naturally, loss of balance increases the risk of falling. Besides causing physical harm, injuries from falls can trigger psychological problems, leading to losses in self-confidence and hastening dependency and a move to a long-term care facility or nursing home.

Falls may be accidental and caused by environmental factors, such as poor lighting, slippery throw rugs, or highly waxed floors. But frequently, falls result from physiologic factors such as temporary muscle paralysis, vertigo, orthostatic (postural) hypotension, central nervous system lesions, dementia, failing eyesight, or decreased strength and coordination.

In a hospital, an accidental fall can change a short stay for a minor problem into a prolonged stay for serious — and possibly life-threatening — ones. The risk of falling is highest during the first week of a stay in a hospital or nursing home. The adage "An ounce of prevention is worth a pound of cure" is worth remembering

---

Who's at risk for a fall?

Preventing falls begins with identifying the patients at greatest risk. Consider a patient with one or more of the following characteristics to be at risk:
- age 65 or older
- poor general health with a chronic disease
- history of falls
- altered mental status
- decreased mobility
- improperly fitted shoes or slippers
- inappropriate use of restraints
- urinary frequency or diarrhea
- sensory deficits — particularly visual deficits
- taking drugs such as diuretics, strong analgesics, antipsychotics, hypnotics.

---

when working with elderly patients (see *Who's at risk for a fall?*).

Equipment
Stethoscope ■ sphygmomanometer ■ analgesics ■ cold and warm compresses ■ pillows ■ blankets ■ emergency resuscitation equipment (crash cart), as needed ■ electrocardiograph (ECG) monitor, if needed.

Preparation of equipment
If you're helping a fallen patient, send an assistant to collect the assessment or resuscitation equipment you need.

Implementation
• Whether your care plan focuses on preventing a fall or managing one in an elderly patient, you'll need to proceed with patience and caution.

To prevent falls
• Assess your patient's risk of falling at least once each shift. Note any changes in his condition — such as decreased mental status — that increase his chances of falling. If you decide that he's at risk, take steps to reduce the danger.
• Correct potential dangers in the patient's room. Position the call light *so that he can reach it without getting out of bed.* Provide adequate nighttime lighting.
• Place the patient's personal belongings and assistive aids — purse, wallet, books, tissues, urinal, commode, cane or walker — within easy reach.
• Instruct him to rise slowly from a supine position *to avoid possible dizziness and loss of balance.*

• Lower the bed to its lowest position *so the patient can easily reach the floor when he gets out of bed. This also reduces the distance to the floor in case he falls.* Lock the bed's wheels. If side rails are to be raised, observe the patient frequently.

• Advise the patient to wear nonskid footwear.

• Respond promptly to the patient's call light *to help limit the number of times he gets out of bed without help.*

• Check the patient at least every 2 hours. Check a high-risk patient every 30 minutes.

• Alert other caregivers to the patient's risk of falling and define interventions you've implemented.

• Consider other precautions, such as placing two high-risk patients in the same room and having someone with them at all times.

• Encourage the patient to perform active range-of-motion (ROM) exercises *to improve flexibility and coordination.*

To manage falls

• If you're with the patient as he falls, try to break his fall with your body.

• As you gently guide him to the floor, support his body — particularly his head and trunk. If possible, help him to a supine position.

• While guiding the patient, concentrate on maintaining proper body alignment yourself to keep the center of gravity within your support base. Spread your feet to widen your support base. Remember, *the wider the base, the better your balance will be.* Bend your knees — not your back — *to support the patient and to avoid injuring yourself.*

• Remain calm and stay with the patient *to prevent any further injury.*

• Ask another nurse to collect any assessment tools you may need, such as a stethoscope, a sphygmomanometer or, if necessary, an ECG monitor.

• Assess the patient's ABCs (airway, breathing, and circulation) *to be sure the fall wasn't caused by respiratory or cardiac arrest.* If you don't detect respirations or a pulse, call a code and begin emergency resuscitation measures. Also note his level of consciousness (LOC), and assess pupil size, equality, and reaction to light.

• *To determine the extent of injuries,* look for lacerations, abrasions, and obvious deformities. Note any deviations from the patient's baseline condition. Notify the doctor.

• If you weren't present during the fall, ask the patient or a witness what happened. Ask if the patient experienced pain or a change in LOC.

• Don't move the patient until you evaluate his status fully. Provide reassurance as needed, and observe for such signs and symptoms as confusion, tremor, weakness, pain, or dizziness.

• Assess the patient's limb strength and motion. Don't perform any ROM exercises if you suspect a fracture or if the patient complains of any odd sensations or limited movement. If you suspect any disorder, don't move the patient until a doctor examines him. Spinal cord injuries from patient falls are rare, *but if injury has occurred, any movement may cause irreversible spinal damage.*

• While the patient lies on the floor until the doctor arrives, offer pillows and blankets *for comfort.* If you suspect a spinal cord injury, though, don't place a pillow under his head.

• If you don't detect any problems, return the patient to his bed with the help of another staff member. Never try to lift a patient alone *because you may injure yourself or the patient.*

• Take steps to control bleeding (if indicated) and to obtain an X-ray if you suspect a fracture. Provide first aid for minor injuries as needed. Then monitor the patient's status for the next 24 hours.

• Even if the patient shows no signs of distress or has sustained only minor injuries, monitor his vital signs every 15 minutes for 1 hour, then every 30 minutes for 1 hour, then every hour for 2 hours or until his condition stabilizes. Notify the doctor if you note any change from the baseline.

• Perform necessary measures to relieve the patient's pain and discomfort. Give analgesics as ordered. Apply cold compresses for the first 24 hours, and warm compresses thereafter, to reduce any pain and swelling.

• Reassess the patient's environment and his risk of falling. Talk to him about the fall — why it occurred and how he thinks it could have been prevented. Review the events that preceded the fall. Did the patient change position abruptly? Does he wear corrective lenses? Was he wearing them when he fell? Review medications, such as tranquilizers and narcotics, that may have contributed to the fall. Assess gait disturbances or improper use of canes, crutches, or a walker as well.

Special considerations

After a fall, review the patient's medical history *to determine if he's at risk for other complications.* For instance, if he hit his head, check his history to see if he takes anticoagulants. If he does, he's at greater risk for intracranial bleeding, and you'll need to monitor him accordingly.

Consider beginning a fall prevention program in your hospital if you don't already have one.

Devise an alternative to restraints for a high-risk patient. For example, investigate using a device, such as a pressure-pad alarm. The pressure sensor pad lies under the bed linens. The reduced pressure that results as the patient gets out of bed triggers an alarm at the nurses' station. One such system consists of a lightweight plastic sensor sheet and a control unit. The system adapts to both bed and chair, and setting it up according to the manufacturer's directions prevents false alarms. An alternative alarm device can be worn by the patient just above the knee. The alarm sounds when the patient moves his leg to a vertical position.

To promote additional patient safety, consider drawing a red arrow next to the patient's room number on the call-light console and making a red dot on the AT RISK card on the patient's door. Also add an appropriate notation to the Kardex and chart.

Provide emotional support whether you're managing a fall or preventing one. Let the elderly patient know that you recognize his limitations and acknowledge his fears. Point out measures that you'll take to provide a safe environment.

Teach the patient how to fall safely. Show him how to protect his hands and face. If the patient uses a walker or a wheelchair, demonstrate how to cope with and recover from a fall, should one occur. Teach him to survey the room for a low, sturdy, supportive piece of furniture (for example, a coffee table). Then review the proper procedure for lifting himself off the floor and either standing up with the walker or getting into the wheelchair.

Home care

Before discharge, teach the patient and his family how to prevent accidental falls at home by correcting common household hazards. Encourage them to take steps to ensure safety (see *Promoting safety in the home*).

As needed, refer the patient to the local visiting nurse association so that nursing services can continue after discharge and during convalescence.

Documentation

After a fall, complete an incident report that provides a detailed account in case the patient takes legal action. Primarily for your hospital's insurance carrier, this report isn't considered part of the patient's record. A copy, however, will go to the hospital's administrator who will evaluate care given in the unit and propose new safety policies, as appropriate.

The incident report should include where and when the fall occurred, how the patient was discovered, and his position when he was found. Include the events leading up to the fall, the names of any witnesses, the patient's emotional response to the fall, and a detailed description of his condition, based on assessment findings. Note any interventions taken and the names of other staff members who helped care for the patient after the fall. Record the doctor's name, and the date and time that he was notified. Include a copy of the doctor's report. Note too if the patient was sent for any diagnostic tests or transferred to another unit.

HOME CARE

Promoting safety in the home

Before your patient leaves the hospital, review these tips for ensuring a safe home environment.

• Secure all carpets and floor coverings around the edges, and tack down worn spots. Never use lightweight, loose mats or rugs on bare floors.

• Make sure potential hazards, such as stairs, are well-lighted. White paint on either side of a staircase can enhance visibility.

• Install strong banisters along all indoor and outdoor steps.

• Use a bedside lamp or low-wattage night-light in the bedroom to avoid having to grope around in the dark when getting out of bed.

• Fit secure handrails in convenient places in the shower, bathtub, and toilet. Use nonskid mats both inside and alongside every tub or shower.

• Minimize clutter. Store children's toys, especially those on wheels, when not in use.

• Walk carefully if a pet, such as a dog or cat, is present.

• Secure wires from electrical appliances to walls or moldings.

• Store frequently used clothing and other items in places where they can be reached without standing on a stool or chair.

• Reduce the risk of accidental slips and falls by selecting well-fitting shoes with nonskid soles, by avoiding long robes, and by wearing glasses if needed.

• Sit on the edge of a bed or chair for a few minutes before rising.

• Use a walking stick, cane, or walker whenever an unsteady feeling arises.

Include all this information in the patient's record. Also note the patient's vital signs. If you're monitoring the patient for a severe complication, record this as well.

Selected references

Blakeslee, J.A., et al. "Making the Transition to Restraint-Free Care," *Journal of Gerontological Nursing* 17(2):4-8, 32-34, February 1991.

Brower, H.T. "The Alternatives to Restraints," *Journal of Gerontological Nursing* 17(2):18-22, 32-34, February 1991.

Burnside, I.M. *Nursing and the Aged: A Self Care Approach,* 3rd ed. New York: McGraw-Hill Book Co., 1988.

Ebersole, P. *Toward Healthy Aging: Human Needs and Nursing Response,* 3rd ed. St. Louis: Mosby-Year Book, Inc., 1990.

Ellickson, E.B. "Bowel Management Plan for the Homebound Elderly," *Journal of Gerontological Nursing* 14(1):16-19, 40-42, January 1988.

Fletcher, K.R. "Restraints Should Be a Last Resort," *RN* 53(1):52-56, 59, January 1990.

Morton, D. "Five Years of Fewer Falls," *AJN* 89(2):204-05, February 1989.

Newman, D.K., and Smith, D.A. "Incontinence: The Problem Patients Won't Talk About," *RN* 52(3):42-45, March 1989.

Rader, J. "Modifying the Environment to Decrease Use of Restraints," *Journal of Gerontological Nursing* 17(2):9-13, 32-34, February 1991.

Scherer, Y.K., et al. "The Nursing Dilemma of Restraints," *Journal of Gerontological Nursing* 17(2):14-17, 32-34, February 1991.

Spellbring, A.M., et al. "Improving Safety for Hospitalized Elderly," *Journal of Gerontological Nursing* 14(2):31-37, 46-47, February 1988.

Stilwell, E.M. "Nurses' Education Related to the Use of Restraints," *Journal of Gerontological Nursing* 17(2):23-26, 32-34, February 1991.

Strumpf, N.E., and Evans, L.K. "The Ethical Problems of Prolonged Physical Restraint," *Journal of Gerontological Nursing* 17(2):27-30, 32-34, February 1991.

Yurick, A., et al. *The Aged Person and the Nursing Process,* 3rd ed. Norwalk, Conn.: Appleton & Lange, 1989.

INDEX

i refers to illustration; t refers to table

i refers to illustration; t refers to table

i refers to illustration; t refers to table

i refers to illustration; t refers to table